HANDBOOK OF PHYSIOLOGY

Section 7: The Endocrine System
Volume I: Cellular Endocrinology

HANDBOOK OF PHYSIOLOGY

A critical, comprehensive presentation of
physiological knowledge and concepts

Section 7: The Endocrine System

VOLUME I: Cellular Endocrinology

Volume Editor

P. MICHAEL CONN

Oregon Regional Primate Research Center
Beaverton, Oregon, and
Oregon Health Sciences University
Portland, Oregon

Section Editor

H. MAURICE GOODMAN

Department of Physiology
University of Massachusetts Medical Center
Worcester, Massachusetts

New York   Oxford
Published for the American Physiological Society
by Oxford University Press
1998

Oxford University Press

Oxford   New York
Athens   Auckland   Bangkok   Bogota
Bombay   Buenos Aires   Calcutta   Cape Town
Dar es Salaam   Delhi   Florence   Hong Kong   Istanbul
Karachi   Kuala Lumpur   Madras   Madrid
Melbourne   Mexico City   Nairobi   Paris
Singapore   Taipei   Tokyo   Toronto   Warsaw

and associated companies in
Berlin   Ibadan

Published for the American Physiological Society by Oxford University Press, Inc.
198 Madison Avenue, New York, New York 10016

Oxford is a registered trademark of Oxford University Press

Library of Congress Cataloging-in-Publication Data
The endocrine system / edited by P. Michael Conn.
   p.   cm. — (Handbook of physiology ; section 7)
Includes bibliographical references and index.
Contents: v. 1. Cellular endocrinology
ISBN 0-19-510935-X
1. Endocrine glands—Physiology.   I. Conn, P. Michael.
I. Conn, P. Michael.
II. Series: Handbook of physiology (Bethesda, Md.) ; section 7.
QP6.H25   1977 sect. 7
[QP187]
571 s
[573.4]—DC21   98-12003
                                                     CIP

9 8 7 6 5 4 3 2 1
Printed in the United States of America
on acid-free paper

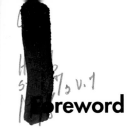

Foreword

Nearly twenty-five years have passed since the first volumes devoted to endocrinology were published as part of the *Handbook of Physiology*. According to the editors, those volumes "constituted the most comprehensive treatment of this bodily system ever undertaken." The present volumes build upon the solid foundation laid down in the initial endocrinology sections of the *Handbook*, and are not designed to replace them or repeat the fundamentals they cover so well. Rather, the current volumes focus primarily on advances made in the seventies, eighties, and nineties and the insights and interpretations these advances provide for unraveling some of the unresolved mysteries.

The previous *Handbook* volumes devoted to endocrinology were arranged morphologically according to the glands of origin of hormones in a manner that is both historically faithful to the way information was obtained and that provides a logical format for organizing the large body of information encompassed by endocrinology. As our understanding has advanced, however, common themes and mechanisms have become apparent, and there is growing awareness of the mechanistic implications of the fact that hormones seldom act alone or that cells are ever free of the influences of multiple regulatory factors. Additionally, with the emergence of exquisitely sensitive techniques, we have learned that hormones and their receptors may be synthesized in rather unexpected places and may serve unanticipated functions. We have therefore chosen to adopt a process-oriented approach to the physiology of the endocrine system and have organized these volumes along the lines of endocrine contributions to the solution of such physiological problems as regulating energy metabolism (Volume 2), regulating salt and water balance (Volume 3), coping with the environment (Volume 4), and regulating growth (Volume 5). Cellular and subcellular mechanisms common to the formation, secretion, and actions of most hormones are dealt with in Volume 1. We have decided not to devote a volume to reproductive endocrinology at this time, largely because it would be duplicative of the wealth of up-to-date works already in print. That we have been able to adopt such an organizational scheme is testimony to the rapid progress that has been made in recent decades. In their preface to the section on endocrinology in the previous *Handbook* series, Roy Greep and Ted Astwood lamented that they "were forced to conclude that this body of information does not readily lend itself to integrated presentation at this time." While an integrative approach still falls somewhat short of ideal, it should nevertheless be helpful to students, teachers, and investigators grappling with a huge and rapidly expanding volume of information on endocrine physiology. Furthermore, the functional rather than morphological orientation provides a framework for organizing emerging concepts and data as experimental biology inevitably evolves from the reductionist mode that has proved so fruitful, to a holistic view of complex systems.

When the original nine volumes on endocrinology in the *Handbook of Physiology* were prepared, the newly introduced radioimmunoassay technology had revolutionized thinking about the regulation of hormone secretion, and even the brain had begun to yield its "releasing factors" to the biochemists' persistence. Since then the concepts and tools of molecular biology have brought astounding advances that have changed even further the way we think about hormones and how they act. A host of old questions has given way to the unprecedented onslaught of new technologies, and new questions undreamt of in the 1970s have not only been asked, but answered. In the mid 1970s overwhelming evidence supported the likely existence of perhaps six or seven hypothalamic releasing factors, but only the thyrotropin releasing hormone (TRH), the luteinizing hormone releasing hormone (LHRH)—now better known as the gonadotropin releasing hormone (GnRH)—and somatostatin had been isolated and characterized. The long-sought corticotropin releasing hormone (CRH), growth hormone releasing hormone (GHRH), and such other hormones as inhibin, leptin, and the atrial natriuretic hormone awaited discovery. Diurnal patterns of hormone secretion were known, and although higher frequency pulsatile secretion had been observed, its significance in preserving or regulating responsiveness of target cells was unknown. By the time the current volumes were planned, not only had the remaining hypophysiotropic factors been isolated and the genes that encode them cloned, but also a host of other peptides, neuro- and otherwise, had been similarly characterized. Although the biochemical mechanisms through which hormones elicit responses in their target cells were already subjects of intense investigation in the 1970s, receptors that occupy so prominent a role in current endocrine research appeared as index terms in only four of the nine earlier volumes. In the early 1970s, growth factors resided almost exclusively in the province of the developmental biologist, and were only beginning to attract the interest of endocrinologists. The terms "paracrine" and "autocrine" helped to define nonendocrine mechanisms, rather than to describe components of hormonal action.

Enormous progress in understanding both secretory and target cells has issued from the ever-widening application of the powerful tools of molecular biology. Beyond the intimidating technology and terminology of the "new biology," classical endocrinologists will still recognize the questions and strategies of the "old biology." Whereas studies in an earlier era focused on the morphology of cells and organs, more attention is being focused on the morphology of molecules, their cellular locations, and on the shapes, sizes, and electrical charges of their interacting surfaces. Whereas earlier studies focused on the isolation of hormones and the characterization of their chemical structure, more recent studies have been aimed at isolating and sequencing the genes that encode them and their receptors. Whereas the classical approach to studying the function of a gland or secretion involved ablation and replacement, current studies of function use gene knockout and transgenic technology to ablate and replace molecules. As this century draws to a close, endocrinology is exploding beyond the classical glands of internal secretion and their products to include studies of the secretions of cells in brain, the heart, the kidneys, the immune system, and virtually all other organs and tissues. The twenty-first century will surely witness further expansion of our understanding of the processes that govern cell function and will undoubtedly provide the tools to manipulate these processes to benefit the health and well-being of humankind.

Our purpose in preparing this section of the *Handbook of Physiology* is to provide a comprehensive resource in contemporary endocrinology for teachers, advanced students, and investigators. Our aims are twofold: *(1)* to provide background, perspective, and information in endocrinology to those whose training was primarily in cellular and molecular biology; and *(2)* to foster an understanding of, and appreciation for, the powerful tools of modern cellular and molecular biology for those whose training was in classical endocrinology. It is our hope that these volumes will contribute to exciting developments that are yet to come.

Worcester, Mass.   H.M.G.
June 1997

Preface

A striking difference between this group of volumes and the previous endocrine section of the *Handbook of Physiology* is that it begins with a molecular orientation. As available techniques increase in resolution and analytical capacity, we recognize that diverse cells share commonalities of action, and it is the goal of this volume to identify these underlying cellular and molecular aspects. It is here that we find justification for this volume: valuable lessons learned from one system are applicable to others.

The volume was written for a range of readers, from students who need a general introduction to bench scientists who need to learn what is known about endocrine systems other than the one they work on. The chapters describe studies conducted in well-established systems. Some deal with conceptual fundamentals (receptor identification, receptor structure, gene expression, signaling, and second messenger systems), while others address newly appreciated concepts in receptor and gene regulation. Still others cover physiological principles such as secretion, steroidogenesis, and apoptosis. Targeted hormone delivery is also included. The authors are all recognized scientists, active in the areas about which they write. They were selected for their skill in "telling the story," which should make the book more readable and more generally applicable than would be the case if it were only a series of reviews on esoteric topics.

I am indebted to Maurice Goodman for his efforts in organizing this section of the *Handbook of Physiology* and inviting this contribution.

Beaverton, Ore.   P.M.C.
June 1997

Contents

Contributors

Robert S. Bar, M.D.
Veterans Administration Medical Center
Department of Internal Medicine
Diabetes and Endocrinology Research Center
The University of Iowa
Iowa City, Iowa

Jeffrey L. Benovic, Ph.D.
Departments of Biochemistry and Molecular Pharmacology,
    Microbiology, and Immunology
Kimmel Cancer Institute
Thomas Jefferson University
Philadelphia, Pennsylvania

Yibang Chen, Ph.D.
Department of Pharmacology
Mount Sinai School of Medicine of the City University
    of New York
New York, New York

P. Michael Conn, Ph.D. (Editor)
Divisions of Neuroscience and Reproductive Services
Oregon Regional Primate Research Center
Beaverton, Oregon
and Department of Physiology and Pharmacology
Oregon Health Sciences University
Portland, Oregon

Priscilla S. Dannies, Ph.D.
Department of Pharmacology
Yale University School of Medicine
New Haven, Connecticut

Carl Denef, M.D., Ph.D.
Laboratory of Cell Pharmacology
School of Medicine
University of Leuven
Leuven, Belgium

Ngozi E. Erondu, Ph.D.
Veterans Administration Medical Center
Department of Internal Medicine
Diabetes and Endocrinology Research Center
The University of Iowa
Iowa City, Iowa

John H. Exton, M.D., Ph.D.
Howard Hughes Medical Institute and Department
    of Molecular Physiology and Biophysics
Vanderbilt University School of Medicine
Nashville, Tennessee

Kevin Ferreri, Ph.D.
VivoRx
Santa Monica, California

Peter F. Hall, M.D., Ph.D.
Department of Endocrinology and Metabolism
Division of Medicine
Prince of Wales Hospital
Randwick, New South Wales, Australia

Sheau Yu Hsu, Ph.D.
Division of Reproductive Biology
Department of Gynecology and Obstetrics
Stanford University Medical School
Stanford, California

Aaron J. W. Hsueh, Ph.D.
Division of Reproductive Biology
Department of Gynecology and Obstetrics
Stanford University Medical School
Stanford, California

Cliff Hurd, Ph.D.
Department of Biological Sciences
and The Institute for Biochemistry and Biotechnology
Oakland University
Rochester, Michigan

Ravi Iyengar, Ph.D.
Department of Pharmacology
Mount Sinai School of Medicine of the City University
    of New York
New York, New York

Barbara M. Judy, Ph.D.
Department of Veterinary Biomedical Sciences
University of Missouri-Columbia
Columbia, Missouri

Karen L. Leach, M.D.
Cell Biology and Inflammation Research
Pharmacia & Upjohn, Inc.
Kalamazoo, Michigan

Lee E. Limbird, Ph.D.
Department of Pharmacology
Vanderbilt University Medical Center
Nashville, Tennessee

Pierre-Marie Lledo, Ph.D.
C.N.R.S.
Institut A. Fessard
Gif-sur-Yvette, France

W. T. Mason, Ph.D.
Department of Molecular Signalling
Babraham Institute
Babraham, Cambridge, United Kingdom

Marc Montminy, M.D., Ph.D.
The Clayton Foundation Laboratories for Peptide Biology
The Salk Institute
La Jolla, California

Harvey Motulsky, M.D.
GraphPad Software, Inc.
San Diego, California

V. K. Moudgil, Ph.D.
Department of Biological Sciences and The Institute
    for Biochemistry and Biotechnology
Oakland University
Rochester, Michigan

Rosalind P. Murray-McIntosh, Ph.D.
Institute of Molecular Biosciences
Massey University
Palmerston North, New Zealand

V. Nebes, Ph.D.
The Thyroid Eye Disease Research Laboratory
Department of Ophthalmology
Allegheny General Hospital
Pittsburgh, Pennsylvania

William M. Pardridge, M.D.
Department of Medicine
University of California at Los Angeles
School of Medicine
Los Angeles, California

Raymond B. Penn, Ph.D.
Departments of Biochemistry and Molecular Pharmacology, Micro-
    biology, and Immunology
Kimmel Cancer Institute
Thomas Jefferson University
Philadelphia, Pennsylvania

Marjan Rupnik, Ph.D.
Institute of Pathophysiology
School of Medicine
Ljubljana, Slovenia

Stuart C. Sealfon, M.D.
Fishberg Research Center in Neurobiology and Department of Neu-
    rology
Mount Sinai School of Medicine of the City University
    of New York
New York, New York

Stanko S. Stojilkovic, Ph.D.
Endocrinology and Reproduction Research Branch
National Institute of Child Health and Human Development
National Institutes of Health
Bethesda, Maryland

Alfredo Ulloa-Aguirre, M.D., Ph.D.
Department of Reproductive Biology
Instituto Nacional de la Nutrición "Salvador Zubirán"
Mexico City, D.F., Mexico
and Divisions of Neuroscience and Reproductive Sciences
Oregon Regional Primate Research Center
Beaverton, Oregon

J. Wall, M.D., Ph.D.
The Thyroid Eye Disease Research Laboratory
Department of Medicine
Allegheny University of the Health Sciences
Pittsburgh, Pennsylvania

Wade V. Welshons, Ph.D.
Department of Veterinary Biomedical Sciences
University of Missouri-Columbia
Columbia, Missouri

Gezhi Weng, Ph.D.
Department of Pharmacology
Mount Sinai School of Medicine of the City University
    of New York
New York, New York

Robert Zorec, Ph.D.
Institute of Pathophysiology
School of Medicine
Ljubljana, Slovenia

HANDBOOK OF PHYSIOLOGY

Section 7: The Endocrine System
Volume I: Cellular Endocrinology

1. Cell biology of secretion

PRISCILLA S. DANNIES | *Department of Pharmacology, Yale University School of Medicine, New Haven, Connecticut*

MOST PROTEINS THAT ARE SECRETED FROM THE CELL are synthesized on membranes of the endoplasmic reticulum and transported through the membrane into its lumen. Secretory proteins are then transferred, through a series of membrane-enclosed compartments in which various processing and sorting events occur, to the cell surface (Fig. 1.1). A compartment may be defined by its function and by its luminal and membrane components; various subdivisions of major compartments, such as the Golgi complex, have been proposed. The exact number of distinct compartments may not yet be resolved, but proteins must go through several, including three major ones in the Golgi complex, on their way to the outside of the cell (118, 164).

INTRACELLULAR TRANSPORT IN VESICLES

Transport from one compartment to the next occurs by budding of transport vesicles that carry cargo and then fusing of the vesicles to the next site (Fig. 1.2). This process maintains the orientation of transmembrane molecules toward the lumen, and ultimately the exterior of the cell, while transporting the molecules through separate cellular compartments. The result of vesicular transport is that proteins that have passed through the membrane as they are made need not do so again to be secreted; passage through membranes is an energetically unfavorable process.

Continuous transport of membrane that is part of the vesicles to the surface of the cell would result in depletion of the endoplasmic reticulum and expansion of the cell surface, were it not prevented by transport in the opposite direction based on the same principles, that is, budding and fusion of vesicles in the reverse direction. Membrane retrieval is as important as forward movement.

Ensuring that vesicles fuse to the correct targets is also crucial. If lysosomes were not maintained separately from other compartments, such as the endoplasmic reticulum or secretory granules, basic functions of the cells would collapse. The recognition of the correct target membrane by each vesicle is essential for the viability of the cell.

Endocrine and neuronal cells that secrete protein and peptide hormones concentrate them into secretory granules (79, 80, 137), which may be regarded as a specialized form of membrane-bound transport vesicle. Secretory granules transport hormones to the cell surface, but differ from most vesicular transport in that they serve as a storage depot. Release from these granules occurs when the vesicles fuse with the plasma membrane in response to a stimulus, which may be a neurotransmitter or another hormone. Over 40 years ago it was recognized that what the different stimulating agents have in common is that they stimulate exocytosis by increasing intracellular Ca^{2+} concentrations (48, 89). Therefore, exocytosis can be regarded as a form of vesicular transport that is specialized, with a requirement for high Ca^{2+} concentrations in order for fusion to occur.

Since Ca^{2+} was identified as important, much effort has been put into understanding how intracellular Ca^{2+} triggers hormone release. In recent years, increasing amounts of evidence have shown that knowledge from very different sources—nerve terminals, secretion in yeast, and in vitro assays for intra-Golgi transport—

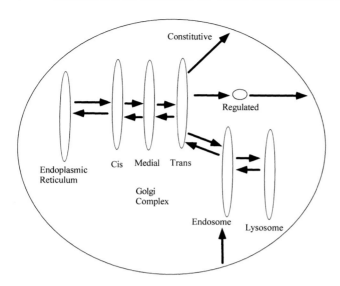

FIG. 1.1. Transport among membrane-enclosed compartments in the cell. Proteins, after synthesis and transport into endoplasmic reticulum, undergo various sorting and processing procedures, and are transported through various compartments. In most cases, soluble proteins are only transported forward, but there is retrograde transport to return membrane components, including membrane proteins that belong in a previous compartment. Membrane and membrane proteins that arrive at the cell surface by constitutive or regulated secretion are returned by endocytosis to endosomes.

is directly relevant both to vesicle fusion and hormone release from endocrine cells and to endocytosis and membrane budding. Transport from yeast endoplasmic reticulum to the Golgi complex and the release of transmitters from neuronal axons have elements in common with formation and fusion of secretory granules in endocrine cells, and the explosion of knowledge in the field is a result of the convergence of these investigations.

MEMBRANE FUSION AND EXOCYTOSIS

Investigations in Synaptic Vesicles

Synaptic vesicles of uniform shape and size are found at presynaptic nerve endings at a high density. They store neurotransmitters that they release when action potentials depolarize the cells opening voltage-dependent Ca^{2+} channels and increasing intracellular Ca^{2+} concentrations. Exocytotic release of neurotransmitters is very fast, occurring after a lag of 200–300 μs (110). The membrane components of these vesicles are retrieved by endocytosis, and the vesicles refill with neurotransmitter in the synaptic terminal to be used again (78).

The high concentration of synaptic vesicles in the neuronal terminals, and of neuronal terminals in the brain, make protein purification feasible. Sudhof and Jahn (185) have pointed out that if synaptic vesicles were single molecules, their concentration in the brain would be micromolar; the proteins in them account for 7% of the total brain protein. Since these vesicles do not contain protein or peptide neurotransmitters, the proteins that are present in the synaptic vesicle membrane are all associated with the function of the vesicles. Several proteins in the nerve terminals, some associated with or located in the membrane of the vesicles, were purified and characterized. Powerful evidence that some of the proteins isolated this way are directly involved in exocytosis comes from the knowledge of how certain neurotoxins work.

Tetanus toxin and botulinum toxins are clostridial neurotoxins that effectively inhibit neurotransmitter release (125). Each is produced as a single chain precursor and cleaved to form two chains connected by disulfide bonds. The heavy chain of each toxin causes specific binding to and entry into neuronal cells. In the cytoplasm, reduction of disulfide bonds activates the light chains, which are highly specific zinc peptidases. Three neuronal proteins are substrates for three toxins (74). Tetanus toxin and botulinum neurotoxin A both cleave synaptobrevin, an integral membrane protein of synaptic vesicles (also called VAMP, vesicle associated membrane protein) in a specific site, between glutamine 76 and phenylalanine 77 (104, 173). Botulinum neurotoxins D and F also cleave synaptobrevin at separate specific sites (18, 175). Botulinum C cleaves syntaxin (23), a transmembrane protein in the neuronal plasma membrane and in synaptic vesicles. Finally, botulinum toxins A and E both cleave SNAP-25 (synaptosomal-

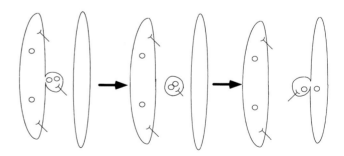

FIG. 1.2. Vesicular transport between compartments. Transport between the compartments, shown in Figure 1.1, is mediated through small membrane-bound vesicles that bud off one compartment, diffuse to the next, and fuse with that compartment. In the example shown, the vesicle is transporting soluble proteins (circles) and membrane receptors (⅄). Transport in the opposite direction occurs through similar vesicles.

associated protein, 25,000 kD) (18, 22, 175), a protein found in high concentrations in nerve terminals, associated with the plasma membrane, and originally thought to be involved in neurite formation (136). In the nerve terminals, these neurotoxin proteases are specific for these substrates. The neurotoxins that cleave synaptobrevin also cleave cellubrevin, a homologous protein with a ubiquitous distribution unlike synaptobrevin, which is only in nerve terminals (74). The other toxins appear to cleave only the proteins indicated. The specificity of these proteases allow a direct link to be made between cleavage of these proteins and inhibition of exocytosis.

Investigations in Yeast

Other groups of researchers, beginning with Schekman and coworkers in the late 1970s (170), used yeast to determine what gene products are necessary for secretion. The use of genetic tools in yeast is powerful, and a number of gene products involved in secretion were identified. Secretion in yeast is a constitutive process; yeast do not store proteins, and therefore can not release proteins that are already synthesized in response to a stimulus. When these studies were begun, it was not thought that they would bear any relationship to the investigation of neurotransmitter release in the brain.

The secretion mutants initially identified, called *sec* (for yeast, *SEC1* is the wild-type gene, *sec1* is the mutant, and Sec1p, the protein coded by *SEC1*), are temperature-sensitive mutants. A temperature-sensitive mutant is caused by a mutation that allows the protein to function at a normal temperature, but makes the protein unstable at higher temperatures. To isolate *sec* mutants, mutagenized cells that became denser at high temperatures, detected by sedimentation on gradients, were screened for secretion of acid phosphatase and invertase (129), to determine if the increased density was caused by accumulation of proteins that could not be secreted. Those that did not secrete the enzymes were characterized further, and twenty-three complementation groups were identified (129).

Subsequently, various other selection procedures have been developed. One example is a screen for genes necessary for transport of proteins to appropriate locations. Carboxypeptidase Y is normally transported to vacuoles in yeast, as is a hybrid of carboxypeptidase Y and invertase. Invertase activity of this hybrid was used as a marker to screen cells expressing this protein to detect those with invertase activity on the surface of the cells. These mutants are *vps* (vacuolar protein sorting) mutants (11, 158, 165). Other genes have been identified because they compensated, when expressed

in high amounts, for mutants that cause lethal defects in transport. These genes usually provide a function related to the defect that they suppress, and therefore provide a genetic way of detecting interactions among the identified genes. A second way of detecting interactions among gene products is called synthetic lethality; when two temperature-sensitive mutants are co-expressed, the combination may be lethal at the permissive temperature, although either expressed alone is not. Such a result strongly indicates that the two gene products interact.

The proof that the product of a gene identified by any means is involved in transport is that deletion of the gene blocks transport; in some cases, genes have redundant functions and more than one gene must be deleted to affect transport.

Combining these genetic techniques with biochemical techniques, reconstitution assays, and effects on morphology has led to the identification of genes necessary for vesicle-mediated protein transport from the endoplasmic reticulum to the Golgi complex, for sorting vacuolar proteins from secretory proteins, and for transporting proteins from the Golgi complex to the plasma membrane (150).

Reconstituted Systems of Transport

A prime example of an extensively investigated cell-free system of transport is that which occurs between Golgi cisternae. Such transport was demonstrated by Rothman and coworkers by incubating a Golgi preparation containing the G protein of vesicular stomatitis virus from cells deficient in an enzyme that adds N-acetylglucosamine to the viral protein with a Golgi preparation from cells that had the enzyme (9, 55, 163). When cytosol and adenosine triphosphate (ATP) were added to this mixture, transfer of G protein from the Golgi preparation lacking the enzyme to the one that had it was measured by addition of radioactive N-acetylglucosamine to the G protein. In this cell-free system, incubation of Golgi membranes with cytosol and ATP also induced the formation of small membrane-enclosed vesicles containing the G protein, which behaved as would be expected if they were intermediates in conveying the VSV G protein from one Golgi cisterna to another; when transport, measured by G protein–modification, was blocked, the vesicles accumulated (10, 133, 163). One way to block transport is to treat cytosol with N-ethylmaleimide (NEM), a reagent that alkylates free sulfhydryl groups (111); transport was recovered when untreated cytosol was added (24, 59, 163). The ability to restore transport inhibited by treatment with NEM was used as an assay to purify the protein that NEM was affecting called NEM-sensitive fusion protein (NSF) (24).

Convergence of Separate Approaches

When NSF was sequenced, it was found to be homologous to the yeast protein Sec18p, one of the yeast proteins identified as necessary for transport from the endoplasmic reticulum to the Golgi complex. Sec18p could be substituted for NSF in the mammalian cell-free fusion assay (206), work that indicates that fusion processes in quite different organisms have common themes.

Rothman and coworkers continued to purify components necessary for fusion in reconstituted systems. Purified NSF does not bind to vesicles or membranes when added by itself, but does when added with cytosol (163). The ability to cause purified NSF to bind to allow fusion provided a new assay used to purify proteins called SNAPs (soluble NSF attachment factors, not to be confused with SNAP-25, isolated independently from nerve terminals and mentioned above). Two proteins, α- and γ-SNAP, are necessary for NSF binding and the transfer assay (34, 35, 181). α-SNAP is homologous to yeast protein Sec17p (61); and Sec17p and Sec18p, the NSF homologue, have been shown to interact genetically (85).

SNAPs bind to Golgi membranes and vesicles with NSF, but NSF does not bind without SNAPs. The next step in this cascade of purifications was to purify the proteins to which SNAPs bind. These proteins are called SNAP receptors, or SNAREs. Rothman predicted that the specificity in fusing vesicles to the right compartment, absolutely essential for viability, would reside in different sets of SNARES for different stages in the transport process (163). Characterization in yeast indicated that Sec17p and Sec18p, and therefore, by analogy, α-SNAP and NSF, could not supply the specificity because they participate in fusion steps in multiple places in the secretory pathway including endoplasmic reticulum to Golgi complex, Golgi complex to plasma membrane, and in endocytosis (60, 85, 156). Instead, sets of SNAREs, one set on a vesicle and one set on the membrane to which the vesicle is to fuse, bind specifically to each other, and then the complex of SNAREs are recognized by the more general factors, SNAPs and NSF, which in turn bind to form a complex that is capable of leading to fusion of the membranes. The prediction that receptors for SNAPs, or SNAREs, should be many places led Rothman's group to start to purify these receptors from the brain, since Rothman predicted they would be there in high concentrations because the concentration of vesicles is so high (185). They purified three proteins on the basis of their ability to bind to the SNAP–NSF complex. These proteins, when characterized, turned out to be previously identified proteins: syntaxin, SNAP-25, and synaptobrevin, proteins already discussed because of their specific susceptibility to neurotoxins (181), and, therefore, their importance in neurotransmitter release. These three proteins also have homologous proteins in yeast that participate in endoplasmic to Golgi complex, Golgi complex to vacuole, and Golgi complex to plasma membrane transport (17, 52). The finding that constitutive transport of vesicles from the endoplasmic reticulum to the Golgi complex in yeast have components in common with the highly specialized, rapid, and regulated release of neurotransmitters from synaptic vesicles in mammalian brain was dramatic. It indicated that fusion processes would be similar throughout the species, and that similar components would be present in fusion processes in many parts of the secretory pathway.

The basic finding is summarized as follows. Synaptobrevin is in the synaptic vesicle membrane and syntaxin is in the plasma membrane of the neuron where it is associated with SNAP-25. These three proteins form a complex in solution (31); the complex may supply the specificity to attach the vesicle to the right membrane before fusion and therefore these proteins are SNAREs. α- and γ-SNAP bind this complex, and NSF then binds in the presence of ATP. NSF hydrolyses ATP, and does not dissociate in the presence of a non-hydrolyzable analog (181). A problem with reconstitution assays is demonstrating that what happens in the assay happens in the intact cells. The evidence from yeast and toxins makes clear that the proteins that were isolated from the reconstitution assay and led to the isolation of NSF and SNAPs have functions in the secretion process in mammalian brains and in yeast, and therefore the proteins must be physiologically relevant. The challenge is now to determine what the exact function is of the complex in docking and fusion, and how fusion occurs.

Calcium Dependence of Stimulated Neurotransmitter Release

Regulated release of neurotransmitter depends on Ca^{2+} in localized concentrations that are quite high, 100 μM or greater (110). A relatively simple way to envision how constitutive release in yeast can use the same components to fuse membranes as regulated exocytosis in brain is to postulate that there is a block added in regulated exocytosis—some component that prevents constitutive fusion from occurring until a Ca^{2+} signal releases the inhibition.

A natural candidate for such a calcium sensor is present in synaptotagmin. Synaptotagmin had been isolated from synaptic vesicles and characterized, and was found to have two Ca^{2+}–binding domains, similar to those in protein kinase C (144, 145), and to change conformation when it binds Ca^{2+} (28). In solution, it competes with α-SNAP for binding to the complex of synaptobrevin, syntaxin, and SNAP-25 (180). One model was that Ca^{2+} would cause dissociation of synaptotagmin from the complex, allowing α- and γ-SNAP and NSF to bind and fusion to proceed (163), but dissociation stimulated by Ca^{2+} has not been demonstrated. These experiments were done with α-SNAP, which is ubiquitous. More recently, a brain-specific form of SNAP, β-SNAP, has been shown to form a complex with synaptotagmin that then binds NSF (174), but the role for Ca^{2+} has not been defined in this complex. If Ca^{2+}-stimulated release occurs because a protein prevents release until Ca^{2+} concentrations increase, a Ca^{2+} sensor and a protein that prevents fusion are necessary. It is not clear that synaptotagmin is the molecule that prevents fusion as well as acting as the sensor for Ca^{2+} (90).

The data generated by knockout mice and expression of mutant synaptotagmin in *Drosophila* do support the role of synaptotagmin as a Ca^{2+} sensor (90, 172). Mice that expressed a truncated mutant synaptotagmin at 5% of wild-type levels had normal nerve terminals in terms of morphology, but the fast component of neurotransmitter release in response to Ca^{2+} was gone (58). *Drosophila*-expressing mutants of synaptotagmin had decreased release of neurotransmitter in response to Ca^{2+} (107). Since terminals were not depleted of vesicles, the simplest interpretation is that synaptotagmin is an important Ca^{2+} sensor, but not the active inhibitor of fusion needed to prevent regulated release from becoming constitutive. Interpretations of knockout experiments, however, are complicated by the existence of multiple isoforms of synaptotagmin that may be overexpressed to compensate for the loss of a particular form (39, 57, 69, 73, 119, 144, 192), and so a role for synaptotagmin in exocytosis in addition to sensing Ca^{2+} cannot be ruled out.

Docking Vesicles to the Correct Membrane

NSF was named NEM-sensitive fusion protein because it was necessary to detect fusion in a reconstituted system. This protein has ATPase activity, and an attractive possibility initially was that the energy provided by the ATP hydrolysis was used to drive the fusion process. Work with yeast, however, suggests that the primary role of NSF may be in targeting. SEC18 is the yeast homologue of NSF. *Sec18* mutants accumulate transport vesicles at the restricted temperature; vesicles do not fuse when the mutant phenotype is expressed. When the vesicles containing the mutant were produced at the per-

missive temperature, they subsequently fused at either the restrictive or the permissive temperature, indicating that the protein may be important in docking, or bringing about the association of the membranes before fusion, but that once docked, the protein is not necessary for subsequent fusion (155). Docking must involve selection, since, as mentioned above, it is essential that only correct fusions occur. The proteins predicted to show the specificity are the SNAP receptors on the membranes, and some specificity has been demonstrated. In solution, α- and γ-SNAPs and NSF bind to SNAP-25, syntaxin, and synaptobrevin, which is consistent with the docking and targeting role. There are multiple forms of syntaxin, as there are of synaptotagmin (16, 75). Evidence for specificity is that synaptobrevin (VAMP) interacts with syntaxins 1 and 4, not 2 and 3, and the ability to form a tight complex with α- and γ-SNAP, NSF, SNAP-25 and synaptobrevin is most pronounced only with syntaxin 1 (15, 31, 147). The model, as it now stands, predicts that there are molecules other than synaptobrevin to which 2 and 3 will bind, and that when bound to their correct partners, SNAPs and NSF will bind to those complexes.

It is clear that many more proteins are probably involved in all processes of transport, docking, and fusion. Knowledge of another family of proteins that must be involved in transport, and most likely in correct targeting, comes from yeast. *SEC4*, which is required for transport from Golgi to the plasma membrane, was determined to encode a *ras*-like protein, which bound and hydrolyzed guanosine triphosphate (GTP) (53, 168, 170). Proteins in the Ras superfamily bind GTP, and in this state bind to membranes and activate effectors. Hydrolysis of GTP reduces the ability of these proteins to remain bound to the membranes and to the effectors, and therefore terminates the activity. *YPT1* was originally found as a gene essential for yeast viability, whose function was not known, but it was of interest because of its homology with *ras* (56). It has now been established that Ypt1p functions in transport from the endoplasmic reticulum to the Golgi apparatus (6, 7, 53, 128). *YPT1* was also shown to be necessary for correct delivery, but not fusion, of transport vesicles to the Golgi complex, and, as would be predicted from the homology with *ras,* to bind and hydrolyze GTP (155).

The discovery that these GTP-binding proteins were important in transport in yeast led to detection of homologous genes in mammalian cells that were more similar to *SEC4* and *YPT1* than *ras* (53, 128, 170). These genes, called *rab*, are a large family of over 30 members, and the products of many have been localized to specific membranes and locations in the cell (177). Rab 5, for example, is found on early endosomes and the plasma membrane (30), and Rab3a is found on secretory vesicles (52). These proteins are found in the cytosol, and binding to membranes is coupled to the nucleotide exchange reaction of guanosine diphosphate (GDP) for GTP (53); the hydrolysis of GTP may play a role in vesicle targeting. The specific locations and the large number of these proteins made them appealing candidates for molecules involved in selecting the correct membrane for transport vesicles. An important question is how Rab family members interact with the docking activities of NSF and γ- and α-SNAP, and with the SNARE proteins on the transport vesicles and target membranes that confer specificity. Two groups have used yeast systems to demonstrate that Rab proteins are necessary to obtain SNAREs capable of binding NSF and the SNAPs (101, 179). The means by which the Rab proteins do this may be indirect, rather than by direct binding, which has not been demonstrated. It is reasonable that something should have to activate SNAREs before they function in targeting, so that they do not direct inappropriate fusion when they are not in the correct position (128), for example, when they are synthesized in the endoplasmic reticulum, or when they are being recycled.

The number of proteins involved in transport to the correct site will continue to become more complex. Rab proteins interact with several other proteins that affect their function (128, 149). Although Rab proteins hydrolyze GTP, the rate of hydrolysis and the exchange of GTP and GDP is slow. The rates are regulated by other proteins. GAP (GTPase-activating protein) increases hydrolysis of GTP; GEF (guanine-nucleotide exchange factor) enhances nucleotide exchange; GDI (guanine-nucleotide dissociation inhibitor) decreases exchange; GDF (GDI-displacement factor) decreases association of GDI with Rab; rabphilin binds Rab in its GTP-bound form and may be a receptor or effector (128, 149). There are therefore many ways in which Rab function may be regulated. GDI, which keeps GDP from dissociating, keeps Rab in an inactive form, and has been used as a tool to show that Rabs are necessary for appropriate membrane fusion in permeabilized cell systems (1).

The success in going from yeast genes to mammalian proteins in the case of Rab has led to other searches for mammalian equivalents of yeast genes known to be necessary for secretion, and these may be equally informative (70, 88, 96, 148).

Other Fusion Mechanisms

Is SNARE/SNAP/NSF all there is? The answer to this question seems to be no. The fusions discussed above have been those involved in vectorial transport between compartments, but there is also homotypic fusion, in which fusion occurs within a compartment. Endoplasmic reticulum tubules may fuse with each other; these homotypic fusion mechanisms do not involve NSF (96, 117, 207), but instead require a cell division cycle gene. *CDC48* is necessary for homotypic endoplasmic reticulum fusion in yeast (95). A mammalian Cdc48p homologue, valosin-containing peptide (VCP), appears to be required from some Golgi fusion steps in mammalian cells (1, 151), steps that do not require SNAP.

A second example that may be even more interesting has come from investigations of MDCK cells, which have distinct mechanisms of transport to the apical and to basolateral cell membranes. Ikonen et al. (76) have investigated transport from the endoplasmic reticulum to the Golgi complex, from the Golgi complex to the basolateral membrane, and from the Golgi complex to the apical membrane. Transport of the first two kinds is stimulated by adding α-SNAP, inhibited by antibodies to NSF, inhibited by Rab-GDI, and inhibited by toxins that cleave cellubrevin (a ubiquitous analog of synaptobrevin [52]). All of these results are consistent with the kind of transport and fusion process mediated through NSF and SNAPs discussed above. Apical transport is not inhibited by any of these treatments. This system is satisfying because of the internal controls. Golgi to plasma membrane transport may be considered heterotypic fusion, but the pathway that appears to apply in so many cells, and so many locations in cells, does not apply here, and so other fusion mechanisms must exist, although at this time they are not well characterized.

Evidence for SNAP–NSF–Mediated Docking/Fusion With Dense Core Granules

Although it seemed highly likely that release from dense core granules is mediated by the SNAP/NSF complex as a step in the process in endocrine cells, it could not be regarded as a given, especially since alternate systems exist. Obtaining evidence that these components were involved was not as straight-forward as might be imagined. If dense core vesicles dock and fuse by the same mechanisms as small synaptic vesicles, then synaptotagmin and synaptobrevin should be present on membrane vesicles, and syntaxin and SNAP-25 present on plasma membranes in endocrine cells. Determining if these proteins are present was complicated by two factors: multiplicity of isoforms of some proteins, and the presence of small synaptic-like microvesicles in endocrine cells. There are at least eight isoforms of synaptotagmin (13, 39, 57, 69, 73, 112, 119, 192, 193, 201) and syntaxin (16, 42, 75, 77, 88, 100, 123), and so reports that synaptotagmin I was only present in some cells of the pituitary gland could not be interpreted to mean that the others used a different way of sensing Ca^{2+}. The absence of a protein may only mean that the correct isoform has not yet been identified. In addition to demonstrating the presence of these proteins, they should be shown to be on the dense core secretory granules, because they may be present on other vesicles. Endocrine cells contain small vesicles with many of the synaptic vesicle membrane proteins (or isoforms of these proteins) (47). These vesicles do not contain proteins as dense core vesicles do, but, at least in some cases, they contain neurotransmitters. In β-cells of the pancreas, these small vesicles contain GABA (47), and in adrenal chromaffin cells, they contain acetylcholine (14). Although the function of these vesicles isn't clear, they do have the components predicted for SNAP/NSF targeting and fusion.

The presence of these proteins on secretory granules in neuroendocrine cells is not sufficient to prove the same kind of docking/fusion procedure is involved. The most dramatic proof that these proteins are involved in exocytosis in neurons came from the work with toxins, in which the neurotoxins inhibited neurotransmitter release by each specifically cleaving one of these proteins. Neurotoxins bind to receptors on neurons and then may enter the cell; non-neural cells lack these receptors, and so the neurotoxins can not simply be added to cultures of viable endocrine cells to determine the effects. The usual way that the experiments have been performed is to permeabilize cells in various ways, add the toxin, and measure effects on Ca^{2+}–stimulated release. Measuring hormone release in a solubilized cell system is measuring the change in hormone from a state that can be sedimented to a state that is soluble. Fusion of a secretory granule membrane with the plasma membrane and release of the contents is one way to make vesicle contents soluble, but there are other ways, such as disruption of the granule membrane, that have the same effect. A requirement for ATP and Ca^{2+} to stimulate release is important, since Ca^{2+} stimulates release in intact cells, but Ca^{2+} also activates proteases and phospholipases, agents that may increase leakage of vesicle contents instead of fusion of membranes, so the requirement for Ca^{2+} is not sufficient to demonstrate that exocytosis is what is making the hormone soluble. It is therefore very satisfying when a toxin is shown to cleave its specific substrate and to prevent release in a permeabilized cell system. It demonstrates that hormone release resembles synaptic neurotransmitter release, and, that the release measured in the permeabilized system is likely to occur by a fusion mechanism rather than leakage. The absence of inhibition by toxin is less conclusive; there may be an alternative fusion system, the release measured may be leakage induced by Ca^{2+}, or the toxin may not have cleaved all the substrate, which may be present in excess over the amounts necessary to stimulate release. Synaptobrevin is not cleaved by tetanus toxin if it is in the complex with SNAP and NSF (142), and a pool of docked vesicles may therefore be protected from toxin but still be capable of bona fide release through the SNARE complex after stimulation with Ca^{2+}.

With these complications, it is therefore not surprising that there were initially some differences in the literature, but the pattern seems to be consistent with SNAP/NSF involvement in dense core vesicle docking, or fusion, or both. Syntaxin, synaptobrevin, SNAP-25, and synaptotagmin are all present in endocrine cells (16, 19, 20, 25, 71, 77, 132, 162, 166, 186, 193, 204), and synaptotagmin and synaptobrevin are present on dense core granules (33, 50, 54, 71, 138, 201). (Syntaxin is somewhat anomalous; it is supposed to be in the target membrane for vesicles, according to predictions about how SNARES cause vesicles to fuse to the correct membrane [163], and it is on the plasma membrane in endocrine cells [77], but it is also found on synaptic vesicles and chromaffin granules [186, 200]. Its function there is not known.) In permeabilized cell systems of chromaffin cells or islet cells, or neuroendocrine cell lines, toxins cleave appropriate substrates and usually inhibit release (19, 25, 71, 98, 166, 193, 204). In one case, intact chromaffin cells were intoxicated with botulinum neurotoxin B by incubating the cells with the toxin in hypotonic conditions; the toxin cleaved synaptobrevin and inhibited catecholamine release (54). (Chromaffin cells have both protein and catecholamines in their dense core granules.) Adding α-SNAP to permeabilized chromaffin cells enhances release (121). Anti-syntaxin antibodies inhibit release from permeabilized chromaffin cells (62), reinforcing the experiments with toxins. In addition, the three proteins, syntaxin, synaptobrevin and SNAP-25, form the same kind of complexes in solution as were isolated from the brain with SNAPs and NSF (132, 162).

Rab proteins, which are important for fusion of SNAP/NSF–directed vesicles, and secretion in yeast (128), and which are associated with synaptic vesicles in the brain (52), also appear to be important for hormone release in neuroendocrine cells (109). Rab3a is the major form associated with vesicles in the brain, but Rab3b is the predominant form in the rat anterior pituitary gland. Antisense nucleotides to Rab3b injected into pituitary cells reduces expression of the protein, and in the injected cells, Ca^{2+}-stimulated exocytosis, measured by increases in membrane capacitance, was reduced (109). Other investigators have used peptides with the same sequence as parts of Rab3 to detect effects; since the same amino composition in a different sequence can give the same results as the Rab-specific sequence, these experiments are less conclusive (49).

Therefore, the components that are involved in NSF and SNARE–mediated docking and fusion are present in endocrine cells. Disrupting the function of these proteins in various ways disrupts the exocytotic function in several different systems, indicating that this fusion system plays an important role in endocrine cells.

Exocytosis in Endocrine Cells

It is difficult to do biochemistry on dense core granules, because they are not present in high concentrations, as synaptic vesicles are, and they can not be manipulated genetically in yeast. There is one major advantage that these granules have, and that is that they are large enough to cause a change in the area of the membrane surface of the cells when they fuse with the plasma membrane. Capacitance, or the ability of a membrane to store an electric charge, is a function on the area of the membrane, and measurements of capacitance have been used to directly measure hormone release. Early measurements were dramatic, because they were performed with mast cells from *beige* mice; these mutant mice have a few (or even one) very large secretory granules, and so the change in capacitance is large and can be correlated visibly with release (64, 143, 211). These investigations also show that there are capacitance flickers, brief reversible changes in capacitance, which indicates that the early stages of fusion are reversible and the pore can close shortly after it opens without releasing the contents of the vesicle (103).

As the large secretory granules of mast cells fuse with the plasma membrane, they also generate a transient electrical current, in addition to the increase in capacitance (26, 64, 182). The current occurs as the vesicle discharges its membrane potential through the fusion pore, and has been used to obtain information about the pore (103). There are two components to the current, one fast, followed by a slower one. The size of the initial pore may be estimated from the fast component, and is no larger than a large ion channel (26, 182). In addition, there is a marked temperature dependence for the opening, which is consistent with protein components forming the initial pore, rather than just lipid.

The use of capacitance measurements have also been applied to endocrine cells as more sensitive methods were developed. The use of capacitance together with a quantitative analysis of the morphology of granules in cells has given a clear analysis of the last stages of

hormone release (139). It had been known for years that release is dependent on Ca^{2+}, but little was known beyond that. An important tool in further characterizing the Ca^{2+}-dependence of exocytosis was demonstrated using capacitance for melanotrophs and adrenal chromaffin cells (72, 189, 198); the investigations revealed a rapid burst of exocytosis, which occurs within 10 ms, followed by a slower rate of exocytosis. The interpretation of these results was ambiguous because Ca^{2+} in the cytosol was increased by causing Ca^{2+} entry through channels in the plasma membrane, which will result in large gradients of Ca^{2+}, highest near the channels (157). Thus, heterogeneity in times of release could reflect differences in exposure to Ca^{2+} concentrations rather than discrete classes of release. To overcome this problem, a photolabile Ca^{2+} chelator, DN-nitrophen [1-(2-nitro-4,5-dimethoxyphenyl)-1,2-diamino-ethane-N,N, N′,N′-tetraacetic acid] (87) was used to cause rapid uniform increases in Ca^{2+} in the cytoplasm. By attaching a pipette to the cell, the chelator and a Ca^{2+} indicator were exchanged with the cytoplasm, so that changes in Ca^{2+} could be followed as well as changes in capacitance. These investigations confirmed that there is a secretory burst followed by slower release from melanotrophs and chromaffin cells (67, 190). In melanotrophs, the first burst lasts 50 ms after a delay of about 10 ms, followed by a slower rate of release lasting one s, which is followed by a still slower rate of release (190, 191). The slow release is inhibited by reducing the cytosolic pH to 6.2, and the slower release phase occurs much more rapidly at temperatures above 30° C than at room temperature, and may be inhibited by dropping the temperature (191). The ability to inhibit the two slow phases meant that it was possible to measure the exocytotic burst alone, which allowed Almers and coworkers to determine the Ca^{2+}-dependence of the exocytotic burst; the rate increases steeply with increasing Ca^{2+} concentrations, and is half-maximal at $[Ca^{2+}]i = 27$ μM, with at least three Ca^{2+} ions required to trigger exocytosis (191). The affinity of the final step for fusion is lower than might be predicted from some of the pemeabilized cell systems. In chromaffin cells, the maximum Ca^{2+} required is usually about 10 μM. These permeabilized systems may be measuring more than one Ca^{2+}-sensitive step, and not just the last step. There is evidence in yeast that fusion that is not regulated also requires Ca^{2+} (7); fusion does not occur in a reconstituted system in the absence of Ca^{2+}. The difference between Ca^{2+}-stimulated release of neurotransmitters and hormones and constitutive fusion in yeast may occur because the release process is less sensitive to Ca^{2+} than other kinds of vesicle fusion, rather than that Ca^{2+} sensitivity is added. Vesicles travelling from the endoplasmic reticulum to the Golgi complex may have high affinity sites for Ca^{2+} that detect amounts present in the cytosol under normal conditions to cause fusion, and vesicles that release after stimulation have lower affinity receptors that only cause fusion when Ca^{2+} concentrations are higher.

The interpretation of the exocytotic burst in melanotrophs and chromaffin cells is that the burst results from the release of docked vesicles, vesicles that are located next to the plasma membrane, and that it represents a very late, most likely the last, stage in exocytosis (190, 191). Counting the number of granules present at the membrane indicated that only a small subset of granules at the plasma membrane actually participate in this final stage of exocytosis in melanotrophs and adrenal chromaffin cells.

The use of DN-nitrophen also suggested that ATP was not necessary for these last steps, including the slower stages after the most rapid exocytotic burst, because the photolysis of Ca-DN-nitrophen, which releases Ca^{2+}, allows the chelator to bind Mg^{2+}, and would be expected to decrease cytosolic Mg^{2+} concentrations below the levels necessary to support ATP hydrolysis. Almers and coworkers confirmed this finding by measuring changes in capacitance after they had demonstrated that the ATP had diffused out of the cell into the attached pipette used to add Ca-DN-nitrophen and Ca^{2+} indicators (139). When ATP is gone, Ca^{2+}-stimulated exocytosis still occurs and continues for minutes; only the release at later times (more than 1 min) is increased by the presence of ATP (139).

The total amount of ATP-independent release, including the slower stages after the exocytotic burst

estimated from the increase in membrane area, is quite similar to vesicles found near the plasma membrane. Ca^{2+} stimulates release of 2700 granules in a melanotroph, where 3300 are next to the membrane, and 840 granules in a chromaffin cell, where 830 are next to the membrane (139). The very rapid exocytotic burst uses a much smaller proportion. Almers and coworkers have proposed the model in Figure 1.3. Vesicles dock through NSF and the SNAP proteins, and ATP hydrolysis occurs. After this step, ATP is no longer required, and the vesicles are considered docked. Ca^{2+} is required, and there are several stages after ATP hydrolysis before the final fusion stage, recognized by susceptibility to temperature or pH. If the energy from ATP hydrolysis by NSF participates in the fusion process itself, it must be stored in the complex for at least 6 min (139). This clear definition of the last stages of hormone release has many unanswered questions; two of the most compelling are: What actually forms the fusion pore detected by the transient electrical current and capacitance flicker? and Now that the role of Ca^{2+} has been tracked to the very last step, what does it do there?

Exocytosis of dense core granules has also been investigated in permeabilized cell systems. Such systems rundown because necessary cytosolic factors leak from the cell. The addition of cytosolic proteins to the permeabilized cells functions as a reconstitution assay. In these systems, release is stimulated by Ca^{2+} and ATP. Using such an assay, various proteins have been identified that regulate Ca^{2+}-stimulated release (121), including protein kinase C (64, 120, 126), protein kinase A (122), annexin II (2, 3, 169), 14–3–3 proteins (208),

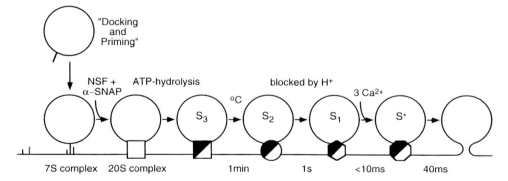

FIG. 1.3. Possible sequence of steps in exocytosis in endocrine cells. Endocrine secretory granules approach the plasma membrane; synaptobrevin on the secretory granule membrane forms a complex with syntaxin and SNAP-25 on the plasma membrane; this complex ensures the vesicle is docking to the correct membrane. These three proteins form a 7S complex in solution. When these three proteins, and possibly more not yet identified, have formed a complex, NSF and α-SNAP bind, to form a larger 20S complex, followed by ATP hydrolysis. At this point, ATP is no longer required, so other steps that require ATP for priming are also complete. Several stages after ATP hydrolysis can be distinguished on the basis of temperature sensitivity (S_3 to S_2), pH sensitivity (S_2 to S_1), and response to Ca^{2+} (S_1 to S^*), which finally leads to release. [Taken from Parsons et al. (139), with permission.]

p145 (126, 202) and phosphatidylinositol transfer protein (66). Release from these systems is measured over minutes and may not always be comparable to what is measured in single cells using capacitance, where the earliest events are detected in milliseconds but there are some good correspondences. In chromaffin cells permeabilized with digitonin, there is an ATP-dependent component of catecholamine release, and an ATP-independent component, which only needs Ca^{2+}; Bittner and Holz found a temperature-sensitive step that occurs after the ATP-dependent step (21).

The ATP-dependent step has been identified in one permeabilized cell system. In PC12 cells, adrenal chromaffin tumor cells, permeabilized by a ball homogenizer, the ATP-requiring step for catecholamine release is formation of phosphatidylinositol 4, 5-bisphosphate by phosphatidylinositol 4-phosphate-5-kinase, and requires a phosphatidylinositol transfer protein (65, 66). This step is referred to as priming the cell for Ca^{2+}-induced release. The relationship of priming to docking is at this time unclear. Formation of phosphatidylinositol 4,5-bisphosphate may be a step necessary to prepare the membranes for fusion of docked vesicles and permeabilized systems may be primarily measuring the release of vesicles that have been previously docked, or secured to the plasma membrane. The method of permeabilizing the cells may also affect what vesicle populations exist, and the states of the membranes involved, making comparisons among systems difficult.

In intact cells, Ca^{2+} is likely to regulate more than the final step. Release from intact cells has been known for a long time to have several different pools or components; prolactin is just one example (41). At least one other step has been demonstrated by capacitance investigations in chromaffin cells. Pretreatment with Ca^{2+} increases the size of the pool that is available to be most rapidly released in the exocytotic burst (198). The physical identity of these pools has not been completely characterized, but at least one step is likely to involve actin. There is a network of actin filaments that run parallel to the plasma membrane in chromaffin cells (124) that may regulate accessibility of secretory vesicles to the plasma membrane, and therefore the ability of these vesicles to dock. Vitale and coworkers showed that phorbol myristol acetate disrupted the actin network, increased the number of granules close to the plasma membrane, and increased the number of vesicles that rapidly fused with the membrane, measured by membrane capacitance changes, when cells were depolarized (196). There may be other stages that may be regulated as well in the transport of the vesicles from the Golgi complex, not yet elucidated.

In some endocrine cells, hormone release stimulated by Ca^{2+} may be inhibited. Dopamine prevents prolactin release in response to Ca^{2+} (40, 97), and epinephrine and somatostatin have the same effect on insulin secretion (194, 195). In insulin–producing cells, this inhibition was shown to occur in permeabilized cells, indicating it was at the later stages of secretion (195). Whether this inhibition is at the very last step of the Ca^{2+} response, past the docking step, or at some earlier step necessary to dock or prime vesicles has yet to be determined, and may be useful in determining what stages can be regulated in endocrine cells.

MEMBRANE BUDDING AND ENDOCYTOSIS

Evidence from yeast and mammalian cells also suggests that the elements that participate in vesicle budding are similar; there are, however, several different systems that have been characterized. In addition, there are several kinds of evidence for the involvement of phospholipids in different ways.

Budding Involving Clathrin

Clathrin was shown early on to be involved in receptor-mediated endocytosis and also in the transport of lysosomal or vacuolar proteins from the Golgi complex (140). Clathrin is a protein with a triskelion structure that binds to coated pits on the plasma membrane, where it forms a basket-like structure that drives vesicle invagination (45, 140, 171). The same structures involved in receptor endocytosis are also involved in synaptic vesicle recycling in the brain, and, again, the extremely high amount of activity in the brain and high concentration of proteins has made this a useful system to investigate the process biochemically. Clathrin is in the nervous system in large amounts concentrated in nerve terminals (113, 187). Clathrin binds to the plasma membrane through protein complexes called adaptors (140); there are separate sets of adaptors for the plasma membrane and the trans-Golgi network (140, 205). The adaptor complexes, AP1 and AP2, are heterotetramers; AP1 is associated with the trans-Golgi network, and involved in the sorting of lysosomal enzymes (140), and AP2 is present in high concentrations in the brain, and implicated in synaptic vesicle endocytosis (45). There are two brain-specific proteins, AP180 and auxilin, which also stimulate clathrin assembly (160). Binding of clathrin to adaptors in isolated systems does not yet mimic binding seen in intact cells completely, as binding in intact cells only occurs at specific locations (159, 171); the binding is likely to be regulated by many factors not yet fully characterized.

Although clathrin is ideally suited to deforming planar membranes into buds, it does not appear to sever the budding vesicle from the membrane. That function is supplied by dynamin; this protein as a GTPase, first discovered as a protein that binds to microtubules (130). In *Drosophila*, the *shibire* gene is identical to dynamin, and temperature-sensitive mutants of this gene lead to a block in synaptic endocytosis at the stage of invaginated pits (91), with an electron dense ring around the neck of the pits. In an in vitro assay for endocytosis in synaptic vesicles, using GTPγS, a nonhydrolyzable analog, multiple rings appeared at the neck of these pits that stained positively for dynamin by immunocytochemistry (187). The current model is that dynamin rings form at the neck of clathrin–coated pits, and GTP hydrolysis drives a change that leads to the fusion reaction and formation of a vesicle from the membrane (45). Support for dynamin involvement in all clathrin–coated vesicle fusion comes from *VSPI*, a gene in yeast required from transport from the Golgi complex to vacuoles, a pathway that requires clathrin (51, 205); *VSP1* is a dynamin homologue. The form in the brain is a neurospecific form of dynamin, dynamin I. As is the case for so many of the proteins discussed here, there are isoforms with tissue specificity. The tissue specificity in this case may reflect the need for very rapid recycling of components in a nerve terminal compared to the speed necessary for endocytosis of receptors and other processes of membrane retrieval. The forms of dynamin that participate in budding from the cell surface, rather than from the Golgi region, have a proline-rich C-terminus that will bind to proteins with an SH3 (Sarc homology 3) domain in them. A number of proteins with these domains have been found—to determine which ones are important, investigators looked for those present in high concentration in the brain. A major SH3 domain–containing protein, amphiphysin, is found in large amounts in nerve terminals (44, 102). Amphiphysin also interacts with the clathrin adaptor, AP2, and is colocalized with dynamin (43, 114). A third protein, also present in nerve terminals and colocalized with amphiphysin, and which also interacts with SH3 domains, is synaptojanin (114, 115). Synaptojanin is closely related to a type II 5-phosphatase, which will dephosphorylate inositol polyphosphates and the phospholipids, phosphatidylinositol 4,5-bisphosphate and phosphatidylinositol 3,4,5-trisphosphate (63, 81, 210). Synaptojanin and dynamin are phosphorylated themselves and rapidly dephosphorylated after neurotransmitter release in vivo and in solution by the Ca^{2+}-dependent phosphatase, calcineurin (45, 160). Stimulation of neurotransmitter release **in vivo** leads to a rapid dephosphorylation of dynamin, a decrease in GTPase activity, and more bound and less soluble dynamin (108, 161). Inducing

exocytosis may therefore at the same time induce compensating endocytosis by activating dynamin and other necessary proteins. Regulation of endocytosis involves phosphorylation and dephosphorylation of lipids and protein, as do so many other regulated processes. The clathrin adaptor complex, AP2, binds to synaptotagmin (209), and mutants of synaptotagmin in *Caenorhabditis elegans* do not recycle synaptic vesicles properly (83). Synaptotagmin therefore may play a role, possibly related to its ability to bind Ca^{2+}, in endocytosis as well as exocytosis.

Clathrin–coated vesicles carry enzymes from the trans-Golgi network to lysosomes in mammalian cells, and from the trans-Golgi network to vacuoles, the equivalent of lysosomes, in yeast. Vps1p, a protein necessary for this transport in yeast, is also a GTPase, and the sequence is closely related to dynamin (37). The evidence is consistent with dynamin functioning in yeast, as it does in neural tissue, to cause the clathrin-induced invagination to bud, and supports the evidence obtained by biochemistry in the brain.

Other evidence implicates phospholipids. Vsp34p is necessary for correct sorting of the hybrid invertase to the vacuole (37, 183). Vsp34p phosphorylates phosphatidylinositol to form phosphatidylinositol 3'-phosphate, and is recruited to the Golgi membrane by binding a serine–threonine protein kinase, Vps15p (37, 46, 184); this complex is necessary for proper sorting of at least some proteins. A homologous complex that appears to be involved in lysosomal sorting has been found in mammalian cells (197). In addition, proper sorting, but not receptor internalization from the plasma membrane, of the PDGF (platelet-derived growth factor) receptor is affected in mutants of the receptor that can not bind phosphoinositide 3'-kinase, because proper sorting after the endosomes does not occur (86). Whether phosphatidylinositol 3'-phosphate is necessary for correct sorting of all proteins or only a subset is not yet known. Finally, *SEC14* is necessary for proper sorting from the Golgi complex in yeast, and this protein is a phosphatidylinositol transfer protein that exchanges phosphatidylinositol for phosphocholine in the Golgi membranes (105). There is, therefore, evidence that phospholipids are important. So far in the case of transport to lysosomes from the Golgi complex, it is phosphorylation of lipids that has been implicated, whereas with endocytosis from the plasma membrane, it is dephosphorylation. The story is likely to become further complicated.

Budding Involving COPI/ARF

The initial reconstitution system for investigating intra-Golgi vesicular traffic in vitro contained, using electron microscopy, vesicles that were coated, not with clathrin, but with a different fuzzy dense coat, unlike the lattice structure made by clathrin. This system, like the clathrin–coated vesicles, has also been studied extensively. These coated vesicles accumulated in the presence of a non-hydrolyzable analog of GTP, GTPγS (163). In the presence of GTP, rather than the analog, uncoated vesicles were produced which fused in an NEM-sensitive manner (111, 116, 134, 163). These vesicles were purified, and the proteins that form the coat characterized; they include the coat proteins (or COPs) α, β, β', γ, δ, ϵ, and ζ, collectively referred to as coatamer and present in equimolar amount (163, 203), and a protein called ARF (adenosine diphosphate-ribosylation factor) (84, 203), which is a GTPase. ARF was originally discovered as a cofactor necessary for cholera toxin-mediated AD-ribosylation of the $G_{S\alpha}$ subunit of heterotrimeric G proteins.

ARF is soluble in its GDP-bound form but associates with membranes in the GTP-bound form, and the GTP-bound form of ARF triggers attachments of the coat proteins. Although ARF was initially proposed to bind coat proteins directly, and the binding of coat proteins provide the force that drives the budding, it is now known that the role of ARF is more complex involving phospholipids. ARF activates a Golgi–localized phospholipase D, and this reaction, as well as GTP hydrolysis, is stimulated by phosphatidylinositol 4,5-bisphosphate (29, 105, 154). Brefeldin, a drug that blocks binding of ARF to Golgi membranes, and which has profound effects on secretion pathways, causing the separation between the Golgi complex and the endoplasmic reticulum to collapse, inhibits stimulation of phospholipase D by ARF (92). A current model is that ARF changes the phospholipid structure so that coat proteins may bind; in addition, changing the phospholipid structure may also increase membrane curvature to facilitate or cause vesicle budding (46, 92, 105).

Any action that changes the phospholipid composition of a membrane in a manner that affects its physical properties would have to be extremely well controlled for the cell to survive. Phospholipase D in the Golgi membrane generates phosphatidic acid, primarily from phosphatidylcholine. Phosphatidic acid activates a phosphatidyl 4-phosphate 5-kinase to generate phosphatidylinositol 4,5-bisphosphate, which causes amplification of the phospholipase D activity (29, 36, 46, 82, 106, 146). Phosphatidylinositol 4,5-bisphosphate and phosphatidic acid also, however, stimulate the activity of a GAP for ARF, which may provide the way to inactivate ARF and break the cycle (154).

There is nothing known aboout these COPI–coated vesicles that is analogous to dynamin, which seems so

clearly involved in causing the invaginated clathrin-coated pit to close and separate from the membrane. Whether there are similar proteins to separate COPI–coated buds yet to be discovered, or whether the budding off process is a completely different mechanism, and even whether it can be so cleanly separated from invagination in this case as it is in the clathrin coats, is not yet known.

The vesicles coated with these COPIs were assumed to be vesicles involved in forward transport from the endoplasmic reticulum to and through the Golgi complex. The bulk of the evidence however, indicates that these vesicles are actually involved in retrograde transport from the Golgi cisternae to the endoplasmic reticulum (99, 141, 171). Two coatamer subunits, α and β', bind the amino acid sequence, KKXX, on the cytoplasmic tail of proteins responsible for proteins that reside in the endoplasmic reticulum being returned there if they escape (38).

The vesicles that mediate transport in the forward direction from the endoplasmic reticulum to the Golgi complex are coated with a different set of proteins, COPII proteins (99, 141, 171), that have recently been isolated, and which were discovered from analysis of the transport pathways in yeast. These COPII vesicles require GTP hydrolysis, and a small GTP-binding protein, Sar1p (12, 68, 167). Homologous proteins have been discovered in mammalian cells, and so the same system exits there (93, 135, 176). COPII vesicles have not been as extensively studied. The enrichment that occurs by combining investigations in mammalian cells with those in yeast has continued to pay off in transport studies.

There may be at least one more type of coated vesicle. Electron micrographs have demonstrated that lacy-coated vesicles, different from the dense coats of COPs or the lattice of clathrin, bud from different regions of the trans-Golgi network than clathrin-coated vesicles do (94).

The reason for apparently different budding mechanisms, certainly with different machinery, in different parts of the cell may be related to differences in membrane composition. Although cholesterol is made in the endoplasmic reticulum, it is present in low amounts there, and in high amounts in the plasma membrane; sphingolipids are synthesized in the cis-Golgi region and therefore not present earlier in the pathway (27). Changes in the composition of the membrane affect its thickness and the flexibility, so that the plasma membrane is thicker and less flexible than the membrane in the endoplasmic reticulum (27). The differences in these properties may require different methods of handling the membrane to make it invaginate and bud.

Endocytosis in Endocrine Cells

All cells have clathrin–mediated endocytosis, and, as discussed above, neuronal cells have neuronal-specific proteins associated with the ubiquitous components that may adapt the machinery to the specialized needs of synaptic terminals. Endocrine cells certainly have clathrin–coated vesicles that participate in endocytosis, but there may be other means specialized for the large granules that store hormone. Capacitance measurements have demonstrated endocytosis that is triggered by Ca^{2+} and released by photolysis of Ca-DM-nitrophen in melanotrophs and adrenal chromaffin cells (67, 188). Endocytosis was detected as a decrease in membrane capacitance that was easily detectable in some cells that did not have extended exocytosis. When extended exocytosis was inhibited by lowering the pH of the cytoplasm, endocytosis was detectable in all cells (188). This Ca^{2+}–induced mechanism is rapid, and retrieves up to 20% of the cell surface area within 10 s at 20° to 26° C (188). This membrane retrieval mechanism is unlikely to be clathrin–mediated, because it is not inhibited by low cytosolic pH or lack of K^+, conditions that inhibit clathrin-mediated endocytosis in other cells (188). In addition, some of the decreases in membrane capacitance occur in clearly resolvable steps. The size of these steps indicates that some retrieval vesicles must be as large or larger than 0.8 μm in diameter—larger than the 100-nm clathrin–coated vesicles, and also larger than secretory granules in melanotrophs (300 nm). Almers and coworkers have suggested the intriguing possibility that exocytosis leads to retrieval of vesicles of sizes similar to secretory granules because it is the secretory granule membrane itself that is being retrieved, at least some of the time (188). A pore opens to the outside for a few seconds and the contents of the granule diffuses out, but the secretory granules membrane does not flatten into the plasma membrane and mix with those components. It remains curved and separate from the plasma membrane, ready to be retrieved. Almers and coworkers suggested that in some cases there may be fusion of secretory granule membranes, resulting in the intake of a membrane area larger than the size of one vesicle. Whether the retrieval mechanism involves a ring formed by dynamin or a similar protein, or whether it proceeds by an entirely different mechanism is not known at this time.

The necessity for increases in Ca^{2+} to trigger this system ensures that it will be ready for membrane removal after exocytosis. Vacuoles the size of secretory granules have been detected in neuroendocrine cells after exocytosis was stimulated, and these vacuoles formed within seconds (4, 5, 8, 127), evidence that supports the rapid retrieval of these relatively large areas of membrane. Unlike the synaptic vesicle membranes that, once retrieved, refill with neurotransmitters by transporters incorporated into the membranes, these vacuoles can not refill with peptide and protein hormones; the components must be recycled through the Golgi to be part of a new filled secretory granule.

Formation of Secretory Granules in Endocrine Cells

Formation of dense core secretory granules in endocrine cells may differ from many other processes in which membrane–enclosed vesicles are generated in the cells, because the formation of secretory granules has an entirely different morphology (153). This morphology was clearly shown for rat prolactin by Rambourg and coworkers (153), who used three-dimensional electron microscopy to obtain the structures. They found that the Golgi complex exists as a layered ribbon in which dense aggregations of prolactin occur in the trans-Golgi cisternae (Fig. 1.4). The dense cores do not bud off of the trans-Golgi region, leaving that region intact. Instead, the last layer of the trans-Golgi ribbon becomes progressively vesiculated. The number of small vesicles in the area is consistent with the vesiculation of the trans-Golgi cisternae being caused by the budding off of the numerous small vesicles, many clathrin–coated. Howell and coworkers examined three-dimensional constructions of the Golgi complex in non-endocrine cells, and also found massive synchronous budding along the tubules of the trans-Golgi network. It is not obvious from these electron micrographs that any special budding mechanism may be necessary to form secretory granules; they may be what is left when all the membrane vesicles enclosing soluble proteins have budded off. The clathrin–coated vesicles, for example, would remove the lysosomal enzymes that are found with prolactin in the early stages of secretory granule formation (178). Since the insoluble dense cores of prolactin have already formed, further budding can not occur when the soluble proteins are removed. In this view, immature secretory granules are ones still linked to the trans-Golgi network, because budding of smaller vesicles is not complete.

Using this mechanism, the last leaf of the trans-Golgi ribbon would completely disintegrate and need to be regenerated (153). Rambourg and Claremont have made the prediction that the last leaf disintegrates based on three-dimensional constructions of several tissues in addition to endocrine tissues (152). This view of secretory granule formation is consistent with results of von Zostrow and Castle with insulin–containing granules. They demonstrated that vesicles bud off of immature secretory granules, removing soluble proteins

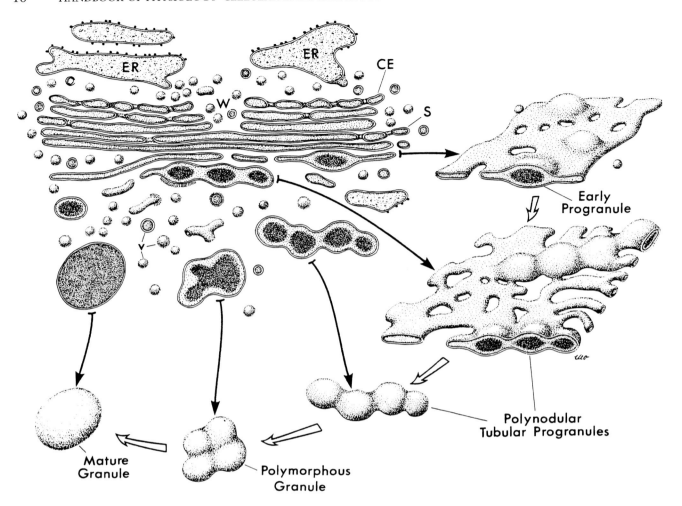

FIG. 1.4. Representation of a portion of the Golgi ribbon of a prolactin cell, developed from three dimensional electron microscopy. Prolactin is made on the endoplasmic reticulum (ER), and transported to the *cis*-Golgi (*cis*-element, CE). The Golgi ribbon is not continuous in the early section; there are gaps (wells, W) with small vesicles near these wells. The Golgi cisternae or saccules (S) and secretory granules are shown in cross section and the *trans*-Golgi region and secretory granules again in three dimensions. Large aggregates of prolactin are seen in the *trans*-Golgi region, which becomes progressively less solid. As the layer vesiculates, prolactin dense cores that have not yet separated merge to form larger cores. Budding of smaller vesicles, many with bristle coats, likely clathrin, continues until the large secretory granules are no longer attached to the layer. [Taken from Rambourg et al. (153) with permission.]

and leaving the insoluble insulin core (199). In the simplest model, the secretory granule pathway would be regarded almost as a default pathway; proteins that were not carried into the small vesicles that budded off would be left in the remaining residue, which becomes the granule. More complicated models are possible.

Two groups have investigated the formation of secretory granules in permeabilized cells, and have used the ability of the small dense secretory granules to be rapidly sedimented as a tool. Huttner and colleagues have found that phosphatidylinositol transfer protein, the protein necessary in yeast for vesicle formation from the Golgi complex, is necessary for secretory granule formation in permeabilized PC12 cells (131).

Chen and Shields showed that ARF, the protein necessary to make vesicles with COPI proteins, enhanced secretory vesicle formation in permeabilized pituitary tumor cells, GH3 cells (32). These results may be interpreted in two ways. Either these factors are necessary for secretory granule formation as an active process on its own, or the factors are necessary for other membrane vesicles to bud off from the complex, leaving the contents of secretory granules in small and dense enough packages so that they can be separated from other parts of the secretory pathway by centrifugation. There is no analogous process in yeast, and therefore it will require different approaches to formation of these vesicles than the approaches that have been used so successfully for dissecting other stages of vesicle formation.

This work was supported by NIH grants HD-11487 and DK-46807.

REFERENCES

1. Acharya, U., R. Jacobs, J. M. Peters, N. Watson, M. G. Farquhar, and V. Malhotra. The formation of Golgi stacks from vesiculated Golgi membranes requires two distinct fusion events. *Cell* 82: 895–904, 1995.

2. Ali, S. M., and R. D. Burgoyne. The stimulatory effect of calpactin (annexin II) on calcium-dependent exocytosis in chromaffin cells: requirement for both the N-terminal and core domains of p36 and ATP. *Cell Signal* 2: 265–276, 1990.

3. Ali, S. M., M. J. Geisow, and R. D. Burgoyne. A role for calpactin in calcium-dependent exocytosis in adrenal chromaffin cells. *Nature* 340: 313–315, 1989.

4. Back, N., S. Soinila, and I. Virtanen. Endocytotic pathways in the melanotroph of the rat pituitary. *Histochem. J.* 25: 133–139, 1993.

5. Back, N., M. Tyynela, M. M. Portier, I. Virtanen, and S. Soinila. Distribution of neurofilament proteins and peripherin in the rat pituitary gland. *Neurosci. Res.* 22: 267–275, 1995.

6. Bacon, R. A., A. Salminen, H. Ruohola, P. Novick, and S. Ferro-Novick. The GTP-binding protein Ypt1 is required for transport in vitro: the Golgi apparatus is defective in ypt1 mutants. *J. Cell. Biol.* 109: 1015–1022, 1989.

7. Baker, D., L. Wuestehube, R. Schekman, D. Botstein, and N. Segev. GTP-binding Ypt1 protein and Ca^{2+} function independently in a cell-free protein transport reaction. *Proc. Natl. Acad. Sci. USA* 87: 355–359, 1990.

8. Baker, P. F., and D. E. Knight. Calcium control of exocytosis and endocytosis in bovine adrenal medullary cells. [Review]. *Phil. Trans. R. Soc. Lond. B. Biol. Sci.* 296: 83–103, 1981.

9. Balch, W. E., W. G. Dunphy, W. A. Braell, and J. E. Rothman. Reconstitution of the transport of protein between successive compartments of the Golgi measured by the coupled incorporation of N-acetylglucosamine. *Cell* 39(2 Pt 1): 405–416, 1984.

10. Balch, W. E., B. S. Glick, and J. E. Rothman. Sequential intermediates in the pathway of intercompartmental transport in a cell-free system. *Cell* 39(3 Pt 2): 525–536, 1984.

11. Bankaitis, V. A., L. M. Johnson, and S. D. Emr. Isolation of yeast mutants defective in protein targeting to the vacuole. *Proc. Natl. Acad. Sci. USA* 83: 9075–9079, 1986.

12. Barlowe, C., C. d'Enfert, and R. Schekman. Purification and characterization of SAR1p, a small GTP-binding protein required for transport vesicle formation from the endoplasmic reticulum. *J. Biol. Chem.* 268: 873–879, 1993.

13. Bauerfeind, R., R. Jelinek, and W. B. Huttner. Synaptotagmin I- and II-deficient PC12 cells exhibit calcium-independent, depolarization-induced neurotransmitter release from synaptic-like microvesicles. *FEBS Lett.* 364: 328–334, 1995.

14. Bauerfeind, R., A. Regnier-Vigouroux, T. Flatmark, and W. B. Huttner. Selective storage of acetylcholine, but not catecholamines, in neuroendocrine synaptic-like microvesicles of early endosomal origin. *Neuron* 11: 105–121, 1993.

15. Bennett, M. K. SNAREs and the specificity of transport vesicle targeting. [Review]. *Curr. Opin. Cell. Biol.* 7: 581–586, 1995.

16. Bennett, M. K., J. E. Garcia-Arraras, L. A. Elferink, K. Peterson, A. M. Fleming, C. D. Hazuka, and R. H. Scheller. The syn-taxin family of vesicular transport receptors. *Cell* 74: 863–873, 1993.

17. Bennett, M. K., and R. H. Scheller. The molecular machinery for secretion is conserved from yeast to neurons. [Review]. *Proc. Natl. Acad. Sci. USA* 90: 2559–2563, 1993.

18. Binz, T., J. Blasi, S. Yamasaki, A. Baumeister, E. Link, T. C. Sudhof, R. Jahn, and H. Niemann. Proteolysis of SNAP-25 by types E and A botulinal neurotoxins. *J. Biol. Chem.* 269: 1617–1620, 1994.

19. Bittner, M. A., B. R. DasGupta, and R. W. Holz. Isolated light chains of botulinum neurotoxins inhibit exocytosis. Studies in digitonin-permeabilized chromaffin cells. *J. Biol. Chem.* 264: 10354–10360, 1989.

20. Bittner, M. A., and R. W. Holz. Effects of tetanus toxin on catecholamine release from intact and digitonin-permeabilized chromaffin cells. *J. Neurochem.* 51: 451–456, 1988.

21. Bittner, M. A., and R. W. Holz. A temperature-sensitive step in exocytosis. *J. Biol. Chem.* 267: 16226–16229, 1992.

22. Blasi, J., E. R. Chapman, E. Link, T. Binz, S. Yamasaki, P. De Camilli, T. C. Sudhof, H. Niemann, and R. Jahn. Botulinum neurotoxin A selectively cleaves the synaptic protein SNAP-25 [see comments]. *Nature* 365: 160–163, 1993.

23. Blasi, J., E. R. Chapman, S. Yamasaki, T. Binz, H. Niemann, and R. Jahn. Botulinum neurotoxin C1 blocks neurotransmitter release by means of cleaving HPC-1/syntaxin. *EMBO J.* 12: 4821–4828, 1993.

24. Block, M. R., B. S. Glick, C. A. Wilcox, F. T. Wieland, and J. E. Rothman. Purification of an N-ethylmaleimide-sensitive protein catalyzing vesicular transport. *Proc. Natl. Acad. Sci. USA* 85: 7852–7856, 1988.

25. Boyd, R. S., M. J. Duggan, C. C. Shone, and K. A. Foster. The effect of botulinum neurotoxins on the release of insulin from the insulinoma cell lines HIT-15 and RINm5F. *J. Biol. Chem.* 270: 18216–18218, 1995.

26. Breckenridge, L. J., and W. Almers. Currents through the fusion pore that forms during exocytosis of a secretory vesicle. *Nature* 328: 814–817, 1987.

27. Bretscher, M. S., and S. Munro. Cholesterol and the Golgi apparatus. [Review]. *Science* 261: 1280–1281, 1993.

28. Brose, N., A. G. Petrenko, T. C. Sudhof, and R. Jahn. Synaptotagmin: a calcium sensor on the synaptic vesicle surface. *Science* 256: 1021–1025, 1992.

29. Brown, H. A., S. Gutowski, C. R. Moomaw, C. Slaughter, and P. C. Sternweis. ADP-ribosylation factor, a small GTP-dependent regulatory protein, stimulates phospholipase D activity [see comments]. *Cell* 75: 1137–1144, 1993.

30. Bucci, C., R. G. Parton, I. H. Mather, H. Stunnenberg, K. Simons, B. Hoflack, and M. Zerial. The small GTPase rab5 functions as a regulatory factor in the early endocytic pathway. *Cell* 70: 715–728, 1992.

31. Calakos, N., M. K. Bennett, K. E. Peterson, and R. H. Scheller. Protein-protein interactions contributing to the specificity of intracellular vesicular trafficking. *Science* 263: 1146–1149, 1994.

32. Chen, Y. G., and D. Shields. ADP-ribosylation factor-1 stimulates formation of nascent secretory vesicles from the trans-Golgi network of endocrine cells. *J. Biol. Chem.* 271: 5297–5300, 1996.

33. Chilcote, T. J., T. Galli, O. Mundigl, L. Edelmann, P. S. McPherson, K. Takei, and P. De Camilli. Cellubrevin and synaptobrevins: similar subcellular localization and biochemical properties in PC12 cells. *J. Cell Biol.* 129: 219–231, 1995.

34. Clary, D. O., I. C. Griff, and J. E. Rothman. SNAPs, a family of NSF attachment proteins involved in intracellular membrane fusion in animals and yeast. *Cell* 61: 709–721, 1990.

35. Clary, D. O., and J. E. Rothman. Purification of three related peripheral membrane proteins needed for vesicular transport. *J. Biol. Chem.* 265: 10109–10117, 1990.

36. Cockcroft, S., G. M. Thomas, A. Fensome, B. Geny, E. Cunningham, I. Gout, I. Hiles, N. F. Totty, O. Truong, and J. J. Hsuan. Phospholipase D: a downstream effector of ARF in granulocytes. *Science* 263: 523–526, 1994.

37. Conibear, E., and T. H. Stevens. Vacuolar biogenesis in yeast: sorting out the sorting proteins. [Review]. *Cell* 83: 513–516, 1995.

38. Cosson, P., and F. Letourneur. Coatomer interaction with dilysine endoplasmic reticulum retention motifs. *Science* 263: 1629–1631, 1994.

39. Craxton, M., and M. Goedert. Synaptotagmin V: a novel synaptotagmin isoform expressed in rat brain. *FEBS Lett.* 361: 196–200, 1995.

40. Cui, Z. J., F. S. Gorelick, and P. S. Dannies. Calcium/calmodulin-dependent protein kinase-II activation in rat pituitary cells in the presence of thyrotropin-releasing hormone and dopamine. *Endocrinology* 134: 2245–2250, 1994.

41. Dannies, P. S. Prolactin: multiple intracellular processing routes plus several potential mechanisms for regulation. [Review]. *Biochem. Pharmacol.* 31: 2845–2849, 1982.

42. Dascher, C., J. Matteson, and W. E. Balch. Syntaxin 5 regulates endoplasmic reticulum to Golgi transport. *J. Biol. Chem.* 269: 29363–29366, 1994.

43. David, C., P. S. McPherson, O. Mundigl, and P. De Camilli. A role of amphiphysin in synaptic vesicle endocytosis suggested by its binding to dynamin in nerve terminals. *Proc. Natl. Acad. Sci. USA* 93: 331–335, 1996.

44. David, C., M. Solimena, and P. De Camilli. Autoimmunity in stiff-man syndrome with breast cancer is targeted to the C-terminal region of human amphiphysin, a protein similar to the yeast proteins, Rvs167 and Rvs161. *FEBS Lett.* 351: 73–79, 1994.

45. De Camilli, P. The eighth Datta Lecture. Molecular mechanisms in synaptic vesicle recycling. [Review]. *FEBS Lett.* 369: 3–12, 1995.

46. De Camilli, P., S. D. Emr, P. S. McPherson, and P. Novick. Phosphoinositides as regulators in membrane traffic. [Review]. *Science* 271: 1533–1539, 1996.

47. De Camilli, P., and R. Jahn. Pathways to regulated exocytosis in neurons. [Review]. *Ann. Rev. Physiol.* 52: 625–645, 1990.

48. Douglas, W. W. Stimulus-secretion coupling: the concept and clues from chromaffin and other cells. [Review]. *Br J Pharmacol* 34: 453–474, 1968.

49. Edwardson, J. M., C. M. MacLean, and G. J. Law. Synthetic peptides of the rab3 effector domain stimulate a membrane fusion event involved in regulated exocytosis. *FEBS Lett.* 320: 52–56, 1993.

50. Egger, C., R. Kirchmair, S. Kapelari, R. Fischer-Colbrie, R. Hogue-Angeletti, and H. Winkler. Bovine posterior pituitary: presence of p65 (synaptotagmin), PC1, PC2 and secretoneurin in large dense core vesicles. *Neuroendocrinology* 59: 169–175, 1994.

51. Ekena, K., and T. H. Stevens. The Saccharomyces cerevisiae MVP1 gene interacts with VPS1 and is required for vacuolar protein sorting. *Mol. Cell. Biol.* 15: 1671–1678, 1995.

52. Ferro-Novick, S., and R. Jahn. Vesicle fusion from yeast to man. [Review]. *Nature* 370: 191–193, 1994.

53. Ferro-Novick, S., and P. Novick. The role of GTP-binding proteins in transport along the exocytic pathway. [Review]. *Annu. Rev. Cell Biol.* 9: 575–599, 1993.

54. Foran, P., G. Lawrence, and J. O. Dolly. Blockade by botulinum neurotoxin B of catecholamine release from adrenochromaffin

cells correlates with its cleavage of synaptobrevin and a homologue present on the granules. *Biochemistry* 34: 5494–5503, 1995.

55. Fries, E., and J. E. Rothman. Transport of vesicular stomatitis virus glycoprotein in a cell-free extract. *Proc. Natl. Acad. Sci. USA* 77: 3870–3874, 1980.

56. Gallwitz, D., C. Donath, and C. Sander. A yeast gene encoding a protein homologous to the human c-has/bas proto-oncogene product. *Nature* 306: 704–707, 1983.

57. Geppert, M., B. T. Archer 3d., and T. C. Sudhof. Synaptotagmin II. A novel differentially distributed form of synaptotagmin. *J. Biol. Chem.* 266: 13548–13552, 1991.

58. Geppert, M., Y. Goda, R. E. Hammer, C. Li, T. W. Rosahl, C. F. Stevens, and T. C. Sudhof. Synaptotagmin I: a major Ca^{2+} sensor for transmitter release at a central synapse. *Cell* 79: 717–727, 1994.

59. Glick, B. S., and J. E. Rothman. Possible role for fatty acyl-coenzyme A in intracellular protein transport. *Nature* 326: 309–312, 1987.

60. Graham, T. R., and S. D. Emr. Compartmental organization of Golgi-specific protein modification and vacuolar protein sorting events defined in a yeast sec18 (NSF) mutant. *J. Cell. Biol.* 114: 207–218, 1991.

61. Griff, I. C., R. Schekman, J. E. Rothman, and C. A. Kaiser. The yeast SEC17 gene product is functionally equivalent to mammalian alpha-SNAP protein. *J. Biol. Chem.* 267: 12106–12115, 1992.

62. Gutierrez, L. M., J. L. Quintanar, S. Viniegra, E. Salinas, F. Moya, and J. A. Reig. Anti-syntaxin antibodies inhibit calcium-dependent catecholamine secretion from permeabilized chromaffin cells. *Biochem. Biophys. Res. Commun.* 206: 1–7, 1995.

63. Hansen, C. A., R. A. Johanson, M. T. Williamson, and J. R. Williamson. Purification and characterization of two types of soluble inositol phosphate 5-hosphomonoesterases from rat brain. *J. Biol. Chem.* 262: 17319–17326, 1987.

64. Hartmann, J., and M. Lindau. A novel Ca^{2+}-dependent step in exocytosis subsequent to vesicle fusion. *FEBS Lett.* 363: 217–220, 1995.

65. Hay, J. C., P. L. Fisette, G. H. Jenkins, K. Fukami, T. Takenawa, R. A. Anderson, and T. F. Martin. ATP-dependent inositide phosphorylation required for Ca^{2+}-activated secretion. *Nature* 374: 173–177, 1995.

66. Hay, J. C., and T. F. Martin. Phosphatidylinositol transfer protein required for ATP-dependent priming of Ca^{2+}-activated secretion. *Nature* 366: 572–575, 1993.

67. Heinemann, C., R. H. Chow, E. Neher, and R. S. Zucker. Kinetics of the secretory response in bovine chromaffin cells following flash photolysis of caged Ca^{2+}. *Biophys. J.* 67: 2546–2557, 1994.

68. Hicke, L., T. Yoshihisa, and R. Schekman. Sec23p and a novel 105-kDa protein function as a multimeric complex to promote vesicle budding and protein transport from the endoplasmic reticulum. *Mol. Biol. Cell.* 3: 667–676, 1992.

69. Hilbush, B. S., and J. I. Morgan. A third synaptotagmin gene, Syt3, in the mouse. *Proc. Natl. Acad. Sci. USA* 91: 8195–8199, 1994.

70. Hodel, A., T. Schafer, D. Gerosa, and M. M. Burger. In chromaffin cells, the mammalian Sec1p homologue is a syntaxin 1A-binding protein associated with chromaffin granules. *J. Biol. Chem.* 269: 8623–8626, 1994.

71. Hohne-Zell, B., A. Ecker, U. Weller, and M. Gratzl. Synaptobrevin cleavage by the tetanus toxin light chain is linked to the inhibition of exocytosis in chromaffin cells. *FEBS Lett.* 355: 131–134, 1994.

72. Horrigan, F. T., and R. J. Bookman. Releasable pools and the

kinetics of exocytosis in adrenal chromaffin cells. *Neuron* 13: 1119–1129, 1994.

73. Hudson, A. W., and M. J. Birnbaum. Identification of a nonneuronal isoform of synaptotagmin. *Proc. Natl. Acad. Sci. USA* 92: 5895–5899, 1995.

74. Huttner, W. B. Cell biology. Snappy exocytoxins [news; comment]. *Nature* 365: 104–105, 1993.

75. Ibaraki, K., H. P. Horikawa, T. Morita, H. Mori, K. Sakimura, M. Mishina, H. Saisu, and T. Abe. Identification of four different forms of syntaxin 3. *Biochem. Biophys. Res. Commun.* 211: 997–1005, 1995.

76. Ikonen, E., M. Tagaya, O. Ullrich, C. Montecucco, and K. Simons. Different requirements for NSF, SNAP, and Rab proteins in apical and basolateral transport in MDCK cells. *Cell* 81: 571–580, 1995.

77. Jacobsson, G., A. J. Bean, R. H. Scheller, L. Juntti-Berggren, J. T. Deeney, P. O. Berggren, and B. Meister. Identification of synaptic proteins and their isoform mRNAs in compartments of pancreatic endocrine cells. *Proc. Natl. Acad. Sci. USA* 91: 12487–12491, 1994.

78. Jahn, R., and T. C. Sudhof. Synaptic vesicles and exocytosis. [Review]. *Annu. Rev. Neurosci.* 17: 219–246, 1994.

79. Jamieson, J. D., and G. E. Palade. Intracellular transport of secretory proteins in the pancreatic exocrine cell. I. Role of the peripheral elements of the Golgi complex. *J. Cell. Biol.* 34: 577–596, 1967.

80. Jamieson, J. D., and G. E. Palade. Intracellular transport of secretory proteins in the pancreatic exocrine cell. II. Transport to condensing vacuoles and zymogen granules. *J. Cell. Biol.* 34: 597–615, 1967.

81. Jefferson, A. B., and P. W. Majerus. Properties of type II inositol polyphosphate 5-phosphatase. *J. Biol. Chem.* 270: 9370–9377, 1995.

82. Jenkins, G. H., P. L. Fisette, and R. A. Anderson. Type I phosphatidylinositol 4-phosphate 5-kinase isoforms are specifically stimulated by phosphatidic acid. *J. Biol. Chem.* 269: 11547–11554, 1994.

83. Jorgensen, E. M., E. Hartwieg, K. Schuske, M. L. Nonet, Y. Jin, and H. R. Horvitz. Defective recycling of synaptic vesicles in synaptotagmin mutants of *Caenorhabditis elegans*. *Nature* 378: 196–199, 1995.

84. Kahn, R. A., and A. G. Gilman. The protein cofactor necessary for ADP-ribosylation of Gs by cholera toxin is itself a GTP binding protein. *J. Biol. Chem.* 261: 7906–7911, 1986.

85. Kaiser, C. A., and R. Schekman. Distinct sets of SEC genes govern transport vesicle formation and fusion early in the secretory pathway. *Cell* 61: 723–733, 1990.

86. Kapeller, R., R. Chakrabarti, L. Cantley, F. Fay, and S. Corvera. Internalization of activated platelet-derived growth factor receptor-phosphatidylinositol-3' kinase complexes: potential interactions with the microtubule cytoskeleton. *Mol. Cell. Biol.* 13: 6052–6063, 1993.

87. Kaplan, J. H., and G. C. Ellis-Davies. Photolabile chelators for the rapid photorelease of divalent cations. *Proc. Natl. Acad. Sci. USA* 85: 6571–6575, 1988.

88. Katagiri, H., J. Terasaki, T. Murata, H. Ishihara, T. Ogihara, K. Inukai, Y. Fukushima, M. Anai, M. Kikuchi, J. Miyazaki, et al. A novel isoform of syntaxin-binding protein homologous to yeast Sec1 expressed ubiquitously in mammalian cells. *J. Biol. Chem.* 270: 4963–4966, 1995.

89. Katz, B. *Nerve, Muscle, and Synapse*. New York: McGraw-Hill, 1966.

90. Kelly, R. B. Neural transmission. Synaptotagmin is just a calcium sensor. [Review]. *Curr. Biol.* 5: 257–259, 1995.

91. Koenig, J. H., and K. Ikeda. Disappearance and reformation of

synaptic vesicle membrane upon transmitter release observed under reversible blockage of membrane retrieval. *J. Neurosci.* 9: 3844–3860, 1989.

92. Ktistakis, N. T., H. A. Brown, P. C. Sternweis, and M. G. Roth. Phospholipase D is present on Golgi-enriched membranes and its activation by ADP ribosylation factor is sensitive to brefeldin A. *Proc. Natl. Acad. Sci. USA* 92: 4952–4956, 1995.

93. Kuge, O., C. Dascher, L. Orci, T. Rowe, M. Amherdt, H. Plutner, M. Ravazzola, G. Tanigawa, J. E. Rothman, and W. E. Balch. Sar1 promotes vesicle budding from the endoplasmic reticulum but not Golgi compartments. *J. Cell. Biol.* 125: 51–65, 1994.

94. Ladinsky, M. S., J. R. Kremer, P. S. Furcinitti, J. R. McIntosh, and K. E. Howell. HVEM tomography of the trans-Golgi network: structural insights and identification of a lace-like vesicle coat. *J. Cell. Biol.* 127: 29–38, 1994.

95. Latterich, M., K. U. Frohlich, and R. Schekman. Membrane fusion and the cell cycle: Cdc48p participates in the fusion of ER membranes. *Cell* 82: 885–893, 1995.

96. Latterich, M., and R. Schekman. The karyogamy gene KAR2 and novel proteins are required for ER-membrane fusion. *Cell* 78: 87–98, 1994.

97. Law, G. J., J. A. Pachter, and P. S. Dannies. Dopamine has no effect on thyrotropin-releasing hormone mobilization of calcium from intracellular stores in rat anterior pituitary cells. *Mol. Endocrinol.* 2: 966–972, 1988.

98. Lawrence, G. W., U. Weller, and J. O. Dolly. Botulinum A and the light chain of tetanus toxins inhibit distinct stages of Mg.ATP-dependent catecholamine exocytosis from permeabilised chromaffin cells. *Eur. J. Biochem.* 222: 325–333, 1994.

99. Lewis, M. J., and H. R. Pelham. SNARE-mediated retrograde traffic from the Golgi complex to the endoplasmic reticulum. *Cell* 85: 205–215, 1996.

100. Li, C., B. Ullrich, J. Z. Zhang, R. G. Anderson, N. Brose, and T. C. Sudhof. Ca^{2+}-dependent and -independent activities of neural and non-neural synaptotagmins. *Nature* 375: 594–599, 1995.

101. Lian, J. P., S. Stone, Y. Jiang, P. Lyons, and S. Ferro-Novick. Ypt1p implicated in v-SNARE activation. *Nature* 372: 698–701, 1994.

102. Lichte, B., R. W. Veh, H. E. Meyer, and M. W. Kilimann. Amphiphysin, a novel protein associated with synaptic vesicles [published erratum appears in EMBO J. 1992 Oct 11(10):3809]. *EMBO J.* 11: 2521–2530, 1992.

103. Lindau, M., and W. Almers. Structure and function of fusion pores in exocytosis and ectoplasmic membrane fusion. [Review]. *Curr. Opin. Cell Biol.* 7: 509–517, 1995.

104. Link, E., L. Edelmann, J. H. Chou, T. Binz, S. Yamasaki, U. Eisel, M. Baumert, T. C. Sudhof, H. Niemann, and R. Jahn. Tetanus toxin action: inhibition of neurotransmitter release linked to synaptobrevin proteolysis. *Biochem. Biophys. Res. Commun.* 189: 1017–1023, 1992.

105. Liscovitch, M., and L. C. Cantley. Signal transduction and membrane traffic: the PITP/phosphoinositide connection. [Review]. *Cell* 81: 659–662, 1995.

106. Liscovitch, M., V. Chalifa, P. Pertile, C. S. Chen, and L. C. Cantley. Novel function of phosphatidylinositol 4,5-bisphosphate as a cofactor for brain membrane phospholipase D. *J. Biol. Chem.* 269: 21403–21406, 1994.

107. Littleton, J. T., M. Stern, M. Perin, and H. J. Bellen. Calcium dependence of neurotransmitter release and rate of spontaneous vesicle fusions are altered in *Drosophila* synaptotagmin mutants. *Proc. Natl. Acad. Sci. USA* 91: 10888–10892, 1994.

108. Liu, J. P., K. A. Powell, T. C. Sudhof, and P. J. Robinson. Dynamin I is a Ca^{2+}-sensitive phospholipid-binding protein

with very high affinity for protein kinase C. *J. Biol. Chem.* 269: 21043–21050, 1994.

109. Lledo, P. M., P. Vernier, J. D. Vincent, W. T. Mason, and R. Zorec. Inhibition of Rab3B expression attenuates Ca^{2+}-dependent exocytosis in rat anterior pituitary cells. *Nature* 364: 540–544, 1993.

110. Llinas, R., I. Z. Steinberg, and K. Walton. Relationship between presynaptic calcium current and postsynaptic potential in squid giant synapse. *Biophys. J.* 33: 323–351, 1981.

111. Malhotra, V., L. Orci, B. S. Glick, M. R. Block, and J. E. Rothman. Role of an N-ethylmaleimide-sensitive transport component in promoting fusion of transport vesicles with cisternae of the Golgi stack. *Cell* 54: 221–227, 1988.

112. Marqueze, B., J. A. Boudier, M. Mizuta, N. Inagaki, S. Seino, and M. Seagar. Cellular localization of synaptotagmin I, II, and III mRNAs in the central nervous system and pituitary and adrenal glands of the rat. *J. Neurosci.* 15(7 Pt 1): 4906–4917, 1995.

113. Maycox, P. R., E. Link, A. Reetz, S. A. Morris, and R. Jahn. Clathrin-coated vesicles in nervous tissue are involved primarily in synaptic vesicle recycling. *J. Cell Biol.* 118: 1379–1388, 1992.

114. McPherson, P. S., E. P. Garcia, V. I. Slepnev, C. David, X. Zhang, D. Grabs, W. S. Sossin, R. Bauerfeind, Y. Nemoto, and P. De Camilli. A presynaptic inositol-5–phosphatase. *Nature* 379: 353–357, 1996.

115. McPherson, P. S., K. Takei, S. L. Schmid, and P. De Camilli. p145, a major Grb2–binding protein in brain, is co-localized with dynamin in nerve terminals where it undergoes activity-dependent dephosphorylation. *J. Biol. Chem.* 269: 30132–30139, 1994.

116. Melancon, P., B. S. Glick, V. Malhotra, P. J. Weidman, T. Serafini, M. L. Gleason, L. Orci, and J. E. Rothman. Involvement of GTP-binding "G" proteins in transport through the Golgi stack. *Cell* 51: 1053–1062, 1987.

117. Mellman, I. Enigma variations: protein mediators of membrane fusion. [Review]. *Cell* 82: 869–872, 1995.

118. Mellman, I., and K. Simons. The Golgi complex: in vitro veritas? [Review]. *Cell* 68: 829–840, 1992.

119. Mizuta, M., N. Inagaki, Y. Nemoto, S. Matsukura, M. Takahashi, and S. Seino. Synaptotagmin III is a novel isoform of rat synaptotagmin expressed in endocrine and neuronal cells. *J. Biol. Chem.* 269: 11675–11678, 1994.

120. Morgan, A., and R. D. Burgoyne. Interaction between protein kinase C and Exo1 (14–3–3 protein) and its relevance to exocytosis in permeabilized adrenal chromaffin cells. *Biochem. J.* 286(15 Sep Pt 3): 807–811, 1992.

121. Morgan, A., and R. D. Burgoyne. A role for soluble NSF attachment proteins (SNAPs) in regulated exocytosis in adrenal chromaffin cells. *EMBO J.* 14: 232–239, 1995.

122. Morgan, A., M. Wilkinson, and R. D. Burgoyne. Identification of Exo2 as the catalytic subunit of protein kinase A reveals a role for cyclic AMP in Ca^{2+}-dependent exocytosis in chromaffin cells. *EMBO J.* 12: 3747–3752, 1993.

123. Nagamatsu, S., T. Fujiwara, Y. Nakamichi, T. Watanabe, H. Katahira, H. Sawa, and K. Akagawa. Expression and functional role of syntaxin 1/HPC-1 in pancreatic beta cells. Syntaxin 1A, but not 1B, plays a negative role in regulatory insulin release pathway. *J. Biol. Chem.* 271: 1160–1165, 1996.

124. Nakata, T., and N. Hirokawa. Organization of cortical cytoskeleton of cultured chromaffin cells and involvement in secretion as revealed by quick-freeze, deep-etching, and double-label immunoelectron microscopy. *J. Neurosci.* 12: 2186–2197, 1992.

125. Niemann, H. Molecular biology of clostridial neurotoxins. In: *Sourcebook of Bacterial Toxins,* edited by J. E. Alair, and J. H. Freer. New York: Academic Press, 1991, p. 303–348.

126. Nishizaki, T., J. H. Walent, J. A. Kowalchyk, and T. F. Martin. A key role for a 145–kDa cytosolic protein in the stimulation of Ca^{2+}-dependent secretion by protein kinase C. *J. Biol. Chem.* 267: 23972–23981, 1992.

127. Nordmann, J. J., and J. C. Artault. Membrane retrieval following exocytosis in isolated neurosecretory nerve endings. *Neuroscience* 49: 201–207, 1992.

128. Novick, P., and P. Brennwald. Friends and family: the role of the Rab GTPases in vesicular traffic. [Review]. *Cell* 75: 597–601, 1993.

129. Novick, P., C. Field, and R. Schekman. Identification of 23 complementation groups required for post-translational events in the yeast secretory pathway. *Cell* 21: 205–215, 1980.

130. Obar, R. A., C. A. Collins, J. A. Hammarback, H. S. Shpetner, and R. B. Vallee. Molecular cloning of the microtubule-associated mechanochemical enzyme dynamin reveals homology with a new family of GTP-binding proteins [see comments]. *Nature* 347: 256–261, 1990.

131. Ohashi, M., K. Jan de Vries, R. Frank, G. Snoek, V. Bankaitis, K. Wirtz, and W. B. Huttner. A role for phosphatidylinositol transfer protein in secretory vesicle formation. *Nature* 377: 544–547, 1995.

132. Oho, C., S. Seino, and M. Takahashi. Expression and complex formation of soluble N-ethyl-maleimide-sensitive factor attachment protein (SNAP) receptors in clonal rat endocrine cells. *Neurosci. Lett.* 186: 208–210, 1995.

133. Orci, L., B. S. Glick, and J. E. Rothman. A new type of coated vesicular carrier that appears not to contain clathrin: its possible role in protein transport within the Golgi stack. *Cell* 46: 171–184, 1986.

134. Orci, L., V. Malhotra, M. Amherdt, T. Serafini, and J. E. Rothman. Dissection of a single round of vesicular transport: sequential intermediates for intercisternal movement in the Golgi stack. *Cell* 56: 357–368, 1989.

135. Orci, L., M. Ravazzola, P. Meda, C. Holcomb, H. P. Moore, L. Hicke, and R. Schekman. Mammalian Sec23p homologue is restricted to the endoplasmic reticulum transitional cytoplasm. *Proc. Natl. Acad. Sci. USA* 88: 8611–8615, 1991.

136. Osen-Sand, A., M. Catsicas, J. K. Staple, K. A. Jones, G. Ayala, J. Knowles, G. Grenningloh, and S. Catsicas. Inhibition of axonal growth by SNAP-25 antisense oligonucleotides in vitro and in vivo [see comments]. *Nature* 364: 445–448, 1993.

137. Palade, G. Intracellular aspects of the process of protein synthesis. [Review]. *Science* 189: 347–358, 1975.

138. Papini, E., O. Rossetto, and D. F. Cutler. Vesicle-associated membrane protein (VAMP)/synaptobrevin-2 is associated with dense core secretory granules in PC12 neuroendocrine cells. *J. Biol. Chem.* 270: 1332–1336, 1995.

139. Parsons, T. D., J. R. Coorssen, H. Horstmann, and W. Almers. Docked granules, the exocytic burst, and the need for ATP hydrolysis in endocrine cells. *Neuron* 15: 1085–1096, 1995.

140. Pearse, B. M., and M. S. Robinson. Clathrin, adaptors, and sorting. [Review]. *Annu. Rev. Cell. Biol.* 6: 151–171, 1990.

141. Pelham, H. R. About turn for the COPs? [Review]. *Cell* 79: 1125–1127, 1994.

142. Pellegrini, L. L., V. O'Connor, and H. Betz. Fusion complex formation protects synaptobrevin against proteolysis by tetanus toxin light chain. *FEBS Lett.* 353: 319–323, 1994.

143. Penner, R., and E. Neher. The patch-clamp technique in the study of secretion. [Review]. *Trends Neurosci.* 12: 159–163, 1989.

144. Perin, M. S., N. Brose, R. Jahn, and T. C. Sudhof. Domain structure of synaptotagmin (p65) [published erratum appears in J. Biol. Chem. 1991 May 25;266(15):10018]. *J. Biol. Chem.* 266: 623–629, 1991.

145. Perin, M. S., V. A. Fried, G. A. Mignery, R. Jahn, and T. C. Sudhof. Phospholipid binding by a synaptic vesicle protein homologous to the regulatory region of protein kinase C. *Nature* 345: 260–263, 1990.

146. Pertile, P., M. Liscovitch, V. Chalifa, and L. C. Cantley. Phosphatidylinositol 4,5–bisphosphate synthesis is required for activation of phospholipase D in U937 cells. *J. Biol. Chem.* 270: 5130–5135, 1995.

147. Pevsner, J., S. C. Hsu, J. E. Braun, N. Calakos, A. E. Ting, M. K. Bennett, and R. H. Scheller. Specificity and regulation of a synaptic vesicle docking complex. *Neuron* 13: 353–361, 1994.

148. Pevsner, J., S. C. Hsu, and R. H. Scheller. n-Sec1: a neural-specific syntaxin-binding protein. *Proc. Natl. Acad. Sci. USA* 91: 1445–1449, 1994.

149. Pfeffer, S. R. Rab GTPases: master regulators of membrane trafficking. [Review]. *Curr. Opin. Cell Biol.* 6: 522–526, 1994.

150. Pryer, N. K., L. J. Wuestehube, and R. Schekman. Vesicle-mediated protein sorting. [Review]. *Annu. Rev. Biochem.* 61: 471–516, 1992.

151. Rabouille, C., T. P. Levine, J. M. Peters, and G. Warren. An NSF-like ATPase, p97, and NSF mediate cisternal regrowth from mitotic Golgi fragments. *Cell* 82: 905–914, 1995.

152. Rambourg, A., and Y. Clermont. Three-dimensional electron microscopy: structure of the Golgi apparatus. [Review]. *Eur. J. Cell Biol.* 51: 189–200, 1990.

153. Rambourg, A., Y. Clermont, M. Chretien, and L. Olivier. Formation of secretory granules in the Golgi apparatus of prolactin cells in the rat pituitary gland: a stereoscopic study. *Anat. Rec.* 232: 169–179, 1992.

154. Randazzo, P. A., and R. A. Kahn. GTP hydrolysis by ADP-ribosylation factor is dependent on both an ADP-ribosylation factor GTPase-activating protein and acid phospholipids [published erratum appears in *J. Biol. Chem.* 1994 Jun 10; 269(23):16519]. *J. Biol. Chem.* 269: 10758–10763, 1994.

155. Rexach, M. F., and R. W. Schekman. Distinct biochemical requirements for the budding, targeting, and fusion of ER-derived transport vesicles. *J. Cell Biol.* 114: 219–229, 1991.

156. Riezman, H. Endocytosis in yeast: several of the yeast secretory mutants are defective in endocytosis. *Cell* 40: 1001–1009, 1985.

157. Roberts, W. M., R. A. Jacobs, and A. J. Hudspeth. Colocalization of ion channels involved in frequency selectivity and synaptic transmission at presynaptic active zones of hair cells. *J. Neurosci.* 10: 3664–3684, 1990.

158. Robinson, J. S., D. J. Klionsky, L. M. Banta, and S. D. Emr. Protein sorting in Saccharomyces cerevisiae: isolation of mutants defective in the delivery and processing of multiple vacuolar hydrolases. *Mol. Cell. Biol.* 8: 4936–4948, 1988.

159. Robinson, M. S. The role of clathrin, adaptors and dynamin in endocytosis. [Review]. *Curr. Opin. Cell. Biol.* 6: 538–544, 1994.

160. Robinson, P. J., J. P. Liu, K. A. Powell, E. M. Fykse, and T. C. Sudhof. Phosphorylation of dynamin I and synaptic-vesicle recycling. [Review]. *Trends Neurosci.* 17: 348–353, 1994.

161. Robinson, P. J., J. M. Sontag, J. P. Liu, E. M. Fykse, C. Slaughter, H. McMahon, and T. C. Sudhof. Dynamin GTPase regulated by protein kinase C phosphorylation in nerve terminals [see comments]. *Nature* 365: 163–166, 1993.

162. Roth, D., and R. D. Burgoyne. SNAP-25 is present in a SNARE complex in adrenal chromaffin cells. *FEBS Lett.* 351: 207–210, 1994.

163. Rothman, J. E. Mechanisms of intracellular protein transport. [Review]. *Nature* 372: 55–63, 1994.

164. Rothman, J. E., and L. Orci. Molecular dissection of the secretory pathway. [Review]. *Nature* 355: 409–415, 1992.

165. Rothman, J. H., and T. H. Stevens. Protein sorting in yeast: mutants defective in vacuole biogenesis mislocalize vacuolar proteins into the late secretory pathway. *Cell* 47: 1041–1051, 1986.

166. Sadoul, K., J. Lang, C. Montecucco, U. Weller, R. Regazzi, S. Catsicas, C. B. Wollheim, and P. A. Halban. SNAP-25 is expressed in islets of Langerhans and is involved in insulin release. *J. Cell Biol.* 128: 1019–1028, 1995.

167. Salama, N. R., T. Yeung, and R. W. Schekman. The Sec13p complex and reconstitution of vesicle budding from the ER with purified cytosolic proteins. *EMBO J.* 12: 4073–4082, 1993.

168. Salminen, A., and P. J. Novick. A ras-like protein is required for a post-Golgi event in yeast secretion. *Cell* 49: 527–538, 1987.

169. Sarafian, T., L. A. Pradel, J. P. Henry, D. Aunis, and M. F. Bader. The participation of annexin II (calpactin I) in calcium-evoked exocytosis requires protein kinase C. *J. Cell Biol.* 114: 1135–1147, 1991.

170. Schekman, R. Genetic and biochemical analysis of vesicular traffic in yeast. [Review]. *Curr. Opin. Cell Biol.* 4: 587–592, 1992.

171. Schekman, R., and L. Orci. Coat proteins and vesicle budding. [Review]. *Science* 271: 1526–1533, 1996.

172. Scheller, R. H. Membrane trafficking in the presynaptic nerve terminal. [Review]. *Neuron* 14: 893–897, 1995.

173. Schiavo, G., F. Benfenati, B. Poulain, O. Rossetto, P. Polverino de Laureto, B. R. DasGupta, and C. Montecucco. Tetanus and botulinum-B neurotoxins block neurotransmitter release by proteolytic cleavage of synaptobrevin [see comments]. *Nature* 359: 832–835, 1992.

174. Schiavo, G., M. J. Gmachl, G. Stenbeck, T. H. Sollner, and J. E. Rothman. A possible docking and fusion particle for synaptic transmission. *Nature* 378: 733–736, 1995.

175. Schiavo, G., O. Rossetto, S. Catsicas, P. Polverino de Laureto, B. R. DasGupta, F. Benfenati, and C. Montecucco. Identification of the nerve terminal targets of botulinum neurotoxin serotypes A, D, and E. *J. Biol. Chem.* 268: 23784–23787, 1993.

176. Shaywitz, D. A., L. Orci, M. Ravazzola, A. Swaroop, and C. A. Kaiser. Human SEC13Rp functions in yeast and is located on transport vesicles budding from the endoplasmic reticulum. *J. Cell. Biol.* 128: 769–777, 1995.

177. Simons, K., and M. Zerial. Rab proteins and the road maps for intracellular transport. [Review]. *Neuron* 11: 789–799, 1993.

178. Smith, R. E., and M. G. Farquhar. Lysosome function in the regulation of the secretory process in cells of the anterior pituitary gland. *J. Cell Biol.* 31: 319–347, 1966.

179. Sogaard, M., K. Tani, R. R. Ye, S. Geromanos, P. Tempst, T. Kirchhausen, J. E. Rothman, and T. Sollner. A rab protein is required for the assembly of SNARE complexes in the docking of transport vesicles. *Cell* 78: 937–948, 1994.

180. Sollner, T., M. K. Bennett, S. W. Whiteheart, R. H. Scheller, and J. E. Rothman. A protein assembly-disassembly pathway in vitro that may correspond to sequential steps of synaptic vesicle docking, activation, and fusion. *Cell* 75: 409–418, 1993.

181. Sollner, T., S. W. Whiteheart, M. Brunner, H. Erdjument-

Bromage, S. Geromanos, P. Tempst, and J. E. Rothman. SNAP receptors implicated in vesicle targeting and fusion [see comments]. *Nature* 362: 318–324, 1993.

182. Spruce, A. E., L. J. Breckenridge, A. K. Lee, and W. Almers. Properties of the fusion pore that forms during exocytosis of a mast cell secretory vesicle. *Neuron* 4: 643–654, 1990.

183. Stack, J. H., D. B. DeWald, K. Takegawa, and S. D. Emr. Vesicle-mediated protein transport: regulatory interactions between the Vps15 protein kinase and the Vps34 PtdIns 3–kinase essential for protein sorting to the vacuole in yeast. *J. Cell Biol.* 129: 321–334, 1995.

184. Stack, J. H., P. K. Herman, P. V. Schu, and S. D. Emr. A membrane-associated complex containing the Vps15 protein kinase and the Vps34 PI 3–kinase is essential for protein sorting to the yeast lysosome-like vacuole. *EMBO J.* 12: 2195–2204, 1993.

185. Sudhof, T. C., and R. Jahn. Proteins of synaptic vesicles involved in exocytosis and membrane recycling. [Review]. *Neuron* 6: 665–677, 1991.

186. Tagaya, M., S. Toyonaga, M. Takahashi, A. Yamamoto, T. Fujiwara, K. Akagawa, Y. Moriyama, and S. Mizushima. Syntaxin 1 (HPC-1) is associated with chromaffin granules. *J. Biol. Chem.* 270: 15930–15933, 1995.

187. Takei, K., P. S. McPherson, S. L. Schmid, and P. De Camilli. Tubular membrane invaginations coated by dynamin rings are induced by GTP-gamma S in nerve terminals [see comments]. *Nature* 374: 186–190, 1995.

188. Thomas, P., A. K. Lee, J. G. Wong, and W. Almers. A triggered mechanism retrieves membrane in seconds after Ca^{2+}-stimulated exocytosis in single pituitary cells. *J. Cell Biol.* 124: 667–675, 1994.

189. Thomas, P., A. Surprenant, and W. Almers. Cytosolic Ca^{2+}, exocytosis, and endocytosis in single melanotrophs of the rat pituitary. *Neuron* 5: 723–733, 1990.

190. Thomas, P., J. G. Wong, and W. Almers. Millisecond studies of secretion in single rat pituitary cells stimulated by flash photolysis of caged Ca^{2+}. *EMBO J.* 12: 303–306, 1993.

191. Thomas, P., J. G. Wong, A. K. Lee, and W. Almers. A low affinity Ca^{2+} receptor controls the final steps in peptide secretion from pituitary melanotrophs. *Neuron* 11: 93–104, 1993.

192. Ullrich, B., C. Li, J. Z. Zhang, H. McMahon, R. G. Anderson, M. Geppert, and T. C. Sudhof. Functional properties of multiple synaptotagmins in brain. *Neuron* 13: 1281–1291, 1994.

193. Ullrich, B., and T. C. Sudhof. Differential distributions of novel synaptotagmins: comparison to synapsins. *Neuropharmacology* 34: 1371–1377, 1995.

194. Ullrich, S., and C. B. Wollheim. Expression of both alpha 1- and alpha 2-adrenoceptors in an insulin-secreting cell line. Parallel studies of cytosolic free Ca^{2+} and insulin release. *Mol Pharmacol* 28: 100–106, 1985.

195. Ullrich, S., and C. B. Wollheim. GTP-dependent inhibition of insulin secretion by epinephrine in permeabilized RINm5F cells. Lack of correlation between insulin secretion and cyclic AMP levels. *J. Biol. Chem.* 263: 8615–8620, 1988.

196. Vitale, M. L., E. P. Seward, and J. M. Trifaro. Chromaffin cell cortical actin network dynamics control the size of the release-ready vesicle pool and the initial rate of exocytosis. *Neuron* 14: 353–363, 1995.

197. Volinia, S., R. Dhand, B. Vanhaesebroeck, L. K. MacDougall, R. Stein, M. J. Zvelebil, J. Domin, C. Panaretou, and M. D. Waterfield. A human phosphatidylinositol 3–kinase complex related to the yeast Vps34p-Vps15p protein sorting system. *EMBO J.* 14: 3339–3348, 1995.

198. von Ruden, L., and E. Neher. A Ca-dependent early step in the release of catecholamines from adrenal chromaffin cells. *Science* 262: 1061–1065, 1993.

199. von Zastrow, M., and J. D. Castle. Protein sorting among two distinct export pathways occurs from the content of maturing exocrine storage granules. *J. Cell Biol.* 105(6 Pt 1): 2675–2684, 1987.

200. Walch-Solimena, C., J. Blasi, L. Edelmann, E. R. Chapman, G. F. von Mollard, and R. Jahn. The t-SNAREs syntaxin 1 and SNAP-25 are present on organelles that participate in synaptic vesicle recycling. *J. Cell Biol.* 128: 637–645, 1995.

201. Walch-Solimena, C., K. Takei, K. L. Marek, K. Midyett, T. C. Sudhof, P. De Camilli, and R. Jahn. Synaptotagmin: a membrane constituent of neuropeptide-containing large dense-core vesicles. *J. Neurosci.* 13: 3895–3903, 1993.

202. Walent, J. H., B. W. Porter, and T. F. Martin. A novel 145 kd brain cytosolic protein reconstitutes Ca^{2+}-regulated secretion in permeable neuroendocrine cells. *Cell* 70: 765–775, 1992.

203. Waters, M. G., T. Serafini, and J. E. Rothman. 'Coatomer': a cytosolic protein complex containing subunits of non-clathrin-coated Golgi transport vesicles. *Nature* 349: 248–251, 1991.

204. Wheeler, M. B., L. Sheu, M. Ghai, A. Bouquillon, G. Grondin, U. Weller, A. R. Beaudoin, M. K. Bennett, W. S. Trimble, and H. Y. Gaisano. Characterization of SNARE protein expression in beta cell lines and pancreatic islets. *Endocrinology* 137: 1340–1348, 1996.

205. Wilsbach, K., and G. S. Payne. Vps1p, a member of the dynamin GTPase family, is necessary for Golgi membrane protein retention in *Saccharomyces cerevisiae*. *EMBO J.* 12: 3049–3059, 1993.

206. Wilson, D. W., C. A. Wilcox, G. C. Flynn, E. Chen, W. J. Kuang, W. J. Henzel, M. R. Block, A. Ullrich, and J. E. Rothman. A fusion protein required for vesicle-mediated transport in both mammalian cells and yeast. *Nature* 339: 355–359, 1989.

207. Wilson, K. L. NSF-independent fusion mechanisms. [Review]. *Cell* 81: 475–477, 1995.

208. Wu, Y. N., N. D. Vu, and P. D. Wagner. Anti-(14–3-3 protein) antibody inhibits stimulation of noradrenaline (norepinephrine) secretion by chromaffin-cell cytosolic proteins. *Biochem. J.* 285(1 Aug Pt 3): 697–700, 1992.

209. Zhang, J. Z., B. A. Davletov, T. C. Sudhof, and R. G. Anderson. Synaptotagmin I is a high affinity receptor for clathrin AP-2: implications for membrane recycling. *Cell* 78: 751–760, 1994.

210. Zhang, X., A. B. Jefferson, V. Auethavekiat, and P. W. Majerus. The protein deficient in Lowe syndrome is a phosphatidylinositol-4,5-bisphosphate 5-phosphatase. *Proc. Natl. Acad. Sci. USA* 92: 4853–4856, 1995.

211. Zimmerberg, J., M. Curran, F. S. Cohen, and M. Brodwick. Simultaneous electrical and optical measurements show that membrane fusion precedes secretory granule swelling during exocytosis of beige mouse mast cells. *Proc. Natl. Acad. Sci. USA* 84: 1585–1589, 1987.

2. Synthesis, internalization, recycling, and regulation of peptide hormone receptors

STUART C. SEALFON | *Fishberg Research Center in Neurobiology and Department of Neurology, Mount Sinai School of Medicine of the City University of New York, New York, New York*

CHAPTER CONTENTS

THE SYSTEMIC COORDINATION that is necessary for the adaptation and survival of the complex organism is provided by the capacity of the endocrine system to regulate cellular function by means of circulating hormones. The reproductive cycle in mammals, for example, requires an orchestration of peptide and glycoprotein hormone biosynthesis and release that involves cells in the hypothalamus, anterior pituitary and gonads. Only when diverse cells attain responses of the correct magnitude and in the proper temporal relationship can homeostasis be maintained. Disturbing this inter-related pattern of hormonal secretion leads to a failure of normal function. The disruption of normal function due to regulatory responses elicited by some hormonal drugs underlie their effects, such as the suppression of the gonads caused by high dose gonadotropin-releasing hormone (GnRH) analogs (30).

The ultimate effect of hormones on the target tissues depends on two fundamental factors. The first is the specificity of interaction of these hormones with the membrane receptors on the target tissues. Peptides and glycoproteins are advantageous in this respect, as they provide complex and highly unique ligands for the target receptors that help ensure signalling specificity. Peptides tend to provide agonists of higher affinity than do neurotransmitters, and more importantly, of greater selectivity for their specific target receptor. Perhaps it is because of this specificity that peptides have been retained throughout evolution for so many aspects of endocrine signalling despite their relatively high bioenergetic cost of production in comparison to neurotransmitters.

The other crucial factor determining the precise response of the target cell is the readiness of the receptor to mediate signal transduction and of the post receptor signalling intermediates to manifest a response. The regulatory mechanisms influencing receptor expression and responsivity have been studied in many peptide receptor systems (14, 20, 21, 28, 32, 46, 67, 141, 142, 152). The goal of this chapter is to provide an understanding of the biosynthetic, processing and modulatory loci at which the localization and level of expression of a receptor is regulated and of the experimental approaches by which these phenomena are studied. Because the purpose of this chapter is to elucidate the principles and practices of the field, not all peptide receptors will be discussed. The regulatory mechanisms of peptide G protein–coupled peptide receptors (GPCR) will receive particular emphasis and aspects of certain receptor systems that are well-characterized or that illustrate unusual mechanisms will be described in detail. The synthesis or processing of peptide and protein receptors outside of the GPCR group will also be described where appropriate, as will the literature concerning non-peptide receptors. From these examples it is hoped that this chapter will provide the background necessary to critically evaluate the studies of the regulatory control mechanisms of any peptide receptor.

CLASSIFICATION OF PEPTIDE RECEPTORS

The regulatory adaptations employed by various receptor systems depend in part on the structure and sequence motifs of each receptor and on the specific signal transduction pathways utilized. Receptors that

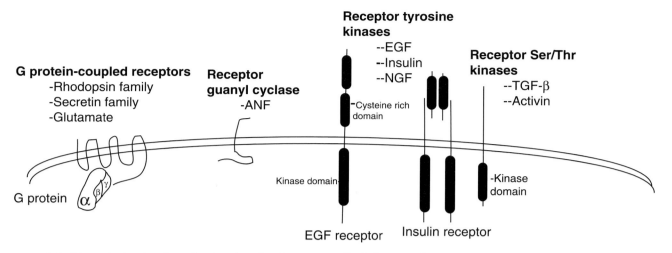

FIG. 2.1. Schematic showing the major domains of various structurally distinct peptide receptors.

signal by coupling to G proteins have an overlapping yet distinct series of potential regulatory responses available as compared to receptors that cause tyrosine phosphorylation. Before discussing the specific regulatory mechanisms, it is useful to provide an overview of the various classes of peptide receptors. The recent cloning of a large number of receptors has revealed that many of these membrane proteins can be categorized according to the presence of related sequence and/or structural motifs. In Figure 2.1, a schematic illustrating the basic structural features of several of the major groups of receptors is presented.

The majority of peptide receptors signal via interaction with heterotrimeric G proteins. These receptors all have seven hydrophobic domains and are believed to be heptahelical in structure. The heptahelical receptors fall into three groups based on specific sequence motifs within the transmembrane domains that are highly conserved within members of each group, but which are not conserved among the three groups. The three groups, referred to according to the first receptor cloned in each, are the rhodopsin family, the secretin family and the metabotropic glutamate family. The rhodopsin family of GPCRs is the largest family and encompasses several hundred distinct receptors. Included in this group are most G protein–coupled neurotransmitter receptors (adrenergic, dopaminergic, serotonergic, muscarinic), the majority of peptide receptors (including receptors for GnRH, thyrotropin releasing hormone [TRH], arginine vasopressin, tachykinins and opioid peptides), and the glycoprotein hormone receptors (luteinizing hormone[LH]/chorionic gonadotropin, thyroid stimulating hormone and follicle stimulating hormone). Members of the rhodopsin family can be

identified by the presence of characteristic amino acids or sequence motifs at corresponding positions, such as an asparagine in helix 1 and an aspartate-arginine-tyrosine motif at the bottom of helix 3 (4, 126).

The binding sites of the various rhodopsin-family receptors show considerable variation. The neurotransmitters bind entirely within a pocket formed by the transmembrane helix domains, the small peptides bind in a pocket formed of both extracellular loops and transmembrane helix domains and the glycoprotein hormones bind to a large amino terminus domain consisting of leucine rich repeat segments.

The secretin receptor family, while similiar to the rhodopsin family in having seven hydrophobic domains, is identified by its own unique shared sequence motifs. Included in this group are the receptors for corticotropin-releasing factor, vasoactive intestinal polypeptide and parathyroid hormone. The last family of G protein–coupled receptors consists of the closely related G protein–coupled "metabotropic" receptors for the neurotransmitter glutamate and does not at present include any peptide receptors.

Other peptide/protein receptors are not G protein coupled. The atrial natriuretic factor receptor consists of a single polypeptide chain encompassing the peptide binding site, a single transmembrane domain and the guanylyl cyclase domain. Activation of this receptor stimulates catalytic activity of the guanylyl cyclase domain leading to formation of the second messenger cyclic guanosine monophosphate (GMPhate). Most of the growth factor receptors have a single transmembrane domain and form dimers during activation, such as the receptor for epidermal growth factor (EGF). Following dimerization, the activated receptor autophosphorylates tyrosine side chains and then interacts with intracellular signal mediators. The insulin and insulin-like growth factor receptors are tetramers with two transmembrane domains and, after activation and autophosphorylation, cause phosphorylation of a signal mediator, the insulin receptor substrate-1. The serine/threonine kinase receptors, including receptors for transforming growth factor-β and for activin, have a single transmembrane domain and intracellular kinase domains.

OVERVIEW OF REGULATORY MECHANISMS

A variety of mechanisms are involved in the control of the response mediated by a receptor. Because the terminology is utilized somewhat variably, it is useful to settle on operational definitions. Desensitization refers to the attenuation of the magnitude of the monitored response following activation of a receptor. The type of response that is monitored can vary for different receptors or experimental systems or even for the same receptor in the same system. For example, the responses to stimulation of the pituitary GnRH receptor includes phosphoinositol hydrolysis, calcium mobilization, calcium influx, MAP kinase activation and gonadotropin release. These different responses may show different patterns of desensitization. Desensitization can occur at the level of the receptor, for example, following receptor phosphorylation (91, 92), decreased cell surface receptor expression (sequestration), or decreased number of receptors (down-regulation). However, desensitization of the monitored response can also occur due to regulation of post receptor signaling components, for example G proteins (36, 42, 49, 51, 52, 129, 144, 145, 154) channels (81, 101), calcium pools (100, 175), inositol trisphophate receptors (176, 178–180), protein kinases (1, 2, 99, 115, 146) and phospholipases (16, 17, 111, 143).

Down-regulation refers to the loss of receptor number in the cell and up-regulation to an increase in receptor number. Receptor number is usually determined by saturation radioligand binding. Changes in receptor number are induced by an imbalance in the rate of receptor biosynthesis compared to the rate of receptor degradation. It follows that modulation of biosynthetic rate, degradation rate, or both can lead to receptor up- or down-regulation. Several regulatory mechanisms have been found to contribute to modulation of receptor number. The rate of biosynthesis, for example, can be altered by regulation of gene transcription, RNA processing, mRNA stability and mRNA translation. Regulation of receptor respon-

siveness or number can occur following agonist activation of the receptor or following stimulation of other receptor systems. The former is termed homologous and the latter heterologous.

Thus there are a large number of potential regulatory loci for a particular receptor system. For most receptors, the various regulatory processes proceed simultaneously with different time courses. Thus at one point in time receptor number may be decreasing due to increased degradative rate. However, at the same point in time, the steady state receptor mRNA level may increase, anticipating a subsequent increase in receptor biosynthesis. Because it is not feasable to measure all receptor regulatory processes at all time points, one must remain cautious about making assumptions about causal relationships between the regulatory changes monitored in any given study.

RECEPTOR BIOSYNTHESIS

The synthesis, processing and membrane insertion of receptors provides many potential loci for regulation of their expression. The majority of GPCRs contain consensus sequences (Asn-X-Ser/Thr) for N-linked glycosylation (80) within their amino terminus domains and mutational analysis of neurotransmitter (44, 128, 170), peptide (34) and glycoprotein hormone receptors (94, 135) are consistent with glycosylation of these sites. The biological role of glycosylation may vary in different receptors. A specific glycosylation site is required for proper cell surface localization of the chorionic gonadotropin receptor (94). The muscarinic m2 receptor does not require glycosylation for either cell surface localization or for proper level of expression (170). The GnRH receptor shows decreased receptor expression with elimination of glycosylation sites, but no evidence of altered membrane targeting. This pattern is consistent with increased receptor degradation in the absence of glycosylation (34).

Interestingly, the human and mouse gonadotropin-releasing hormone receptors differ in the number of amino terminus glycosylation sites and in their level of expression. The mouse receptor has an increased level of expression in transfected cells and has two glycosylation sites in comparison to a single site in the human receptor. Introducing this second site into the human receptor has been found to improve the level of receptor expression, presumably by decreasing receptor degradation (35).

Glycosylation and phosphorylation may be required for activity of the atrial natriuretic peptide receptor type A, a receptor-guanylyl cyclase. Mutants that are inactive are not phosphorylated and are only partly glycosylated (79).

Several GPCRs have been shown to be palmitoylated on cysteine residues located in the carboxy-terminus domain of these receptors (102). The functional role of receptor palmitoylation is not known and may vary in different receptors. For some receptors, palmitoylation of intracellular cysteines in the carboxy terminus domain serves to anchor this segment of the receptor to the membrane. This hypothesis is supported by fluorescent studies of the location and membrane accessibility of the palmitoylation sites of rhodopsin, which indicate that the palmitoylation sites are situated in the membrane and thereby form a fourth cytoplasmic loop of the receptor (103). In some GPCRs, such as the β_2 adrenergic receptor, elimination of the palmitoylated cysteine by site-directed mutagenesis caused signficant receptor uncoupling from G proteins (104, 114) and a high degree of basal phosphorylation (104). In other GPCRs, including the gastrin-releasing peptide receptor (12) and α_{2A} adrenergic receptor (75), elimination of the palmitoylation site did not affect receptor coupling. One GPCR, the gonadotropin-releasing hormone receptor, lacks an intracellular carboxy terminal domain and the potentially palmitoylated cysteines found in other receptors (166).

GPCRs are also phosphorylated and dephosphorylated. This important regulatory modification is involved in desensitization and receptor trafficking (see below).

ENDOCYTOTIC CYCLE

The dynamic trafficking between the plasmalemma and intracellular vesicles can contribute to ligand degradation, receptor degradation, or desensitization of various receptors. Much insight into the mechanisms underlying receptor translocation comes from studies of the rapid cycling nutrient receptors, such as the receptors for transferrin and low density lipoproteins (48, 161). Ligand-activated receptors have not been as well studied and are thought to share similar internalization mechanisms, although the precise pathways of internalization may be distinct (174). Whereas nutrient receptors are constitutively internalized, however, ligand-activated receptors require agonist binding for efficient aggregation and internalization.

Following ligand binding, receptors aggregate and internalize via invaginations coated with the protein clathrin or internalize via smooth, non–clathrin, coated pits. The basic components of the clathrin-coated internalization pathway are illustrated in Figure 2.2. These invaginations pinch off to form intracellular

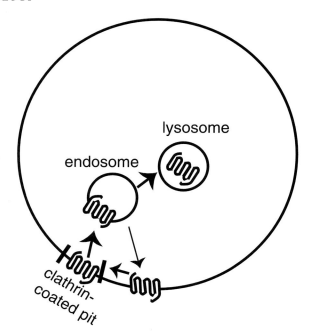

FIG. 2.2. Cartoon showing the clathrin-coated pit mediated endocytotic cycle.

vesicles that transport the receptors to sorting endosomes from which they can be directed to the Golgi complex and back to the cell surface or to the lysosomes for degradation. Different internalization pathways can be differentiated experimentally. For example, saturation of the internalization pathway of the EGF receptor does not affect transferrin internalization (174).

Coated and smooth endocytotic vesicles have distinct electron microscopic appearances (119, 133). Coated pits are approximately 100 nm in diameter. Clathrin forms a polygonal shell for the coated pit and is associated with adaptor proteins that serve to recognize and trap the transmembrane proteins (120). The aggregation of receptors into coated pits involves an interaction between adaptins and specific cytoplasmic or juxtamembrane receptor sequences (see below). The adaptins can be different in different coated pits and will determine which membrane proteins are trapped. Internalization can also occur via smooth pits (37, 56, 84). A marker for certain smooth pits, which are called caveolae, is the protein caveolin (134). Non-caveolin associated smooth vesicles are also found and may provide an alternative route for internalization when the coated vesicle system is disrupted (84). The internalization via clathrin-coated vesicles and caveolae can be distinguished by selected inhibition. Coated pit internalization is inhibited by high sucrose concentration, potassium depletion, acidification of the cytoplasm, or exposure to chlorpromazine, whereas the internalization of caveolae is selectively blocked by filipin, cytochalasin D, phorbol esters and okadaic acid (84). All mechanisms of internalization are temperature sensitive and are slowed at 4° C. Mathematical models to describe the kinetics of receptor cycling have been developed (88).

The EGF receptor requires tyrosine kinase activity for rapid internalization. Internalization of the EGF receptor is blocked by a tyrosine kinase inhibitor, whereas internalization of the transferrin receptor is less affected (83). Studies of a kinase-deficient mutant of the EGF receptor found that the internalization of the mutant was reduced to the rate of unoccupied wild-type receptors (85). Mutagenesis studies of the fibroblast growth factor receptor (151) and platelet-derived growth factor receptor (105) indicate that in both cases an autophosphorylated C-terminal tyrosine residue is required for internalization.

Following invagination of the pits and pinching off of vesicles, the coats of clathrin-coated vesicles are removed. Multiple vesicles fuse to form the sorting endosomes (136). At the level of the sorting endosome, the internalization pathways of coated and non-coated pits converge (159). In the acidic environment of these endosomes, the ligand may dissociate from some peptide receptors and proceed to the lysosomes for degradation. In the sorting endosome, the destination of the endocytosed receptor is determined. It can proceed either to the lysosomes for degradations or to the transgolgi reticulum for recycling to the membrane. The processes underlying this crucial targeting for expression or degradaton are not well understood. Some studies indicate that the receptors directed for recycling to the membrane converge with the secretory vesicles of newly synthesized receptors (77, 153). Further discussion of receptor mediated endocytosis may be found elsewhere in this volume (5).

RECEPTOR SEQUESTRATION

Sequestration refers to removal of receptors from the cell surface, leading, as noted above, to the trafficking of receptors into the lysosomes or to the recycling of receptors to the cell surface. The receptors targeted to the lysosomes are degraded, contributing to receptor down-regulation. Receptors that are recycled to the plasmalemma may be dephosphorylated during transit, thereby providing a potential mechanism for resensitizing receptors that have been desensitized through phosphorylation (41, 124, 181).

Sequestration of peptide receptors has been studied by the use of modified analogs to allow detection by microscopy or autoradiography, by anti-receptor antibodies and by the introduction of detection sequences into the receptors followed by immunocytochemistry. Various phases of agonist stimulated sequestration have been observed. Following agonist stimulation, the receptors are seen to aggregate into small patches followed by accumulation into a large mass, a change referred to as capping. Patching and capping are associated with receptor internalization.

Studies of the GnRH receptor illustrate the various ligand-based detection strategies that have been developed. Agonist-induced receptor capping and endocytosis of the GnRH receptor has been visualized using a ferritin-coupled GnRH analog allowing detection by electron-microscopy (62). Fluorescently labeled GnRH analogs allowed receptor aggregation and internalization to be visualized in living cells (109). Upon stimulation of the GnRH receptor at 37° C, GnRH receptors aggregate and are internalized into endocytoic vesicles (59). Ligand internalization and stimulation of LH release are independent processes, as shown by the finding that patching and capping are inhibited with vinblastin while agonist-stimulated luteinizing hormone release is not affected (31). The time course of internalization has been followed by ligand autoradiography and light and electron microscopy in rat pituitary sections (121). After 10–30 min, grains are localized to the golgi and at 1–3 h labeling is found in the golgi, lysosomes and secretory granules (70). Receptor trafficking can be hormonally regulated. Castration of female rats, for example, increases the rate of migration of GnRH receptors. Immunohistochemical detection of a biotinylated GnRH analog has also been utilized to follow capping and patching of receptors (27). Internalization of the GnRH receptor is temperature dependent, occuring at 37° C but not at 4° C (57), as has been found for other receptors (108).

The association of internalized label both with lysosomes and with secretory granules suggests that the internalized GnRH receptors can be either degraded or recycled to the membrane (57). Consistent with this view is the finding that GnRH receptor sequestration and down-regulation are separable phenomena. Chloroquine and methylamine, which make lysosomes less acidic, and monensin, a proton ionophore, decrease degradation but do not block recycling to the surface. These results are consistent with the view that receptors that internalize with agonist enter a separate pool, the sorting endosome (see Fig. 2.2), and they can either proceed to lysosomes or recycle to the cell surface (138).

Processing of the GnRH receptor is not entirely agonist dependent as antagonist also shows uptake into intracellular compartments (58, 71). However the time course of internalization of agonist and antagonist differs. The internalization of antagonist is slower than that of agonist. Internalization of labeled antagonist most likely reflects the basal rate of receptor processing whereas rapid internalization requires receptor activation (183).

The mechanisms and pathways of internalization may be cell type specific for the same receptors. GnRH receptor processing has been compared in pituitary cells and in ovarian granulosa cells using a biotinylated ligand. In both cell types, internalization is seen within 3 min. However, In ovarian cells, labeling is intially localized over endosomes and no early staining is observed over the Golgi. In contrast, in the pituitary cells the Golgi cisternae begin to show label at 3 min (26). Different receptor processing in different cell types has also been found with other peptide receptors. The cholecystokinin (CCK) receptor is internalized via clathrin-dependent and independent pathways in Chinese hamster ovary (CHO) cells (132), but is immobilized on the cell surface in pancreatic acinar cells (131). The processing of thrombin receptors differs in a megakaryoblastic cell line (15, 63) and in endothelial cells (181).

In some experimental systems, receptor sequestration may require agonist occupancy of the receptor. Bradykinin receptors are sequestered in smooth muscle cells following exposure to bradykinin. However, while exposure to phorbol esters desensitizes the receptor, this treatment does not lead to sequestration (107). Receptor phosphorylation plays a role in the internalization for some GPCRs. Agonist-stimulated internalization of the α_1 adrenergic receptors occurs with a time course similar to that of serine and threonine phosphorylation in smooth muscle cells (90). In addition, this receptor also appears to require occupancy by agonist for internalization. This conclusion comes from studies of heterologous phosphorylation of the α_1 adrenergic receptor. While phosphorylation can be induced by phorbol esters or by activation of bradykinin receptors on these cells, neither of these treatments leads to a loss of cell surface receptor (90). The requirement of agonist occupancy for sequestration of some receptors suggests that phosphorylation by G protein–coupled receptor kinases may be required for efficient internalization of some receptors. These kinases, which utilize G protein–coupled receptors as their substrates, require agonist occupancy of the receptors for activity (25, 91, 92). A number of peptide receptors can be phosphorylated by G protein–coupled receptor kinases (43, 68, 82, 127).

Studies of the CCK receptor show that the pathway of internalization can determine the ultimate fate of the sequestered receptor. Internalization of the agonist occupied CCK receptor occurs via both clathrin-dependent and independent pathways in a CCK recep-

tor–expressing cell line. The clathrin-dependent internalization leads to endosomal and lysosomal localization as well as to receptor recycling to the membrane. The clathrin-independent internalization, however, leads to localization in a caveola-like smooth vesicular compartment (132). Agonist stimulation of the pancreatic CCK receptor leads to phosphorylation on serines (78) and receptor kinase and phosphatase activity are hormone regulated (97). It has been proposed that the classical clathrin-mediated internalization serves predominantly to allow lysosomal targeting and downregulation of the CCK receptor whereas the caveola-like smooth vesicular compartment allows dephosphorylation and rapid receptor resensitization (132). Notably, in pancreatic acinar cells, instead of internalization, agonist stimulation leads to receptor immobilization on the membrane surface (131).

Studies of mutant and deletion GPCRs indicate that sequestration can allow resensitization of receptors that have been desensitized by phosphorylation. For example, a mutation of the β_2 adrenergic receptor that eliminates sequestraton also eliminates receptor resensitization (7). Studies of other neurotransmitter and peptide receptors support a role for recycling in receptor resensitization (41, 124, 187).

The internalization of the TRH receptor has been studied using a fluorescent TRH analog and an epitope-tagged recombinant receptor. No internalization of receptor is detected in the absence of agonist. Agonist binding at 37° C leads to rapid receptor internalization via clathrin-coated vesicles and to subsequent recycling to the cell surface following removal of agonist. This internalization required the carboxy terminus domain of the receptor (3). With increased duration of agonist exposure, progressively less TRH receptor is recycled to the plasmalemma. The proportion of receptor and ligand diverted to the non-cycling pathway differs, suggesting that the ligand and receptor dissociate and are processed independently (123).

For many GPCRs, agonist-mediated internalization requires coupling to signal transduction. A receptor containing a mutation in helix 2 that causes an uncoupled TRH receptor also causes a marked reduction in receptor internalization (113). Chimeric bombesin/m3 muscarinic receptors that are deficient in coupling also show diminished internalization (162).

The molecular events involved in sorting receptors following sequestration either to the lysosomes for degradation or back to the plasma membrane are not well understood. Autophosphorylation of the platelet-derived growth factor receptor leads to the development of high affinity binding for a number of cellular proteins, including phosphatidylinositol 3–kinase. Using mutant receptors, it has been shown that elimination of these kinase binding sites does not interfere with internalization but does eliminate diversion of the receptor to the degradative pathway (72).

Sequestration Motifs and Domains

The sequence and structural motifs required for internalization have been investigated for many receptors (161). Studies of nutrient receptors suggest that some internalization sequences form a characteristic structure. Sequences related to the internalization sequences of the transferrin receptor (Tyr-Thr-Arg-Phe) and of the low density lipoprotein (LDL) receptor (Asn-Pro-Val-Tyr) are found to promote tight turns in proteins (161). The ability to restore internalization to internalization-deficient mutants by transplanting one receptor's internalization motif into a different receptor (29, 69, 160) indicates that the internalization motifs comprise interchangeable and self-contained domains.

Deletion studies indicated that the internalization sequences of the EGF receptor were contained within the receptor's carboxyl terminal domain. Progressive truncation of this domain of the EGF receptor decreases the rate of ligand-mediated internalization, indicating that this domain contains the receptor's internalization signals. Using an internalization-deficient truncated receptor, internalization was restored by the introduction of either of two short C-terminal sequences (QQGFF, FYRAL) (24). These EGF receptor sequences were both able to replace the internalization sequence of the transferrin receptor. However, EGF receptor internalization required both the presence of an appropriate internalization sequence and functional intrinsic tyrosine kinase activity of the receptor. Other growth factor internalization motifs have been identified, such as the dileucine motifs of the insulin receptor. The insulin receptor has two dileucine signals, one located juxta-membrane and the other in the tyrosine kinase domain. When fused to a reporter antigen, the dileucine segments from the insulin receptor directs the chimera to the lysosomes. Elimination of the juxta-membrane leucines by mutation to alanine reduces internalization (54).

Rhodopsin class GPCRs have a conserved Asn-Pro $(X)_{2-3}$Tyr sequence located at the cytoplasmic side of transmembrane helix seven. Because of the apparent similarity of this sequence to the Asn-Pro-X-Tyr internalization sequence of the LDL receptor, the effect of mutation of the tyrosine was investigated in several GPCRs. The results of these studies indicate that an intact Asn-Pro $(X)_{2-3}$Tyr domain is required for internalization of some receptors, but suggest that this sequence does not represent a specific sequestration motif for seven helix transmembrane receptors. In the β_2 adrenergic receptor, mutation of the tyrosine in this domain to alanine causes a loss of internalization.and a reduction of coupling to adenylate cyclase (6, 7). Significantly, this mutation also eliminated resensitization, supporting the hypothesis that recycling can provide a means of dephosphorylating and resensitizing receptors. However, the sequestation inhibiting effect of mutating this tyrosine was not shared by other related GPCRs. Mutation of this cognate tyrosine of the gastrin-releasing peptide receptor (147) or of the angiotensin II (AT1) receptor (66) did not affect internalization, indicating that the tyrosine does not form part of a general sequestration signal. Furthermore, mutation of other residues in this domain in the β_2 adrenergic receptor interfered with diverse aspects of receptor function, including sequestration, coupling and agonist-stimulated phosphorylation (6). These results most likely reflect a more general role for this domain than providing a signal for sequestration. Consistent with this view are double mutation studies of the GnRH receptor (188) and of the serotonin 5–HT$_{2A}$ receptor (139) that suggest that the Asn present in this domain in most GPCRs interacts with a conserved Asp in helix 2 to facilitate the conformational changes underlying receptor activation.

Deletion studies of several GPCRs have revealed the importance of particular receptor regions to internalization. C terminal truncations and deletions inhibit agonist mediated internalization of the angiotension II receptor (AT$_{1A}$) but have no effect on desensitization (23, 158). The carboxy-terminus of the α_{1B}-adrenergic receptor (87) and the β_2 adrenergic receptor (93) were also implicated in sequestration. Ser and Thr domains in the carboxy-terminus of the gastrin-releasing peptide receptor have been implicated in sequestration mediated by protein kinase C and non-protein kinase C phosphorylation (11, 12). Deletion studies of the angiotensin$_{1A}$ receptor showed that a 17 amino acid region of the carboxy terminus domain was required for internalization (23). In the muscarinic m1 receptor, the sequestration signal is located in the third intracellular loop (86). Bombesin and CCK receptors show a much greater degree of agonist-stimulated internalization than do m3 muscarinic receptors when expressed in CHO cells. Study of chimeric receptors in which the carboxy-terminus tail has been interchanged indicated that for these receptors the carboxy-terminus domain contains signals that augment both agonist-stimulated internalization and receptor recycling (163). The C terminus domain has been implicated as critical for TRH receptor internalization (112). In contrast, deletion of the distal portion of the luteinizing hormone/chorionic gonadotropin receptor caused an enhancement of receptor internalization (130).

While receptor internalization requires coupling to signal transduction for many receptors, coupling is not sufficient for internalization. Efficient internalization of the TRH receptor has been shown to require two distinct domains in the C terminus of the receptor (112). A C terminus domain-truncated TRH receptor, while still coupled to signal transduction, shows no agonist stimulated internalization (3). Down-regulation of G protein–coupled receptors may require specific domains of the receptor. Splice variants of the mouse somatostatin$_2$ receptor, for example, differ in their C terminal domains and in their agonist stimulated down regulation (171).

Intracellular Ser-Thr rich sequences have been implicated in internalization of several GPCRs. Point mutations of the m1 muscarinic receptor demonstrates the third intracellular loop sequence Glu-Ser-Leu-Thr-Ser-Ser-Glu is required for receptor internalization and that the Thr-Ser-Ser is crucial (106). A Ser-Thr-Leu sequence in the carboxy terminus of the angiotensin II receptor has also been found to be required for internalization (65). Serine and threonine residues of the gastrin-releasing peptide receptor have been shown to be required for internalization (12). Two specific residues of the carboxy-terminus of the neurotensin receptor, Thr-422 and Tyr-424 are critical for agonist-stimulated receptor internalization (22).

RECEPTOR REGULATION

Receptor regulation refers to an alteration in the number of receptors. Two types of receptor regulation can be differentiated. Regulation induced by activation of the receptor itself is termed homologous regulation. Examples of homologous regulation of peptide receptors include regulation of thyrotropin-releasing hormone (45) or GnRH receptors (96) by agonist. Many peptide receptors show down-regulation following agonist exposure, such as the vasopressin, bombesin and neurotensin receptors in cell lines (17, 184). The GnRH receptor, as discussed below, shows an unusual biphasic regulation with agonist. Regulation caused by activation of other receptor systems is termed heterologous regulation, such as the regulation of GnRH receptor number by gonadal steroids. Homologous and heterologous mechansims can also be identified in receptor desensitization (91, 92).

Receptor number can be altered by modulation of the rate of biosynthesis and/or of degradation. Receptor biosynthesis can be regulated at many potential loci, including gene transcription, mRNA processing, mRNA stability and rate of translation. Because all of these processes are studied in different experimental systems, one must be cautious in evaluating the physiological relevance of the various regulatory events described. The promotors of many G protein–coupled receptors have been shown to be highly regulated. The β_3 adrenergic receptor, for example, has multiple cAMP response elements that cause its mRNA to be up-regulated by agonist stimulation (157). Glucocorticoids have been shown to down-regulate β_1-adrenergic receptor expression by suppressing transcription of the receptor gene (76). Agonist stimulation can also lead to receptor sequestration (see above) and receptor trafficking to lysosomes for degradation.

Homologous down-regulation of TRH receptors in cell lines has been well-studied and the results illustrate a posttranscriptional biosynthetic regulatory mechanism. The number of thyrotropin-releasing hormone receptors in culture decreases markedly following agonist exposure. Exposure of cells to 100 nM TRH for 24 h causes a 70% decrease in the number of receptors (45). The TRH receptor also shows heterologous regulation following exposure to thyroid hormones, estrogen or EGF (47, 61, 122).

The mechansim underlying homologous down-regulation of TRH receptors was initially studied using a *Xenopus laevis* oocyte-based mRNA activity assay. These experiments were done prior to the cloning of a cDNA for the TRH receptor. When *Xenopus* oocytes are injected with heterologous mRNA encoding a receptor, they synthesize and insert the receptor encoded. The number of receptors is reflected in the size of the currents detected electrophysiologically upon exposure of the oocytes to ligand. For this assay, cells can be treated to achieve regulation. RNA is then extracted and injected into oocytes. Subsequently, the TRH receptor mRNA activity is assessed by measuring the response of the oocytes to TRH. Using this technique, it was found that, following exposure to TRH, TRH receptor mRNA activity manifested a very rapid decrease to 15% of control values within 3 h (117). Following cloning of the TRH receptor (155), it was confirmed that this loss of mRNA activity in the oocyte assay reflected a decrease in the amount of TRH receptor mRNA and was found to be mediated by protein kinase C activation (40, 185, 186). This rapid decrease induced by TRH is due, at least in part, to an increase in the rate of TRH receptor mRNA degradation (39) caused by an increase in RNAse activity (110). By studying regulation of transfected receptors, it was demonstrated that the mRNA sequences mediating this regulated degradation are located in the 3'-untranslated region of the receptor mRNA (110).

Agonist-stimulated receptor mRNA destabilization has also been observed for the β_2-adrenergic receptor and for the thrombin receptor. Exposure of DDT 1

MF-2 cells, which express the β_2-adrenergic receptor, to the agonist isoproterenol leads to a reduction in the level of receptor mRNA as detected by solution hybridization/nuclease protection assay (50). In contrast to the effects of dexamethone, which increases β_2-adrenergic receptor mRNA levels by increasing the transcription rate of the receptor gene (53), the reduction in mRNA levels caused by isoproterenol is not accompanied by any change in transcription rate. Instead, isoproterenol was found to promote degradation of the β_2-adrenergic receptor mRNA, reducing the half-life from 12 h in control cells to 5 h in treated cells (53). Covalent UV catalyzed cross-linking was utilized to identify a 35,000 M_r protein that bound selectively to mRNAs that, like the β_2-adrenergic receptor mRNA, contain uracil-rich regions with AUUUA pentamers (125). The level of this protein was induced by adrenergic receptor stimulation and correlated inversely with the level of β_2-adrenergic receptor mRNA (125). By studying interaction of this protein, called β-ARB, with defined sequences, it was determined that both the AUUUA pentamer and flanking poly(U) regions were required for binding (64). These results suggest that this inducible protein binds to specific 3'-untranslated sequences and promotes receptor degradation. The level and half-life of thrombin receptor mRNA levels in a cell line is also decreased by thrombin and by activation of adenylate cyclase (156). The thrombin receptor, like the β_2-adrenergic receptor, contains 3'-untranslated poly(U) flanked AUUUA pentamers that are sensitive to β-ARB–mediated destabilization.

The GnRH receptor shows a complex regulatory reponse to agonist exposure. Exposure of dispersed rat pituitary cells to low concentrations of GnRH (0.1– 2.5 nM) induces a biphasic modulation of GnRH receptor number. Over the first several hours receptor number is decreased. Subsequently, receptor number recovers to exceed control levels by 6–9 h (33, 95, 96). The GnRH receptor is unusual in being capable of manifesting either down- or up-regulation in response to GnRH, depending on the duration and level of GnRH exposure. Whereas low concentrations of GnRH increase receptor number after 6 h, higher concentrations of GnRH decrease receptor number at all time points (33, 95). The up-regulation of the GnRH receptor in rat pituitary primary cultures requires both protein and RNA synthesis (33, 96), whereas the down-regulation induced by high GnRH concentrations does not (33).

The mechanisms underlying homologous GnRH receptor regulation have been studied in dispersed pituitary cells and in the gonadotrope cells line, αT3–1 cells (177). In dispersed rat pituitary cells, homologous up-regulation is accompanied by a significant increase in the levels of GnRH receptor mRNA as determined by northern blot analysis (73). A similar up-regulation in the number of GnRH receptors following exposure to low concentration of agonist is observed in the gonadotrope cell line αT3–1 cells (165). However, in contrast to the increase in mRNA levels observed with up-regulation in pituitary primary cultures, in these cells no change in mRNA levels is observed by nuclease protection assay or by northern blot analysis (165). In addition, when pure RNA from regulated αT3–1 cells is injected into *Xenopus* oocytes and the number of receptors synthesized is assayed by the electrophysiological response to GnRH, the ability of the RNA to direct the expression of receptors in oocytes is regulated in concert with the regulation that occurs in the αT3–1 cells. These results suggest that an RNA distinct from the GnRH receptor mRNA is regulated and affects the level of receptor expression.

αT3–1 cells also demonstrate down-regulation of the number of GnRH receptors following exposure to high levels of GnRH for 24 h. The down-regulation in αT3–1 cells is accompanied by a slight (98) or absent (164) decrease in the level of GnRH receptor mRNA. However, the polysome pattern of GnRH receptor mRNA is shifted with down-regulation from denser to less dense polysomes, suggesting that decreased translation contributes to the down regulation observed (164).

In other experimental systems, changes in GnRH receptor mRNA induced by GnRH exposure have been reported. Exposure of LβT2 gonadotrope cells to four 15-minute pulses of 10 nM GnRH for 3 days induces a significant increase in steady state GnRH receptor mRNA levels (167). Pulsatile GnRH treatment up-regulates GnRH receptor and GnRH receptor mRNA levels in sheep (169) and chronic GnRH agonist treatment decreases GnRH receptor mRNA levels relative to controls in sheep both in vivo (18) and in vitro (182). In contrast to the effects seen in pituitary, in ovarian granulosa cells in culture no change is seen in GnRH receptor mRNA levels following low level GnRH exposure, and an increase is observed with exposure to 1–10 μM GnRH for 24 h (116). In ovariectomized sheep, GnRH administration was found to increase the levels of the mRNAs of the immediate early genes *c-fos* and *c-jun* in the pituitary; these results raise the possiblity that immediate early genes are involved in GnRH induced regulation in this system (118).

In addition to its regulation by agonist, GnRH receptor levels also show heterologous regulation in response to a variety of hormonal manipulations. Activin A increases GnRH mRNA levels in αT3–1 cells, in part by increasing the rate of transcription (38). GnRH receptor mRNA levels show cyclical variation with the estrous cycle in sheep (19, 118) and in rats (8, 9).

Steroid replacement studies in ovariectomized rats suggest that the up-regulation seen during proestrus is largely due to estrogens (10). mRNA levels in rats progressively increase following gonadectomy (73, 74). While estradiol administration causes a marked decrease in GnRH receptor mRNA levels in female gonadectomized rats, testosterone causes only a small decrease in male gonadectomized rats (73). In contrast to the results in rats, in ewes, estradiol causes an increase the level of GnRH receptor mRNA levels following ovariectomy (55). Lactating rats show a decrease in GnRH receptor binding sites (148, 149) and in mRNA levels, with the suppression reversed by pup removal (150). These changes may be due to alterations in the pattern of GnRH secretion. Estradiol and inhibin increase the level of GnRH receptor mRNA and receptor number in primary cultures from sheep pituitary (89, 140, 182) while progesterone has the opposite effect (140, 182). Luteolysis induced in sheep by $PGF_{2\alpha}$ administration causes an increase in GnRH receptor mRNA levels, most likely due to accompanying decrease in progesterone levels (168). Estradiol and dexamethasone have been shown to increase the steady-state level of GnRH receptor mRNA in the $L\beta T2$ gonadotrope cell line (167).

The thrombin receptor, with its unique mechanism of activation, provides an interesting system for regulatory control. Activation of the thrombin receptor occurs by an irreversible proteolytic modification of the receptor's amino terminus. The thrombin receptor is unique among G protein–coupled receptors in that it is activated by a segment of the amino terminus that is masked in the unactivated receptor. Thrombin is a proteolytic enzyme that recognizes a specific sequence within the amino terminus domain of the receptor. Mutation of the thrombin cleavage site causes of loss of receptor activation by thrombin (172), and alteration of the thrombin recognition site to the sequence specifying enterokinase cleavage results in a receptor that can be activated by enterokinase, but not by thrombin (173). Studies of peptides corresponding to the amino terminus created by thrombin cleavage demonstrate that this domain, when exposed by cleavage, can mediate receptor activation (137, 173).

Once the tethered agonist is unmasked by thrombin, it cannot dissociate. The receptors are rapidly inactivated. The processing of thrombin receptors varies in different cell lines. In a megakaryoblastic cell line, thrombin causes internalization via coated pits of nearly all receptors within several minutes. While most receptors are shuttled to lysosomes and degraded, a significant portion of these internalized receptors is recycled to the cell surface. The recycled receptors do not signal spontaneously, despite the presence of an exposed tethered ligand (15, 63). This may be due to phosphorylation by a G protein–coupled receptor kinase (13, 68). Restoration of the reponse to thrombin requires synthesis of new receptors (15, 63). In contrast, in endothelial cells, both rapid and slow internalization occurs and the internalized receptors do not recycle. The recovery of the response to thrombin is not dependent on protein synthesis and occurs by expression on the cell surface of an intracellular pool of receptors (181). Comparison of the processing of thrombin receptors with that of β_2 adrenergic receptors in transfected fibroblasts showed that, in contrast to adrenergic receptors, in unstimulated cells a pool of thrombin receptors is localized to the Golgi apparatus. While the adrenergic receptors recycle, the thrombin receptors are all degraded and the intracellular pool is translocated to the membrane (60).

In addition to reiterating the cell specific differences in regulatory mechanisms, thrombin receptor studies also demonstrate how homologous and heterologous regulation can occur via different mechanisms. Homologous thrombin receptor regulation in mesangial cells occurs by receptor degradation without altered mRNA levels whereas heterologous down-regulation via phorbol ester or adenylyl cyclase stimulation causes a decrease in steady state receptor mRNA expression and the down-regulation is due to decreased biosynthesis (13).

CONCLUSIONS

The cloning of the majority of peptide receptors has facilitated the elucidation of the regulatory mechanisms underlying the expression of these receptors. We can appreciate the rich variety of mechanisms available to the cell to control the response mediated by a particular receptor system. Yet even as our understanding of the detailed mechanisms of receptor regulation continues to grow, so does the challenge to correctly judge the physiological relevance of these various regulatory phenomena. One striking feature of the literature on peptide regulation is the degree to which each receptor and experimental system is unique. One must be exceedingly cautious in generalizing from receptor to receptor or even from one experimental system to another for the same receptor. It is often impossible to be certain of the causative role of a particular regulatory event that is characterized, such as altered mRNA levels, in determining the physiological changes observed in vivo in the responsivity of that receptor system. While there is a definable set of instruments in the regulatory orchestra, each receptor and each experimental system can utilize a different tempo and melody.

REFERENCES

1. Akita, Y., S. Ohno, Y. Yajima, Y. Konno, T. C. Saido, K. Mizuno, K. Chida, S. Osada, T. Kuroki, S. Kawashima, et al. Overproduction of a Ca(2+)-independent protein kinase C isozyme, nPKC epsilon, increases the secretion of prolactin from thyrotropin-releasing hormone-stimulated rat pituitary GH4C1 cells. *J. Biol. Chem.* 269: 4653–4660, 1994.

2. Akita, Y., S. Ohno, Y. Yajima, and K. Suzuki. Possible role of Ca2(+)-independent protein kinase C isozyme, nPKC epsilon, in thyrotropin-releasing hormone-stimulated signal transduction: differential down-regulation of nPKC epsilon in GH4C1 cells. *Biochem. Biophys. Res. Commun.* 172: 184–189, 1990.

3. Ashworth, R., R. Yu, E. J. Nelson, S. Dermer, M. C. Gershengorn, and P. M. Hinkle. Visualization of the thyrotropin-releasing hormone receptor and its ligand during endocytosis and recycling. *Proc. Natl. Acad. Sci. USA* 92: 512–516, 1995.

4. Baldwin, J. M. Structure and function of receptors coupled to G proteins. *Curr. Opin. Cell Biol.* 6: 180–190, 1994.

5. Erondu, N. E., and Bar, R. S. Receptor-mediated endocytosis of polypeptide hormones by vascular endotaelium Endocrinology. Volume I: Cellular Mechanisms, edited by Michael P. Conn. New York: Oxford etc. In: *Handbook of Physiology*, Section 7: 1998.

6. Barak, L. S., L. Menard, S.S.G. Ferguson, A. Colapietro, and M. G. Caron. The conserved seven-transmembrane sequence NP(X)2,3Y of the G-protein coupled receptor superfamily regulates multiple properties of the β2–adrenergic receptor. *Biochemistry* 34: 15407–15414, 1995.

7. Barak, L. S., M. Tiberi, N. J. Freedman, M. M. Kwatra, R. J. Lefkowitz, and M. G. Caron. A highly conserved tyrosine residue in G protein-coupled receptors is required for agonist-mediated beta 2–adrenergic receptor sequestration. *J. Biol. Chem.* 269: 2790–2795, 1994.

8. Bauer-Dantoin, A. C., A. N. Hollenberg, and J. L. Jameson. Dynamic regulation of gonadotropin-releasing hormone receptor mRNA levels in the anterior pituitary gland during the rat estrous cycle. *Endocrinology* 133: 1911–1914, 1993.

9. Bauer-Dantoin, A. C., and J. L. Jameson. Gonadotropin-releasing hormone receptor messenger ribonucleic acid expression in the ovary during the rat estrous cycle. *Endocrinology* 136: 4432–4438, 1995.

10. Bauer-Dantoin, A. C., J. Weiss, and J. L. Jameson. Roles of estrogen, progesterone, and gonadotropin-releasing hormone (GnRH) in the control of pituitary GnRH receptor gene expression at the time of the preovulatory gonadotropin surges. *Endocrinology* 136: 1014–1019, 1995.

11. Benya, R. V., M. Akeson, J. Mrozinski, R. T. Jensen, and J. F. Battey. Internalization of the gastrin-releasing peptide receptor is mediated by both phospholipase C-dependent and -independent processes. *Mol. Pharmacol.* 46: 495–501, 1994.

12. Benya, R. V., Z. Fathi, J. F. Battey, and R. T. Jensen. Serines and threonines in the gastrin-releasing peptide receptor carboxyl terminus mediate internalization. *J. Biol. Chem.* 268: 20285–20290, 1993.

13. Brass, L. F. Homologous desensitization of HEL cell thrombin receptors. Distinguishable roles for proteolysis and phosphorylation. *J. Biol. Chem.* 267: 6044–6050, 1992.

14. Brass, L. F., M. Ahuja, E. Belmonte, N. Blanchard, S. Pizarro, A. Tarver, and J. A. Hoxie. Thrombin receptors: turning them off after turning them on. *Semin. Hematol.* 31: 251–260, 1994.

15. Brass, L. F., S. Pizarro, M. Ahuja, E. Belmonte, N. Blanchard, J. M. Stadel, and J. A. Hoxie. Changes in the structure and function of the human thrombin receptor during receptor activation, internalization, and recycling. *J. Biol. Chem.* 269: 2943–2952, 1994.

16. Briscoe, C. P., R. Plevin, and M. J. Wakelam. Rapid desensitization and resensitization of bombesin-stimulated phospholipase D activity in Swiss 3T3 cells. *Biochem. J.* 298: 61–67, 1994.

17. Briscoe, C. P., and M. J. Wakelam. Heterologous desensitization of bombesin- and vasopressin-stimulated phospholipase D activity in Swiss 3T3 fibroblasts. *FEBS Lett.* 361: 162–166, 1995.

18. Brooks, J., and A. S. McNeilly. Regulation of gonadotrophin-releasing hormone receptor mRNA expression in the sheep. *J. Endocrinol.* 143: 175–182, 1994.

19. Brooks, J., W. J. Struthers, and A. S. McNeilly. GnRH-dependent and -independent components of FSH secretion after actue treatment of anoestrous ewes with ovine follicular fluid and a GnRH antagonist. *J. Reprod. Fertil.* 98: 591–595, 1993.

20. Carpentier, J.L. Robert Feulgen Prize Lecture 1993. The journey of the insulin receptor into the cell: from cellular biology to pathophysiology. *Histochemistry* 100: 169–184, 1993.

21. Carpentier, J. L. Insulin receptor internalization: molecular mechanisms and physiopathological implications. *Diabetologia* 37: S117–S124, 1994.

22. Chabry, J., J.M. Botto, D. Nouel, A. Beaudet, J.P. Vincent, and J. Mazella. Thr-422 and Tyr-424 residues in the carboxyl terminus are critical for the internalization of the rat neurotensin receptor. *J. Biol. Chem.* 270: 2439–2442, 1995.

23. Chaki, S., D.F. Guo, Y. Yamano, K. Ohyama, M. Tani, M. Mizukoshi, H. Shirai, and T. Inagami. Role of carboxyl tail of the rat angiotensin II type 1A receptor in agonist-induced internalization of the receptor. *Kidney Int.* 46: 1492–1495, 1994.

24. Chang, C. P., C. S. Lazar, B. J. Walsh, M. Komuro, J. F. Collawn, L. A. Kuhn, J. A. Tainer, I. S. Trowbridge, M. G. Farquhar, M. G. Rosenfeld, et. al. Ligand-induced internalization of the epidermal growth factor receptor is mediated by multiple endocytic codes analogous to the tyrosine motif found in constitutively internalized receptors. *J. Biol. Chem.* 268: 19312–19320, 1993.

25. Chen, C. Y., S. B. Dion, C. M. Kim, and J. L. Benovic. Beta-adrenergic receptor kinase. Agonist-dependent receptor binding promotes kinase activation. *J. Biol. Chem.* 268: 7825–7831, 1993.

26. Childs, G. V., E. Hazum, A. Amsterdam, R. Limor, and Z. Naor. Cytochemical evidence for different routes of gonadotropin-releasing hormone processing by large gonadotropes and granulosa cells. *Endocrinology* 119: 1329–1338, 1986.

27. Childs, G. V., Z. Naor, E. Hazum, R. Tibolt, K. N. Westlund, and M. B. Hancock. Localization of biotinylated gonadotropin releasing hormone on pituitary monolayer cells with avidin-biotin-peroxidase complexes. *J. Histochem. Cytochem.* 31: 1422–1425, 1983.

28. Clayton, R. N., and K. J. Catt. Gonadotropin-releasing hormone receptors: characterization, physiological regulation, and relationship to reproductive function. *Endocr. Rev.* 2: 186–209, 1981.

29. Collawn, J. F., L. A. Kuhn, L. F. Liu, J. A. Tainer, and I. S. Trowbridge. Transplanted LDL and mannose-6–phosphate

receptor internalization signals promote high-efficiency endocytosis of the transferrin receptor. *EMBO J.* 10: 3247–3253, 1991.

30. Conn, P. M., and W. Crowley, Jr. Gonadotropin-releasing hormone and its analogs. *Annu. Rev. Med.* 45: 391–405, 1994.

31. Conn, P. M., and E. Hazum. Luteinizing hormone release and gonadotropin-releasing hormone (GnRH) receptor internalization: independent actions of GnRH. *Endocrinology* 109: 2040–2045, 1981.

32. Conn, P. M., J. A. Janovick, D. Stanislaus, d. Kuphal, and L. Jennes. Molecular and cellular bases of gonadotropin-releasing hormone action in the pituitary and central nervous system. *Vitam. Horm.* 50: 151–214, 1995.

33. Conn, P. M., D. C. Rogers, and S. G. Seay. Biphasic regulation of the gonadotropin-releasing hormone receptor by receptor microaggregation and intracellular Ca^{2+} levels. *Mol. Pharmacol.* 25: 51–55, 1984.

34. Davidson, J. S., C. Flanagan, W. Zhou, I. Becker, R. Elario, W. Emeran, S. C. Sealfon, and R. P. Millar. Identification of N-glycosylation sites in the gonadotropin-releasing hormone receptor: role in receptor expression but not ligand binding. *Mol. Cell. Endocrinol.* 107: 241–245, 1995.

35. Davidson, J. S., C. A. Flanagan, P. D. Davies, J. Hapgood, D. Mybrugh, R. Elario, R. P. Millar, W. Forrest-Owen, and C.A. McArdle. Incorporation of an additional glycosylation site enhances expression of functional human gonadotropin-releasing hormone receptor. *Endocrine*, 4:207–212, 1996.

36. Eason, M. G., and S. B. Liggett. Subtype-selective desensitization of alpha 2–adrenergic receptors. Different mechanisms control short and long term agonist-promoted desensitization of alpha 2C10, alpha 2C4, and alpha 2C2. *J. Biol. Chem.* 267: 25473–25479, 1992.

37. Feger, J., S. Gil-Falgon, and C. Lamaze. Cell receptors: definition, mechanisms and regulation of receptor-mediated endocytosis. *Cell. Mol. Biol.* 40: 1039–1061, 1994.

38. Fernandez-Vasquez, G., U. B. Kaiser, C. R. Albarracin, and W. W. Chin. Transcriptional activation of the gonadotropin-releasing hormone receptor gene by activin A. *Mol. Endocrinol.* 10: 356–366, 1996.

39. Fujimoto, J., C. S. Narayanan, J. E. Benjamin, M. Heinflink, and M. C. Gershengorn. Mechanism of regulation of thyrotropin-releasing hormone receptor messenger ribonucleic acid in stably transfected rat pituitary cells. *Endocrinology* 130: 1879–1884, 1992.

40. Fujimoto, J., R. E. Straub, and M. C. Gershengorn. Thyrotropin-releasing hormone (TRH) and phorbol myristate acetate decrease TRH receptor messenger RNA in rat pituitary GH3 cells: evidence that protein kinase-C mediates the TRH effect. *Mol. Endocrinol.* 5: 1527–1532, 1991.

41. Garland, A. M., E. F. Grady, M. Lovett, S. R. Vigna, M. M. Frucht, J. E. Krause, and N. W. Bunnett. Mechanisms of desensitization and resensitization of G protein-coupled neurokinin1 and neurokinin2 receptors. *Mol. Pharmacol.* 49: 438–446, 1996.

42. Gasic, S., and A. Green. Gi down-regulation and heterologous desensitization in adipocytes after treatment with the alpha 2–agonist UK 14304. *Biochem. Pharmacol.* 49: 785–790, 1995.

43. Gates, L. K., C. D. Ulrich, and L. J. Miller. Multiple kinases phosphorylate the pancreatic cholecystokinin receptor in an agonist-dependent manner. *Am. J. Physiol.* 264 *(Gastrointest. Liver Physiol.* 33*)*: G840–G847, 1993.

44. George, S. T., A. E. Ruoho, and C. C. Malbon. N-glycosylation in expression and function of beta-adrenergic receptors. *J. Biol. Chem.* 261: 16559–16564, 1986.

45. Gershengorn, M. C. Bihormonal regulation of the thyrotropin-releasing hormone receptor in mouse pituitary thyrotropic tumor cells in culture. *J. Clin. Invest.* 62: 937–943, 1978.

46. Gershengorn, M. C. Thyrotropin-releasing hormone receptor: cloning and regulation of its expression. *Recent Prog. Horm. Res.* 48: 341–363, 1993.

47. Gershengorn, M. C., B. E. Marcus-Samuels, and E. Geras. Estrogens increase the number of thyrotropin-releasing hormone receptors on mammotropic cells in culture. *Endocrinology* 105: 171–176, 1979.

48. Goldstein, J. L., M. S. Brown, R. G. Anderson, D. W. Russell, and W. J. Schneider. Receptor-mediated endocytosis: concepts emerging from the LDL receptor system. *Annu. Rev. Cell Biol.* 1: 1–39, 1985.

49. Gupta, S. K., and R. K. Mishra. Desensitization of D1 dopamine receptors down-regulates the Gs alpha subunit of G protein in SK-N-MC neuroblastoma cells. *J. Mol. Neurosci.* 4: 117–123, 1993.

50. Hadcock, J. R., and C. C. Malbon. Down-regulation of beta-adrenergic receptors: agonist-induced reduction in receptor mRNA levels. *Proc. Natl. Acad. Sci. USA* 85: 5021–5025, 1988.

51. Hadcock, J. R., and C. C. Malbon. Agonist regulation of gene expression of adrenergic receptors and G proteins. *J. Neurochem.* 60: 1–9, 1993.

52. Hadcock, J.R., M. Ros, D.C. Watkins, and C.C. Malbon. Cross-regulation between G-protein-mediated pathways. Stimulation of adenylyl cyclase increases expression of the inhibitory G-protein, Gi alpha 2. *J. Biol. Chem.* 265: 14784–14790, 1990.

53. Hadcock, J. R., H. Y. Wang, and C. C. Malbon. Agonist-induced destabilization of beta-adrenergic receptor mRNA. Attenuation of glucocorticoid-induced up-regulation of beta-adrenergic receptors. *J. Biol. Chem.* 264: 19928–19933, 1989.

54. Haft, C. R., R. D. Klausner, and S. I. Taylor. Involvement of dileucine motifs in the internalization and degradation of the insulin receptor. *J. Biol. Chem.* 269: 26286–26294, 1994.

55. Hamernik, D. L., C. M. Clay, A. Turzillo, E. A. Van Kirk, and G. E. Moss. Estradiol increases amounts of messenger ribonucleic acid for gonadotropin-releasing hormone receptors in sheep. *Biol. Reprod.* 53: 179–185, 1995.

56. Hansen, S. H., K. Sandvig, and B. van Deurs. The preendosomal compartment comprises distinct coated and noncoated endocytic vesicle populations. *J. Cell Biol.* 113: 731–741, 1991.

57. Hazum, E., Y. Koch, M. Liscovitch, and A. Amsterdam. Intracellular pathways of receptor-bound GnRH agonist in pituitary gonadotropes. *Cell Tissue Res.* 239: 3–8, 1985.

58. Hazum, E., R. Meidan, M. Liscovitch, D. Keinan, H. R. Lindner, and Y. Koch. Receptor-mediated internalization of LHRH antagonists by pituitary cells. *Mol. Cell. Endocrinol.* 30: 291–301, 1983.

59. Hazum, E., and A. Nimrod. Photoaffinity-labeling and fluorescence-distribution studies of gonadotropin-releasing hormone receptors in ovarian granulosa cells. *Proc. Natl. Acad. Sci. USA* 79: 1747–1750, 1982.

60. Hein, L., K. Ishii, S. R. Coughlin, and B. K. Kobilka. Intracellular targeting and trafficking of thrombin receptors. A novel mechanism for resensitization of a G protein-coupled receptor. *J. Biol. Chem.* 269: 27719–27726, 1994.

61. Hinkle, P. M., E. d. Shanshala, and Z. F. Yan. Epidermal growth factor decreases the concentration of thyrotropin-releasing hormone (TRH) receptors and TRH responses in pituitary GH4C1 cells. *Endocrinology* 129: 1283–1288, 1991.

62. Hopkins, C. R., and H. Gregory. Topographical localization of the receptors for luteinizing hormone-releasing hormone on the

surgace of dissociated pituitary cells. *J. Cell Biol.* 75: 528–540, 1977.

63. Hoxie, J. A., M. Ahuja, E. Belmonte, S. Pizarro, R. Parton, and L. F. Brass. Internalization and recycling of activated thrombin receptors. *J. Biol. Chem.* 268: 13756–13763, 1993.

64. Huang, L. Y., B. G. Tholanikunnel, E. Vakalopoulou, and C. C. Malbon. The M(r) 35,000 beta-adrenergic receptor mRNA-binding protein induced by agonists requires both an AUUUA pentamer and U-rich domains for RNA recognition. *J. Biol. Chem.* 268: 25769–25775, 1993.

65. Hunyady, L., M. Bor, T. Balla, and K. J. Catt. Identification of a cytoplasmic Ser-Thr-Leu motif that determines agonist-induced internalization of the AT1 angiotensin receptor. *J. Biol. Chem.* 269: 31378–31382, 1994.

66. Hunyady, L., M. Bor, A. J. Baukal, T. Balla, and K. J. Catt. A conserved NPLFY sequence contributes to agonist binding and signal transduction but is not an internalization signal for the type 1 angiotensin II receptor. *J. Biol. Chem.* 270: 16602–16609, 1995.

67. Inagami, T., N. Iwai, K. Sasaki, D. F. Guo, Y. Furuta, Y. Yamano, S. Bardhan, S. Chaki, N. Makito, and K. Badr. Angiotensin II receptors: cloning and regulation. *Arzneimittelforschung* 43: 226–228, 1993.

68. Ishii, K., J. Chen, M. Ishii, W. J. Koch, N. J. Freedman, R. J. Lefkowitz, and S. R. Coughlin. Inhibition of thrombin receptor signaling by a G-protein coupled receptor kinase. Functional specificity among G-protein coupled receptor kinases. *J. Biol. Chem.* 269: 1125–1130, 1994.

69. Jadot, M., W. M. Canfield, W. Gregory, and S. Kornfeld. Characterization of the signal for rapid internalization of the bovine mannose 6–phosphate/insulin-like growth factor-II receptor. *J. Biol. Chem.* 267: 11069–11077, 1992.

70. Jennes, L., W. E. Stumpf, and P. M. Conn. Intracellular pathways of electron-opaque gonadotropin-releasing hormone derivatives bound by cultured gonadotropes. *Endocrinology* 113: 1683–1689, 1983.

71. Jennes, L., W. E. Stumpf, and P. M. Conn. Receptor-mediated binding and uptake of GnRH agonist and antagonist by pituitary cells. *Peptides* 5: 215–220, 1984.

72. Joly, M., A. Kazlauskas, and S. Corvera. Phosphatidylinositol 3–kinase activity is required at a postendocytic step in platelet-derived growth factor receptor trafficking. *J. Biol. Chem.* 270: 13225–13230, 1995.

73. Kaiser, U. B., A. Jakubowiak, A. Steinberger, and W. W. Chin. Regulation of rat pituitary gonadotropin-releasing hormone receptor mRNA levels in vivo and in vitro. *Endocrinology* 133: 931–934, 1993.

74. Kakar, S. S., K. Grantham, L. C. Musgrove, D. Devor, J. C. Sellers, and J. D. Neill. Rat gonadotropin-releasing hormone (GnRH) receptor: Tissue expression and hormonal regulation of its mRNA. *Mol. Cell. Endocrinol.* 101: 151–157, 1994.

75. Kennedy, M. E., and L. E. Limbird. Mutations of the alpha 2A-adrenergic receptor that eliminate detectable palmitoylation do not perturb receptor-G-protein coupling. *J. Biol. Chem.* 268: 8003–8011, 1993.

76. Kiely, J., J. R. Hadcock, S. W. Bahouth, and C. C. Malbon. Glucocorticoids down-regulate beta 1–adrenergic-receptor expression by suppressing transcription of the receptor gene. *Biochem. J.* 302: 397–403, 1994.

77. Klausner, R. D. Sorting and traffic in the central vacuolar system. *Cell* 57: 703–706, 1989.

78. Klueppelberg, U. G., L. K. Gates, F. S. Gorelick, and L. J. Miller. Agonist-regulated phosphorylation of the pancreatic cholecystokinin receptor. *J. Biol. Chem.* 266: 2403–2408, 1991.

79. Koller, K. J., M. T. Lipari, and D. V. Goeddel. Proper glycosylation and phosphorylation of the type A natriuretic peptide receptor are required for hormone-stimulated guanylyl cyclase activity. *J. Biol. Chem.* 268: 5997–6003, 1993.

80. Kornfeld, R., and S. Kornfeld. Assembly of asparagine-linked oligosaccharides. *Annu. Rev. Biochem.* 54: 631–664, 1985.

81. Kovoor, A., D. J. Henry, and C. Chavkin. Agonist-induced desensitization of the mu opioid receptor-coupled potassium channel (GIRK1). *J. Biol. Chem.* 270: 589–595, 1995.

82. Kwatra, M. M., D. A. Schwinn, J. Schreurs, J. L. Blank, C. M. Kim, J. L. Benovic, J. E. Krause, M. G. Caron, and R. J. Lefkowitz. The substance P receptor, which couples to Gq/11, is a substrate of beta-adrenergic receptor kinase 1 and 2. *J. Biol. Chem.* 268: 9161–9164, 1993.

83. Lamaze, C., T. Baba, T. E. Redelmeier, and S. L. Schmid. Recruitment of epidermal growth factor and transferrin receptors into coated pits in vitro: differing biochemical requirements. *Mol. Biol. Cell* 4: 715–727, 1993.

84. Lamaze, C., and S. L. Schmid. The emergence of clathrin-independent pinocytic pathways. *Curr. Opin. Cell Biol.* 7: 573–580, 1995.

85. Lamaze, C., and S. L. Schmid. Recruitment of epidermal growth factor receptors into coated pits requires their activated tyrosine kinase. *J. Cell. Biol.* 129: 47–54, 1995.

86. Lameh, J., M. Philip, Y. K. Sharma, O. Moro, J. Ramachandran, and W. Sadee. Hm1 muscarinic cholinergic receptor internalization requires a domain in the third cytoplasmic loop. *J. Biol. Chem.* 267: 13406–13412, 1992.

87. Lattion, A. L., D. Diviani, and S. Cotecchia. Truncation of the receptor carboxyl terminus impairs agonist-dependent phosphorylation and desensitization of the alpha 1B-adrenergic receptor. *J. Biol. Chem.* 269: 22887–22893, 1994.

88. Lauffenburger, D. A., and J. J. Linderman. Receptors: Models for binding, trafficking and signaling. New York: *Oxford University Press*, 1993. p. 73–124.

89. Laws, S. C., J. C. Webster, and W. L. Miller. Estradiol alters the effectiveness of gonadotropin-releasing hormone (GnRH) in ovine pituitary cultures: GnRH receptors versus responsiveness to GnRH. *Endocrinology* 127: 381–386, 1990.

90. Leeb-Lundberg, L. M., S. Cotecchia, A. De Blasi, M. G. Caron, and R. J. Lefkowitz. Regulation of adrenergic receptor function by phosphorylation. I. Agonist-promoted desensitization and phosphorylation of alpha 1-adrenergic receptors coupled to inositol phospholipid metabolism in DDT1 MF-2 smooth muscle cells. *J. Biol. Chem.* 262: 3098–3105, 1987.

91. Lefkowitz, R. J. G protein-coupled receptor kinases. *Cell* 74: 409–412, 1993.

92. Lefkowitz, R. J., J. Inglese, W. J. Koch, J. Pitcher, H. Attramadal, and M. G. Caron. G-protein-coupled receptors: regulatory role of receptor kinases and arrestin proteins. *Cold Spring Harb. Symp. Quant. Biol.* 57: 127–133, 1992.

93. Liggett, S. B., N. J. Freedman, D. A. Schwinn, and R. J. Lefkowitz. Structural basis for receptor subtype-specific regulation revealed by a chimeric beta 3/beta 2–adrenergic receptor. *Proc. Natl. Acad. Sci. USA* 90: 3665–3669, 1993.

94. Liu, X., D. Davis, and D. L. Segaloff. Disruption of potential sites for N-linked glycosylation does not impair hormone binding to the lutropin/choriogonadotropin receptor if Asn-173 is left intact. *J. Biol. Chem.* 268: 1513–1516, 1993.

95. Loumaye, E., and K. J. Catt. Homologous regulation of gonadotropin-releasing hormone receptors in cultured pituitary cells. *Science* 215: 983–985, 1982.

96. Loumaye, E., and K. J. Catt. Agonist-induced regulation of pituitary receptors for gonadotrophin-releasing hormone: Disso-

ciation of receptor recruitment from hormone release in cultured gonadotrophs. *J. Biol. Chem.* 258: 12002–12009, 1983.

97. Lutz, M. P., D. I. Pinon, L. K. Gates, S. Shenolikar, and L. J. Miller. Control of cholecystokinin receptor dephosphorylation in pancreatic acinar cells. *J. Biol. Chem.* 268: 12136–12142, 1993.

98. Mason, D. R., K. K. Arora, L. M. Mertz, and K. J. Catt. Homologous down-regulation of gonadotropin-releasing hormone receptor sites and messenger ribonucleic acid transcripts in alpha T3–1 cells. *Endocrinology* 135: 1165–1170, 1994.

99. McArdle, C. A., W. R. Huckle, L. A. Johnson, and P. M. Conn. Enhanced responsiveness of gonadotropes after protein kinase-C activation: postreceptor regulation of gonadotropin releasing hormone action. *Endocrinology* 122: 1905–1914, 1988.

100. McArdle, C. A., and A. Poch. Dependence of gonadotropin-releasing hormone-stimulated luteinizing hormone release upon intracellular Ca^{2+} pools is revealed by desensitization and thapsigargin blockade. *Endocrinology* 130: 3567–3574, 1992.

101. Mestek, A., J. H. Hurley, L. S. Bye, A. D. Campbell, Y. Chen, M. Tian, J. Liu, H. Schulman, and L. Yu. The human mu opioid receptor: modulation of functional desensitization by calcium/calmodulin-dependent protein kinase and protein kinase C. *J. Neurosci.* 15: 2396–2406, 1995.

102. Milligan, G., M. Parenti, and A. I. Magee. The dynamic role of palmitoylation in signal transduction. *Trends Pharm. Sci.* 20: 181–186, 1995.

103. Moench, S. J., J. Moreland, D. H. Stewart, and T. G. Dewey. Fluorescence studies of the location and membrane accessibility of the palmitoylation sites of rhodopsin. *Biochemistry* 33: 5791–5796, 1994.

104. Moffett, S., B. Mouillac, H. Bonin, and M. Bouvier. Altered phosphorylation and desensitization patterns of a human beta 2–adrenergic receptor lacking the palmitoylated Cys341. *EMBO J.* 12: 349–356, 1993.

105. Mori, S., L. Ronnstrand, L. Claesson-Welsh, and C. H. Heldin. A tyrosine residue in the juxtamembrane segment of the platelet-derived growth factor beta-receptor is critical for ligand-mediated endocytosis. *J. Biol. Chem.* 269: 4917–4921, 1994.

106. Moro, O., J. Lameh, and W. Sadee. Serine- and threonine-rich domain regulates internalization of muscarinic cholinergic receptors. *J. Biol. Chem.* 268: 6862–6865, 1993.

107. Munoz, C. M., S. Cotecchia, and L. M. Leeb-Lundberg. B2 kinin receptor-mediated internalization of bradykinin in DDT1 MF-2 smooth muscle cells is paralleled by sequestration of the occupied receptors. *Arch. Biochem. Biophys.* 301: 336–344, 1993.

108. Munoz, C. M., and L. M. Leeb-Lundberg. Receptor-mediated internalization of bradykinin. DDT1 MF-2 smooth muscle cells process internalized bradykinin via multiple degradative pathways. *J. Biol. Chem.* 267: 303–309, 1992.

109. Naor, Z., D. Atlas, R. N. Clayton, D. S. Forman, A. Amsterdam, and K. J. Catt. Interaction of fluorescent gonadotropin-releasing hormone with receptors in cultured pituitary cells. *J. Biol. Chem.* 256: 3049–3052, 1981.

110. Narayanan, C. S., J. Fujimoto, R. E. Geras, and M. C. Gershengorn. Regulation by thyrotropin-releasing hormone (TRH) of TRH receptor mRNA degradation in rat pituitary GH3 cells. *J. Biol. Chem.* 267: 17296–17303, 1992.

111. Nieto, M., E. Kennedy, D. Goldstein, and J. H. Brown. Rapid heterologous desensitization of muscarinic and thrombin receptor-mediated phospholipase D activation. *Mol. Pharmacol.* 46: 406–413, 1994.

112. Nussenzveig, D. R., M. Heinflink, and M. C. Gershengorn. Agonist-stimulated internalization of the thyrotropin-releasing hormone receptor is dependent on two domains in the receptor carboxyl terminus. *J. Biol. Chem.* 268: 2389–2392, 1993.

113. Nussenzveig, D. R., M. Heinflink, and M. C. Gershengorn. Decreased levels of internalized thyrotropin-releasing hormone receptors after uncoupling from guanine nucleotide-binding protein and phospholipase-C. *Mol. Endocrinol.* 7: 1105–1111, 1993.

114. O'Dowd, B. F., M. Hnatowich, M. G. Caron, R. J. Lefkowitz, and M. Bouvier. Palmitoylation of the human B$_2$-adrenergic receptor. *J. Biol. Chem.* 264: 7564–7569, 1989.

115. Ohno, S., Y. Konno, Y. Akita, A. Yano, and K. Suzuki. A point mutation at the putative ATP-binding site of protein kinase C alpha abolishes the kinase activity and renders it down-regulation-insensitive. A molecular link between autophosphorylation and down-regulation. *J. Biol. Chem.* 265: 6296–6300, 1990.

116. Olofsson, J. I., C. C. Conti, and P. C. Leung. Homologous and heterologous regulation of gonadotropin-releasing hormone receptor gene expression in preovulatory rat granulosa cells. *Endocrinology* 136: 974–980, 1995.

117. Oron, Y., R. E. Straub, P. Traktman, and M. C. Gershengorn. Decreased TRH receptor mRNA activity precedes homologous downregulation: assay in oocytes. *Science* 238: 1406–1408, 1987.

118. Padmanabhan, V., A. Dalkin, M. Yasin, D. J. Haisenleder, J. C. Marshall, and T. D. Landefeld. Are immediate early genes involved ion gonadotropin-releasing hormone receptor gene regulation? Characterization of changes in GnRH receptor (GnRH-R), c-fos and c-jun messenger ribonucleic acids during the ovine estrous cycle. *Biol. Reprod.* 53: 263–269, 1995.

119. Palade, G. E. A small particulate component of the cytoplasm. *J. Biophys. Biochem. Cytol.* 1:59–68, 1955.

120. Pearse, B. M. and M. S. Robinson. Clathrin, adaptors, and sorting. *Annu. Rev. Cell Biol.* 6: 151–171, 1990.

121. Pelletier, G., D. Dube, J. Guy, C. Seguin, and F. A. Lefebvre. Binding and internalization of a luteinizing hormone-releasing hormone agonist by rat gonadotrophic cells. A radioautographic study. *Endocrinology* 111: 1068–1076, 1982.

122. Perrone, M. H. and P. M. Hinkle. Regulation of pituitary receptors for thyrotropin-releasing hormone by thyroid hormones. *J. Biol. Chem.* 253: 5168–5173, 1978.

123. Petrou, C. P., and A. Tashjian, Jr. Evidence that the thyrotropin-releasing hormone receptor and its ligand are recycled dissociated from each other. *Biochem. J.* 306: 107–113, 1995.

124. Pippig, S., S. Andexinger, and M. J. Lohse. Sequestration and recycling of beta 2–adrenergic receptors permit receptor resensitization. *Mol. Pharmacol.* 47: 666–676, 1995.

125. Port, J. D., L. Y. Huang, and C. C. Malbon. Beta-adrenergic agonists that down-regulate receptor mRNA up-regulate a M(r) 35,000 protein(s) that selectively binds to beta-adrenergic receptor mRNAs. *J. Biol. Chem.* 267: 24103–24108, 1992.

126. Probst, W. C., L. A. Snyder, D. I. Schuster, J. Brosius, and S. C. Sealfon. Sequence alignment of the G-protein coupled receptor superfamily. *DNA Cell Biol.* 11: 1–20, 1992.

127. Prossnitz, E. R., C. M. Kim, J. L. Benovic, and R. D. Ye. Phosphorylation of the N-formyl peptide receptor carboxyl terminus by the G protein-coupled receptor kinase, GRK2. *J. Biol. Chem.* 270: 1130–1137, 1995.

128. Rands, E., M. R. Candelore, A. H. Cheung, W. S. Hill, C. D. Strader, and R. A. F. Dixon. Mutational analysis of β-

adrenergic receptor glycosylation. *J. Biol. Chem.* 265: 10759–10764, 1990.

129. Rapiejko, P. J., D. C. Watkins, M. Ros, and C. C. Malbon. Thyroid hormones regulate G-protein beta-subunit mRNA expression in vivo. *J. Biol. Chem.* 264: 16183–16189, 1989.

130. Rodriguez, M. C., Y. Xie, H. Wang, K. Collison, and D. L. Segaloff. Effects of truncations of the cytoplasmic tail of the luteinizing hormone/chorionic gonadotropin receptor on receptor-mediated hormone internalization. *Mol. Endocrinol.* 6: 327–336, 1992.

131. Roettger, B., F., R. U. Rentsch, E. M. Hadac, E. H. Hellen, T. P. Burghardt, and L. J. Miller. Insulation of a G protein-coupled receptor on the plasmalemmal surface of the pancreatic acinar cell. *J. Cell Biol.* 130: 579–590, 1995.

132. Roettger, Cerrab B. F., R. U. Rentsch, D. Pinon, E. Holicky, E. Hadac, J. M. Larkin, and L. J. Miller. Dual pathways of internalization of the cholecystokinin receptor. *J. Cell Biol.* 128: 1029–1041, 1995.

133. Roth, T. E., and K. R. Porter. Yolk protein uptake in the oocyte of the mosquito Aedes aegypti L. *J. Cell Biol.* 20: 313–330, 1964.

134. Rothberg, K. G., J. E. Heuser, W. C. Donzell, W. S. Ying, J. R. Glenney, and R. G. W. Anderson. Caveolin, a protein component of caveolae membrane coats. *Cell* 68: 673–682, 1992.

135. Russo, D., G. D. Chazenbalk, Y. Nagayama, H. L. Wadsworth, and B. Rapoport. Site-directed mutagenesis of the human thyrotropin receptor: Role of asparagine-linked oligosaccharides in the expression of a functional receptor. *Mol. Endocrinol.* 5: 29–33, 1991.

136. Salzman, N. H., and F. R. Maxfield. Intracellular fusion of sequentially formed endocytic compartments. *J. Cell Biol.* 106: 1083–1091, 1988.

137. Scarborough, R. M., M. A. Naughton, W. Teng, D. T. Hung, J. Rose, T. K. Vu, V. I. Wheaton, C. W. Turck, and S. R. Coughlin. Tethered ligand agonist peptides. Structural requirements for thrombin receptor activation reveal mechanism of proteolytic unmasking of agonist function. *J. Biol. Chem.* 267: 13146–13149, 1992.

138. Schvartz, I., and E. Hazum. Internalization and recycling of receptor-bound gonadotropin-releasing hormone agonist in pituitary gonadotropes. *J. Biol. Chem.* 262: 17046–17050, 1987.

139. Sealfon, S. C., L. Chi, B. J. Ebersole, V. Rodic, D. Zhang, J. A. Ballesteros, and H. Weinstein. Related contribution of specific helix 2 and 7 residues to conformational activation of the serotonin 5–HT$_{2A}$ receptor. *J. Biol. Chem.* 270: 16683–16688, 1995.

140. Sealfon, S. C., S. C. Laws, J. C. Wu, B. Gillo, and W. L. Miller. Hormonal regulation of gonadotropin-releasing hormone receptors and messenger RNA activity in ovine pituitary culture. *Mol. Endocrinol.* 4: 1980–1987, 1990.

141. Sealfon, S. C., and R. P. Millar. The gonadotropin-releasing hormone receptor: structural determinants and regulatory control. In: *Oxford Reviews of Reproductive Biology*, edited by H. M. Charlton. ed. Oxford, England: Oxford University Press, 1994, p. 255–283.

142. Segaloff, D. L., and M. Ascoli. The lutropin/choriogonadotropin receptor . . . 4 years later. *Endocr. Rev.* 14: 324–347, 1993.

143. Servant, M., G. Guillemette, and J. Morisset. Pancreatic acinar-cell desensitization alters InsP3 production and Ca2 + mobilization under conditions where InsP3 receptor remains intact. *Biochem. J.* 305: 103–110, 1995.

144. Shah, B. H., and G. Milligan. Activation of the gonadotrophin

releasing hormone receptor of alpha T3 cells results in downregulation of the alpha subunits of both Gq/G11. *Biochem. Soc. Trans.* 21: 4995, 1993.

145. Shah, B. H., and G. Milligan. The gonadotrophin-releasing hormone receptor of alphaT3-1 pituitary cells regulates cellular levels of both of the phosphoinositidase C-linked G proteins, Gqalpha and G11alpha, equally. *Mol. Pharmacol.* 46: 1–7, 1994.

146. Shraga-Levine, Z., D. Ben-Menahem, and Z. Naor. Activation of protein kinase C beta gene expression by gonadotropin-releasing hormone in alpha T3–1 cell line. Role of Ca^{2+} and autoregulation by protein kinase C. *J. Biol. Chem.* 269: 31028–31033, 1994.

147. Slice, L. W., H. C. Wong, C. Sternini, E. F. Grady, N. W. Bunnett, and J. H. Walsh. The conserved NPXnY motif present in the gastrin-releasing peptide receptor is not a general sequestration sequence. *J. Biol. Chem.* 269: 21755–21761, 1994.

148. Smith, M. S. Effects of the intensity of the suckling stimulus and ovariasn steriods on pituitary gonadotropin-releasing hormone receptors during lactation. *Biol. Reprod.* 31: 548–555, 1984.

149. Smith, M. S., and L.-R. Lee. Modulation of pituitary gonadotropin-releasing hormone receptors during lactation in the rat. *Endocrinology* 124: 1456–1461, 1989.

150. Smith, M. S., and J. Reinhart. Changes in pituitary gonadotropin-releasing hormone receptor messenger ribonucleic acid content during lactation and after pup removal. *Endocrinology* 133: 2080–2084, 1993.

151. Sorokin, A., M. Mohammadi, J. Huang, and J. Schlessinger. Internalization of fibroblast growth factor receptor is inhibited by a point mutation at tyrosine 766. *J. Biol. Chem.* 269: 17056–17061, 1994.

152. Stojilkovic, S. S., J. Reinhart, and K. J. Catt. Gonadotropin-releasing hormone receptors: structure and signal transduction pathways. *Endocr. Rev.* 15: 462–499, 1994.

153. Stoorvogel, W., H. J. Geuze, J. M. Griffith, and G. J. Strous. The pathways of endocytosed transferrin and secretory protein are connected in the trans-Golgi reticulum. *J. Cell Biol.* 106: 1821–1829, 1988.

154. Strassheim, D., and C. C. Malbon. Phosphorylation of Gi alpha 2 attenuates inhibitory adenylyl cyclase in neuroblastoma/glioma hybrid (NG-108–15) cells. *J. Biol. Chem.* 269: 14307–14313, 1994.

155. Straub, R. E., G. C. Frech, R. H. Joho, and M. C. Gershengorn. Expression cloning of a cDNA encoding the mouse pituitary thyrotropin-releasing hormone receptor. *Proc. Natl. Acad. Sci. USA* 87: 9514–9518, 1990.

156. Tholanikunnel, B. G., J. G. Granneman, and C. C. Malbon. The Mr 35,000 β-adrenergic receptor mRNA-binding protein binds transcripts of G-protein linked receptors which undergo agonist-induced destabilization. *J. Biol. Chem.* 270: 12787–12793, 1995.

157. Thomas, R. F., B. D. Holt, D. A. Schwinn, and S. B. Liggett. Long-term agonist exposure induces upregulation of beta 3–adrenergic receptor expression via multiple cAMP response elements. *Proc. Natl. Acad. Sci. USA* 89: 4490–4494, 1992.

158. Thomas, W. G., T. J. Thekkumkara, T. J. Motel, and K. M. Baker. Stable expression of a truncated AT1A receptor in CHO-K1 cells. The carboxyl-terminal region directs agonist-induced internalization but not receptor signaling or desensitization. *J. Biol. Chem.* 270: 207–213, 1995.

159. Tran, D., J. L. Carpentier, F. Sawano, P. Gorden, and L. Orci. Ligands internalized through coated or noncoated invaginations follow a common intracellular pathway. *Proc. Natl. Acad. Sci. USA* 84: 7957–7961, 1987.

160. Trowbridge, I. S., and J. F. Collawn. Structural requirements for high efficiency endocytosis of the human transferrin receptor. *J. Inorg. Biochem.* 47: 209–217, 1992.

161. Trowbridge, I. S., and J. F. Collawn. Signal-dependent membrane protein trafficking in the endocytic pathway. *Annu. Rev. Cell Biol.* 9: 129–161, 1993.

162. Tseng, M. J., S. Coon, E. Stuenkel, V. Struk, and C. D. Logsdon. Influence of second and third cytoplasmic loops on binding, internalizatio n, and coupling of chimeric bombesin/m3 muscarinic receptors. *J. Biol. Chem.* 270: 17884–17891, 1995.

163. Tseng, M. J., K. Detjen, V. Struk, and C. D. Logsdon. Carboxyl-terminal domains determine internalization and recycling characteristics of bombesin receptor chimeras. *J. Biol. Chem.* 270: 18858–18864, 1995.

164. Tsutsumi, M., S. C. Laws, V. Rodic, and S. C. Sealfon. Translational regulation of the gonadotropin-releasing hormone receptor in alpha T3–1 cells. *Endocrinology* 136: 1128–1136, 1995.

165. Tsutsumi, M., S. C. Laws, and S. C. Sealfon. Homologous up-regulation of the gonadotropin-releasing hormone receptor in alpha T3–1 cells is associated with unchanged receptor messenger RNA (mRNA) levels and altered mRNA activity. *Mol. Endocrinol.* 7: 1625–1633, 1993.

166. Tsutsumi, M., W. Zhou, R. P. Millar, P. L. Mellon, J. L. Roberts, C. A. Flanagan, K. Dong, B. Gillo, and S. C. Sealfon. Cloning and functional expression of a mouse gonadotropin-releasing hormone receptor. *Mol. Endocrinol.* 6: 1163–1169, 1992.

167. Turgeon, J. L., Y. Kimura, D. W. Waring, and P. L. Mellon. Steroid and pulsatile gonadotropin-releasing hormone (GnRH) regulation of luteinizing hormone and GnRH receptor ina novel gonadotrope cell line. *Mol. Endocrinol.* 10: 439–450, 1996.

168. Turzillo, A. M., C. E. Campion, C. M. Clay, and T. M. Nett. Regulation of gonadotropin-releasing hormone (GnRH) receptor messenger ribonucleic acid and GnRH receptors during the early preovulatory period in the ewe. *Endocrinology* 135: 1353–1358, 1994.

169. Turzillo, A. M., J. L. Juengel, and T. M. Nett. Pulsatile gonadotropin-releasing hormone (GnRH) increases concentrations of GnRH receptor messenger ribonucleic acid and numbers of GnRH receptors during luteolysis in the ewe. *Biol. Repro.* 53: 418–423, 1995.

170. van Koppen, C. J. and N. M. Nathanson. Site-directed mutagenesis of the m2 muscarinic acetylcholine receptor. Analysis of the role of N-glycosylation in receptor expression and function. *J. Biol. Chem.* 265: 20887–20892, 1990.

171. Vanetti, M., G. Vogt, and V. Hollt. The two isoforms of the mouse somatostatin receptor (mSSTR2A and mSSTR2B) differ in coupling efficiency to adenylate cyclase and in agonist-induced receptor desensitization. *FEBS Lett.* 331: 260–266, 1993.

172. Vu, T. K., D. T. Hung, V. I. Wheaton, and S. R. Coughlin. Molecular cloning of a functional thrombin receptor reveals a novel proteolytic mechanism of receptor activation. *Cell* 64: 1057–1068, 1991.

173. Vu, T. K., V. I. Wheaton, D. T. Hung, I. Charo, and S. R. Coughlin. Domains specifying thrombin-receptor interaction. *Nature* 353: 674–677, 1991.

174. Wiley, H. S. Anomalous binding of epidermal growth factor to A431 cells is due to the effect of high receptor densities and a saturable endocytic system. *J. Cell Biol.* 107: 801–810, 1988.

175. Willars, G. B. and S. R. Nahorski. Heterologous desensitization of both phosphoinositide and Ca^{2+} signaling in SH-SY5Y neuroblastoma cells: a role for intracellular Ca^{2+} store depletion? *Mol. Pharmacol.* 47: 509–516, 1995.

176. Willems, P. H., B. A. Van den Broek, C. H. Van Os, and J. J. De Pont. Inhibition of inositol 1,4,5-trisphosphate-induced Ca^{2+} release in permeabilized pancreatic acinar cells by hormonal and phorbol ester pretreatment. *J. Biol. Chem.* 264: 9762–9767, 1989.

177. Windle, J. J., R. I. Weiner, and P. L. Mellon. Cell lines of the pituitary gonadotrope lineage derived by targeted oncogenesis in transgenic mice. *Mol. Endocrinol.* 4: 597–603, 1990.

178. Wojcikiewicz, R. J. Type I, II, and III inositol 1,4,5-trisphosphate receptors are unequally susceptible to down-regulation and are expressed in markedly different proportions in different cell types. *J. Biol. Chem.* 270: 11678–11683, 1995.

179. Wojcikiewicz, R. J., T. Furuichi, S. Nakade, K. Mikoshiba, and S. R. Nahorski. Muscarinic receptor activation down-regulates the type I inositol 1,4,5-trisphosphate receptor by accelerating its degradation. *J. Biol. Chem.* 269: 7963–7969, 1994.

180. Wojcikiewicz, R. J., and S. R. Nahorski. Chronic muscarinic stimulation of SH-SY5Y neuroblastoma cells suppresses inositol 1,4,5-trisphosphate action. Parallel inhibition of inositol 1,4,5-trisphosphate-induced Ca^{2+} mobilization and inositol 1,4,5-trisphosphate binding. *J. Biol. Chem.* 266: 22234–22241, 1991.

181. Woolkalis, M. J., M. T. De, Jr., N. Blanchard, J. A. Hoxie, and L. F. Brass. Regulation of thrombin receptors on human umbilical vein endothelial cells. *J. Biol. Chem.* 270: 9868–9875, 1995.

182. Wu, J. C., S. C. Sealfon, and W. L. Miller. Gonadal hormones and gonadotropin-releasing hormone (GnRH) alter messenger ribonucleic acid levels for GnRH receptors in sheep. *Endocrinology* 134: 1846–1850, 1994.

183. Wynn, P. C., C. A. Suarez-Quian, G. V. Childs, and K. J. Catt. Pituitary Binding and internalization of radioiodinated gonadotropin-releasing hormone agoinst and antagoinst ligands *in vitro* and *in vivo*. *Endocrinology* 119: 1852–1863, 1986.

184. Yamada, M., M. Yamada, and E. Richelson. Further characterization of neurotensin receptor desensitization and down-regulation in clone N1E-115 neuroblastoma cells. *Biochem. Pharmacol.* 45: 2149–2154, 1993.

185. Yang, J. and A. Tashjian, Jr. Regulation of endogenous thyrotropin-releasing hormone (TRH) receptor messenger RNA by TRH in GH4C1 cells. *Mol. Endocrinol.* 7: 753–758, 1993.

186. Yang, J., and A. Tashjian, Jr. Regulation of endogenous thyrotropin-releasing hormone receptor messenger RNA in GH4C1 cells: roles of protein and RNA synthesis. *Mol. Endocrinol.* 7: 1144–1150, 1993.

187. Yu, S. S., R. J. Lefkowitz, and W. P. Hausdorff. Beta-adrenergic receptor sequestration. A potential mechanism of receptor resensitization. *J. Biol. Chem.* 268: 337–341, 1993.

188. Zhou, W., C. Flanagan, J. A. Ballesteros, K. Konvicka, J. S. Davidson, H. Weinstein, R.P. Millar, and S.C. Sealfon. A reciprocal mutation supports helix 2 and helix 7 proximity in the gonadotropin-releasing hormone receptor. *Mol. Pharmacol.* 45: 165–170, 1994.

3. Receptor-mediated endocytosis of polypeptide hormones by vascular endothelium

NGOZI E. ERONDU
ROBERT S. BAR

Veterans Administration Medical Center, Department of Internal Medicine, Diabetes and Endocrinology Research Center, The University of Iowa, Iowa City, Iowa

CHAPTER CONTENTS

THE VASCULAR ENDOTHELIUM, in vivo, occupies a critical anatomical and physiological position as the initial fixed surface with which the circulation comes in contact. The endothelial cells, which form the single cell intimal lining of the vasculature, have several critical functions, including the regulation of the transport of hormones across the vessel wall to the tissue site(s) of action (67). The egress of polypeptide hormones from the circulation to subendothelial tissues occurs primarily through capillaries. To accomplish this function while presumably allowing tissue specificity of transendothelial transport, the microcirculation manifests several types of interendothelial cell junctions that have been classified as continuous, fenestrated, or discontinuous; within each type of junction, there are differences involving the occurrence, type, and frequency of basic cellular components such as vesicles, channels, and surface receptors (55).

Both physiological and morphological approaches have been used to study the mechanisms that mediate the transendothelial passage of proteins. Perfusion experiments have led to the "pore" model (46, 47), which predicts the existence of two populations of pores with diameters ~4–8 nm and ~36–100 nm, the latter constituting the pathway for the transport of macromolecules having the size of most proteins. In spite of a large number of morphological studies, no cellular structures corresponding to these pores has been identified with certainty. However, electron microscopic studies have revealed a number of subcellular structures potentially involved in endothelial transcytosis (movement of substances from luminal to abluminal surface of the cell) (54). As shown in Figure 3.1, these include intercellular junctions, fenestrae, plasmalemmal vesicles and transendothelial channels. The "tightness" of endothelial junctions vary from tissue to tissue and, in general, have low permeability under normal physiological conditions (54). During inflammation, numerous small gaps have been noted in certain junctions leading to increased permeability (15, 26, 39, 49, 54, 66). Fenestrae are large gaps between endothelial cells in the capillaries of some organs such as the kidney, choroid plexus, endocrine glands, and the ciliary bodies (54). They may be diaphragmed (closed) or nondiaphragmed (open) and their large size a priori would be expected to permit easy and unregulated access to the movement of macromolecules. However, the luminal aspect of the fenestral diaphragm is highly negatively charged, being rich in heparan sulfate, thereby limiting passage of proteins which are also anionic (54). Plasmalemmal vesicles are small membrane-bound vesicles (~70 nM in diameter) that have been proposed to mediate the fluid phase transport of macromolecules by shuttling between the luminal and abluminal surfaces of endothelial cells (55). Transendothelial channels are postulated to be produced by the fusion of several plasmalemmal vesicles (56). However, they occur so rarely that their role in transendothelial transport is thought to be quite limited (54, 18). The uptake and transport of a given macromolecule across the endothelium are influenced by *(1)* its net charge, size, and shape, *(2)* the size and net charge of the endothelial structures involved in transport, and *(3)* the prevailing hemodynamic forces, such as hydrostatic or oncotic pressure (54). The transport pathways described above depend mostly on diffusion mechanisms, are therefore only effective for macromolecules present at high concentrations in the circulation, and are likely to be less

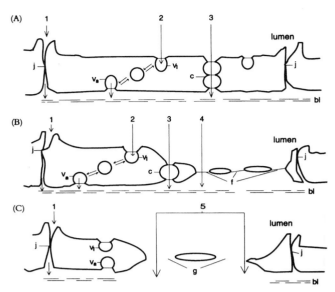

FIG. 3.1. Schematic representation of the three basic types of blood capillaries. Organelles and routes involved in the non-specific (bulk-phase) transport of plasma proteins *(A)*, continuous capillary; *(B)*, fenestrated capillary; *(C)*, discontinuous capillary (sinusoid). *(1)* transport via endothelial junctions (j) effective in inflammatory conditions); *(2)* vesicular transport (the main transport mechanism in continuous and fenestrated capillary endothelia); *(3)* transport via transendothelial channels (c) (minor contribution to the transport due to their scarcity); *(4)* transport through the diaphragmed fenestrae (f) (minor contribution to plasma protein transport due to their negative charge); *(5)* diffusion through the endothelial gaps (g) (effective and efficient transport but only in sinusoids). bl, basal lamina; v_a, abluminal plasmalemmal vesicle; v_l, luminal plasmalemmal vesicle. [Reproduced with permission from (27).]

effective for polypeptide hormones that circulate in a lower concentration.

It has been demonstrated that endothelial cells possess specific binding sites (receptors) on their surface for a number of macromolecules including hormones (21, 22, 30–32, 58, 63, 64). Available data indicate that these binding sites play an important role in the passage of these macromolecules into and across the vascular endothelium (54). We will use studies on the endothelial transport of insulin, insulin-like growth factors (IGF-I and IGF-II), gonadotropins, and glucagon to review available data on the structures and mechanisms involved in the receptor-mediated endocytosis and transcytosis of protein hormones by the vascular endothelium.

INSULIN

Several laboratories have demonstrated the presence of insulin receptors on endothelial cells (4, 24, 37, 45, 62). Unlike most target cells for insulin action where

receptor-bound insulin is slowly degraded after internalization, cultured endothelial cells were shown to rapidly transfer receptor-bound insulin to an intracellular compartment from which the hormone is quickly released extracellularly in an intact, biologically active form (21, 22, 33). Mono A_{14}–[^{125}I]-iodoinsulin was incubated with cultured endothelial cells. Unbound insulin removed by rapid washing and the processing of cell-bound insulin was evaluated by examining the nature of the radioactivity released into the media by trichloroacetic acid (TCA) precipitation, gel filtration, and high performance liquid chromatography. As shown in Figure 3.2 for bovine pulmonary artery endothelial cells, approximately 95% of cell-bound insulin was dissociated from the cells in less than 15 min and greater than 80% of this insulin was biologically intact. Similar results have been reported from cultured endothelial cells derived from bovine aorta, bovine microvessels, rat epididymal endothelium, and human umbilical vein (10, 12, 29). For these experimental observations to have physiological relevance, it had to be shown that endothelial cells in vitro and in vivo possess the appropriate vectorial polarity such that insulin is internalized via receptor-mediated endocytosis on the luminal surface and released in an intact form on the abluminal surface from where it will reach the target tissue.

In 1985, King's laboratory directly measured [^{125}I]-labeled insulin transport through the use of dual chambers separated by a monolayer of cultured bovine aortic endothelial cells (37). This study demonstrated that the transendothelial transport of insulin was both saturable and temperature sensitive. More importantly, transport of ^{125}I-insulin was inhibited by unlabeled insulin and by antibodies to the insulin receptor in direct proportion to the ability of these substances to inhibit insulin binding to its receptor. Unrelated polypeptides, such as nerve growth factor, did not inhibit the transport of insulin or the binding of labeled insulin by the endothelial cells. Nonreceptor-mediated transport was estimated to be 10%–30% using [^{14}C]-labeled inulin which was remarkably similar to the proportion of [^{125}I]insulin transported in the presence of excess unlabeled insulin. Subsequently, this group used this nucleopore-filter monolayer model to show that leupeptin, a lysosomal protease inhibitor, had no effect on the transport or release of [^{125}I]insulin (2). However, monensin, a proton ionophore, decreased both the release and transport of [^{125}I]insulin in capillary and aortic endothelial cells, suggesting that the receptor mediated transport of insulin involves a compartment that requires acidification for its function (2).

We have utilized the isolated, perfused, beating rat

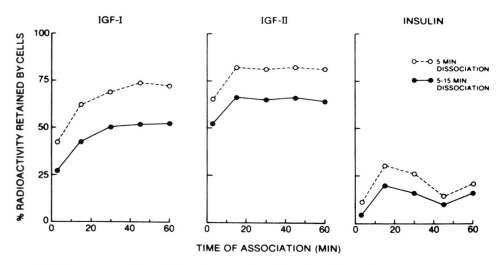

FIG. 3.2. Time course of dissociation of receptor-bound insulin and IGFs from cultured endothelial cells. [Reproduced with permission from (7).]

heart (Langendorff preparation) as a model system to study the transport of insulin across the continuous capillary endothelium to cardiac muscle (4, 6). The perfused vascular system in this preparation is composed of over 99% microvascular endothelium, with occluding or tight intercellular junctions (17). In these experiments, the beating hearts were perfused with [^{125}I]insulin followed by perfusion with unlabeled insulin, proinsulin, or other unrelated peptides such as glucagon, albumin and adrenocorticotrophic hormone. As illustrated in Figure 3.3, unlabeled insulin displaced

the bound [^{125}I] insulin in a concentration dependent fashion. On the other hand, proinsulin was only ~1% as potent as unlabeled insulin, consistent with the known insulin receptor reactivity and bioactivity of proinsulin. Unrelated peptides had no effect. Autoradiographic analysis of ^{125}I silver grains over blood vessels, which were shown to represent intact insulin, confirmed the specificity of the insulin binding to endothelial cells. Co-perfusion of [^{125}I]insulin with unlabeled insulin caused a dose-dependent decrease in the number of silver grains over capillaries and over cardiac muscle (Fig. 3.4). When this experiment was repeated using ^{125}I-desoctapeptide (DOP) insulin, an insulin analog with little affinity for insulin receptors, there was no effect of unlabeled insulin on ^{125}I-DOP insulin binding to the capillaries or its appearance over

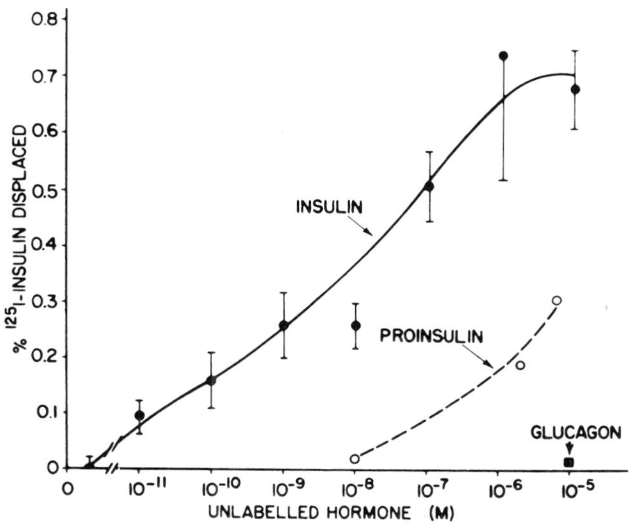

FIG. 3.3. Displacement of [^{125}I]insulin, pro-insulin, and glucagon in the perfused heart. [Reproduced with permission from (9).]

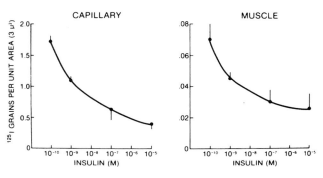

FIG. 3.4. ^{125}I grains over capillary endothelium *(left)* and cardiac muscle *(right)* in intact hearts perfused with [^{125}I]insulin alone or [^{125}I]insulin and varying concentrations of unlabeled insulin. [Reproduced with permission from (6).]

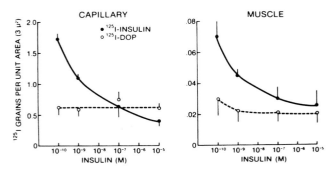

FIG. 3.5. Localization of ^{125}I grains in intact hearts perfused with either [^{125}I]insulin or [^{125}I]desoctapeptide (DOP) insulin alone or coperfused with varying concentrations of unlabeled insulin. [Reproduced with permission from (6).]

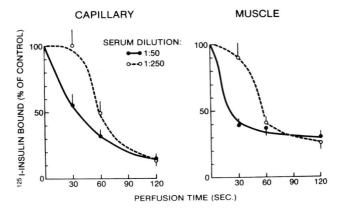

FIG. 3.7. Effect of anti-insulin receptor antibody, perfused at two dilutions (1:50 and 1:250) on the subsequent appearance of [^{125}I]insulin in capillary endothelium and cardiac muscle. [Reproduced with permission from (6).]

cardiac muscle (Fig. 3.5). Further support for the role of the insulin receptor in the transendothelial transport of insulin in this model system was obtained in experiments using trypsin and anti-insulin receptor antibodies. These studies showed a decreased appearance of perfused [^{125}I]insulin in cardiac muscle that was proportional to the degree of receptor loss by trypsin or receptor occupancy by antireceptor antibody. The proportionality of receptor loss/blockade to subsequent appearance of insulin in cardiac muscle suggested that insulin binding to capillary insulin receptors was not only important, but may be rate-limiting in the transport of insulin from the circulation to cardiac muscle (Figs. 3.6 and 3.7). These findings are consistent with an important role of the insulin receptor in the passage of the hormone across the vascular endothelium.

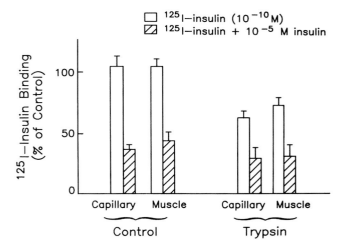

FIG. 3.6. Effect of trypsin treatment on subsequent appearance of [^{125}I]insulin in capillary endothelium and cardiac muscle. [Reproduced with permission from (6).]

The interaction of insulin with endothelial cells has also been investigated morphologically. Some groups have reported that [^{125}I]insulin is endocytosed by coated vesicles and pits (14, 44) while others have suggested the involvement of non-coated pits and vesicles (57, 59). Recent studies have, however, implicated both pathways in the receptor-mediated transport of insulin by the vascular endothelium. Roberts and Sandra (48) applied the techniques of freeze-fracture gold immunochemistry and pre-embedding indirect immunocytochemistry to investigate insulin uptake by endothelial cells cultured from the bovine pulmonary artery. Both techniques yielded similar results demonstrating that both coated and non-coated vesicles are involved in insulin transport by these cells, with the latter accounting for about 70% of the insulin that was endocytosed. Stitt et al. (61), used transmission electron microscopic studies of cultured bovine retinal vascular endothelial cells (RVECs) to investigate the intracellular trafficking of insulin conjugated to gold particles. They showed that the first step is the binding of insulin to its receptor as demonstrated by the ability of preincubation with antiinsulin receptor antibody or excess unconjugated insulin to significantly inhibit (up to 89%) the binding of the insulin–gold conjugate to the endothelial surface. Subsequently, the receptor-bound insulin was internalized mostly in clathrin-coated pits and vesicles, finally localizing in uncoated cytoplasmic vesicles corresponding to early and late endosomes or multivesicular bodies. However, there was evidence for the transcytosis of a small, but significant (23%), proportion of the gold–insulin conjugate. It is not clear whether these morphological studies can be extrapolated to the in vivo situation vis a vis the relative contributions of coated vs. non-coated vesicles in the receptor-mediated transport of insulin by the vasculature. For one, endothelial cells may undergo phenotypic alteration when placed in culture, for example, in the density of non-coated vesicles in cultured endothelial cells vs. in situ endothelium (52). Secondly, the number, type, and distribution of these vesicles can be affected by artifacts such as those caused by tissue/cell preparation and fixation (52). However, the fact that insulin can be endocytosed by both clathrin-coated and non-coated vesicular pathways in the endothelium has important consequences. The clathrin pathway usually involves endocytosis into lysosomes and is thus degradative, while caveolae (noncoated vesicles) have been postulated to mediate transcytosis (55). Thus, it makes at least teleological sense that endothelial cells which internalize insulin not only for degradation but transcytosis should utilize both pathways. It is therefore, interesting that filipin, a sterol-binding agent which preferentially disassembles caveolae, inhibited the transcytosis of insulin by bovine lung microvascular cells without diminishing insulin degradation (50).

It should be noted that the receptor-mediated transendothelial transport of insulin is not universally accepted. Knutson and colleagues were unable to demonstrate receptor mediated transport of insulin across a monolayer derived from bovine aortic endothelial cells (41), despite the similarity of this model system to that successfully used by the King group (37). Recently, Steil et al. (60) performed euglycemic glucose clamps on anesthetized dogs in which both physiological and pharmacological doses of insulin were infused. They demonstrated that insulin transport into muscle interstitial fluid increased 41% with pharmacological change in insulin concentration. They concluded from these results that insulin transport is not saturable in vivo and is therefore not receptor mediated. However, this study is confounded by at least two factors: (1) the observed increase in diffusionary capacity with pharmacological doses of insulin, presumably a result of capillary dilation and/or recruitment, and (2) the insulin receptor down regulation that should occur under these conditions (19, 40). Interestingly, this group has also published data using a similar in vivo model which showed that insulin transport across the capillary endothelium of the brain is saturable and therefore is suggested to be receptor mediated (51).

INSULIN-LIKE GROWTH FACTORS

The insulin-like growth factors, IGF-I and II, are peptides of approximately 7500 daltons that possess both mitogenic and insulin-like activity in a wide variety of cell types (1, 13, 35, 53). Unlike insulin, the IGFs normally circulate in blood in association with six distinct IGF-binding proteins (IGFBPs). The possible role of the IGFPBs in the transendothelial transport of the IGFs will be discussed below.

Data from a number of laboratories have shown that both micro-and macrovascular endothelial cells express IGF receptors (2–5, 7, 12, 25, 28). These studies demonstrated that in cultured endothelial cells, the processing of IGFs differed from that of insulin. For example, about 20%–30% of cell bound ^{125}I-IGF was rapidly released from cultured endothelial cells vs. 50%–70% of internalized insulin that was released over the same time period (Fig. 3.2). Analysis of this released material by TCA precipitation, gel filtration, and high-performance liquid chromatography (HPLC) showed it to be intact IGF-I and IGF-II. However, in the IGF studies, following 10 more min of dissociation, an additional 20% of the ^{125}I was released from the cells, of which 70% represented intact IGF-I and only 30% was intact IFG-II. Similar results were obtained by King and colleagues and this led to the conclusion that the predominant pathway for IGF-I processing (as is the case with insulin) is nondegradative while IGF-II is channeled to a greater extent to the degradative (lysosomal) pathway (25, 28). It is pertinent to note that transgenic and knock-out mouse experiments suggest that the IGF-II (cation-independent mannose-6-phosphate) receptor may function primarily as a degradative pathway to remove IGF-II from the extracellular environment (20, 23).

We have also examined the endothelial transport of IGFs using the perfused heart model (4, 5). Coperfusion of ^{125}I-IGF with increasing amounts of unlabeled IGF yielded progressively less ^{125}I-IGF that remained associated with both the capillary endothelial cells and cardiac muscle (Figs. 3.8 and 3.9). The specificity of this binding was shown in studies in which varying concentrations of unlabeled insulin was perfused. Insulin competed with IGF-I binding at a much lower affinity but did not compete for IGF-II binding. This result is consistent with the fact that insulin binds with low affinity to the IGF-I receptor but does not compete for binding to the IGF-II receptor (1, 13, 34).

Since endothelial cells produce IGFBPs (42, 68, 69), we have been interested in investigating their role, if any, in the transendothelial transport of IGFs. We showed that in the perfused rat heart IGFs can cross the capillary endothelium when attached to circulating IGFBPs (8). However, in the same model, the transcapillary transport of free IGF-I was greater than that of IGF-I cross linked to an IGFBP. We proposed a mechanism for endothelial transcytosis that takes into consideration the presence in the circulation of IGF–IGFBP complexes, most of which (80%) are in a 140 kDa

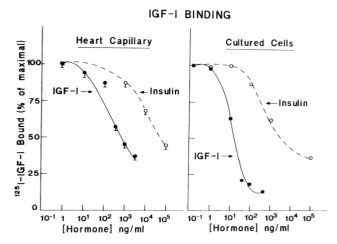

FIG. 3.8. IGF-I binding to capillary endothelium of the perfused heart *(left)*. For comparison, IGF-I binding to cultured microvessel endothelial cells is shown *(right)*. [Reproduced with permission from (4).]

complex, composed of IGF-I, an IGFBP-3, and an acid labile subunit that cannot cross the vascular endothelium and therefore prolongs the half-life of IGF in the circulation (1, 13, 34, 42). In this hypothetical scheme, dissociation of the IGFs from the IGFBPs will occur at the luminal surface of the endothelial cell, a process that may be enhanced by either the interaction of these IGF–IGFBP complexes with cell surface integrins or endothelial-surface IGFBP-3 proteases, such as plasmin or thrombin (16, 35, 38). The freed IGFs would then bind to their endothelial membrane receptors for IGF-I/II followed by internalization of the IGF-I/receptor complexes. Subsequently, the internalized IGFs would

associate with intracellular IGFBPs and finally be secreted from the abluminal endothelial cell surface into the interstitial space. There has not been any published morphological studies of endothelial IGF transport to date. Thus, whether subcellular structures such as coated pits/vesicles, caveolae, or multivesicular bodies are involved is presently not known.

HUMAN CHORIONIC GONADOTROPIN (hCG)

Ghinea et al. (26) used both biochemical and morphological approaches to determine the transendothelial route of hCG transport to its target tissue—Leydig cells in rat testis. They examined (by electron microscopy) arteriolar, capillary, and venular endothelial cells isolated from testes that were collected at various times following perfusion of the rats with hCG conjugated to gold particles. hCG first bound to specific receptors expressed on the luminal surface of the endothelial cells. This was followed by concentration of hCG in coated pits with transfer of hCG to the endosomal compartment via coated vesicles. Subsequently, the hormone-receptor complexes were transported to the abluminal side of the cell by means of smooth vesicles that apparently pinched off from tubular extensions of the endosomes. Finally, following insertion of these vesicles into the abluminal plasma membrane, the hormone was released into the subendothelial space. Presumably, recycling of the receptor occurred by its reinternalization on the endothelial abluminal surface by means of coated pits and vesicles. These results are summarized in Figure 3.10.

The authors used a number of experimental approaches to establish the specificity of the observed transendothelial transport of hCG. First, the transport of both radiolabeled [^{125}I]hCG and hCG–gold conjugate was saturable and temperature sensitive. Second, when BSA–gold particles without hCG were perfused, even at a 20-fold higher concentration than that used for hCG, only minimal uptake occurred, and that only by plasmalemmal vesicles rather than coated vesicles. Third, there was no uptake of hCG in coated pits and vesicles in nontarget organs such as the heart, lung, diaphragm, and epididymal fat.

A number of questions remain. Although there was co-localization of hCG–gold particles and LH/hCG receptor antibodies in the same vesicles, this does not constitute proof of direct involvement of the receptor in the transport phenomenon described. It would have been interesting to show that there was significant loss of hCG transcytosis in the presence of excess amounts of receptor-blocking antibody. Analogs of hCG that do not bind to the hCG receptor can also be powerful tools in such experiments. If the receptor is indeed

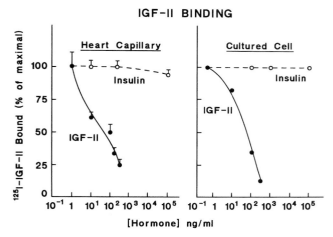

FIG. 3.9. IGF-II binding to capillary endothelium of the perfused heart *(left)* and to cultured microvessel endothelial cells *(right)*. [Reproduced with permission from (5).]

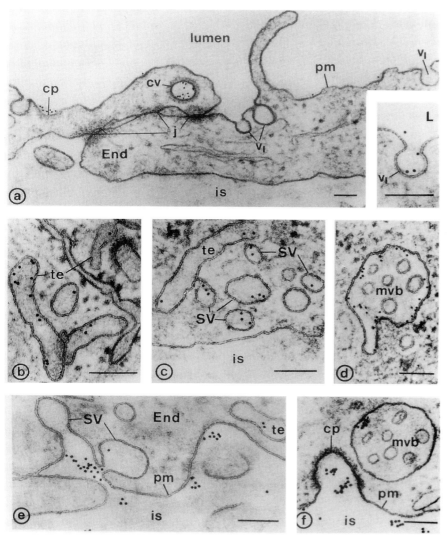

FIG. 3.10. Transcytosis of hCG-AU$_{5\ nm}$ through the endothelial cells of rat testicular capillaries. (a) After 5 min of perfusion with hCG-AU$_{5nm}$ the tracer marks the luminal plasma membrane (pm), the coated pits (cp), and the coated vesicles (cv), but fails to label the plasmalemmal vesicles (v$_1$) open to the capillary lumen and the endothelial junctions (j). (b–d) After 15 min of perfusion the gold-labeled hormone is detected in the tubular (te) and vesicular (ve) endosomes (b) and in large smooth vesicles (SV) located near the abluminal side of the endothelium (c). Some hormone is present in the multivesicular bodies (mvb) (d). (e, f) After 20 min of perfusion hCG-Au$_{5\ nm}$ is delivered into the interstitial space (is) via smooth vesicles (SV) (e). Some of the tracer is associated with the plasma membrane (pm) and the coated pits (cp) of the abluminal cell surface of the endothelium (f). (Inset) Control perfusion with BSA-AU$_{5nm}$. The gold-labeled albumin was perfused for 5 min at a concentration 20-fold higher than the concentration of hCG-AU$_{5\ nm}$ (A$_{540\ nm}^{1\ cm}$ = 2 and A$_{540\ nm}^{1\ cm}$ = 0.1 respectively). Some gold particles are present in the plasmalemmal vesicles (v$_1$) open to the capillary lumen (L). End, endothelial cell. Bar, 0.1 μm. [Reproduced with permission from (26).]

involved, the mechanism of the dissociation of the hormone receptor complex on the abluminal surface is yet to be determined. As speculated by the authors, possibilities include covalent modifications, such as phosphorylation of the receptor as well as possible differences in the intravesicular pH vs. the interstitial fluid that would induce a conformational change in the receptor molecule that causes release of the hormone from the hormone/receptor complex. To these possibilities one may add proteolysis of the receptor, as has been suggested in other models of transcytosis (43).

GLUCAGON

Unlike the protein hormones discussed above, the endothelial cells through which glucagon must traverse to reach its major site of action (the liver) are discontinuous. As already stated in the introduction, the gaps in discontinuous capillary endothelium in hepatic sinusoids, despite their large size, do not permit necessarily the free movement of proteins. Electron microscopic studies by Watanabe et al. (65) indicated that the transfer of glucagon–gold complexes across sinusoidal endothelial cells involved coated pits located on the luminal surface. These complexes were subsequently delivered into the subendothelial space via smooth vesicles. No diffusion of the conjugate was noted through either the gaps or the intercellular junctions. These workers also showed that the binding and transport of the glucagon–gold conjugate were inhibited in the presence of excess unlabeled glucagon. Although the presence of putative glucagon receptors on these endothelial cells was demonstrated by studies with [^{125}I]glucagon (65), the receptor-mediated transcytosis of glucagon in this system needs confirmation, at a minimum, by the use of antiglucagon receptor antibodies in immunocytochemical studies.

This work was supported by NIH grants DK25421 and DK25295, and by research funds from the Veterans Administration.

REFERENCES

1. Bach, L. A., and M. M. Rechler. Insulin-like growth factor binding proteins. *Diabetes Rev.* 3: 38–61, 1995.
2. Banskota, N. K., J.-L. Carpenter, and G. L. King. Processing and and release of insulin and insulin-like growth factor I by macro- and microvascular endothelail cells. *Endocrinology* 119: 1904–1913, 1986.
3. Bar, R. S., and M. Boes. Distinct receptors for IGF-I, IGF-II, and insulin are present on bovine capillary endothelial cells and large vessel endothelial cells. *Biochem. Biophys. Res. Commun.* 124: 203–209, 1984.
4. Bar, R. S., M. Boes, and A. Sandra. Receptors for insulin-like growth factor-I (IGF-I) in myocardial capillary endothelium of the intact perfused heart. *Biochem. Biophys. Res. Commun.* 133: 724–730, 1985.
5. Bar, R. S., M. Boes, and A. Sandra. IFG receptors in myocardial capillary endothelium: Potntial regulation of IGF-I transport to cardiac muscle. *Biochem. Biophys. Res. Commun.* 152: 93–98, 1988.
6. Bar, R. S., M. Boes, and A. Sandra. Vascular transport of insulin to rat cardiac muscle: Central role of the capillary endothelium. *J. Clin. Invest.* 81: 1225–1233, 1988.
7. Bar, R. S., M. Boes, and M. Yorek. Processing of insulin-like growth factors I and II by capillary and large vessel endothelial cells. *Endocrinology* 118: 1072–1080, 1986.
8. Bar, R. S., D. R. Clemmons, M. Boes, W. H. Busby, B. A. Booth, B. L. Dake, and A. Sandra. Transcapillary permeability and subendothelial distribution of endothelial and amniotic fluid insulin-like growth factor binding proteins in the rat heart. *Endocrinology* 127: 1078–1086, 1990.
9. Bar, R. S., A. DeRose, A. Sandra, M. L. Peacock, and W. G. Owen. Insulin binding to microvascular endothelium in intact heart: A kinetic and morphometric analysis. *Am. J. Physiol.* 244 (*Endocrinol. Metab.* 13): E447–E452, 1983.
10. Bar. R. S., S. Dolash, B. L. Dake, and M. Boes. Cultured capillary endothelial cells from bovine adipose tissue: A model for insulin binding and action in microvascular endothelium. *Metabolism* 35: 317–322, 1986.
11. Bar, R. S., J. C. Hoak, and M. L. Peacock. Insulin receptors in human endothelial cells: Identification and characterization. *J. Clin. Endocrinol. Metab.* 47: 699–702, 1978.
12. Bar, R. S., K. Siddle, S. Dolash, M. Boes, and B. Dake. Actions of insulin and insulin-like growth factors I and II in cultured capillary endothelial cells from bovine adipose tissue. *Metabolism* 37: 714–720, 1988.
13. Baxter, R. C., and J. L. Martin: Binding proteins for the insulin-like growth factors: Structure, regulation and function. *Prog. Growth Factor Res.* 1: 49, 1989.
14. Bergeron, J. J., R. Silkstrom, R. R. Hand, and B. I. Posner. Binding and uptake of [^{125}I] insulin into rat liver hepatocytes and endothelium. *J. Cell Biol.* 80: 427–443, 1979.
15. Bjork, J., K. E. Arfors, S. E. Dahlen, and P. Hedqvist. Effects of leukotrienes on vascular permeability and leukocyte adhesion. In: *The Inflammatory Process,* edited by P. Venge and A. Lindborn. Stockholm: Almqvist and Wiksell, 1981, p. 103–112.
16. Booth, B. A., M. Boes, and R. S. Bar. IGFBP-3 proteolysis by plasmin, thrombin, serum: Heparin binding, IGF binding and structure of fragments. *Am. J. Physiol.* 271 (*Endocrinol. Metab.* 34) E465–E470, 1996.
17. Bruns, R. R., and G. E. Palade. Studies in blood capillaries. *J. Cell. Biol.* 37: 244–276, 1968.
18. Bundgaard, M., J. Frokjaer-Jensen, and C. Crone. Endothelial plasmalemmal vesicular profiles as elements in a system of branching invaginations from the cell surface. *Proc. Natl. Acad. Sci. USA* 76: 6439–6442, 1979.
19. Carpenter, J.-L. Insulin receptor internalization: Molecular mechanisms and physiopathological implications. *Diabetologia* 37(Suppl 2): S117–S124, 1994.
20. DeChiara, T. M., A. Efstratiadis, and E. J. Robertson. A growth-deficiency phenotype in heterozygous mice carrying an insulin-like growth factor II gene disrupted by targeting. *Nature* 345: 78–80, 1990.
21. Dernovsek, K. D., and R. S. Bar. Processing of cell bound insulin by capillary and macrovascular endothelial cells in culture. *Am. J. Physiol.* 248 (*Endocrinol. Metab.* 17)248: E244–E251, 1985.
22. Dernovsek, K. D., R. S. Bar, B. H. Ginsberg, and M. N. Lioubin. Rapid transport of biologically intact insulin through cultured endothelial cells. *J. Clin. Endocrinol. Metab.* 58: 761–763, 1984.
23. Filson, A. J., A. Louvi, A. Efstratiadis, and E. J. Robertson. Rescue of the T-associated maternal effect in mice carrying null mutaitons in Igf-2 and Igf-2r, two reciprocally imprinted genes. *Development* 118: 731–736, 1993.
24. Frank, H.J.L., and W. M. Partridge. A direct *in vitro* demonstration of insulin binding to isolated brain microvessels. *Diabetes* 30: 757–761, 1981.
25. Frank, H.J.L., W. M. Pardridge, W. L. Morris, R. G. Rosenfeld, and T. B. Choi. Binding and internalization of insulin and insulin-like growth factors by isolated brain microvessels. *Diabetes* 35: 654–661, 1986.
26. Ghinea, N., M.T.V. Hai,. M.-T. Groyer-Picard, and E. Milgrom. How protein hormones reach their target cells. Receptor-mediated transcytosis of hCG through endothelial cells. *J. Cell. Biol.* 125: 87–97, 1994.
27. Ghinea, N., and E. Milgrom. Transport of protein hormones through the vascular endothelium. *J. Endocrinol.* 145: 1–9, 1995.
28. Hachiya, H. L., J.-L. Carpenter, and G. L. King. Comparative studies on insulin-like growth factor II and insulin processing by vascular endothelial cells. *Diabetes* 35: 1065–1072, 1986.
29. Hachiya, H. L., P. A. Halban, and G. L. King. Intracellular pathways of insulin transport across vascular endothelial cells. *Am. J. Physiol.* 255 (*Cell Physiol.* 24): C459–C464, 1988.
30. Hashida, R., C. Anamizu, J. Kimura, S. Ohkuma, Y. Yoshida, and T. Takano. Transcellular transport of lipoprotein through arterial endothelial cells in monolayer culture. *Cell. Struct. Funct.* 11: 31–42, 1986.
31. Heltianu, C., M. Simionescu, and N. Simionescu. Histamine receptors of the microvascular endothelium revealed in situ with a histamine-ferritin conjugate: Characteristic high affinity binding sites in venules. *J. Cell Biol.* 93: 357–364, 1982.
32. Jefferies, W. A., M. R. Brandon, S. V. Hunt, A. F. Williams, K. C. Gatter, and D. Y. Mason. Transferrin receptor on endothelium of brain capillaries. *Nature* 312: 162–163, 1984.
33. Jialal, I., G. L. King, and S. Buchwald. Processing of insulin by bovine endothelial cells in culture: Internalization without degradation. *Diabetes* 33: 794–800, 1984.

34. Jones, J. I., and D. R. Clemmons. Insulin-like growth factors and their binding proteins: Biological actions. *Endocr. Rev.* 16: 3–34, 1995.

35. Jones, J. I., A. Gockerman, W. H. Busby, Y. G. Wright, and D. R. Clemmons. Insulin-like growth factor binding protein-1 stimulates cell migration and binds to the $\alpha_5\beta_1$ intergrin by means of its Arg-Gly-Asp sequence. *Proc. Natl. Acad. Sci. USA* 90: 10553–10557, 1993.

36. King, G. L., I. Jialal, S. Buchwald, and S. Johnson. Receptor-mediated uptake and transport of insulin by endothelial cells. *Diabetes* 33(Suppl. 1): 9A, 1984.

37. King, G. L., and S. M. Johnson. Receptor-mediated transport of insulin across endothelial cells. *Science* 227: 1583–1586, 1985.

38. Lassarc, C., and M. Binoux. Insulin-like growth factor binding protein-3 is functionally altered in pregnancy plasma. *Endocrinology* 134: 1254–1262, 1994.

39. Majno, G., and G. E. Palade. Studies on inflammation. I. The effect of histamine and serotonin on vascular permeability: An electron microscopic study. *J. Biophys. Biochem. Cytol.* 11: 607–626, 1961.

40. McClain, D. A. Mechanism and role of insulin receptor endocytosis. *Am. J. Med. Sci.* 304: 192–201, 1992.

41. Milton, S. G., and V. P. Knutson. Comparison of the function of the tight junctions of endothelial cells and epithelial cells in regulating the movement of electrolytes and macromolecules across the cell monolayer. *J. Cell. Physiol.* 144: 4; 98–504, 1990.

42. Moser, D. R., W. L. Lowe, Jr., B. L. Dake, B. A. Booth, M. Boes, D. R. Clemmons, and R. S. Bar. Endothelial cells express insulin-like growth factor binding proteins 2 to 6. *Mol. Endocrinol.* 6: 1805–1814, 1992.

43. Mostov, K. E., and N. E. Simister. Transcytosis. *Cell* 43: 389–390, 1985.

44. Pilch, P. F., M. A. Shia, R. J. J. Benson, and R. E. Fine. Coated vesicles participate in the receptor-mediated endocytosis of insulin. *J. Cell Biol.* 96: 133–138, 1983.

45. Pillion, D. J., J. F. Haskell, and E. Meezan. Cerebral cortical microvessels: An insulin sensitive tissue. *Biochem. Biophys. Res. Commun.* 104: 686–692, 1982.

46. Renkin, E. M. Transport pathways and processes. In: *Endothelial Cell Biology in Health and Disease,* edited by N. Simionescu and M. Simionescu. New York: Plenum, 1988, p. 51–67.

47. Rippe, B., and B. Haroldson. Transport of macromolecules across microvascular walls: The two-pore theory. *Physiol. Rev.* 74: 163–219, 1994.

48. Roberts, R. L., and A. Sandra. Receptor-mediated endocytosis of insulin by cultured endothelial cells. *Tissue Cell* 24: 603–611, 1992.

49. Royall, J. A., R. L. Berkow, J. S. Beckman, M. K. Cunningham, S. Matalon, and B. A. Freeman. Tumor necrosis factor and interleukin-1 alpha increase vascular endothelial permeability. *Am. J. Physiol.* 257 (*Lung Physiol.* 24): L399–L410, 1989.

50. Schnitzer, J. E., P. Oh, E. Pinney, and J. Allard. Filipin sensitive caveolae-mediated transport in endothelium: Reduced transcytosis, scavenger endocytosis, and capillary permeability of select macromolecules. *J. Cell Biol.* 127: 1217–1232, 1994.

51. Schwartz, M. W., R. N. Bergman, S. E. Kahn, G. J. Taborsky, L. D. Fisher, A. J. Sipols, S. C. Woods, G. M. Stiel, and D. J. Porte, Jr. Evidence for entry of plasma insulin into cerebrospinal fluid through an intermediate compartment in dogs. Quantitative aspects and implications for transport. *J. Clin. Invest.* 88: 1272–1281, 1991.

52. Severs, N. J. Caveolae: Static inpocketings of the plasma membrane, dynamic vesicles or plain artifacts? *J. Cell Sci.* 99: 341–348, 1988.

53. Shimasaki, S., and N. Ling. Identification and molecular characterization of insulin-like growth factor binding proteins (IGFBP-1, -2, -3, -4, -5 and -6). *Prog. Growth Factor Res.* 3: 253–266, 1991.

54. Simionescu, M. Receptor mediated transcytosis of plasma molecules by vascular endothelium. In: *Endothelial Cell Biology in Health and Disease,* edited by N. Simionescu and M. Simionescu. New York: Plenum, 1988, p. 69–104.

55. Simionescu, M., and N. Simionescu. Endothelial transport of macromolecules: Transcytosis and endocytosis. A look from cell biology. *Cell Biol. Rev.* 25: 1–78, 1991.

56. Simionescu, N., M. Simionescu, and G. E. Palade. Permeability of muscle capillaries to small heme-peptides. Evidence for the existence of patent transendothelial channels. *J. Cell Biol.* 64: 586–607, 1975.

57. Smith, R. M., and L. Jarett. Receptor-mediated endocytosis and intracellular processing of insulin: Ultrastructural and biochemical evidence for specific heterogeneity and distinction from non-hormonal ligands. *Lab. Invest.* 58: 613–629, 1988.

58. Soda, R., and M. Tavassoli. Liver endothelium and not hepatocytes or Kupffer cells have transferrin receptors. *Blood* 63: 270–276, 1984.

59. Solenski, N. J, and S. K. Williams. Insulin binding and vesicular ingestion in capillary endothelium. *J. Cell Physiol.* 124: 87–95, 1985.

60. Steil, G. M., M. Ader, D. M. Moore, K. Rebrin, and R. N. Bergman. Transendothelial insulin transport is not saturable *in vivo.* *J. Clin. Invest.* 97: 1497–1503, 1996.

61. Stitt, A. W., H. R. anderson, T. A. Gardiner, J. R. Bailie, and D. B. Archer. Receptor-mediated endocytosis and intracellular trafficking on insulin and low-density lipoprotein by retinal vascular endothelial cells. *Invest. Ophthalmol. Vis. Sci.* 35: 3384–3392, 1994.

62. VanHouten, M., and B. I. Posner. Insulin binds to brain blood vessels *in vivo.* *Nature* 282: 623–625, 1979.

63. Vasile, E., G. Popescu, M. Simionescu, and N. Simionescu. Enhanced transcytosis and accumulation of β14–very low density lipoproteins in the aorta of rabbits with experimental hyperlipidemia. In: *XVIth International Congress of the International Academy of Pathology.* Vienna, 1986, Abstracts Volume, p. 68.

64. Vasile, E., M. Simionescu, and N. Simionescu. Visualization of the binding, endocytosis and transcytosis of low-density lipoprotein in the arterial endothelium in situ. *J. Cell. Biol.* 96: 1677–1689, 1983.

65. Watanabe, J., K. Kanai, and S. Kanamura. Glucagon receptors in endothelial and Kupffer cells of mouse liver. *J. Histochem. Cytochem.* 36: 1081–1089, 1988.

66. Wu, N. Z., and A. L. Baldwin. Transient venular permeability increase and endothelial gap formation induced by histamine. *Am. J. Physiol.* 262 (*Heart Circ. Physiol.* 31): H1238–H1247, 1992.

67. Zetter, B. R. The endothelial cells of large and small blood vessels. *Diabetes* 30: 24–28, 1981.

68. Zhou, J., and C. B. Bondy. Anatomy of the insulin-like growth factor system in the human testis. *Fertil. Steril.* 60: 897–904, 1993.

69. Zimmerman, E. M., J. Cohen, M. Pardo, E. Hoyt, S. N. Lichtman and P. K. Lund. The cell specific expression of adult rat liver IGF binding proteins. In: *Endocrine Society Program of the 75th Annual Meeting of the Endocrine Society,* Las Vegas, NV, 1993, p. 480, Abstract 1718B.

4. Receptor identification and characterization

LEE E. LIMBIRD

HARVEY MOTULSKY

Department of Pharmacology, Vanderbilt University Medical Center, Nashville, Tennessee

GraphPad Software, Inc., San Diego, California

RECEPTORS are bifunctional molecules that recognize and bind a molecule of biological interest and, as a consequence of that binding, mediate changes in physiological response, presumably via ligand-induced conformational changes.

Receptors may exist on the cell surface or in any number of intracellular compartments. Receptors on the cell surface often evoke signal transduction cascades via protein–protein interactions, activation of chemical second messenger pathways, or modulation of changes in cation or anion movements that set up electrical signaling pathways. However, other cell surface receptors, in response to receptor occupancy, serve to bring nutrients into the cell. Examples include the transferrin receptor that transports iron, and the low density lipoprotein (LDL) receptor that transports cholesterol into cells containing LDL particles. Receptors inside the cytosolic or nuclear compartment interact with metabolic or gonadal steroids, retinoic acid, and other agents that are freely permeable to the surface bilayer. These receptors form an important family of molecules that binds ligands and thereby regulates transcriptional events. (Whether or not these membrane-permeable agents also have surface membrane transporters for regulated uptake of these ligands has yet to be rigorously established.) One should also expect, as well, the discovery of a family of molecules that regulates translational events in response to extracellular cues.

Receptors often serve as targets for drugs. However, drug targets are not always bifunctional, receptor molecules, as defined above. For example, important therapeutic agents targeted to the central nervous system block the function of neurotransmitter transporters, but these transporters, at least based on our current understandings, are not bifunctional receptor molecules. This chapter focuses on the identification and characterization of receptors that bind ligand and then elicit effects.

Agents that interact with receptors can be characterized in terms of the receptor-elicited response they evoke following binding to the receptor. *Agonists* mimic the role of endogenous hormones, neurotransmitters, autocoids, or other effectors. Agonists are "doers," whether or not the ultimate physiological function is stimulatory or inhibitory. *Antagonists* block the action of agonists. Classically, antagonists have been conceptualized as having no intrinsic activity in their own right, but instead block the binding pocket occupied by agonists. It is now clear that some antagonists can also block agonist-independent activity of receptors. Such antagonists are referred to as *negative antagonists* or, alternatively, *inverse agonists*. *Partial agonists* activate a physiological process, be it stimulatory or inhibitory in its net effect, but require more encounters than agonists with the receptor in order to elicit the same net response. In the simplest example, partial agonists are agents that, even at maximal receptor occupancy, are not able to elicit the same maximal response as a "full agonist." However, in a more sophisticated receptor theory first introduced by Stephenson (20), it was understood that "weak" agonists exist and that they elicit the same maximal response as "strong" agonists, but nonetheless require greater fractional occupancy of the receptor population than a "strong" agonist to elicit that response.

IDENTIFICATION OF RECEPTORS BASED ON FUNCTIONAL PROPERTIES

The initial identification of a "receptor" is based on the observation that an agent elicits a concentration-dependent effect on a biological response. Further characterization of a receptor would include investigating the specificity of a response by determining the breadth of target tissues that respond in a similar way and the ability of chemically similar agents to elicit the same response or to block the response of the parent molecule. It is important to appreciate that the relationship between receptor occupancy and response is rarely linear. This is shown schematically in Figure 4.1.

Because of the probable amplification between receptor occupancy and ultimate physiological response, the characterization of receptors based simply on the order of agonist potency is potentially misleading, particularly if the agonists evaluated have different efficacies in different target tissues such that they require differing levels of receptor occupancy to elicit the same response in varying settings. Classifying receptors by the order of potency of antagonists (when available) is much more definitive. If one is dealing with an antagonist with no negative intrinsic activity, that is, an antagonist that blocks response simply by preventing agonist occupancy, then the K_d value that defines the potency of each antagonist is independent of the tissue evaluated or of the agonist eliciting the response in different settings. Determination of this K_d value can be accomplished using Schild analysis (7, 17).

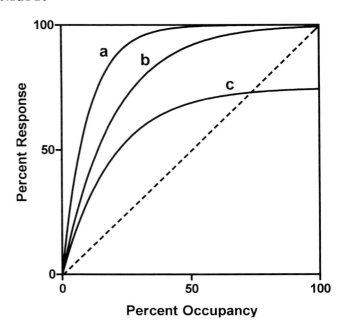

FIG. 4.1. Dose-response curves. With many full agonists, such as *a*, occupation of a small fraction of receptors elicits a nearly maximal response. A partial agonist can either be an agent such as *b*, where higher occupancy is required to elicit a response, or an agent such as *c*, which does not elicit the maximum response even at very high concentrations. Stephenson (20) would have referred to agonist *a* as a "strong" agonist.

Schild Analysis

A classical experimental strategy for determining the K_d values for competitive antagonists in physiological settings is to examine the agonist concentration—response relationship for the function of interest in the presence of antagonist, as shown schematically in Figure 4.2*A*

In the presence of a competitive antagonist the dose response curve for an agonist is shifted to the right. The agonist can still elicit the same maximal response, but it takes a higher concentration, that is, the antagonism is said to be surmountable. The dose ratio is defined as the concentration of agonist required to elicit a response in the presence of antagonist divided by the concentration of agonist needed to elicit that same response in the absence of antagonist. Typically, the agonist dose ratio in the presence of varying concentrations of antagonist is determined at a concentration of agonist that elicits half-maximal effect. The dose ratio is influenced by the concentration of antagonist and its affinity for the receptor. The dissociation constant for antagonist binding to the receptor, K_d, can be calculated from a single concentration of antagonist using the relationship $K_d = [antagonist] / DR - 1$.

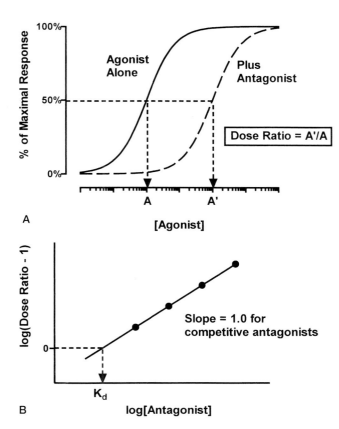

FIG. 4.2. Schild regression. In the presence of a competitive antagonist *(dashed line)* the dose-response curve for an agonist is shifted to the right. The agonist can still elicit the same maximal response, but it takes a higher concentration. *A* demonstrates the definition of the dose ratio. It is the concentration of agonist required to elicit a response in the presence of antagonist divided by the concentration of agonist needed to elicit that same response in the absence of antagonist. *B:* a Schild regression. Each *circle* represents a dose ratio of agonist in the presence of a different concentration of antagonist. If the drug is a competitive antagonist, the slope of the Schild regression line must equal 1.0. The intercept when log (dose ratio − 1) equals zero (that is, when dose ratio = 2) is the K_d of the antagonist. The term pA_2 sometimes is used to refer to the K_d for a competitive antagonist; $pA_2 = -\log K_d$ for the antagonist.

This calculation assumes that the interaction is competitive. Determination of the agonist dose-ratio in the presence of several concentrations of the antagonist is needed to test that assumption. A Schild regression plots the lot (dose ratio − 1) as a function of the logarithm of antagonist concentration (Fig. 4.2B) (7, 17). If the drug interacts in a competitive manner, the slope of the Schild regression line must equal 1.0. The intercept when the log (dose ratio − 1) equals zero (that is, when the dose ratio equals 2) is the K_d of the antagonist.

IDENTIFICATION OF RECEPTORS WITH RADIOLIGAND BINDING

A *radioligand* is a radioactively labeled agent that can associate with a receptor of physiological importance. The term ligand derives from the Latin (*ligo*, verb, to tie or bind) indicating the role of this agent in being recognized by and bound to a receptor site. What motivates an investigator to characterize receptors via radioligand binding strategies is an interest in more directly characterizing the molecule that mediates a particular physiological response. Consequently, the criteria for evaluating whether or not the binding detected reflects interaction with physiologically relevant receptors evolve from a prior understanding of the functional properties of the receptor of interest.

Choosing the Biological Preparation

The identification of a receptor of biological interest typically starts with refining an understanding of receptor function in a particular physiological setting. For example, if one wishes to identify receptors for an agent that regulates the rapidity of cardiac contractions, the tissue selected for initial radioligand binding studies would be the heart. If, on the other hand, one is trying to understand the mechanisms by which a newly classified agent influences bone growth or maturation, studies with isolated osteoblasts would be more appropriate. If sufficient information exists to understand that the receptor is at the cell surface, particulate preparations derived from cell lysates would permit more facile receptor characterization. On the other hand, if there is reason to believe that the agent under study is freely permeable to membranes and might elicit its effects in the cytosol or in an as yet uncharacterized cellular compartment, intact cells or unfractionated cell lysates would represent useful initial starting materials for identifying the receptor of interest.

Choosing a Radioligand

The choice of the radioligand for receptor identification is a practical consideration that often is limited by commercial availability or ease of synthesis. The radioactive properties of various isotopes are given in Table 4.1. ^{14}C has an extremely long half-life but low energy so that it emits too few counts to make it practical

TABLE 4.1. *Radioisotopes Commonly Used to Detect Receptors*

Isotope	Half life	k_{decay}	Specific Radioactivity, Ci/mmol
^{3}H	12.43 yr	0.056 yr^{-1}	28.7
^{125}I	59.6 days	0.0116 day^{-1}	2190
^{32}P	14.3 days	0.0485 day^{-1}	9128
^{35}S	87.4 days	0.0079 day^{-1}	1493

The specific radioactivity is calculated assuming that each molecule is labeled with a single radioactive atom. It is common to label molecules with 2 or 3 tritium atoms, which raises the specific radioactivity.

for identification of physiologically relevant receptors. Tritium (^{3}H) is commonly used to label ligands for receptor identification. Its half–life is long enough that radioactive decay over time is negligible, but it is of high enough energy to emit sufficient counts to typically permit reliable detection of receptors. It is possible to synthesize molecules with two or three tritium atoms, raising the specific radioactivity of the ligand further. A disadvantage of tritium is that the equipment needed to synthesize tritiated ligands is beyond that available in most laboratories, so that investigators are limited to commercially available or custom-synthesized ligands. ^{32}P is useful when the ligand of interest contains a phosphorous atom (for example, ATP or GTP). ^{125}I-labeled ligands are extremely popular, as they have high energy (2125 Ci/mmol specific radioactivity) and a reasonably long half–life (60 days). Ligands also can be iodinated using standard laboratory equipment. Iodinated radioligands are definitely preferable to tritiated ligands when limited amounts of biological tissue are available, such as discrete regions of the brain or primary cell cultures. A potential disadvantage to iodinated radioligands in receptor identification, however, is that an ^{125}I atom introduces a structural substitution the approximate size of a benzene ring; thus, for small molecules, the introduction of ^{125}I may severely perturb the structure and alter biological activity. In such cases, the binding sites identified using the ^{125}I-labeled compound may not reflect binding to the physiologically relevant receptor. This can be evaluated by confirming the bioactivity of the corresponding ^{127}I (nonradioactive)-labeled compound.

Before using a radioligand to identify receptors, it is important to first establish that the radioisotopically-labeled molecule retains the biological activity characteristic of the native molecule. Without ascertaining that the biological activity of the molecule to be used as the receptor probe is retained, it is senseless to

proceed. Binding sites are not necessarily reflective of physiologically relevant receptors; it would be impossible to identify a biologically important receptor with a radioligand that has lost its bioactivity either as an agonist, antagonist, partial agonist, or inverse agonist at the receptor.

Separating Bound From Free Radioligand

Binding incubations typically are allowed to proceed until steady–state is reached, that is, a point in time when no net change in binding occurs. Steady–state is not necessarily synonymous with equilibrium, as the steady–state might be achieved by an increase in binding that directly compensates for loss of receptors due to degradation or, alternatively, loss of ligand due to metabolism.

The incubation is terminated by separating bound from free radioligand. To detect the small amount of binding achieved relative to the amount of radioligand added, successful separation of bound from free radioligand must occur without significant dissociation of the ligand from the receptor. For ligand–receptor interactions of low affinity ($K_d > 10$ nM or so), the radioligand–receptor complex of interest may not be successfully trapped by most common methods of separating bound from free, as shown in Table 4.2. Frequently utilized strategies for separation of free ligand from binding to membrane-bound receptors include vacuum filtration and centrifugation through dense media (10). Resolving bound from free ligand for receptors that are not tethered to membranes is experimentally more cumbersome, but often involves gradient centrifugation protocols, such as those used

TABLE 4.2. *Relationship Between Equilibrium Dissociation Constant (K_d) and Allowable Separation Time of Ligand–Receptor Complex*

K_d (M)	Allowable Separation Time (0.15 $t\frac{1}{2}$)[1]
10^{-12}	1.2 days
10^{-11}	2.9 h
10^{-10}	17.0 min
10^{-9}	1.7 min
10^{-8}	10.0 s
10^{-7}	0.10 s
10^{-6}	0.01 s

[From Yamamura, H. I., S. J. Enna, and M. J. Kuhar. *Neurotransmitter Receptor Binding*, 2nd ed. New York: Raven Press, 1985.]

for the identification of cytosolic and nuclear receptors for steroids, retinoic acid, and their metabolites (18).

An alternative to using a radiolabeled ligand is to use a fluorescent ligand, and to distinguish bound and free ligand by fluorescence enhancement (for example, via energy transfer) or fluorescent quenching. This approach permits the termination of receptor binding in real time, as has been achieved successfully for interaction of Formyl-met-leu-phe with the chemotactic receptor of human neutrophils (19). However, fluorescence-based strategies currently are available only in a limited number of experimental settings, and usually require considerable methodology development. Consequently, they will not be further discussed in this chapter.

Irrelevant Binding

Not all binding detected as "bound ligand" at the termination of a binding incubation represents binding to the physiologically relevant receptor. Binding of interest to the investigator is defined as "specific" binding. Binding not of interest to the investigator is referred to as "nonspecific" binding, although operationally defined nonspecific binding can indeed reflect binding to a biological entity, such as the binding of catecholamines to metabolic enzymes or to neurotransmitter transporters rather than to adrenergic receptors. Nonspecific binding also refers to binding to generalized membrane or cytosolic sites due to interactions often driven by chemical properties of the ligands, such as charge or hydrophobicity. Means for resolving specific versus nonspecific binding will be dealt with in more detail in the discussion of the analysis of radioligand binding data.

Establishing That the Radioligand Binding Detected Reflects Interaction With the Physiologically Significant Receptor

Minimal criteria that demonstrate that a radioligand is interacting with a physiologically relevant receptor include:

1. Specific binding must be saturable, as you expect that a finite number of receptors exists. This is assessed by a saturation binding curve, as discussed later. In contrast, nonspecific binding is anticipated to increase linearly with increasing concentrations of radioligand, since one imagines that nonspecific sites would be infinite in number relative to the discrete number of physiological receptor sites.

2. Unlabeled drugs must compete for radioligand binding with potencies (or at least order of potency)

that match those observed in receptor-elicited physiological events. Competitive binding assays and their analyses are discussed below.

3. The kinetics of radioligand association and dissociation should reflect rates expected from the onset and reversal of effects elicited by the occupied receptors.

Analysis of Radioligand Binding Data Based on the Law of Mass Action

The chemical details of how a ligand binds to a receptor are not known in most cases. Binding is a complicated event involving conformational changes and multiple noncovalent bonds. However, radioligand binding experiments usually are analyzed based on a very simple model of binding, called the law of mass action:

$$\text{Ligand} + \text{Receptor} \rightleftharpoons \text{Ligand} \cdot \text{Receptor}$$

The model is based on these simple ideas:

1. Binding occurs when ligand and receptor collide due to diffusion, and when the collision has the correct orientation and enough energy. The rate of association (number of binding events per unit of time) equals $[\text{Ligand}] \cdot [\text{Receptor}] \cdot k_{on}$, where k_{on} is the association rate constant in units of $M^{-1}min^{-1}$.

2. Once binding has occurred, the ligand and receptor remain bound together for a random amount of time influenced by the affinity of the receptor and ligand for one another. The rate of dissociation (number of dissociation events per unit time) equals $[\text{ligand} \cdot \text{receptor}] \cdot k_{off}$, where k_{off} is the dissociation rate constant expressed in units of min^{-1}.

3. After dissociation, the ligand and receptor are the same as they were before binding.

4. Equilibrium is reached when the rate at which new ligand·receptor complexes are formed equals the rate at which the ligand·receptor complexes dissociate.

At equilibrium, ligand·receptor complexes form at the same rate that they dissociate:

$$[\text{Ligand}] \cdot [\text{Receptor}] \cdot k_{on} = [\text{Ligand} \cdot \text{Receptor}] \cdot k_{off}$$

$$(4\text{--}1)$$

The relationship can be rearranged to define the equilibrium dissociation constant, K_d.

$$K_d = \frac{k_{off}}{k_{on}} = \frac{[\text{Ligand}][\text{Receptor}]}{[\text{Ligand} \cdot \text{Receptor}]} \quad (4\text{--}2)$$

The K_d, expressed in units of moles/liter or molar, is the concentration of ligand which occupies half of the receptors at equilibrium. A small K_d means that the receptor has a high affinity for the ligand. A large K_d means that the receptor has a low affinity for the ligand.

Fractional Occupancy

The law of mass action predicts the fractional receptor occupancy at equilibrium as a function of ligand concentration. Fractional occupancy is the fraction of all available receptors that are bound to ligand.

$$\text{Fractional Occupancy} = \frac{[\text{Ligand} \cdot \text{Receptor}]}{[\text{Receptor}]_{\text{total}}} = \quad (4\text{--}3)$$

$$\frac{[\text{Ligand} \cdot \text{Receptor}]}{[\text{Receptor}] + [\text{Ligand} \cdot \text{Receptor}]}$$

Algebraic rearrangement yields a useful equation:

$$\text{Fractional occupancy} = \frac{[\text{Ligand}]}{[\text{Ligand}] + K_d} \quad (4\text{--}4)$$

When [Ligand] = 0, the occupancy equals zero. When [Ligand] is very high (many times K_d), the fractional occupancy approaches 1.00. When [Ligand] = K_d, fractional occupancy is 0.50. The approach to saturation as [ligand] increases is slower than many investigators appreciate. When the ligand concentration equals four times its K_d, it will only occupy 80% of the receptors at equilibrium. The occupancy rises to 90% when the ligand concentration equals nine times the K_d. It takes a concentration equal to 99 times the K_d to occupy 99% of the receptors at equilibrium.

Assumptions Inherent in the Law of Mass Action

Although termed a "law," the law of mass action is simply a model based on these assumptions:

1. All receptors are equally accessible to ligands.
2. All receptors are either free or bound to ligand. The model ignores any states of partial binding.
3. Neither ligand nor receptor are altered by binding.
4. Binding is reversible.
5. Only a small fraction of the ligand added actually binds to the receptors, so that the concentration of free ligand can be assumed to equal the concentration added.

If these assumptions are not met, the investigator has two choices. One choice is to develop a more complicated model, beyond the scope of this chapter. For example, if ligand depletion occurs, and the experimental protocol cannot be changed to minimize ligand depletion, mathematical accounting for depletion is appropriate (21). The other choice is to analyze the data using this simple model, but treat the values obtained merely as empirical descriptors of the data and not as rigorous thermodynamic parameters.

SATURATION BINDING STUDIES

Saturation binding experiments measure specific binding at equilibrium at various concentrations of the radioligand, and are used to determine receptor number and affinity, as shown schematically in Figure 4.3A.

The analysis of saturation-binding studies depends on the assumption that the incubation has achieved equilibrium. This can take anywhere from a few minutes to many hours, depending on the ligand, receptor, temperature, and other experimental conditions. Since lower concentrations of radioligand take longer to equilibrate, the lowest concentration of radioligand to be used in the saturation analyses should be used in preliminary studies to ascertain how long it will take to achieve equilibrium in the saturation binding experiments.

Defining Nonspecific Binding in a Radioligand Binding Assay

As mentioned earlier, nonspecific binding is defined as binding to sites other than the physiologically relevant receptor under study. This definition will always be somewhat arbitrary, and should be refined as increasing information is obtained about the receptor under study. Several approaches can be used at the outset to estimate nonspecific binding.

1. Nonspecific binding often is defined as that binding not competed for by unlabeled ligand present at concentrations that represent $100 \times K_d$ for the unlabeled agent. However, a limitation to this practice is that if the radioligand is present at concentrations in excess of its K_d, which can occur in early steps of receptor characterization, then the competitor will not successfully block radioligand binding to all relevant receptors. Another limitation to this approach is that if the unlabeled ligand used in this analysis is structurally identical to the radioligand, then radioligand binding will be decreased simply by radioisotopic dilution, whether or not the binding identifies the physiologically relevant receptor. In some circumstances, only a single compound is available, so the radioligand and unlabeled agent have the same structure. The potential misleading nature of the nonspecific binding obtained using this strategy (that is, isotope dilution rather than competition for the physiologically relevant receptor) should be appreciated by the investigator.

2. An alternate method for estimating nonspecific binding is to add increasing concentrations of a presumed competitor to incubations containing a single

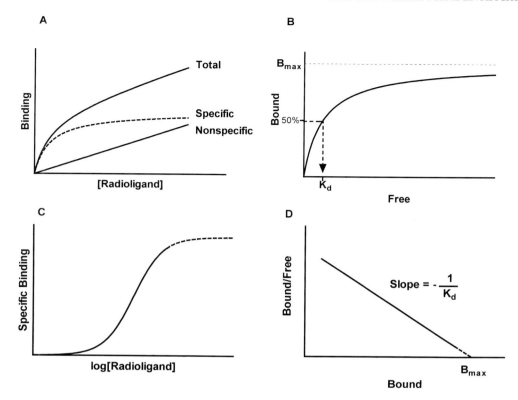

FIG. 4.3. Saturation binding. *A:* total and nonspecific binding at equilibrium as a function of increasing concentrations of radioligand. The difference, also shown, is specific binding. *B:* specific binding only. Note the definition of B_{max} (the maximal amount of binding extrapolated to infinite radioligand concentration) and K_d (the concentration of radioligand that occupies half the receptors at equilibrium). *C:* the same data, but plotting the concentration of radioligand on a logarithmic axis. The solid part of the curve in C corresponds to the curve in B; the dotted portion is extrapolated. *D:* the same data transformed into a Scatchard plot.

concentration of radioligand until the decrease in radioligand binding as a function of the unlabeled agent reaches a plateau. The concentration of competitor where the curve becomes asymptotic with a horizontal line reflects the concentration of competitor that fully occupies receptor sites under the incubation conditions. This approach is most valid when the competitor selected is chemically different from the radioligand, assuring that the decrease in radioligand binding is not simply due to isotopic dilution. If multiple agents that are expected to interact with the same physiological receptor decrease radioligand binding to the same plateau, then confidence in using those "saturating" concentrations of competitors to define nonspecific binding is enhanced.

3. A third approach for defining nonspecific binding is mathematical, rather than experimental, and will be more intuitive after reading further to learn of methods for computer-assisted analysis of radioligand binding. The mathematical model on which computer-based analysis is based includes an algebraic description of saturable binding (a rectangular hyperbola) plus a component of binding that increases linearly with increasing ligand concentrations, that is, nonspecific binding. Fitting the data with these models can provide an estimate of nonspecific binding.

No estimate of nonspecific binding is fail-safe. The investigator should objectively evaluate both experimental and mathematical approaches and re-evaluate the operational definition of nonspecific binding in the laboratory as more information regarding the receptor under study accrues.

Figure 4.3C shows the specific binding again on a graph with a logarithmic x axis. The saturation binding curve plotted on a log axis looks like the familiar sigmoidal dose–response curve. The dotted curve in Figure 4.3A represents the specific binding detected over the same range of radioligand concentrations. The dotted portion of the curve in Figure 4.3C shows extrapolation of binding at higher radioligand concentrations. These high concentrations are used rarely, due to the cost of radioligands and increased amounts of nonspecific binding, leading to a larger fraction of the total binding detected.

Equilibrium specific binding at a particular radioligand concentration, [L], equals fractional occupancy times the total receptor number (B_{max}):

$$\text{Specific Binding} =$$
$$\text{Fractional Occupancy} \cdot B_{max} = \frac{B_{max} \cdot [L]}{K_d + [L]} \quad (4\text{-}5)$$

This equation for the binding isotherm describes a rectangular hyperbola. The Y axis of the plot is [LR], or amount bound as a function of [L], the concentration of free radioligand, plotted on the X axis (see Fig. 4.3A) B_{max} is the total number of receptors expressed in the same units as the [LR] values (that is, cpm, sites/cell or fmol/mg protein) and K_d is the equilibrium dissociation constant (expressed in the same units as [L], usually nM). Typical values might be a B_{max} of 10–1000 fmol binding sites per milligram of crude membrane protein (corresponding to about one receptor per square micron of surface membrane) and a K_d between 10 pM and 10 nM.

To determine the B_{max} and K_d, the data are fit to the Equation 4–5 using nonlinear regression. This analysis is based on several assumptions:

1. Binding follows the law of mass action and has attained equilibrium.
2. There is only one population of receptors.
3. Only a small fraction of the radioligand binds so that the free concentration is essentially identical to the concentration added.
4. There is no cooperativity. Binding of a ligand to one binding site does not alter the affinity of another binding site. In other words, the K_d is constant during the experiment.

Before nonlinear regression programs were widely available, scientists transformed data to make a linear graph, and then analyzed the transformed data with linear regression. There are several ways to linearize binding data, but Scatchard analysis is used most often (16); the plots derived from this analysis are more accurately attributed to Rosenthal (14). For these plots, the X axis is specific binding (usually labeled "bound") and the Y axis is the ratio of specific binding to concentration of free radioligand (usually labeled "bound/free"). B_{max} is the X intercept; K_d is the negative reciprocal of the slope (Fig. 4.3D).

The Y axis of this plot should be expressed as a unitless fraction, that is, cpm bound/cpm free. If the highest Y value is large (greater than 0.10), then the free concentration will be substantially less than the added concentration of radioligand, and the analyses will yield inaccurate parameters of B_{max} and K_d. In such situations, the experimental protocol should be revised to reduce ligand depletion. If the experimental protocol cannot easily be revised, special analysis methods that deal with ligand depletion should be employed (21).

While linear transformations are very useful for visualizing data, they are not the most accurate way to analyze data. Linear regression assumes that the scatter of points around the line follows a Gaussian distribution and that the standard deviation is the same at every value of X. These assumptions are not true with the transformed data. Secondly, the value of X (bound) is used to calculate Y (bound/free) in a Rosenthal (see attached) plot, violating the assumptions of linear regression. Consequently, the B_{max} and K_d values determined by linear regression of transformed data are likely to be further from their true values than the B_{max} and K_d determined by nonlinear regression. Although it is inappropriate to analyze data by performing linear regression on a Scatchard plot, it often is helpful to display data as a Rosenthal (Scatchard) plot, as it can be easier to visually interpret linear plots than binding curves, especially when comparing results from different experimental treatments.

DEFINING THE SPECIFICITY OF RADIOLIGAND BINDING USING COMPETITIVE BINDING ANALYSIS

Competitive binding experiments measure the binding of a single concentration of labeled ligand in the presence of various concentrations of unlabeled ligand. They are used to:

1. *Define the specificity of radioligand binding.* Demonstrating that drugs compete for radioligand binding with the expected potencies, or at least order of potency, characteristic of functional studies helps document that the radioligand has identified the receptor of functional interest. This kind of experiment is crucial to confirm the physiological significance of the binding site under study.

2. Determine whether an agent binds to the receptor. This use has value both in characterizing a novel receptor preparation as well as in screening a library of compounds to identify agents that bind to the receptor. Radioligand binding assays typically are faster and easier than other screening methods for receptor identification and assessment of receptor specificity.

3. Investigate the interaction of low affinity drugs with receptors. Binding assays are only useful when

the radioligand has a high affinity ($K_d \leq 10$ nM; see Table 4.2), since a radioligand with low affinity generally has a fast dissociation rate constant and dissociates from the receptor during the separation of bound from free radioligand. To study the binding of a low affinity agent, it is evaluated as an unlabeled competitor of high affinity radioligand binding.

4. Determine receptor number and affinity by using the same compound as both the labeled and unlabeled ligand. This use is described in more detail later under Homologous Competitive Binding Curves. . . .

Competitive binding experiments, as noted above, are performed with a single concentration of radioligand. The amount of radioligand to use is not dogma; many investigators choose a concentration approximately equal to about the K_d of the radioligand for binding to the receptor, but this is neither universal nor necessary. The incubation must be carried out for a duration that permits equilibrium to be reached. This will be considerably longer than it takes the radioligand to reach equilibrium in the absence of competitor. The incubation theoretically should extend for 4–5 times the half-life for receptor dissociation, determined in an off-rate experiment, if such information is available. Typically, investigators use 12–24 concentrations of unlabeled compound spanning about 5–6 orders of magnitude to evaluate the potency of the competitor.

Analyzing Competitive Binding Data

Figure 4.4 provides a schematic diagram of data obtained in a competitive binding study.

The top of the curve is a plateau at a value equal to total radioligand binding in the absence of the competing unlabeled agent. The bottom of the curve is a plateau equal to nonspecific binding (NS). The difference between the top and bottom plateaus is the specific binding. The concentration of unlabeled drug that decreases *specific* radioligand binding by half is called the IC$_{50}$ (inhibitory concentration, 50%; see Fig. 4.4*A*) or the EC$_{50}$ (effective concentration 50%). When a series of agents is evaluated, the order of potency of competing agents, that is, a > b > c in Figure 4.4*B*, is determined. These assessments are critical for defining the *specificity* of radioligand binding.

If the labeled and unlabeled ligand compete for a single binding site, the steepness of the competitive binding curve is determined by the law of mass action. The curve descends from 90% specific binding to 10% specific binding with an 81-fold increase in the concentration of the unlabeled drug. More simply, nearly the entire curve will cover two log units (100-fold change in concentration), as shown in Figure 4.4*C*.

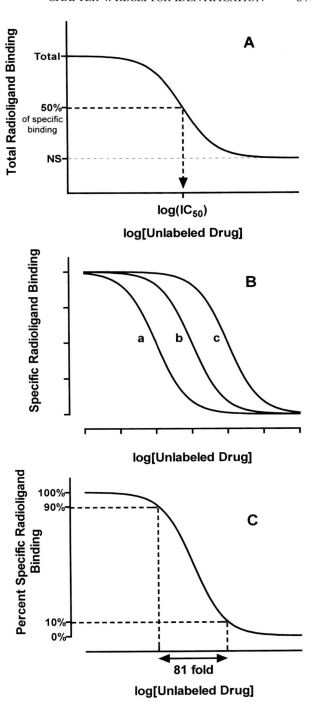

FIG. 4.4. Competitive binding experiments. *A*: definition of the IC$_{50}$ as the concentration of unlabeled drug that competes for half of specific radioligand binding at equilibrium. *B*: competition by three different drugs. The IC$_{50}$ is lowest for drug *a*, so drug *a* has the highest affinity. The order of potency is *a>b>c*. *C*: an 81-fold increase in the concentration of unlabeled drug makes the curve descend from 90% to 10% occupancy. If the curve is shallower or steeper than this, then the radioligand and competitor do not compete for binding to a single class of binding sites with unchanging affinity for radioligand and competitor.

Competitive binding data are analyzed by fitting to the equation:

$$Binding = Nonspecific + \frac{Specific}{1 + \frac{[D]}{IC_{50}}} = \qquad (4-6)$$

$$\frac{(Total - Nonspecific)}{1 + 10^{\log[D] - \log(IC50)}}$$

The Y axis represents the total binding measured in the presence of various concentrations of the unlabeled drug, and log[D] is the logarithm of the concentration of competitor plotted on the X axis. Nonspecific binding is defined as binding in the presence of a saturating concentration of an agent known to interact with the biologically relevant receptor (as described above), and Total is the binding in the absence of competitor. The values of total and nonspecific binding are all expressed in the same units, such as cpm, fmol/mg, or sites/cell. (Total-nonspecific binding is defined as specific binding.)

Calculating the K_i From the IC_{50}

The value of the IC_{50} is influenced by three factors, as follows:

1. *The K_i of the receptor for the competing drug.* The K_i is the equilibrium dissociation constant for binding of the unlabeled drug—the concentration of the unlabeled drug that will bind to half maximally occupy the binding sites at equilibrium in the absence of radioligand or other competitors. The K_i is proportional to the IC_{50}. If the K_i is low (that is, the affinity is high), the IC_{50} will also be low.

2. *The concentration of the radioligand.* It will take a larger concentration of unlabeled drug to compete for the binding of a higher concentration of radioligand than a lower concentration of radioligand. Thus, increasing the concentration of radioligand increases the IC_{50}, although the equilibrium binding constant, K_i is not changed.

3. *The affinity of the radioligand for the receptor (K_d).* It takes more unlabeled drug to compete for a high affinity radioligand than for a lower affinity radioligand. Using a radioligand with a lower K_d (higher affinity) will increase the IC_{50} of the competitor.

Under some circumstances, the K_i can be directly calculated from the IC_{50}, using the equation of Cheng and Prusoff (2).

$$K_i = \frac{IC_{50}}{1 + \frac{[Radioligand]}{K_d}} \qquad (4-7)$$

The ability to use this equation to calculate K_i from IC_{50} is based on several assumptions.

1. Only a small fraction of both the labeled and unlabeled ligand has bound. This means that the free concentration is virtually the same as the added concentration. (See the discussion concerning "ligand depletion," earlier, to learn about methods that don't rely on this assumption.)

2. The receptors are homogeneous and all have the same affinity for the radioligand and competing ligands, that is, there is only one value for K_i of the competitor and K_d of the radioligand.

3. The K_d of the radioligand has been evaluated directly in a saturation-binding experiment performed under incubation conditions similar to those utilized in the competitive binding experiment.

4. There is no cooperativity—binding to one binding site does not alter affinity at another site.

5. The experiment has reached equilibrium.

6. Binding is reversible and follows the law of mass action.

Homologous Competitive Binding Curves Permit an Assessment of Both K_d and B_{max}

A competitive binding experiment is termed *homologous* when the same compound is used as the radioactive and unlabeled ligand. The term *heterologous* is used when radioligand and competing ligands differ. Homologous competitive binding experiments represent a special case of competitive binding experiments that can be used to determine the affinity of a ligand for the receptor and the receptor number. In other words, such an experiment has the same goals as a saturation binding curve. Because homologous competitive binding experiments use a single concentration of radioligand (which can be low), they consume less radioligand and are thus more practical when radioligands are expensive or difficult to synthesize.

To analyze a homologous competitive binding curve, certain assumptions must be met:

1. The receptor has identical affinity for the labeled and unlabeled ligand. Since iodination often changes the binding properties of ligands, it may be wise to use an iodinated unlabeled compound, that is, ^{127}I-ligand, as competitor.

2. There is no cooperativity.

3. No ligand depletion occurs during the incubation. In other words, the analysis assumes that the free concentration of ligand is equal to the concentration that is added. There is only one class of binding sites. It is difficult to detect a second class of binding sites

unless the number of lower affinity sites vastly exceeds the number of higher affinity receptors (because the single low concentration of radioligand used in the experiment will bind to only a small fraction of low affinity receptors).

4. A homologous competitive binding curve is analyzed using the same equation used for a one-site heterologous competitive binding curve to determine the top and bottom plateaus and the IC_{50}. The Cheng and Prussoff equation permits calculation of the K_i from the IC_{50}. In a homologous competitive binding experiment, it is assumed that the radioactive and competing ligand have identical affinities so that K_d and K_i are the same. Knowing that, simple algebra converts the equation to:

$$K_d = K_i = IC_{50} - [Radioligand] \qquad (4-8)$$

The concentration of radioligand is set by the experimental design, and IC_{50} is determined from nonlinear regression. The difference between the two is the K_d of the ligand (again assuming hot and cold ligands bind the same).

To determine the B_{max} in homologous competitive binding assays, the specific binding is divided by the fractional occupancy, calculated from the K_d and the concentration of radioligand.

$$B_{max} = \frac{Top - Bottom}{Fractional\ Occupancy} =$$
$$\frac{Top - Bottom}{[Radioligand] \Big/ (K_d + [Radioligand])} \qquad (4-9)$$

KINETIC ANALYSIS OF RADIOLIGAND BINDING EXPERIMENTS

Studies of Radioligand Dissociation

Since the rate of receptor occupancy often is diffusion limited, differences in receptor affinity typically are reflected by variable rate constants for dissociation from the receptor. To measure the rate of dissociation, ligand and receptor are first permitted to bind, most conveniently to steady–state. At that point, *further binding* of radioligand to receptor is prevented using one of two strategies:

1. Excess unlabeled competitor: Add a very high concentration of an unlabeled ligand that instantly binds to all, or nearly all, of the unoccupied receptors and thus competes for further binding of the radioligand as well as for rebinding of dissociated ligand.

2. Infinite dilution: Dilute the incubation by a large factor sufficient to eliminate new binding of radioligand and rebinding of dissociated radioligand due to dilution of both radioligand and receptor. Typically, a 100-fold dilution (for example, 100 μl to 10.0 ml) is sufficient.

The utility of these two strategies in differentiating among various explanations for complex binding phenomena will be emphasized later in this chapter. After the dissociation phase of the experiment is initiated, binding is measured over time to determine how rapidly the ligand dissociates from the receptors.

As shown in Figure 4.5, decreases in ligand binding due to dissociation from a single LR complexes follows an exponential decay as a function of time, and can be described by equation 4-10.

$$Total\ Binding = NS + (Total - NS) \cdot e^{-k_{off}} \qquad (4-10)$$

Total binding and nonspecific binding (NS) are expressed in cpm, fmol/mg protein, or sites/cell. Time *(t)* usually is expressed in minutes. The dissociation rate constant (k_{off}) is expressed in units of inverse time, usually min^{-1}. Since it is difficult to think in those units, it helps to calculate the half–life for dissociation, termed the $t_{1/2}$ (Fig. 4.5A).

$$t_{1/2} = \frac{ln(2)}{k_{off}} = \frac{0.693}{k_{off}} \qquad (4-11)$$

In one half–life, half of the radioligand will have dissociated. In two half–lives, three quarters of the radioligand will have dissociated, etc. Dissociation data often are shown on a semi-log plot of $ln(B_t/B_0)$ vs. time, B_t is the specific binding at time *t*; B_0 is specific binding at time zero. If the system follows the law of mass action with a single affinity state, the semi-log plot will be linear with a slope equal to $-k_{off}$. Note that this analysis utilizes the specific (not total) binding in the calculations and must use natural logs (not log base 10), in order for the slope to equal $-k_{off}$. If an investigator instead plots $log_{10}(B_t/B_0)$ vs. time, the slope $= -2.303\ k_{off}$ (Fig. 4.5B).

Typically the dissociation rate constant of useful radioligands is between 0.001 and 0.1 min^{-1}. If the dissociation rate constant were any faster, it would be difficult to perform radioligand binding experiments as the radioligand would dissociate from the receptors during the separation of bound from free radioligand (see Table 4.2).

Studies of Radioligand Association

Association binding experiments are performed by adding radioligand and measuring specific binding at vari-

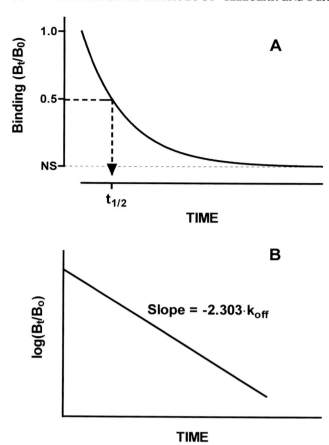

FIG. 4.5. Dissociation kinetics. *A:* before the first time point on the graph, binding was allowed to occur, perhaps to equilibrium. At time zero on the graph, dissociation was initiated by infinite dilution or by addition of an excess of unlabeled drug. Under either condition, the radioligand cannot rebind after dissociating from the receptor; consequently the total amount of binding decreases over time. The half-life ($t_{1/2}$) is the time when half of the specific binding has dissociated. *B:* the same data on a log plot, which linearizes the dissociation data.

2. *The concentration of radioligand.* The system equilibrates faster at higher concentrations of radioligand and k_{ob} will be larger.

3. *The dissociation rate constant, k_{off}.* Investigators often are surprised to realize that the observed rate of association depends in part on the dissociation rate constant. This makes sense when you realize that an association experiment doesn't directly measure how long it takes radioligand to bind, but rather measures how long it takes the binding to reach equilibrium. Equilibrium is reached when the rate of the forward binding reaction equals the rate of the reverse dissociation reaction. If the radioligand dissociates quickly from the receptor, equilibrium will be reached faster, but there will be less binding at equilibrium. If the radioligand dissociates slowly, equilibrium will be reached more slowly and there will be more binding at equilibrium.

To calculate the association rate constant, usually expressed in units of Molar^{-1} min^{-1}, equation 4–13 is employed. (For greater experimental detail in assessing k_{ob} and k_{on}, see ref. 10.) Typically ligands have association rate constants of about 10^8 M^{-1} min^{-1}. The association rate depends mostly on diffusion, so most ligands tend to have similar "on rates."

$$k_{on} = \frac{k_{ob} - k_{off}}{[\text{Radioligand}]} \quad (4\text{–}13)$$

The separately determined k_{on} (min^{-1}M^{-1}) and k_{off} (min^{-1}) values can be combined to estimate the K_d of receptor binding:

$$K_d = \frac{k_{off}}{k_{on}} \quad (4\text{–}14)$$

ous times thereafter, as shown schematically in Figure 4.6. Specific binding data as a function of time follows the one-phase exponential association equation given in equation 4–12. The specific binding achieved at equilibrium depends on the concentration of radioligand.

$$\text{Specific Binding} = \text{Top}(1 - e^{-k_{ob} \cdot t}) \quad (4\text{–}12)$$

The observed rate constant, k_{ob}, is expressed in units of inverse time, usually min^{-1}. It is a measure of how quickly the incubation reaches equilibrium; the k_{ob} is determined by three factors, as follows:

1. *The association rate constant, k_{on}.* If k_{on} is larger (faster), k_{ob} will be larger as well.

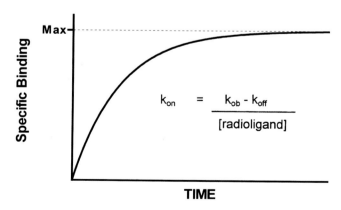

FIG. 4.6. Association kinetics. Radioligand binding was added at time zero, and the graph shows the increase in specific binding thereafter.

If binding follows the law of mass action, the K_d calculated based on the ratio of on and off rate constants should be the same as the K_d calculated from a saturation binding curve measured at steady state.

COMPLEX BINDING PHENOMENA

Competitive Binding Experiments With Two (or More) Receptor Sites

Tissues often contain two or more classes of binding sites for a radioligand, for example, two or more subtypes of a given receptor. In the simplest case, when radioligand has identical affinity at both receptor populations, the K_d for each site and their related abundance can be determined by fitting the data to equation 4–15.

$$\text{Binding} = \text{NS} + (\text{Total} - \text{NS})$$
$$\left[\frac{F}{1 + 10^{\log[D] - \log(IC_{50} - 1)}} + \frac{1 - F}{1 + 10^{\log[D] - \log(IC_{50} - 2)}}\right]$$
$$(4\text{–}15)$$

This equation has five variables: the total and nonspecific binding (the top and bottom binding plateaus), the fraction of binding to receptors of the first type of receptor (F), and the IC_{50} values of the unlabeled ligand for each type of receptor. If you know the K_d of the labeled ligand and its concentration, you can convert the IC_{50} values to K_i values (see earlier discussion of Cheng and Prusoff analysis, equation 4–7). A more complicated equation is needed when the two classes of receptors have different affinities for the labeled ligand, as well as different affinities for the unlabeled ligand (13).

In situations where two or more receptor populations with different affinities exist, investigators might expect to see a biphasic competitive binding curve. However, an obviously biphasic curve occurs only in cases where the affinities of the receptor subpopulations for the competing ligand are extremely different (4). More often, a smooth but shallow curve is detected (Fig. 4.7A). Figure 4.7B shows the competitive binding profile for a competitor interacting with two equally abundant sites that have a tenfold (one log unit) difference in IC_{50} for competitor. Although the curve is shallow (it takes more than two log units to go from 90% to 10% competition), two distinct components cannot readily be detected by eye. Nonlinear regression is needed to estimate the affinity of the competitor at each receptor population and the relative density of receptors in each of the two subpopulations.

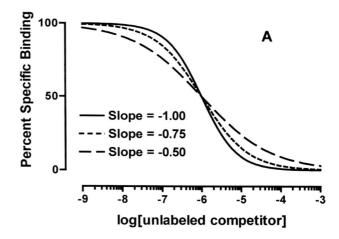

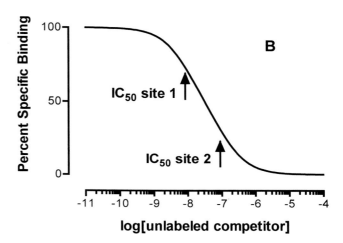

FIG. 4.7. Complex competitive binding curves. A: the meaning of the slope factor. A fractional slope factor (such as −0.5) means that the curve is shallow. A normal competitive binding curve (single binding site, no cooperativity) has a slope factor of −1.0, as shown in the solid curve. B: competition for two different binding sites. The radioligand binds identically to both sites, but the competitor has a tenfold difference in affinity. Although the curve is shallow, it is not obviously biphasic.

Saturation Binding Experiments With Two Receptor Sites

When radioligand binds to two classes of receptors, the data can be analyzed by using equation 4–16, which is simply the sum of two rectangular hyperbolas (8).

$$\text{Specific Binding} = \frac{B_{max1} \cdot [L]}{K_{d1} + [L]} + \frac{B_{max2} \cdot [L]}{K_{d2} + [L]} \quad (4\text{–}16)$$

Panel A in Figure 4.8 shows specific binding to two classes of receptors present in equal quantities and whose K_d values differ tenfold. Panel *B* shows the transformation to a Scatchard (Rosenthal) plot. In both graphs, the dotted and dashed lines show binding to the two individual receptor populations that sum to the solid curves.

Two points are worthy of mention: *(1)* the graph of specific binding to both receptor sites (the solid line) is not obviously biphasic, as it is very hard to see the existence of two receptor binding affinities by visual inspection. The best way to detect the second site is to fit data to one- versus two-sites, and let the nonlinear regression program compare the two fits, *(2)* on the Scatchard plot, the data are not linear (solid curve), although experimental scatter might obscure the curvature. An important surprise in examining the two components of a biphasic Scatchard are that the solid and dashed line are *not* asymptotes of the curve. This realization emphasizes the importance of using nonlin-

ear regression to define properties of the multiple receptors that contribute to complex binding phenomena.

Comparing One- and Two-Site Models

A two-site model almost always fits the data better than a one-site model. A three-site model fits even better, and a four-site model better yet! As more variables (sites) are added to the equation, the curve becomes "more flexible" and gets closer to the points. Consequently, it is essential to use statistical calculations to determine if the improvement in fit between two-site and one-site models is statistically valid. However, before thinking about statistical comparisons, the investigator should consider whether the results make sense. For example, a two-site fit should be disregarded when the two IC_{50} or K_d values are almost identical or, alternatively, if one of the IC_{50} or K_d values is outside of the range of the raw data. A two-site fit also should be disregarded if one of the sites has a very small fraction of the receptors, or the best-fit values for the bottom and top plateaus are far from the range of Y values observed in a competitive binding experiment.

If the two-site fit seems reasonable, then the investigator should test whether the improvement is statistically significant. This is accomplished by calculating an F ratio which quantifies the relationship between the relative increase in sum-of-square (SS) and the relative increase in degrees of freedom (DF).

$$F = \frac{(SS1 - SS2)/SS2}{(DF1 - DF2)/DF2} \qquad (4-17)$$

If the one-site model is correct, the F ratio will usually be near 1.0. If the ratio is much greater than 1.0, there are two possibilities. One possibility is that the two-site model is correct. The other possibility is that the one-site model is correct, but random scatter led the two-site model to fit better by chance. F corresponds with a *P* value that provides an estimate of how rarely this coincidence would occur. The *P* value answers this question: If the one-site model is really correct, what is the chance that data that fit the two-site model so much better could be obtained randomly? If the *P* value is small, it can be concluded that the two-site model is significantly better than the one-site model. Most scientists reach this conclusion when *P* is 0.05, but the threshold *P* value is arbitrary.

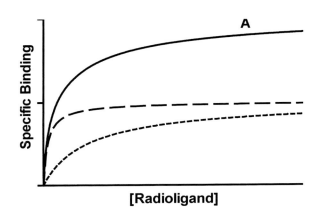

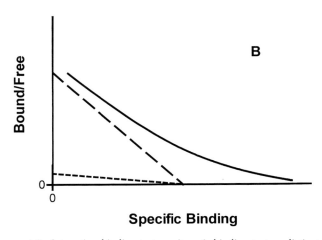

FIG. 4.8. Saturation binding to two sites. *A:* binding to two distinct receptor types indicated by *dotted* and *dashed curves*. The two sum to the *solid curve*. Experimental data will follow the solid curve, and computer analysis is needed to find the B_{max} and K_d of the two components. *B:* the same data as represented on a Scatchard plot.

The Slope Factor of a Competitive Binding Curve

Many competitive binding curves are shallower than predicted by law of mass action for binding to a single site. One explanation for a shallow competitive binding curve is a mixture of two receptor types, as discussed above. Another explanation is negative cooperativity. Regardless of the biological explanation, the steepness of a binding curve can be quantified with a slope factor. The slope factor is determined by fitting competitive binding data curve to Equation 4–18:

$$\text{Binding} = \text{Nonspecific} + \frac{(\text{Total} - \text{Nonspecific})}{1 + 10^{(\log(\text{IC}_{50}) - (\log[D]) \cdot \text{Slope Factor}}}$$

$$(4\text{–}18)$$

A one-site competitive binding curve that follows the law of mass action has a slope of -1.0. If the curve is more shallow, the slope factor will be a negative fraction (that is, -0.85 or -0.60). (The slope factor is negative because the curve goes downhill.) The slope factor is a number that describes the steepness of the curve (see Fig. 4.7A). In most situations, there is no way to interpret the value in terms of chemistry or biology. However, if the slope factor differs significantly from 1.0, then the binding does not follow the expectations for interaction of the ligand with a single receptor population possessing a single and unchanging affinity for ligand.

Using Dissociation Experiments to Investigate Complex Binding

The data from a dissociation experiment frequently deviate from a simple exponential decay, resulting in a semi-log plot that is nonlinear. This occurs when there are multiple independent receptor populations, multiple interchangeable affinity states, or cooperative interactions among receptors.

Distinguishing Between Independent Receptor Subtypes and Negative Cooperativity

To distinguish between multiple independent binding sites and negative cooperativity among receptors, dissociation rates are compared after initiating dissociation by infinite dilution and, in separate incubations, by saturating with an unlabeled ligand. If the radioligand is bound to multiple, independent receptor subtypes, the dissociation curve observed will be indistinguishable whether dissociation is initiated by excess unlabeled ligand or by "infinite dilution" (Fig. 4.9A), as each receptor is "naive" about interactions occurring at the other receptors and thus is not influenced by whether other receptors are occupied by ligand or not.

In contrast, when radioligand is bound to receptors which exhibit negative cooperativity, that is, overall binding affinity decreases as occupancy increases, the dissociation curves will differ depending on how dissociation is initiated (Fig. 4.9B). If dissociation is initiated by infinite dilution, the dissociation rate will change over time, the results will not follow a simple exponential decay, and a semi-log graph will not be linear. In contrast, if dissociation is initiated by adding an unlabeled ligand, the increased receptor occupancy leads to a decrease in receptor affinity and an increase in dissociation rate; since the receptors are always fully occupied (as labeled ligands fall off they are replaced

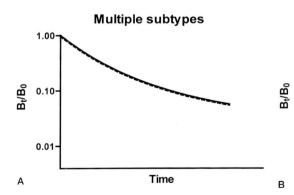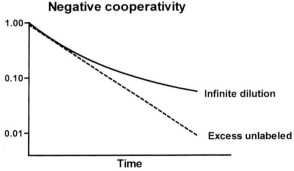

FIG. 4.9. Distinguishing between multiple subtypes *(A)* and negative cooperativity *(B)* by dissociation kinetic strategies. If the binding sites are independent (no cooperativity, *right panel*) the rate of dissociation will be identical when dissociation is initiated by infinite dilution *(solid curve)* or addition of excess unlabeled drug *(dashed curve)*. If the binding sites are cooperative, then the dissociation curve will differ depending on how dissociation was initiated. When

monitoring of the dissociation phase is initiated by adding an excess of unlabeled drug, all of the binding sites are always occupied by either labeled or unlabeled drug. With infinite dilution, there is no rebinding and the number of occupied sites decreases over time. After radioligand dissociates from one site, the affinity at another site will increase and the observed rate of dissociation will slow.

by unlabeled ligand), dissociation always occurs at the maximal rate and the dissociation will follow an exponential decay with a linear semi-log graph (see Fig. 4.9B). The k_{off} value calculated from the slope will correspond to the K_d of the receptor at maximal occupancy, that is, its lowest affinity state.

Evaluating Allosteric Phenomena

Dissociation experiments also can be used to investigate allosteric regulation of ligand binding by heterotopic agents, that is, agents acting via binding to an allosteric site on the receptor, or to another molecule associated with the receptor. Examples of allosteric regulation include effects of anesthetic agents on binding at the nicotinic cholinergic receptor (3), of Mg^{++} and glycine on glutamate binding to the ligand-gated NMDA receptor–ion channel (11), of monovalent cations on G protein–coupled receptors (6), and of GTP on agonist binding to G protein–coupled receptors due to interaction with receptor-associate heterotrimeric G proteins (15). The nature of the overall experimental design to reveal the existence of allosteric regulation is shown schematically in Figure 4.10. Evaluation of allosteric phenomena is performed as follows:

1. For convenience, radioligand binding is allowed to proceed until steady state is achieved; binding at this time is defined as "time 0" binding.

2. Monitoring of the dissociation phase is initiated by adding excess unlabeled ligand. To be absolutely confident that enough unlabeled agent has been added to prevent rebinding, a higher concentration of the same agent, or another agent known to act at the same binding site, should be tested to assure that it does not accelerate dissociation. At this point in the incubation, the investigator can be reasonably confident that the binding pocket of the receptor under study is fully occupied, either by the radioligand or unlabeled ligand.

3. The putative allosteric modifier is added into one set of tubes, and the rate of dissociation with and without the allosteric agent is compared. Assuming that the allosteric modifier of interest influences receptor affinity for radioligand at least in part by altering k_{off}, the introduction of the modifier into the incubation will change the observed rate of dissociation. Modulators can either increase or decrease the rate, depending on whether they decrease or increase receptor affinity (see Fig. 4.10). This experimental strategy has been exploited in a number of systems, but with particular success in characterizing the multiple, independent allosteric sites that exist on voltage-gated Ca^{++} channels for functionally distinct Ca^{2+} channel blockers (5).

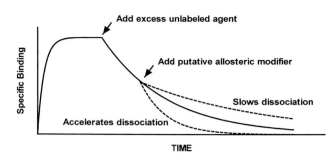

FIG. 4.10. Evaluating allosteric regulation. Radioligand is allowed to bind to a site, and then dissociation begins when an excess of unlabeled agent is added. Addition of an allosteric modified can accelerate or slow the rate of dissociation.

Obtaining Independent Data to Clarify the Biological Origin of Complex Binding Phenomena

When investigators detect complex binding phenomena, it is important to pursue and clarify the biological origins of the complexity. Complex radioligand binding data often result from binding to two or more independent binding sites or to two or more interconvertible affinity states. Independent binding sites usually are the product of distinct genes or of distinct transcripts of a single gene. The proportion of binding to each site, therefore, will differ depending on which tissue or cell line and which subcellular fraction is investigated. The relative proportions may also vary with age or stage of development. Ideally, pharmacological data about receptors with different affinities will match biochemical data about different receptor subtypes.

Complex binding also can result from interconvertible affinity states that are "trapped" in one or another state under the conditions of the incubation. The simplest model would be a receptor that is in equilibrium between two states, R and R*, and the ligand binds to both states of the receptor, but with different affinities. This form of complexity will only be detected before equilibrium is reached, or if the receptors are heterogenous so that not all can make the transition between R or R*. The most studied example of complex binding is the interaction of agonists with receptors linked to G proteins.

Agonist Binding and the Ternary Complex

The extended ternary complex model accounts for the properties of the binding of agonists, antagonists, partial agonists, and inverse agonists as well as data with mutant receptors that stimulate effectors even in the absence of agonist (9, 15). In the extended ternary complex model, the receptor exists in two interconvertible states, R and R* (Fig. 4.11). The latter form preferentially interacts with G proteins, which then are activated to bind GTP, and dissociate into α_{GTP} and $\beta\gamma$ subunits, either of which can stimulate or inhibit effectors. Even without agonist, some receptors can be in the R* form. When this unoccupied R* form associates and activates the G protein, agonist-independent stimulation of the effector occurs, sometimes referred to as basal effector activation. Basal stimulation is blocked by drugs that bind preferentially to the R form, and thus push the equilibrium away from R*. These drugs are known as inverse agonists or negative antagonists. (Basal stimulation is enhanced by receptor structures that stabilize the R* form, that is, agonists.) Recent studies suggest that multiple receptor subtypes in a single receptor family can possess differing degrees of agonist-independent activity (1, 12). In addition, some disease states arise because a receptor mutation has occurred that renders a receptor constitutively active, even in the absence of agonists (9).

In the extended ternary complex model, binding of agonist (or hormone) to a receptor fosters the transition from R to R*. Since only the R* form can interact with a G protein, binding of an agonist indirectly promotes interaction of receptor with the G protein.

The interaction of receptor with G proteins can be studied indirectly by comparing agonist competition curves in the absence and presence of GTP or its hydrolysis resistant analogues GTPγS or Gpp(NH)p. In the absence of GTP, agonist competition curves are usually complex and have shallow slopes. This complexity occurs because some receptors interact with G protein and others do not. It is not known whether this is due to a limited concentration of G protein, heterogeneity in R, or compartmentation in the membrane restricting access of some receptors to G. If all of the receptors were able to interact with G, and G were present in excess, the competitive binding curves would be of normal steepness (slope factor = -1) but with high affinity. In the presence of GTP or one of its analogues, the binding curve is of normal steepness, but manifests a lower affinity. The explanation for these guanine nucleotide–regulated receptor affinity states for agonist is as follows: agonist binds to R and facilitates interaction with G; the G protein lowers its affinity for bound GDP, which dissociates and is replaced by GTP; the G protein complex is unstable and dissociates into its α and $\beta\gamma$ subunits; the receptor is again uncoupled from G. The cycle occurs quickly. Consequently, when GTP or its analogs are present in the incubation, the fraction of receptors coupled to G at any point in time is tiny, so no binding to the high-affinity state is detectable experimentally. Instead, all of the receptors appear to bind agonists with low affinity and are uncoupled from G.

Although the extended ternary complex model has proven to be a very useful conceptual model, it is not very useful for analyzing data, since there are too many variables. Even the simpler ternary complex model where receptors exist in two states (R and RG) has proven to be difficult to use for data analysis. The

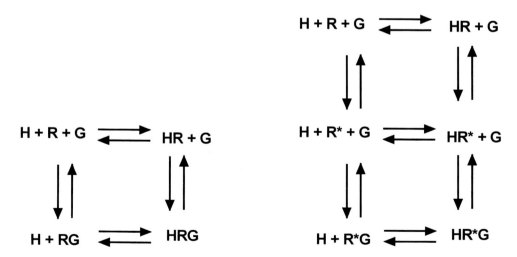

FIG. 4.11. The extended ternary complex model. The *left panel* shows the simple ternary complex model. Receptors can be coupled or uncoupled from G. Agonist or hormone *(H)* binding facilitates the interaction of R with R. The *right panel* shows the extended ternary complex model. Receptors exist in interconvertible R and R* states. Binding of agonist promotes transition to the R* state. Only the R* state can interact with G proteins. (see refs. 9, 15).

extended ternary complex allows for three forms of receptor (R, R*, and R*G) or four (if RG is included too) making it even less useful for day-to-day analyses. Instead, many investigators fit agonist binding data to a simpler model where receptors exist in two nonconvertible affinity states. In this model, in the absence of GTP, some receptors are coupled to a G protein and these have high affinity for agonist. Other receptors are not coupled to a G protein and these have low affinity for agonists. This model (which the Ligand program is based upon (13)) is very simplistic, as it does not allow the coupling of receptors to a G protein to be altered by agonist binding. Since we know that agonist receptor–G interactions are more complicated than this, the high- and low-affinity dissociation constants estimated from these competitive bind experiments performed in the absence or presence of guanine nucleotides should be considered to be empirical descriptions of the data, and should not be thought of as true molecular equilibrium dissociation constants.

As emphasized above, the properties of agonist binding to G protein–coupled receptors often are explored by evaluating the interaction of agonist with the receptor through competitive binding for a radiolabeled antagonist. An alternative is to study the binding of radiolabeled agonist directly. In many cases, the lower affinity interaction of agonist with receptors cannot be observed in direct agonist binding, since the dissociation rate from the lower affinity state is too fast and binding does not persist through the steps used to separate bound and free ligand. In these circumstances, measurements of radiolabeled agonist binding only detect the higher affinity binding of receptors coupled to G proteins. Adding GTP (or other guanine nucleotides) will reduce the number of receptors in this state and will thus reduce steady state binding or accelerate the dissociation of radiolabeled agonist measured using kinetic strategies (see Fig. 4.10). These strategies can be used to test whether ligand binding to a receptor is influenced by guanine nucleotides, thus suggesting the possibility that the receptor of interest elicits its effects via heterotrimeric G proteins as signal transducers.

SUMMARY

This chapter has attempted to provide an overview of the means for receptor identification based on characterization of receptor-mediated functional responses and direct identification by radioligand binding. Criteria for confirming that the radioligand binding detected indeed reflects interaction with the physiological receptor of interest are outlined, as are the methods for determining receptor affinity and density. Binding data do not always follow the expectations for binding to a single receptor population with unchanging affinity for ligand. Means for analyzing complex binding data as well as for determining, using both steady state and kinetic strategies, if the complexity is due to multiple independent receptor populations, interchangeable affinity states, negative cooperativity, or allosteric modulation are described. Hopefully these insights will be of value in fully characterizing the already-identified receptors discussed in the other chapters of this volume, as well as for revealing the existence of novel receptor populations.

REFERENCES

1. Barker, E. L., R. S. Westphal, D. Schmidt, and E. Sanders-Bush. Constitutively active 5-hydroxytryptamine 2c receptors reveal novel inverse agonist activity of receptor ligands. *J. Biol. Chem.* 260: 11607–11690, 1994.
2. Cheng, Y. and W. H. Prusoff. Relationship between the inhibition constant (K_i) and the concentration of an inhibitor that causes a 50% inhibition (I_{50}) of an enzymatic reaction. *Biochem. Pharmacol.* 22: 3099–3108, 1973.
3. Cohen, J. B., M. Weber, J -P. Changeaux. Effects of local anesthetics and calcium on the interaction of cholinergic ligands with the nicotinic receptor protein from *Torpedo marmorata*. *Mol. Pharmacol.* 10: 904–932, 1974.
4. DeLean, A., A. A. Hancock, and R. J. Lefkowitz. Validation and statistical analysis of the computer modeling method for quantitative analysis of radioligand binding data for mixtures of pharmacological subtypes. *Mol. Pharmacol.* 21: 5–16, 1982.
5. Garcia, M. L., V. F. King, P. K. S. Siegl, J. P. Reuben, and G. J. Kaczorowski. Binding of Ca^{++} entry blockers to cardiac sarcolemmal membrane vesicles: Characterization of diltiazem-binding sites and their interaction with dihydropyridine and aralkylamine receptors. *J. Biol. Chem.* 261: 8146–8157, 1986.
6. Horstman, D. A., S. Brandon, A. L. Wilson, C. A. Guyer, E. J. Cragoe, Jr., and L. E. Limbird. An aspartate conserved among G protein–coupled receptors confers allosteric regulation of α_2-adrenergic receptors by sodium. *J. Biol. Chem.* 365(35): 21590–21595, 1990.
7. Kenakin, R. P., R. A. Bond, and T. I. Bonner. Definition of pharmacological receptors. *Pharm. Rev.* 44: 351–362, 1992.
8. Klotz, I. M. and D. L. Hunston. Mathematical models for ligand-receptor binding: Real sites, ghost sites. *J. Biol. Chem.* 259: 10060–10062, 1984.
9. Lefkowitz, R. J., S. Cotecchia, P. Samama, and T. Costa. Constitutive activity of receptors coupled to guanine nucleotide regulatory proteins. *Trends Pharmacol. Sci.* 14: 303–307, 1993.
10. Limbird, L. E. *Cell Surface Receptors: A Short Course on Theory and Methods,* Second Edition. Boston: Kluwer Academic Publishers, 1996.
11. Monaghan, D. T., H. J. Olverman, L. Nguyen, and J. C. Watkins. Two classes of N-methyl-D-aspartate recognition sites and differential distribution and differential regulation by glycine. *Proc. Natl. Acad. Sci. USA* 85: 9836–9840, 1988.
12. Prezeau, L., J. Gomez, S. Ahern, S. Mary, T. Galvez, J. Bockaert, and J -P. Pin. Changes in the carboxyl-terminal domain of metabotropic glutamate receptor 1 by alternative splicing gener-

ates receptors with differing agonist-independent activity. *Mol. Pharmacol.* 49: 422–429, 1996.

13. Rodbard, D. A graphic method for the determination and presentation of binding parameters in complex systems. *Anal. Biochem.* 20: 525–532, 1973.

14. Rosenthal, H. E. A graphic method for the determination and presentation of binding parameters in complex systems. *Anal. Biochem.* 20: 525–532, 1967.

15. Samama, P., S. Cotecchia, T. Costa, and R. J. Lefkowitz. A mutation-induced activated state of the β_2-adrenergic receptor: extending the ternary complex model. *J. Biol. Chem.* 268: 4625–4636, 1993.

16. Scatchard, G. The attractions of proteins for small molecules and ions. *Ann. N.Y. Acad. Sci.* 51: 660–672, 1949.

17. Schild, H. O. pA, a new scale for the measurement of drug antagonism. *Brit. J. Pharm.* 2: 189–206, 1947.

18. Simons, S. S., Jr. and W. B. Pratt. Glucocorticoid receptor thiols and steroid-binding activity. *Methods Enzymol.* 257: 406–422, 1995.

19. Sklar, L. Signal transduction and ligand-receptor dynamics in the human neutrophil. Transient response and occupancy-response relations at the formyl peptide receptor. *J. Biol. Chem.* 260: 1461–1467, 1985.

20. Stephenson, R. P. A modification of receptor theory. *Br. J. Pharm.* 11: 379–393, 1956.

21. Swillens, S. Interpretation of binding curves obtained with high receptor concentrations; practical aid for computer analysis. *Mol. Pharmacol.* 47: 1197–1203, 1985.

5. Mediation of secretory cell function by G protein–coupled receptors

PIERRE-MARIE LLEDO | C.N.R.S., Institut A. Fessard, Gif-sur-Yvette, France

ROBERT ZOREC
MARJAN RUPNIK | Institute of Pathophysiology, School of Medicine, Ljubljana, Slovenia

W. T. MASON | Department of Molecular Signalling, Babraham Institute, Babraham, Cambridge, United Kingdom

CHAPTER CONTENTS

THE EUKARYOTIC CELL is divided into a number of compartments bounded by membranes, including the nuclear envelope, endoplasmic reticulum, Golgi apparatus, lysosomes, various classes of endosomes, and a number of still poorly defined organelles. Membranes compartmentalize but also isolate cells from their immediate environment. The process of exocytosis is an important means to overcome such isolation since secretory products may be released into the external milieu through both constitutive and regulated secretion.

It is now well known that the flow of material through successive organelles of the secretory and endocytotic pathways is mediated by transport vesicles. These lipid vesicles are formed by budding of "donor" compartments and are precisely targeted to the membrane of the "acceptor" compartment, with which they fuse. Clearly, membrane fusion must be a specific and carefully controlled process, otherwise the vesicle "cargo" will be delivered to an incorrect acceptor compartment. Such a situation would destroy the highly differentiated, compartmentalized structure of the eukaryotic cell and disrupt the ordered, vectorial, sequential processing and trafficking of newly synthesized products. The means by which eukaryotic cells achieve such a degree of fidelity has been recently the topic of intense investigations which have highlighted the role of low molecular weight GTPases. Their functions depend on their ability to alternate between inactive and active forms and on their localization. Through these functions, they have been proposed to ensure fidelity in the process of docking and/or fusion of vesicles with their correct acceptor compartment.

The patch–clamp technique offers a number of tools to study the signal pathways involved in regulated secretion. First, it allows the recording of whole-cell currents that are involved in the control of the internal calcium concentration ($[Ca^{2+}]_i$). Second, in favorable cases it provides an assay for the secretory process itself through membrane capacitance measurements by providing direct measurement of surface area. The technique has such high-quality resolution that fusion events of even single vesicles can be recorded. Thirdly, it is readily combined with the measurement of $[Ca^{2+}]_i$ by the calcium indicator dyes (that is, Fura-2, Indo-1, Fluo-3). Finally, it allows introduction of solutions of known composition into the cell interior, since there is rapid diffusional exchange between a patch pipette milieu and a small cell compartment, in the tight-seal whole-cell recording configuration (49).

Recent work has established that despite the high degree of specialization, secretory vesicle membrane traffic shares many basic properties with other intracellular membrane pathways. In the following sections, we will discuss the molecular mechanisms by which exocytosis may be regulated in anterior pituitary and chromaffin cells. From these data, a concrete relationship between constitutive and triggered exocytosis can be established showing that secretory mechanisms are evolutionarily well conserved and therefore that universal biochemical mechanisms underlie aspects of constitutive and regulated membrane fusion. However, our data also demonstrate that this ubiquitous process can be well adapted to the cell physiology and therefore could have very different functions in different cell types (for reviews covering various aspects of vesicular trafficking, readers are also referred to the following: 7, 12, 38, 61, 64, 70, 76, 77).

THE IMPACT OF MOLECULAR BIOLOGY ON CELL PHYSIOLOGY

The traditional genetic approach to regulation of protein expression involves chemicals or radiation to delete or alter genes randomly. The treated organisms or cells and their progeny can then be observed, and mutated individuals that display characteristics of interest to the experimentalist can be used. This approach has been tremendously successful with microorganisms, some plants, and certain invertebrate animals but less successful with vertebrates. Because of the long generation times and because most intriguing mutations are usually lethal, traditional genetic mutation studies are poorly suited to studies of vertebrates. Another shortcoming of any genetic approach is that the observable effect of a mutation may not reveal precisely the mechanisms of the mutation.

With the advent in the past decade of technology for cloning genes, it is now possible to turn off or to modify the activity of targetted genes. One method, using antisense oligonucleotides, is in principle, remarkably simple. The basic idea of antisense approaches is to interfere with the information flow from gene to protein, and in a very specific manner. Briefly, reagents that bind to single- or double-stranded nucleic acids are potential candidates for powerful tools targeted at specific genes; at the level of either messenger RNA (mRNA) or double-stranded DNA. Using oligo-

deoxynucleotides in antisense orientation (antisense DNA) leads to hybridization with specific mRNA, and an RNA duplex is formed. This duplex is either rapidly degraded, it may impair mRNA nuclear processing, or it may specifically block the translation into protein (see ref. 87). Such a strategy was inspired by naturally occurring antisense RNA molecules first found in viruses and bacteria, which regulate some genes during their life cycles. Today, such an approach is straightforward enough for investigators to apply antisense probes as tools to a broad range of problems.

The purpose of this paper is thus to present an experimental strategy employing antisense oligodeoxynucleotide molecules in combination with patch–clamp techniques to assign biological function of GTP-binding proteins in calcium entry and in control of exocytotic machinery of adenohypophyseal cells.

SECRETORY CELL PHYSIOLOGY

Adenohypophyseal cells secrete a number of hormones controlling bodily functions including growth, lactation in mammals, responses to stress, and reproduction. Lactotrophs secrete prolactin; corticotrophs, adrenocorticotropic hormone (ACTH); gonadotrophs, luteinizing and follicle stimulating hormones; melanotrophs, β-endorphin, α-melanocyte stimulating hormone, and other peptides; and somatotrophs, growth hormone. Most of these secretory cell types are triggered to release hormones following binding of bloodborne hypothalamic factors to the plasmalemma. In addition, the activity of melanotrophs is controlled by neuromodulators and transmitters released from innervating nerve terminals (for a review, see ref. 8). It has been thought for more than 30 yrs that the events following the occupancy of plasma membrane receptors involve a change in cytosolic calcium homeostasis leading to augmented exocytosis of secretory granules. This primary response may be modulated at two levels—(1) at the site of calcium entry and (2) at the site of exocytosis—but detailed knowledge about the molecular events is fragmental, since the major obstacle to elucidation of these mechanisms is the relative inaccessibility of the cytosol, especially if we consider studying responses at cellular level. In this paper, experiments performed mainly on lactotrophs are reviewed. This cell can be separated from other cell types employing sedimentation techniques (34, 35) and cultured by standard techniques. Rat melanotrophs, on the other hand, can easily be separated by dissecting anatomically defined pars intermedia, which consists mainly of melanotrophs [> 95% of cells are melanotrophs (see ref. 47)].

MECHANISMS OF ACTION OF ANTISENSE OLIGONUCLEOTIDES

Antisense RNA molecules were initially used to inactivate specific genes such as mutations could, but with a higher selectivity (for a review see ref. 89). However, antisense RNA are not the only antisense molecules that can hybridize with messenger RNA and prevent the translation of protein. Short complementary strands of DNA can also hybridize with messenger RNA. Antisense oligodeoxynucleotides, strands of DNA only 12–20 bases long, can be introduced into cells where they will have inhibitory effects on information flow similar to those of antisense RNA. Antisense DNA technology, which was used before the development of antisense RNAs, was first applied in an attempt to inhibit Rous sarcoma virus from transforming cultured chicken cells into a cancerous state (91).

There are several points one has to consider before using antisense oligodeoxynucleotides in experiments (see refs. 15, 18, 73, 83, 87, 88). Briefly, one of these points is selectivity of the oligodeoxynucleotides employed. The specificity of an antisense oligonucleotide depends on its length. The longer an oligonucleotide is, the more likely it is to bind to one and only one DNA or RNA target.

The action of oligodeoxynucleotides can be explained by traditional receptor theory. The affinity of oligodeoxynucleotides for their nucleic acids receptor results from hybridization interactions that depend upon hydrogen bonding and base stacking in the double helix that is formed. A minimum level of affinity is required for the desired specific interaction and this can be achieved with an oligodeoxynucleotide that is 11–15 nucleotides in length (15). Computational approaches have been designed (see refs. 75, 85) to help predict antisense oligodeoxynucleotide efficacy; however, it is imperative that every oligonucleotide sequence is checked for similarities with other sequences present in gene databases.

LIFETIMES OF ANTISENSE PROBES IN LIVING CELLS

An additional point to be considered is the stability of these compounds since the half-life of the oligodeoxynucleotide probe should exceed that of the targeted protein to be effective. The stability of the duplex increases with oligomer length (48). However, in general, work from many laboratories has demonstrated that phosphodiester oligodeoxynucleotides are rapidly degraded [within less than 1 h (see ref. 15)]. For this, a wide range of modifications of the oligodeoxynucleotide backbone has been introduced to increase stability.

For example, phosphorothiorate oligodeoxynucleotide probes (sulfur atoms substituted for oxygen atoms in the sugar phosphate backbone) have half-lifs of more than 24 h in serum media and inside cells (15). There are also nonionic methylphosphonate analogues which are extremely stable to nucleases but more easily enter the cytosol in comparison to the charged oligodeoxynucleotides.

ANTISENSE SITES OF ACTION

The site of action of oligodeoxynucleotides is intracellular. The mechanism of uptake of oligodeoxynucleotides is largely unknown but it may involve endocytosis (see ref. 15). The concentration of oligodeoxynucleotides administered may be toxic to cells. Under in vitro conditions, the addition of oligodeoxynucleotides to the extracellular medium or intracellular injection may be toxic if the concentration is above about 10 μM (see ref. 15). When these probes are injected into cells by the patch–clamp technique, effective concentrations are a few orders of magnitude below toxicity (see below). Thus the patch–clamp approach is an attractive technique to administer specific oligodeoxynucleotides intracellularly.

The oligodeoxynucleotide strategy clearly has a number of important advantages, but there are also disadvantages (88). Apart from occasional nonspecific or toxic actions, the greatest drawback may be the incomplete effect of oligodeoxynucleotide treatment. For example, if a biological function requires only a few molecules for a full response, but in the cell these are synthesized redundantly, oligodeoxynucleotide treatment may result as "functionally" silent.

The mechanisms of potential antisense oligonucleotide interactions with target nucleic acids are complex, possibly relating to many sites along the sequence of events leading from DNA to protein synthesis, and this is beyond the scope of this review (see refs. 15, 88). We focus mainly on the experimental use of antisense oligodeoxynucleotide targeted to a messenger RNA. Figure 5.1 shows the possible mechanisms by which the association of a messenger RNA with a complementary sequence could specifically block the synthesis of the encoded protein. Most of the results obtained with antisense DNA were explained by the RNase–H activity known to induce hydrolysis of messenger RNA binding to DNA (Fig. 5.1) (15). In the nucleus, this enzyme cleaves the RNA moiety of DNA/RNA hybrids during DNA replication. In the antisense approach, the cleaved messenger RNA no longer supports translation, whereas the antisense DNA will act catalytically for the RNase-H activity by binding to messenger RNA,

.1) Induction of mRNA hydrolysis

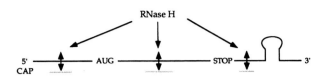

2) Blockade of translation by ribosomes

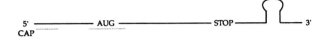

3) Modification of the mRNA metabolism

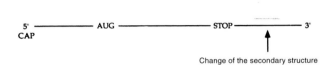

Change of the secondary structure

4) Duplex mRNA not exported from the nucleus

FIG. 5.1. Mechanisms of action of antisense oligonucleotides. The antisense oligodeoxynucleotide probes are illustrated by the shaded lines, AUG is the initiation codon, and STOP is the stop codon of a targeted messenger RNA. *(1)* Inhibition of target protein production may be initiated by RNase-H cleavage of hybridized mRNA. RNaseH acts as an amplifier of the antisense action since it cleaves only duplex mRNA, and not antisense DNA, which can therefore induce the degradation of multiple transcript. It is noteworthy that the majority of modified oligonucleotides is unable to elicit RNase-H activity. *(2)* Physical block of the translation by impeding the binding of the initiation complex that scans the 5' leader of the MRNA. It has been claimed that CAP and AUG regions constitute the best targets for antisense oligonucleotides. *(3)* By changing the secondary structure of the messenger RNA, the antisense probe may induce an increase in messenger RNA degradation. *(4)* The duplex mRNA can no longer be exported from the nucleus. Note that mechanism 2 would not affect the total level of mRNA in the cytosol.

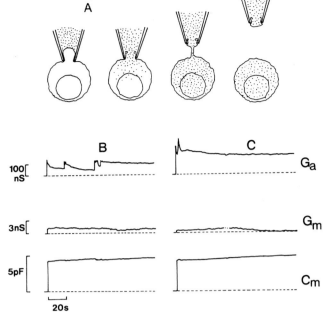

FIG. 5.2. *(A)* Diagrammatic representation showing establishment of a cell-attached recording and a whole-cell recording by the patch–clamp technique. Antisense probe molecules are depicted as dots in the recording pipette lumen. Note the diffusional exchange of these molecules upon establishing whole-cell recording (removal of the membrane around the rim of pipette tip). Withdrawal of the pipette results in trapping of the antisense molecules inside the cytoplasm. *(B)* Time-dependent changes in membrane capacitance (C_m), parallel combination of leak and membrane conductance (G_a), and access conductance (G_m). Pipette solution contained 2.7×10^{-8} pM N63 antisense probe. Bathing solution consisted of the following (mM): NaCl (127), KCl (5), $MgCl_2$ (2), $CaCl_2$ (5), NaH_2PO_4 (0.5), $NaHCO_3$ (5), HEPES (10), D-glucose (10), pH 7.25/NaOH. *(C)* Time-dependent changes in C_m., G_a., *and* G_m recorded in the same cell as in B, but 48 h later.

therefore inducing its hydrolysis. Another way to arrest the translation machinery results from a physical block to binding of the initiation complex (the 40S subunit) at the AUG initiation codon or at the region that covered the ribosome binding site, upstream of the initiation codon (close to the cap region) (see Fig. 5.2). Binding of antisense oligodeoxynucleotides may also have two other consequences: an increase in the catabolism rate of the targeted messenger RNA due to a change of its secondary structure (Fig. 5.3) and the arrest of exportation of the messenger RNA from the nucleus to the cytoplasm (Fig. 5.4). A major advantage

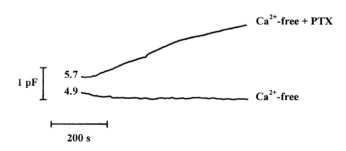

FIG. 5.3. Patch–clamp recordings in a secretory cell. Representative changes in C_m, recorded in a control *(bottom)* and a pertussis toxin pretreated cell (250 ng/ml, 7 h) *(top)*. Pipette and bath solutions as in Rupnik and Zorec (65). The noncompensated method of membrane capacitance measurements was used (44, 92, 93).

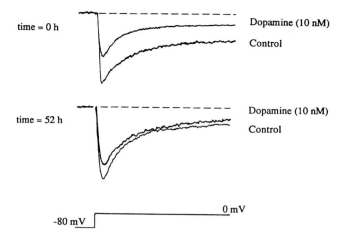

FIG. 5.4. Dopamine-induced responses to voltage-activated calcium current recorded during and after loading a lactotroph cell with an antisense oligonucleotide probe directed to messenger RNA α_O. The voltage-activated calcium current was recorded under the same experimental conditions as in Table I. Compare the slight reduction (10%) in calcium current induced by dopamine, 52 h after antisense loading, with the 55% decrease at time 0.

of this antisense oligodeoxynucleotide approach is that the simple synthesis and testing of a number of oligodeoxynucleotides enable a screening process before their use. A "trial-and-error" approach must be performed to determine whether translated messenger RNA regions (including among them the initiation codon) as well as 5' (for example, capping-region)- or 3'-untranslated messenger RNA regions can be targeted. Most of our antisense oligodeoxynucleotides (nonmodified) have been designed to bind to the translation initiation codon or its immediate vicinity after having tested them in vitro.

THE WHOLE CELL PATCH–CLAMP TECHNIQUE AND LOADING CELLS WITH ANTISENSE OLIGONUCLEOTIDE PROBES

The introduction of patch–clamp techniques a decade ago (30) provided new possibilities to study single-cell membrane conductances by measuring currents through single channels and through whole-cell membranes (49). The consequence of exocytosis is a net change in surface area, which can be monitored by whole-cell membrane capacitance (Cm) measurements. The electrical capacity of the cell membrane is linearly related to the surface of the membrane (56). Since the membrane surface area increases upon exocytotic addition of vesicular membrane, electrical capacitance is useful in monitoring exocytotic secretion. Thus secre-

tory activity of single cells can be monitored by the patch–clamp technique. The sensitivity of this technique also allows detection of interactions between single secretory organelles and plasmalemma (56, 94). Importantly, an advantage of the patch–clamp techniques is that it provides the means to introduce substances into the cytosol. Molecules, ions, peptides, antibodies, and oligonucleotides, putatively interfering with cytosolic processes, can be dissolved in the pipette-filling solution, and upon the formation of the whole-cell configuration the diffusional barrier between pipette lumen and cytosol is eliminated, allowing an exchange of substances between cytosol and pipette lumen (49, 63, 68).

However, a word of caution is required. Loading large quantities of high molecular weight substances may be impractical since cellular constituents can be lost into the pipette.

In this paper we describe the loading of low molecular weight compounds (2–10 kD) as well as high molecular weight antibodies (over 100 kD) into single cells using the patch–pipette. For example, loading of antisense probes into adenohypophyseal cells can be accomplished by filling the pipette with a solution containing an antisense probe, and by establishing a whole-cell recording for a period of time as shown in Figure 5.2A.

Antisense probes used in most of our work have molecular weights between 6300 and 6600, and it can be estimated that over 11,000 molecules of N63 antisense probe were loaded into the cytoplasm at the end of the 128-s whole-cell recording displayed in Figure 5.2B. At the end of the recording the pipette was removed and the cell membrane resealed. The location of the loaded cell is marked by cutting the bottom of the plastic petri dish with the patch–pipette to identify it and later reexamine it electrophysiologically after a period of time (6–110 h). During this time the interaction between the injected probe and the translation machinery is allowed to take place. After the loading procedure, petri dishes with loaded cells are placed in an incubator and the bathing medium for electrophysiological measurements is replaced with standard culture medium supplemented by antibiotics.

After incubation for hours or days, loaded cells are used in the second electrophysiological experiment, as shown in Figure 5.2C. A second successful recording can usually be obtained in 25% of loaded cells. About half of the loaded cells are lost in the washing of petri dishes with culture and bathing media. Our results suggest that the double-patching procedure, and loading by antisense probes, did not affect the passive electrophysiological parameters of recorded cells.

ANTISENSE OLIGONUCLEOTIDES ASSIGN G PROTEIN SUBTYPES IN THE COUPLING OF DOPAMINE RECEPTORS TO IONIC CHANNELS

Although thought to be involved primarily in the regulation of second-messenger systems, it has become evident that G proteins also are intimately involved in the regulation of ion channels (31, 32, 41). Dopamine receptors are seven transmembrane-segment proteins, and so they are believed to activate heterotrimeric G proteins to achieve their cellular effects. Therefore, G protein activation is likely to be the first step in dopamine-elicited ion channel modulation. G proteins may subsequently interact directly with a given channel in a "membrane delimited" manner. On the other hand, they may also activate an intracellular pathway that secondarily modifies the parameters of ion channel function. The multiplicity of G proteins and other molecules belonging to corresponding signalling pathways is vast and could account for the pleiotropic action of any transmitter to which they are connected (32).

MODELS FOR THE STUDY OF REGULATED SECRETORY EVENTS

The adenohypophysis is an endocrine tissue composed of different cells secreting a variety of hormones. These are stored within the cells in dense core granules and are released by appropriate stimuli. In addition to dense core granules, anterior pituitary cells contain small translucent vesicles, which are very similar to synaptic vesicles not only in their morphological appearance but also with regard to their protein constituents (36, 77). For example, chromogranins and secretogranins found in secretory granules and small vesicles of endocrine cells, have also been detected in their neuronal counterparts (for a review, see ref. 72). It is also noteworthy that membrane proteins from synaptic vesicles such as synaptotagmin, a calcium sensor protein (quoted ref. 72, p. 65), have also been found associated with secretory granule membranes. All of these findings indicate that neurons and endocrine cells are very similar with respect to the composition of their characteristic small vesicles and large secretory granules besides having a variety of molecular, biochemical, and functional similarities (29). Such similarities in the molecular machinery for secretion suggest that processes responsible for secretion of neurotransmitters and hormones are likely to have evolved from the trafficking machinery that controls secretion in more simple cells such as in yeast (9, 64).

PACKAGING AND STORAGE IN DIFFERENT SECRETORY ORGANELLES

There is abundant evidence that small-molecule transmitters are located in vesicles (see refs. 38, 74, 77 for reviews). Vesicular stores constitute a large reserve of transmitter that is protected from intracellular catabolism. These vesicles may contain small-molecule transmitters or neuroactive peptides. Because these latter are synthesized as secretory products, it can be assumed that essentially all of the peptides within an endocrine cell or a neuron are packaged within vesicles. Unlike small-molecule transmitters, none of these peptides are synthesized in the cytosol and no mechanism for regulating their cytoplasmic concentration need exist. The absence of specific enzymes for controlling the intracellular store of these messengers is an important feature.

The means by which secretory vesicles acquire their contents is different between vesicles and granules. Packaging into synaptic vesicles is performed from cytoplasmic pools, hence synaptic vesicle membranes contain (1) electrogenic proton pumps making the inside positive with respect to the outside (24), and (2) chloride channels which dissipate the membrane potential and allow the build-up of an acidic environment inside the vesicles (78). The electrochemical gradient generated by the proton pump drives the accumulation of transmitters via several classes of neurotransmitter transporter. Therefore, after releasing their contents, the secretory vesicles reform and fill with transmitter from the cytoplasmic pools.

On the other hand, since secretory granules contain protein, they cannot refill in the cytoplasm after undergoing exocytosis. Hence, packaging into secretory granules occurs in the cytoplasm rather than at the trans Golgi network.

MEMBRANE CAPACITANCE REVEALS EXOCYTOTIC AND ENDOCYTOTIC ACTIVITIES

Incorporation of membrane vesicles into the plasma membrane is a consequence of the process of exocytosis. As a result, the total cell surface may increase concomitantly with the secretory activity, depending on the number of fusing vesicles and the respective rate of both exocytotic membrane fusion and endocytotic membrane retrieval. Therefore, one may estimate the secretory activity of a single cell by quantifying the cell membrane capacitance that is proportional to the membrane surface area.

As early as 1776, long before the nature of electricity was understood, the English physicist, Henry Cavendish, wondered whether the thin membranes of the cells in the electric organ of *Torpedo* (the electric ray) might not function like the glass walls of Leiden jars, which were used at that time to store electricity. Today, we know that because cell membranes are able to maintain a difference of electrical potential, they exhibit the property of electrical capacitance. Depending on the desired resolution, various methods can be used to assess membrane capacitance: *(1)* the pseudo-random binary sequence technique uses the transfer function of a given stimulation to obtain membrane capacitance (21); *(2)* the time-domain technique determines capacitance from the current relaxation in response to a voltage step (44); and *(3)* the two-phase lock-in amplifier technique derives passive membrane parameters by delivering a sinusoidal voltage command and measuring the resulting current response at two orthogonal phases (56). Only the last of these methods allows capacitance to be monitored in real time whilst providing the highest resolution.

Measurements of C_m have been applied to the investigation of the influence of $[Ca^{2+}]_i$ on exocytosis of cultured lactotrophs (92, 93). Intracellular $[Ca^{2+}]$ was modified by either dialyzing the cytosol with different calcium-containing pipette solutions or changing the membrane potential. High calcium resulted in a large C_m increase demonstrating a role for $[Ca^{2+}]_i$ in stimulus-secretion coupling as previously suggested in pituitary cells (79). Tonic calcium influx through voltage-gated calcium channels, seen to occur at resting membrane potential, was found to play a major role in secretory activity monitored by C_m.

More recently, a number of other signaling pathways have been suggested to modulate hormonal release from pituitary cells. In gonadotropes, breakdown of polyphosphoinositides induces calcium oscillations which trigger rhythmic exocytosis (84). In lactotrophs, cAMP was found to increase the magnitude and rate of calcium-induced exocytosis. In contrast, cAMP had no detectable effect on C_m when intracellular calcium was low (69). It can therefore be concluded that cAMP facilitates calcium-induced secretion by acting directly on the secretory apparatus of anterior pituitary cells. The role of GTP-binding proteins on calcium-induced exocytosis has also been investigated in lactotrophs using nonhydrolyzable GTP analogues (GTP-γ-S and GMP-PNP) to irreversibly activate all GTPases. In this way, two distinct effects of G protein activation could be distinguished: the maximum C_m increase due to intracellular calcium injection was diminished, while the rate of C_m increase $\Delta C_m/\Delta t$ was facilitated, revealing a converse stimulatory role of G proteins in the translocation of secretory granules to the fusion sites (67).

HOMEOSTASIS OF THE INTRACELLULAR-FREE CALCIUM CONCENTRATION

Among intracellular processes that regulate $[Ca^{2+}]_i$, calcium-binding proteins play a central role because of their high and fast buffering capacity, their relatively high mobility within the cytoplasm, and their high affinity for calcium. In this respect, parvalbumin and the M_r 28,000 protein calbindin-D_{28K} are believed to play an important role in controlling $[Ca^{2+}]_i$ (14). We have used calbindin-transfected GH_3 cell lines to examine the effect of calbindin on ionic channel activities and $[Ca^{2+}]_i$ homeostasis. Because ionic channel activities are very susceptible to alterations during the whole-cell recording technique, the patch was perforated with the pore-forming antibiotic nystatin (33) in these experiments to enable recording of ionic currents. This allowed us to measure ionic currents and $[Ca^{2+}]_i$ levels simultaneously, without outward diffusion of cytoplasmic constituents and without introducing alien calcium buffers into the cell. Thus, we were able to measure calcium entry through voltage-sensitive calcium channels and to assess simultaneously the $[Ca^{2+}]_i$ level. Interestingly, only about 1/100th of the calcium influx through the plasma membrane of anterior pituitary cells was seen as free calcium at the peak of the $[Ca^{2+}]_i$ transient, revealing that most of the calcium (>99%) that enters through calcium channels binds to endogenous calcium buffers.

This percentage is in reasonable agreement with the value used by Smith and Zucker (71) to fit arsenazo III signals in *Aplysia* neurons. We have also examined the direct effects of introducing purified calbindin and other synthetic products known to be calcium buffers, by recording responses in the whole-cell configuration. Our findings from these different experimental approaches indicate that the presence of calbindin affects both calcium influx through voltage-dependent calcium channels and $[Ca^{2+}]_i$ homeostasis. Therefore, this protein exhibits the characteristics of both a "buffer" protein, by binding internal calcium, and a "trigger" protein by affecting calcium-regulating proteins such as calcium channels or the plasma membrane Ca^{2+}/Mg^{2+}-ATPase. Through such a dual effect, calcium-binding proteins may play an important role in regulating exocytosis, and could act as molecular switches whose "on" and "off" states are triggered by binding and release of calcium. Conserved structure and mechanism in myriad versions of the switch (from bacteria to vertebrates) suggest that they all derive from a single primordial protein, repeatedly modified in the course of evolution to perform a large variety of functions.

As reported above, the role of calcium release from internal pools has recently been demonstrated to regulate exocytosis in anterior pituitary cells. Tse and colleagues have shown that gonadotropin-releasing hormone induced the rhythmic release of calcium from an inositol 1,4,5–triphosphate (IP$_3$)-sensitive store, in pituitary gonadotropes (84). Exocytosis measured in single gonadotropes revealed that each elevation of $[Ca^{2+}]_i$ induced a burst of exocytosis. From this finding, it was concluded that agonist-induced oscillations of $[Ca^{2+}]_i$ in secretory cells may be a mechanism to optimize the secretory output while avoiding the toxic effects of sustained elevation of $[Ca^{2+}]_i$.

THE EXOCYTOTIC MACHINERY IS REGULATED BY INTRACELLULAR CALCIUM CONCENTRATION

The role of the intracellular calcium concentration in secretion from endocrine cells has been studied in three ways: *(1)* the effect of elevated $[Ca^{2+}]_i$ on secretion rate has been measured in permeabilized cells (4, 26); *(2)* the average $[Ca^{2+}]_i$ has been assessed during secretion triggered by depolarization or release of calcium from internal stores and finally, *(3)* the secretion stimulated by perfusion of cells with solutions of different calcium concentrations through a whole-cell patch pipette has been monitored. These studies have shown that there is a threshold level of peak $[Ca^{2+}]_i$ for hormone release to occur. More interestingly, the release of hormones and neurotransmitters has been found to be linearly related to the time integral of $[Ca^{2+}]_i$ elevation above this threshold (60).

With dialysis and perfusion of calcium buffers, the rate of secretion achieved for a given $[Ca^{2+}]_i$ is substantially less pronounced than that observed in response to a brief depolarization. This could be taken to indicate that depolarizing pulses open calcium channels such that $[Ca^{2+}]_i$ is locally elevated near release sites to levels substantially higher than the average $[Ca^{2+}]_i$ recorded with photometric techniques. Consistent with such a hypothesis, even at high cytoplasmic $[Ca^{2+}]_i$ (300–1000 nM), secretion rates during dialysis always remained clearly lower than those obtained during voltage pulses. Several other means of rapidly elevating $[Ca^{2+}]_i$ also yield higher secretion rates. Conversely, the total amount of secretion is always much larger with calcium dialysis than with rapid calcium elevation using caged calcium ions or depolarization-induced calcium entry. These observations may be related to the existence of multiple pools of hormone, that is, a relatively small, rapidly releasable pool and a larger reserve pool. In this respect, both movement of vesicles between pools and secretion have recently been shown to be sensitive to the intracellular calcium level (57, 80, 81).

THE ROLE OF SMALL GTP-BINDING PROTEINS IN EXOCYTOSIS

The superfamily of Ras-related small GTP-binding proteins has been found to regulate a large spectrum of elementary cellular processes. Among them, the *Rab* gene subfamily have in common not only their structural features, but also their ability to regulate intracellular vesicle traffic and sorting at the plasma membrane (62, 86).

By analogy with other guanine nucleotide-binding proteins, the Rab proteins are considered inactive in their GDP-bound form. This form is stabilized by guanine nucleotide dissociation inhibitors (GDI). Upon stimulation by a guanine nucleotide releasing protein (GNRP), the GDP is exchanged for GTP, and the Rab proteins switch to their active, GTP-bound form. This state is quasi-irreversible until the Rab proteins hydrolyze the bound GTP to GDP, this effect being stimulated by a GTPase activating protein (GAP). Thus, the proteins become inactivated, allowing the process to be repeated. Hence, as with other G proteins, Rab proteins behave as molecular switches cycling from an active (GTP-bound) to an inactive (GDP-bound) conformation (10, 28). Since the general role of G proteins is to control the specificity and the temporal coherence of intermolecular recognition processes, it is very likely that Rab proteins act as regulators of vesicular targeting from an upstream to a downstream compartment.

SEC4 is a protein present on the membrane vesicles in yeast known to control exocytosis (27, 66). A search for the mammalian counterparts of SEC4 has led to the identification of a large number of Ras-related proteins termed Rab proteins (for "Ras-like proteins from rat brain").

It is now clear that each Rab family member has distinct subcellular locations within cells and most of the organelles involved in exocytosis or endocytosis possess at least one distinct member (13, 77). Depending essentially upon the sequence of their C-terminus, each member of the Rab protein family seems to be associated with a particular vesicular compartment (see ref. 62 for a review). In addition, a posttranslational isoprenylation of cysteine residues at the C-terminus of the Rab proteins is required for their functional association with the vesicular membrane (39, 55). Although most of the Rab family members are uniformly distributed in mammalian cells, they could also be involved in more differentiated secretory or compartmentalized processes specific to neurons, endocrine, or epithelial cells. In this respect, it has been reported that Rab3A is specifically expressed in neurons (16, 51, 52), where it could control the recruitment of synaptic vesicles and their fusion with the plasma membrane during exocytosis (22, 23, 58). Other members of the Rab3 subfamily, termed Rab3B and Rab3C (50, 82, 90) are thought to be associated with the membrane of secretory vesicles or granules, although this has not yet been demonstrated. In this respect, we have found that Rab3B is the major form found in rat anterior and intermediate pituitary gland, in contrast to Rab3A which is highly expressed in selected brain areas like hippocampus, cerebellum, or thalamic nuclei (2, 54, 73a). Some overlap expression for Rab3A and Rab3B mRNA also exists in the olfactory tubercle or striatum. More recently, Baldini and colleagues reported the cloning of Rab3D from mouse which is proposed to control insulin-induced exocytosis in adipocytes (6). This latter protein is homologous to the rat Rab16 protein which is mainly expressed in lung but also many other peripheral and neuronal tissues (20). Whether the different Rab3 proteins are functionally identical proteins expressed in different cell types, or proteins associated with different kind of secretory vesicles awaits further investigation.

IDENTIFICATION OF SPECIFIC G PROTEINS CONTROLLING IONIC CHANNEL ACTIVITIES

Several criteria, either direct or indirect, have to be fulfilled to attribute G protein intervention to the modulation of ion channels by receptors. The requirements for a G protein–dependent phenomenon can be explored by injecting into the cell poorly hydrolyzable GTP or GDP analogues. These molecules either activate (GTP-γ-S) or inactivate (GDP-β-S) the G proteins of the cells in a relatively irreversible manner. The use of toxins [cholera toxin (CTX) and *Bordetella pertussis* toxin (PTX)] has also helped to distinguish among several species of G proteins. Cholera toxin activates G_a by ADP-ribosylation, while other G proteins, including G_i and G_i, have been found to be covalently altered by PTX-dependent ADP-ribosylation, resulting in a loss of response to agonist.

Reconstitution experiments using D2 dopamine receptors partially purified from the bovine anterior pituitary demonstrated that different G proteins can be associated with these receptors. Thus, bearing in mind *(1)* the varied signaling systems affected by dopamine receptor activation, *(2)* the diversity of G protein subunits, and *(3)* the implications of both and subunits in multiple physiological functions, the question has arisen which G protein is involved in the specific coupling of dopamine receptor to a particular effector.

Four approaches have recently been employed to address these questions. The first approach is a broad-brush one, using for example PTX to inactivate endogenous G proteins, then testing for a specific function. This approach is often used for initial screening, but because PTX inactivates virtually all G proteins, its use is limited from the standpoint of identifying a role for a specific G protein.

The second approach consists of reconstituting the coupling of receptors to ionic channels using purified G_α subunits after inactivation of endogenous G proteins with PTX (11). However, reconstitution experiments with purified G proteins must be carefully interpreted. One potential shortcoming of these experiments is that the heterogeneity of purified G protein fractions such as these can resist resolution, even after multiple chromatographic steps. Unless the coupled G protein is identified unambiguously, these experiments only give an indication of which protein is capable of mediating the channel response, and not direct evidence of which one mediates the response in the normal cell.

A third approach is the use of specific antibodies to different G proteins which disrupt the link with the receptor (45). The whole-cell recording method affords the advantage of introducing large molecules such as antibodies into the cell. For example, we have used a patch–pipette filled either with polyclonal antibodies raised against purified bovine G_o or with affinity-purified antibodies raised against synthetic decapeptides corresponding to the carboxy-terminal sequence of the subunits of either G_o, G_{i3}, or $G_{i1,2}$.

A fourth approach is the use of antisense oligonucleotides. Oligodeoxynucleotides corresponding to the antisense orientation of messenger RNAs coding for the different G_α subunits can be synthesized and will specifically block the translation of the corresponding message into proteins. The introduction of oligonucleotides into the cells can be accomplished either by microinjection (see for example, refs. 37, 40) or by diffusion from the patch–pipette into the cytoplasm (3, 46). In the latter approach, a sequential patch–clamp procedure allowed recording from the same cell, at several-day intervals, as shown in Figure 5.2A. The advantages over antibody quenching of a target protein function are threefold. First, the risks of channel run-down are much lower with the sequential patch–clamp technique, since an additional 10 min is required for the dialysis of the larger antibody proteins. Second, oligonucleotides are far easier to produce and more specific than antibodies. Finally, distinction between the protein subtypes is greater at the nucleic acid level than in the translated protein subtypes. Further major advantages of the antisense oligodeoxynucleotide strategy is the reversibility of the effect; other advantages include the possibility to study any product of a cloned gene from any species; the low cost to the laboratory, and finally, the fact that little specialized equipment is required.

USE OF PERTUSSIS TOXIN TO IDENTIFY A ROLE FOR G PROTEINS IN CELL FUNCTION

Heterotrimeric GTP-binding proteins may as well play a role in exocytosis (43). However, the characterization of these GTP-binding proteins may prove to be difficult, since there are more than 16 different α subunits of heterotrimeric GTP-binding proteins (10). In addition, as was found for the GTP-binding proteins involved in the control of voltage-gated Ca^{2+} channels, different β subunits bound to α subunits may determine the functional role of the heterotrimeric GTP-binding proteins (40). Aridor et al. (1) have analyzed the pertussis-sensitive (PTX) heterotrimeric GTP-binding proteins in mast cells, as potential G_e candidates, since pertussis toxin pretreatment of these cells inhibits exocytosis. They found an activation of exocytosis by the heterotrimeric GTP-binding protein G_{i3}.

To see whether secretory activity of a single adenohypophyseal cell is sensitive to pertussis toxin, rat melanotrophs were pretreated with PTX (250 ng/ml, 7 h) and recorded secretory responses by monitoring changes in membrane capacitance using the patch–clamp technique (92, 93). As shown in Figure 5.3, in PTX pretreated cells Ca^{2+}-insensitive secretory activity was recorded, suggesting that a step downstream of other calcium-dependent steps requires a PTX-sensitive heterotrimeric GTP-binding protein for vesicle fusion to take place. This activity was blocked by GDP-β-S (65), which indicates that the PTX treatment might lock the heterotrimeric GTP-binding protein in the GTP bound state.

In contrast to nonexcitable cells (1), PTX pretreatment of excitable melanotrophs resulted in increased secretory activity. This may indicate that a PTX sensitive heterotrimeric GTP-binding protein is coupled to the exocytotic control pathway of melanotrophs in a stimulatory sense, whereas in mast cells it may have an inhibitory role.

USE OF ANTISENSE OLIGONUCLEOTIDES TO STUDY α_O-MEDIATED CALCIUM CURRENT RESPONSES TO DOPAMINE IN LACTOTROPH CELLS

The activation of D_2 dopamine receptor in anterior pituitary prolactin-secreting cells (lactotrophs) has been reported to decrease two voltage-activated calcium currents and simultaneously to increase two voltage-activated potassium currents (45). We have used the antisense oligodeoxynucleotide approach to identify the G protein subtypes involved in the coupling of D_2 dopamine receptor with these ionic channels. The antisense oligodeoxynucleotides were complementary to partial cDNA sequences for rat neuroepithelial G protein subunits. These antisense probes were aimed at sequences overlapping the translation initiation site and were designed to maximize the number of mismatches to nontargeted mRNAs. On day 1, lactotrophs in culture were dialyzed with antisense oligodeoxynucleotides (15 nM–1.5 μM) or vehicle (control) by recording voltage-activated calcium current with patch–pipettes in the whole-cell recording mode. The cell dialysis lasted an average of 160 s. The effectiveness and specificity of action of six types of antisense were determined by their effects on the in vitro translation of α_o, α_{i1}, α_{i2}, α_{i3}, and α_s. Figure 5.4 shows that during the loading of cells with antisense DNA directed against the α_o messenger RNA, dopamine application (10 nM) induces a 50% reduction of calcium current, while 52 h later, a second application of dopamine (10 nM) onto the same cell induces only a slight reduction even when the dopamine concentration was raised to 1 μM. This further indicates that the reduction of dopamine efficiency was not due to loss of dopamine receptor affinity to antisense, as the response to dopamine remained slight (about a 10% decrease). The reduced response was not due to nonspecific effects of time or culture conditions, since after vehicle dialysis or loading cells with antisense DNA directed to α_s, α_{i1}, α_{i2}, α_{i3} messenger RNAs, cells respond to a similar extent before and after loading with antisense DNA (see Table 5.1). We have also used scrambled analogues of the presumably active oligodeoxynucleotide molecules, as well as mismatched analogues maintaining the same base composition as the antisense molecule, for more stringent control experiments. Also, an important control for specificity of the active antisense that we used is to identify another nonoverlapping antisense oligodeoxynucleotide able to induce similar inhibition of the dopamine response. To check the effects of "knocking out" the expression of the α_o subunit by the antisense approach, we also visualized cells by immunofluorescence microscopy after loading with different sense or antisense probes. Only cells loaded with α_o antisense DNA for 42–52 h showed a dramatic reduction of the immunostaining for the α_o subunit.

TIME DEPENDENCE OF ANTISENSE ACTION IN SINGLE-CELL STUDIES

Figure 5.5 illustrates that after loading lactotrophs with α_o antisense DNA, inhibition of calcium current induced by dopamine is reduced in a time-dependent

TABLE 5.1. *Calcium Current Inhibition by Dopamine in Lactotrophs Loaded With Antisense Oligodeoxynucleotide Directed Against mRNAs Encoding α Subunits*

Treatment	Mean ± SE (%) dopamine response	Number of cells tested
Control	54 ± 9	18
+ AS α_O	15 + 8	7
+ AS α_s	50 ± 12	6
+ AS α_{i1}	51 ± 8	5
+ AS α_{i2}	49 ± 14	6
+ AS α_{i3}	57 ± 11	8

Voltage-activated calcium current was recorded every 5 sec in response to 200 msec depolarization steps from a holding potential of −80 to −10 mV. To isolate calcium current, the pipette-filling solution contained the following (mM): CsCl (130), tetraethylammonium-Cl (20), MgCl$_2$ (1), HEPES (10), EGTA (10.25), CaCl$_2$ (1), cAMP (0.1), ATP (2), GTP (0.4), pH 7.25/CsOH. Control denotes vehicle-dialyzed cells; AS α_O (CCC CGG TGG TAC CCT ACA) is an antisense probe overlapping the translation initiation codon of MRNA α_O; AS α_s (CGG CGG antisense probe overlapping the mRNA α_s; AS α_{i1} (TGG TAC antisense probe overlapping the MRNA α_{i1}; AS α_{i2} (TCC TAC CCG ACG TGG CAC), an antisense probe overlapping the translation initiation codon of MRNA α_{i2}; and AS α_{i3} (CAG TAC CCG ACG TGC AAC), an antisense probe overlapping the translation initiation codon of mRNA α_{i3}. All these sequences are oriented 3' to 5'.

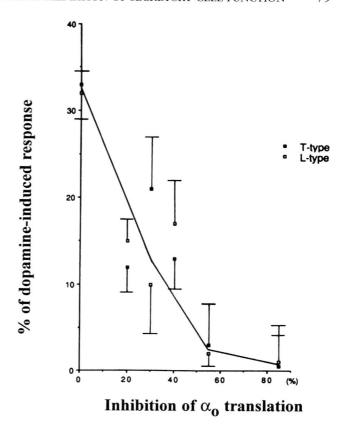

Inhibition of α_O translation

FIG. 5.6. Percentage of dopamine (10 nM)-induced response of voltage-activated calcium current as a function of percentage inhibition of in vitro translation of the α_O subunit. The mRNAs used in the in vitro translation were transcribed from α_O, α_{i1}, α_{i2}, and α_{i3} cDNA of R. Reed that were subcloned into p1B131 and from α_s CDNA of L. Birnbaumer. Translation was performed using rabbit reticulocyte lysate. The gel autoradiographs were scanned and analyzed on a BioImage Analyzer (Visage 4000, Millipore, Ann Arbor, MI). Zero percentage of inhibition of α_O translation was obtained with a vehicle, and then the increase in inhibition of in vitro α_O translation was obtained using different oligonucleotides (see ref. 3).

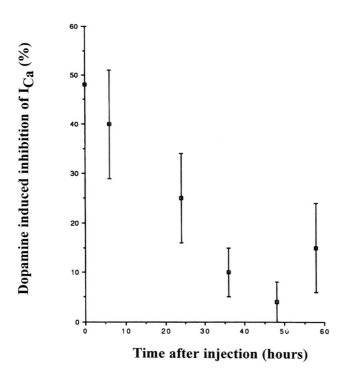

Time after injection (hours)

FIG. 5.5. Time course of calcium current inhibition by dopamine (10 nM) in lactotroph cells injected with antisense to α_O. Mean values from six different cells are shown and bars represent standard errors of the means.

manner. This reduction of dopamine response parallels the disappearance of α_O immunoreactivity. Interestingly after 48 h of cell loading, the response of calcium current to dopamine is largely restored, indicating that antisense suppression of gene expression can be overcome. The 48-h period required for near abolition of the calcium current response would be compatible with a half-life of α of 28 h measured in the GH$_4$ pituitary tumor cell line (69).

Using a panel of different antisense DNA probes, it is also possible to establish a correlation between the extent of inhibition of calcium currents (both the T- and the L-type calcium current) induced by 10 nM dopamine and inhibition of in vitro translation of the α_O subunit (Fig. 5.6). The effects of antisense on in vivo translation were quantified by image analysis of the gel autoradiographs. In linear single regressions fitting to the data, the percentage inhibition of calcium currents inversely correlated with the inhibition of in vivo translation of α_o .

USE OF ANTISENSE OLIGONUCLEOTIDES TO ESTABLISH A ROLE FOR RAB3B SMALL GTP-BINDING PROTEIN IN CALCIUM-INDUCED EXOCYTOSIS OF ANTERIOR PITUITARY CELLS

A GTP-binding protein has been postulated to be involved in the biochemical machinery controlling the fusion process named G_e (26). Sikdar et al. (67) have shown that GTP-binding proteins are involved in the regulation of secretory activity of single adenohypophyseal cells. However, it was not clear which proteins might mediate the responses recorded. Both heterotrimeric and monomeric may play a role in the control of exocytosis.

An indication for a role of monomeric GTP-binding proteins in exocytosis comes from experiments where putative effector–domain peptides of rab3A were introduced into mast cells, chromaffin cells, pancreatic cells, and insulin-secreting cells (for a review, see ref. 5), which induced exocytosis in the absence of calcium. If these peptides were presented to a cell-free system (19), exocytotic fusion was stimulated as well. On the other hand, rab3A peptides were found to be inhibitory (17) or had no effect (53, 59) on exocytotic fusion recorded in permeabilized or patch-clamped cells. Moreover, a mastoparan-like effect of these peptides was described as well (42). Therefore the results obtained by the application of effector domain peptides should be considered critically.

To study whether control of exocytosis in adenohypophyseal cells involves monomeric GTP-binding proteins, the more specific approach of inhibition of expression of rab3 proteins by antisense probes is used. It has thus been shown that rab3B proteins are required for the Ca^{2+}-induced secretory activity of adenohypophyseal cells (46). Preloading of cells with antisense DNA probes engineered against the 5' part of the translation initiation codon of rab3B mRNA resulted in an attenuation of Ca^{2+}-induced secretory responses monitored by the membrane capacitance technique (see Table 5.2). Secretory responses determined as relative changes in resting capacitance (displayed in Table 5.2) were determined 450 s after establishing the whole-cell recording. However, in four cells, recordings were longer than 1000 s, and in three of these the responses were characterized by a biphasic time course (Fig. 5.7, lower trace). These results suggest that the early attenuated response in antisense-loaded cells is proba-

TABLE 5.2. *Secretory Activity of Control and Treated (Preloaded With Antisense Probes) Single Adenohypophyseal Cells Determined as Relative Changes in Membrane Capacitance (%) With Respect to Resting Capacitance, 450 s After the Start of Cytosol Dialysis With a High-Ca^{2+} Containing Pipette-Filling Solution*

Treatment	Mean ± SE (%) secretory response	Number of cells tested
Control	33 + 4	34
+N63	12 ± 3*	5
+PT3	30 ± 8	3
+N62	26 + 8	5
+N61	27 ± 4	4

The solution contained the following (rnM): KCl (150), MgCl, (2), HEPES (10), EGTA (10.25), CaCl$_2$ (9), cAMP (0.1), GTP (0.4), pH 7.25/KOH. The calcium activity of this solution was calculated to be close to 1000 nM, assuming an apparent dissociation constant for the Ca-EGTA complex of 150 nM. Controls are represented by responses of nonloaded cells. +N63 (AGT TAC TGA GGC CAT CTC GGA T) denotes addition of an antisense probe overlapping the translation initiation codon of MRNA rab3B; +PT3 (TGT GGC TGA GGC CAT CTF GCC C), addition of an antisense probe overlapping the translation initiation codon of MRNA rab3A, +N61 (GAA GCA GAG GAG AAG TGG GC); +N62, addition of a sense probe corresponding to the nucleotides 188 to 208, relative to the first ATG in this coding region of rab3B (ACA GTT TAC CGT CCA TGA GAA GC). Sequences of antisense and sense probes are oriented 5' to 3'.* $P < 0.02$, Fischer's test.

bly due to the small remaining population of rab3B in cells. Once the fusion competent vesicles (possibly associated with rab3B) are exhausted, no exoytosis occurs and the membrane capacitance signal is dominated by endocytosis (94). These results also suggest that rab3B may be required for docking of new secretory granules to the plasmalemma or it may be required for translocation of these from cytoplasm to plasmalemma. The attenuation of secretory responses in cells preloaded with antisense probe B63 is specific. If a sense probe to a coding region of mRNA or an antisense probe to a noncoding region of mRNA were preloaded into cells, secretory responses were not significantly different from controls (Table 5.2). Similarly, if an antisense probe directed against mRNA rab3A was used, the recorded responses were not different from controls. Such a distinction in assigning the function of rab3 isoforms would be difficult or impossible with other methods, since specific non-crossreacting antibodies are not yet available.

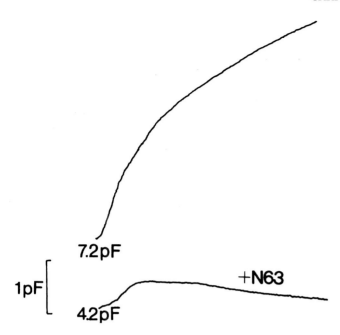

7.2 pF

1 pF

4.2 pF

+N63

FIG. 5.7. *Top:* Representative long-term recording of membrane C_m in a control adenohypophyseal cell dialyzed with a pipette filling solution containing 1000 nM free Ca^{2+} (solutions as in Table 5.2, and the caption to Fig. 5.2). *Bottom:* A different cell dialyzed by a pipette solution as in the top trace but loaded 48 h earlier by the N63 antisense probe.

DISCUSSION

Neurons and endocrine cells are very similar with respect to the composition of their characteristic small vesicles and large secretory granules, besides having a variety of functional similarities. However, more recent morphological and biochemical observations indicate that synaptic transmission differs in many respects from glandular release. Release by endocrine cells mainly involves the large dense-cored granules that contain high concentrations of hormonal products; these large vesicles interact slowly with the plasma membrane of the gland cell. In nerve endings, the small vesicles contain little if any core proteins, whilst the large vesicles contain both low molecular weight amine transmitters, core proteins, and peptides. Since all the neuropeptides are found primarily, or even perhaps exclusively, in larger vesicles of neurons, nerve terminals would seen to maintain the more "primitive" mechanism of release used by gland cells.

Membrane trafficking along the exocytotic and the endocytotic pathways is mediated by a number of vesicular intermediates. This vesicular transport is vectorial since each step is mediated by specific targeting, docking, and fusion events. Among these processes, calcium and GTP-regulated exocytosis lead to the final

stage of the secretory pathway. The combination of yeast genetics, biochemistry of synaptic proteins, and in vitro reconstitution of vesicular transport have provided convincing evidence for a common mechanism which involves elements conserved through evolution such as calcium-sensor proteins and GTP-binding proteins.

Assigning biological function to proteins at the cellular level is a difficult task, because cells are small and experimentally relatively inaccessible. Moreover, some proteins are present in the cell as isoforms, with a very similar structure, but their function may be distinctly different. For example, rab3B and rab3A, products of different genes, coexist in a number of cells (73a). In adenohypophyseal cells rab3B is the predominant species, although rab3A is present as well. The primary sequence homology of these proteins is 76%, thus, currently the approach of choice to distinguish the function between two isomeric proteins is to employ antisense probes directed at messenger RNA sequences unique to the two species. The patch–clamp technique, on the other hand, allows the use of this approach at the cellular level, since it can be used to load antisense probes into cells and can also be used to assay the function and activity of single cells. The advantages of patch–pipette dialysis of antisense over nuclear microinjections of antisense are twofold. First, the cell under study may be functionally identified during the first recording. Second, the cell may be dialyzed using a known concentration of antisense molecules in the patch–pipette.

Many important refinements of antisense technology are still needed, and many important questions must still be answered. It should be possible, for example, to modify antisense oligonucleotides chemically so that they can be introduced into cells more efficiently or be bound with their targets more effectively. In addition, certain parts of messenger RNA may be more susceptible than others to inhibition by antisense DNA. As these parameters become better understood, it should be possible to design more effective antisense DNA molecules. New methods should also be able to maintain high levels of antisense oligonucleotides in single cells.

A better understanding of the precise mechanisms whereby antisense DNA inhibits the production of proteins is also essential. Research suggests that antisense RNA can act both within the cell's nucleus as well as in the cytoplasm and that it may arrest protein translation by hybridizing with messenger RNA, preventing it from being spliced and modified in essential ways leading to expression. A difficulty in all studies with antisense oligonucleotides is the independent demonstration of the effectiveness and specificity of antisense in single cells. Theoretically, it may be possible to perform in situ hybridization to detect the mRNA remaining after antisense treatment. However, the inhibition of target protein production may be initiated not only by RNase-H cleavage of hybridized mRNA or by inhibition of transcription and splicing, but also by hybridization arrest of translation at the ribosomes. The quantification of remaining mRNA would therefore be inappropriate.

The challenge to develop new ways to manipulate the activity of cellular genes is spurring the development of antisense technology and other techniques such as gene targeting. No doubt with more information, more sophisticated technology, and additional imagination, new approaches will emerge that will complement those already in use. The new field of "reverse genetics" is rapidly providing inroads into the understanding of gene function; with luck it will eventually enhance medicine's ability to understand and treat disease.

SUMMARY

A basic function of nearly every cell type is the exocytotic release of synthesized molecules, stored and packaged into intracellular vesicles or granules. Although many efforts have been used to elucidate the pathways which lead to exocytosis, the nature of the process that ultimately induces membrane fusion is not yet known. This review presents the application of molecular and electrophysiological approaches to single secretory cells which have led to new knowledge of the cellular mechanisms controlling hormone and neurotransmitter release from endocrine cells and neurones respectively, with a special focus on calcium and second messengers. Intracellular calcium, known to be a key facilitator of exocytosis, acts in concert with other compounds such as small G proteins to regulate secretion. Increases in $[Ca^{2+}]_i$ are due both to release from intracellular stores and entry from the extracellular space via voltage- and agonist-gated ion channels. Here, we examine how calcium entry is modulated by neurotransmitters, and how calcium buffering processes (for example, calbindin, endoplasmic reticulum) and small G proteins control exocytotic activity. New approaches enabling study of these microscopic processes provide compelling evidence demonstrating two new functions played by the rab3 protein found in a variety of cell types. Using endocrine cells, electrophysiological experiments have shown that rab3b catalyses the molecular processes which control the interaction between exocytotic organelles and the plasma membrane. In contrast, in

chromaffin cells used as a neuronal model, it was found that rab3a is intrinsically programmed to keep fusion switched off until an appropiate signal triggers the release of the locked vesicles. In this way, synaptic vesicles can be docked at the presynaptic membrane to ensure a rapid response, with final control being effected by small G proteins.

It can be conclued that exocytosis from endocrine cells reflects constitutive secretion and that regulated secretion, observed in neurones, uses a similar molecular machinery necessary for constitutive fusion events but in which an inhibitory component(s) prevents fusion from occurring. Finally, insights into secretory vesicles will not only be relevant for understanding vesicular trafficking but also for our concepts of higher nervous functions.

REFERENCES

1. Aridor, M., G. Rajmilevich, M. A. Beaven, and R. Sagi-Eisenberg. Activation of exocytosis by the heterotrimeric G protein G_{i3}. *Science* 262:1572–1579, 1993.
2. Ayala, J., B. Olofsson, A. Tavitian, and A. Prochiantz. Developmental and regional regulation of *rab3* a new brain specific *ras*-like gene. *J. Neurosci. Res.* 22: 241–246, 1989
3. Baertschi, A. J., Y. Audigier, P. -M. Lledo, J. M. Israel, J. Bockaert, and J. D. Vincent. Dialysis of lactotropes with antisense oligonucleotides assigns G protein subtypes to their channel effectors. *Mol. Endocrinol.* 6: 2257–2265, 1992.
4. Baker, P. F. and D. E. Knight. Calcium-dependent exocytosis in bovine adrenal medullary cells with leaky plasma membranes. *Nature* 276: 620–622, 1978.
5. Balch, W. E., J. M. Fernandez, and H. Plutner. In: *Methods: A Companion to Methods in Enzymology, Vol 5,* New York: Academic Press, pp. 258–263, 1993.
6. Baldini, G., T. Hohl, H. Y. Lin, and H. F. Lodish. Cloning of a *Rab3* isotype predominantly expressed in adipocytes. *Proc. Natl. Acad. Sci. USA.* 89: 5049–5052, 1992.
7. Bark, C. and M. Wilson. Regulated vesicular fusion in neurons: snapping together the details. *Proc. Natl. Acad. Sci. USA* 91: 4621–4624, 1994.
8. Ben-Jonathan, N., M. Laudon, and P. A. Garris. Novel aspects of posterior pituitary function: Regulation of prolactin secretion. *Front. Neuroendocrinol.* 12:231–277, 1991.
9. Bennett, M. K. and R. H. Scheller. The molecular machinery for secretion is conserved from yeast to neurons. *Proc. Natl. Acad. Sci. USA* 90: 2559–2563, 1993.
10. Bourne, H. R., D. A. Sanders, and F. McCormick. The GTPase superfamily: a conserved switch for diverse cell functions. *Nature* 348: 125–132, 1990.
11. Brown, D. A. G proteins and potassium currents in neurons. *Annu. Rev. Physiol.* 52:215–242, 1990.
12. Calakos, N. and R. H. Scheller. Synaptic vescile Biogenesis, docking, and fusion: A molecular description. *Physiol. Rev.* 76: 1–29, 1996.
13. Chavrier, P., J. P. Gorvel, E. Stelzer, K. Simons, J. Gruenberg, and M. Zerial. Hypervariable C-terminal domain of *rab* proteins acts as a targeting signal. *Nature* 353: 769–772, 1991.
14. Christakos, S., C. Gabrielides, and W. B. Rhoten. Vitamin D-dependent calcium binding proteins: chemistry, distribution,

functional considerations and molecular biology. *Endocrinol Rev.* **10**: 3–26, 1989.

15. Crooke, S.T. Therapeutic applications of oligonucleotides. *Annu. Rev. Pharmacol. Toxicol.* **32**:329–376, 1992.

16. Darchen, F., A. Zahraoui, F. Hammel, M. -P. Monteils, A. Tavitian, and D. Scherman. Association of the GTP-binding protein *Rab3A* with bovine adrenal chromaffin granules. *Proc. Natl. Acad. Sci. USA.* **87**: 5692–5696, 1990.

17. Davidson, J. S., A. Eales, R. W. Roeske, and R. P. Millar. Inhibition of pituitary hormone exocytosis by a synthetic peptide related to the effector domain. *FEBS Lett.* **326**:219–221, 1993.

18. Dolnick, B.J. Antisense agents in pharmacology. *Biochem. Pharmacol.* **40**:671–675, 1990.

19. Edwardson, J. M., C. M. MacLean, and G. J. Law. Synthetic peptides of the *rab3* effector domain stimulate a membrane fusion event in regulated exocytosis. *FEBS Lett.* **320**: 52–56, 1993.

20. Elferink, L. A., K. Anzai and R. H. Sheller. *Rab 15*, a novel low molecular weight GTP-binding protein specifically expressed in the rat brain. *J. Biol. Chem.* **267**: 5768–5775, 1992.

21. Fernandez, J. M., F. Bezanilla and R. E. Taylor. Distribution and kinetics of membrane dielectric polarization. *J. Gen. Physiol.* **79**: 41–67, 1982.

22. Fischer von Mollard, G., G. A. Mignery, M. Baumert, M. S. Perin, T. J. Hanson, P. M. Burger, R. Jahn, and T. C. Südhof. *Rab3* is a small GTP-binding protein exclusively localized to synaptic vesicles. *Proc. Natl. Acad. Sci. USA.* **87**: 1988–1992, 1990.

23. Fischer von Mollard, T. C. Südhof, and R. Jahn. A small GTP-binding protein dissociates from synaptic vesicles during exocytosis. *Nature* **349**: 79–81, 1991.

24. Floor, E., P. S. Leventhal and S. F. Schaeffer. Partial purification and characterization of the vacuolar H^+-ATPase of mammalian synaptic vesicles. *J. Neurochem.* **55**: 1663–1670, 1990.

25. Gomperts, B.D. G_E: a GTP-binding protein mediating exocytosis. *Annu. Rev. Physiol.* **52**:591–606, 1990

26. Gomperts, B. D. and J. M. Fernandez. Technique for membrane permeabilization. *Trends Biochem. Sci.* **10**: 414–417, 1985.

27. Goud, B., A. Salminen, N. C. Walworth, and P. J. Novick. A GTP-binding protein required for secretion rapidly associates with secretory vesicles and the plasma membrane in yeast. *Cell* **53**: 753–768, 1988.

28. Grand, R. J. and D. Owen. The biochemistry of *ras* p21. *Biochem J.* **279**: 609–631, 1991.

29. Gratzl, M. and O. K. Langley. (eds.) *Markers for neurons and neuroendocrine cells. Molecular and cell biology, diagnostic applications.* Weinheim: VCH-Verlagsgesellschaft, 1991.

30. Hamill, O. P., A. Marty, E. Neher, B. Sakmann, and F. J. Sigworth. Improved patch-clamp techniques for high-resolution current recording from cells and cell-free membrane patches. *Pflugers Arch.* **391**:85–100, 1981.

31. Hepler, J. R., and A. G. Gilman. G proteins. *Trends Biochem. Sci.* **17**:383–387, 1992.

32. Hille, B. G protein-coupled mechanisms and nervous signalling. *Neuron* **9**:187–195, 1992.

33. Horn, R. and A. Marty,. Muscarinic activation of ionic currents measured by a new whole-cell recording method. *J. Gen. Physiol.* **92**: 145–159, 1988.

34. Ingram, C. D., R. J. Bicknelland W. T. Mason. Intracellular recordings from bovine interior pituitary cells: Modulation of spontaneous activity by regulators of prolactin secretion. *Endocrinology* **119**:2508–2518., 1986.

35. Israel, J. M., C. Kirk, and J. D. Vincent. Electrophysiological responses to dopamine of rat hypophysial cells in lactotroph-enriched primary cultures. *J. Physiol.* **309**:1–22, 1987.

36. Jahn, R. and P. De Camilli,. Membrane proteins of synaptic vesicles: Markers for neurons and neuroendocrine cells; tools for the study of neuroscretion. In: Gratzl, M. and K. Langley, eds. *Markers for Neurons and Neuroendocrine Cells. Molecular and Cell Biology, Diagnostic Applications.* Weinheim: VCH-Verlagsgesellschaft, pp 25–92, 1991.

37. Johannes, L., P. -M. Lledo, M. Roa, J. -D.Vincent, J. -P. Henry, and F. Darchen The GTPase Rab3a negatively controls calcium dependent exocytosis in neuroednocrine cells. *EMBO J.* **13**:2029–2037, 1994.

38. Kelly, R. B. Storage and release of neurotransmitters. *Cell / Neuron (Suppl.)* **72**: 43–53, 1993.

39. Khosravi-Far, R., G. J. Clark, K. Abe, A. D. Cox, T. McLain, R. J. Lutz, M. Sinenski, and C. J. Der. Ras (CXXX) and rab (CC/CXC) prenylation signal sequences are unique and functionally distinct. *J. Biol. Chem.* **267**: 24363–24368., 1992.

40. Kleuss, C., J. Hescheler, C. Ewel, W. Rosenthal, G. Schultz, and B. Wittig. Assignment of G protein subtypes to specific receptors inducing inhibition of calcium currents. *Nature* **353**:43–48, 1991.

41. Kleuss, C., J. Scherübl, J. Hescheler, G. Schultz, and B. Wittig. Different α-subunits determine G protein interaction with transmembrane receptors. *Nature* **358**: 424–426., 1992.

42. Law, G. J., A. Northrop, and W. T. Mason. rab3–peptide stimulates exocytosis from mast cells via a pertussis toxin-sensitive mechanism. *FEBS Letters* **333**:56–60, 1993.

43. Lillie, T. H. W. and B. D. Gomperts. Nucleotides and divalent cations as effectors and modulators of exocytosis in permeabilized rat mast cells. *Phil. Trans. R. Soc. Lond. B* **336**:25–34., 1992.

44. Lindau, M. and E. Neher. Patch-clamp techniques for time-resolved capacitance measurements in single cells. *Pflugers Archiv. Ges. Physiol.* **411**: 137–146, 1988.

45. Lledo, P. M., V. Homburger, J. Bockaert and J. D. Vincent. Differential G protein-mediated coupling of D2 dopamine receptors to K^+ and Ca^{2+} currents in rat anterior pituitary cells. *Neuron* **8**:455–460, 1992.

46. Lledo, P. M., P. J. D. Vernier, W. T. Vincent, W. T. Mason, and R. Zorec. Inhibition of Rab3b expression attenuates calcium-dependent exocytosis in rat anterior pituitary cells. *Nature* **364**:540–544., 1993.

47. Mains, R. E., and B. A. Eipper. Synthesis and secretion of corticotropins, melanotropins, and endorphins by rat intermediate pituitary cells. *J. Biol. Chem.* **254**:7885–7894, 1979.

48. Marcus-Sakura, C. J., A. M. Woerner, K. Shinozuka, G. Zon, G. and G. V. Quinnan Jr. Comparative inhibition of chloramphenicol acetyltransferase gene expression by antisense oligonucleotide analogues having alkyl phospotriester, methylphosphonate and phosphorotioate linkages. *Nucleic Acids Res.* **15**:5749–5759, 1987.

49. Marty, A. and E. Neher. Tight-seal whole-cell recording. In: B. Sakmann and E. Neher, Eds, *Single-Channel Recording* Plenum Press, New York, pp. 107–121, 1983.

50. Matsui, Y., A. Kikuchi, J. Kondo , T. Hishida, Y. Teranishi, and Y. Takai. Nucleotide and deduced amino acid sequences of a GTP-binding protein family with molecular weights of 25,000 from bovine brain. *J. Biol. Chem.* **263**: 11071–11074, 1988.

51. Matteoli, M., K. Takei, R. Cameron, P. Hurlbut, P. A. Johnston, T. C. Südhof, R. Jahn, and P. De Camilli. Association of *Rab3A* with synaptic vesicles at late stages of the secretory pathway. *J. Cell. Biol.* **3**: 625–633, 1991.

52. Mizoguchi, A., S. Kim, T. Ueda, A. Kikuchi, H. Yorifuji, N. Hirokawa, and Y. Takai . Localization and subcellular distribution of smg p25A, a ras p21–like GTP-binding protein, in rat brain. *J. Biol. Chem.* **265:** 11872–11879, 1990.

53. Morgan, A. and R. D. Burgoyne. A synthetic peptide of the N-terminus of ADP-rybosilation factor (ARF) inhibits regulated exocytosis in adrenal chromaffin cells. *FEBS Lett.* 329:121–124, 1993.

54. Moya, K. L., B. Tavitian, A. Zahraoui, and A.Tavitian. Localization of the ras-like *rab3*A protein in the adult rat brain. *Brain Res.* 590: 118–127, 1992.

55. Musha, T., M. Kawata, and Y. Takai. The geranylgeranyl moiety but not the methyl moiety of the smg-25A/*rab*3A protein is essential for the interaction with membrane and its inhibitory GDP/GTP exchange protein. *J. Biol. Chem.* 267: 9821–9825, 1992.

56. Neher, E. and A. Marty. Discrete changes of cell membrane capacitance observed under conditions of enhanced secretion in bovine adrenal chromaffin cells. *Proc. Natl. Acad. Sci. USA* 79:6712–6716, 1982.

57. Neher, E. and R. Zucker. Multiple calcium-dependent processes related to secretion in bovine chromaffin cells. *Neuron* 10: 21–30, 1983.

58. Oberhauser, A. F., J. R. Monck,, W. E. Balch and J. M. Fernandez. Exocytotic fusion is activated by *Rab*3A peptides. *Nature* 360: 270–273., 1992.

59. Okano, K., J. R. Monck and J. M. Fernandez. GTP-✓-S stimulates exocytosis in patch-clamped rat melanotrophs. *Neuron* 11: 165–172, 1993.

60. Peng, Y. Y. and R. S. Zucker. Release of LHRH is linearly related to the time integral of presynaptic calcium elevation above a threshold level in bullfrog sympathetic ganglia. *Neuron* 10: 465–473., 1993.

61. Pevsner J. and R. H. Scheller. Mechanisms of vesicle docking and fusion: insight from the nervous system. *Curr. Opin. Cell Biol.* 6: 555–560, 1994.

62. Pfeffer, S. R. GTP-binding proteins in intracellular transport. *Trends Cell Biol.* 2:41–46, 1992.

63. Pusch, M., and E. Neher. Rates of diffusional exchange between small cells and a measuring pipette. *Pflugers Arch.* 411:204–211, 1988.

64. Rothman J. E. Mechanisms of intracellular protein transport. Nature 372: 55–63, 1994.

65. Rupnik, M. and R. Zorec. Heterotrimeric GTP-binding proteins control Ca^{2+}-independent secretory activity of rat melanotrophs. *J. Physiol* 475:142P, 1994.

66. Salminen, A. and P. J. Novick. A ras-like protein is required for a post-Golgi event in yeast secretion. *Cell* 47: 527–538, 1987.

67. Sikdar, S. K., R. Zorec, D. Brown and Mason, W. T. Dual effects of G protein activation on calcium-dependent exocytosis in bovine lactotrophs. *FEBS Lett.* **253:** 88–92, 1989.

68. Sikdar, S. K., R. Zorec and W. T. Mason. cAMP directly facilitates calcium-induced exocytosis in bovine lactotrophs. *FEBS Lett.* 273: 150–154, 1990 1989.

69. Silbert, S., T. Michel, R. Lee and E. J. Neher. Differential degradation rate of G protein α_o in cultured cardiac and pituitary cells. *J. Biol. Chem.* 265:3102–3105, 1990.

70. Simmons, K., and M. Zerial. Rab proteins and the road maps for intracellular transport. *Neuron* 11:789–799, 1993.

71. Smith, S. J., and R. S. Zucker. Aequorin response facilitation and intracellular calcium accumulation in molluscan neurones. *J. Physiol.* 300: 167–196, 1980.

72. Somogyi P., A. J., Hodgson, R. W. DePotter, R. Fischer-Colbrie, M. Schober, H. Winkler, and I. W. Chubb. Chromogranin immunoreactivity in the central nervous sytem. Immunochemical characterization, distributuion and relationship to catecholamine and enkephalin pathways. *Brain Res. Rev.* 8: 193–230, 1984.

73. Stein, C. A. Anti-sense oligodeoxynucleotides - Promises and pitfalls. *Leukemia* 6:967–974., 1992.

73a. Stettler,)., Nothias, F., Tavitian, B. and P. Vernier. Double in situ hybridization reveals overlapping nevronal populations expressing the low molecular weight GTPases Rab 3a and Rab 3b. *Env. J. Neuroui.*

74. *Stevens, C. F. Quantal release of neurotransmitter and long-term potentiation. Cell /Neuron (Suppl.) 72: 55–64, 1993.*

75. Stull, R. A., L. A. Taylor and F. C. Szoka, Jr. Predicting antisense oligonucleotide inhibitory efficacy: A computation approach using histograms and thermodynamic indices. *Nucleic Acids Res.* 20:3501–3508, 1992.

76. Südhof, T. C. The synaptic vesicle cycle: a cascade of proteins interactions. *Nature* 375: 645–653, 1995.

77. Südhof, T. C. and R. Jahn. Proteins of synaptic vesicles involved in exocytosis and membrane recycling. *Neuron* 6: 665–677, 1991.

78. Tabb, J. S., P. E. Ksh, R. Van Dyke and T. Ueda. Glutamate transport into synaptic vesicles: Roles of membrane potential, pH gradient and intravesicular pH. *J. Biol. Chem.* 267: 15412–15418, 1992.

79. Taraskevich, P. S. and W. W. Douglas. Electrical activity in adenohypophyseal cells and effects of hypophyseotropic substances. *Federation Proc. Federation Am. Socs. Exp. Biol.* 43: 2373–2378, 1984

80. Thomas, P., A. Surprenant and W. Almers. Cytosolic Ca2 +, exocytosis, and endocytosis in single melanotrophs of the rat pituitary. *Neuron* 5: 723–733., 1990.

81. Thomas, P., J. G. Wong, and W. Almers. Millisecond studies of secretion in single rat pituitary cells stimulated by flash photolysis of caged calcium. *EMBO J.* **12:** 303–306, 1993.

82. Touchot, N., P. Chardin, and A. Tavitian. Four additional members of the *ras* gene superfamily isolated by an oligonucleotide strategy: molecular cloning of YPT-related cDNAs from a rat brain library. *Proc. Natl. Acad. Sci. USA.* **84:** 8210–8214, 1987.

83. Toulme, J. J. and C. Helene. Antimessenger oligodeoxyribonucleotides: An alternative to antisense RNA for artificial regulation of gene expression. *Gene* 7:51–58, 1988.

84. Tse, A., F.W. Tse, W. Almers and B. Hille. Rhytmic exocytosis stimulated by GnRH-induced calcium oscillations in rat gonadotropes. *Science* 260: 82–84, 1993.

85. TsÕ, P.O.P., P. S., Miller, L., Aurelian, A., Murakami, C., Argris, K. R., Blake, S. B., Lin, B. L., Lee, and C. C. Smith. An approach to chemotherapy based on base sequence information and nucleic acid chemistry. Biological approaches to the controlled delivery of drugs. *Ann. N.Y.Acad. Sci.* 507:220–241, 1987.

86. Valencia, A., P. Chardin, A. Wittinghofer and C. Sander. The ras protein family: evolutionary tree and role of conserved amino acids. *Biochemistry* 30: 4637–4648, 1991.

87. van der Krol, A. R., J. N. M., Mol, and A. R. Stuitje. Modulation of eukaryotic gene expression by complementary RNA or DNA sequences. *Biotechniques* 6:958–978, 1993.

88. Wahlestedt, C. Antisense oligonucleotide strategies in neuropharmacology. *Trends Pharmacol. Sci.* 15:42–46, 1994.

89. Weintraub, H., J. G. Izant and Harland, R. M. Anti-sense RNA as a molecular toll for genetic analysis. *Trends Genet.* 1:23–25, 1985.

90. Zahraoui, A., N. Touchot, P. Chardin, and A. Tavitian. Complete coding sequences of the ras related *rab*3 and 4 cDNAs. *Nucleic Acids Res.* 16: 1204, 1988.

91. Zamecnik, P. C., and M. L. Stephenson. Inhibition of Rous sarcoma virus replication and cell transformation by a specific oligonucleotide. *Proc. Natl. Acad. Sci. USA* 75:280–284, 1978.

92. Zorec, R., F. Henigman, W. T. Mason and M. Kordas. Electrophysiological study of hormone secretion by single adenohypophyseal cells. *Methods Neurosci.* **4**: 194–210, 1991a.

93. Zorec, R., S. K. Sikdar, and W. T. Mason. Increased cytosolic calcium stimulates exocytosis in bovine lactotrophs. *J. Gen. Physiol.* **97**: 473–497, 1991b.

94. Zupancic, G., L. Kocmur, P. Veranic, S. Grilc, M. Kordas and R. Zorec. The separation of exocytosis from endocytosis in membrane capacitance records. *J. Physiol.* 4803:539–552, 1994.

6. G Protein–coupled receptors and the G protein family

ALFREDO ULLOA-AGUIRRE

Department of Reproductive Biology, Instituto Nacional de la Nutrición "Salvador Zubirán," Mexico City, D. F., Mexico, and Divisions of Neuroscience and Reproductive Sciences, Oregon Regional Primate Research Center, Beaverton, Oregon

P. MICHAEL CONN

Divisions of Neuroscience and Reproductive Sciences, Oregon Regional Primate Research Center, Beaverton, Oregon, and Department of Physiology and Pharmacology, Oregon Health Sciences University, Portland, Oregon

CHAPTER CONTENTS

CELLS COMMUNICATE WITH EACH OTHER and respond to their environment through chemical signals. Signaling molecules bind to specific receptors located in the target cell. For water-soluble signaling molecules, the complementary receptors are localized usually on the surface membrane of the target cell they influence. Upon binding, the signaling molecules activate receptor proteins, which act as signal transducers for specific extracellular messengers. An intracellular signal is then generated, initiating a cascade of amplified events that eventually culminates in a particular biological response (402). Thus, the primary function of cell-surface receptors is to discriminate the specific signaling molecule or ligand from among a large array of chemically diverse extracellular substances and to activate an effector system that triggers an intracellular signal and eventually a biological effect.

There are three main classes of cell-surface receptor: ion channel–linked receptors, enzyme-coupled receptors, and G protein–coupled receptors (GPCRs) (13, 105, 114, 283, 450, 483). G protein-linked cell-surface receptors mediate their intracellular actions through the activation of one or more guanine nucleotide–binding signal-transducing proteins (G proteins) (27, 154, 184, 322, 344, 430, 441). G proteins are heterotrimeric molecules composed of three subunits; in the presence of a specific agonist, receptors activate specific G proteins by catalyzing the exchange of the α-subunit-bound guanosine-diphosphate (GDP) for guanosine-5′-triphosphate (GTP) (27, 31, 32, 66, 403). This exchange leads to dissociaton of the subunit complex into a $\beta\gamma$-dimer and the free α-subunit (184, 322, 403, 430). Although initially the GTP-activated $G\alpha$-subunit alone was considered to be the main promoter of effector activation (for example, the membrane-associated enzymes adenylyl cyclase and phospholipase $C\beta$ or the Ca^{2+} channels) (24–26, 81), the $\beta\gamma$-dimer also may play a major role in signal transduction (62, 77, 117, 208, 209, 516).

Hundreds of receptors signal through G proteins. These receptors, which consist of a single polypeptide chain of variable length that threads back and forth across the lipid bilayer seven times to form characteristic transmembrane helices, form a large and functionally diverse superfamily (13, 105, 450). Based on nucleotide and amino-acid sequence similarities, these protein receptor molecules can be separated further into three main families. The large rhodopsin/β-adrenergic group, to which the majority of GPCRs identified to date belong (13, 105, 383, 450), is the best studied from structural and functional points of view; it is comprised of receptors that respond to a large variety of stimuli, including photons (341, 342) and odorants (365, 396), as well as hormones and neurotransmitter agonists of variable molecular structure, ranging from small biogenic amines [catecholamines and histamine (100, 110, 147, 155, 252)] to peptides [substance P and gonadotropin-releasing hormone (GnRH) (186, 232, 233, 397)] and complex glycoproteins [such as the gonadotropic hormones, luteinizing hormone (LH) and follicle-stimulating hormone (FSH) (159, 182, 259, 298, 315, 325, 422, 481, 482); Fig. 6.1]. Because of the large variability in the

structure of the ligands that bind these receptors, both the NH$_2$- and the COOH-termini, but not the transmembrane domains, may be highly variable in length (Fig. 6.1). The metabotropic glutamate receptor family, which is comprised of at least six closely related subtypes, binds glutamate, the major excitatory neurotransmitter in the central nervous system; all receptor subtypes exhibit long NH$_2$-terminal domains but

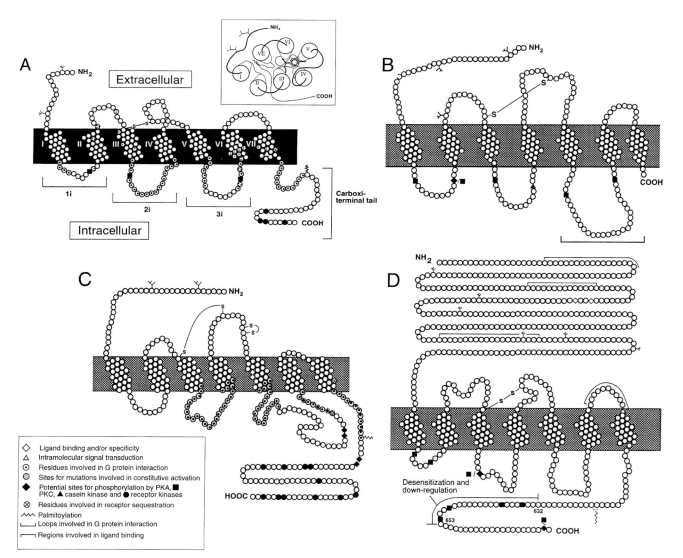

FIG. 6.1. Putative membrane topography of G protein–coupled receptors (GPCRs). *A:* Proposed seven-transmembrane-spanning domains of a prototypic GPCR belonging to the rhodopsin/β-adrenergic family, showing some structural characteristics, including putative glycosylation sites *(branched-like structures)* as well as some amino-acid residues involved in signal transduction, receptor phosphorylation, sequestration, and palmitoylation. The structure also shows the location of some spontaneously occurring mutations leading to constitutive activation of the receptor (for example, thyrotropin, melanocyte-stimulating hormone, luteinizing hormone, rhodopsin, and adrenergic receptors) (250, 263, 281, 370, 398, 409, 427, 492). A region in the NH$_2$-terminal end of the first intracellular loop *(1i)* in-

volved in effector activation by the human calcitonin receptor also is shown (355). *Inset:* Proposed arrangement for the transmembrane helices of the β$_2$-adrenergic receptor, depicting the binding site for epinephrine. Note the proximity between helices 2 and 7, which is characteristic of this family of GPCRs. [Reproduced from Ostrowski et al. (363) with permission]. *B, C, D:* Putative membrane topographies of the rat gonadotropin-releasing hormone receptor (232), the β-adrenergic receptor (363), and the luteinizing hormone/choriogonadotropin receptor (421), respectively, showing some particular structure–function relationships (11, 13a, 21, 33, 153, 175, 176, 193, 405, 420, 421, 473, 501a, 538–540). *PKA,* protein kinase A; *PKC,* protein kinase C.

COOH-terminal domains of variable length (306, 338, 466). Although the calcium-sensing receptor exhibits only modest identity in its amino-acid sequence with the metabotropic glutamate receptor (18%–24%), it shares striking topological similarity and, thus, may be included as a member of this restricted GPCR family (42, 54). Finally, the secretin/vasointestinal peptide (VIP) class—which binds several neuropeptides, including vasointestinal polypeptide (212) and pituitary adenylyl cyclase–activating peptide (392, 438), as well as several peptide hormones such as calcitonin (287), parathyroid hormone (3, 230, 414), secretin (211, 371), glucagon (220), glucagon-like peptide 1 (477, 514), growth hormone–releasing hormone (308), and corticotropin-releasing hormone (57) receptors—exhibits none of the fingerprint residues characteristic of the rhodopsin/β-adrenergic receptor family, with the exception of the putative disulfide bridge between the third transmembrane domain (or the COOH-terminal end of the first extracellular loop) and the second extracellular loop (see STRUCTURE OF G PROTEIN–COUPLED RECEPTORS, below). These receptors are characterized by a large NH$_2$-terminus with at least six highly conserved Cys residues conceivably involved in ligand binding (450).

Even though the receptor–G protein system is a highly efficient means through which the cell responds to a wide variety of extracellular stimuli, in some abnormal conditions "loss-of-function" or "gain-of-function" mutations in the G proteins or the receptor molecule may modify the activity of the signal-transduction pathways and lead to altered cell function, including abnormal growth and tumorigenesis (75, 97, 111, 263, 273, 281, 370, 439, 486).

STRUCTURE OF G PROTEIN–COUPLED RECEPTORS

General Features

Within each GPCR subfamily there is considerable structural homology. Cloning and sequence determination as well as hydrophobic analysis of the primary sequences of at least 300 members of the main family of receptor proteins show the characteristic existence of seven stretches of 20–25 predominantly hydrophobic amino acids [Fig. 6.1; (13, 105, 136, 383, 451)]. By extrapolation from the structure of bacteriorhodopsin [a seven-transmembrane-domain protein from *Halobacterium halobium* which is not coupled to G proteins (183)], these stretches are predicted to form α-helical membrane–spanning domains, connected by alternating extracellular and intracellular loops (which are predicted to be between ten and 40 amino acids in length, with the exception of the third intracellular loop, which may exhibit more than 150 residues) ori-

ented to form a ligand-binding pocket (12, 13, 136, 413, 451). The seven transmembrane domains are thought to form a barrel shape, oriented roughly perpendicular to the plane of the membrane, the extracellular NH$_2$- and the intracellular COOH-termini, and the three extracellular and intracellular connecting loops (Fig. 6.1A). Most of the primary sequence homology among the different subclasses of this type of protein receptor is contained within the hydrophobic transmembrane domain (100, 105, 244, 252, 363, 454). Residues which are highly conserved among the members of this receptor family (and probably among members of other families) apparently represent essential determinants of receptor structure and function. For example, in the majority of the receptors belonging to the rhodopsin/β-adrenergic family, two highly conserved residues are an Asp in transmembrane domain 2 and an Asn in transmembrane domain 7 (22, 200, 224, 349, 420, 451, 456, 500); the exact locations of and interaction between these residues seem to be essential to keep helices 2 and 7 in close proximity and to allow receptor activation and signal transduction [Fig. 6.1A; (22, 61, 200, 224, 349, 363, 420, 463, 500, 537)]. On the other hand, binding specificity requires differences in residues between receptor subclasses but a high degree of conservation for subtypes of receptors with related ligands (137, 155, 451, 454). This is the case of several receptors, such as the muscarinic (45, 454, 508), adrenergic (98, 453, 454, 456), dopaminergic (79), and serotonin (198) receptors, which exhibit a highly conserved third transmembrane domain Asp residue that facilitates the formation of an ionic interaction with the corresponding ligands (Fig. 6.2). Alternately, the hydrophilic loops connecting the transmembrane segments as well as the NH$_2$- and COOH-termini may vary substantially. Thus, the NH$_2$-terminus may be formed by a relatively short peptide chain, such as in the photoreceptor rhodopsin (244, 341) and β_2-adrenergic receptors (100, 110, 155); by medium-length chains, as in the members of the secretin/VIP receptor subfamily (211, 212, 371); or by a very long chain, such as the gonadotropic hormone receptors (182, 259, 482), the metabotropic glutamate receptors (306, 338, 466), and the calcium-sensing receptor [Fig. 6.1; (42, 54)]. Although most GPCRs exhibit a COOH-terminal domain rich in Ser and Thr residues (which are potential sites for phosphorylation by kinases that induce GPCR desensitization), in some rare instances, such as in the GnRH receptor, there is a complete absence of the intracellular COOH-terminal domain in several species [Fig. 6.1B; (232, 233, 397)].

The general structural homology (primary and tertiary) shared by the large family of receptors belonging to the rhodopsin/β-adrenergic class reflects their common mechanism of action (100, 105, 136, 383, 450).

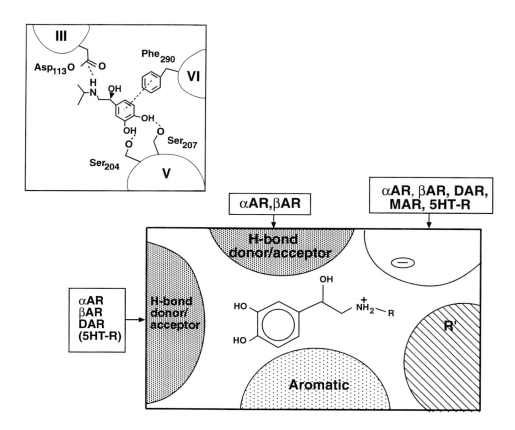

FIG. 6.2. Pharmacophore map of the catecholamine-binding site of the β-adrenergic receptor. A catecholamine ligand is shown in a hypothetical binding site intercalated among the transmembrane helices of the receptor. Each of the large semicircles represents a transmembrane helix of the receptor, inscribed with the type of binding interaction expected. Other G protein–coupled receptors expected to have similar interactions with their specific ligands are designated in boxes next to each helix. *αAR,* α-adrenergic receptor; *βAR,* β-adrenergic receptor; *DAR,* dopaminergic receptor; *MAR,* muscarinic acetylcholine receptor; *5HT-R,* 5-hydroxytryptamine (serotonin) receptor. *Inset:* Model for the ligand-binding site of the β-adrenergic receptor showing key interactions with the agonist isoproterenol. [Reproduced from Strader et al. (450, 454) with permission.]

For example, the rod photoreceptor cell bears the photosensitive rhodopsin receptor molecule (115, 244, 458). Upon activation by photons of light, its covalently linked ligand, all-*cis*-retinal, isomerizes to the all-*trans* isomer; this structural change in retinal forces a series of conformational modifications in rhodopsin, which in turn binds the trimeric retinal G protein transducin (G_t) (244, 267, 354, 391, 435). The α-subunit of rhodopsin-activated transducin activates the effector enzyme cyclic guanosine monophosphate (cGMP) phosphodiesterase, which hydrolyzes GMP, with a consequent decrease in intracellular GMP levels, closure of GMP-gated membrane Na^+-specific channels, hyperpolarization of the plasma membrane, and reduction of the rate of neurotransmitter release from the synaptic region; this sequence of intracellular events allows light to free the neurons from neurotransmitter

inhibition and excite them (144, 238, 266, 458, 513). A similar pathway of GPCR-mediated signal transduction has been characterized for the adrenergic receptors (87, 105, 451). These relatively widely distributed receptors interact with the endogenous catecholamines epinephrine and norepinephrine, as well as with a large number of synthetic agonists and antagonists (450, 454). Upon specific agonist binding, β-adrenergic receptors (including subtypes β_1, β_2, and β_3) activate a stimulatory G protein (G_s), which in turn activates the effector adenylyl cyclase (16, 26, 118); this enzyme is responsible for cyclic adenosine 3′,5′-monophosphate (AMP) formation, one of the main intracellular mediators of extracellular signals (417, 468).

G protein–coupled receptors contain a variable number of Cys residues. Conserved Cys residues in the NH_2-terminus and the extracellular loops (particularly in the first and second) may form disulfide bonds that stabilize the structure of the functional protein (Fig. 6.1). Employing site-directed mutagenesis, substitution of either of the Cys residues present in the first (Cys_{106}) and the second (Cys_{184}) extracellular loops of the β_2-adrenergic receptor resulted in destabilization of the tertiary structure of the protein and alterations in the binding properties of the receptor (101, 104); similar results were obtained with substitutions performed in Cys_{110} and Cys_{187} of rhodopsin (235). For receptors in which the principal determinants of ligand binding reside within a large extracellular NH_2-terminal domain (see *Ligand-Binding Domain,* below), such as the calcium-sensing receptor and the metabotropic glutamate receptors, the numerous conserved Cys residues located within the extracellular domain may help to organize this region into a binding pocket appropriate for interaction with small charged ligands, such as glutamate or Ca^{2+} (42, 54, 306, 338). Most GPCRs exhibit one or two Cys residues in the membrane-proximal portion of the COOH-terminus; these residues are particularly important because they are susceptible to palmitoylation, that is, reversible thioesterification of the C_{16} fatty acid palmitate (34) (Fig. 6.1). Palmitoylation of a number of GPCRs has been documented. These include rhodopsin (the first GPCR shown to be modified by palmitoylation) (234, 364), β_2- and α_{2A}-adrenergic (242, 356), D_1-dopaminergic (351), $5-HT_{1B}$-serotonergic (350), and luteinizing hormone/choriogonadotropin (239, 540) receptors. All of these receptors have in common the presence of one or two Cys residues in the membrane-proximal domain of the COOH-terminus. Since fatty acylation of several soluble proteins promotes their association with the inner surface of the plasma membrane, it is thought that palmitoylation of Cys residues in the membrane-proximal portion of the COOH-terminus facilitates the formation of an anchoring that creates a fourth intracellular loop (Fig. 6.1A). Although a strict consensus sequence that determines the occurrence of covalent S-palmitoylation of the Cys residues present in the proximal segment of the COOH-terminus tail of these receptors has not yet been identified, the consensus sequence $F/Y(X)n_1B(X)n_2C^P$ . . . (where B is a hydrophobic residue, n_1 and n_2 are residues that may vary between between 0 and 4, and C^P is the palmitoylated Cys), based on the primary sequence of the palmitoylated receptors mentioned above (34), has been proposed. Modulation of receptor palmitoylation by agonist has been documented for the β_2- and α_{2A}-adrenergic receptors and for the D_1-dopamine receptor (241, 329, 351); these studies have suggested that stimulation of a receptor by its specific signaling molecule affects the turnover rate of the palmitate moiety

linked to the receptor by increasing its relative rate of depalmitoylation (34, 329). The physiological significance of receptor palmitoylation remains to be fully understood; however, mutations that prevent palmitoylation of the β_2-adrenergic receptor promote the functional uncoupling of the receptor and, consequently, a loss of G protein activation (356). Palmitoylation increases the hydrophobicity of a protein and may favor redistribution to the membrane compartment. Since prevention of palmitoylation of the β_2-adrenergic receptor is accompanied by an increased protein kinase A (PKA)–dependent phosphorylation of the receptor (326, 329), it has been proposed that in receptors harboring phosphorylation sites near potentially palmitoylated Cys residues, there is a close relationship between palmitoylation, phosphorylation, and receptor desensitization (34) (see REGULATORY MECHANISMS, below). Although uncoupling of G proteins after mutation of a palmitoylated Cys residue also has been observed for the μ opiate receptor (227), for other receptors, such as rhodopsin (234, 328), α_{2A}-adrenergic (242), M_2 muscarinic (489), and luteinizing hormone/choriogonadotropin (540), abolition of palmitoylation has no effect on G protein and effector activation. Nevertheless, the fact that the presence of Cys residues susceptible to palmitoylation is highly conserved among this GPCR subfamily strongly suggests that this posttranslational modification is important for the function of these receptors.

Another posttranslational modification found in most GPCRs is the presence of one or more consensus sequences (Asn-Xaa-Ser/Thr) for N-linked glycosylation (17, 29, 103, 150, 173, 180, 418, 445, 535). Heterogeneity in the glycosylation pattern contributes to the anomalous migration of these glycoproteins on gel electrophoresis (82). The N-linked oligosaccharides usually are located near the NH_2-terminus of the receptor molecule, though for some receptors there may be glycosylation sites in the first and second extracellular loops as well (232) (Fig. 6.1). For some receptors (for example, β-adrenergic receptor, rhodopsin, luteinizing hormone/choriogonadotropin, and GnRH receptors), prevention of glycosylation, either by inhibiting post-translational glycosylation or by site-directed mutagenesis, led to decreased cell-surface receptor expression without any significant change in binding or functional activity (83, 106, 150, 225, 294, 389, 469), whereas incorporation of an additional glycosylation site on the human GnRH receptor resulted in an enhancement of both binding affinity and the level of cell-surface expression of the receptor (82). Thus, it seems that for this type of receptor glycosylation is functionally important for membrane insertion and expression. GPCRs may exhibit a certain degree of heterogeneity or variability in the type of oligosaccharide residues attached to the NH_2-terminal domain (86, 181, 445). The impact of such microheterogeneity on receptor function and/or expression remains to be clearly defined.

The diversity among receptor subtypes may be explained by alternate splicing (1, 87, 158, 159, 194, 308). Even though not all mRNA spliced variants of a given receptor may be expressed as receptor proteins, when this occurs, the receptor isoform either may or may not exhibit distinct functional characteristics (87, 126, 172, 194, 308, 339, 346, 347, 465). For example, two isoforms of the related growth hormone–releasing hormone receptor may be generated by in-frame insertion of 123 base pairs in the third intracellular loop without detectable functional consequences (308). Likewise, alternative splicing of the human α_{1C}-adrenergic receptor produced three isoforms differing in the COOH-terminal domain but exhibiting no differences in functional parameters when expressed in Chinese hamster ovary (CHO) cells (194). In other instances, divergent structures of the receptor may alter profoundly ligand binding or G-protein activation (126, 172, 339, 346, 347, 465). For instance, the prostaglandin E type EP_3 receptor gene may produce at least four receptor isoforms by alternate mRNA splicing that differ only in the sequence of the COOH-terminus (339, 465): EP_{3A} couples to the G_i/G_o proteins; EP_{3B} and EP_{3C} to $G\alpha_S$ and EP_{3D} more permissively to $G\alpha_i/G\alpha_o$, $G\alpha_S$, and $G\alpha_q/G\alpha_{11}$ (172, 339, 346). These receptor variants also exhibit different abilities to undergo agonist-induced desensitization (347). Thus, diversity in receptor isoform expression may influence the specificity, sensitivity, and magnitude of response of a given receptor–G protein system.

Ligand-Binding Domain

The specific receptor region at which the ligand binds to the receptor varies depending on the receptor subfamily as well as on the size and chemical structure of the ligand (50, 450, 508). For example, receptors for small ligand molecules, such as the biogenic amines and small peptides, characteristically bind the ligand through a "pocket" involving highly conserved residues located in the middle and extracellular third of hydrophobic transmembrane helices (50, 99, 160, 205, 375, 455, 456, 508, 525). However, in the calcium-sensing and the metabotropic glutamate receptors, the principal determinants of the corresponding binding pockets reside in the NH_2-terminus (54, 466). For larger ligands, such as moderate-sized and large peptides and complex glycoproteins, the binding site usually resides in both the extracellular and the trans-

membrane domains or within the extracellular NH_2-terminus alone (21, 91, 131, 151, 199, 202, 240, 272, 292, 464, 473, 480, 498, 539). Receptors which bind large ligands usually exhibit a long NH_2-terminus. For example, in the parathyroid hormone/calcitonin receptor subfamily, an approximately 100-residue extracellular NH_2-terminus contains regions critical for ligand binding (231); and the luteinizing hormone/choriogonadotropin receptor has a long NH_2-terminus (Fig. 6.1D), comprised of 338 amino-acid residues, which exhibits high affinity and specificity for its ligands even when the receptor is expressed in the absence of the transmembrane domains or when it is expressed in a chimeric form with transmembrane and COOH-terminal domains from other G-protein receptors (21, 330, 421, 473).

The receptor ligand-binding determinants for small molecules (such as retinal and the biogenic amines) which bind to the rhodopsin/β-adrenergic family of receptors have been studied extensively (99, 102, 121, 244, 407, 455, 456, 474, 525, 541). Experiments involving construction of chimeric receptors, specific amino-acid residue substitutions (site-directed mutagenesis), and affinity labeling of ligands have indicated that no single transmembrane domain is the dominant contact site for ligand binding to these receptors. The rhodopsin ligand 11-cis-retinal is linked as a protonated Schiff base to the ϵ-amino group of Lys_{296} in transmembrane domain 7 (a major determinant in wavelength regulation of retinal-based pigments is the protonation state of the retinylidene Schiff base); this base is stabilized by a counterion, the Glu_{113} carboxylate group at transmembrane domain 3 (340, 407, 408, 474, 541). The interaction between Glu_{113} and the protonated base at Lys_{296} requires that the seven helices in rhodopsin fold to bring transmembrane domains-3 and 7 into apposition [Fig. 6.1A; (244, 413)]. Additional sites of retinal binding to rhodopsin have been identified in transmembrane domain 5 as well (105), indicating the involvement of multiple transmembrane helices to form the binding pocket for this particular ligand. In fact, the retinal-binding pocket in the membrane-embedded transmembrane domain of this receptor must contain approximately 20 amino acids that interact with the chromophore retinal (244). Another structural feature of rhodopsin essential for normal binding of its ligand is the presence of a disulfide bridge between Cys_{110} and Cys_{187} that connects transmembrane domain 3 to the second extracellular loop (235, 244, 413); replacement of these Cys residues results in an inability to bind 11-cis-retinal (235).

The discovery that binding of agonists or antagonists to the β_2-adrenergic receptor was not affected by deletion of the hydrophilic extra- and intracellular loops of the receptor suggested that the binding domain for these small molecules also was localized within the transmembrane domain of the protein receptor (98, 99). Similar to rhodopsin, whose binding site for retinal is buried within the core of the receptor protein, studies employing chimeras of the α_2- and β_2-adrenergic receptors have indicated that various sites in several of the hydrophobic transmembrane domains contribute to forming the binding pocket for catecholamines [Fig. 6.1A; (99, 160, 456, 474, 478, 525)]. Employing site-directed mutagenesis, it has been shown that two particular residues (Ser_{204} and Ser_{207}) in transmembrane domain 5 of the β_2-adrenergic receptor, both of which are highly conserved among the receptors for catecholamines (451, 500), are required for normal binding of agonists, but not of antagonists (noncatechol), to the catecholamine receptors, thus indicating that the catechol hydroxyl groups of the agonist form hydrogen bonds with the side chains of the two Ser residues (448). Another important binding determinant in these receptors is the Phe_{290} residue in transmembrane domain 6; whereas the catechol hydroxyl groups of the agonist form hydrogen bonds with the side chains of the two Ser residues at transmembrane domain 5, the catechol-containing aromatic ring interacts with the side chain of Phe_{290} in transmembrane domain 6 [Fig. 6.2; (102, 451, 454)]. Analogous to the Glu_{113} residue in transmembrane domain 3 of rhodopsin (407), systematic mutagenesis of the negatively charged residues in the transmembrane domain of the β-adrenergic receptor has disclosed that Asp_{113} in transmembrane domain 3 acts as the counterion for the basic amines in both agonists and antagonists (448, 456). In contrast to the interaction of ligand with residues in transmembrane domain 5 and 6, which is important for both binding and receptor activation, the ionic interaction in transmembrane domain 3, while important as a source of binding energy between ligand and the receptor protein, is not essential for receptor activation (448, 452, 453, 456). Mutagenesis analysis of other receptors for biogenic amines (dopamine, α_2-adrenergic, muscarinic, serotonin, and histamine receptors) has demonstrated the importance of these key amino-acid positions in ligand binding and receptor activation, albeit with the expected variations in specific residues according to the chemical structure of the ligand (137, 146, 205, 437, 451, 500, 508). For example, a Phe residue at the position analogous to Phe_{290} of the β-adrenergic receptor in transmembrane domain 6 is conserved in all other receptors for biogenic amines but not in the muscarinic receptor (for example, the rat M_3-muscarinic receptor), in which a Tyr_{506} is essential for high-affinity binding (508, 511). Other residues important for receptor binding in this subclass include two Thr residues at positions 231 and 234 (transmembrane domain 5); three Tyr residues at positions 148 (transmembrane domain 3), 529, and 533 (transmembrane domain 7); and an Asp residue at position 147 (transmembrane domain 3) (23, 78, 137, 267, 508, 511). As with other receptors from this family, the highly conserved Asp_{113} (in transmembrane domain 2 of the muscarinic receptors) plays a pivotal role in mediating the conformational changes associated with receptor activation (452, 453, 456, 508). In the histamine receptor, Ser_{204} and Ser_{207} in transmembrane domain 5 of the β-adrenergic receptor (448) [Thr_{231} and Thr_{234} in the M_3-muscarinic receptor (511)] are replaced by Asp_{186} and Thr_{190}, respectively; substitution of these residues leads to a significant reduction in binding affinity of the ligand (146). The overall data indicate that binding of small ligands (such as the biogenic amines) to their corresponding receptors is characterized by a complex network of interactions involving several transmembrane domains, in which key residues in transmembrane domains 5 and 6 are essential to form a binding pocket critical for ligand binding, with the specificity for agonist recognition determined by the particular chemical nature of the side chains of these residues. Based on the combination of mutagenesis, amino-acid replacements, medicinal chemistry, and molecular modeling, it has been possible to generate a pharmacophore map from which specific interactions between biogenic amines and the transmembrane domains of the receptor may be inferred based on specific amino-acid residues present within the transmembrane receptor domains and the particular chemical structure of the ligand [Fig. 6.2; (454)]. However, similar to rhodopsin, the existence of disulfide bonds within the extracellular hydrophobic domains appears to be necessary to stabilize the correctly folded conformation of the adrenergic receptors and thus to preserve normal ligand-binding characteristics [Fig. 6.1; (101, 104)].

In contrast to cationic neurotransmitter receptors, the ligand-binding site has not been defined clearly for GPCRs which bind small peptide ligands. Residues located in the transmembrane domains at positions corresponding to the monoamine-binding pocket (see above) do not always affect the binding of peptide ligands (202, 480). However, mutations in extracellular domains often lead to significant decreases in peptide binding (130, 199, 204). These data suggest that the binding site for peptide ligands involves a larger surface area, comprising the extracellular or the transmembrane domains of the receptor or both. For example, the binding pocket for the tripeptide thyrotropin-releasing hormone is localized within the transmembrane domains of the receptor and involves specific residues in transmembrane domains 3 (Tyr_{106}, Asn_{110}), 6 (Arg_{283}), and 7 (Arg_{306}) (375). Binding of the decapeptide GnRH requires, in addition to the proximity of helices 2 and 7, an ionic interaction between Arg_8 of the decapeptide and the carboxylate side chain of Glu_{301} in the third extracellular loop (122, 538, 539). These two transmembrane domains possess two highly conserved residues; however, whereas most GPCRs exhibit an Asp or Glu residue at a conserved position in domain 2 and a conserved Asn residue in domain 7, in the GnRH receptor these residues are exchanged so that Asn_{87} is located in helix 2 and Asp_{318} in helix 7 (232, 233, 538). Mutating the Asn_{87} in domain 2 to an Asp abolished agonist binding, whereas a second mutation in domain 7, replacing Asp_{318} by Asn, led to restoration of high-affinity ligand binding (420, 538). Further, when these mutations were introduced in a pituitary-derived lactotrope cell line expressing the rat GnRH receptor, they abolished the initial down-regulation of the receptor and impaired its interaction with the G proteins involved in inositol phosphate production (11). Site-directed mutagenesis on the neurokinin-1 (NK_1) receptor, which binds substance P, has shown that three residues in the first extracellular segment (Asn_{23}, Gln_{24}, and Phe_{25}) and two in the second (Asp_{96} and His_{108}) are required particularly for ligand binding (130); several residues in the second and the seventh transmembrane domains of this receptor (Asn_{85}, Asn_{89}, Tyr_{92}, and Asn_{96} in domain 2 and Tyr_{287} in domain 7) are also important in determining the affinity of the receptor for its ligand (128, 533). The residues in domain 2 are predicted to be positioned on the same face of the α-helical region, thus indicating that their side chains may form a hydrogen-bonding surface projecting into the ligand-binding site. In other peptide-binding receptors, such as the angiotensin, vasopressin, oxytocin, and neuropeptide Y receptors, the ligands also bind to determinants located in both the first extracellular loop and several transmembrane domains (domains 2–7) (480), emphasizing the importance of the transmembrane domains in the binding of peptide ligands to GPCRs.

In many cases, the sites required for high-affinity binding of antagonists of these peptide ligands may be distinct from those of the naturally occurring ligands. This is exemplified by the tachykinin NK_1 receptor, in which nonpeptide antagonists do not interact with the extracellular domain but rather with residues located in transmembrane domains 4 (Gln_{165}), 5 (His_{197}), 6 (Tyr_{272} and His_{265}), and 7 ($Tyre_{287}$), some of which do not participate in binding of the natural peptide ligand (127, 129, 202, 203) (see above); these antagonists may exhibit up to a 100-fold difference in affinity between species homologous to the NK_1 receptor, in

contrast to the similar affinities of the endogenous ligands (129). Another example is the GnRH receptor. Molecular modeling of this receptor predicts a Lys_{121} residue in transmembrane domain 3 [positioned at a locus that corresponds to the conserved Asp_{113} of the cationic amine receptors (448, 456)] that contributes to the ligand-binding pocket (Fig. 6.1B); substitution of this charge-strengthened hydrogen bond donor by Gln resulted in considerable loss of agonist binding without any significant effect in antagonist binding (539). Employing photoaffinity-labeling techniques and enzymatic digestion of the labeled GnRH receptor, it has been demonstrated that agonists and antagonists bind to different regions of the receptor and, therefore, are likely to be oriented differently with respect to the receptor (219).

The NH_2-terminus of receptors for other relatively larger peptide ligands and glycoprotein molecules plays a major role in determining high-affinity binding to the corresponding ligands. In the secretin/VIP receptor subfamily, there is a sequence conservation in the NH_2-terminus that strongly suggests a role of this region in mediating receptor–ligand interactions (199, 212, 231, 287, 414). For example, it has been shown that the NH_2-terminal extracellular regions of the parathormone and secretin receptors contain domains that largely determine the binding affinity of these hormones (199, 231). Nevertheless, some of these ligands also may interact with other extracellular domains; although the first ten residues of the NH_2-terminus of the secretin receptor are critical for ligand binding, other extracellular domains located at the COOH-terminus of the first extracellular loop as well as at the NH_2-terminal half of the second loop also provide critical determinants (199). Other receptors in which the NH_2-terminal region appears to be critical in determining ligand binding include the interleukin-8 (272, 464), the C5a (91), the glycoprotein hormone [luteinizing hormone/choriogonadotropin, FSH, and thyroid-stimulating hormone (TSH) (21, 473, 498)], and the thrombin (151, 292) receptors. Glycoprotein receptors have large extracellular domains (300–400 amino acids in length) and bind complex ligands with molecular weights ranging from 28 to 38 kd. These receptors exhibit an extraordinary amino-acid homology (30%–50%) in the extracellular domains, where multiple discontinuous segments spanning the entire domain contribute to the binding site and ligand specificity (5, 21, 336, 337, 473, 498). The extracellular domain of the luteinizing hormone/choriogonadotropin receptor exhibits multiple ($n = 14$) Leu-rich repeats (421, 473); in particular, composite regions encompassed by Leu-rich repeats 1–6 are involved in high-affinity binding and binding specificity (473). Some studies employing mutant receptors have pointed toward the existence of an additional site important for the binding affinity of luteinizing hormone/choriogonadotropin located in the second transmembrane domain (Asp_{383}) as well as a low-affinity ligand-binding site in a specific region of the third extracellular connecting loop (Lys_{583}) [Fig. 6.1D; (153, 405)]. Apparently, this binding site is critical for activating specific transmembrane conductors that eventually lead to the generation of particular intracellular signals, such as cAMP (153). Finally, the thrombin receptor exhibits in its NH_2-terminus a unique mechanism for ligand binding and receptor activation. In this receptor, the ligand is a protease and its extracellular NH_2-terminus contains both a ligand-specific anion-binding site and a specific proteolytic cleavage substrate site; it is activated by binding its tethered ligand domain, which is unmasked upon receptor cleavage by thrombin (151, 292).

G Protein–Coupling Domain

G protein–coupled receptors characteristically bind G proteins, which in turn act as mediators of receptor-induced effector activation (120, 184, 344, 430). The nature of the second-messenger pathways activated in response to agonist binding to a GPCR essentially is determined by the type of G protein(s) coupled to each particular receptor. As can be expected from both the general topography of these receptors and the fact that GPCRs couple and interact with a number of distinct G proteins (at least 17 different species of $G\alpha$ genes coding for four main classes and their numerous corresponding subtypes have been identified, see THE HETEROTRIMERIC G-PROTEIN FAMILY, below), the G protein-coupling domains lie within the divergent sequences of the intracytoplasmic domains of the receptor (59, 80, 195, 258, 301, 355, 357, 510). When a particular ligand binds to its receptor, the molecular perturbation is relayed from the membrane-embedded helices to the cytoplasmic face of the protein molecule (291). These intracellular domains, particularly the regions closest to the plasma membrane, as well as some specific regions located in the intracellular ends of the transmembrane domain helices and in the membrane-proximal portion of the COOH-terminus, are important for receptor–G protein coupling, interaction, and specificity determination [Fig. 6.1; (11, 60, 137, 253, 357, 449)]. Segments of the intracellular loops are important not only in determining the selectivity and relative affinity of the receptor to different G proteins but also in activating the receptor and transmitting the signal generated following agonist binding (see REGULATORY MECHANISMS, below).

Within members of the various GPCR families there are some receptor classes with corresponding subtypes that may show particular preference or specificity toward a particular G-protein class [G_s, G_i/G_o, G_q, or G_{12}, though specificity of the receptor for this latter class remains to be determined fully (96, 344)] (20, 369, 433, 523). This is the case, for example, of the muscarinic receptor class, in which the M_2 and M_4 receptors preferentially couple to proteins of the G_i/G_o class, which are sensitive to pertussis toxin (see THE HETEROTRIMERIC G-PROTEIN FAMILY, below), whereas the M_1, M_3, and M_5 receptors predominantly stimulate pertussis toxin–insensitive proteins of the G_q/G_{11} class (20, 369, 433). The different subclasses of the serotoninergic (5-HT) receptors ($5-HT_1$–$5-HT_7$) with their corresponding subtypes (for example, $5-HT_{1A}$, $5-HT_{1B}$, etc.) also show particular preferences: $5-HT_1$ receptors bind preferentially to G_i/G_o proteins, whereas the $5-HT_2$ and $5-HT_4$ and the $5-HT_6$ and $5-HT_7$ subtypes are coupled to members of the G_q/G_{11} and G_s protein classes, respectively (116, 331, 376, 395). In the metabotropic glutamate receptor (mGluR) family, the $mGluR_1$ (including its splice variants $mGluR_{1\alpha}$, $mGluR_{1\beta}$, and $mGluR_{1C}$) and $mGluR_5$ types are associated with effects most likely mediated by the G_q/G_{11} class (185, 534), whereas the $mGluR_2$, $mGluR_3$, $mGluR_4$, and $mGluR_6$ classes exhibit some preference toward the G_i/G_o class (378, 537). An additional level of complexity in receptor–G protein coupling is the fact that certain receptors in a given family may show a strong preference for a particular member of a G-protein class; for example, the C5A receptor prefers G_{16} to other members of the G_q class (277). Finally, there are receptors that couple normally to different G-protein classes. The receptors for glycoprotein hormones (luteinizing hormone/choriogonadotropin, TSH, and FSH) stimulate (albeit not to the same extent) both cAMP and inositol phosphate production throughout the pathways defined by G_s and G_q proteins, respectively (195, 260, 386, 490).

Experiments employing specifically directed mutagenesis, chimeric receptors, peptides corresponding to different positions of the receptor sequence, and antibodies against various cytoplasmic domains of specific G proteins have been used to characterize the sites of contact as well as some of the sequences involved in activation and specificity determination (59, 60, 80, 133, 195, 258, 301, 355, 363, 524). These studies have led to the recognition of the importance of the second and third intracellular loops as well as the membrane-proximal region of the COOH-terminus of several GPCRs in G-protein coupling. This issue has been explored deeply in some members of the rhodopsin/β-adrenergic family. In rhodopsin, the second and third intracellular loops, as well as the fourth loop created by palmitoylation of Cys residues in the membrane-proximal portion of the COOH-terminus, are involved in the interaction between the receptor and G_t; synthetic peptides derived from these loops were able to interact, either alone or in several combinations, with transducin (133). However, at least two sites, one in the second and another in the third intracellular loop, are required for activation of bound transducin (133), which indicates that determinants present in several intracellular domains are important for receptor–G protein interaction. In the muscarinic and catecholamine receptors (and presumably in other receptors for biogenic amines and peptide hormones), both the NH_2- and the COOH-terminal portions of the third intracellular loop appear to be critical determinants of G-protein binding and activation (74, 178, 265, 268, 275, 303, 425, 509, 510). Data from studies of deletions in limited regions of the NH_2-terminal (residues 222–229) and the COOH-terminal (residues 258–270) portions of the third intracellular loop in the β_2-adrenergic receptor (which is coupled to the G_s protein) as well as construction of chimeric α_1/β_2-adrenergic receptors and several β_2-adrenergic receptor mutants have indicated that these particular regions are necessary for the β_2-adrenergic receptor–mediated activation of adenylyl cyclase [Fig. 6.1C; (74, 253, 286, 357, 449)]. Apparently, in the β-adrenergic receptor, the COOH-terminal region of this loop is more important for G-protein coupling specificity than the opposite NH_2-terminal region of the same loop since substitution of residues 216–237 in the latter with the corresponding residues from the α_2-adrenergic receptor (which is coupled to the G_q/G_{11} class) failed to affect the ability of the β_2 receptor to couple G_s, whereas substitution of residues 263–274 corresponding to the COOH-terminal region of the loop resulted in a severe impairment of coupling (286). Similar results have been found in the D_{1A}-dopamine and the α_1-adrenergic receptors (60, 73, 301). In these receptors, co-expression of the entire third intracellular loop of the α_{1B} receptor or domains involving both restricted NH_2- and COOH-terminal regions of this loop with its parent receptor significantly decreased inositol phosphate production, presumably through specific competitive inhibition of G-protein (G_q/G_{11}) binding (60, 301). However, some chimeric studies also have indicated that a restricted region, composed of 27 amino-acid residues of the NH_2-terminal region from the third intracellular loop of the α_{1B}-receptor, plays a major role in determining the selectivity for receptor–G_q/G_{11} protein coupling (74). In all of these receptors, both specific amino-acid residues from the NH_2- and the COOH-terminal

portions of the third intracellular loop and the secondary structure of these regions, which form amphipathic helical extensions of the adjacent transmembrane domains, play crucial roles in determining coupling specificity, selectivity, and efficiency to activate a particular class of G protein (G_i, G_s, or G_q) (59, 60, 188, 253).

For several GPCRs, the importance of the second intracellular loop in G-protein coupling and specificity has been well documented (74, 80, 244, 314, 357, 360, 361). The amino-acid sequence of this loop is among the most highly conserved in the GPCR superfamily, and substitutions in some of its highly conserved residues may severely impair G-protein coupling. The second intracellular loop is essential for maintaining the configuration of the G-protein binding site and, thus, for the normal interaction between the β_2-adrenergic receptor and G_s (357, 524). Construction of a chimeric α_{1B}/β_2-adrenergic receptor, in which the third intracellular loop of the α_1-adrenergic receptor replaced the corresponding loop in the β_2 receptor, resulted in a chimeric receptor capable of activating both the G_q/G_{11} and the G_s pathways (74), thus suggesting the existence of determinants for G_s specificity in regions other than the third intracellular loop, probably in the second loop. Similar findings have been reported for the M_2-muscarinic receptor, which normally couples to the G_i protein class; replacement of the third intracellular loop of this receptor with the corresponding loop of the β_2-adrenergic receptor resulted in a chimeric receptor species coupled to both G_i and G_s (314). Other lines of evidence strongly suggest that the second intracellular loop is involved in G-protein coupling and selectivity (135, 361, 500, 508). Mutational analysis of the M_1-muscarinic receptor has shown that a highly conserved Asp residue located at the beginning of the second intracellular loop is important for efficient G-protein coupling (508). In addition, specific regions located in the COOH-terminal region of this loop in the M_2- and M_4-muscarinic receptors are involved in selection and activation of G_i (314, 361). The importance of the second intracellular loop in receptor interaction with G proteins also is exemplified in rhodopsin (134, 244, 258), the angiotensin II receptor (360), and the interleukin-8 receptor (80). In this latter receptor, four specific residues in the second intracellular loop (Tyr_{136}, Leu_{137}, Ile_{139}, and Val_{140}) are critical for coupling to the G_i protein (80).

The COOH-terminal domain of GPCRs may be involved in G-protein coupling and activation (195, 258, 357). In rhodopsin, a synthetic polypeptide from the fourth intracellular loop is capable of interacting with G_t (258). In the β_2-adrenergic receptor, substitution of residues forming the fourth intracellular loop with the corresponding residues from the α_2 receptor has resulted in a reduced efficiency of coupling to the corresponding G protein (357). In this receptor, substitution of the conserved Cys residue (Cys$_{341}$) within the NH$_2$-terminal segment of the cytoplasmic tail produces a significant reduction in its ability to stimulate adenylyl cyclase (356); as mentioned above, palmitoylation of this residue may induce anchoring of this portion of the COOH-terminus to the cell membrane, leading to formation of a short fourth intracellular loop, which in turn may facilitate receptor–G protein coupling. For other receptors of the same family, this structural feature might not be important for G-protein coupling. Mutations of this highly conserved Cys residue in α_2-adrenergic receptors (241, 242), as well as in the luteinizing hormone/choriogonadotropin (540) and M$_1$- and M$_2$-muscarinic (489) receptors, had no effect on agonist-mediated activation of the corresponding second messengers. Similarly, mutations in the Cys$_{322}$ and/or Cys$_{323}$ residues of bovine opsin which resulted in complete abolition of palmitoylation did not affect activation of G$_t$ (234). These data indicate that this shared structural motif plays differing roles in different receptor–G protein interactions.

Although there is little evidence indicating that the first intracellular loop is involved in G-protein binding, one study employing chimeric calcitonin receptors has shown that substitution with the first intracellular loop of a particular isoform of the human calcitonin receptor, containing a unique insertion of 16 amino acids in this loop, completely abolished production of inositol phosphates while allowing stimulation of the cAMP pathway by the host porcine receptor (355).

The overall data indicate that many intracellular domains are involved in receptor–G protein coupling. The most important domains lie within the membrane-proximal regions of the second and third intracellular loops. Although these domains are crucial for high-affinity binding, coupling specificity, and activation of specific G proteins, other regions or particular residues located in the transmembrane helices or even in some extracellular loops play major roles in signal transduction and G-protein activation [Fig. 6.1A, C; (11, 137, 153, 263, 273, 405)].

THE HETEROTRIMERIC G-PROTEIN FAMILY

General Features

Heterotrimeric G proteins are signal-transducing molecules belonging to a superfamily regulated by guanine nucleotides (25, 96, 120, 184, 344, 430, 441). These signal-carrying proteins are heterotrimers, individually termed α- (molecular weight 39–52 kd), β- (35–37 kd), and γ- (6–10 kd) subunits, which are encoded by distinct genes (38, 39, 124, 214, 228, 318, 430). The most diverse genes are those encoding for the α-subunits; in fact, molecular cloning has revealed the existence of at least 17 Gα genes which encode different members of the four main classes of Gα-subunit (G$_s$, G$_i$, G$_q$, and G$_{12}$) grouped on the basis of amino-acid identity and effector regulation (15, 26, 38, 96, 120, 174, 184, 430, 457). Figure 6.3 shows the structural relationship between the different G-protein α-subunits and Table 6.1 lists the different classes of Gα-subunit and some of their specific effects on their corresponding effectors. The tissue distribution of Gα-subunits is highly variable; it may be ubiquitous (or nearly ubiquitous, as in the case of Gα_s and some members of the G$_i$ and G$_q$ classes) or expressed in selected tissues [Gα_{t1} in photoreceptor rod outer segments, Gα_{olf} in

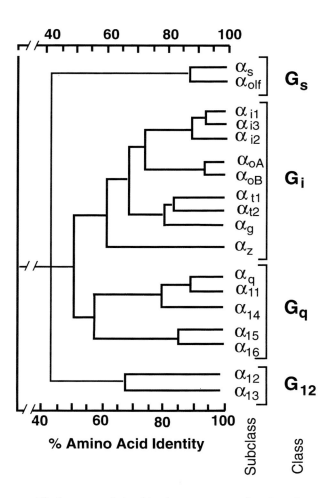

FIG. 6.3. Sequence relationships between mammalian Gα-subunits and family groupings. [Reproduced from Hepler and Gilman (184) and Simon et al. (430) with permission.]

TABLE 6.1. *Characteristics of Mammalian Gα-Subunits*

Gα-Subunit	Size (kd)	Effect(s)	Sensitivity to Toxins	Tissue Distribution
G_s class				
$G\alpha_{s1-4}$	45–52	↑ Adenylyl cyclase, regulation of Ca^{2+} channels	CTX*	Ubiquitous Olfactory neurons
G_i class				
$G\alpha_{i1-3}$	40–41	↓ Adenylyl cyclase	PTX*	Ubiquitous
$G\alpha_{o1,2}$	39	↓ Ca^{2+} channels	PTX	Neural, endocrine
$G\alpha_{t1,2}$	39–40	↑cGMP-PDE*	PTX/CTX	Retina
$G\alpha_{gust}$	41	↑cGMP-PDE	PTX	Taste buds
$G\alpha_z$	41	↓ Adenylyl cyclase, ↓K^+ channel, cell growth	—	Neural, platelets
G_q class				
$G\alpha_q$	41–43	↑ Phospholipase Cβ	—	Ubiquitous
$G\alpha_{11}$			—	Ubiquitous
Ga_{14}			—	Liver, lung, kidney
$G\alpha_{15}$			—	Blood cells
$G\alpha_{16}$			—	
G_{12} class				
Ga_{12}	44	Na^+–H^+ antiporter?, cell growth	—	Ubiquitous
$G\alpha_{13}$			—	

*cGMP-PDE, cyclic guanosine monophosphate–dependent phosphodiesterase; CTX, cholera toxin; PTX, pertussis toxin.

the olfactory neuroepithelium, $G\alpha_g$ (gusducin) in the taste buds, and $G\alpha_{15}$ and $G\alpha_{16}$ in some hematopoietic cells] (7, 44, 96, 120, 142, 184, 201, 228, 316, 396, 521). The $G\alpha_s$ class includes $G\alpha_s$ and $G\alpha_{olf}$, and it is involved in the activation of the various types (I–VIII) of the enzyme adenylyl cyclase to enhance the synthesis of the second-messenger cAMP, which in turn activates PKA; in some tissues, this G-subunit also participates in the regulation of Ca^{2+} and Na^+ channels (154, 216, 307, 419, 462, 515, 530). The $G\alpha_i$ class includes $G\alpha_{gust}$, $G\alpha_t$ ($G\alpha_{t1}$ and $G\alpha_{t2}$), $G\alpha_{i1}$–$G\alpha_{i3}$, $G\alpha_o$ ($Ga2_{o1}$ and $G\alpha_{o2}$), and $G\alpha_z$; they mediate different effects, such as stimulation of cGMP-phosphodiesterase ($G\alpha_t$) (238, 266, 267, 318, 354, 459), inhibition of adenylyl cyclase and activation of K^+ channels ($G\alpha_i$ class) (56, 66, 470, 499, 526, 527, 531), and Ca^+ channel closure and inhibition of inositol phosphate turnover ($G\alpha_o$) (178, 399, 515). The $G\alpha_q$ class includes $G\alpha_q$, $G\alpha_{11}$, and $G\alpha_{14}$–α_{16}; they are associated predominantly with activation of the enzyme phospholipase $C\beta_{1-4}$, which catalyzes the hydrolysis of the lipid phosphatidylinositol-4,5-biphosphate to form two second messengers, inositol-1,4,5-triphosphate (IP_3) and diacylglycerol, and activation of protein kinase C (PKC) (107, 112, 120, 353, 359, 457, 528). Finally, the $G\alpha_{12}$ class, defined by the α-subunits of G_{12} and G_{13}, constitutes the fourth and the most recent family to be identified; although the downstream effector systems for this G protein remain to be demonstrated, studies have indicated that the signaling pathways regulated by these G proteins include modulation of the ubiquitous sodium–proton exchanger NHE_1 and regu-

lation of cell growth and differentiation (96, 358, 496).

$G\beta$- and γ-subunits are also diverse, and at least five different β-subunits and eight γ-subunits have been identified [Table 6.2; (62, 184, 209, 393, 430, 435, 493, 503)]. Although this diversity in β- and γ-subunits theoretically may yield 30 or more different $\beta\gamma$-complexes, not all of the possible pairs can combine and some β-subunits are more able to interact and form stable combinations with particular γ-subunits than others (416). This specific dimerization raises the possibility of differential effector regulation by unique $G\beta\gamma$-complexes; in fact, some studies have localized regions on both subunits which are important in defining dimerization specificity (43, 149, 435, 442, 499). In this regard, chimeras of $G\gamma_1/G\gamma_2$ have shown Phe_{40} of $G\gamma_t$ to be particularly important for discriminating between dimer combinations (276); $G\gamma_t$ will not bind Gβ-subunits other than $G\beta_t$, whereas different Gγ-subunits with smaller side chains in this position will bind $G\beta_t$ (435). Thus, diversity of α-, β-, and γ-subunits theoretically would allow a limit of nearly 1000 oligomeric combinations between the three components comprising G proteins; such a high number of possible combinations not only facilitates the transduction of signals with a high degree of specificity but also helps to define receptor and effector signal sorting and specificity. $G\beta\gamma$-subunits confer distinct functional roles of this complex on effector activation (62, 113, 381, 462, 493). Some of these effects are described below (see *Gβγ Structure and Function*, below).

As discussed above, G proteins interact with the intracellular elements (loops and the COOH-terminal

TABLE 6.2. *Characteristics of Mammalian Gβ- and Gγ-Subunits*

Subunit	Size (kd)	Gβγ Effectors	Tissue Distribution
β_1	36	K$^+$ channel (I_{KACh}); phospholipase A2; Adenylyl cyclases I, II, and IV; phospholipase Cβ_{1-3}; GRK * (β-adrenergic); c-Src kinase	Ubiquitous
β_2	35		Ubiquitous
β_3	36		Retina
β_4	37		Ubiquitous
β_5	39		Neural
γ_1	8		Retina
γ_2	6		Neural, endocrine
γ_3	7		Neural, endocrine
γ_4	7		Kidney, retina?
γ_5	7		Ubiquitous
γ_6	7		Neural
γ_7	7		Ubiquitous
γ_{10}	7		Ubiquitous
γ_{11}	7		Ubiquitous

* GRK, G protein–coupled receptor kinase.

domain) of the receptor, which implies that they must be associated in some way with the plasma membrane. Despite the fact that G proteins do not bear strongly hydrophobic membrane-spanning domains, they usually are tightly associated with the cytoplasmic surface of the plasma membrane (440). Membrane anchoring of G-protein heterotrimers is mediated, in large part, by co- and posttranslational modifications of the α-subunits and βγ-complexes (51, 62, 191, 209, 256, 507). Some α-subunits (for example, α_t, α_i, α_o, α_{gust}, and α_z) possessing the MGXXXS consensus sequence are co-translationally myristoylated at the corresponding NH$_2$-terminus (27, 156, 518). Mutations that prevent permanent myristoylation of these subunits also prevent membrane localization (229, 333). Observations of the pheromone-responsive yeast Gα protein (447) and of Gα$_o$ (289) strongly suggest that myristoylation of some particular α-subunits is also essential for high-affinity interaction with βγ-dimers. The basis for membrane association of other Gα-subunits, such as α_s and α_q, is posttranslational palmitoylation at Cys$_3$ or another Cys residue (for example, Cys$_9$ and Cys$_{10}$ in Gα$_q$) located near the NH$_2$-terminus (288, 367, 507). Myristoylation and palmitoylation of Gα-subunits not only allow for subunit anchoring to the plasma membrane but also influence the activity of the G protein (145, 470, 507). For example, only the myristoylated form of recombinant Gα$_i$ inhibits adenylyl cyclase in vitro (27, 470). Replacement of Cys$_3$ by Ser in α_s prevents its palmitoylation and produces both loss of membrane localization and reduction in receptor-mediated activation of adenylyl cyclase (90, 507); likewise, mutation of Cys$_9$ and Cys$_{10}$ to Ser in α_q

interferes with its capacity to activate phosphoinositide breakdown (507). In contrast to myristoylation, palmitoylation is reversible and can be regulated dynamically (89, 334, 507). Further, this modification is closely related to the functional state and localization of some Gα monomers; agonist or cholera toxin activation of the β-adrenergic receptor–G$_s$ protein complex leads to dramatic changes in the palmitoylation status of Gα$_s$, causing its release from the plasma membrane and either its reversible redistribution along the inner surface of the plasma membrane and/or into the cytoplasm or its degradation (89, 505, 506). Similar results have been observed with receptors coupled to the G$_q$/G$_{11}$ class of proteins (218, 443, 507). Thus, control of Gα palmitoylation by receptor activation might be an additional mechanism regulating the rate and intensity of signal transduction and effector activation.

Even though the primary amino-acid sequences of G protein β- and γ-subunits do not predict regions of high hydrophobicity, their isolation requires detergent extraction, which implies that they are associated tightly with the membrane. Although no specific posttranslational lipidation has been described for the Gβ-subunits, the γ-subunits have at their COOH-terminus a CAAX consensus polyisoprenylation signal and are isoprenylated (51, 64, 141, 191, 332, 410, 411, 431). Processing of Gγ involves polyisoprenylation at the Cys at −4 followed by a protease cleavage of the AAX residues and carboxylation of the isoprenylated Cys (64, 411). In this way, Gγ-subunits may be either farnesylated [for example, the rod photoreceptor γ-subunit (γ1)] or geranyl-geranylated [for example, the brain γ-subunits (Gγ$_{2-4}$)] depending on the nature of the amino acid in the X position (141, 191, 440). Although this lipophilic modification in the γ-subunit is not important for β–γ association, it is essential for co-localization and orientation of the subunits on the inner membrane surface as well as for high-affinity interactions of the dimer with both Gα subunits and effectors (210, 431).

Some types of Gα-subunit and Gβγ-complex can be phosphorylated in vivo and in vitro (81, 120, 177, 299). Even though Gα-subunit phosphorylation on Ser or Thr residues does not change the activity of the protein, it may modify its association with other proteins (254). In some systems (for example, human leukemia cells), the Gβγ-subunits may be phosphorylated on His residues (517), though the functional significance of this modification remains to be ascertained.

G Protein–Regulatory Cycle

Association and interaction of a receptor with a G protein promotes the development of a high-affinity binding state of the receptor for its corresponding agonist (280, 282, 409). Agonist binding and activation of a receptor exhibiting a high-affinity binding state are followed by a conformational change in the receptor and by activation of the trimeric $G\alpha\beta\gamma$ protein complex by guanine nucleotide (see REGULATORY MECHANISMS, below). The $G\alpha$-subunits have a single high-affinity binding site for the guanine nucleotides, which is within a highly conserved amino-acid sequence that forms a guanine nucleotide–binding pocket (66, 249, 267, 354). The GDP–$G\alpha$ complex binds tightly to the $\beta\gamma$-dimer and as such is inactive (that is, in an "off" state). Receptor-promoted and Mg^{2+}-dependent GDP→GTP exchange within the $G\alpha$ guanine nucleotide–binding site leads to a conformational change of the subunit that causes G-protein activation and dissociation of the trimeric complex into $G\alpha$–GTP and $G\beta\gamma$ ("on" state), allowing their interaction with, and activation of, different effector enzymes or ion channels [Fig. 6.4; (31, 32, 66, 190, 217, 354)]. De-

tailed structural analysis of G_t strongly suggests that $G\alpha$ activation occurs through its nucleotide-dependent structural reorganization, whereas $G\beta\gamma$ activation is solely a consequence of its release from the $G\alpha\beta\gamma$-complex (267, 354, 436). This raises the interesting possibility that $G\alpha$ acts as a negative regulator of $G\beta\gamma$ by restricting its degrees of freedom and/or masking sites on the surface of $G\beta$ that interact with downstream signaling components (27, 435). G-protein activation and subunit dissociation mediated by GTP are accompanied by separation of the protein from the receptor, whose ligand-binding state is then switched to the low-affinity state (see below) (280, 409). Intrinsic GTPase activity of the α-subunit leads to hydrolysis of the terminal phosphate of bound GTP to yield GDP, release of inorganic phosphate, dissociation of the $G\alpha$-subunit from effector, reassociation with the $\beta\gamma$-dimer, and switching of the G-protein complex to the "off" membrane-associated state (Fig. 6.4). Hydrolysis of GTP is a relatively slow process that contrasts with the rapid termination of signaling observed in many tissues. For $G\alpha_s$, $G\alpha_i$, $G\alpha_o$, and $G\alpha_t$, GTP-bound α-subunits exhibit in vitro an average activated $t_{1/2}$ of ~ 10–20 s (37, 189, 190, 343), whereas $G\alpha_q$ and $G\alpha_z$ are even slower, with activated $t_{1/2}$ values of ~1 min and more than 10 min, respectively (19, 20, 52). Despite the slow in vitro rates for GTP hydrolysis by these $G\alpha$-subunits, some effectors, such as the myocardial $G\alpha_i$-activated K^+ channel and the $G\alpha_t$cGMP phosphodiesterase, are deactivated with extraordinarily short $t_{1/2}$ values (for example, ~0.2 s for the myocardial K^+ channel) (9, 40, 41, 497), which implies that at least some cells possess alternative mechanisms to accelerate $G\alpha$-subunit deactivation by GTP hydrolysis. The effector enzyme phospholipase $C\beta_1$, which is activated by the G_q/G_{11} protein class, can stimulate the steady-state GTPase activity of G_q up to 50-fold when GTP–GDP exchange is catalyzed by the activated M_1-muscarinic receptor (19, 20), thus acting as a GTPase-activating protein (GAP) specific for the members of this particular heterotrimeric G-protein class. There is also evidence for a GAP effect of the retinal cGMP phosphodiesterase on $G\alpha_t$ (8, 366).

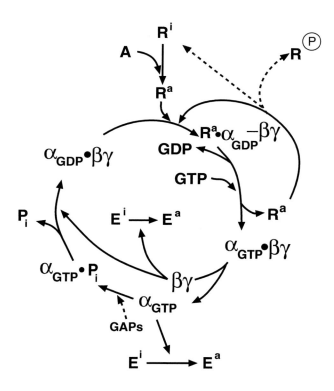

FIG. 6.4. Basic regulatory cycle of a G protein involving both GTP-induced activation and subunit dissociation and GTPase-dependent inactivation and subunit reassociation. The unoccupied receptor *(R^i)* interacts with a specific agonist *(A)*, leading to activation of the receptor *(R^a)*, which interacts with the trimeric $G\alpha\beta\gamma$ protein complex, promoting Mg^{2+}-dependent GDP→GTP exchange and subunit dissociation, allowing their interaction with effectors *(E^i)*. GAPs, GTPase-activating proteins; *R^®*, phosphorylated receptor; *E^a*, activated effector.

Structural and Functional Relationships of $G\alpha$-Subunit

$G\alpha$-subunits that bind GTP are the main effector activators. The predicted primary structures of cloned $G\alpha$ family members disclose a consistent pattern of conserved and divergent sequences. The α-subunits are at least 45%–80% similar in amino-acid sequence (Fig. 6.3); the regions of higher identity lie mainly in the domains that form the guanine nucleotide–binding pocket (96, 430, 457). Whereas the conserved regions apparently perform similar functions in the various Gα-subunits, the variable domains reflect unique properties, such as interaction with a specific receptor, effector, and Gβγ complex (see below). Although the three-dimensional structure in the majority of the Gα proteins is still unknown, the structures of Gα$_t$ and Gα$_{i1}$ suggest mechanisms for GTP hydrolysis and reveal the conformational changes occurring during the transition from the inactive to the active state (66, 267, 354, 499). Basically, Gα$_t$ consists of two domains separated by a deep guanine nucleotide–binding cleft [Fig. 6.5; (267, 354)]. One domain (the GTPase domain) contains the GTP-binding motif whose core consists of a six-stranded β-sheet, in which five strands are parallel and one is antiparallel; this β-sheet is surrounded by five α-helices (267, 354, 399). The domain contains the consensus sequences involved in GTP binding of all of the GTPases (95, 169, 249, 274), the phosphate-binding loop (Gα$_t$ residues 36–43; consensus GXXXXGKS/T), the Mg^{2+}-binding domain (residues 196–199, between strands β$_2$ and β$_3$; DXXG), and the guanine ring–binding region (residues 264–268; NKXD) (267, 327, 399). It also contains a second guanine ring–binding site (TCAT) and another region

involved in binding Mg^{2+} and the phosphates (RXXT) (267, 399). The second is an entirely α-helical domain consisting of a long central helix surrounded by five shorter helices (267). The overall architecture of α$_{i1}$ is similar to that of Gα$_t$, albeit with some differences when comparing the conformational change between the GDP (inactive) and the GTP (active) forms (66, 499).

For some G proteins, the COOH-terminus (and some regions of the α$_5$ helix) of the Gα-subunit is involved in the interaction and specificity of the protein with its cognate receptor (67, 170, 171, 344). Binding of antibodies against the COOH-terminus of G proteins as well as mutagenesis of Gα in this region disrupts receptor–G protein interactions (163, 196, 432, 461), and a COOH-terminal Gα$_t$ peptide (residues 340–350) can bind to and directly stabilize activated rhodopsin (108, 171). Specificity may involve additional sites since several Gα-subunits (for example, Gα$_{oA}$ and Gα$_{oB}$) interact with different receptors despite being identical at their extreme COOH-termini (251). These possible additional regions have been described for Gα$_t$ (171, 267, 354). The COOH-terminus is also essential for Gα interactions with effectors (18, 213, 354, 391).

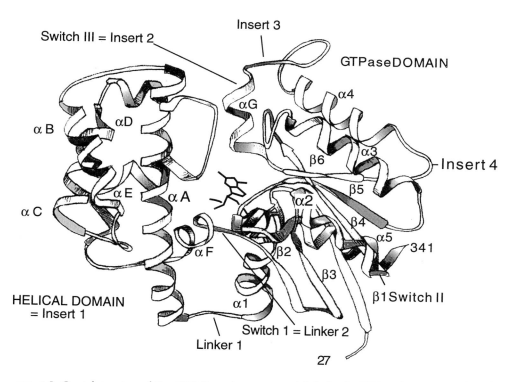

FIG. 6.5. Crystal structure of Gα$_t$-GDP. Secondary structure labels for the GTPase domain were derived from the numerical designations used to describe the homologous *ras* p21 domains. Additional unique helices in Gα$_t$ are labeled *A–G*. Locations of inserts, linkers, and switch regions also are labeled (354). [Reproduced from Rens-Domiano and Hamm (399) with permission.]

Construction of $G\alpha_i/G\alpha_s$ chimeras and mutational studies have demonstrated that the adenylyl cyclase–activating region is contained in the COOH-terminus of $G\alpha_s$, corresponding to residues 235–356 (213, 362). For $G\alpha_t$, studies employing synthetic peptides have indicated that residues 293–314, which are adjacent to the receptor-activation domain, are important for $G\alpha_t$-regulated cGMP–phosphodiesterase activation (391); another region, corresponding to the phosphate-binding loop, undergoes a significant conformational change between the active (GTP-bound) and inactive (GDP-bound) crystal structures and, thus, also may be important for effector activation (267, 354). The crystal structure of $G\alpha_{i2}$ suggests the existence of an additional region located in its α-helical domain which is also important for its interaction with the effector (66, 499). Finally, the NH_2-terminus of the $G\alpha$-subunit, particularly its first 60 amino-acid residues, appears to be one of the sites of interaction with the $G\beta\gamma$-dimer (67, 93, 143, 399). Apparently, the $G\alpha$-subunit is able to interact with both the β- and the γ-subunits (267). Monoclonal antibody 4A directed against the NH_2-terminus of $G\alpha_t$ causes dissociation from the $\beta\gamma$-dimer (309, 310); likewise, limited proteolysis and expression of NH_2-terminally truncated $G\alpha$-subunits indicate that the myristoylated NH_2-terminus and a region within the first 25 residues of the $G\alpha$-subunit are essential for interaction with $G\beta\gamma$ (93, 143, 399). Another possible site of $G\alpha$-subunit interaction with the $G\alpha\gamma$-dimer lies within the switch regions [that is, regions that undergo nucleotide-dependent conformational changes (Fig. 6.5) of the subunit], specifically in the switch II region (amino-acid residues 199–216 in $G\alpha_{i1}$ and 195–215 in $G\alpha_t$) (267, 499). The $G\beta\gamma$-dimer may bind to a hydrophobic pocket present in $G\alpha$-GDP, but it may be closed by the GTP-dependent conformational change (267, 399); this pocket is made up of the switch II region and the β-sheet hydrophobic core (267). A Cys in this switch region (Cys_{215} in $G\alpha_o$, cognate to Cys_{210} in $G\alpha_t$) can be chemically cross-linked to $\beta\gamma$ (475), and the Gly_{226}-to-Ala mutation in $G\alpha_s$ that impairs the GTP-induced conformational changes in the switch II region also prevents dissociation of the $G\alpha$-subunit from the $\beta\gamma$-dimer (279, 320).

Certain subclasses of the $G\alpha$-subunit are adenosine diphosphate (ADP)–ribosylated by bacterial toxins from *Bordetella pertusis* (pertussis toxin or PTX) and *Vibrio cholerae* (cholera toxin or CTX) (2, 53, 488, 512). Cholera toxin catalyzes ADP-ribosylation of an Arg residue present within the GTP-binding domain of $G\alpha_s$ and $G\alpha_{olf}$ in a ligand-independent fashion and of $G\alpha_t$ and $G\alpha_i$ in a ligand-dependent manner (2, 53, 488). This CTX-induced modification of the $G\alpha$-subunit considerably decreases the intrinsic GTPase

activity, causing constitutive activation of the protein. Mutation of the same Arg residue also inhibits GTPase activity, leading to a comparable constitutive activation (139). $G\alpha_i$, $G\alpha_t$, $G\alpha_{gust}$, and $G\alpha_o$ can be ADP-ribosylated by PTX on the fourth Cys residue from the COOH-terminus (335, 512); this modification, which is enhanced by the presence of the $G\alpha\beta\gamma$-dimer (that is, the presence of the G-protein heterotrimeric state), leads to uncoupling of the G protein from the receptor without modifying other functions, such as guanine nucleotide exchange or GTPase activity (67, 388).

$G\beta\gamma$ Structure and Function

$G\beta\gamma$-subunits are bound tightly to each other through noncovalent hydrophobic interactions (62, 209, 435); the complex is resistant to tryptic cleavage and can be dissociated only by treatment with denaturing agents. Separate expression of these subunits leads to unstable $G\beta$-subunits and unfolded $G\gamma$-subunits (191). The $G\beta$-subunits display 58%–90% identity, whereas the $G\gamma$-subunits are more diverse (430, 503). This probably accounts for the high degree of specificity for subunit association; $G\beta_1$ can associate with $G\gamma_1$ or $G\gamma_2$, whereas $G\beta_2$ can associate with $G\gamma_2$ but not with $G\gamma_1$, and $G\beta_3$ does not associate with either $G\gamma_1$ or $G\gamma_2$ (384, 416). Primary structures of the cloned $G\beta$-subunits as well as the crystal structure of the heterotrimeric $G\alpha_i\beta_1\gamma_2$ protein and the transducin $\beta\gamma$-dimer indicate the existence of two distinct domains. The relatively conserved NH_2-terminal domain forms an amphipathic α-helical coiled coil that lies closely parallel to, and interacts with, the NH_2-terminal helix of $G\gamma$ (300); the existence of this proximity is supported by the fact that Cys residues located in both subunits (Cys_{25} of $G\beta_1$ and Cys_{37-38} of $G\gamma_1$) can be chemically cross-linked and Glu_{10} of $G\beta$ is necessary for $G\beta\gamma$ dimerization (43, 149, 435, 499). The second domain of $G\beta$ consists of seven 40 to 43-residue repetitive segments that contain a characteristic tryptophan–aspartic acid pair, termed WD40, which may be found in a variety of apparently functionally unrelated proteins engaged in a variety of functions, including signal transduction, cell division, transcription, cytoskeletal assembly, and vesicle function (62, 430, 435). The WD repeat regions in $G\beta$ may be involved in the regulation of selectivity of the β-subunit to dimerize with a particular γ-subunit as well as in the capacity of the β-subunits to adopt multiple conformations, which in turn could greatly expand the number of protein–protein interactions (for example, with the β-adrenergic receptor kinase; see REGULATORY MECHANISMS, below) and signaling pathways (62, 345, 501). However, $G\gamma$-subunits are largely α-helical, and their selectivity for the various β-subunits is determined by a stretch of 14 amino acids located in the middle of the γ-subunit (300, 435, 442); this region contains the Cys residue that is susceptible to cross-linking with the β-subunit (see above) (43, 149). In some systems, this subunit appears to be critical for determining the function of the Gβγ-dimer. For example, the function of $G\beta_1\gamma_1$ (localized in the retina) is quite different from that of $G\beta_1\gamma_2$ (found in the brain and other tissues); since the Gβ-subunits are the same, the functional differences between the two dimers are probably due to the different γ-subunits (62). On the contrary, in other systems, the Gβ-subunits appear to determine effector selectivity (519, 536); this effect of Gβ has been demonstrated by in vitro studies, showing that while both $G\beta_1$ and $G\beta_5$ were able to activate phospholipase-$C\beta_2$ in a γ_2-dependent manner, $G\beta_5$, unlike β_1, did not stimulate the mitogen-activated protein kinase (MAPK) or the cJun NH_2-terminal kinase (JNK) pathways (536).

The association of the Gβγ-dimer with Gα is the best defined protein–protein interaction of the dimer. The Gβγ-dimer is associated with the α-subunit through direct interactions between the prenylated form of the Gγ-subunit and Gα(387, 532); the Gβ- and Gα-subunits are in close proximity, but apparently they do not interact independently of the Gγ-subunit (267, 435, 532). The association of Gβγ with Gα increases the affinity of the latter subunit for GDP by about 100-fold, stabilizing the inactive state of the protein (190). However, the Gβγ-complex associates with its cognate receptor through the COOH-terminus of the γ-subunit, which becomes physically available for such interaction during the course of receptor–Gαβγ-complex coupling (62, 247, 248, 377). Thus, it seems that the Gγ-subunit plays a key role in conferring the specificity of the G-protein interaction with receptors. The presence of the Gβγ-dimer is a prerequisite for effective interaction of the G_t protein with rhodopsin and, hence, for receptor-catalyzed nucleotide exchange (62, 123, 248, 428).

The Gβγ-dimer is required for efficient association of the Gα-subunit with the plasma membrane and for an effective interaction of the Gα-subunit with the receptor (see above) (197, 247, 248, 377). In addition to this well-known effect, the Gβγ-complex regulates the activity of many effectors (62, 161, 209, 290, 296, 467, 529, 536). It is involved in adenylyl cyclase types II and IV activation and type I inhibition (27, 119, 414, 467, 471). The extent of activation of these isoforms may vary depending on the specific βγ-dimer involved; the type II isoform is activated effectively by $G\beta_1\gamma_2$, $G\beta_2\gamma_2$, and $G\beta_2\gamma_3$, whereas the activation induced by transducin $G\beta_1\gamma_1$ is about one-tenth as effective as that mediated by the other dimers (210).

The activity of the other adenylyl cyclase types is not altered by the Gβγ-complex (462). The Gβγ-dimer also activates isoforms 1–3 of phospholipase Cβ (28, 36, 47, 48, 161, 236, 290); the stimulation is, however, subtype-specific, with a rank order of effect of phospholipase $C\beta_3 \geq \beta_2 >> \beta_1$, which is different from that of $G\alpha_{q/11}$ (27, 223, 368, 434, 528). Gβγ does not modify the activity of phospholipase $C\beta_4$ (278). Another important role of the Gβγ-complex is regulation of the muscarine-gated K^+ channels; after years of controversy over the role of the Gα-subunit vs. the Gβγ-dimer in cardiac muscarinic K^+ channel activation, the bulk of evidence strongly indicates that the Gβγ-dimer activates this particular channel more effectively than $G\alpha_i$ (295, 296, 516). Gβγ-subunits also activate phospholipase A_2, the enzyme responsible for arachidonic acid formation (221, 245); although arachidonic acid and its metabolites have been implicated in the activation of muscarine-dependent cardiac K^+ channels (264), their effect is weaker than that elicited by the Gβγ-complex (62). In contrast to the members of the $G\alpha_i$ family, the dimer does not influence significantly the activity of the cardiac ATP-sensitive K^+ channel (215). The Gβγ-dimer produces a 10-fold increase in the agonist-dependent phosphorylation of purified β_2-adrenergic receptor (207, 379); this increase, which leads to receptor desensitization, occurs through a mechanism that involves interaction of the dimer with a specific region of the pleckstrin homology domain of the β-adrenergic receptor kinase (208, 382) and translocation of the kinase from the cytosol to the plasma membrane by the prenylated Gβγ-subunit, allowing the enzyme to recognize and interact with those intracellular elements of the receptor susceptible to modification by phosphorylation (see Receptor Desensitization, below). In this vein, it is interesting that rhodopsin kinase (the analog of the β-adrenergic receptor kinase in the retina) is farnesylated at its COOH-terminus and does not require Gβγ to phosphorylate the receptor (138).

In addition to the actions of the Gα-subunit and the Gβγ-dimer described above, all classes of G protein may mediate long-term effects on gene expression and cell growth induced by mitogenic hormones that bind to GPCRs (10, 30, 96, 97, 117, 208, 381, 486). The best established pathway by which heterotrimeric G proteins transduce signals destined to phosphorylate nuclear transcription factors and thus promote the transcription of genes controlling cellular growth is the G protein–activated/*Ras*-regulated MAPK cascade, a series of protein–protein interactions and phosphorylations (84, 352, 374, 381). *Ras* proteins are low-molecular-weight GTPases involved in mitogenesis and differentiation triggered by activated enzyme (tyrosine kinase)–linked receptors (167, 317); they belong to the superfamily of monomeric small G proteins which embraces the Rho proteins (*Rho, Rac,* and cdc42) involved in cytoskeletal rearrangements (31, 32, 168). Activated (GTP-bound) *Ras* binds to and activates the *Raf-1* Ser/Thr kinase, which in turn promotes the phosphorylation of a second kinase, MEK (mitogen-activated/extracellular signal–regulated kinase) (271). This kinase specifically activates, through dual phosphorylation of Tyr and Thr residues, the classical MAPKs, which are then translocated from the cytoplasm to the nucleus, where they phosphorylate a variety of transcription factors [Fig. 6.6; (65, 84)]. The activity of MAPKs can be regulated by PTX-sensitive and -insensitive heterotrimeric G proteins in a *Ras*-dependent manner (6, 92, 269, 487, 522). Certain G_i-linked receptors [for example, the M_2-muscarinic (522) and α_2-adrenergic (6) receptors] trigger the *Ras*–MAPK cascade through a complex mechanism which may involve stimulation of Src tyrosine kinase activity by

the G$\beta\gamma$-dimer (117, 179, 255). In turn, Src kinase phosphorylates several substrates, including tyrosine kinase receptors (for example, epidermal growth factor or platelet-derived growth factor receptors) and/or the Shc adapter molecule, which binds to a second adapter, the Grb2 protein, through Src-homology 2 (SH2) domains (58, 254, 406, 479, 485); since Grb2 and the guanosine nucleotide exchange factor Sos1 are associated constitutively, the G$\beta\gamma$-mediated recruitment of Grb2 to activated (tyrosine-phosphorylated) Shc augments the Shc-associated guanine nucleotide exchange factor activity, leading to GDP→GTP exchange and activation of *Ras* (429). However, G_q-linked receptors may activate MAPK by their corresponding Gα proteins through either *Ras*-dependent or -independent pathways [Fig. 6.6; (179, 257, 406)]. *Ras*-independent activation of MAPKs involves Gα_q activation of PKC, which in turn phosphorylates and activates *Raf-1*, whereas the *Ras*-dependent mechanism involves Gα_q-triggered activation of downstream signals that lead

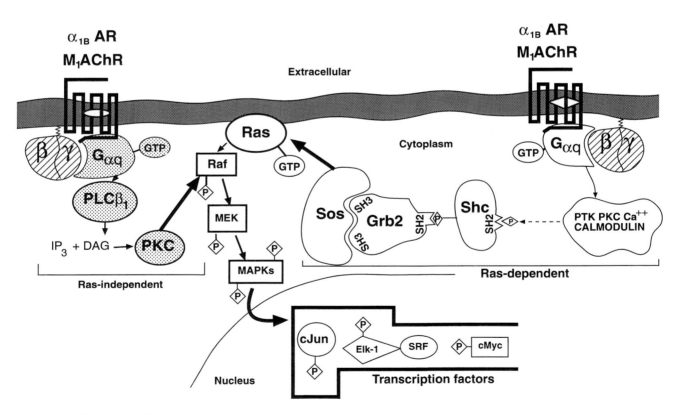

FIG. 6.6. *Ras*-dependent *(right)* and -independent *(left)* pathways of mitogen-activated protein kinase *(MAPK)* activation by G protein–coupled receptors [for example, α_{1B}-adrenergic receptor *(α_{1B} AR)* and muscarinic M_1-acetylcholine receptor *(M_1AChR)*] coupled to pertussis toxin–insensitive *(Gα_q)* G proteins. Gα_q activates phospholipase Cβ_1 *(PLCβ_1)*, resulting in the conversion of phosphatidylinositol-4,5-biphosphate to inositol-1,4,5-triphosphate

(IP$_3$) and diacylglycerol *(DAG)*, which in turn contributes to the activation of protein kinase C *(PKC)*, which then activates *Raf* kinase by a still poorly understood mechanism. Activated Gα_q also interacts with other intracellular signaling molecules [PKC, protein tyrosine kinases *(PTK)*, etc.] to activate the *Ras*-regulated MAPK cascade. *MEK,* mitogen-activated/extracellular signal–regulated kinase.

to formation of the Shc–Grb2–Sos signaling complex [probably through a PKC- and/or a Ca^{2+}-activated, PYK2-mediated Shc phosphorylation mechanism (284)] and the subsequent activation of *Ras*. Other studies suggest that MAPK activation by G_q proteins may be modulated further by the contribution of their $G\beta\gamma$-subunits (77, 385). Another effector pathway whereby heterotrimeric G proteins may transduce signals to the nucleus involves activation of *JNK*, a kinase related to MAPK but differentially regulated (70, 85, 96). Activation of *JNK* proceeds through a cascade of protein–protein interactions, triggered by the low-molecular-weight cdc42 and Rac G proteins, that involve the activation of several kinases, including the p21-activated kinase (PAK), MEK kinase (MEKK-1), and JNK kinase (JNKK) (71, 94, 271, 324); JNK, like MAPK, phosphorylates and increases the activity of several transcription factors (162, 324). Activation of M_1-muscarinic receptors as well as expression of constitutively active $G\alpha_q$, $G\alpha_{12}$, or $G\alpha_{13}$ result in increased JNK activity (70, 96, 491). Finally, although cAMP is not mitogenic in most cell types, G_s activation may induce growth responses in some in vitro and in vivo systems (117, 140, 270, 302, 484). Constitutively active mutants of the G_s-linked TSH and growth hormone receptors have been isolated from thyroid and pituitary tumors (270, 302). In other systems, however, G_s appears to be involved in inhibition of nuclear transduction signals (69, 76, 423). In isoproterenol-stimulated COS-7 cells, G_s-coupled receptors may mediate simultaneous but opposing effects (76), with the $G\beta\gamma$-subunits inducing MAPK activation and the cAMP generated through $G\alpha$-stimulated adenylyl cyclase inhibiting such effects. Thus, it appears that the intensity of the response in these β-adrenergic stimulated cells is determined by the balance between the two differing signals.

REGULATORY MECHANISMS

From this discussion, it is clear that the function of the GPCRs involves the concerted action of several control mechanisms operating at different levels, including the receptor molecule, the G protein, and the effector levels. However, our current understanding of the exact mechanisms that allow for a highly specific and equilibrated function of the receptor–G protein–effector system is still limited and further complicated by the existence of several factors and potential down- and upstream pathways or loops that may influence receptor availability and rates of activation and deactivation, the specificity of receptor–G protein interaction and signal transduction, and the intensity of G protein-mediated activation of a given effector (394). Some of these mechanisms are discussed briefly in this section.

Mechanisms that Regulate Receptor Function

Several feedback mechanisms that control the functional status of GPCRs have been explored extensively. Among these, three are worthy of particular consideration; the first mechanism involves changes in the dynamic state of the receptor triggered by conformational changes in the receptor molecule and its interaction with its coupled G proteins, whereas the other two are involved with desensitization.

Receptor Conformation and Signaling. The GPCRs exist in several dynamic states, as disclosed by marked shifts in agonist affinity (125, 280, 282, 409). Receptors are assumed to exist in an equilibrium between an inactive (R) and an active (R*) conformation. Binding of agonists exhibiting a preferentially higher affinity for R* promotes an isomerization step that stabilizes the receptor in a "relaxed" state and shifts the equilibrium toward the R* conformation, promoting its interaction with G proteins and allowing the formation of a highly efficient ternary complex (agonist–R*–G protein) that stabilizes the R* state and triggers G-protein activation (88). The requirement of such an isomerization step in the receptor molecule to switch into the R* conformation was unmasked by the particular behavior exhibited by a series of mutant adrenergic receptors, disclosing that certain intracellular regions of the receptor are critical for maintaining the receptor in a relatively constrained, "unrelaxed" state in the absence of agonist (282, 409). Mutations in specific amino-acid residues in the COOH-terminus of the third intracellular loop of the α_{1B}- and α_{2A}-adrenergic receptors (coupled to the G_q–phospholipase $C\beta$ and the G_i–adenylyl cyclase pathways, respectively), as well as in the same loop of its relative, the G_s-coupled β_2-adrenoreceptor, resulted, in all instances, in elevated basal, agonist-independent signaling activity, as well as in a supersensitivity to agonists [Fig. 6.1C; (250, 282, 398, 409)]. Thus, the mutations introduced allowed for conformational changes that led to a high level of constitutive receptor activation and interaction with the G proteins in the unliganded state, recreating the R* state promoted in intact wild receptors only by agonist binding (152). Although the exact nature of the conformational changes that lead to the R* state are still unknown, analysis of several spontaneously occurring gain-of-function mutations that induce constitutive receptor hyperactivity suggests that multiple regions of the receptor molecule, including the extracellular, intracellular, and transmembrane domains, are involved in the molecular mechanisms that constrain the G-protein coupling of the receptor, a constraint normally relieved upon agonist occupancy [Fig. 6.1A, C; (250, 263, 281, 370, 390, 401, 409, 427, 492)]. Several physiological implications arise from this mechanism of receptor activation. The equilibrium between R and R* implies that at any time a certain proportion of receptors resides in a constitutively active state even in the absence of an activating ligand. This, in fact, occurs, and some endogenous GPCRs exhibit demonstrable activity even in the absence of agonist (72, 409). Thus, different receptor isoforms that bind the same ligand and activate the same effector may vary in their ability to spontaneously isomerize into the active state and, therefore, in their affinity for endogenous agonists. In this setting, it is expected that agonists acting through receptor variants with an elevated constitutive isomerization rate will have a higher potency, whereas those acting through variants with a low isomerization rate will provoke a more graded range of responses (409). Such differences in intrinsic capacity to isomerize could be accounted for by alterations of one or more critically placed amino-acid residues and could reasonably explain the existence of distinct receptor subtypes for a single ligand (282). In addition, the existence of naturally occurring, constitutively active GPCRs may allow for certain antagonistic drugs and endogenous ligands to elicit negative activity or inverse agonism (that is, lowering the basal activity); as opposed to agonists, which are presumed to have a high affinity for R*, inverse agonists exhibit a high affinity for R and, therefore, decrease the R*/R ratio (323).

Receptor Desensitization. Continuous or prolonged stimulation of a cell generally results in progressively attenuated responses to subsequent stimulation by the same agonist. This decrease in cellular sensitivity to further stimulation, or desensitization, may be considered one of the most important mechanisms to protect the cell from excessive stimulation, particularly under conditions of high agonist exposure. Phosphorylation-mediated deactivation of rhodopsin exemplifies the paramount importance of this protective mechanism; in this system, signaling is inactivated rapidly (high millisecond–second time scale) following exposure to light, thereby preventing a brief flash of light from being perceived as continuous illumination (35, 476, 520). Transgenic mice bearing a mutation in rhodopsin that prevents short-term desensitization exhibit a marked prolongation of light-evoked electrical responses from single rods, leading to retinal degeneration (55). Thus, for many cells bearing GPCRs the functional status of such receptors is determined by the phosphorylation state (33, 175, 176, 192, 351, 386, 400, 519).

Early receptor desensitization occurs rapidly, in seconds to minutes of agonist exposure, and involves phosphorylation of intracellular domains of the stimulated receptors by second messenger–dependent activated kinases (PKA or PKC) (138, 243) and/or by a special class of Ser/Thr-specific kinases called G protein–coupled receptor kinases (GRK1–6) (382), with the subsequent uncoupling of the receptors from their respective G proteins and loss of downstream signaling events (138). Homologous short-term desensitization occurs very rapidly, with a half-life from milliseconds to a few seconds, and is observed when the cell's response decreases after high receptor occupancy by a specific agonist (138, 176, 192, 386, 404, 415); heterologous desensitization (nonagonist-specific) is observed after several minutes of low amounts of agonist exposure and usually occurs when a cell's response to various agonists acting through different receptors decreases after receptor activation by a particular agonist (63, 132, 138). Whereas homologous desensitization may be mediated through receptor phosphorylation triggered by both second messenger–activated protein kinases and GRKs, heterologous desensitization generally involves phosphorylation by second messenger–dependent kinases (63, 138, 192, 193, 386).

Several GPCRs desensitize through phosphorylation (176, 192, 386, 400, 476). The molecular basis of agonist-induced phosphorylation has been studied particularly in the biogenic amine receptors (for example, the β-adrenergic receptor) and rhodopsin (132, 176, 519, 520). In these receptors, GRK-mediated Ser/Thr phosphorylation and subsequent G-protein uncoupling involve several steps. In unstimulated cells, GRKs are located primarily in the cytoplasm; upon agonist-induced receptor activation, GRKs translocate to the plasma membrane, a process that involves receptor–GRK interactions as well as isoprenylation [for example, farnesylation of rhodopsin kinase (206, 207)], palmitoylation [as in GRK4 and GRK6 (446)], or interaction of the GRK with the membrane-anchored $G\beta\gamma$-complex and phosphatidylinositol-4,5-biphosphate through its COOH-terminal pleckstrin homology domain [such as the β-adrenergic receptor kinase (382)] (208). Once the receptor is phosphorylated near the sites required for G-protein interaction [for example, in at least seven and eleven sites located within 10- and 59-amino-acid stretches of the COOH-terminal domains of rhodopsin and the β_2-adrenergic receptor, respectively (33, 175, 520); Fig. 6.1C], the subsequent binding of a group of inhibitory proteins, the arrestins, amplifies the desensitization process initiated by phosphorylation and turns off the receptor by impeding its coupling to G proteins (297, 444). Although the available studies do not allow unambiguous clarification of the in vivo specificity of the several GRK and arrestin isoforms, it is possible that, with few exceptions, short-term desensitization of GPCRs is regulated by more than one GRK or arrestin isoform.

It has been shown that short-term desensitized receptors are resensitized by a complex process that involves arrestin-mediated receptor sequestration into endosomes, where they become dephosphorylated by a particular group of membrane-associated receptor Ser/Thr phosphatases (380, 494, 495). For the β_2-adrenergic receptor and the NK_1 receptor, resensitization requires vesicular acidification and subsequent changes in receptor conformation to become accessible to the Ser/Thr phosphatases (148, 157, 261). Whether this tightly regulated resensitization mechanism is applicable to other members of the GPCR superfamily remains to be investigated.

A more profound deactivation process, long-term desensitization, is observed after hours or days of high levels of agonist exposure and involves a decrease in the net complement of receptors specific for a particular agonist, without detectable changes in receptor affinity (46, 68, 164, 176, 226, 305, 312, 426, 460). This type of cellular desensitization is subserved by several biochemically distinct mechanisms, including receptor down-regulation (that is, loss in total cellular content of functional receptors) and internalization (loss of surface receptors) (68, 176, 222, 305, 312). Although this type of desensitization does not require previous phosphorylation of the receptor, in some systems it amplifies the loss of functional receptors initiated by short-term deactivation (176, 502). For certain GPCRs, the net loss in receptor number and/or function involves the occurrence of various receptor and postreceptor events, including internalization, sequestration, and degradation of the receptor (222, 261, 305, 319), as well as changes in the rate of receptor synthesis by alterations in receptor mRNA levels or function (164–166). In others, down-regulation does not require immediate changes in protein synthesis and decreased receptor mRNA levels are observed only after prolonged exposure to agonist (68). The overall process leads to a significant reduction in the number of functionally available receptors on the cell surface, where they could interact with agonist and activate signaling. Finally, in certain cells bearing GPCRs, loss of ability to respond to prolonged agonist stimulation also may be achieved by mechanisms related not to the receptor itself but to downstream and negative feedback mechanisms involving inactivation of Gα-subunits or loss of functional activity of effectors. An example of these postreceptor mechanisms is the GnRH-responsive cell, in which loss of responsiveness is due, on the one hand, to receptor loss (68, 222) and, on the other, to the action of GAPs or RGS (regulators of G-protein signaling) proteins (104a, 109, 348, 504), decreased functional activity of the Ca^{2+} ion channel, and reduced efficiency of mobilization by IP_3 of Ca^{2+} from the intracellular pool (313).

G Protein–Mediated Regulatory Mechanisms

As discussed above, G proteins are the molecules that transduce the signal triggered by receptor activation (see THE HETEROTRIMERIC G-PROTEIN FAMILY, above). In addition to the particular characteristics of the individual α- and βγ-subunits that allow for some degree of selectivity for interaction with each other, with the receptor, and with their corresponding effectors, there are other mechanisms that tightly regulate the selectivity and intensity of the signal transduced by these molecules. Thus, in some systems, activation of particular effectors by the Gβγ-complex is conditioned by Gα priming [for example, stimulation of adenylyl cyclase types II and IV (119, 467)], whereas in others it seems to be independent [for example, activation of phospholipase $C\beta_{1-3}$ (62, 368, 434)]. However, whereas in certain systems the effects mediated by the Gβγ-dimer are the opposite of those triggered by Gα [for example, activation of type I adenylyl cyclase by the latter and inhibition by the former (119, 467, 470, 472, 527)], in others stimulation of the same effector (for example, activation of the acetylcholine-regulated cardiac K^+ channels) occurs as a result of the activation of convergent pathways triggered independently by both elements (295, 296, 515, 516, 531). Activation of divergent G protein–dependent pathways leading to stimulation of different effectors also may occur, as exemplified by phospholipase Cβ activation by PTX-sensitive G proteins (G_i and G_o) through their corresponding Gβγ-complexes (28, 113, 236). Thus, the existence of convergent, divergent, and opposite pathways for effector activation, as well as of differences in selectivity for protein–protein interactions [activation and selectivity being accomplished by differences in affinity or efficacy of interaction of the G-protein subunits with the receptor, effector, and themselves (20, 74, 116, 253, 277, 384, 416, 433, 534); compartmentation of particular activators and effectors (49, 412); and tissue distribution and expression of the different classes and subclasses of each G protein and effector (142, 228, 237, 316, 393, 459)] among the G proteins, allows for the different, fine-tuning mechanisms through which the cells may regulate the specificity of the signal conveyed by these effector-activating protein molecules.

Cells also limit their extent of response to external stimuli by decreasing the levels of specific G proteins involved in the signal transduction triggered by an agonist-activated GPCR (246, 285, 321, 424). Receptor-mediated down-regulation of G proteins is thus another mechanism through which cells may desensitize. G-protein down-regulation has been demonstrated in several in vitro systems in which a specific receptor is expressed at high levels. For example, NG108-15 cells (a neuroblastoma–glioma hybrid cell line) transfected to express the β_2-adrenergic receptor at high levels and exposed to the agonist isoprenaline responded with a significant decrease in intracellular levels of $G\alpha_s$ (but not of $G\alpha_{i/o}$ or $G\alpha_q/G\alpha_{11}$) compared to clones with a low expression level of the same receptor (4). Down-regulation of $G\alpha_i$ and $G\alpha_q/G\alpha_{11}$ also has been documented (246, 321, 424). Further, this desensitization apparently is not mediated by changes at the transcriptional or translational levels but rather by an agonist-promoted enhancement of turnover of the specific G proteins (424).

Another interesting mechanism that regulates the activity of G proteins is mediated through the phosphoprotein phosducin, which originally was purified from retina, as a complex with the $G\beta\gamma$-subunit ($\beta_1\gamma_1$) of transducin, and from the pineal gland (14, 62). This protein inhibits retinal cGMP phosphodiesterase in vitro probably by preventing the association of G-protein subunits with activated rhodopsin (14). Phosducin mRNA is present in a variety of tissues, including brain, heart, kidney, liver, lung, spleen, and skeletal muscle (14). In vitro, recombinant phosducin inhibits the GTPase activity of $G\alpha_s$ and $G\alpha_i/G\alpha_o$ as well as $G\alpha_s$-mediated adenylyl cyclase activation, in a PKA-regulated manner. In this setting, the regulation of effector activity promoted by phosducin may be achieved through the formation of a complex between phosducin and the trimeric G protein, thus inhibiting G protein–mediated signaling either by preventing the formation of an activated state after GTP-binding or by sterically interfering with G protein–effector interaction (14, 62).

In addition to the receptor- and G protein–dependent mechanisms described above, the selectivity and intensity of the signal triggered upon agonist-induced receptor activation may be influenced by other factors, such as the functional expression of receptor splice variants (or isoforms) exhibiting different sensitivities and specificities to ligands and G proteins (237, 339, 346, 347, 373); receptor coupling to more than one G-protein class (195, 260, 386); and cross-talk between different G protein–transduced signals (293, 311, 372), different GPCRs (304), or even different receptor systems [GPCRs and enzyme (tyrosine kinase)–linked receptors] (92, 300a, 486). Thus, the mechanisms controlling activation of a particular GPCR by a determined ligand, the specificity of receptor–G protein–effector interaction, and the intensity and duration of the signal are highly complex and multifactorial.

A.U.-A. is a visiting scientist in receipt of a fellowship award from NICHD/Fogarty (HD00668) and CONACyT, Mexico (250010); P.M.C. received support from HD19899, HD00668, HD18185 (P30) 1, and RR00163.

REFERENCES

1. Aatsinki, J. T., E. M. Pietilä, J. T. Lakkakorpi, and H. J. Rajaniemi. Expression of the LH/CG receptor gene in rat ovarian tissue is regulated by an extensive alternative splicing of the primary transcript. *Mol. Cell. Endocrinol.* 84: 127–135, 1992.
2. Abood, M. E., J. B. Hurley, M.-C. Pappone, H. R. Bourne, and L. Stryer. Functional homology between signal-coupling proteins. Cholera toxin inactivates the GTPase activity of transducin. *J. Biol. Chem.* 257: 10540–10543, 1982.
3. Abou-Samra, A. B., H. Jüppner, T. Force, M. W. Freeman, X. F. Kong, E. Schipani, P. Urena, J. Richards, J. V. Bonventre, J. T. Potts, Jr., H. M. Kronenberg, and G. V. Segre. Expression cloning of a parathyroid hormone/parathyroid hormone–related peptide receptor from rat osteoblast-like cells: a single receptor stimulates intracellular accumulation of both cAMP and inositol triphosphates and increases intracellular free calcium. *Proc. Natl. Acad. Sci. U.S.A.* 89: 2732–2736, 1992.
4. Adie, E. J., and G. Milligan. Agonist regulation of cellular levels of the stimulatory guanine nucleotide-binding protein, G_s, in wild-type transfected neuroblastoma-glioma hybrid NG108–15 cells. *Biochem. Soc. Trans.* 21: 432–435, 1993.
5. Akamizu, T., D. Inoue, S. Kosugi, T. Ban, L. D. Khon, H. Imura, and T. Mori. Chimeric studies of the extracellular domain of the rat thyrotropin (TSH) receptor: aminoacids (268–304) in the TSH receptor are involved in ligand high affinity binding, but not in TSH receptor-specific signal transduction. *Endocr. J.* 40: 363–372, 1993.
6. Alblas, J., E. J. van Corven, P. L. Hordijk, G. Milligan, and W. H. Moolenaar. G_i-mediated activation of the p21[ras]-mitogen-activated protein kinase pathway by α_2-adrenergic receptors expressed in fibroblasts. *J. Biol. Chem.* 268: 22235–22238, 1993.
7. Amatruda, T. T. I., D. A. Steele, V. Z. Slepak, and M. I. Simon. $G\alpha_{16}$, a G protein α subunit specifically expressed in hematopoietic cells. *Proc. Natl. Acad. Sci. U.S.A.* 88: 5587–5591, 1991.
8. Arshavsky, V. Y., and M. D. Bownds. Regulation of deactivation of photoreceptor G protein by its target enzyme and cGMP. *Nature* 357: 416–417, 1992.
9. Arshavsky, V. Y., M. P. Gray-Keller, and M. D. Bownds. cGMP suppresses GTPase activity of a portion of transducin equimolar to phosphodiesterase in frog rod outer segments. Light-induced cGMP decreases as a putative feedback. *J. Biol. Chem.* 266: 18530–18537, 1991.
10. Ashkenazy, A., E. G. Peralta, J. W. Winslow, J. Ramachandran, and D. J. Capon. Functional diversity of muscarinic receptor subtypes in cellular signal transduction and growth. *Trends Pharmacol. Sci.* (Suppl.) 16–21, 1989.
11. Awara, W. M., C.-H. Guo, and P. M. Conn. Effects of Asn[318] and Asp[87] Asn[318] mutations on signal transduction by the gonadotropin-releasing hormone receptor and receptor regulation. *Endocrinology* 137: 655–662, 1996.

12. Baldwin, J. M. The probable arrangement of the helices in G protein-coupled receptors. *EMBO J.* 12: 1693–1703, 1993.

13. Baldwin, J. M. Structure and function of receptors coupled to G proteins. *Curr. Opin. Cell Biol.* 6: 180–190, 1994.

13a. Barak, L. S., M. Tiberi, N. J. Freedman, M. M. Kwatra, R. J. Lefkowitz, and M. G. Caron. A highly conserved tyrosine residue in G protein–coupled receptors is required for agonist-mediated β_2-adrenergic receptor sequestration. *J. Biol. Chem.* 269: 2790–2795, 1994.

14. Bauer, P. H., S. Müller, M. Puzicha, S. Pippig, B. Obermaier, E. J. M. Helmreich, and M. J. Lohse. Phosducin is a protein kinase A–regulated G-protein regulator. *Nature* 358: 73–76, 1992.

15. Beals, C. R., C. B. Wilson, and R. M. Perlmutter. A small multigene family encodes G_i signal transduction. *Proc. Natl. Acad. Sci. U.S.A.* 84: 7886–7889, 1987.

16. Benovic, J. L., M. Bouvier, M. G. Caron, and R. J. Lefkowitz. Regulation of adenylyl cyclase–coupled β-adrenergic receptors. *Annu. Rev. Cell Biol.* 4: 405–428, 1988.

17. Benovic, J. L., C. Staniszewski, R. A Cerione, J. Codina, R. J. Lefkowitz, and M. G. Caron. The mammalian β-adrenergic receptor: structural and functional characterization of the carbohydrate moiety. *J. Recep Res.* 7: 257–281, 1987.

18. Berlot C. H., and H. R. Bourne. Identification of effector-activating residues of $G_{s\alpha}$. *Cell* 68: 911–922, 1992.

19. Berstein, G., J. L. Blank, D.-Y. Jhon, J. H. Exton, S. G. Rhee, and E. M. Ross. Phospholipase Cβ1 is a GTPase-activating protein for $G_{q/11}$, its physiological regulator. *Cell* 70: 411–418, 1992.

20. Berstein, G., J. L. Blank, A. V. Smrcka, T. Higashijima, P. C. Sternweis, J. H. Exton, and E. M. Ross. Reconstitution of agonist-stimulated phosphatidylinositol 4,5-biphosphate hydrolysis using purified m1 muscarinic receptor, $G_{q/11}$, and phospholipase Cβ1. *J. Biol. Chem.* 267: 8081–8088, 1992.

21. Bhowmick, N., J. Huang, D. Puett, N. W. Isaacs, and A. J. Lapthorn. Determination of residues important in hormone binding to the extracellular domain of the luteinizing hormone/choriogonadotropin receptor by site-directed mutagenesis and modeling. *Mol. Endocrinol.* 10: 1147–1159, 1996.

22. Bihoreau, C., C. Monnot, E. Davies, B. Teutsch, K. E. Berstein, P. Corvol, and E. Clauser. Mutation of Asp74 of the rat angiotensin II receptor confers changes in antagonist affinities and abolishes G-protein coupling. *Proc. Natl. Acad. Sci. U.S.A.* 90: 5133–5137, 1993.

23. Birdsall, N. J. M., F. Cohen, S. Lazareno, and H. Matsui. Allosteric regulation of G-protein-linked receptors. *Biochem. Soc. Trans.* 23: 108–111, 1995.

24. Birnbaumer, L. Which G protein subunits are the active mediators in signal transduction? *Trends Pharmacol. Sci.* 8: 209–211, 1987.

25. Birnbaumer L. G proteins in signal transduction. *Annu. Rev. Pharmacol. Toxicol.* 30: 675–705, 1990.

26. Birnbaumer, L., J. Abramowitz, and A. M. Brown. Receptor–effector coupling by G proteins. *Biochim. Biophys. Acta* 1031:163–224, 1990.

27. Birnbaumer, L., and M. Birnbaumer. Signal transduction by G proteins: 1994 edition. *J. Recept. Signal Transduction Res.* 15: 213–252, 1995.

28. Blank, J. L., K. A. Brattain, and J. H. Exton. Activation of cytosolic phosphoinositide phospholipase C by G-protein $\beta\gamma$ subunits. *J. Biol. Chem.* 267: 23069–23075, 1992.

29. Boege, F., M. Ward, R. Jurss, M. Hekman, and E. J. M. Helmreich. Role of glycosylation for β_2-adrenoceptor function in A431 cells. *J. Biol. Chem.* 263: 9040–9049, 1988.

30. Bokoch, G. M. Interplay between Ras-related and heterotrimeric GTP binding proteins: lifestyles of the BIG and little. *FASEB J.* 10: 1290–1295, 1996.

31. Bourne, H. R., D. A. Sanders, and F. McCormick. The GTPase superfamily: a conserved switch for diverse cell functions. *Nature* 348: 125–132, 1990.

32. Bourne, H. R., D. A. Sanders, and F. McCormick. The GTPase superfamily: conserved structure and molecular mechanism. *Nature* 349: 117–127, 1990.

33. Bouvier, M., W. P. Hausdorff, A. De Blasi, B. F. O'Dowd, B. K. Kobilka, M. G. Caron, and R. J. Lefkowitz. Removal of phosphorylation sites from the β_2-adrenergic receptor delays onset of agonist-promoted desensitization. *Nature* 333: 370–373, 1988.

34. Bouvier, M., T. P. Loisel, and T. H. Hebert. Dynamic regulation of G-protein coupled receptor palmitoylation: potential role in receptor function. *Biochem. Soc. Trans.* 23: 577–581, 1995.

35. Bownds, D., J. Dawes, J. Miller, and M. Sthalman. Phosphorylation of frog photoreceptor membranes induced by light. *Nature* 237: 125–127, 1972.

36. Boyer, J. L., G. L. Waldo, and T. K. Harden. $\beta\gamma$-Subunit activation of G-protein-regulated phospholipase C. *J. Biol. Chem.* 267: 25451–25456, 1992.

37. Brandt, D. R., and E. M. Ross. GTPase activity of the stimulatory GTP-binding regulatory protein of adenylate cyclase, Gs. Accumulation and turnover of enzyme-nucleotide intermediates. *J. Biol. Chem.* 260: 266–272, 1985.

38. Bray, P., A. Carter, V. Guo, C. Puckett, J. Kamholz, A. Spiegel, and M. Nirenberg. Human cDNA clones for an α subunit of G_i signal-transduction protein. *Proc. Natl. Acad. Sci. U.S.A.* 84: 5115–5119, 1987.

39. Bray, P., A. Carter, C. Simons, V. Guo, C. Puckett, J. Kamholz, A. Spiegel, and M. Nirenberg. Human cDNA clones for four species of Gαs signal transduction protein. *Proc. Natl. Acad. Sci. U.S.A.* 83: 8893–8897, 1986.

40. Breitwieser, G. E., and G. Szabo. Uncoupling of cardiac muscarinic and β-adrenergic receptors from ion channels by a guanine nucleotide analogue. *Nature* 317: 538–540, 1985.

41. Breitwieser, G. E., and G. Szabo. Mechanism of muscarinic receptor-induced K^+ channel activation as revealed by hydrolysis-resistant GTP analogues. *J. Gen. Physiol.* 91: 469–493, 1988.

42. Brown, E. M., G. Gamba, D. Riccardi, M. Lombardi, R. Butters, O. Kifor, A. Sun, M. A. Hediger, J. Lytton, and S. C. Hebert. Cloning and characterization of an extracellular Ca^{2+}-sensing receptor from bovine parathyroid. *Nature* 366: 575–580, 1993.

43. Bubis, J., and H. C. Khorana. Sites of interaction in the complex between β- and γ-subunits of transducin. *J. Biol. Chem.* 265: 12995–12999, 1990.

44. Buck, L. B. The olfactory multigene family. *Curr. Opin. Neurobiol.* 2: 282–288, 1992.

45. Burgen, A. S. V. Some considerations of receptor specificity. *Trends Pharmacol. Sci.* (Suppl.) 1–3, 1989

46. Campbell, P. T., M. Hnatowich, B. F. O'Dowd, M. G. Caron, R. J. Lefkowitz, and W. P. Hausdorff. Mutations of the human β_2-adrenergic receptor that impair coupling to Gs interfere with receptor down-regulation but not sequestration. *Mol. Pharmacol.* 39: 192–198, 1991.

47. Camps, M., C. Hou, D. Sidiropoulus, J. B. Stock, K. H. Jakobs, and P. Gierschik. Stimulation of phospholipase C by guanine-nucleotide-binding protein $\beta\gamma$ subunits. *Eur. J. Biochem.* 206: 821–831, 1992.

48. Camps, M. C., A. Carozzi, P. Schnabel, P. Scheer, P. J. Parker, and P. Gierschik. Isoenzyme selective stimulation of phospholi-

pase C-β2 by G protein βγ subunits. *Nature* 360: 684–686, 1992.

49. Carrasco, M. A., J. Sierralta, and P. DeMazancourt. Characterization and subcellular distribution of G-proteins in highly purified skeletal muscle fractions from rabbit and frog. *Arch. Biochem. Biophys.* 310: 76–81, 1994.

50. Cascieri, M. A., T. Ming Gong, and C. D. Strader. Molecular characterization of a common binding site for small molecules within the transmembrane domain of G-protein coupled receptors. *J. Pharmacol. Toxicol. Methods* 33: 179–185, 1995.

51. Casey, P. J. Lipid modifications of G proteins. *Curr. Opin. Cell Biol.* 6: 219–225, 1994.

52. Casey, P. J., H. K. W. Fong, M. I. Simon, and A. G. Gilman. Gz, a guanine nucleotide-binding protein with unique biochemical properties. *J. Biol. Chem.* 265: 2383–2390, 1990.

53. Cassel, D., and Z. Selinger. Mechanism of adenylate cyclase activation by cholera toxin. Inhibition of GTP hydrolysis at the regulatory site. *Proc. Natl. Acad. Sci. U.S.A.* 74: 3307–3311, 1977.

54. Chattopadhyay, N., A. Mithal, and E. M. Brown. The calcium-sensing receptor: a window into the physiology and pathophysiology of mineral ion metabolism. *Endocr. Rev.* 17: 289–307, 1996.

55. Chen, C. K., J. Inglese, R. J. Lefkowitz, and J. B. Hurley. Ca^{2+}-dependent interaction of recoverin with rhodopsin. *J. Biol. Chem.* 270: 18060–18066, 1995.

56. Chen, J. Q., and R. Iyengar. Inhibition of cloned adenylyl cyclases by mutant-activated $G_{i\alpha}$ and specific suppression of type-2 adenylyl cyclase inhibition by phorbol ester treatment. *J. Biol. Chem.* 268: 12253–12256, 1993.

57. Chen, R., K. A. Lewis, M. H. Perrin, and W. W. Vale. Expression cloning of a human corticotropin-releasing-factor receptor. *Proc. Natl. Acad. Sci. U.S.A.* 90: 8967–8971, 1993.

58. Chen, Y., D. Gral, A. E. Salcini, P. G. Pelicci, J. Pouyssegur, and E. Van Obberghen-Schilling. Shc adaptor proteins are key transducers of mitogenic signaling mediated by the G protein-coupled thrombin receptor. *EMBO J.* 15: 1037–1044, 1996.

59. Cheung, A. H., R. R. Huang, M. P. Graziano, and C. D. Strader. Specific activation of Gs by synthetic peptides corresponding to an intracellular loop of the β-adrenergic receptor. *FEBS Lett.* 279: 277–280, 1991.

60. Cheung, A. H., R. R. Huang, and C. D. Strader. Involvement of specific hydrophobic, but not hydrophilic amino acids in the third intracellular loop of the β-adrenergic receptor in the activation of G_s. *Mol. Pharmacol.* 41: 1061–1065, 1992.

61. Chung, F.-Z., C.-D. Wang, P. C. Potter, J. C. Venter, and C. M. Fraser. Site-directed mutagenesis and continuous expression of human β-adrenergic receptors. *J. Biol. Chem.* 263: 4052–4055, 1988.

62. Clapham, D. E., and E. J. Neer. New roles for G-protein βγ-dimers in transmembrane signalling. *Nature* 365: 403–406, 1993

63. Clark, R. B., J. Friedman, R. A. Dixon, and C. D. Strader. Identification of a specific site required for rapid heterologous desensitization of the β-adrenergic receptor by cAMP-dependent protein kinase. *Mol. Pharmacol.* 36: 343–348, 1989.

64. Clarke, S. Protein isoprenylation and methylation at carboxy-terminal cysteine residues. *Annu. Rev. Biochem.* 61: 355–386, 1992,

65. Cobb, M. H., and E. J. Goldsmith. How MAP kinases are regulated. *J. Biol. Chem.* 270: 14843–14846, 1995.

66. Coleman, D. E., A. M. Berghuis, E. Lee, M. E. Linder, A. G. Gilman, and S. R. Sprang. Structures of active conformations of $G_{i\alpha1}$ and the mechanism of GTP hydrolysis. *Science* 265: 1405–1412, 1994.

67. Conklin, B. R., and H. R. Bourne. Structural elements of Gα subunits that interact with Gβγ, receptors and effectors. *Cell* 73: 631–641, 1993.

68. Conn, P. M., D. C. Rogers, and S. G. Seay. Biphasic regulation of the gonadotropin-releasing hormone receptor by receptor microaggregation and intracelullar Ca^{2+} levels. *Mol. Pharmacol.* 25: 51–55, 1984.

69. Cook, S. J., and F. McCormick. Inhibition by cAMP of Ras-dependent activation of Raf. *Science* 262: 1069–1072, 1993.

70. Coso, O. A., M. Chiariello, G. Kalinec, L. M. Kyriakis, J. Woodgett, and J. S. Gutkind. Transforming G protein–coupled receptors potently activate JNK (SAPK). Evidence for a divergence from the tyrosine kinase signaling pathway. *J. Biol. Chem.* 270: 5620–5624, 1995.

71. Coso, O. A., M. Chiariello, J. C. Yu, H. Teramoto, P. Crespo, N. Xu, T. Miki, and J. S. Gutkind. The small GTP binding proteins Rac1 and Cdc42 regulate the activity of the JNK/SAPK signaling pathway. *Cell* 81: 1137–1146, 1995.

72. Costa, T., Y. Ogino, P. J. Munson, H. O. Onaran, and D. Rodbard. Drug efficacy at guanine nucleotide-binding regulatory protein-linked receptors: thermodynamic interpretation of negative antagonism and of receptor activity in the absence of ligand. *Mol. Pharmacol.* 41: 549–560, 1992.

73. Cotecchia, S., S. Exum, M. G. Caron, and R. J. Lefkowitz. Regions of the α_1-adrenergic receptor involved in coupling to phosphatidylinositol hydrolysis and enhanced sensitivity of biological function. *Proc. Natl. Acad. Sci. U.S.A.* 87: 2896–2900, 1990.

74. Cotecchia, S., J. Ostrowski, M. A. Kjelsberg, M. G. Caron, and R. J. Lefkowitz. Discrete amino acid sequences of the α1–adrenergic receptor determine the selectivity of coupling to phosphatidylinositol hydrolysis. *J. Biol. Chem.* 267: 1633–1639, 1992.

75. Coughlin, S. R. Expanding horizons for receptors coupled to G proteins: diversity and disease. *Curr. Opin. Cell Biol.* 6: 191–197, 1994

76. Crespo, P., T. G. Cachero, N. Xu, and J. S. Gutkind. Dual effect of β-adrenergic receptors on mitogen-activated protein kinase. Evidence for a βγ-dependent activation and a Gαs-cAMP-mediated inhibition. *J. Biol. Chem.* 270: 25259–25265, 1995.

77. Crespo, P., W. F. Simonds, and J. S. Gutkind. Ras-dependent activation of MAP kinase pathway mediated by G-protein βγ subunits. *Nature* 369: 418–420, 1994.

78. Curtis C. A. M., M. Wheatley, S. Bansal, N. J. Birdsall, P. Eveleigh, E. K. Pedder, D. Poyner, and E. C. Hulme. Propylbenzilylcholine mustard labels an acidic residue in transmembrane helix 3 of the muscarinic receptor. *J. Biol. Chem.* 264: 489–495, 1989.

79. Dahl, S. G., O. Edvardsen, and I. Sylte. Molecular dynamics of dopamine at the D_2 receptor. *Proc. Natl. Acad. Sci. U.S.A.* 88: 8111–8115, 1991.

80. Damaj, B. B., S. R. McColl, K. Neote, N. Songqing, K. T. Ogborn, C. A. Hébert, and P. H. Naccache. Identification of G-protein binding sites of the human interleukin-8 receptors by functional mapping of the intracellular loops. *FASEB J.* 10: 1426–1434, 1996.

81. Daniel-Issakani, S., A. M. Spiegel, and B. Strulovici. Lipopolysaccharide response is linked to the GTP binding domain, G_{i-2}, in the promonocytic cell line U937. *J. Biol. Chem.* 264: 20240–20247, 1989.

82. Davidson, J. S., C. A. Flanagan, P. D. Davies, J. Hapgood, D. Myburgh, R. Elario, R. P. Millar, W. Forrest-Owen, and C. A. McArdle. Incorporation of an additional glycosylation site enhances expression of functional human gonadotropin-releasing hormone receptor. *Endocrine* 4: 207–212, 1996.

83. Davidson, J. S., C. A. Flanagan, W. Zhou, I. I. Becker, R. Elario, W. Emeran, S. C. Seaflon, and R. P. Millar. Identification of N-glycosylation sites in the gonadotropin-releasing hormone receptor: role in receptor expression but not ligand binding. *Mol. Cell. Endocrinol.* 107: 241–245, 1995.

84. Davis, R. J. The mitogen-activated protein kinase signal transduction pathway. *J. Biol. Chem.* 268: 14553–14556, 1993.

85. Davis, R. J. MAPKs: new JNK expands the group. *Trends Biochem. Sci.* 19: 470–473, 1994.

86. De Almeida Catanho, M.-T. J., A. Bérault, M. Théoleyre, and M. Jutisz. Solubilization and partial purification of the high-affinity gonadoliberin receptor from the bovine pituitary gland. *Arch. Biochem. Biophys.* 225: 535–542, 1983.

87. De la Peña, P., L. M. Delgado, D. Del Camino, and F. Barros. Two isoforms of the thyrotropin-releasing hormone receptor generated by alternative splicing have indistinguishable functional properties. *J. Biol. Chem.* 267: 25703–25708, 1992.

88. De Lean, A., J. M. Stadel, and R. J. Lefkowitz. A ternary complex model explains the agonist-specific binding properties of the adenylate cyclase–coupled β-adrenergic receptor. *J. Biol. Chem.* 255: 7108–7117, 1980.

89. Degtyarev, M. Y., A. M. Spiegel, and T. L. Z. Jones. Increased palmitoylation of the G_s protein α subunit after activation by the β-adrenergic receptor or cholera toxin. *J. Biol. Chem.* 268: 23769–23772, 1993.

90. Degtyarev, M. Y., A. M. Spiegel, and T. L. Z. Jones. The G protein $α_s$ subunit incorporates [^{3}H]-palmitic acid and mutation of cysteine-3 prevents this modification. *Biochemistry* 32: 8057–8061, 1993.

91. DeMartino, J. A., G. V. Riper, S. J. Siciliano, C. J. Molineaux, Z. D. Konteatis, H. Rosen, and M. S. Springer. The amino terminus of the human C5a receptor is required for high affinity C5a binding and for receptor activation by C5a but not C5a analogs. *J. Biol. Chem.* 269: 14446–14450, 1994.

92. Denhardt, D. T. Signal-transducing protein phosphorylation cascades mediated by Ras/Rho proteins in the mammalian cell: the potential for multiplex signalling. *Biochem J.* 318: 729–747, 1996.

93. Denker, B. M., E. J. Neer, and C. J. Schmidt. Mutagenesis of the amino terminus of the α subunit of the G protein, G_o: in vitro characterization of $α_oβγ$ interactions. *J. Biol. Chem.* 267: 6272–6277, 1992.

94. Derijard, B., M. Hibi, I. Wu, T. Barret, B. Su, T. Deng, M. Karin, and R. J. Davis. JNK1: a protein kinase stimulated by UV light and Ha-Ras that binds and phosphorylates the c-Jun activation domain. *Cell* 76: 1025–1037, 1994.

95. Dever, T. E., M. J. Glynias, and W. C. Merrick. The GTP-binding domain: three consensus sequence elements with distinct spacing. *Proc. Natl. Acad. Sci. U.S.A.* 84: 1814–1818, 1987.

96. Dhanasekaran, N., and J. M. Dermott. Signaling by the G_{12} class of G proteins. *Cell. Signal.* 8: 235–245, 1996.

97. Dhanasekaran, N., I. E. Heasley, and G. L. Johnson. G protein-coupled receptor systems involved in cell growth and oncogenesis. *Endocr. Rev.* 16: 259–270, 1995.

98. Dixon, R. A., I. S. Sigal, M. R. Candelore, R. B. Register, E. Rands, and C. D. Strader. Structural features required for ligand binding to the β-adrenergic receptor. *EMBO J.* 6: 3269–3275, 1987.

99. Dixon, R. A., I. S. Sigal, E. Rands, R. B. Register, M. R. Candelore, A. D. Blake, and S. D. Strader. Ligand binding to the β-adrenergic receptor involves its rhodopsin-like core. *Nature* 326: 73–77, 1987.

100. Dixon, R. A. F., B. K. Kobilka, D. J. Strader, J. L. Benovic, H. G. Dohlman, T. Frielle, M. A. Bolanowsky, C. D. Bennet, E. Rands, R. E. Diehl, R. A. Mumford, E. E. Slater, I. S. Sigal, M. G. Caron, R. J. Lefkowitz, and C. D. Strader. Cloning the gene and cDNA for mammalian β-adrenergic receptor and homology with rhodopsin. *Nature* 321: 75–79, 1986.

101. Dixon, R. A. F., I. S. Sigal, M. R. Candelore, R. B. Register, W. Scattergood, E. Rands, and C. D. Strader. Structural features required for ligand binding to the β-adrenergic receptor. *EMBO J.* 11: 3269–3275, 1987.

102. Dixon, R. A. F., I. S. Sigal, and C. D. Strader. Structure–function analysis of the β-adrenergic receptor. *Cold Spring Harb. Symp. Quant. Biol.* 53: 487–497, 1988.

103. Dohlman, H. G., M. Bouvier, J. L. Benovic, M. G. Caron, and R. J. Lefkowitz. The multiple membrane spanning topography of the $β_2$-adrenergic receptor. Localization of the sites of binding, glycosylation and regulatory phosphorylation by limited proteolysis. *J. Biol. Chem.* 262: 14282–14288, 1987.

104. Dohlman, H. G., M. G. Caron, A. DeBlasi, T. Frielle, and R. J. Lefkowitz. Role of extracellular disulfide-bonded cysteines in the ligand binding function of the $β_2$-adrenergic receptor. *Biochemistry* 29: 2335–2342, 1990.

104a. Dohlman, H. G., and J. Thorner. RGS proteins and signaling by hetrotrimeric G proteins. *J. Biol. Chem.* 272: 3871–3874, 1997.

105. Dohlman, H. G., J. Thorner, M. G. Caron, and R. J. Lefkowitz. Model systems for the study of seven-transmembrane-segment receptors. *Annu. Rev. Biochem.* 60: 653–688, 1991.

106. Doss, R. C., N. R. Kramarcy, T. K. Harden, and J. P. Perkins. Effects of tunicamycin on the expression of beta-adrenergic receptors in human astrocytoma cells during growth and recovery from agonist-induced down-regulation. *Mol. Pharmacol.* 27: 507–516, 1985.

107. Downes, C. P. G protein–dependent regulation of phospholipase C. *Trends Pharmacol. Sci.* (Suppl.): 39–42, 1989.

108. Dratz, E. D., J. E. Fursteneau, C. G. Lambert, D. L. Threault, H. Rarick, T. Schepers, S. Pakhlevaniants, and H. E. Hamm. NMR structure of receptor-bound G-protein peptide. *Nature* 363: 276–280, 1993.

109. Druey, K. M., K. J. Blumer, V. H. Kang, and J. H. Kehrl. Inhibition of G-protein-mediated MAP kinase activation by a new mammalian gene family. *Nature* 379: 742–746, 1996.

110. Emorine, L. J., S. Maurullo, C. Delavier-Klutchko, S. V. Kaveri, O. Durieu-Trautmann, and A. D. Strosberg. Structure of the gene encoding for human $β_2$-adrenergic receptor: expression and promoter characterization. *Proc. Natl. Acad. Sci. U.S.A.* 84: 6995–6999, 1987.

111. Esapa, C., S. Foster, S. Johnson, J. L. Jameson, P. Kendall-Taylor, and P. E. Harris. G protein and thyrotropin receptor mutations in thyroid neoplasia. *J. Clin. Endocrinol. Metab.* 82: 493–496, 1997.

112. Exton, J. H. Phosphoinositide phospholipases and G proteins in hormone action. *Annu. Rev. Physiol.* 56: 349–369, 1994.

113. Exton, J. H. Regulation of phosphoinositide phospholipases by hormones, neurotransmitters, and other agonists linked to G proteins. *Annu. Rev. Pharmacol. Toxicol.* 36: 481–509, 1996.

114. Fantl, W. J., D. E. Johnson, and L. T. Williams. Signaling by receptor tyrosine kinases. *Annu. Rev. Biochem.* 62: 453–481, 1993.

115. Farahbakhsh, Z. T., K. Hideg, and W. L. Hubbell. Photoactivated conformational changes in rhodopsin: a time-resolved spin label study. *Science* 262: 1416–1419, 1993.

116. Fargin, A., J. R. Raymond, J. W. Regan, S. Cotecchia, R. J. Lefkowitz, and M. G. Caron. Effector coupling mechanisms of the cloned 5-HT$_{1A}$ receptor. *J. Biol. Chem.* 264: 14848–14852, 1989.

117. Faure, M. A., A. Voyno-Yasenetskaya, and H. R. Bourne. cAMP and $\beta\gamma$ subunits of heterotrimeric G proteins stimulate the mitogen-activated protein kinase pathway in COS-7 cells. *J. Biol. Chem.* 269: 7851–7854, 1994.

118. Feder, D., M. J. Im, H. W. Klein, M. Hekman, A. Holzhofer, C. Dees, A. Levitzki, E. J. Helmreich, and T. Pfeuffer. Reconstitution of β_1-adrenoceptor-dependent adenylate cyclase from purified components. *EMBO J.* 5: 1509–1514, 1986.

119. Federman, A. D., B. R. Conklin, K. A. Schrader, R. R. Reed, and H. R. Bourne. Hormonal stimulation of adenylyl cyclase through G_i-protein $\beta\gamma$ subunits. *Nature* 356: 159–161, 1992.

120. Fields, T. A., and P. J. Casey. Signalling functions and biochemical properties of pertussis toxin–resistant G-proteins. *Biochem. J.* 321: 561–571, 1997.

121. Findlay, J. B., and D. J. Pappin. The opsin family of proteins. *Biochem J.* 238: 625–642, 1986.

122. Flanagan, C. A., I. I. Becker, J. S. Davidson, I. K. Wakefield, W. Zhou, S. C. Seaflon, and R. P. Millar. Glutamate301 of the mouse gonadotrophin releasing hormone receptor determines the specificity for Arginine8 of the mammalian gonadotrophin releasing hormone. *J. Biol. Chem.* 269: 22636–22641, 1994.

123. Florio, V. A., and P. C. Sternweis. Mechanisms of muscarinic receptor action on G_o in reconstituted phospholipid vesicles. *J. Biol. Chem.* 264: 3909–3915, 1989.

124. Fong, H. K. W., K. K. Yoshimoto, P. Eversole-Cire, and M. I. Simon. Identification of a GTP-binding protein α-subunit that lacks an apparent ADP-ribosylation site for pertussis toxin. *Proc. Natl. Acad. Sci. U.S.A.* 85: 3066–3070, 1988.

125. Fong, T. M. Mechanistic hypothesis for the activation of G-protein-coupled receptors. *Cell. Signal.* 8: 217–224, 1996.

126. Fong, T. M., S. A. Anderson, H. Yu, R.-R. C. Huang, and C. D. Strader. Differential activation of intracellular effector by two isoforms of human neurokinin-1 receptor. *Mol. Pharmacol.* 41: 24–30, 1991.

127. Fong, T. M., R. R. Huang, and C. D. Strader. Localization of agonist and antagonist binding domains of the human neurokinin-1 receptor. *J. Biol. Chem.* 267: 25664–25667, 1992.

128. Fong, T. M., R. R. Huang, H. Yu, and C. D. Strader. Mapping the ligand binding site of the NK-1 receptor. *Regul. Pept.* 46: 43–48, 1993.

129. Fong, T. M., R. C. Huang, H. Yu, C. J. Swain, D. Underwood, M. A. Cascieri, and C. D. Strader. Mutational analysis of neurokinin receptor function. *Can. J. Physiol. Pharmacol.* 73: 860–865, 1995.

130. Fong, T. M., H. Yu, R. R. C. Huang, and C. D. Strader. The extracellular domain of the neurokinin-1 receptor is required for high-affinity binding of peptides. *Biochemistry* 31: 11806–11811, 1992.

131. Fong, T. M., H. Yu, and C. D. Strader. The extracellular domain of substance P (NK1) receptor comprises part of the ligand binding site. *Biophys. J.* 62: 59–60, 1992.

132. Fowles, C., R. Sharma, and M. Akhtar. Mechanistic studies on the phosphorylation of photoexcited rhodopsin. *FEBS Lett.* 238: 56–60, 1988.

133. Franke, R. R., B. Koning, T. P. Sakmar, H. G. Khorana, and K. P. Hofmann. Rhodopsin mutants that bind but fail to activate transducin. *Science* 250: 123–125, 1990.

134. Franke, R. R., T. P. Sakmar, R. M. Graham, and H. G. Khorana. Structure and function of rhodopsin. Studies of the interaction between rhodopsin cytoplasmic domain and transducin. *J. Biol. Chem.* 267: 14757–14774, 1992.

135. Fraser, C. M., F. Z. Chung, C. D. Wang, and J. C. Venter. Site-directed mutagenesis of human β-adrenergic receptors: substitution of aspartic acid-130 by aspargine produces a receptor with high-affinity agonist binding that is uncoupled from adenylate cyclase. *Proc. Natl. Acad. Sci. U.S.A.* 85: 5478–5482, 1988.

136. Fraser, C. M., N. H. Lee, S. M. Pellegrino, and A. R. Kerlavage. Molecular properties and regulation of G-protein-coupled receptors. *Prog. Nucleic Acid Res. Mol. Biol.* 49: 113–155, 1994.

137. Fraser, C. M., C.-D. Wong, D. A. Robinson, J. D. Gocayne, and J. C. Venter. Site directed mutagenesis of m1 muscarinic acetylcholine receptors: conserved aspartic acids play important roles in receptor function. *Mol. Pharmacol.* 36: 840–847, 1990.

138. Freedman, N. J., and R. J. Lefkowitz. Desensitization of G protein–coupled receptors. *Recent Prog. Horm. Res.* 51: 319–353, 1996.

139. Freissmuth, M., and A. G. Gilman. Mutations of $G_s\alpha$ designed to alter the reactivity of the protein with bacterial toxins. Substitutions at Arg187 result in loss of GTPase activity. *J. Biol. Chem.* 264: 21907–21914, 1989.

140. Frodin, M., P. Peraldi, and E. Van Obberghen. Cyclic AMP activates the mitogen-activated protein kinase cascade in PC12 cells. *J. Biol. Chem.* 269: 6207–6214, 1994.

141. Fukada, Y., T. Takao, H. Ouguro, T. Yoshizawa, T. Akino, and Y. Shimonishi. Farnesylated γ subunit of photoreceptor G protein indispensable for GTP-binding. *Nature* 346: 658–660, 1992.

142. Fung, B. K. Characterization of transducin from bovine retinal rod outer segments. I. Separation and reconstitution of the subunits. *J. Biol. Chem.* 258: 10495–10502, 1983.

143. Fung, B.K.-K., and C. R. Nash. Characterization of transducin from bovine retinal rod outer segments. II. Evidence for distinct binding sites and conformational changes revealed by limited proteolysis with trypsin. *J. Biol. Chem.* 258: 10503–10510, 1983.

144. Fung, B.K.-K., and L. Stryer. Photolyzed rhodopsin catalyzes the exchange of GTP for bound GDP in retinal rod outer segments. *Proc. Natl. Acad. Sci. U.S.A.* 77: 2500–2504, 1980.

145. Gallego, C., S. K. Gupta, S. Winitz, B. J. Eisfelder, and G. L. Johnson. Myristoylation of the $G\alpha_{is}$ polypeptide, a G protein α subunit, is required for its signaling and transformation functions. *Proc. Natl. Acad. Sci. U.S.A.* 89: 9695–9699, 1992.

146. Gantz, I., J. DelValle, L. Wang, T. Tashiro, G. Munzert, Y.-J. Guo, Y. Konda, and T. Yamada. Molecular basis for the interaction of histamine with the histamine H2 receptor. *J. Biol. Chem.* 267: 20840–20843, 1992.

147. Gantz, I., J. M. Schaffer, J. DelValle, C. Logsdon, V. Campbell, M. Uhler, and T. Yamada. Molecular cloning of a gene encoding the histamine H2 receptor. *Proc. Natl. Acad. Sci. U.S.A.* 88: 429–433, 1991.

148. Garland, A. M., E. F. Grady, M. Lovett, S. R. Vigna, M. M. Frucht, J. E. Krause, and N. W. Bunnet. Mechanisms of desensitization and resensitization of G protein–coupled neurokinin 1 and neurokinin 2 receptors. *Mol. Pharmacol.* 49: 438–446, 1996.

149. Garritsen, A., P. J. M. van Galen, and W. F. Simonds. The N-terminal coiled-coil domain of β is essential for γ association: a model for G-protein $\beta\gamma$ subunit interaction. *Proc. Natl. Acad. Sci. U.S.A.* 90: 7706–7710, 1993.

150. George, S. T., A. E. Ruoho, and C. C. Malbon. N-Glycosylation in expression and function of β-adrenergic receptors. *J. Biol. Chem.* 261: 16559–16564, 1986.

151. Gerszten, R. E., J. Chen, M. Ishii, K. Ishii, L. Wang, T. Nanevicz, C. W. Turck, T.-K. H. Vu, and S. R. Coughlin. Specificity of the thrombin receptor for agonist peptide is

defined by its extracellular surface. *Nature* 368: 648–651, 1994.

152. Gether, U., J. A. Ballesteros, R. Seifert, E. Sanders-Bush, H. Weinstein, and B. K. Kobilka. Structural instability of a constitutively active G protein–coupled receptor. Agonist-independent activation due to conformational flexibility. *J. Biol. Chem.* 272: 2587–2590, 1997.

153. Gilchrist, R.L., K.-S. Ryu, I. Ji, and T. H. Ji. The luteinizing hormone/chorionic gonadotropin receptor has distinct transmembrane conductors for cAMP and inositol phosphate signals. *J. Biol. Chem.* 271: 19283–19287, 1996.

154. Gilman, A. F. G proteins: transducers of receptor-generated signals. *Annu. Rev. Biochem.* 56: 615–649, 1987.

155. Gocayne, J., D. A. Robinson, M. G. Fitz-Gerald, F.-Z. Chung, A. R. Kerlavage, K.-W. Lentes, J. Lai, Ch.-D. Wang, C. M. Fraser, and J. C. Venter. Primary structure of rat β-adrenergic and muscarinic cholinergic receptors obtained by automated DNA sequencing analysis: further evidence for a multigene family. *Proc. Natl. Acad. Sci. U.S.A.* 84: 8296–8300, 1987.

156. Gordon, J. I., R. J. Duronio, D. A. Rudnick, S. P. Adams, and G. W. Goke. Protein N-myristoylation. *J. Biol. Chem.* 266: 8647–8650, 1991.

157. Grady, E. F., A. M. Garland, P. D. Gamp, M. Lovett, D. G. Payan, and N. W. Bunnet. Delineation of the endocytic pathway of substance P and its seven-transmembrane domain NK1 receptor. *Mol. Biol. Cell* 6: 509–524, 1995.

158. Graves, P. N., Y. Tomer, and T. F. Davies. Cloning and sequencing of a 1.3 kb variant of human thyrotropin receptor mRNA lacking the transmembrane domain. *Biochem. Biophys. Res. Commun.* 187: 1135–1143, 1992.

159. Gromoll, J., T. Guderman, and E. Nieschlag. Molecular cloning of a truncated isoform of the human follicle stimulating hormone receptor. *Biochem. Biophys. Res. Commun.* 188: 1077–1083, 1992.

160. Guan, X. M., A. Amend, and C. D. Strader. Determination of structural domains for G protein coupling and ligand binding in β3-adrenergic receptor. *Mol. Pharmacol.* 48: 492–498, 1995.

161. Guo, C.-H., J. A. Janovick, D. Kuphal, and P. M. Conn. Transient tranfection of GGH3-1' cells [GH3 cells stably transfected with the gonadotropin-releasing hormone (GnRH) receptor complementary deoxyribonucleic acid] with the carboxi-terminal of β-adrenergic receptor kinase 1 blocks prolactin release: evidence for a role of the G protein βγ-subunit complex in GnRH signal transduction. *Endocrinology* 136: 3031–3036, 1995.

162. Gupta, S., D. Campbell, B. Derijard, and R. J. Davis. Transcription factor ATF2 regulation by the JNK signal transduction pathway. *Science* 267: 389–393, 1995.

163. Gutowski, S., A. Smrcka, L. Nowac, D. Wu, M. Simon, and P. C. Sternweis. Antibodies to the αq subfamily guanine nucleotide–binding regulatory protein α subunits attenuate activation of phosphatidylinositol 4,5-biphosphate hydrolysis by hormones. *J. Biol. Chem.* 266: 20519–20524, 1991.

164. Hadcock, J. R., and C. C. Malbon. Down-regulation of β-adrenergic receptors: agonist-induced reduction in receptor mRNA levels. *Proc. Natl. Acad. Sci. U.S.A.* 85: 5021–5025, 1988.

165. Hadcock, J. R., M. Ros, and C. C. Malbon. Agonist regulation of β-adrenergic receptor mRNA. *J. Biol. Chem.* 264: 13956–13961, 1989.

166. Hadcock, J. R., H.-Y. Wang, and C. C. Malbon. Agonist-induced desestabilization of β-adrenergic receptor mRNA. Attenuation of glucocorticoid-induced up-regulation of β-adrenergic receptors. *J. Biol. Chem.* 264: 19928–19933, 1989.

167. Hall, A. Ras-related proteins. *Curr. Opin. Cell Biol.* 5: 265–268, 1993.

168. Hall, A. Small GTP-binding proteins and the regulation of the actin cytoskeleton. *Annu. Rev. Cell Biol.* 10: 31–54, 1994.

169. Halliday, K. R. Regional homology in GTP-binding proto-oncogene products and elongation factors. *J. Cyc. Nucl. Protein Phos. Res.* 9: 435–448, 1984.

170. Hamm, H. E. Molecular interactions between the photoreceptor G-protein and rhodopsin. *Cell. Mol. Neurobiol.* 11: 563–578, 1991.

171. Hamm, H. E., D. Deretic, A. Arendt, P. A. Hargrave, B. Koenig, and K. P. Hoffman. Site of G-protein binding to rhodopsin mapped with synthetic peptides from the α subunit. *Science* 241: 832–835, 1988.

172. Harazono, A., Y. Sugimoto, A. Ichikawa, and M. Negishi. Enhancement of adenylate cyclase stimulation by prostaglandin E receptor EP3 subtype isoforms with different efficiencies. *Biochem. Biophys. Res. Commun.* 201: 340–345, 1994.

173. Hargrave, P. A., J. H. McDowell, R. J. Feldman, P. H. Atkinson, J. K. Mohana Rao, and P. Argos. Rhodopsin's protein and carbohydrate structure: selected aspects. *Vision Res.* 24: 1487–1499, 1984.

174. Harhammer, R., B. Nürnberg, C. Harteneck, D. Leopoldt, T. Exner, and G. Schultz. Distinct biochemical properties of the native members of the G12 G-protein subfamily. Characterization of Gα12 purified from rat brain. *Biochem. J.* 319: 165–171, 1996.

175. Hausdorff, W. P., M. Bouvier, B. F. O'Dowd, G. P. Irons, M. G. Caron, and R. J. Lefkowitz. Phosphorylation sites on two domains of the β2-adrenergic receptor are involved in distinct pathways of receptor desensitization. *J. Biol. Chem.* 264: 12657–12665, 1989.

176. Hausdorff, W. P., M. G. Caron, and R. J. Lefkowitz. Turning off the signal: desensitization of β-adrenergic receptor function. *FASEB J.* 4: 2881–2889, 1990.

177. Hausdorff, W. P., J. A. Pitcher, D. K. Luttrell, M. E. Linder, H. Kurose, S. J. Parsons, M. G. Caron, and R. J. Lefkowitz. Tyrosine phosphorylation of G protein α subunits by pp60c-src. *Proc. Natl. Acad. Sci. U.S.A.* 89: 5720–5724, 1992.

178. Hawes, B. E., L. M. Luttrell, S. T. Exum, and R. J. Lefkowitz. Inhibition of G protein–coupled receptor signaling by expression of cytoplasmic domains of the receptor. *J. Biol. Chem.* 269: 15776–15785, 1994.

179. Hawes, B. E., T. van Biesen, W. J. Koch, L. M. Luttrell, and R. J. Lefkowitz. Distinct pathways of Gi- and Gq-mediated mitogen-activated protein kinase activation. *J. Biol. Chem.* 270: 17148–17153, 1995.

180. Hazum, E. GnRH-receptor of rat pituitary is a glycoprotein: differential effect of neuraminidase and lectins on agonist and antagonist binding. *Mol. Cell. Endocrinol.* 26: 217–222, 1982.

181. Hazum, E., I. Schvartz, Y. Waksman, and D. Keinan. Solubilization and purification of rat pituitary gonadotropin-releasing hormone receptor. *J. Biol. Chem.* 261: 13043–13048, 1986.

182. Heckert, L. L., I. J. Daley, and M. D. Griswold. Structural organization of the follicle-stimulating hormone receptor gene. *Mol. Endocrinol.* 6: 70–80, 1992.

183. Henderson, R., J. M. Baldwin, T. A. Ceska, F. Zemlin, E. Beckmann, and K. H. Downing. Model for the structure of bacteriorhodopsin based on high-resolution electron cryomicroscopy. *J. Mol. Biol.* 213: 899–929, 1990.

184. Hepler, J. R., and A. G. Gilman. G Proteins. *Trends Pharmacol. Sci.* 17: 383–387, 1992.

185. Herrero, I., M. T. Miras-Portugal, and J. Sanchez-Prieto. Rapid desensitization of the metabotropic glutamate receptor that

facilitates glutamate release in rat cerebrocortical nerve terminals. *Eur. J. Neurosci.* 6: 115–120, 1994.

186. Hershey, A. D., and J. E. Krause. Molecular characterization of a functional cDNA encoding the rat substance P receptor. *Science* 247: 958–962, 1990.

187. Hescheler, J., W. Rosenthal, W. Trautwein, and G. Schultz. The GTP-binding protein, G_o, regulates neuronal calcium channels. *Nature* 325: 445–447, 1987.

188. Higashijima, T., J. Burnier, and E. M. Ross. Regulation of G_i and G_o by Mastoparan, related amphiphilic peptides and hydrophobic amines. *J. Biol. Chem.* 265: 14176–14186, 1990.

189. Higashijima, T., K. M. Ferguson, P. C. Sternweis, E. M. Ross, M. D. Smigel, and A. G. Gilman. The effect of activating ligands on the intrinsic fluorescence of guanine nucleotide-binding regulatory proteins. *J. Biol. Chem.* 262: 752–756, 1987.

190. Higashijima, T., K. M. Ferguson, P. C. Sternweis, M. D. Smigel, and A. G. Gilman. Effects of M^{2+} and the $\beta\gamma$ subunit complex on the interactions of guanine nucleotides with G proteins. *J. Biol. Chem.* 262: 762–766, 1987.

191. Higgins, J. B., and P. J. Casey. In vitro processing of recombinant G-protein γ subunits. *J. Biol. Chem.* 269: 9067–9073, 1994.

192. Hipkin, R. W., J. Sánchez-Yagüe, and M. Ascoli. Phosphorylation of the luteinizing hormone/choriogonadotropin receptor expressed in a stably transfected cell line. *Mol. Endocrinol.* 7: 823–832, 1993.

193. Hipkin, R. W., Z. Wang, and M. Ascoli. Human chorionic gonadotropin (CG)– and phorbol ester–stimulated phosphorylation of the luteinizing hormone/CG receptor maps to serines 635, 639, 649, and 652 in the C-terminal cytoplasmic tail. *Mol. Endocrinol.* 9: 151–158, 1995.

194. Hirisawa, A., K. Shibata, K. Horie, Y. Takei, K. Obika, T. Tanaka, N. Muramoto, K. Takagaki, J. Yano, and G. Tsujimoto. Cloning, functional expression and tissue distribution of human α_{1C}-adrenoceptor splice variants. *FEBS Lett.* 363: 256–260, 1995.

195. Hirsch, B., M. Kudo, F. Naro, M. Conti, and A. J. W. Hsueh. The C-terminal third of the human luteinizing hormone (LH) receptor is important for inositol phosphate release: analysis using chimeric human LH/follicle-stimulating hormone receptors. *Mol. Endocrinol.* 10: 1127–1137, 1996.

196. Hirsch, J. P., C. Dietzel, and J. Kurjan. The carboxyl terminus of Scg1, the Gα subunit involved in yeast mating, is implicated in interactions with the pheromone receptors. *Genes Dev.* 5: 467–474, 1991.

197. Hirschman, J. E., G. S. De Zutter, W. F. Simonds, and D. D. Jenness. The G$\beta\gamma$ complex of the yeast pheromone response pathway. Subcellular fractionation and protein–protein interactions. *J. Biol. Chem.* 272: 240–248, 1997.

198. Ho, B. Y., A. Karchiin, T. Branchek, N. Davidson, and H. A. Lester. The role of conserved aspartate and serine residues in ligand binding and in function of the 5–HT$_{1A}$ receptor: a site-directed mutation study. *FEBS Lett.* 312: 259–262, 1992.

199. Holtmann, M. H., S. Ganguli, E. M. Hadac, V. Dolu, and L. J. Miller. Multiple extracellular loop domains contribute critical determinants for agonist binding and activation of the secretin receptor. *J. Biol. Chem.* 271: 14944–14949, 1996.

200. Horstman, D. A., S. Brandon, A. L. Wilson, C. A. Guyer, E. J. Cragoe, and L. E. Limbird. An aspartate conserved among G-protein receptors confers allosteric regulation of α_2-adrenergic receptors by sodium. *J. Biol. Chem.* 265: 21590–21595, 1992.

201. Houamed, K. M., J. L. Kuijper, T. L. Gilbert, B. A. Haldeman,
P. J. O'Hara, E. R. Mulvihill, W. Almers, and F. S. Hagen. Cloning, expression and gene structure of a G-protein coupled glutamate receptor from rat brain. *Science* 252: 1318–1321, 1991.

202. Huang, R. R., P. P. Vicario, C. D. Strader, and T. M. Fong. Identification of residues involved in ligand binding to the neurokinin-2 receptor. *Biochemistry* 34: 10048–10055, 1995.

203. Huang, R. R., H. Yu, C. D. Strader, and T. M. Fong. Interaction of substance P with the second and seventh transmembrane domains of the neurokinin-1 receptor. *Biochemistry* 33: 3007–3013, 1994.

204. Huang, R. R., H. Yu, C. D. Strader, and T. M. Fong. Localization of the ligand binding site of the neurokinin-1 receptor: interpretation of chimeric mutations and single-residue substitutions. *Mol. Pharmacol.* 45: 690–695, 1994.

205. Hulme, E. C., C. A. M. Curtis, M. Wheatley, A. Aitken, and A. C. Harris. Localization and structure of the muscarinic receptor ligand binding site. *Trends. Pharmacol. Sci.* (Suppl.): 22–25, 1989.

206. Inglese, J., J. F. Glickman, W. Lorenz, M. G. Caron, and R. J. Lefkowitz. Isoprenylation of a protein kinase: requirement of farnesylation/α-carboxy methylation for full enzymatic activity of rhodopsin kinase. *J. Biol. Chem.* 267: 1422–1425, 1992.

207. Inglese, J., W. J. Koch, M. G. Caron, and R. J. Lefkowitz. Isoprenylation in the regulation of signal transduction by G-protein-coupled receptor kinases. *Nature* 359: 147–150, 1992.

208. Inglese, J., W. J. Koch, K. Touhara, and R. J. Lefkowitz. G$\beta\gamma$ interactions with PH domains and Ras-MAPK signaling pathways. *Trends Biochem. Sci.* 20: 151–156, 1995.

209. Iñiguez-Lluhi, J., C. Kleuss, and G. Gilman. The importance of G-protein $\beta\gamma$ subunits. *Trends Cell. Biol.* 3: 230–236, 1993.

210. Iñiguez-Lluhi, J. A., M. I. Simon, J. D. Robishaw, and A. G. Gilman. G-protein $\beta\gamma$ subunits synthesized in Sf9 cells. Functional characterization and the significance of prenylation of γ. *J. Biol. Chem.* 267: 23409–23417, 1992.

211. Ishigara, T., S. Nakamura, Y. Kaziro, T. Takahashi, K. Takahashi, and S. Nagata. Molecular cloning and expression of a cDNA encoding the secretin receptor. *EMBO J.* 10: 1635–1641, 1991.

212. Ishigara, T., R. Shigemoto, K. Mori, K. Takahashi, and S. Nagata. Functional expression and tissue distribution of a novel receptor for vasoactive intestinal polypeptide. *Neuron* 8: 811–819, 1992.

213. Ito, H., and A. G. Gilman. Expression and analysis of $G_{s\alpha}$ mutants with decreased ability to activate adenylyl cyclase. *J. Biol. Chem.* 266: 16226–16231, 1991.

214. Itoh, H., R. Toyama, T. Kazana, T. Tsukamoto, M. Matsuoka, and Y. Kaziro. Presence of three distinct molecular species of G_i protein α subunit: structure of rat cDNAs and human genomic DNAs. *J. Biol. Chem.* 263: 6656–6664, 1988.

215. Ito, H., R. T. Tung, T. Sugimoto, I. Kobayashi, K. Takahashi, T. Katada, M. Ui, and Y. Kurachi. On the mechanism of G protein $\beta\gamma$ subunit activation of the muscarinic K^+ channel in guinea pig atrial cell membrane. *J. Gen. Physiol.* 99: 961–983, 1992.

216. Iyengar, R. Molecular and functional diversity of mammalian G_s-stimulated adenylyl cyclases. *FASEB J.* 7: 768–775, 1993.

217. Iyengar, R., and L. Birnbaumer. Hormone receptors modulate the regulatory component of adenylyl cyclases by reducing its requirement for Mg^{2+} ion and enhancing its extent of activation by guanine nucleotides. *Proc. Natl. Acad. Sci. U.S.A.* 79: 5179–5183, 1982.

218. Janovick, J. A., S. P. Brothers, and P. M. Conn. GnRH agonist stimulates net loss in immunoassayable $G_{q/11}$ proteins. In:

Program, 79th Annual Meeting of the Endocrine Society, Minneapolis. 1997, p. 168.

219. Janovick, J. A., Haviv, F., T. D. Fitzpatrick, and P. M. Conn. Differential orientation of a GnRH agonist and antagonist in the pituitary GnRH action. *Endocrinology* 133: 942–945, 1993.

220. Jelinek, L. J., S. Lok, G. B. Rosenberg, R. A. Smith, F. J. Grant, S. Biggs, P. A. Bensch, J. L. Kuijper, P. O. Sheppard, C. A. Sprecher, P. J. O'Hara, D. Foster, K. M. Walker, L. H. J. Chen, P. A. McKernan, and W. Kindsvogel. Expression cloning and signaling properties of the rat glucagon receptor. *Science* 259: 1614–1616, 1993.

221. Jelsema, C. L., and J. Axelrod. Stimulation of phospholipase A2 activity in bovine rod outer segments by the $\beta\gamma$ subunits of transducin and its inhibition by the α subunit. *Proc. Natl. Acad. Sci. U.S.A.* 84: 3623–3627, 1987.

222. Jennes, L., W. E. Stumpf, and P. M. Conn. Receptor-mediated binding and uptake of GnRH agonist and antagonist by pituitary cells. *Peptides* 5 (Suppl. 1): 215–220, 1984.

223. Jhon, D.-Y., H.-H. Lee, D. Park, C.-W. Lee, K.-H. Lee, and O. J. Yoo. Cloning, sequencing, purification and G_q-dependent activation of phospholipase C-β_3. *J. Biol. Chem.* 268: 6654–6661, 1993.

224. Ji, I., and T. Ji. Asp^{383} in the second transmembrane domain of the lutropin receptor is important for high affinity hormone binding and cAMP production. *J. Biol. Chem.* 266: 14953–14957, 1991.

225. Ji, I., R. G. Slaughter, and T. H. Ji. N-linked oligosaccharides are not required for hormone binding of the lutropin receptor in a Leydig tumor cell line and rat granulosa cells. *Endocrinology* 127: 494–496, 1990.

226. Jinnah, H. A., and P. M. Conn. GnRH-stimulated LH release from rat anterior pituitary cells in culture: refractoriness and recovery. *Am. J. Physiol.* 249 (*Endocrinol. Metab.* 12): E619–E625, 1985.

227. Johnson, P. S., C. K. Surrat, B. K. Seideleck, C. J. Blaschak, J. B. Wang, and G. R. Uhl. μ Opiate receptor: site-directed mutagenesis produces differential effect on second messenger systems. In: *Program, 24th Annual Meeting of the Society for Neuroscience, Miami, FL.* 1994, p. 745.

228. Jones, D. T., and R. R. Reed. Molecular cloning of five GTP-binding protein cDNA species from rat olfactory neuroepithelium *J. Biol. Chem.* 262: 14241–14249, 1987.

229. Jones, R. L. Z., W. F. Simonds, J. J. Merendino, M. R. Brann, and A. M. Spiegel. Myristoylation of an inhibitory GTP-binding protein α subunit is essential for its membrane attachment. *Proc. Natl. Acad. Sci. U.S.A.* 87: 568–572, 1990.

230. Jüppner H., A. B. Abou-Amra, M. W. Freeman, X. F. Kong, E. Schipani, J. Richards, L. F. Kolakowski, Jr., J. Hock, J. T. Potts, Jr., H. M. Kronenberg, and G. V. Segre. A G protein-linked receptor for parathyroid hormone and parathyroid hormone-related peptide. *Science* 254: 1024–1026, 1991.

231. Jüppner, H., E. Schipani, F. R. Bringhurst, I. McClure, H. T. Keutmann, J. T. Potts, H. M. Kronenberg, A. B. Abou-Samra, G. V. Segre, and T. J. Gardella. The extracellular amino-terminal region of the parathyroid hormone (PTH)/PTH-related peptide receptor determines the binding affinity for carboxyl-terminal fragments of PTH-(1-34). *Endocrinology* 134: 879–884, 1994.

232. Kaiser, U. B., D. Zhao, G. R. Cardona, and W. Chin. Isolation and characterization of cDNAs encoding the rat pituitary gonadotropin-releasing hormone receptor. *Biochem. Biophys. Res. Commun.* 189: 1645–1652, 1992.

233. Karkar, S. S., L. C. Musgrove, D. C. Devor, J. C. Sellers, and J. D. Neil. Cloning, sequencing and expression of human gonadotropin releasing hormone (GnRH) receptor. *Biochem. Biophys. Res. Commun.* 189: 289–295, 1992.

234. Karnik, S., K. Ridge, S. Bhattacharya, and G. H. Khorana. Palmitoylation of bovine opsin and its cystein mutants in COS cells. *Proc. Natl. Acad. Sci. U.S.A.* 90: 40–44, 1993.

235. Karnik, S. S., J. P. Sakmann, H. B. Chen, and H. G. Khorana. Cysteine residues 110 and 187 are essential for the formation of correct structure in bovine rhodopsin. *Proc. Natl. Acad. Sci. U.S.A.* 85: 8459–8463, 1988.

236. Katz, A., D. Wu, and M. I. Simon. Subunits $\beta\gamma$ of heterotrimeric G protein activate $\beta2$ isoform of phospholipase C. *Nature* 360: 686–689, 1992.

237. Kaupmann, K., C. Burns, D. Hoyer, K. Seuwen, and H. Lübbert. Distribution and second messenger coupling of four somatostatin receptor subtypes expressed in brain. *FEBS Lett.* 331: 53–59, 1993.

238. Kaupp, U. B., and K. W. Koch. Role of cGMP and Ca^{2+} in vertebrate photoreceptor excitation and adaptation. *Annu. Rev. Physiol.* 54: 153–176, 1992.

239. Kawate, N., and K. M. Menon. Palmitoylation of luteinizing hormone/human choriogonadotropin receptors in transfected cells. *J. Biol. Chem.* 269: 30651–30658, 1994.

240. Kennedy, K., V. Gigoux, Ch. Escrieut, B. Maigret, J. Martinez, L. Moroder, D. Fréhel, D. Gully, N. Vaysse, and D. Fourmy. Identification of two amino acids of the human cholecystokinin-A receptor that interact with the N-terminal moiety of cholecystokinin. *J. Biol. Chem.* 272: 2920–2926, 1997.

241. Kennedy, M., and L. E. Limbird. Palmitoylation of the α_{2A}-adrenergic receptors. *J. Biol. Chem.* 269: 31915–31922, 1994.

242. Kennedy, M. E., and L. E. Limbird. Mutations of the α_{2A}-adrenergic receptor that eliminate detectable palmitoylation do not perturb receptor–G-protein coupling. *J. Biol. Chem.* 268: 8003–8011, 1993.

243. Kennelly, P. J., and E. G. Krebs. Consensus sequences as substrate specificity determinants for protein kinases and protein phosphatases. *J. Biol. Chem.* 266: 15555–15558, 1991.

244. Khorana, H. G. Rhodopsin, photoreceptor of the rod cell. An emerging pattern for structure and function. *J. Biol. Chem.* 267: 1–4, 1992.

245. Kim, D., D. L. Lewis, L. Graziadei, E. J. Neer, D. Bar-Sagi, and D. E. Clapham. G-protein $\beta\gamma$-subunits activate the cardiac muscarinic K$^+$ channel via phospholipase A2. *Nature* 337: 557–560, 1989.

246. Kim, G.-D., I. C. Carr, L. A. Anderson, J. Zabavnik, K. A. Eidne, and G. Milligan. The long isoform of the rat thyrotropin-releasing hormone receptor down-regulates G_q proteins. *J. Biol. Chem.* 269: 19933–19940, 1994.

247. Kisselev, O., and N. Gautman. Specific interaction with rhodopsin is dependent on the γ subunit type in a G-protein. *J. Biol. Chem.* 268: 24519–24552, 1993.

248. Kisselev, O., A. Pronin, M. Ermolaeva, and N. Gautman. Receptor–G protein coupling is established by a potential conformational switch in the $\beta\gamma$ complex. *Proc. Natl. Acad. Sci. U.S.A.* 92: 9102–9106, 1995.

249. Kjeldgaard, M., J. Nyborg, and B. F. C. Clark. The GTP binding motif: variations on a theme. *FASEB J.* 10: 1347–1368, 1996.

250. Kjelsberg, M. A., S. Cotecchia, J. Ostrowski, M. G. Caron, and R. J. Lefkowitz. Constitutive activation of the α_{1B}-adrenergic receptor by all amino acid substitutions at a single site. *J. Biol. Chem.* 267: 1430–1433, 1992.

251. Kleuss, C. J., C. Hescheler, W. Ewel, G. Rosenthal, G. Schultz,

and B. Wittig. Assignment of G-protein subtypes to specific receptors inducing inhibition of calcium channels. *Nature* 353: 43–48, 1991.

252. Kobilka, B. K., R. A. F. Dixon, T. Frielle, H. G. Dohlman, M. A. Bolanowski, I. S. Sigal, T. L. Yang-Feng, U. Francke, M. G. Caron, and R. J. Lefkowitz. cDNA for the human β-adrenergic receptor: a protein with multiple membrane spanning domains and a chromosomal location shared with the PDGF receptor gene. *Proc. Natl. Acad. Sci. U.S.A.* 84: 46–50, 1987.

253. Kobilka, B. K., T. S. Kobilka, K. W. Daniel, J. W. Regan, M. G. Caron, and R. J. Lefkowitz. Chimeric α_2-, β_2-adrenergic receptors: delineation of domains involved in effector coupling and ligand binding specificiy. *Science* 249: 1310–1316, 1988.

254. Koch, C. A., D. Anderson, M. F. Moran, C. Ellis, and T. Pawson. SH2 and SH3 domains: elements that control interactions of cytoplasmic signaling proteins. *Science* 252: 668–674, 1991.

255. Koch, W. J., B. E. Hawes, L. F. Allen, and R. J. Lefkowitz. Direct evidence that Gi-coupled receptor stimulation of mitogen-activated protein kinase is mediated by G $\beta\gamma$ activation of p21ras. *Proc. Natl. Acad. Sci. U.S.A.* 91: 12706–12710, 1994.

256. Kokame, K., Y. Fukada, T. Yoshizawa, T. Takao, and Y. Shimonishi. Lipid modification of the N-terminus of photoreceptor G-protein α-subunit. *Nature* 359: 749–752, 1992.

257. Kolch, W., G. Heidecker, G. Kochs, R. Hummel, H. Vahidi, H. Mischak, G. Finkenzeller, D. Marme, and U. R. Rapp. Protein kinase Cα activates RAF-1 by direct phosphorylation. *Nature* 364: 249–252, 1993.

258. Konig, B., A. Arendt, J. H. McDowell, M. Kahlert, P. A. Hargrave, and K. P. Hofmann. Three cytoplasmic loops of rhodopsin interact with transducin. *Proc. Natl. Acad. Sci. U.S.A.* 86: 6878–6882, 1989.

259. Koo, Y. B., I. Ji, R. G. Slaughter, and T. H. Ji. Structure of the luteinizing hormone receptor gene and multiple exons of the coding sequence. *Endocrinology* 128: 2297–2308, 1991.

260. Kosugi, S., F. Okajima, T. Ban, A. Hidaka, A. Shenker, and L. D. Kohn. Mutation of alanine 623 in the third cytoplasmic loop of the rat thyrotropin (TSH) receptor results in a loss in the phosphoinositide but not the cAMP signal induced by TSH and receptor antibodies. *J. Biol. Chem.* 267: 24153–24156, 1992.

261. Krueger, K. M., Y. Daaka, J. A. Pitcher, and R. J. Lefkowitz. The role of sequestration in G protein–coupled receptor resensitization. *J. Biol. Chem.* 272: 5–8, 1997.

262. Kubo, T., H. Bujo, I. Akiba, J. Nakai, M. Mishina, and S. Numa. Location of a region of the muscarinic acetylcholine receptor involved in selective effector coupling. *FEBS Lett.* 241: 119–125, 1988.

263. Kudo, M., Y. Osuga, B. K. Kobilka, and A.J.W. Hsueh. Transmembrane regions V and VI of the human luteinizing hormone receptor are required for constitutive activation by a mutation in the third intracellular loop. *J. Biol. Chem.* 271: 22470–22478, 1996.

264. Kurachi, Y., H. Ito, T. Sugimoto, T. Shimizu, I. Miki, and M. Ui. Arachidonic acid metabolites as intracellular modulators of the G protein–gated cardiac K$^+$ channel. *Nature* 337: 555–557, 1989.

265. Kurtenbach, E., C.A.M. Curtis, E. K. Pedder, A. Aitken, A.C.M. Harris, and E. C. Hulme. Muscarinic acetylcholine receptors. Peptide sequencing identifies residues involved in antagonist binding and disulfide bond formation. *J. Biol. Chem.* 265: 13702–13708, 1990.

266. Lagnado, L., and D. Baylor. Signal flow in visual transduction. *Neuron* 8: 995–1002, 1992.

267. Lambright, D. G., J. Sondek, A. Bohm, N. P. Skiba, H. E. Hamm, and P. B. Sigler. The 2.0 Å crystal structure of a heterotrimeric G protein. *Nature* 379: 311–319, 1996.

268. Lameh, J., M. Philip, Y. K. Sharma, O. Moro, J. Ramachandran, and W. Sadee. Hm1 muscarinic cholinergic receptor internalization requires a domain in the third cytoplasmic loop. *J. Biol. Chem.* 267: 13406–13412, 1992.

269. LaMorte, V. J., E. D. Kennedy, L. R. Collins, D. Goldstein, A. T. Harootunian, J. H. Brown, and J. R. Feramisco. A requirement for Ras protein function in thrombin-stimulated mitogenesis in astrocytoma cells. *J. Biol. Chem.* 268: 19411–19415, 1993.

270. Landis, C. A., S. B. Masters, A. Spada, A. M. Pace, H. R. Bourne, and L. Vallar. GTPase inhibiting mutations activate the α chain of G$_s$ and stimulate adenylyl cyclase in human pituitary tumors. *Nature* 340: 692–696, 1989.

271. Lange-Carter, C. A., C. M. Pleiman, A. M. Gardner, K. J. Blumer, and G. L. Johnson. A divergence in the MAP kinase regulatory network defined by MEK kinase and Raf. *Science* 260: 315–319, 1993.

272. LaRosa, G. J., K. M. Thomas, M. E. Kaufmann, R. Mark, M. White, L. Taylor, G. Gray, D. Witt, and J. Navarro. Amino terminus of the interleukin-8 receptor is a major determinant of receptor subtype specificity. *J. Biol. Chem.* 267: 25402–25406, 1992.

273. Laue, L. L., W. Shao-Ming, M. Kudo, C. J. Bourdony, G. B. Cutler, A. J. W. Hsueh, and W.-Y. Chan. Compound heterozygous mutations of the luteinizing hormone receptor gene in Leydig cell hypoplasia. *Mol. Endocrinol.* 10: 987–997, 1996.

274. Leberman, R., and U. Egner. Homologies in the primary structure of GTP-binding proteins: the nucleotide binding site. *EMBO J.* 4: 339–341, 1984.

275. Lechleiter, J., R. Hellmiss, K. Duerson, D. Ennulat, N. David, D. Clapham, and E. Peralta. Distinct sequence elements control the specificity of G-protein activation by muscarinic acetylcholine receptor subtypes. *EMBO J.* 9: 4381–4390, 1990.

276. Lee, C., T. Murakami, and W. F. Simonds. Identification of a discrete region of the G protein γ subunit conferring selectivity in βγ complex. *J. Biol. Chem.* 270: 8779–8784, 1995.

277. Lee, C. H., A. Katz, and M. I. Simon. Multiple regions of Gα_{16} contribute to the specificity of activation by the C5A receptor. *Mol. Pharmacol.* 47: 218–223, 1995.

278. Lee, C.-W., D. J. Park , K.-H. Lee, C. G. Kim, and S. G. Rhee. Purification, molecular cloning, and sequencing of phospholipase C-β4. *J. Biol. Chem.* 268: 21318–21327, 1993.

279. Lee, E., R. Taussig, and A. G. Gilman. The G226A mutant of G$_{s\alpha}$ highlights the requirement for dissociation of G protein subunits. *J. Biol. Chem.* 267: 1212–1218, 1992.

280. Leff, P. The two-state model of receptor activation. *Trends Pharmacol. Sci.* 16: 89–97, 1995.

281. Lefkowitz, R. J. Turned on to ill effect. *Nature* 365: 603–604, 1993.

282. Lefkowitz, R. J., S. Cotecchia, P. Samama, and T. Costa. Constitutive activity of receptors coupled to guanine nucleotide regulatory proteins. *Trends Pharmacol. Sci.* 14: 303–307, 1993.

283. Lester, H. A. The permeation pathway of neurotransmitter-gated ion channels. *Annu. Rev. Biophys. Biomol. Struct.* 21: 267–292, 1992.

284. Lev, S., H. Moreno, R. Martinez, P. Canoll, E. Peles, J. M. Musacchio, G. D. Plowman, B. Rudy, and J. Schlessinger. Protein tyrosine-kinase PYK2 involved in Ca^{2+}-induced regula-

tion of ion channel and MAP kinase functions. *Nature* 376: 737–745, 1995.

285. Levis, M. J., and H. R. Bourne. Activation of the α subunit of G_s in intact cells alters its abundance, rate of degradation, and membrane avidity. *J. Cell Biol.* 119: 1297–1307, 1992.

286. Liggett, S. B., M. G. Caron, R. J. Lefkowitz, and M. Hnatowich. Coupling of a mutated form of the human β_2-adrenergic receptor to G_i and G_s. *J. Biol. Chem.* 266: 4816–4821, 1991.

287. Lin, H. Y., T. L. Harris, M. S. Flannery, A. Aruffo, E. H. Kaji, A. Gorn, L. F. Kolafowski, Jr., H. F. Lodish, and S. R. Goldring. Expression cloning of an adenylate cyclase–coupled calcitonin receptor. *Science* 254: 1022–1024, 1991.

288. Linder, M. E., P. Middleton, J. R. Hepler, R. Taussig, A. G. Gilman, and S. M. Mumby. Lipid modification of G-proteins: α subunits are palmitoylated. *Proc. Natl. Acad. Sci. U.S.A.* 90: 3675–3579, 1993.

289. Linder, M. E., I.-H. Pang, R. J. Duronio, J. I. Gordon, P. C. Sternweis, and A. G. Gilman. Lipid modifications of G protein subunits. Myristoylation of $G_{o\alpha}$ increases its affinity for $\beta\gamma$. *J. Biol. Chem.* 266: 4654–4659, 1991.

290. Litosch, I. G-protein inhibition of phospholipase C-β_1 in membranes: role of G-protein $\beta\gamma$ subunits. *Biochem. J.* 319: 173–178, 1996.

291. Liu, J., N. Blin, B. R. Conklin, and J. Wess. Molecular mechanisms involved in muscarinic acetylcholine receptor–mediated G protein activation studied by insertion mutagenesis. *J. Biol. Chem.* 271: 6172–6178, 1996.

292. Liu, L.-W., T.-K. H. Vu, C. T. Esmon, and S. R. Coughlin. The region of the thrombin receptor resembling hirudin binds to thrombin and alters enzyme specificity. *J. Biol. Chem.* 266: 16977–16980, 1991.

293. Liu, M., and M. I. Simon. Regulation by cAMP-dependent protein kinase of a G-protein-mediated phospholipase C. *Nature* 382: 83–87, 1996.

294. Liu, X. B., D. Davis, and D. L. Segaloff. Disruption of potential sites for N-linked glycosylation does not impair hormone binding to the lutropin/choriogonadotropin receptors if Asn-173 is left intact. *J. Biol. Chem.* 268:1513–1516, 1993.

295. Logothetis, D. E., D. Kim, J. K. Northrup, E. J. Neer, and D. E. Clapham. Specificity of action of guanine nucleotide-binding regulatory protein on the cardiac muscarinic K^+. *Proc. Natl. Acad. Sci. U.S.A.* 85: 5815–5818, 1988.

296. Logothetis, D. E., Y. Kurachi, J. Galper, E. J. Neer, and D. E. Clapham. The $\beta\gamma$ subunits of GTP-binding proteins activate the muscarinic K^+ channel in heart. *Nature* 325: 321–326, 1987.

297. Lohse, M. J., J. L. Benovic, M. G. Caron, and R. J. Lefkowitz. β-Arrestin: a protein that regulates β-adrenergic receptor function. *Science* 248: 1547–1550, 1990.

298. Loosfelt, H. M., M. Misrahi, M. Atger, R. Salesse, M. T. Vu Hai-Luu Thi, A. Jolivet, A. Guiochon-Mantel, S. Sar, B. Jalla, J. Garnier, and E. Milgrom. Cloning and sequencing of porcine LH-hCG receptor cDNA: variants lacking transmembrane domain. *Science* 245: 525–528, 1989.

299. Lounsbury, K. M., P. J. Casey, L. F. Brass, and D. R. Manning. Phosphorylation of G_z in human platelets: selectivity and site of modification. *J. Biol. Chem.* 266: 22051–22056, 1991.

300. Lupas, A. N., J. M. Lupas, and J. B. Stock. Do G protein subunits associate via a three-stranded coiled coil? *FEBS Lett.* 314: 105–108, 1992.

300a. Luttrell, L. M., J. Della Rocca, T. van Biesen, D. K. Lutterll, and R. J. Lefkowitz. G$\beta\gamma$ subunits mediate Src-dependent phosphorylation of the epidermal growth factor receptor. *J. Biol. Chem.* 272: 4637–4644, 1997.

301. Luttrell, L. M., J. Ostrowski, S. Cotecchia, H. Kendall, and R. J. Lefkowitz. Antagonism of catecholamine receptor signaling by expression of cytoplasmic domains of the receptors. *Science* 259: 1453–1457, 1993.

302. Lyons, J., C. A. Landis, G. Harsh, L. Vallar, K. Grunewald, H. Feichtinger, Q.-Y. Suk, O. H. Clark, E. Kawasaki, and H. R. Bourne. Two G protein oncogenes in human endocrine tumors. *Science* 249: 655–659, 1990.

303. Maeda, S., J. Lameh, W. G. Mallet, M. Philip, J. Ramachandran, and W. Sadee. Internalization of the Hm1 muscarinic cholinergic receptor involves the third cytoplasmic loop. *FEBS Lett.* 269: 386–388, 1990.

304. Maggio, R., Z. Vogel, and J. Wess. Coexpression studies with mutant muscarinic/adrenergic receptors provide evidence for intermolecular "cross-talk" between G-protein-linked receptors. *Proc. Natl. Acad. Sci. U.S.A.* 90: 3103–3107, 1993.

305. Mahan, L. C., A. M. Koachman, and P. A. Insel. Genetic analysis of β-adrenergic receptor internalization and down-regulation. *Proc. Natl. Acad. Sci. U.S.A.* 82: 129–133, 1985.

306. Masu, M., Y. Tanabe, K. Tsuchida, R. Shigemoto, and S. Nakanishi. Sequence and expression of a metabotropic glutamate receptor. *Nature* 349: 760–765, 1991.

307. Mattera, R., M. P. Graziano, A. Yatani, Z. Zhou, R. Graf, J. Codina, L. Birnbaumer, A. G. Gilman, and A. M. Brown. Splice variants of the α subunit of the G protein G_s activate both adenylyl cyclase and calcium channels. *Science* 243: 804–807, 1989.

308. Mayo, K. E. Molecular cloning and expression of a pituitary-specific receptor for growth hormone-releasing hormone. *Mol. Endocrinol.* 6: 1734–1744, 1992.

309. Mazzoni, M. R., and H. E. Hamm. Effect of monoclonal antibody binding on α–$\beta\gamma$ subunit interactions in the rod outer segment G protein, G_t. *Biochemistry* 28: 9873–9880, 1989.

310. Mazzoni, M. R., J. A. Malinksi, and H. E. Hamm. Structural analysis of rod GTP-binding protein, G_t: limited proteolytic digestion pattern of G_t with four proteases defines monoclonal antibody epitope. *J. Biol. Chem.* 266: 14072–14081, 1991.

311. McArdle, C. A., and R. Countis. GnRH and PACAP action in gonadotropes. Cross-talk between phosphoinositidase C and adenylyl cyclase mediated signaling pathways. *Trends Endocrinol. Metab.* 7: 168–175, 1996.

312. McArdle, C. A., W. C. Gorospe, W. R. Huckle, and P. M. Conn. Homologous down-regulation of gonadotropin-releasing hormone receptors and desensitization of gonadotropes: lack of dependence on protein kinase C. *Mol. Endocrinol.* 1: 420–429, 1987.

313. McArdle, C. A., G. B. Willars, R. C. Fowkes, S. R. Nahorski, J. S. Davidson, and W. Forrest-Owen. Desensitization of gonadotropin-releasing hormone action in αT3–1 cells due to uncoupling of inositol 1,4,5-triphosphate generation and Ca^{2+} mobilization. *J. Biol. Chem.* 271: 23711–23717, 1966.

314. McClue, S. J., B. M. Baron, and B. A. Harris. Activation of G_i protein by peptide of the muscarinic M_2 receptor second intracellular loop. *Eur. J. Pharmacol.* 267: 185–193, 1994.

315. McFarland, K. C., R. Sprengel, H. S. Phillips, M. Kohler, N. Rosemblit, K. Nikolics, D. L. Segaloff, and P. H. Seeburg. Lutropin-choriogonadotropin receptor: an unusual member of the G protein receptor family. *Science* 245: 494–499, 1989.

316. McLaughlin, S. K., P. J. McKinnon, and R. F. Margoolskee. Gustducin is a taste-cell-specific G protein closely related to the transducins. *Nature* 357: 563–569, 1992.

317. Medema, R. H., and Bos, J. L. The role of p21ras in receptor tyrosine kinase signaling. *Crit. Rev. Oncog.* 4: 615–661, 1993.

318. Medynski, D., S. K. Sullivan, D. Smith, C. VanDop, F.-H.

Chang, B. K.-K. Fung, P. H. Seeburg, and H. R. Bourne. Amino acid sequence of the α subunit of transducin deduced from the cDNA sequence. *Proc. Natl. Acad. Sci. U.S.A.* 82: 4311–4315, 1985.

319. Ménard, L., S. S. G. Ferguson, L. S. Barak, L. Bertrand, R. T. Premont, A.-M. Colapietro, R. L. Lefkowitz, and M. G. Caron. Members of the G protein–coupled receptor kinase family that phosphorylate the β₂-adrenergic receptor facilitate sequestration. *Biochemistry* 35: 4155–4160, 1996.

320. Miller, R. T., S. B. Masters, K. A. Sullivan, B. Beiderman, and H. R. Bourne. A mutation that prevents GTP-dependent activation of the α chain of Gₛ. *Nature* 334: 712–715, 1988.

321. Milligan, G. Agonist regulation of cellular G protein levels and distribution: mechanisms and functional implications. *Trends Pharmacol. Sci.* 14: 405–410, 1993.

322. Milligan, G. Signal sorting by G-protein-linked receptors. *Adv. Pharmacol.* 32: 1–29, 1995.

323. Milligan, G., R. A. Bond, and M. Lee. Inverse agonism: pharmacological curiosity or potential therapeutic strategy? *Trends Pharmacol. Sci.* 16: 10–13, 1995.

324. Minden, A., A. Lin, F.-X. Claret, A. Abo, and M. Karin. Selective activation of the JNK signaling cascade and c-Jun transcriptional activity by the small GTPases Rac abd Cdc42. *Cell* 81: 1147–1157, 1995.

325. Minegishi, T., K. Nakamura, Y. Takakura, K. Miyamoto, Y. Hasegawa, Y. Ibuki, and M. Igarashi. Cloning and sequencing of human LH/hCG receptor cDNA. *Biochem. Biophys. Res. Commun.* 172: 1049–1054, 1990.

326. Moffett, S., B. Mouillac, H. Bonin, and M. Bouvier. Altered phosphorylation and desensitization patterns of a human β2-adrenergic receptor lacking the palmitoylated Cys341. *EMBO J.* 12: 349–356, 1993.

327. Möller, W., and R. Amons. Phosphate-binding sequences in nucleotide-binding proteins. *FEBS Lett.* 186: 1–7, 1985.

328. Morrison, D. F., P. J. O'Brien, and D. R. Pepperberg. Depalmitoylation with hydroxylamine alters the functional properties of rhodopsin. *J. Biol. Chem.* 266: 20118–20123, 1991.

329. Mouillac, B., M. Caron, H. Bonin, M. Dennis, and M. Bouvier. Agonist-modulated palmitoylation of β₂-adrenergic receptors in sf9 cells. *J. Biol. Chem.* 267: 21733–21737, 1992.

330. Moyle, W. R., M. P. Bernard, R. V. Myers, O. M. Marko, and C. D. Strader. Lutropin/β-adrenergic receptor chimeras bind choriogonadotropin and adrenergic ligands but are not expressed at the cell surface. *J. Biol. Chem.* 266: 10807–10812, 1991.

331. Mulheron, J. G., S. J. Casanas, J. M. Arthur, M. N. Garnovskaya, T. W. Gettys, and J. R. Raymond. Human 5-HT₁ₐ receptor expressed in insect cells activates endogenous G₀-like G proteins. *J. Biol. Chem.* 269: 12954–12962, 1994.

332. Mumby, S. M.P.J. Casey, A. G. Gilman, S. Gutowski, and P. C. Stemweis. G protein γ subunits contain a 20-carbon isoprenoid. *Proc. Natl. Acad. Sci. U.S.A.* 87: 5873–5877, 1990.

333. Mumby, S. M., R. O. Heukeroth, J. E. Gordon, and A. G. Gilman. G-protein α-subunit expression, myristoylation, and membrane association in COS cells. *Proc. Natl. Acad. Sci. U.S.A.* 87: 728–733, 1990.

334. Mumby, S. M., C. Kleuss, and A. G. Gilman. Receptor regulation of G-protein palmitoylation. *Proc. Natl. Acad. Sci. U.S.A.* 91: 2800–2804, 1994.

335. Murayama, T., and M. Ui. Loss of the inhibitory function of the guanine nucleotide regulatory component of adenylate cyclase due to its ADP ribosylation by islet-activating protein, pertussis toxin, in adipocyte membranes. *J. Biol. Chem.* 258: 3319–3326, 1983.

336. Nagayama, Y., D. Russo, H. L. Wadsworth, G. D. Chazenbalk, and B. Rapoport. Eleven amino acids (Lys-201 to Lys-211) and 9 amino acids (Gly-222 to Leu-230) in the human thyrotropin receptor are involved in ligand binding. *J. Biol. Chem.* 266: 14926–14930, 1991.

337. Nagayama, Y., H. L. Wadsworth, G. D. Chazenbal, D. Russo, P. Seto, and B. Rapoport. Thyrotropin-luteinizing hormone/chorionic gonadotropin-receptor extracellular domain chimeras as probes for thyrotropin receptor function. *Proc. Natl. Acad. Sci. U.S.A.* 88: 902–905, 1991.

338. Nakanishi, S. Molecular diversity of glutamate receptors and implications for brain function. *Science* 258: 597–603, 1992.

339. Namba T. Y. Sugimoto, M. Negishi, A. Irie, F. Ushikubi, A. Kakisuka, S. Ito, A. Ichikawa, and S. Narumiya. Splicing of C-terminal tail of prostaglandin E receptor subtype EP3 determines G-protein specificity. *Nature* 365: 155–170, 1993.

340. Nathans, J. Determinants of visual pigment absorbance: identification of the retinylidene Schiff's base counterion in bovine rhodopsin. *Biochemistry* 29: 9746–9752, 1990.

341. Nathans, J., and D. S. Hogness. Isolation and nucleotide sequence of the gene encoding human rhodopsin. *Proc. Natl. Acad. Sci. U.S.A.* 81: 4851–4855, 1984.

342. Nathans, J., and D. S. Hogness. Isolation, sequence analysis, and intron–exon arrangement of the gene encoding bovine rhodopsin. *Cell* 34: 807–814, 1983.

343. Navon, S. E., and B. K.-K. Fung. Characterization of transducin from bovine retinal rod outer segments. Mechanism and effects of cholera toxin–catalyzed ADP-ribosylation. *J. Biol. Chem.* 259: 6686–6693, 1984.

344. Neer, E. J. Heterotrimeric G proteins: organizers of transmembrane signals. *Cell* 80: 249–257, 1995.

345. Neer, E. J., C. J. Schmidt, R. Nambudripad, and T. F. Smith. The ancient regulatory-protein family of WD-repeat proteins. *Nature* 371: 297–300, 1994.

346. Negishi, M., T. Namba, Y. Sugimoto, A. Irie, T. Katada, S. Narumiya, and A. Ichikawa. Opposite coupling of prostaglandin E receptor EP3C with Gₛ and G₀. *J. Biol. Chem.* 268: 26067–26070, 1993.

347. Negishi, M., Y. Sugimoto, A. Arie, S. Narumiya, and A. Ichikawa. Two isoforms of prostaglandin E receptor EP3 subtype. Different COOH-terminal domains determine sensitivity to agonist-induced desensitization. *J. Biol. Chem.* 268: 9517–9523, 1993.

348. Neill, J. D., L. W. Duck, J. C. Sellers, L. C. Musgrove, A. Scheschonka, K. M. Druey, and J. H. Kherl. Potential role for a regulator of G protein signaling (RGS2) in gonadotropin releasing hormone (GnRH) stimulated desensitization. *Endocrinology* 138: 843–846, 1997.

349. Neve, K. A., B. A. Cox, R. A. Henningsen, A. Spanoyannis, and R. L. Nerve. Pivotal role for aspartate-80 in the regulation of dopamine D₂ receptor affinity for drugs and inhibition of adenylyl cyclase. *Mol. Pharmacol.* 39: 733–739, 1991.

350. Ng, G. Y., S. R. George, R. L. Zastawny, M. Caron, M. Bouvier, M. Dennis, and F. O. O'Dowd. Human serotonin 1B receptor expression in Sf9 cells: phosphorylation, palmitoylation, and adenylyl cyclase inhibition. *Biochemistry* 32: 11727–11733, 1993.

351. Ng, G. Y., B. Mouillac, S. R. George, M. Caron, M. Dennis, M. Bouvier, and B. F. O'Dowd. Desensitization, phosphorylation and palmitoylation of the human dopamine D1 receptor. *Eur. J. Pharmacol.* 267: 7–19, 1994.

352. Nishida, E., and Y. Gotoh. The MAP kinase cascade is essential for diverse signal transduction pathways. *Trends Biochem. Sci.* 18: 128–130, 1993.

353. Nishizuka, Y. Studies and perspectives of protein kinase C. *Science* 233: 305–312, 1986.

354. Noel, J. P., H. E. Hamm, and P. B. Sigler. The 2.2 Å crystal structure of transducin-α complexed with GTPγs. *Nature* 366: 654–662, 1993.

355. Nussenzveig, D. R., C. N. Thaw, and M. C. Gershengorn. Inhibition of inositol phosphate second messenger formation by intracellular loop one of a human calcitonin receptor. *J. Biol. Chem.* 269: 28123–28129, 1994.

356. O'Dowd, B. F., M. Hnatowich, M. G. Caron, R. J. Lefkowitz, and M. Bouvier. Palmitoylation of the human β₂-adrenergic receptor. Mutation of Cys341 in the carboxyl tail leads to an uncoupled nonpalmitoylated form of the receptor. *J. Biol. Chem.* 264: 7564–7569, 1989.

357. O'Dowd, B. F., M. Hnatowich, J. W. Regan, W. M. Leader, M. G. Caron, and R. J. Lefkowitz. Site-directed mutagenesis of the cytoplasmic domains of the human β₂-adrenergic receptor. *J. Biol. Chem.* 263: 15985–15992, 1988.

358. Offermanns, S., and G. Schultz. What are the functions of the pertussis toxin–insensitive G-proteins G₁₂, G₁₃ and Gz. *Mol. Cell. Endocrinol.* 100: 71–74, 1994.

359. Offermanns, S., and M. I. Simon. Gα₁₅ and Gα₁₆ couple to a wide variety of receptors to phospholipase C. *J. Biol. Chem.* 270: 15175–15180, 1995.

360. Ohyama, K., Y. Yamano, S. Chaki, T. Kondo, and T. Inagami. Domains for G-protein coupling in angiotensin II receptor type I: studies by site-directed mutagenesis. *Biochem. Biophys. Res. Commun.* 189: 677–683, 1992.

361. Okamoto, T., and I. Nishimoto. Detection of G protein-activator regions in M₄ subtype muscarinic cholinergic, and α₂-adrenergic receptors based upon characteristics in primary structure. *J. Biol. Chem.* 267: 8342–8346, 1992.

362. Osawa, S., N. Dhanasekaran, C. W. Woon, and G. L. Johnson. Gαi-Gαs chimeras define the function of α chain domains in control of G-protein activation and βγ subunit complex interactions. *Cell* 63: 697–706, 1990.

363. Ostrowski, J., M. A. Kjelsberg, M. G. Caron, and R. J. Lefkowitz. Mutagenesis of the β₂-adrenergic receptor: how structure elucidates function. *Annu. Rev. Pharmacol. Toxicol.* 32: 167–183, 1992.

364. Ovchinnikov, Y. A., N. G. Abdulaev, and A. S. Bogachuk. Two adjacent cysteine residues in the C-terminal cytoplasmic fragment of bovine rhodopsin are palmitoylated. *FEBS Lett.* 230: 1–5, 1988.

365. Pace, U., E. Hanski, Y. Salomon, and D. Lancet. Odorant-sensitive adenylate cyclase may mediate olfactory reception. *Nature* 316: 255–258, 1985.

366. Pages F., P. Deterre, and C. Pfister. Enhanced GTPase activity of transducin when bound to cGMP phosphodiesterase in bovine retinal rods. *J. Biol. Chem.* 267: 22018–22021, 1992.

367. Parenti, M., M. A. Vigano, C. M. H. Newman, G. Milligan, and A. I. Magee. A novel N-terminal motif for palmitoylation of G-protein α subunits. *Biochem. J.* 291: 349–353, 1993.

368. Park, D., D.-Y. Jhon, C.-W. Lee, C.-H. Lee, and S. G. Rhee. Activation of phospholipase C isoenzymes by G protein βγ subunits. *J. Biol. Chem.* 268: 4573–4577, 1993.

369. Parker, E. M., K. Kameyama, T. Higashijima, and E. M. Ross. Reconstitutively active G protein–coupled receptors purified from baculovirus-infected insect cells. *J. Biol. Chem.* 266: 519–527, 1991.

370. Parma, J., L. Duprez, J. V. Sande, P. Cochaux, C. Gervy, J. Mokel, J. Dumont, and G. Vassart. Somatic mutations in the thyrotropin receptor gene cause hyperfunctioning thyroid adenomas. *Nature* 365: 649–651, 1993.

371. Patel, D. R., Y. Kong, and S. P. Sreedharan. Molecular cloning and expression of a human secretin receptor. *Mol. Pharmacol.* 47: 467–473, 1995.

372. Paulssen, E. J., R. H. Paulssen, K. M. Gautvik, and J. O. Gordeladze. "Cross-talk" between phospholipase C and adenylyl cyclase involves regulation of G-protein levels in GH₃ rat pituitary cells. *Cell. Signal.* 4: 747–755, 1992.

373. Paulssen, R. H., E. J. Paulssen, K. M. Gautvik, and J. O. Gordeladze. The thyroliberin receptor interacts directly with a stimulatory guanine-nucleotide-binding protein in the activation of adenylyl cyclase in GH₃ rat pituitary tumour cells. Evidence obtained by the use of antisense RNA inhibition and immunoblocking of the stimulatory guanine-nucleotide-binding protein. *Eur. J. Biochem.* 204: 413–418, 1992.

374. Pelech, S. L., and J. S. Sanghera. MAP kinases: charting the regulatory pathways. *Science* 257: 1355–1356, 1992.

375. Perlman, J. H., L. Laakkonen, R. Osman, and M. C. Gershengorn. A model of the thyrotropin-releasing hormone (TRH) receptor binding pocket. *J. Biol. Chem.* 269: 23383–23386, 1994.

376. Peroutka, S. J. 5-Hydroxytryptamine receptors. *J. Neurochem.* 60: 408–416, 1993.

377. Phillips, W. J., and R. A. Cerione. Rhodopsin/transducin interactions. I. Characterization of the binding of the transducin–βγ subunit complex to rhodopsin using fluorescence spectroscopy. *J. Biol. Chem.* 267: 17032–17039, 1992.

378. Pin, J. P., and R. Duvoisin. The metabotropic glutamate receptors: structure and functions. *Neuropharmacology* 34: 1–26, 1995.

379. Pitcher, J. A., J. Inglese, J. B. Higgins, J. L. Arriza, P. J. Casey, C. Kim, J. L. Benovic, M. W. Kwatra, M. G. Caron, and R. J. Lefkowitz. Role of the βγ subunits of G-proteins in targeting the β-adrenergic receptor kinase to membrane-bound receptors. *Science* 257: 1264–1267, 1992.

380. Pitcher, J. A., E. S. Payne, C. Csortos, A. A. DePaoli-Roach, and R. J. Lefkowitz. The G-protein-coupled receptor phosphatase: a protein phosphatase type 2A with a distinct subcellular distribution and substrate specificity. *Proc. Natl. Acad. Sci. U.S.A.* 92: 8343–8347, 1995.

381. Post, G. R., and J. H. Brown. G protein–coupled receptors and signaling pathways regulating growth responses. *FASEB J.* 10:741–749, 1996.

382. Premont, R. T., J. Inglese, and R. L. Lefkowitz. Protein kinases that phosphorylate activated G protein-coupled receptors. *FASEB J.* 9: 175–182, 1995.

383. Probst, W. C., L. A. Snyder, D. I. Schuster, J. Brosius, and S. C. Seaflon. Sequence alignment of the G-protein coupled receptor superfamily. *DNA Cell Biol.* 11: 1–11, 1992.

384. Pronin, A. N., and N. Gautman. Interaction between G-protein β and γ subunit types is selective. *Proc. Natl. Acad. Sci. U.S.A.* 89: 6220–6224, 1992

385. Pumiglia, K. M., H. LeVine, T. Haske, T. Habib, R. Jove, and S. J. Decker. A direct interaction between G-protein βγ subunits and the Raf-1 protein kinase. *J. Biol. Chem.* 270: 14251–14254, 1995.

386. Quintana, J., R. W. Hipkin, J. Sanchez-Yague, and M. Ascoli. Follitropin (FSH) and phorbol ester stimulate the phosphorylation of the FSH receptor in intact cells. *J. Biol. Chem.* 269: 8722–8779, 1994.

387. Rahmatullah, M., and J. D. Robishaw. Direct interaction of the α and subunits of the G-proteins. *J. Biol. Chem.* 269: 3574–3580, 1994.

388. Ramdas, L., R. M. Disher, and T. G. Wensel. Nucleotide exchange and cGMP phosphodiesterase activation by pertussis

toxin inactivated transducin. *Biochemistry* 30: 11637–11645, 1991.

389. Rands, R., M. R. Candelore, A. H. Cheung, W. S. Hill, D. C. Strader, and R. A. F. Dixon. Mutational analysis of β-adrenergic receptor glycosylation. *J. Biol. Chem.* 265: 10759–10764, 1990.

390. Rao, V. R., G. B. Cohen, and D. D. Oprian. Rhodopsin mutation G90D and a molecular mechanism for congenital blindness. *Nature* 367: 639–642, 1994.

391. Rarick, H. M., N. O. Artemyev, and H. E. Hamm. A site on rod G protein α subunit that mediates effector activation. *Science* 256: 1031–1033, 1992.

392. Rawlings, S. R. PACAP, PACAP receptors, and intracellular signaling. *Mol. Cell. Endocrinol.* 101: C5–C9, 1994.

393. Ray, K., C. Kunsch, L. M. Bonner, and J. D. Robishaw. Isolation of cDNA clones encoding eight different human G protein γ subunits, including three novel forms designated the γ_4, γ_{10} and γ_{11} subunits. *J. Biol. Chem.* 270: 21765–21771, 1995.

394. Raymond, J. R. Multiple mechanisms of receptor–G protein signaling specificity. *Am. J. Physiol.* 269 (*Renal Fluid Electrolyte Physiol.* 40): F141–F158, 1995.

395. Raymond, J. R., C. L. Olsen, and T. W. Gettys. Cell-specific physical and functional coupling of human 5–HT$_{1A}$ receptors to inhibitory G protein α subunits and lack of coupling to G$_{s\alpha}$. *Biochemistry* 32: 11064–11073, 1993.

396. Reed, R. R. How does the nose know? *Cell* 60: 1–2, 1990.

397. Reinhart, J., L. M. Mertz, and K. J. Catt. Molecular cloning and expression of cDNA encoding the murine gonadotropin-releasing hormone receptor. *J. Biol. Chem.* 267: 21281–21284, 1992.

398. Ren, Q., H. Kurose, R. J. Lefkowitz, and S. Cotecchia. Constitutively active mutants of the α_2-adrenergic receptor. *J. Biol. Chem.* 268: 16483–16487, 1993.

399. Rens-Domiano, S., and H. E. Hamm. Structural and functional relationships of heterotrimeric G-proteins. *FASEB J.* 9: 1059–1066, 1995.

400. Richardson, R. M., and M. M. Hosey. Agonist-induced phosphorylation and desensitization of human m2 cholinergic receptors in Sf9 insect cells. *J. Biol. Chem.* 267: 22249–22255, 1992.

401. Robbins, L. S., J. H. Nadeau, K. R. Johnson, M. A. Kelly, L. Roselli-Rehfuss, E. Baack, K. G. Mountjoy, and R. D. Cone. Pigmentation phenotypes of variant extension locus alleles result from point mutations that alter MSH receptor function. *Cell* 72: 827–834, 1993.

402. Rodbell, M. Signal transduction: evolution of an idea. *Environ. Health Perspect.* 103: 338–345, 1995.

403. Ross, E. M. G protein GTPase-activating proteins: regulation of speed, amplitude, and signaling selectivity. *Recent Prog. Horm. Res.* 50: 207–221, 1995.

404. Roth, N. S., P. T. Campbell, M. G. Caron, R. J. Lefkowitz, and M. J. Lohse. Comparative rates of desensitization of β-adrenergic receptors by the β-adrenergic receptor kinase and the cyclic AMP–dependent protein kinase. *Proc. Natl. Acad. Sci. U.S.A.* 88: 6201–6204, 1991.

405. Ryu, K.-S., R. L. Gilchrist, I. Ji, S.-J. Kim, and T. H. Ji. Exoloop 3 of the luteinizing hormone/choriogonadotropin receptor. Lys[583] is essential and irreplaceable for human choriogonadotropin (hCG)–dependent receptor activation but not for high affinity hCG binding. *J. Biol. Chem.* 271: 7301–7304, 1996.

406. Sadoshima, J., and S. Izumo. The heterotrimeric Gq protein–coupled angiotensin II receptor activates p21ras via the tyrosine kinase Shc-Grb-Sos pathway in cardiac myocytes. *EMBO J.* 15: 775–787, 1996.

407. Sakmar, T. P., R. R. Franke, and H. G. Khorana. Glutamic acid-113 serves as the retinylidene Schiff base counterion in bovine rhodopsin. *Proc. Natl. Acad. Sci. U.S.A.* 86: 8309–8313, 1989.

408. Sakmar, T. P., R. R. Franke, and H. G. Khorana. The role of the retinylidene Schiff base counterion in rhodopsin in determining wavelength absorbance and Schiff base pKa. *Proc. Natl. Acad. Sci. U.S.A.* 88: 3079–3083, 1991.

409. Samama, P., S. Cotecchia, T. Costa, and R. J. Lefkowitz. A mutation-induced activated state of the β_2-adrenergic receptor. Extending the ternary complex model. *J. Biol. Chem.* 268: 4625–4636, 1993.

410. Sanford, J., J. Codina, and L. Birnbaumer. γ-Subunits of G proteins, but not their α- or β-subunits, are polyisoprenylated. Studies on post-translational modifications using in vitro translation with rabbit reticulocyte lysates. *J. Biol. Chem.* 266: 9570–9579, 1991.

411. Schafer, W. R., and J. Rine. Protein prenylation: genes, enzymes, targets and functions. *Annu. Rev. Genet.* 25: 209–238, 1992.

412. Schelling, J. R., A. S. Hanson, R. Marzen, and S. L. Linas. Cytoskeleton-dependent endocytosis is required for apical-type angiotensin II receptor–mediated phospholipase C activation in cultured rat proximal tubule cells. *J. Clin. Invest.* 90: 2472–2480, 1992.

413. Schertler, G.F.X., C. Villa, and R. Henderson. Projection structure of rhodopsin. *Nature* 362: 770–772, 1993.

414. Schipani, E., H. Karga, A. C. Karaplis, J. T. Potts, Jr., H. M. Kronenberg, G. V. Segre, A. B. Abou-Samra, and H. Jüppner. Identical complementary deoxyribonucleic acids encode a human renal and bone parathyroid hormone (PTH)/PTH-related peptide receptor. *Endocrinology* 132: 2157–2165, 1993.

415. Schleicher, S., I. Boekhoff, J. Arriza, R. J. Lefkowitz, and H. Breer. A β-adrenergic receptor kinase-like enzyme is involved in olfactory signal termination. *Proc. Natl. Acad. Sci. U.S.A.* 90: 1420–1424, 1993.

416. Schmidt, C. J., T. C. Thomas, M. A. Levine, and E. J. Neer. Specificity of G-protein β and γ subunit interaction. *J. Biol. Chem.* 267: 13807–13810, 1992.

417. Schramm, M., and Z. Selinger. Message transmission: receptor controlled adenylate cyclase system. *Science* 225: 1350–1356, 1984.

418. Schvarts, I., and E. Hazum. Tunicamycin and neuraminidase effects of luteinizing hormone (LH)–releasing hormone binding and LH release from rat pituitary cels in culture. *Endocrinology* 116: 2341–2346, 1985.

419. Scott, R. H., and A. C. Dolphin. Activation of a G-protein promotes agonist responses to calcium channel ligands. *Nature* 330: 760–762, 1987.

420. Seaflon, S. C., and R. P. Millar. The gonadotrophin-releasing hormone receptor: structural determinants and regulatory control. *Hum. Reprod. Update* 1: 216–230, 1995.

421. Segaloff, D. L., and M. Ascoli. The lutropin/choriogonadotropin receptor . . . 4 years later. *Endocr. Rev.* 14: 324–347, 1993.

422. Segaloff, D. L., R. Sprengel, K. Nikolics, and M. Ascoli. The structure of the lutropin/choriogonadotropin receptor. *Recent Prog. Horm. Res.* 46: 261–303, 1990.

423. Sevetson, B. R., X. Kong, and J. C. Lawrence, Jr. Increasing cAMP attenuates activation of mitogen-activated protein kinase. *Proc. Natl. Acad. Sci. U.S.A.* 90: 10305–10309, 1993.

424. Shah, B. H., D. J. MacEwan, and G. Milligan. Gonadotrophin-releasing hormone receptor agonist-mediated down-regulation of G$_q\alpha$/G$_{11}\alpha$ (pertusis toxin–insensitive) G proteins in αT3–1 gonadotroph cells reflects increased G protein turnover but not

alterations in mRNA levels. *Proc. Natl. Acad. Sci. U.S.A.* 92: 1886–1890, 1995.

425. Shapiro, R. A., and N. M. Nathanson. Deletion analysis of the mouse m1 muscarinic acetylcholine receptor: effects on phosphoinositide metabolism and down-regulation. *Biochemistry* 28: 8946–8950, 1989.

426. Shear, M., P. A. Insel, K. L. Melmon, and P. Coffino. Agonist-specific refractoriness induced by isoproterenol: studies with mutant cells. *J. Biol. Chem.* 251: 7572–7576, 1976.

427. Shenker, A., L. Laue, S. Kosugl, J. Merendino, Jr., T. Minegishi, and G. B. Cutler. A constitutively activating mutation of the luteinizing hormone receptor in familial male precocious puberty. *Nature* 365: 652–654, 1993.

428. Shinozawa, T., S. Uchida, E. Martin, D. Cafiso, W. Hubbell, and M. Bitensky. Additional component required for activity and reconstitution of light activated vertebrate photoreceptor GTPase. *Proc. Natl. Acad. Sci. U.S.A.* 77: 1408–1411, 1980.

429. Simon, M. A., G. S. Dodson, and G. M. Rubin. An SH3-SH2-SH3 protein is required for p21^{Ras1} activation and binds to sevenless and Sos proteins *in vitro*. *Cell* 73: 169–177, 1993.

430. Simon, M. I., P. Strathmann, and N. Gautam. Diversity of G proteins in signal transduction. *Science* 252: 802–808, 1991.

431. Simonds, W. F., J. E. Butrynski, N. Gautam, C. G. Unsion, and A.M. Spiegel. G-protein $\beta\gamma$ dimers. Membrane targeting requires subunit co-expression and intact γ CAAX domain. *J. Biol. Chem.* 266: 5363–5366, 1991.

432. Simonds, W. F., P. K. Goldsmith, J. Codina, C. G. Unson, and A. M. Spiegel. G_{i2} mediates α_2-adrenergic inhibition of adenylyl cyclase in platelet membranes: in situ identification with Gα C-terminal antibodies. *Proc. Natl. Acad. Sci. U.S.A.* 86: 7809–7813, 1989.

433. Smrcka, A. V., J. R. Helper, K. O. Brown, and P. C. Sternweiss. Regulation of polyphosphoinositide-specific phospholipase C activity by purifed Gq. *Science* 251: 804–807, 1991.

434. Smrcka, A. V., and P. C. Sternweis. Regulation of purified subtypes of phosphatidylinositol-specific phospholipase Cβ by G protein α and $\beta\gamma$ subunits. *J. Biol. Chem.* 268: 9667–9674, 1993.

435. Sondek, J., A. Bohm, D. G. Lambright, H. E. Hamm, and P. B. Sigler. Crystal structure of a G_A protein $\beta\gamma$ dimer at 2.1 Å resolution. *Nature* 379: 369–374, 1996.

436. Sondek, J., D. G. Lambright, J. P. Noel, H. E. Hamm, and P. B. Sigler. GTPase mechanism of G proteins from the 1.7-Å crystal structure of transducin α-GDP-AlF$_4^-$. *Nature* 372: 276–279, 1994.

437. Spalding, T., N. Birdsall, C. Curtis, and E. Hulme. Acetylcholine mustard labels the binding site aspartate in muscarinic acetylcholine receptors. *J. Biol. Chem.* 269: 4092–4097, 1994.

438. Spengler, D., C. Waeber, C. Pantaloni, F. Holsboer, J. Bockaert, P. H. Seburg, and L. Journot. Differential signal transduction by five splice variants of the PACAP receptor. *Nature* 365: 170–175, 1993.

439. Spiegel, A. M. Defects in G protein–coupled signal transduction in human disease. *Annu. Rev. Physiol.* 58: 143–170, 1995.

440. Spiegel, A. M., P. S. Backlund, J. E. Butyrinski, T. L. Z. Jones, and W. F. Simonds. The G protein connection: molecular basis of membrane association. *Trends Biochem. Sci.* 16: 338–341, 1991.

441. Spiegel, A. M., A. Shenker, and L. S. Weinstein. Receptor-effector coupling by G proteins: implications for normal and abnormal signal transduction. *Endocr. Rev.* 13: 536–565, 1992.

442. Spring, D. J., and E. J. Neer. A 14 amino acid region of the G protein γ subunit is sufficient to confer the selectivity of α binding to the β subunit. *J. Biol. Chem.* 269: 22882–22886, 1994.

443. Stanislaus, D., J. A. Janovick, S. Brothers, and P. M. Conn. Regulation of $G_{q/11\alpha}$ by the gonadotropin-releasing hormone receptor. *Mol. Endocrinol.* 11: 738–746, 1997.

444. Sterne-Marr, R., and J. L. Benovic. Regulation of G protein-coupled receptors by receptor kinases and arrestins. *Vitam. Horm.* 51: 193–234, 1995.

445. Stiles, G. L., J. L. Benovic, M. G. Caron, and R. J. Lefkowitz. Mammalian beta-adrenergic receptors, distinct glycoprotein populations containing high mannose or complex type carbohydrate chains. *J. Biol. Chem.* 259: 8655–8663, 1984.

446. Stoffel, R. H., R. R. Randall, R. T. Premont, R. J. Lefkowitz, and J. Inglese. Palmitoylation of G protein–coupled receptor kinase, GRK6: lipid modification diversity in the GRK family. *J. Biol. Chem.* 269: 27791–27794, 1994.

447. Stone, D. E., G. M. Cole, M. De Barros Lopez, M. Goebl, and S. I. Reed. N-Myristoylation is required for function of the pheromone-responsive Gα protein of yeast: conditional activation of the pheromone response by a temperature-sensitive N-myristoyl transferase. *Genes Dev.* 5: 1969–1981, 1991.

448. Strader, C. D., M. R. Candelore, W. S. Hill, I. S. Sigal, and R. A. Dixon. Identification of two serine residues involved in agonist activation of the β-adrenergic receptor. *J. Biol. Chem.* 264: 13572–13578, 1989.

449. Strader, C. D., R. A. Dixon, A. H. Cheung, M. R. Candelore, A. D. Blake, and I. S. Sigal. Mutations that uncouple the β-adrenergic receptor from Gs and increase agonist affinity. *J. Biol. Chem.* 262: 16439–16443, 1987.

450. Strader, C. D., T. M. Fong, M. P. Graziano, and M. R. Tota. The family of G-protein-coupled receptors. *FASEB J.* 9: 745–754, 1995.

451. Strader, C. D., T. M. Fong, M. R. Tota, and D. Underwood. Structure and function of G protein–coupled receptors. *Annu. Rev. Biochem.* 63: 101–132, 1994.

452. Strader, C. D., T. Gaffney, E. E. Sugg, M. R. Candelore, R. Keys, A. A. Patchett, and R.A.F. Dixon. Allele-specific activation of genetically engineered receptors. *J. Biol. Chem.* 266: 5–8, 1991.

453. Strader, C. D., I. S. Sigal, M. R. Candelore, E. Rands, W. S. Hill, and R.A.F. Dixon. Conserved aspartate residues 79 and 113 of the β-adrenergic receptor have different roles in receptor function. *J. Biol. Chem.* 263: 10267–10271, 1988.

454. Strader, C. D., I. S. Sigal, and R.A.F. Dixon. Genetic approaches to the determination of structure–function relationships of G protein–coupled receptors. *Trends Pharmacol. Sci.* (Suppl.): 26–30, 1989.

455. Strader, S. D., I. S. Sigal, and R. A. Dixon. Mapping the functional domains of the β-adrenergic receptor. *Am. J. Resp. Cell Mol. Biol.* 1: 81–86, 1989.

456. Strader, C. D., I. S. Sigal, R. B. Register, M. R. Candelore, E. Rands, and R. A. Dixon. Identification of residues required for ligand binding to the β-adrenergic receptor. *Proc. Natl. Acad. Sci. U.S.A.* 84: 4384–4388, 1987.

457. Strathmann, M., and M. I. Simon. G protein diversity: a distinct class of α subunits is present in vertebrates and invertebrates. *Proc. Natl. Acad. Sci. U.S.A.* 87: 9113–9117, 1990.

458. Stryer, L. Visual excitation and recovery. *J. Biol. Chem.* 266: 10711–10714, 1991.

459. Stryer, L., J. B. Hurley, and B. K. Fung. Transducin and the cyclic GMP phosphodiesterase of retinal rod outer segments. *Methods Enzymol.* 96: 617–627, 1983.

460. Su, Y.-F., T. K. Harden, and J. P. Perkins. Catecholamine-specific desensitization of adenylate cyclase: evidence for a multistep process. *J. Biol. Chem.* 255: 7410–7419, 1980.

461. Sullivan, K. A., R. T. Miller, S. B. Masters, B. Beiderman, W. Heideman, and H. R. Bourne. Identification of receptor contact

site involved in receptor–G protein coupling. *Nature* 330: 758–760, 1987.

462. Sunahara, R. K., C. W. Dessauer, and A. G. Gilman. Complexity and diversity of mammalian adenylyl cyclases. *Annu. Rev. Pharmacol. Toxicol.* 36: 461–480, 1996.

463. Suprenant, A., D. A. Horstman, H. Akbarali, and L. E. Limbird. A point mutation of the α2–adrenoceptor that blocks coupling to potassium but not calcium currents. *Science* 257: 977–980, 1992.

464. Suzuki, H., G. N. Prado, N. Wilkinson, and J. Navarro. The N-terminus of interleukin-8 (IL-8) receptor confers high affinity binding to human IL-8. *J. Biol. Chem.* 269: 18263–18266, 1994.

465. Takeuchi, K., N. Takahashi, T. Abe, and K. Abe. Two isoforms of the rat kidney EP3 receptor derived by alternative RNA splicing: intrarenal expression co-localization. *Biochem. Biophys. Res. Commun.* 199: 834–840, 1994.

466. Tanabe, Y., M. Masu, T. Ishii, R. Shigemoto, and S. Nakanishi. A family of metabotropic glutamate receptors. *Neuron* 8: 169–179, 1992.

467. Tang, W.-J., and A. G. Gilman. Type-specific regulation of adenylyl cyclase by G protein $\beta\gamma$ subunits. *Science* 254: 1500–1504, 1991.

468. Tang, W.-J., and A. G. Gilman. Adenylyl cyclases. *Cell* 70: 869–872, 1992.

469. Tapanainen, J. S., M. Bo, L. Dunkel, H. Billig, E. A. Perlas, I. Boime, and A.J.W. Hsueh. Deglycosylation of the human luteinizing hormone receptor does not affect ligand binding and signal transduction. *Endocr. J.* 1: 219–225, 1993.

470. Taussig, R., J. A. Iñiguez-Lluhi, and A. G. Gilman. Inhibition of adenylyl cyclase by $G_{\alpha i}$. *Science* 261: 218–221, 1993.

471. Taussig, R., L. M. Quarmby, and A. G. Gilman. Regulation of purified type-I and type-II adenylyl cyclases by G protein $\beta\gamma$ subunits. *J. Biol. Chem.* 268: 9–12, 1993.

472. Taussig, R., W.-J. Tang, J. R. Hepler, and A. G. Gilman. Distinct patterns of bidirectional regulation of mammalian adenylyl cyclases. *J. Biol. Chem.* 269: 6093–6100, 1994.

473. Thomas, D., T. G. Rozell, X. Liu, and D. L. Segaloff. Mutational analyses of the extracellular domain of the full-length lutropin/choriogonadotropin receptor suggest leucine-rich repeats 1–6 are involved in hormone binding. *Mol. Endocrinol.* 10: 760–768, 1996.

474. Thomas, D. D., and L. Stryer. Transverse location of the retinal chromophore of rhodopsin in rod outer segment disc membranes. *J. Mol. Biol.* 154: 145–157, 1982.

475. Thomas, T. C., C. J. Schmidt, and E. J. Neer. G protein α_o subunit: mutation of conserved cysteines identifies a subunit contact surface and alters GDP affinity. *Proc. Natl. Acad. Sci. U.S.A.* 90: 10295–10299, 1993.

476. Thompson, P., and J.B.C. Findlay. Phosphorylation of ovine rhodopsin. *Biochem J.* 220: 773–780, 1984.

477. Thorens, B. Expression cloning of the pancreatin β cell receptor for the gluco-incretin hormone glucagon-like peptide. *Proc. Natl. Acad. Sci. U.S.A.* 89: 8641–8645, 1992.

478. Tota, M. R., and C. D. Strader. Characterization of the binding domain of the β-adrenergic receptor with the fluorescent antagonist carazolol. Evidence for a buried ligand binding site. *J. Biol. Chem.* 265: 16891–16897, 1990.

479. Touhara, K., B. E. Hawes, T. van Biesen, and R. J. Lefkowitz. G protein $\beta\gamma$ subunits stimulate phosphorylation of Shc adapter protein. *Proc. Natl. Acad. Sci. U.S.A.* 92: 9284–9287, 1995.

480. Trumpp-Kallmeyer, S., B. Chini, B. Mouillac, C. Barberis, J. Hoflack, and M. Hibert. Towards understanding the role of the first extracellular loop for the binding of peptide hormones

to G-protein coupled receptors. *Pharm. Acta Helv.* 70: 255–262, 1995.

481. Tsai-Morris, C. H., E. Buczko, W. Wang, and M. L. Dufau. Intronic nature of the rat luteinizing hormone receptor gene defines a soluble receptor subspecies with hormone binding activity. *J. Biol. Chem.* 265: 19385–19388, 1990.

482. Tsai-Morris, C. H., E. Buczko, W. Wang, X. Z. Xie, and M. L. Dufau. Structural organization of the rat luteinizing hormone (LH) receptor gene. *J. Biol. Chem.* 266: 11355–11359, 1991.

483. Ullrich, A., and J. Schlessinger. Signal transduction by receptor with tyrosine kinase activity. *Cell* 61: 203–212, 1990.

484. Vaillancourt, R. R., A. M. Gardner, and G. L. Johnson. B-Raf-dependent regulation of the MEK-1/mitogen-activated protein kinase pathway in PC12 cells and regulation by cyclic AMP. *Mol. Cell. Biol.* 14: 6522–6530, 1994.

485. van Biesen, T., B. E. Hawes, D. K. Luttrell, K. M. Krueger, K. Touhara, E. Porfiri, M. Sakaue, L. M. Luttrell, and R. J. Lefkowitz. Receptor-tyrosine-kinase- and G$\beta\gamma$-mediated MAP kinase activation by a common signalling pathway. *Nature* 376: 781–784, 1995.

486. van Biesen, T. M., L. M. Luttrell, B. E. Hawes, and R. J. Lefkowitz. Mitogenic signaling via G protein–coupled receptors. *Endocr. Rev.* 17: 698–714, 1996.

487. van Corven, E. J., P. L. Hordijk, R. H. Medema, J. L. Bos, and W. H. Moolenaar. Pertussis toxin–sensitive activation of p21ras by G protein–coupled receptor agonist in fibroblasts. *Proc. Natl. Acad. Sci. U.S.A.* 90: 1257–1261, 1993.

488. Van Dop, C., M. Tsubokawa, H. R. Bourne, and J. Ramachandran. Amino acid sequence of retinal transducin at the site ADP-ribosylated by cholera toxin. *J. Biol. Chem.* 259: 696–699, 1984.

489. van Koppen, C. J., and N. M. Nathanson. The cysteine residue in the carboxy-terminal domain of the m2 muscarinic acetylcholine receptor is not required for receptor-mediated inhibition of adenylate cyclase. *J. Neurochem.* 57: 1873–1877, 1991.

490. Van Sande, J., E. Raspe, J. Perret, C. Lejeune, C. Maenhaut, G. Vassar, and J. E. Dumont. Thyrotropin activates both the cAMP and the PIP_2 cascades in CHO cells expressing the human cDNA of the TSH receptor. *Mol. Cell. Endocrinol.* 74: R1-R6, 1990.

491. Vara Prasad, M.V.V.S., J. M. Dermott, L. E. Heasley, G. L. Johnson, and N. Dhanasekaran. Activation of Jun kinase/stress-activated protein kinase by GTPase-deficient mutants of $G\alpha_{12}$ and $G\alpha_{13}$. *J. Biol. Chem.* 270: 18655–18659, 1995.

492. Vassart, G., L. Desarnaud, L. Duprez, D. Eggerickx, O. Labbé, F. Libert, C. Mollerau, J. Parma, R. Paschke, M. Tonacchera, P. Vanderhaeghen, J. Van Sande, J. Dumont, and M. Parmentier. The G protein–coupled receptor family and one of its members, the TSH receptor. *Ann. N.Y. Acad. Sci.* 766: 23–30, 1995.

493. Von Weizsäcker, E., M. P. Strathmann, and M. I. Simon. Diversity among the β subunits of heterotrimeric GTP-binding proteins: characterization of a novel β-subunit. *Biochem. Biophys. Res. Commun.* 183: 350–356, 1992.

494. von Zastrow, M., and B. K. Kobilka. Ligand-regulated internalization and recycling of human β_2-adrenergic receptors between the plasma membrane and endosomes containing transferrin receptors. *J. Biol. Chem.* 267: 3530–3538, 1992.

495. von Zastrow, M., R. Link, D. Daunt, G. Barsh, and B. K. Kobilka. Subtype specific differences in the intracellular sorting of G protein–coupled receptors. *J. Biol. Chem.* 268: 763–766, 1993.

496. Voyno-Yasenetskaya, T., B. R. Conklin, R. L. Gilbert, R.

Hooley, H. R. Bourne, and D. L. Barber. Gα_{13} stimulates Na–H exchange. *J. Biol. Chem.* 269: 4721–4724, 1994.

497. Vuong, T. M., and M. Chabre. Deactivation kinetics of the transduction cascade of vision. *Proc. Natl. Acad. Sci. U.S.A.* 88: 9813–9817, 1991.

498. Wadsworth, H. L., G. D. Chazenbalk, Y. Nagayama, D. Russo, and B. Rapoport. An insertion in the human thyrotropin receptor critical for high affinity hormone binding. *Science* 249: 1423–1425, 1990.

499. Wall, M. A., D. E. Coleman, E. Lee, J. A. Iñiguez-Lluhi, B. A. Posner, A. G. Gilman, and S. R. Sprang. The structure of the G protein heterotrimer $G_{i\alpha 1}\beta_1\gamma_2$. *Cell* 83: 1047–1068, 1995.

500. Wang, C. D., M. A. Buck, and C. M. Fraser. Site-directed mutagenesis of α_{2A}-adrenergic receptors: identification of amino acids involved in ligand binding and receptor activation by agonists. *Mol. Pharmacol.* 40: 168–179, 1991.

501. Wang, D. S., R. Shaw, J. C. Winkelmann, and G. Shaw. Binding of PH domains of β-adrenergic receptor kinase and β-spectrin to WD40/β-transducin repeat containing regions of the β-subunit of trimeric G-proteins. *Biochem. Biophys. Res. Commun.* 203: 29–35, 1994.

501a. Wang, Z., R. W. Hipkin, and M. Ascoli. Progressive cytoplasmic tail truncations of the lutropin-choriogonadotropin receptor prevent agonist- or phorbol ester–induced phosphorylation, impair agonist- or phorbol ester–induced desensitization, and enhance agonist-induced receptor down-regulation. *Mol. Endocrinol.* 10: 748–759, 1996.

502. Wang, Z., X. Liu, and M. Ascoli. Phosphorylation of the lutropin/choriogonadotropin receptor facilitates uncoupling of the receptor from adenylyl cyclase and endocytosis of the bound hormone. *Mol. Endocrinol.* 11: 183–192, 1997.

503. Watson, A. J., A. Katz, and M. I. Simon. A fifth member of the mammalian G-protein β-subunit family. *J. Biol. Chem.* 269: 22150–22156, 1994.

504. Watson, N., M. E. Liknder, K. M. Druey, J. H. Kehrl, and K. J. Blumer. RGS family members: GTPase-activating proteins for heterotrimeric G-protein α-subunits. *Nature* 383: 172–177, 1996.

505. Wedegaertner, P. B., and H. R. Bourne. Activation and depalmitoylation of $G_{s\alpha}$. *Cell* 77: 1063–1070, 1994.

506. Wedegaertner, P. B., H. R. Bourne, and M. von Zastrow. Activation-induced subcellular redistribution of $G_{s\alpha}$. *Mol. Biol. Cell* 7: 1225–1233, 1996.

507. Wedegaertner, P. B., D. H. Chu, P. T. Wilson, M. J. Levis, and H. R. Bourne. Palmitoylation is required for signaling functions and membrane attachment of $G_{q\alpha}$ and $G_{s\alpha}$. *J. Biol. Chem.* 268: 25001–25008, 1993.

508. Wess, J. Molecular basis of muscarinic acetylcholine receptor function. *Trends Pharmacol. Sci.* 14: 308–313, 1993.

509. Wess, J., T. I. Bonner, F. Dörje, and M. R. Brann. Delineation of muscarinic receptor domains conferring selectivity of coupling to guanine nucleotide–binding proteins and second messengers. *Mol. Pharmacol.* 38: 517–523, 1990.

510. Wess, J., M. R. Brann, and T. I. Bonner. Delineation of muscarinic receptor domains conferring selectivity of coupling to guanine nucleotide–binding proteins and second messengers. *FEBS Lett.* 358: 133–136, 1994.

511. Wess, J., D. Gdula, and M. R. Brand. Site-directed mutagenesis of the m3 muscarinic receptor: identification of a series of threonine and tyrosine residues involved in agonist but not antagonist binding. *EMBO J.* 10: 3729–3734, 1991.

512. West, R. E., J. Moss, M. Vaughan, T. Lui, and T. Y. Lin. Pertussis toxin–catalyzed ADP-ribosylation of transducin.

513. Wheeler, G. L., and M. W. Bitensky. A light-activated GTPase in vertebrate photoreceptors: regulation of light-activated cyclic GMP phosphodiesterase. *Proc. Natl. Acad. Sci. U.S.A.* 74: 4238–4242, 1977.

514. Wheeler, M. B., M. Lu, J. S. Dillon, X.-H. Leng, C. Cheng, and A. E. Boyd III. Functional expression of the rat glucagon-like peptide-I receptor: evidence for coupling to both adenylyl cyclase and phospholipase C. *Endocrinology* 133: 57–62, 1993.

515. Wickman, K., and D. E. Clapham. Ion channel regulation by G proteins. *Physiol. Rev.* 75: 865–885, 1995.

516. Wickman, K. D., J. Iñiguez-Lluhi, P. Davenport, R. A. Taussig, G. B. Krapivinsky, M. E. Linder, A. Gilman, and D. E. Clapham. Recombinant G$\beta\gamma$ activates the muscarinic-gated atrial potassium channel I_{KACh}. *Nature* 368: 255–257, 1994.

517. Wieland, T., B. Nurnberg, I. Ulibarri, S. Kaldenberg-Stasch, G. Schultz, and K. H. Jakobs. Guanine nucleotide–specific phosphate transfer by guanine nucleotide–binding regulatory protein β-subunits: characterization of the phosphorylated amino acid. *J. Biol. Chem.* 268: 18111–18118, 1993.

518. Wilcox, C., J.-S. Hu, and E. N. Olson. Acylation of proteins with myristic acid occurs cotranslationally. *Science* 238: 1275–1278, 1987.

519. Wilden, U., S. W. Hall, and H. Kuhn. Phosphodiesterase activation by photoexcited rhodopsin is quenched when rhodopsin is phosphorylated and binds the intrinsic 48-kDA protein of rod outer segments. *Proc. Natl. Acad. Sci. U.S.A.* 83: 1174–1178, 1986.

520. Wilden, U., and H. Kuhn. Light-dependent phosphorylation of rhodopsin: number of phosphorylation sites. *Biochemistry* 21: 3014–3022, 1982.

521. Wilkie, T. M., P. A. Scherle, M. P. Strathmann, V. Z. Slepak, and M. I. Simon. Characterization of G-protein α subunits in the G_q class: expression in murine tissues and in stromal and hematopoietic cell lines. *Proc. Natl. Acad. Sci. U.S.A.* 88: 10049–10053, 1991.

522. Winitz, S., M. Russell, N, Qian, A. Gardner, L. Dwyer, and G. L. Johnson. Involvement of Ras and Raf in the Gi-coupled acetylcholine muscarinic m2 receptor activation of mitogen-activated protein (MAP) kinase kinase and MAP kinase. *J. Biol. Chem.* 268: 19196–19199, 1993.

523. Wise, A., M.-A.Watson-Koken, S. Rees, M. Lee, and G. Milligan. Interactions of the α_{2A}-adrenoceptor with multiple G_i-family G-proteins: studies with pertussis toxin–resistant G-protein mutants. *Biochem. J.* 321: 721–728, 1997.

524. Wong, S. K.-F., E. M. Parker, and E. M. Ross. Chimeric muscarinic cholinergic: β-adrenergic receptors that activate G_s in response to muscarinic agonist. *J. Biol. Chem.* 265: 6219–6224, 1990.

525. Wong, S. K.-F., C. Slaughter, A. E. Ruoho, and E. M. Ross. The catecholamine binding site of the β-adrenergic receptor is formed by juxtaposed membrane-spanning domains. *J. Biol. Chem.* 263: 7925–7928, 1988.

526. Wong, Y. H., B. R. Conklin, and H. R. Bourne. G_z-mediated hormonal inhibition of cyclic AMP accumulation. *Science* 255: 339–341, 1992.

527. Wong, Y. H., A. Federman, A. M. Pace, I. Zachary, T. Evans, J. Pouyssegur, and H. R. Bourne. Mutant α subunits of G_{i2} inhibit cyclic AMP accumulation. *Nature* 351: 63–65, 1991.

528. Wu, D., C. H. Lee, S. G. Ree, and M. I. Simon. Activation of phospholipase C by the α subunits of G_q and G_{11} proteins in transfected Cos-7 cells. *J. Biol. Chem.* 267: 1811–1817, 1992.

Cysteine-347 is the ADP ribose acceptor site. *J. Biol. Chem.* 260: 14428–14430, 1985.

529. Yang, K., and N. Gautman. Structural determinants for interaction with three different effectors on the G protein β subunit. *J. Biol. Chem.* 272: 2056–2059, 1997.

530. Yatani, A., J. Codina, Y. Imoto, J. P. Reeves, L. Birnbaumer, and A. M. Brown. A G-protein directly regulates mammalian cardiac calcium channels. *Science* 238: 1288–1292, 1987.

531. Yatani, A., R. Mattera, J. Codina, R. Graf, K. Okabe, E. Padrell, R. Iyenegar, A. M. Brown, and L. Birnbaumer. The G protein–gated atrial K$^+$ channel is stimulated by three distinct G$_i\alpha$ subunits. *Nature* 336: 680–682, 1988.

532. Yi, F., B. M. Denker, and E. J. Neer. Structural and functional studies of cross-linked G$_o$ protein subunits. *J. Biol. Chem.* 266: 2900–3906, 1991.

533. Ykota, Y., C. Akazawa, H. Ohkubo, and S. Nakanishi. Delineation of structural domains involved in the subtype specificity of the tachykinin receptors through chimeric formation of substance P/substance K receptors. *EMBO J.* 11: 3585–3591, 1992.

534. Yuzaki, M., and K. Mikoshiba. Pharmacological and immunocytochemical characterization of metabotropic glutamate receptors in cultured Purkinje cells. *J. Neurosci.* 12: 4253–4263, 1992.

535. Zhang, R., C. H. Tsai-Morris, M. Kitamura, E. Buczko, and M. L. Dufau. Changes in binding activity of luteinizing hormone receptors by site directed mutagenesis of potential glycosylation sites. *Biochem. Biophys. Res. Commun.* 181: 804–808, 1991.

536. Zhang, S., O. A. Coso, C. Lee, J. S. Gutkind, and W. F. Simonds. Selective activation of effector pathways by brain-specific G protein β_5. *J. Biol. Chem.* 271: 33575–33579, 1996.

537. Zheng, F., and J. P. Gallagher. (1S,3R)-1-Aminocyclopentane-1,3-dicarboxylic acid–induced burst firing is mediated by native pertussis toxin–sensitive metabotropic receptor at rat dorsolateral septal nucleus neurons. *Neuroscience* 68: 423–434, 1995.

538. Zhou, W., C. Flanagan, J. A. Ballesteros, K. Konvicka, J. S. Davidson, H. Weinstein, R. P. Millar, and S. C. Seaflon. A reciprocal mutation supports helix 2 and helix 7 proximity in the gonadotropin-releasing hormone receptor. *Mol. Pharmacol.* 45: 165–170, 1994.

539. Zhou, W., V. Rodic, S. Kitanovic, C. A. Flanagan, L. Chi, H. Weinstein, S. Maayani, R. P. Millar, and S. C. Seaflon. A locus of the gonadotropin-releasing hormone receptor that differentiates agonist and antagonist binding sites. *J. Biol. Chem.* 270: 18853–18857, 1995.

540. Zhu, O., A. Wang, and M. Ascoli. The lutropin/choriogonadotropin receptor is palmitoylated at intracellular cysteine residues. *Mol. Endocrinol.* 9: 141–150, 1995.

541. Zhukovsky, E. A., and D. D. Oprian. Effect of carboxylic acid side chains on the absorption maximum of visual pigments. *Science* 246: 928–930, 1989.

7. Regulation of G protein–coupled receptors

RAYMOND B. PENN
JEFFREY L. BENOVIC

Departments of Biochemistry and Molecular Pharmacology, Microbiology, and Immunology, Kimmel Cancer Institute, Thomas Jefferson University, Philadelphia, Pennsylvania

THE CURRENT STUDY of G protein–coupled receptor (GPR) regulation does not appear to suffer from a lack of interest or effort. The almost complete absence of mention of receptor regulation from the preceding endocrinology volumes of the *Handbook of Physiology* in the 1970s underscores the great strides made in this field since that time. While at that time tachyphalaxis to various drugs on a physiological level had been recognized for decades, the cellular events involved in receptor–G protein–effector interactions were largely unknown, and the concept of receptor desensitization was only just emerging. By the mid-1980s the development and application of various pharmacological and biochemical techniques helped identify and characterize many GPRs, G proteins, and effector molecules. Subsequent advances in molecular and cell biology permitted the cloning, expression, and mutagenesis of signal transduction proteins and led to an explosion of knowledge in the field of receptor regulation, facilitat-ing the discovery of new classes of regulatory proteins and providing a means of manipulating receptor function through multiple intracellular targets.

Regulation of GPR signal transduction pathways is defined in this chapter as modulation of the processes by which GPR activation produces stimulation or inhibition of second messenger generation. This modulation involves a modification of the signaling pathway that persists following treatment cessation, thus rendering it distinct from classical pharmacological antagonism or acute inhibition. Desensitization refers to the specific reduction in a GPR pathway's ability to effect changes in second messenger production following exposure to various agents. These agents may be the GPR's own activating ligand or other agents involved in the activation of other signaling pathways. Kakiuchi and Rall (175) in 1968 were the first to describe desensitization in these terms when they reported that exposure of rabbit cerebellar slices to norepinephrine resulted in an initial increase in adenosine 3′,5′-cyclic monophosphate (cAMP) accumulation followed by a progressive decline that could not be explained by phosphodiesterase activity. In addition, prolonged incubation of cerebellar slices with norepinephrine rendered the tissue refractory to subsequent rechallenge with norepinephrine. Su et al. (358) later described conditions under which exposure of astrocytoma cells to prostaglandin E_1 (PGE_1) led to diminished responsiveness to catecholamines, while exposure of cells to catecholamines could also produce a loss of responsiveness to PGE_1. These seminal findings have been supported by hundreds of studies that demonstrate the desensitization of numerous GPRs in a wide variety of cell types.

In this chapter we describe our current understanding of the molecular mechanisms involved in the regulation of GPRs. We emphasize the mechanisms of desensitization of the system at the receptor locus, and the role of receptor kinases and arrestin proteins in these processes. Most of the information presented refers to the beta-adrenergic receptor–stimulatory guanine-nucleotide-binding protein- adenylyl cyclase (βAR-G$_s$-adenylyl cyclase) and the rhodopsin-transducin–guanosine 3′,5′-cyclic monophosphate (cGMP) phosphodiesterase pathways, reflecting the prominence of these systems in the study of GPR regulation. Additional receptors for which mechanisms of regulation have been elucidated are also discussed. A generalized summary of the most prevalent characteristics of GPR regulation is offered in an attempt to provide a conceptual framework within which to view this admittedly complex and diverse phenomenon.

As a prelude to discussing the molecular mechanisms of GPR regulation, we first address the basic features of the transmembrane-signaling components and how these components interact to transduce an extracellular stimulus into an intracellular message.

SIGNALING VIA G PROTEIN–COUPLED RECEPTOR PATHWAYS

The principal components of GPR transmembrane signaling are the receptor, the heterotrimeric guanosine 5′-triphosphate (GTP)-binding protein (G protein), and the effector molecule [Harden (141) provides an excellent history of physical and functional resolution of these three proteins]. Activation of a receptor by ligand (or in the case of rhodopsin, by a photon of light) induces its interaction with and activation of the G protein, which in turn regulates an effector. This generic model, discussed in greater detail below, encompasses the actions of a large and growing number of receptors, G proteins, and effectors whose characteristics have been the focus of intense investigation the last two decades.

G Protein–Coupled Receptors

G protein–coupled receptors comprise a superfamily of proteins capable of transducing a wide range of extracellular signals across the lipid bilayer of the cell. Inclusion into the GPR superfamily requires that the receptor be a polypeptide containing seven predicted hydrophobic transmembrane domains (TMDs) and that it possess the ability to activate G proteins directly upon receptor stimulation. Subdivision of this superfamily into families sharing high degrees of sequence similarity in the seven TMDs distinguishes three major families that include mammalian GPRs: *(1)* receptors related to rhodopsin/β_2AR; *(2)* receptors related to calcitonin and parathyroid hormone receptors; and *(3)* receptors related to metabotropic glutamate receptors (189, 349). Most GPRs identified thus far belong to the rhodopsin/beta-2-adrenergic receptor (β_2AR) fam-

ily, and the majority of studies to date examining GPR structure-function and signaling has been performed using receptors in this family. (A continuously updated database containing a wide range of information on GPRs is presently accessible through on-line computer access via the World Wide Web [http://receptor.mgh.harvard.edu/GCRDBHOME.html]).

Although detailed information from crystal structures is presently lacking, the salient structural features of GPRs have been predicted by hydrophobicity analysis of the primary amino acid sequence and comparison with the structure of bacteriorhodopsin (a seven TMD protein) (151). Recently, electron diffraction studies have also confirmed the presence of seven TMDs in rhodopsin (311). The predicted features of GPRs are evident in the proposed structure of the β_2AR (Fig. 7.1). They include the seven membrane-spanning domains of 20–28 hydrophobic residues, three extracellular, and three or four cytoplasmic loops, an extracellular amino terminus, and a cytoplasmic carboxy terminus. The degree of sequence identity present in the seven TMD regions within a GPR family of related receptors is 20%, reaching as high as 60%–80% for related subtypes of a given receptor (for example, the β_1, β_2, and β_3 adrenergic receptors). The hydrophilic regions of the receptor tend to be less highly conserved. From a functional standpoint, the amphipathic alpha–helical arrangement of the TMDs helps form a hydrophobic "pocket" that confers specificity for ligand binding. Our knowledge in this area has improved to the extent that the class of ligand (for example, biogenic amine, small peptide) capable of activating a cloned receptor can often be predicted on the basis of the primary sequence of the receptor's TMDs. The cytoplasmic loops of GPRs tend to mediate interactions with the G proteins. Studies using deletion and site-directed mutagenesis of the β_2AR have established the role of the third cytoplasmic loop (87, 254, 347) as critical to G protein activation. Similar studies have emphasized the importance of the third cytoplasmic loop of rhodopsin (104–106, 322), the alpha 1b-adrenergic receptor (α_{1b}AR) (148, 230, 399), alpha 2a-adrenergic receptor (α_{2a}AR) (148, 385), the m1–muscarinic receptor (m1AChR)(148, 155, 319), the m2–muscarinic receptor (m2AChR)(149), the m3–muscarinic receptor (m3AChR)(202), and the follicle-stimulating hormone receptor (120) in their respective interactions with G proteins.

G Proteins

The G proteins that link GPRs with effectors are composed of three distinct polypeptides (and as such are distinguished from smaller, single unit G proteins

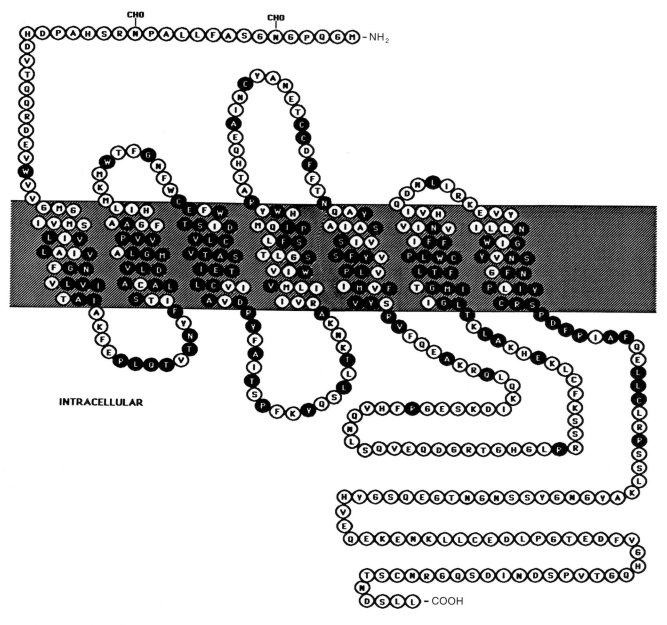

FIG. 7.1. Proposed topology of the human β_2-adrenergic receptor (β_2AR). The amino acid sequence of the human β_2AR, as it is proposed to reside in the plasma membrane, is shown. The amino acids identical in the human β_1-, β_2-, β_3-, and turkey β_1-adrenergic receptors are shaded. [From Gomez and Benovic (119), with permission from Academic Press.]

such as ras) designated as α, β, and γ subunits. To date, 18 different G_α subunits have been identified, being subdivided into four classes ($G_{\alpha s}$, $G_{\alpha i}$, $G_{\alpha q}$, and $G_{\alpha 12/13}$) based on amino acid identity (a summary of these classes and salient characteristics is presented in Table 7.1). In addition, five β subunits and at least nine γ subunits (72, 293) have been identified. Recent resolution of the crystal structures of various nucleotide-bound alpha subunits (72, 73, 209, 337) and the guanosine 5′-diphosphate (GDP)-bound $\alpha i1$–$\beta 1\gamma 2$ complex (388) has contributed greatly to our understanding of G protein structure. A limited but rapidly increasing amount of information exists regarding the regions of G protein subunits responsible for

TABLE 7.1. *Classification of G_α Subunits*[*]

Class	Members	Modifying Toxin	Functions	Localization[†]	Specific Receptors
α_S	α_S, α_{olf}	Cholera	Stimulation of adenylyl cyclase, regulation of Ca^{2+} channels and K^+ channels	α_{olf}-olfactory epithelia	α_{olf}-olfactory
α_i	α_{i-1}, α_{i-2}, α_{i-3}, α_o, α_{t-1}, α_{t-2}, α_{gust}, α_z	Pertussis (except α_z); cholera (α_{t-1})	Inhibition of adenylyl cyclase, stimulation of cGMP phosphodiesterase, regulation of Ca^{2+} and K^+ channels	α_{t-1}-rods; α_{t-2}-cones; α_{gust}-taste epithelia; α_o-brain α_z-platelets, brain	α_{t-1}-rhodopsin α_{t-2}-color opsins
α_q	α_q, α_{11}, α_{14}, α_{15}, α_{16}	—	Stimulation of PLC	α_{16}-hematopoietic cells	
α_{12}	α_{12}, α_{13}	—	Stimulation of Na^+-H^+ exchanger		

[*] For references, see reviews by Gilman (115), Simon et al. (332), Clapham and Neer (66), Rens-Domiano and Hamm (298), and Neer (247, 248).   [†] Widely expressed unless noted.

interactions with receptors, effectors, and each other. [For a review of G protein/subunit structure and function, see Neer (248) and Rens-Domiano and Hamm (298).]

The heterotrimeric complex is linked to the membrane via isoprenylation of the gamma subunit and myristylation and/or palmitoylation of the alpha subunit (392). The β and γ subunits are tightly associated in the cell and for all practical purposes constitute a functional monomer. While the possibility of multiple combinations of different α, β, and γ subunits exist, few have been defined (certain combinations appear not possible (287, 314) and the selectivity of various combinations for linkage with receptors and effector units is therefore largely unknown. For the purpose of describing their roles in the signal transduction process, the general tendency has been to identify the heterotrimeric G proteins based on the known actions of the associated alpha subunit on effectors (for example; G_s and G_i are associated with stimulation and inhibition, respectively, of adenylyl cyclase). While convenient, this approach is rapidly proving too simplistic as the continuing characterization of G proteins and their subunit composition reveals a diversity and complexity in function that belies such classification.

The central role of G proteins in GPR signaling was first articulated in the mid-1970s by Cassell and colleagues in a proposed model of hormonal regulation of adenylyl cyclase (48–50). Today, the basic principles of this model remain essentially correct and extend to all G proteins, although considerably more detail is known. Figure 7.2 depicts our current understanding of the process. G protein activation is initiated by the formation of a ternary complex of ligand, receptor, and the GDP-liganded heterotrimeric G protein. Ternary complex formation is driven by the higher agonist affinity for the receptor–G protein complex versus receptor alone. Agonist binding results in a conformational change in the receptor that promotes a multisite interaction with the GDP-liganded G protein. This interaction in turn induces a structural change in G_α that reduces its affinity for GDP. GDP dissociates from G_α and is replaced by GTP, which typically exists in high intracellular concentrations. GTP binding results in an activated α subunit that dissociates from the receptor and $\beta\gamma$ complex. At this point, the α subunit (and $\beta\gamma$ as well) is capable of regulating an effector. The activated state of G_α persists until the intrinsic GTPase activity of the α subunit hydrolyzes GTP to GDP, returning G_α to an inactive form that reassociates with $\beta\gamma$. The rate of GTP hydrolysis dictates the duration of the active state. This property has been experimentally exploited by persistent activation of G_α subunits through the use of non-hydrolyzable GTP analogs such as guanyl-5′-yl imidodiphosphate (Gpp(NH)p) and GTPγS, and aluminum fluoride, which binds to G_α subunits and mimics the terminal phosphate of GTP rendering the GDP-liganded α subunit active. Cholera toxin, which decreases the intrinsic GTPase activity of $G_{\alpha s}$ via ADP-ribosylation of the subunit, is also a powerful activator of $G_{\alpha s}$. Different α subunits also possess different rates of GTPase activity; moreover, GTPase activity can also be regulated by some effectors (8, 28, 248).

The specific cellular response evoked by GPR activation depends in part on the cell's complement of receptors, G proteins, effectors, and the relative specificity of the potential receptor-G protein, G protein-effector interactions. Since a much greater number of GPRs (>250) than G proteins have been identified, it is not surprising that a given class of G_α proteins can be activated by numerous GPRs. Interestingly, reconstitution of purified components in phospholipid vesicles demonstrates that GPRs may also display only moder-

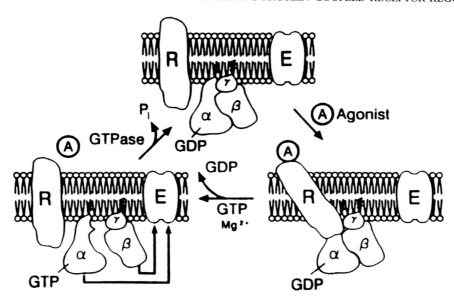

FIG. 7.2. G protein–coupled receptor activation of effector. See text for description. [From Clapham and Neer (66), with permission from *Nature*.]

ate selectivity among G_α subunits (9, 53), particularly with respect to isoforms within a class (52, 239, 318). For example, the βAR preferentially activates $G_{\alpha s}$ but can also activate $G_{\alpha i}$ when components are reconstituted in phospholipid vesicles (9, 53, 305). The serotonin 5–HT1A receptor appears capable of activating several different G_α subtypes, as suggested by its demonstrated ability to inhibit or stimulate adenylyl cyclase, stimulate or inhibit phosphoinositide hydrolysis, and regulate membrane ion channels in a cell-specific manner (146). In addition, a lack of specificity is frequently implicated in intact cell studies in which receptors and/or G proteins are overexpressed and apparent alterations in stoichiometry reveal unexpected coupling between a given receptor and G protein (174, 317). It remains to be determined whether these interactions actually occur in the normal environment of the cell or are simply a consequence of overexpression.

A somewhat lesser degree of promiscuity has been observed with respect to effectors and their selectivity towards G proteins. Adenylyl cyclase can be diametrically regulated by $G_{\alpha s}$ and $G_{\alpha i}$. However, evidence exists of highly specific G_α interactions. Adenylyl cyclase is activated solely by αs, whereas αq/α11 are the only α subunits capable of phospholipase C (PLC)β activation (248). Restricted tissue localization of G proteins and/or effectors may provide clues to the specific G_α-effector interactions that occur in vivo. Localization of $G_{\alpha t-1}$ and $G_{\alpha t-2}$ to retinal rods and cones, respectively, is consistent with reconstitution

experiments demonstrating the restricted selectivity of $G_{\alpha t}$ isoforms for cGMP phosphodiesterase (144).

Early evidence demonstrating that dissociated $G_{\alpha s}$ subunits were capable of activating cGMP phosphodiesterase (110) and adenylyl cyclase (253) led to the widely held assumption that G_α was the subunit responsible for effector regulation. However, Logothetis et al. (223) subsequently demonstrated that $G\beta\gamma$ subunits purified from bovine brain could activate muscarinic-gated cardiac K^+ channels, suggesting that $\beta\gamma$ played a wider role in signaling than was previously believed. Since then, $G\beta\gamma$ has been shown capable of regulating a large number of effectors in conjunction with or independent of G_α. For example, $\beta\gamma$ acts synergistically with αs in the activation of adenylyl cyclase types II and IV, and can act independently in the inhibition of adenylyl cyclase type I (361). $\beta\gamma$ has also been shown to regulate PLC β1–3 [see Clapham and Neer (66) and references therein], phospholipase A_2 (167, 186), the ras-MAP kinase pathway (78), PI-3 kinase (367), and the beta-adrenergic receptor kinase (137, 185, 278) (see later under The Beta-Adrenergic Receptor Kinase).

Effectors

Relative to our understanding of GPRs and G proteins, considerably less is known regarding the associated effector proteins. Among the best characterized are: adenylyl cyclase, whose activation by the beta-adrenergic receptor (βAR) and other G_s-coupled receptors results in the conversion of adenosine 5'-triphosphate (ATP) to cAMP and subsequent activation of the cAMP-dependent protein kinase (PKA), which phosphorylates numerous intracellular proteins to produce a host of cell-specific physiological responses [see Tang and Gilman (362), Taussig and Gilman (364), and Chapter 8 in this *Handbook* for reviews]; cGMP phosphodiesterase, whose activation by opsins-$G_{\alpha t}$ in rod and cone cells results in cell hyperpolarization (143, 144); and PLC, which converts phosphotidylinositol 4,5-bisphosphate (PIP_2) to inositol 1,4,5 trisphosphate (IP_3) and diacylglycerol, important second messengers in the activation of protein kinase C and cellular calcium flux (see Chapter 11 in this *Handbook* for review).

MECHANISMS OF G PROTEIN–COUPLED RECEPTOR REGULATION

Early studies (1968–1975) examining GPR desensitization were essentially descriptive in nature and devoid of mechanistic interpretation. Advances in receptor pharmacology, the use of mutant cell lines, and the application of various cell and molecular biology techniques have since helped to uncover multiple time-dependent mechanisms by which GPRs are desensitized. While each component of the GPR-G protein-effector pathway represents a potential target of modification and regulation, alterations at the receptor locus are the most widely observed. Consequently, the depth of our knowledge of GPR desensitization is exhibited in those mechanisms by which receptors are modified: receptor phosphorylation and uncoupling from G protein; the loss of receptors from the cell surface (sequestration); and the reduction in cellular receptor density (down-regulation). The most intensely investigated of these receptor modifications is receptor phosphorylation/uncoupling, which features the actions of intracellular kinases and arrestin proteins in this most rapid form of GPR desensitization.

Classification of Desensitization

Two basic classes of desensitization have been distinguished in the literature: *homologous* or *agonist-specific*; and *heterologous* (often referred to as nonagonist-specific or agonist-nonspecific). As originally defined by Perkins and coworkers (153, 358, 359), homologous desensitization refers to an agonist-specific phenomenon whereby stimulation of a given receptor reduces the ability of that receptor alone to alter second messenger production. Alternatively, with heterologous desensitization, stimulation of a given receptor also

induces a loss of responsiveness in additional receptors. Su et al. (358, 359) identified conditions in 1321N1 human astrocytoma cells under which each form of desensitization could be discerned. Short-term treatment of astrocytoma cells with β-agonist led to a reduction in responsiveness to beta-agonists, but not to PGE_1. Similarly, treatment with PGE_1 led to a reduction in PGE_1-, but not β-agonist-mediated cAMP production. Heterologous desensitization was observed if cells were treated beyond 30 min; treatment with beta-agonist or PGE_1 resulted in a loss of responsiveness to both β-agonist and PGE_1.

The majority of desensitization studies to date have tended to focus on the regulation of specific receptor pathways (for example, the βAR-G_s-adenylyl cyclase pathway) with less concern for differentiating the effects of agonist exposure on a cell's various receptor populations. As a consequence, the terms homologous and heterologous desensitization have been frequently applied to describe the regulation of a given receptor, as opposed to the degree of specificity of the desensitization process. In this respect, homologous desensitization of a receptor may be defined as the loss of responsiveness that occurs solely as a result of that receptor's activation, whereas heterologous desensitization may be defined as the loss of responsiveness caused by agents that are not specific ligands for the receptor. Somewhat problematic with these definitions is the tendency to imply mechanisms in their usage when it is apparent that both forms of desensitization may include a common mechanism (see below). As will be discussed, homologous desensitization is frequently equated with cAMP-independent mechanisms, while heterologous desensitization is equated with cAMP-dependent mechanisms. While the appropriateness of such definitions is subject to debate, they nonetheless have emerged through the shear force of their pervasive usage. Accordingly, the student of receptor regulation should appreciate the context in which these terms are utilized in order to reconcile apparent disparities in usage.

Based on the latter definitions offered above, a graphical representation of adenylyl cyclase responsiveness in cells exhibiting rapid homologous and heterologous desensitization of the βAR (Fig. 7.3) can be constructed. In this model, cells expressing β_2ARs are pretreated for 30 min with either: *(1)* a high concentration (for example; 10 μM) of isoproterenol; or *(2)* a cAMP-generating agent other than β-agonist such as PGE_1 (assuming the cell responds to PGE_1) or forskolin, which activates adenylyl cyclase independent of receptor activation. Cells are then washed at 4°C to remove the pretreating agent and subsequently rechallenged with isoproterenol in a concentration-dependent manner for 10 min. The reaction is stopped and cAMP

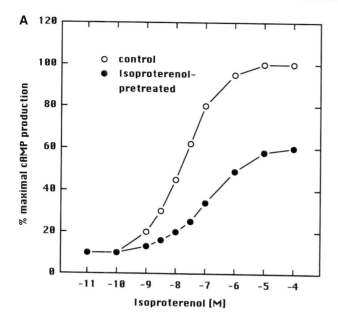

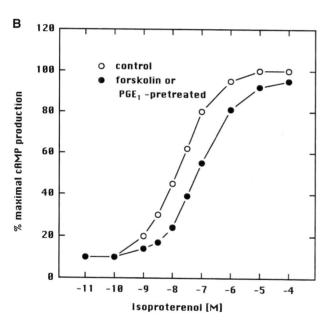

FIG. 7.3. Models of rapid desensitization of β_2AR-mediated cAMP production. *A.* Homologous desensitization. Cells are pretreated with a high concentration of beta-agonist (10 μM isoproterenol) for 30 min, washed extensively with cold phosphate-buffered saline, then re-challenged with isoproterenol in a concentration-dependent manner for 10 min. Reactions are stopped and cAMP is isolated and quantitated by radioimmunoassay. Concentration-dependent response to isoproterenol stimulation exhibits a significant reduction in maximal cAMP accumulation (reduced B_{max}) and a reduction in sensitivity to isoproterenol (increased EC_{50}). *B.* Heterologous desensitization. Experiment identical to that described in *A,* except cells are pretreated for 30 min with a cAMP-generating agent (forskolin or PGE$_1$) other than beta-agonist. Concentration-dependent response to isoproterenol stimulation exhibits a significant increase in EC_{50} with little or no loss in B_{max}.

is isolated and quantitated. Figure 7.3*A* depicts homologous desensitization as a result of the isoproterenol pretreatment. The concentration-dependent response to isoproterenol exhibits a reduction in maximal cAMP accumulation (that is, reduced B_{max}) and a reduction in sensitivity to isoproterenol (increased EC_{50}). The concentration-dependent response to isoproterenol following heterologous desensitization (Figure 7.3*B*) also exhibits an increase in EC_{50} but often (although not always) does not depict a reduction in B_{max} (67). The extent to which alterations in B_{max} and EC_{50} are observed in homologous or heterologous desensitization tends to be cell type- and receptor-specific.

Both homologous and heterologous desensitization are observable, in a cell-specific manner, in intact cells or in plasma membranes prepared following exposure of cells to a desensitizing agent (cell-free assays). In intact cells, cAMP generation may be measured by loading cells with radiolabeled adenine so that radiolabeled cAMP accumulates in the presence of a phosphodiesterase inhibitor upon cell stimulation. Alternatively, cold cAMP can be isolated following intact cell stimulation and quantitated by radioimmunoassay (273). In membrane preparations, adenylyl cyclase activity can be assessed as described by Salomon (307) by examining the rate at which stimulated membranes convert radiolabeled ATP to cAMP. However, two caveats with membrane preparations involve the potential for loss of experimental effects with cell lysis and the artificial nature of the in vitro adenylyl cyclase activity. These potential problems likely account for the failure of early attempts to identify heterologous desensitization in membranes, despite having observed the phenomenon in intact cell assays. Clark and co-workers (69, 71, 171, 173) remedied this enigma in part by discovering that high Mg^{2+} levels frequently employed in the adenylyl cyclase assay obscured the identification of heterologous desensitization (69). Today, both intact cell and cell-free assays tend to be reliable means of assessing adenylyl cyclase responsiveness, the choice depending upon the cell and receptor type being examined, the resources available, and the experimenter's disposition.

The Beta-Adrenergic Receptor and Rhodopsin Signaling Pathways: Model Systems of GPR Signaling and Regulation

Due in part to the early establishment of methods for identifying βARs and assessing βAR function, the βAR-G$_s$ adenylyl cyclase system is perhaps the most widely investigated and most understood GPR signaling pathway. Lands et al. (211) originally subdivided βARs in β_1 and β_2 subtypes based on the organ selectivity of various agonists. Subsequent development of subtype-specific ligands and radioligands facilitated more precise identification, quantification and characterization of these two receptors in tissues and cells. The development of a cell-free assay system capable of measuring adenylyl cyclase activity (307) (described above) enabled a relatively direct assessment of βAR (and other GPRs) function in membrane preparations. Purification of the β_2AR (325) and the turkey β_1AR (326) further substantiated the existence of these receptor subtypes, and ultimately led to the cloning of the hamster β_2AR (86) and the turkey β_1AR (404). Recently, a third βAR subtype, termed the beta-3–adrenergic receptor (β_3AR), has been identified by cloning (96). This receptor shares considerable amino acid homology with the β_1 and β_2 subtypes and is able to stimulate cAMP production in response to beta-agonist, albeit with an agonist profile distinct from that of the β_1AR and β_2AR [for an extensive review of βAR structure and function, see Gomez and Benovic (119) and Strosberg (354)]. Interestingly however, the β_3AR has been shown to be resistant to desensitization in many cell systems (47, 54, 221, 242). Of the three βAR subtypes, the β_2AR is the most extensively characterized, due primarily to its wide distribution in readily obtainable tissues, as well as the relative ease in which it is heterologously expressed and purified.

The basic model of hormonal activation of adenylyl cyclase described above is derived primarily from studies examining the βAR-G_s-adenylyl cyclase system. Interactive sites between the β_2AR and beta-agonists have been localized to specific amino acid residues in the TMDs of the receptor. [For analysis of the specific molecular interactions between ligands and β_2AR, see Strader et al. (348).] In addition, the intracellular loops contribute to ligand binding indirectly via their role in determining receptor–G protein association. Characteristic of GPRs, βARs have a higher affinity for agonist (but not antagonist) when the receptor is associated with G protein.

The β_2AR appears highly selective for G_s, although reconstitution of β_2AR with G_i can demonstrate G_i activation (9, 53, 305), albeit at a relatively low level. As noted above, mutagenesis studies examining β_2AR-G_s interaction have identified the third intracellular loop, particularly the proximal and distal regions of the loop (254, 347), as important for $G_{\alpha s}$ activation. In addition, peptides representing the third intracellular loop of the β_2AR have been shown capable of activating G_s (60, 256) and (indirectly) adenylyl cyclase (256).

Although principally considered as an activator of adenylyl cyclase, the βAR can also directly regulate other effectors via G proteins, including an Na^+-H^+ exchanger in cardiac myocytes (12), cardiac Na^+ channels (316) cardiac L type Ca^{2+} channels (405) and K^+ channels in airway smooth muscle (198, 199). Studies examining βAR regulation have focused on the receptor's activation of adenylyl cyclase; altered responsiveness of other effector functions is largely unexplored.

Adenylyl cyclase responsiveness to βAR activation is subject to acute counter-regulation by signaling systems that activate G proteins other than G_s. The mechanisms by which such inhibition (may) occur include direct inhibition of certain adenylyl cyclases by $G_{\alpha i}$, $G_{o\alpha}$, or $G_{z\alpha}$, and the inhibition of adenylyl cyclase type 1 by $\beta\gamma$ subunits [reviewed by Taussig and Gilman (364)]. In addition, $\beta\gamma$ subunits released via other GPR activation may also serve to potentiate βAR-$G_{\alpha s}$ activation of adenylyl cyclase types II (362) and IV (111). Thus, the cellular stoichiometry of signaling proteins, and the regulatory effect mediated by other cross-regulating signaling pathways will help determine the magnitude of the effect of β_2AR activation on cAMP production.

The majority, if not all, of the physiological effects elicited by β-agonist–stimulated cAMP production are mediated through cAMP activation of PKA. Binding of cAMP to the regulatory subunit of PKA releases the associated catalytic subunit of the protein, which is capable of phosphorylating a host of cellular proteins (116), including enzymes, contractile proteins, membrane pumps, ion channels, and receptors. Multiple targets of phosphorylation frequently exist in a given cell type, and their collective regulation can dictate highly specific cellular responses. For example, PKA-mediated phosphorylation of (1) membrane-bound Ca^{2+} channels, (2) the Ca^{2+} pump located on the sarcoplasmic reticulum (phospholambin), (3) the regulatory Ca^{2+}-binding protein troponin C, and (4) other targets in cardiac myocytes contributes to the precise regulation of rate, duration, and intensity of the contractile state of the cell. Activation of PKA in airway smooth muscle cells results in phosphorylation of several key regulatory proteins, including PLC, myosin light chain kinase, and calcium-sensitive potassium channels, each of which contribute to reducing the cellular level or effects of intracellular calcium and thus promote airway smooth muscle relaxation. Because the activation of PKA represents a point of extreme divergence in signaling, and multiple points of regulation may exist beyond the βAR-G_s-adenylyl cyclase pathway, it is often difficult to link measured alterations in physiological responses with alterations in the βAR-G_s-adenylyl cyclase pathway per se.

Characterization of the signaling and regulation of the rhodopsin-transducin-cGMP phosphodiesterase pathway preceded the similar characterization of the βAR-G_s-adenylyl cyclase system by several years. While initially the similarity of the two systems was not apparent, discoveries in both systems led to the establishment of the paradigm of receptor–G protein–effector signaling, prompting further, informative comparisons. Rhodopsin is the major protein localized in the disk membranes found in the outer segments of rod cells, while the color opsins (red, green, and blue) reside in cone cells. Absorption of a photon of light by rhodopsin results in the isomerization of the covalently-attached chromophore 11-cis retinal to the all-trans conformation, producing a transient active form of rhodopsin, metarhodopsin II. Metarhodopsin II specifically interacts with and promotes activation of the G protein transducin (possessing $G_{\alpha t-1}$ subunits in rods, $G_{\alpha t-2}$ in cones) (identified as $G_{\alpha t-1}\beta 1\gamma 1$ complexes in rods, $G_{\alpha t-2}\beta 1\gamma 1$ complexes in cones). The active (GTP-liganded) transducin specifically activates cGMP phosphodiesterase, which leads to a decrease in intracellular cGMP levels. This reduction in intracellular cGMP causes cGMP to dissociate from the cGMP-gated plasma membrane Na^+ channels and induces channel closing. The resulting reduction in Na^+ flux causes membrane hyperpolarization, which is ultimately integrated into a visual signal. In order to perceive continuous changes in light, the system must be rapidly recycled. Reattainment of photoreceptor function is dependent upon deactivating the rhodopsin signaling pathway and regenerating rhodopsin with 11-cis retinal. This physiological need is served in part by the rapid uncoupling of rhodopsin from transducin effected by the proteins rhodopsin kinase and arrestin.

The early identification of these two proteins facilitated the discovery and characterization of similar proteins operating in the regulation of the βAR and other GPRs. While rhodopsin itself essentially appears to undergo but a single mode of regulation (activation-dependent uncoupling from G protein), rhodopsin signaling nonetheless represents a highly instructive pathway in our understanding of the regulation of GPRs, insomuch as many (and likely most) GPRs appear to be regulated by activation-dependent uncoupling.

Receptor Phosphorylation And Uncoupling: Rapid Desensitization

Early studies in multiple cell types describing homologous desensitization of the βAR demonstrated a rapid loss of catecholamine-stimulated adenylyl cyclase activity with no change in the sodium fluoride (NaF)- or Gpp(NH)p-stimulated activity (101, 166, 170, 303, 356, 357). Further evidence that G protein function is not affected in agonist-specific desensitization was provided by Iyengar et al. (166). G proteins extracted from membranes of desensitized wild-type s49

lymphoma cells and reconstituted in membranes from the cyc- s49 mutant cells (which are deficient in stimulatory G protein activity) fully reestablished responsiveness to catecholamines. Furthermore, Su et al. (357) demonstrated that the rate of G protein activation by Gpp(NH)p in not altered in catecholamine-specific desensitization, although stimulation of the rate of activation by catecholamines (but not PGE_1) is decreased. Collectively, these studies suggested that the lesion in signaling in homologous desensitization is restricted to the receptor locus. Alternatively, heterologous desensitization frequently appeared to be associated with alterations in G protein/adenylyl cyclase activity (see discussion of heterologous desensitization in PKA below).

In several studies (235, 238, 321), homologous desensitization of βAR was shown to be associated with a loss of membrane bound receptors, suggesting that receptor sequestration/internalization may be a possible mechanism of desensitization (see later under Receptor Sequestration). However, this finding was not universal, and when it was noted, the extent of reduction in catecholamine-stimulated adenylyl cyclase activity was substantially greater than the reduction in receptors (166, 170, 177, 321, 356, 357, 374, 387). For example, Su et al. (356, 357) demonstrated rapid βAR desensitization in 1321N1 astrocytoma cells (374) with only a small loss in βAR number. However, desensitization was associated with a large reduction in high-affinity binding of agonist, and the effect of guanine nucleotides on binding was also largely reduced, suggesting an uncoupling of receptor from G protein. Distinctions were ultimately drawn in precise temporal analyses (166, 387) revealing that rapid βAR desensitization could be observed prior to any decrease in βAR number. Further evidence that the initial uncoupling of the βAR was not dependent upon receptor sequestration was provided by Waldo et al. (387), who demonstrated that pretreatment of astrocytoma cells with concanavalin A, a lectin that prevents receptor sequestration, does not prevent the rapid isoproterenol-induced desensitization of the βAR.

In an attempt to substantiate that functional modification of the βAR occurs with agonist-specific desensitization, multiple studies employing reconstitution/cell fusion techniques were performed. Using Sendai virus to fuse βARs from frog erythrocytes (previously desensitized to catecholamines) with G protein/adenylyl cyclase from "fresh" frog erythrocytes, Pike and Lefkowitz (275) demonstrated a decreased responsiveness to isoproterenol in the resulting hybrid. Later studies by Reilly and Blecher (297) using cultured differentiated RL-PR-C hepatocytes and Kassis and Fishman (177) using HeLa membranes and Friend erythroleukemic cells yielded similar results. Although the nature of the apparent modification of the βAR was not known, phosphorylation of the receptor, perhaps by PKA, was strongly suspected. However, in 1976 Shear et al. (321) had demonstrated that isoproterenol-induced desensitization of the βAR occurs in kin- s49 lymphoma mutant cells, which are PKA-defective. This study was later extended by Clark and co-workers (122, 123) who determined that homologous desensitization could be evidenced in membranes from epinephrine-pretreated cyc- s49 lymphoma mutant cells (which lack G_s) that were reconstituted with G protein/adenylyl cyclase from wild-type s49 lymphoma cells. Importantly, these studies suggested that the homologous desensitization of the βAR required neither cAMP accumulation, PKA activity, nor receptor–G protein interaction.

Speculation that covalent modification of the βAR occurred during desensitization was fueled by the observation of Stadel et al. (339) that isoproterenol-induced βAR desensitization was accompanied by a decrease in the mobility of the βAR as assessed by photoaffinity labeling and SDS-polyacrylamide gel electrophoresis. Direct evidence of isoproterenol-induced phosphorylation of turkey βAR was subsequently provided by Stadel et al. (340). Shortly thereafter Sibley et al. (331) demonstrated that phosphorylation of the frog erythrocyte βAR could occur in an agonist-specific manner, that is, treatment with isoproterenol, but not PGE_1, promoted βAR phosphorylation. Supportive of these studies and consistent with the findings of Clark and co-workers was the observation of Strasser et al. (352) that homologous desensitization in wild-type, cyc-, and kin- s49 lymphoma cells was accompanied by a rapid phosphorylation of the βAR. Maximal phosphorylation was achieved within 1–2 min of isoproterenol exposure, with maximal desensitization being observed by 5 min. Thus, homologous desensitization of the βAR was associated with an agonist-specific phosphorylation of the receptor that occurred in the absence of cAMP, was not mediated by PKA, and did not require receptor-G protein coupling.

The Beta-Adrenergic Receptor Kinase. These findings prompted the search for a kinase that specifically phosphorylated the agonist-occupied form of the β_2AR, presumably a kinase similar to the already-identified rhodopsin kinase, which was shown capable of phosphorylating rhodopsin in a light-dependent manner (see below). This kinase, termed the beta-adrenergic receptor kinase (βARK), was initially identified in a crude cytosolic fraction of kin- s49 lymphoma cells (27). [βARK is presently also known as G protein-coupled receptor kinase-2 (GRK2) (200), due to the necessity of classifying several recently-identified ho-

mologs of βARK that share similar but distinct properties—see below]. The kinase activity was shown to be specific for the agonist-occupied form of the β_2AR and was not affected by cAMP, cGMP, cAMP-dependent kinase inhibitor, Ca^{2+}/calmodulin, or Ca^{2+}/phosphatidylserine/phorbol 12-myristate 13-acetate (PMA). Purification of βARK from bovine brain identified a single subunit of 80 kDa that was able to phosphorylate the agonist-occupied form of the β_2AR to a stoichiometry of 8 mol phosphate/mol receptor (21). Subsequent cloning of the βARK cDNA from a bovine brain library (18) revealed a 2167 bp open reading frame encoding a 689 amino acid protein. Salient features include a central catalytic domain [the catalytic domain for protein kinases has been defined by Hanks and Quinn (140)] of 270 amino acids flanked by large amino- and carboxy-terminal domains (184 and 235 amino acids, respectively). The catalytic domain shares considerable homology with the catalytic domains of the yeast ypk1 (43.1% amino acid identity) and ypk2 (42.7%) protein kinases as well as with PKC (33.7%) and PKA (33.1%). Based on comparison with other serine-threonine kinases, specific functions can be ascribed to various regions within the catalytic domain (see below). The amino–terminal region does not share significant homology with other protein kinases, and its function is presently unknown, although mutagenesis studies suggest it may be involved in receptor recognition (Kong and Benovic, unpublished data). The carboxy-terminal region shares, with other proteins, a loosely-defined homology known as a *pleckstrin homology* (PH) domain (114, 241) that is believed to be involved in targeting βARK to the membrane upon receptor activation (see below).

Evidence to date suggests that βARK is ubiquitous, having been found in all tissues and cells examined (21, 261). Northern blot analyses reveal an mRNA of 3.8 kb and suggest a high level of expression in leukocytes (65) as well as in tissues with a high degree of sympathetic innervation (18). βARK demonstrates wide substrate selectivity in vitro; the β_2AR, m2AChR (205), α_2AR (25), substance P receptor (208), and A3 adenosine receptor (264) have been shown to be excellent substrates for βARK. Rhodopsin is a relatively poor substrate, although light-dependent phosphorylation of rhodopsin in vitro remains the most frequently used method of assessing βARK activity based on the relative ease with which rhodopsin can be prepared (17). The kinetics of the phosphorylation reaction suggest a high-affinity interaction between kinase and receptor (261). Analysis of deletion/substitution mutants of the β_2AR has localized the sites phosphorylated by βARK to the carboxy-terminus of the β_2AR (35, 88, 147). Potential sites on the β_1AR are similarly located in the carboxy terminus (119) with one potential site in the third cytosolic loop, while the m2AChR (158) and the α_{2a}AR (94) appear to be phosphorylated by βARK on the third intracellular loop. The β_3AR possesses only three serines in its carboxy tail, none of which appear to be good substrates for βARK, which may explain in part the β_3AR's relative resistance to desensitization. Analyses of in vitro peptide phosphorylation suggest that βARK preferentially phosphorylates serines/threonines that have acidic residues on the amino-terminal side (258). While the stoichiometry of βARK-mediated β_2AR phosphorylation in vitro is 8 mol phosphate/mol receptor, it appears to be considerably lower in intact cells (352). This disparity may reflect a minimal level of receptor phosphorylation required to promote physiological desensitization (68, 129, 132, 327).

The wide substrate selectivity of βARK demonstrated in vitro suggests βARK may play a role in phosphorylating and regulating multiple GPRs. Evidence of intracellular translocation of βARK from the cytosol to the membrane upon stimulation of various cells with β-agonist (351), PGE$_1$ (233, 351), somatostatin (233, 351) and platelet-activating factor (65) suggests that βARK may display wide substrate selectivity in vivo and that agonist-induced translocation of βARK may represent the initial step in homologous desensitization.

Additional evidence of the potential role of βARK in vivo is provided by studies in which the expression of mutagenized β_2ARs lacking putative sites of phosphorylation by βARK eliminates or significantly reduces their agonist-induced phosphorylation and desensitization (35, 88, 147, 220). Recent studies have provided more direct evidence of the role of βARK in vivo. Kong et al. (190) demonstrated that overexpression of a phosphorylation-inactive mutant of βARK could attenuate β_2AR desensitization in human airway epithelial cells. Utilizing this same mutant, Pals-Rylaarsdam et al. (267) were able to reduce both agonist-dependent phosphorylation and acute desensitization of the m2AChR in human embryonic kidney 293 cells. Similar effects of the βARK dominant–negative mutant have recently been demonstrated on the desensitization of the β_1AR (109), δ-opioid receptor (271), κ-opioid receptor (295), and α_{1b}AR receptor (84). Employing a different approach, Shih and Malbon (323) have recently reported that incubation of β_2AR-transfected CHO cells with a βARK antisense oligodeoxynucleotide significantly reduced β_2AR desensitization.

Evidence of a different nature comes from transgenic mice studies by Koch et al. (188), in which cardiac-specific overexpression of βARK resulted in blunted inotropic and chronotropic responsiveness to isoproterenol. The observed physiological alterations were accompanied by reductions in the β_1AR binding affinity for isoproterenol, as well as a reduction in sensitivity and B$_{max}$ of isoproterenol-stimulated adenylyl cyclase in myocardial membranes. The authors imply that each of these indices of diminished β_1AR function could be attributed to increased phosphorylation of the β_1AR in vivo, and that under normal physiological conditions βARK levels may be limiting in desensitization.

Thus, modes of regulation of cellular βARK activity may include both the regulation of βARK protein expression as well as "dynamic" regulation via protein–protein interactions. In a study consistent with the observations of Koch et al., Pippig et al. (276) identified conditions under which cellular levels of βARK may be limiting in homologous desensitization. Overexpression of βARK in CHO cells expressing high levels of β_2AR resulted in a greater desensitization following pretreatment with high concentrations of isoproterenol [similar results have recently been obtained in similar experiments examining the β_1AR (109)]. However, βARK overexpression had little effect on the desensitization produced by pretreatment with low concentrations of isoproterenol. This finding reflects the restricted selectivity of βARK for the *agonist-occupied* receptor and exemplifies the fact that the effects of βARK are most prominent under conditions of *high receptor occupancy* (high agonist concentrations) (71, 147, 226). Accordingly, a cell's reduction in adenylyl cyclase responsiveness that occurs following exposure to low concentrations of agonist may predominately reflect the effects of other (non-βARK-mediated) mechanisms such as those mediated by PKA (see later under Protein Kinase A).

Supportive studies identifying physiological/pathological alterations in βARK expression and the concomitant effects are scarce. Ungerer et al. (378) have determined that failing human myocardium, in which βARs appear markedly desensitized, exhibited ~3–fold higher βARK mRNA levels compared to levels in control (healthy) hearts, as well as increased levels of βARK activity. In light of the findings in transgenic mice, these findings suggest that the apparently increased myocardial βARK levels associated with heart failure may contribute in part to the disease. Presumably, these alterations might be induced by the high levels of circulating catecholamines associated with heart failure. However, the intracellular signal by which increased transcription of βARK mRNA can occur is unclear; no apparently relevant regulatory control regions are evident in the recently-cloned human βARK gene (272), which possesses a 5' regulatory region characteristic of (but not restricted to) constitutively-expressed "housekeeping" genes. Moreover, no studies to date exist which identify specific regulation of βARK expression by exposure to β-agonist, mediators of cAMP generation, or PKA activation, any of which might exert either positive or negative feedback on βARK-mediated desensitization. This lack of findings in light of the results of Lohse et al. emphasizes the potential power and limitations inherent in in vivo studies.

Additional evidence of regulation of βARK expression has recently emerged from studies examining hematopoietic cell activation/differentiation. De Blasi et al. (80) reported that βARK expression is increased threefold in mononuclear leukocytes following 72-h exposure of cells to the T-cell activator phytohemagglutanin, presumably via a PKC-mediated mechanism. Loudon and Benovic (228) have recently determined that differentiation of promyeloid HL60 cells toward myeloid lineage with dimethylsulfoxide or retinoic acid produces a two- to threefold increase in βARK expression, whereas PMA-induced differentiation of the cells towards the monocytic lineage results in an ~5–10 fold decrease in βARK expression.

With regard to acute regulation of βARK, interaction of βARK with regions of the activated receptor distinct from the phosphorylation loci appears to be an important mechanism of βARK activation. Light-activated rhodopsin and agonist-treated $β_2AR$ and m2AChR each activate βARK-mediated phosphorylation of peptides (56, 139). It is likely that interaction of βARK with the first and third intracellular loops of the $β_2AR$ are important in βARK interaction, since peptides representing these regions are potent inhibitors of $β_2AR$ phosphorylation by βARK (22). Similar studies have also described the interaction with rhodopsin kinase by activated rhodopsin (103) and have implicated the first, second, and third intracellular loops of rhodopsin in the interaction with rhodopsin kinase (181, 260, 263).

G protein βγ subunits have also been identified as important regulators of βARK activity. Their primary function in this respect appears to involve their binding to a region of βARK (presently localized to residues 546–670) (187) that overlaps the PH domain, for the purpose of targeting βARK to the membrane. From a teleological perspective this function makes sense, since: (1) βARK is devoid of modifications typically involved in membrane targeting, lacking the CAAX motif in the carboxy terminus that specifies the post-translational isoprenylation of other proteins (including rhodopsin kinase) that is important for their membrane association and function; and (2) release of βγ subunits occurs with receptor activation and thus represents an appropriate, specific signal for the dynamic

regulation of βARK. βγ subunits promote βARK association with phospholipid vesicles and rod outer segments, and increase the initial rate of rhodopsin, $β_2AR$, and m2AChR phosphorylation by βARK approximately 10-fold in in vitro assays (137, 185, 278). Construction of a mutant βARK that undergoes isoprenylation in vitro enables membrane association and activation of the kinase to occur in the absence of βγ subunits (163). Additional evidence from various assay systems suggests βγ subunits may also possess an inherent capacity to activate βARK independent of their ability to promote translocation (138, 185).

Recent studies have indicated that net negatively-charged phospholipids may regulate βARK, apparently by binding to a region in the βγ-binding domain (82, 257, 279). Whether this regulation occurs via the promotion of βARK translocation, a stabilization of the βARK-receptor complex, or by increasing inherent kinase activity is presently unclear. Since substrates for G protein-activated PLC include phospholipids, these findings suggest that another mode of cross-regulation of GPR pathways may exist at the level of βARK.

Acute regulation of βARK activity by PKC has recently been described (63a, 396a). Phosphorylation of βARK in its C-terminus (396a) by PKC resulted in an ~2–3-fold activation of the kinase, presumably by enhancing βARK association with the membrane (63a, 396a). Again, these findings identify another potential mode by which GPR pathways may cross-regulate.

While the role of βARK in mediating rapid agonist-specific desensitization of GPRs has been well established, the recent finding that disruption of the βARK gene in mice by homologous recombination leads to embryonic death (166a) suggests additional, undetermined βARK functions. Attempts to generate βARK "knockout" mice resulted in no homozygous βARK embryos surviving beyond gestation day 15.5, with embryos displaying pronounced hypoplasia of the ventricular myocardium. These findings suggest that βARK plays a prominent role in cardiac development (perhaps via its modulation of a potential convergence of GPR signaling and transcription factors) and will likely extend the study of GRKs well beyond the field of GPR regulation.

The Family of G Protein–Coupled Receptor Kinases.
Early evidence emerged with the cloning of the βARK cDNA that homologs of βARK, distinct from rhodopsin kinase, may exist and thereby identify a multigene family. Southern blots of bovine genomic DNA probed with a catalytic domain fragment of the βARK cDNA revealed five hybridizing bands (18), suggesting the existence of multiple βARK homologs. Soon thereafter, low-stringency hybridization screening of a bovine

brain cDNA library identified a novel kinase, highly homologous to βARK, termed βARK2 (23). βARK2 has been subsequently shown to possess many of the characteristics of βARK (Table 7.2), including receptor specificity, modes of regulation, and tissue distribution, although βARK2 mRNA levels are considerably less than those of βARK in most tissues. Multiple cloning strategies have subsequently resulted in the identifica-

tion of four additional βARK homologs (including rhodopsin kinase), prompting their classification as the family of G protein–coupled receptor kinases (GRKs) within the family of serine/threonine protein kinases. In addition, two *Drosophila* homologs of βARK, designated GPRK1 and GPRK2, have been cloned (51). Inclusion into the GRK family is based on sequence homology within the catalytic domain, basic structural

TABLE 7.2. *Molecular Properties of the GRKs*

Parameter	GRK1 (RK)	GRK2 (βARK)	GRK3 (βARK2)	GRK4 (IT11)	GRK5	GRK6
Polypeptide molecular weight (kDa)	62.9	79.5	79.8	57.6, 61.2, 62.9, 66.5 [a]	67.8	66.1
Amino acids	561	689	688	500, 532, 546, 578	590	576
N-terminal	186	190	190	154, 186	185	185
Catalytic	266	263	263	264	263	263
C-terminal	109	236	235	82, 128	142	128
Receptor substrates [b,c]	Rhodopsin, β_2AR	β_1AR, β_2AR, rhodopsin, SPR, m2 AchR, m3 AchR, α_{2a}AR, α_{2b}AR, δopiod, A3 adenosine	β_2AR, rhodopsin, m2 AchR, m3 AchR, SPR, α_{2a}AR, α_{2b}AR, thrombin	β_2AR, LH/CGR	β_1AR, β_2AR, m2 AchR, rhodopsin	β_2AR, m2 mAChR, rhodopsin
Peptide substrates	Acidic	Acidic	Acidic	?	Neutra > acidic [d]	Neutra > acidic [d]
Tissue distribution	Retina > pineal	Ubiquitous, brain, hematopoietic, skeletal muscle	Ubiquitous, brain, hematopoietic, skeletal muscle, olfactory	Testis >> brain	Ubiquitous, heart, lung, placenta, hematopoietic, retina	Ubiquitous, brain, hematopoietic, skeletal muscle
Autophosphorylation	+++	+	+	—	+++	+
Covalent modifications	Farnesylation	?	?	Palmitoylation	?	Palmitoylation
Activators	Polycations	βγ subunits, PS, PA, PG, PI, PE, PIP$_2$	βγ subunits, PS, PA, PG, PI, PE[e], PIP$_2$	PIP$_2$	Polycations, PC, PE, DAG, fatty acids	Polycations
Inhibitors	Sangivamycin, Recoverin	Polyanions	Polyanions	?	Polyanions	Polyanions
Chromosomal localization [f]	?	11q13	22q11	4p16.3	10q24-qter	5q35, 13pter-q21
mRNA size (kb)	3.1, 5.8	3.8	8	2.5	3	3, 3.6

[a] Splice variants of GRK4 have recently been reported by Sallese et al. (306) and Premont et al. (284). [b] Receptors which can act as phosphoacceptors in a light- or agonist-dependent fashion in vitro (irrespective of efficacy) or implicated as substrates from in vivo experiments. [c] Abbreviations: β_2AR, β_2-adrenergic receptor; α_{2a}AR, α_{2a}-adrenergic receptor; α_{2c}AR, α_{2c}-adrenergic receptor; LH/CGR, leutenizing hormone/chorionic gonadotropin receptor; mAChR, muscarinic cholinergic receptor; SPR, substance P receptor; PS, phosphatidylserine; PA, phosphatidic acid; PG, phosphatidylglycerol; PI, phosphatidylinositol; PE, phosphatidylethanolamine; PC, phosphatidylcholine; DAG, diacylglycerol; PIP$_2$, phosphatidylinositol-4,5-bisphosphate. [d] All peptides contained 3 Arg residues at the N-terminus which aids in the isolation of peptides on phosphocellulose paper. Peptides differed in that nearest neighbors of the phosphoacceptor serine were either neutral (Ala) or acidic (Glu, Asp, phospho-Ser). [e] The effects of phospholipids on βARK2 is presumed to be based on the similarity between βARK and βARK2 in the region thought to be involved in phospholipid binding. [f] See Benovic et al. (26), Calabrese et al. (45), Ambrose et al. (3), Bullrich et al. (43), and Haribabu and Snyderman (145).

[Table modified from Sterne-Marr and Benovic (345), with permission from Academic Press.]

features, and functional similarities. Due to the present inability to clearly establish the receptor selectivity of GRKs, and the uncertain number of family members yet to be discovered, current members of the family have been named according to their order of discovery: rhodopsin kinase (GRK1)(37, 104, 196, 227); βARK1 (GRK2); βARK2 (GRK3); IT11 (GRK4)(3), GRK5 (200); and GRK6 (19).

A comparison of the amino acid sequences of the GRKs suggests that there are two major branches of the GRK family tree (Fig. 7.4). βARK2 and *Drosophila* GPRK-1 appear to be the most similar to βARK with amino acid identities of 84% and 64%, respectively. In contrast, rhodopsin kinase, GRK4, GRK5, GRK6 and *Drosophila* GPRK-2 have significantly lower homology with βARK (35%–40% amino acid identity)

and form a separate branch of the tree. Overall, the common features of the GRKs include a centrally localized catalytic domain of 270 amino acids that shares significant amino acid identity (46%–95%), an N-terminal domain of 184 amino acids (except for GPRK-2), and a variable-length C-terminal domain of 105–233 amino acids. [For a comparison of GRK domain structures, see Inglese et al. (161).]

The hallmark feature of GRKs is their ability to specifically recognize and phosphorylate only the agonist- (or light-) activated form of the receptor. To date, all GRKs have been shown to phosphorylate the β_2AR and/or rhodopsin in an activation-dependent manner. Comparison and characterization of the six known GRKs have recently been reviewed [Sterne-Marr and Benovic (345)]. Therefore, we will restrict our present discussion of GRKs to a synopsis of important features and differences. Table 7.2 offers a summary of these features.

As previously mentioned, rhodopsin kinase (GRK1) was identified prior to the discovery of βARK. Rhodopsin kinase is expressed solely in rods, cones, and (to a much lesser extent) the pineal gland (262, 336). Unlike other GRKs, rhodopsin kinase has clearly defined in vivo substrates—light-activated rhodopsin in rods, and likely the light-activated color opsins in cones. Rhodopsin kinase phosphorylates multiple sites on the carboxy-terminus of metarhodopsin II (37, 104, 196), thereby lowering the affinity of the receptor for transducin while significantly increasing receptor affinity for a 48-kDa protein termed *arrestin*. Arrestin binding to activated, phosphorylated rhodopsin inhibits rhodopsin–transducin interaction, effectively uncoupling the receptor (see below).

The amino acid sequence of rhodopsin kinase terminates with the residues -CVLS, a motif that directs posttranslational farnesylation (C15 isoprenylation) of the cysteine residue (6, 113, 162). Isoprenylation serves to target multiple cellular proteins to membranes, and appears critical to the activation-dependent translocation of rhodopsin kinase to the disk membrane. Like many small G proteins, rhodopsin kinase is not constitutively associated with the membrane and appears to cycle on and off the membrane as dictated by the presence/absence of rhodopsin activation. A mutant rhodopsin kinase that lacks the isoprene moiety does not translocate to membranes in in vitro assays following rhodopsin activation and exhibits diminished kinase activity (162, 163). Moreover, a mutant that possesses a more lipophilic C20 geranylgeranyl group associates with membranes independent of light activation and retains full kinase activity. Thus, isoprenylation appears important in rhodopsin kinase translocation and maximal enzyme activity.

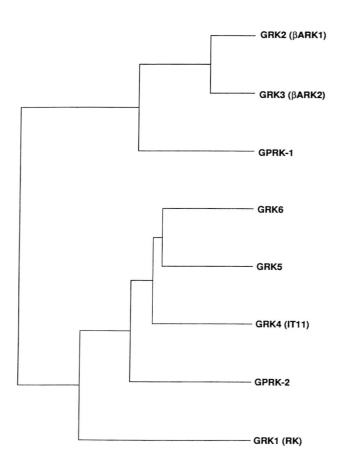

FIG. 7.4. Comparison of the amino acid sequence of related GRKs by dendogram analysis. The PILEUP program in the Wisconsin Genetics Computer Group (GCG) software was used to align and compare amino acid sequences of bovine GRK1 (rhodopsin kinase), GRK2 (βARK1), GRK3 (βARK2), human GRK4 (IT11), GRK5, GRK6, and *Drosophila* GPRK-1 and GPRK-2. See Benovic and Gomez (19) for detailed sequence comparisons. PILEUP uses a progressive pairwise alignment as previously described (97).

Rhodopsin kinase undergoes intramolecular auto-phosphorylation to a stoichiometry of 3–4 mol phosphates/mol kinase (42, 181). Autophosphorylation does not appear to be involved in the translocation or activation of rhodopsin kinase. However, unphosphorylated rhodopsin kinase binds light-activated, phosphorylated rhodopsin much better than does autophosphorylated rhodopsin kinase (42). This finding suggests that autophosphorylation of rhodopsin kinase may function to promote the dissociation of the kinase from the phosphorylated receptor.

βARK2 (GRK3) has the highest homology to βARK among the GRKs, and shares a similar structural architecture with respect to its amino, catalytic, and carboxy domains. Like βARK, βARK2 contains a PH domain in its C-terminal domain and is regulated by βγ subunits. In general, βARK and βARK2 share a similar tissue distribution. However, one important distinction is that βARK2 appears to be the GRK predominately expressed in olfactory epithelium, and mediates, in conjunction with PKA, the desensitization of olfactory receptors (79, 313). In addition, βARK2 has been implicated as the principal GRK involved in the agonist-specific phosphorylation and desensitization of the thrombin receptor when co-expressed with the receptor in *Xenopus* oocytes (165).

GRK4 (originally termed IT11) was identified, in the search for the Huntington's disease locus, on human chromosome 4 using positional cloning in combination with exon amplification (3). GRK4 mRNA is detectable in significant amounts only in testis. Four splice variants of GRK4 (designated α, β, γ, δ) are known to exist (284, 306). When co-expressed with leutenizing hormone/chorionic gonadotropin receptor (LH/CGR) in HEK 293 cells, each of the variants has been shown to reduce agonist-stimulated cAMP production via the LH/CGR (284).

GRK5 has been cloned from both human heart (200) and gustatory (283) cDNA libraries. Although widely distributed among tissues, GRK5 is most prevalent in heart, lung, retina, and hematopoetic cells, and is expressed in relevantly low levels in the brain (200). Autophosphorylation of GRK5 in the C-terminal domain (serine 484 and/or threonine 485) significantly activates the kinase. Substitution of serine 484 and/or threonine 485 with alanine substantially reduces autophosphorylation and results in a dramatic reduction in the ability of the kinase to phosphorylate receptor substrates (201). Autophosphorylation is also stimulated by various lipids (201, 283).

GRK5 associates with rod outer segment membranes in the dark or light in the presence or absence of ATP (283). Thus, unlike rhodopsin kinase and βARK, GRK5 appears to be constitutively localized to membranes, although it does not undergo any known modification by lipid and is not regulated by βγ subunits. GRK5 binding to phospholipid vesicles can be blocked by a fusion protein containing the last 102 amino acids of GRK5, implicating this highly basic region in lipid binding/membrane association.

Recent studies (63b, 287a) have determined that calmodulin can significantly inhibit GRK5 (and to a lesser extent GRK2, 3, and 6) binding to membranes and receptor in a calcium-dependent manner in vitro, and thereby inhibit kinase activity. Interestingly, calmodulin also activates GRK5 autophosphorylation at sites distinct from the two previously determined autophosphorylation sites, and this autophosphorylation serves to inhibit GRK5–receptor interaction. In addition, Pronin and Benovic (286) have recently demonstrated that PKC can phosphorylate GRK5 in vitro, while stimulation of COS-1 cells with PMA results in phosphorylation of transiently expressed GRK5. This phosphorylation results in significant inhibition of GRK5 activity (unlike PKC activation of GRK2) and a reduced capacity to bind rhodopsin-containing membranes. Two major sites of PKC-mediated phosphorylation were localized to the C-terminus. Collectively, these studies suggest that agents that activate Gq-coupled pathways linked to Ca^{2+} mobilization and/or PKC-activating pathways may promote mechanisms that differentially regulate GRKs and help establish GRK specificity (286).

GRK6 is the most recently-cloned GRK. Initial characterization of GRK6 expressed and purified from Sf9 cells identified relatively weak phosphorylation of rhodopsin, the β_2AR, and m2AChRs (229), suggesting that these receptors are either poor substrates for GRK6, or alternatively, that the in vitro phosphorylation assays employed lacked some important regulatory factor. Stoffel et al. (346) subsequently determined that GRK6 is palmitoylated in vivo at one or more cysteine residues in its C terminus. Palmitoylation was apparent only in membrane-bound GRK6, while the soluble fraction of GRK6 was not palmitoylated. These findings suggest that membrane association, and perhaps activation of GRK6 is dependent upon its palmitoylation, and that in vitro assessments of GRK6 activity may have been hampered by difficulties in purifying a palmitoylated, "active" form of the kinase.

Arrestins. The role of arrestins in mediating receptor desensitization has been most extensively studied in the visual system. Retinal arrestin (frequently referred to as simply "arrestin"), also termed the 48 kDa protein or S antigen, was initially identified as a major protein which redistributed (along with rhodopsin kinase) from the cytoplasm to the disk membrane following light activation of rod outer segments (195). In 1984, Kuhn et al. demonstrated that the binding of the 48 kDa protein to photoreceptor membranes was significantly enhanced by the phosphorylation of rhodopsin (197). While phosphorylated rhodopsin has a reduced ability to interact with transducin and stimulate the cGMP phosphodiesterase (PDE), the binding of arrestin to rhodopsin suppresses PDE activation by 98% (394). In contrast, arrestin does not quench the ability of nonphosphorylated rhodopsin to activate PDE. Arrestin was initially purified and characterized from bovine retinas (384) and has been shown to specifically interact with phosphorylated metarhodopsin II with a Kd of 50 nM (312). The cloning of a bovine retinal arrestin cDNA reveals that arrestin has 404 amino acids (45.3 kDa) with several short stretches of amino acid homology with the α subunit of transducin (397, 401). Several studies have demonstrated that while rhodopsin phosphorylation is important to the desensitization process, it is the arrestin binding which effectively blocks rhodopsin activation of transducin (197).

Evidence for the involvement of an arrestin-related protein in the adenylyl cyclase system was initially suggested by studies which demonstrated that β_2AR phosphorylation using crude βARK preparations resulted in substantial uncoupling of the receptor from G_s (20). However, when the receptor was phosphorylated with a highly purified βARK preparation, the β_2AR-G_s interaction remained largely intact. This finding suggested that there was a factor present in the crude βARK preparations that could uncouple the βARK-phosphorylated β_2AR from G_s. When purified retinal arrestin was added to this reconstituted system it was found to specifically impair β_2AR/G_s coupling. However, this effect was observed only when the receptor was phosphorylated by βARK (20). Utilizing low stringency hybridization techniques a cDNA encoding an arrestin homolog was subsequently cloned from a bovine brain library (324). This cDNA encodes a protein, termed β-arrestin, of 418 amino acids (47.1 kDa) which has 58% identity with arrestin and appears to uncouple βARK phosphorylated β_2AR from G_s in a reconstituted system (224, 324) with a 20-fold greater efficiency than that of retinal arrestin. Utilizing various cloning strategies, a third arrestin cDNA was subsequently cloned from human thyroid (292), rat brain (10), and bovine brain (344) libraries. This arrestin, which has been termed hTHY-ARRX, β-arrestin2, or arrestin3, has 79% amino acid identity with β-arrestin and 56% with retinal arrestin. A fourth homolog, termed X-arrestin, C-arrestin, or arrestin4, has recently been cloned and likely plays a role in the visual system since it appears to be localized in cone cells (77, 240). In addition to the mammalian arrestins, two *Drosophila*-arrestin-related genes have also been cloned (160, 334, 400).

Arrestin, β-arrestin, and arrestin3 are each expressed as polypeptide variants that arise as a result of alternative (gene) splicing. Arrestin is predominately expressed in its originally-identified 404-amino acid form. Arrestin is also expressed as a 370-amino-acid form, in which the last 35 residues are replaced by a single alanine, and a 396-residue form that lacks the eight residues (residues 338–345) encoded by exon 13 of the human gene (269, 402). β-arrestin exists as two polypeptide variants—the 418-amino-acid "long" form (β-arrL), and a 410-residue "short" form (β-arrS) that lacks the comparable eight-amino acid stretch that is spliced in arrestin (residues 334–341). Arrestin3 is expressed predominately as a 409-amino-acid protein, although in some tissues a 420-residue form that contains an 11 amino-acid insert following residue 361 is observed (344). A summary of the properties and tissue distribution of the various arrestins is presented in Table 7.3.

Characterization of the localization, receptor specificity, and mechanisms of binding to receptor substrates, and structural similarities of the various arrestins has been recently reviewed in detail (345). We will therefore restrict our discussion to the more salient features of arrestin proteins.

Northern analysis demonstrates that both arrestin (225) and X-arrestin (240) are expressed most abundantly in the retina and pineal gland. PCR analysis has also identified low levels of arrestin in leukocytes, and low levels of both arrestin and X-arrestin in heart, kidney, lung, and skeletal muscle (335). β-arrestin and arrestin3 are widely expressed, with the highest levels of expression in the brain, spleen, and prostate (269, 344). In most tissues examined, β-arrestin appears to be expressed at significantly higher levels than arrestin3. A notable exception is olfactory epithelium, in which arrestin3 is the preferentially expressed arrestin isoform and appears to play a prominent role in the desensitization of odorant receptors (79).

The specificity of the arrestin–rhodopsin interaction, which is inferred from the restricted localization of arrestin to the retina, is suggested by the observation that arrestin binds substantially better to rhodopsin than to other receptors such as the β_2AR or m2AChR (131). Moreover, arrestin is 100-fold more potent than β-arrestin in uncoupling rhodopsin from transducin (224). X-arrestin has been also shown to effectively uncouple activated rhodopsin from transducin in vitro, although the role of X-arrestin relative to that of arrestin in vivo is unclear. β-arrestin and arrestin3 are equally effective at uncoupling the β_2AR from G_s, both being 100-fold more potent than arrestin (10).

TABLE 7.3. *Molecular Properties of the Arrestins*

Parameter	Arrestin	β-arrestin	Arrestin3	X-arrestin
Polypeptide variants (amino acids)	404, 396, 370	418, 410	420, 409	388
Tissue distribution	Retina (rods) > pineal body	Ubiquitous, brain, hematopoietic, prostate	Ubiquitous, brain, hematopoietic, prostate, olfactory cilia	Retina (cones)
mRNA size (kb)	1.5	7.5, 4.1, 1.3	1.7–2.4	1.35
Chromosomal localization*	2q37	11q13	17p13	Xcen-q21
Receptor affinity (K_d) (nM)				
Rhodopsin†	30–50	?	?	?
β_2AR‡	2.1	0.14	0.33	?
m2 AChR‡	7.2	0.48	0.35	?
Uncoupling efficiency	Rhodopsin >> β_2AR	β_2AR >> rhodopsin	β_2AR >> rhodopsin	?
Receptor binding preference	Rhodopsin >> β_2AR ~m2 AChR	m2 AChR > β_2AR ~rhodopsin	m2 AChR~β_2AR ≥ rhodopsin	?

*See Calabrese et al. (44, 45) and Murakami et al. (240).   †Determined by stabilization of metarhodopsin II (312).   ‡Determined by Scatchard analysis using radiolabeled arrestins (129, 131). [Table modified from Sterne-Marr and Benovic (345), with permission from Academic Press.]

However, none of the polypeptide variants of β-arrestin or arrestin3 display significant specificity for binding among rhodopsin, the β_2AR, or the m2AChR (ref). An extensive analysis of the structural features of receptors and arrestins that confer specificity of interactions has been provided by Gurevich et al. (128, 130–132). Figure 7.5 depicts the roles of βARK and β-arrestin in a basic model of the rapid agonist-specific desensitization of the β_2AR.

Multiple studies to date have implicated arrestins in mediating desensitization in intact or permeablized cells. Dawson et al. (79) have demonstrated that arrestin3–specific antibodies are able to block desensitization of odorant receptors in permeabilized olfactory epithelium. Pippig et al. (276) showed that coexpression of β-arrestin with β_2AR in Chinese hamster ovary (CHO) cells significantly enhanced isoproterenol-induced desensitization. In a similar manner, β_1AR desensitization in 293 cells was augmented by overexpression of either β-arrestin or arrestin3 (109), while Diviani et al. (84) demonstrated that coexpression of β-arrestin with α_{1b}AR in containing origin SV40 (COS) cells significantly attenuated α_{1b}AR-mediated phosphoinositide hydrolysis. Most recently, nonvisual arrestins have also been implicated as important mediators of GPR sequestration (see later under Receptor Sequestration).

Protein Kinase A. Several early observations strongly implicated protein kinase A as an important mediator of desensitization, particularly heterologous desensitization. First, PKA activation was shown to result in the phosphorylation and regulation of several key regulatory proteins (116, 194). Similar modifications that inhibit the function of βAR-G_s-adenylyl cyclase signaling components would constitute classical negative-feedback regulation. Secondly, multiple studies demonstrated that incubation of cells with cAMP analogs, or agents such as forskolin that bypass the receptor to stimulate cAMP production, were capable of mimicking heterologous desensitization (13, 329, 333, 358, 365).

Although direct evidence of PKA-mediated phosphorylation of G_s/adenylyl cyclase was lacking, diminution of G_s/adenylyl cyclase activity was frequently observed in studies in which heterologous desensitization was induced via cAMP analogs, forskolin, or phosphodiesterase inhibitors in addition to hormonal activation (177, 333, 338). However, alterations in G_s/adenylyl cyclase activity were not readily apparent in several studies describing heterologous desensitization induced by hormonal activation (11, 68, 191, 252, 299) or PKA-activating agents (11, 191, 252, 299), suggesting that the receptor is a primary locus of PKA-mediated regulation.

Stadel et al. (340) determined that desensitization of turkey erythrocytes with 8-Br-cAMP was accompanied by an altered mobility of purified, photo-affinity labeled βARs, partially mimicking the effect of catecholamine-induced desensitization. In addition, purified turkey βARs were shown to be phosphorylated in vitro by the catalytic subunit of PKA. Sibley et al. (329) subsequently showed that turkey erythrocyte βARs were phosphorylated in vivo by cell treatment with cAMP analogs. Shortly thereafter Benovic et al.

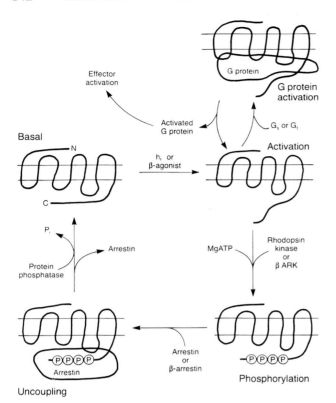

FIG. 7.5. Stimulus-dependent phosphorylation and desensitization of rhodopsin and the β_2AR. Receptor activation, either by light (rhodopsin) or a β-agonist (β_2AR), promotes interaction of the receptor with transducin or G$_s$, respectively, leading to G protein and effector activation. Receptor activation also promotes phosphorylation of the receptor, which is mediated either by rhodopsin kinase or βARK. Phosphorylation of the receptor appears to uncouple it partially from the G protein, but also promotes its interaction with arrestin (for rhodopsin) or β-arrestin (for β_2AR). This interaction further uncouples the receptor from the G protein. Desphosphorylation of rhodopsin requires regeneration with 11-*cis* retinal, which is followed by arrestin dissociation and dephosphorylation of the receptor by phosphatase 2A. The mechanism of β_2AR dephosphorylation remains poorly understood but may involve sequestration of the receptor into a compartment where dephosphorylation can occur. [From Palczewski and Benovic (261), with permission from *Trends in Biochemical Sciences*.]

(24) demonstrated that β_2AR purified from hamster lung was phosphorylated by PKA in vitro to a stoichiometry of 2 mol phosphate/mol receptor. The rate of phosphorylation was stimulated 2–3 fold by agonist-occupancy of the receptor. In addition, functional impairment of the PKA-phosphorylated receptor was revealed in reconstitution studies in which isoproterenol-stimulated GTPase activity was markedly reduced.

More direct evidence of PKA-mediated desensitization has been provided by studies that have employed

either PKA-inhibitors (203, 226) or expression of mutant β_2ARs in which the consensus PKA sites had been ablated (68, 147). PKA is known to preferentially phosphorylate serine and threonine residues in the consensus sequence RRXS (31). [For a review of PKA function and substrate specificity, see Walsh and Van Patten (389).] On the β_2AR, two potential sites of phosphorylation by PKA exist, each having been shown to be substrates in vitro (24). The site in the third intracellular loop (I3, residue 262 in the human β_2AR) appears to represent the preferred site of phosphorylation, while the site in the carboxy terminus (CT, residue 346) is a relatively poorer substrate (32, 34). Hausdorff et al. (147) demonstrated that β_2ARs lacking the I3 PKA site were significantly impaired in their ability to undergo phosphorylation and desensitization mediated by exposure of cells to low concentrations of isoproterenol. [As intimated above, exposure of cells to low concentrations of beta-agonist can produce, despite low βAR occupancy, high levels of intracellular cAMP sufficient to maximally activate PKA (69, 71, 203).] Clark et al. (68) distinguished the respective contributions of the I3 and CT PKA sites in mediating heterologous desensitization in L cells. Following exposure to 50 nM epinephrine, cells expressing β_2ARs lacking the CT site exhibited β_2AR desensitization comparable to that observed in cells expressing wild-type β_2AR. Cells expressing β_2AR lacking the I3 site, however, were unable to undergo desensitization under the same conditions. Similar results were obtained in cell-free assays in which membranes expressing mutant β_2ARs were subject to phosphorylation conditions in the presence of purified PKA (68). Thus, the I3 PKA site of the β_2AR appears to be the principal target through which PKA-mediated desensitization is mediated.

The mechanism by which PKA phosphorylation uncouples or partially uncouples the β_2AR from G protein is unclear although PKA phosphorylation of the β_2AR does not promote arrestin binding to the receptor. Phosphorylation by PKA of a peptide from the third cytoplasmic loop of the β_2AR reduced the potency of the peptide to stimulate GTPγS binding to G$_s$ 100 fold (256). Alterations in charge induced by phosphorylation of the interactive site represent a potential mechanism for reducing receptor-G$_s$ coupling efficiency. However, Yuan et al. (408) recently demonstrated that mutation of serine 262 in the hamster β_2AR (the principle site of PKA-mediated phosphorylation) to aspartic acid did not significantly uncouple the β_2AR, suggesting that charge effects alone cannot sufficiently explain PKA-mediated uncoupling of the β_2AR.

Several studies have attempted to clarify the relative contributions of βARK and PKA in rapid β_2AR desensitization evoked by differing conditions of low and high receptor occupancy. Using permeabilized A431 cells, Lohse et al. (226) assessed the effects of blocking βARK-dependent phosphorylation (by heparin) and PKA-dependent phosphorylation (with PKI, an inhibitory peptide) on desensitization. With high (1 μM) isoproterenol pretreatment for 10 min it was determined by selective blockage that βARK or PKA alone could each mediate significant desensitization. However, desensitization by pretreatment with low (10 nM) isoproterenol appeared specifically mediated by PKA. Studies examining mutant β_2ARs lacking putative βARK and PKA-phopshorylation sites (147, 220) reached similar conclusions asserting the predominant role of PKA in the phosphorylation/desensitization of the β_2AR at low agonist concentrations, and the capacity for both βARK- and PKA-mediated desensitization with high agonist concentrations.

Freedman et al. (109) have recently characterized βARK- and PKA-mediated desensitization of the β_1AR in CHW and HEK 293 cells. One μM isoproterenol-induced rapid β_1AR desensitization was qualitatively similar to that of the β_2AR. Selective inhibition of PKA reduced β_1AR desensitization by 50%. Further analyses suggested that isoproterenol-induced phosphorylation of the β_1AR expressed in HEK 293 cells was mediated equally by βARK and PKA.

Utilizing an approach similar to that employed by Lohse et al. (226), Roth et al. (304) described the kinetics and magnitude of βARK- and PKA-mediated phosphorylation and desensitization in A431 cells. Isoproterenol-induced phosphorylation and desensitization of the β_2AR by βARK exhibited $t_{1/2}$'s of < 20 sec each. PKA-mediated effects were relatively slower for both phosphorylation ($t_{1/2}$ 2 min) and desensitization (3.5 min). In addition, the degree of desensitization mediated by βARK was more than 50% greater than that mediated by PKA. Thus, the authors concluded that βARK-mediated phosphorylation is the most rapid and quantitatively most important process contributing to rapid desensitization. These findings are consistent with the widespread observation in desensitization studies that heterologous desensitization of the βAR typically is observed later and is of a lesser magnitude when compared to homologous desensitization (141).

While the studies mentioned above support βARK as the principal mediator of rapid agonist-specific desensitization, recent studies have suggested that relative contributions of GRKs versus PKA in mediating agonist-specific desensitization may be cell-specific. Utilizing antisense oligonucleotides targeting PKA or βARK in multiple cell types, Shih and Malbon (323) reported that agonist-induced β_2AR desensitization in CHO cells and DDT_1MF-2 smooth muscle cells is largely mediated by βARK, desensitization in rat osteo-

sarcoma cells appears predominately dependent upon PKA activity and PKA and βARK appear equally effective in A431 cells. Using a different approach, Post et al. (281a) demonstrated that high-affinity [^{3}H]forskolin binding (an index of receptor-activated Gs-adenylyl cyclase association) is significantly higher in kin- s49 lymphoma cells compared to wild-type cells following beta-agonist pretreatment, suggesting a prominent role for PKA in the agonist-promoted uncoupling of the β_2AR.

Demonstration of the putative roles of PKA in beta-agonist induced desensitization has contributed to some confusion in the use of the terms agonist-specific, homologous, agonist-nonspecific, and heterologous desensitization, particularly when they are exclusively linked to GRK- or PKA-mediated mechanisms. Clearly, GRKs are powerful (and likely principal) mediators of the rapid desensitization of the agonist-occupied receptor. In many cells PKA appears to be the predominate mediator of heterologous desensitization. However, PKA-mediated effects can clearly occur in the desensitization that results from receptor occupancy; whether one associates PKA-mediated effects with homologous desensitization is largely a question of semantics.

The physiological circumstances under which PKA-mediated and GRK-mediated desensitization of the βAR occurs can be implied from the above studies. Transient elevations in endogenous circulating catecholamines that occur with stress represent conditions in which PKA-mediated desensitization could occur. Alternatively, the existence of higher concentrations of norepinephrine at synaptic clefts, or the acute administration of high-dose beta-agonist inhalants in the management of asthma represent conditions in which GRK-mediated desensitization likely occurs. Accordingly, Arriza et al. (7) have identified relatively high expression of βARK1 and βARK2 by in situ hybridization and immunocytochemistry in axon terminals and postsynaptic densities in rat brain.

Other Protein Kinases (Protein Kinase C, Tyrosine Kinase). Several studies suggest that protein kinase C (PKC) phosphorylation of the βAR (and other GPRs) plays a cell-specific role in heterologous desensitization. Phorbol ester activation of PKC in avian erythrocytes has been shown to promote βAR phosphorylation and desensitization (182, 328). However, the effects of phorbol esters are cell-specific, can produce alterations in both G proteins and adenylyl cyclase, and can result in increases or decreases in adenylyl cyclase responsiveness (85, 171, 179, 250, 371). While phosphorylation of the β_2AR by PKC has been demonstrated in vitro (36), the effect of such phosphorylation in vivo is unclear and difficult to assess. Toward this end, Johnson et al. (171) discerned complex cellular changes associated with the phorbol ester-induced desensitization of the β_2AR in stably-transfected L cells. Results revealed: (1) a 2–3 fold reduction in affinity for beta-agonist simulation but a 2–3 fold increase in B_{max}; and (2) a decrease in G_i-mediated inhibition of forskolin stimulation. Mutational deletion of the PKC phosphorylation site of the third intracellular loop (residues 259–263) ablated the phorbol-ester induced reduction in affinity for β-agonist, but did not alter the B_{max} for β-agonist or the reduction in G_i-mediated inhibition. Deletion of the consensus phosphorylation PKC site in the carboxy terminus (residues 343–348) was without consequence. Thus, in L cells PKC appears capable of desensitizing the β_2AR via phosphorylation of the third intracellular loop, while at the same time enhancing adenylyl cyclase responsiveness through a potential direct effect on G_i.

Additional evidence of the cell-specific effects of PKC has recently been provided by Malbon and co-workers (323). Treatment of cells with antisense oligodeoxynucleotides to the mRNA encoding PKC slightly reduced β agonist–induced β_2AR desensitization in Rat osteosarcoma and CHO cells, yet significantly enhanced β_2AR desensitization in DDT$_1$MF-2 and A431 cells. Use of oligodeoxynucleotides against PKA and βARK mRNA were able to reduce β_2AR desensitization in a cell-specific manner. βARK, PKA, and PKC may therefore all contribute, to different extents in different cells, to the regulation of βAR signaling.

Although numerous studies have demonstrated insulin-mediated effects on Gs, Gi, and cAMP PDE that alter β_2AR-stimulated cAMP accumulation [reviewed in Valiquette et al. (380)], the establishment of tyrosine kinase-mediated phosphorylation and regulation of the β_2AR has remained elusive. Recently, however, Hadcock et al. (134) have reported that exposure of DDT$_1$MF-2 cells to insulin results in desensitization of the hamster β_2AR. The basal state of phosphorylation of the β_2AR was increased twofold by insulin exposure, presumably by receptor phosphorylation by tyrosine kinase. Mutation of β_2AR tyrosyl residues 350 and 354 abolished the effects of insulin (176). In contrast, Valiquette et al. (380) have recently demonstrated that insulin treatment of β_2AR-transfected Chinese hamster fibroblasts results in β_2AR phosphorylation and sensitization of β_2AR-stimulated adenylyl cyclase activity. Phosphorylated tyrosine residues were identified using highly sensitive antiphosphotyrosine antibodies and two-dimensional phopshoamino analysis. Mutation of tyrosine 141 (but not tyrosine 350, 354, or 366) prevented both the tyrosine phosphorylation and supersensitization of the β_2AR induced by insulin treatment. These two studies suggest that tyrosine kinase activity is capable of specifically regulating the β_2AR via phosphorylation, with the effect being either desensitization or sensitization and dependent on cell type.

Receptor Sequestration

Receptor sequestration may be defined as the agonist-induced internalization of receptors to an ill-defined cytosolic compartment, such that receptors are physically "sequestered" from membrane-bound G proteins. Sequestration is an interesting process whose role in the regulation of receptor responsiveness has yet to be clearly established. The rapid redistribution of cell surface βARs was initially recognized by Costa, Chuang and co-workers (63, 64) who noted that β-agonist treatment of bullfrog erythrocytes resulted in a decrease in cell surface βARs with a concomitant increase in "cytosolic" receptors. Sequestration was temperature dependent, occurring at 14°C but not at 4°C, and was blocked by pretreatment of cells with concanavalin A. Perkins and co-workers (142, 387) were the first to discover that sequestered βARs were associated with a "light vesicle" fraction that could be separated from particulate membranes by sucrose gradient fractionation. Application of this technique enabled several important observations regarding the phenomenon of βAR sequestration in human astrocytoma cells. As previously observed by Chuang and Costa (63), sequestered βARs displayed a reduced binding affinity for agonist and no GTP-induced reduction in agonist affinity (142). Sequestration that resulted from 1 μM isoproterenol treatment proceeded with a t$_{1/2}$ of 2 min after a lag of 45–60 s, and was reversed following removal of agonist (387). Light vesicle fractions containing sequestered βARs were essentially devoid of isoproterenol-stimulated adenylyl cyclase activity. Agonist-induced loss of isoproterenol-stimulated adenylyl cyclase activity in plasma membranes preceded sequestration by 1–2 min, and concanavalin A pretreatment of cells prevented receptor sequestration but did not affect the magnitude of rapid βAR desensitization (374, 387). These data distinguish the rapid initial uncoupling of βARs from the sequestration phenomenon. Using similar techniques, Clark and coworkers confirmed and extended these findings in their studies of desensitization of s49 lymphoma cells (70). Rapid desensitization and sequestration of βARs from s49 lymphoma cells displayed similar kinetics to those observed in astrocytoma cells, while binding and functional assays demonstrated that sequestered βARs were uncoupled from G proteins. An apparent requirement for receptor occupancy was implied by the fact that 50 nM epinephrine represented the threshold concentration at which sequestration occurred during a 30-min exposure of cells to agonist. Sequestration was apparently independent of βAR-G protein coupling since it could also be observed in the cyc- and kin- mutant s49 lymphoma lines. Moreover, sequestered βARs from cyc- cells were shown capable of significant adenylyl cyclase stimulation when reconstituted with cholate extracts of wild-type cells.

Results similar to those described above in bullfrog erythrocytes and s49 lymphoma cells were obtained by Stadel et al. (341) in grassfrog erythrocytes in which differential centrifugation was used to separate particulate membrane fractions from light vesicle fractions. As in s49 cells, sequestered receptors from grassfrog erythrocytes appeared to be structurally intact and capable of stimulating adenylyl cyclase when reconstituted in Xenopus laevis erythrocytes (355), which lack endogenous βARs.

Strasser et al. (353) provided evidence of sequestration in an in vivo model of desensitization. Intraperitoneal injection of isoproterenol into rats resulted in rapid βAR desensitization in membranes prepared from lung. This desensitization was accompanied by a translocation of 40% of the βARs from the plasma membrane fraction to the light vesicle fraction.

Additional evidence of receptor sequestration was inferred from studies of βAR antagonist and agonist binding in intact cells. Early binding studies in intact cells demonstrated a progressive loss of high-affinity binding of agonists for the βAR during the course of the binding assay (164, 280, 370). Characteristic of sequestration, the loss of high-affinity binding appeared independent of G protein coupling and PKA activity, having been observed in both cyc- and kin- s49 lymphoma cells. Pretreatment of cells with concanavalin A significantly reduced the loss of high-affinity binding but did not alter isoproterenol-induced desensitization. These findings were interpreted as reflecting the relative inaccessibility of hydrophilic agonists to penetrate the plasma membrane and bind internalized βARs (372). Supporting this hypothesis was the observation that the hydrophilic antagonist CGP-12177 specifically binds cell surface receptors, whereas lipophilic compounds are accessible to all receptors in the cell (342, 343). Selective use of radiolabeled βAR antagonists and CGP-12177 has subsequently become an important strategy in the analysis of βAR sequestration in intact cells.

The collective analyses of βAR distribution in subcellular fractions and intact cells strongly implies the agonist-induced translocation of the βAR from the plasma membrane to intracellular vesicles in which receptors are not degraded, perhaps via the clathrin-coated pit/endosome pathway employed by receptors for epidermal growth factor (EGF), insulin, low-density lipoprotein (LDL), and transferrin. That such an endocytotic process occurs has not been directly established, but is inferred from several findings (204). Light vesicle fractions containing βARs possess distinctive hydrodynamic (142, 387) and permeability (154, 374) properties and are essentially devoid of plasma membrane markers, suggesting physical separation of the βAR from the plasma membrane. Incubation of astrocytoma cells with EGF and isoproterenol results in the comigration of these ligand's receptors to the low density regions of sucrose gradients, suggesting that EGF receptors and βARs are processed in parallel by astrocytoma cells (386). Moreover, the kinetics of β_2AR internalization (204, 387) and externalization (204, 277), the ability to inhibit βAR recycling (internalization or externalization) using phenylarsine oxide (152, 178), sucrose/hypertonicity (277, 407), reduced temperature (64, 156, 373), reduced cellular ATP (218), low intracellular pH (219), and reduced cellular K^+ (219, 277), are all consistent with the involvement of an endocytotic pathway, with some of these properties suggesting clathrin-coated pit involvement.

However, precise subcellular localization of the sequestered βAR suffered for several years from a lack of corroborating immunocytochemical evidence. This evidence was ultimately supplied by van Zastrow and Kobilka (383), who examined the agonist-induced internalization of the human β_2AR in HEK 293 cells. Immunocytochemical localization of the β_2AR by conventional and confocal fluorescence microscopy showed a rapid agonist-induced translocation of the β_2AR into the cytosol that temporally paralleled the sequestration measured by radioligand binding. Within 2 min of agonist exposure β_2ARs were shown to redistribute in small, punctate accumulations. Moreover, internalized β_2ARs colocalized with transferrin receptors, suggesting that sequestered β_2ARs undergo processing through endosomal membranes in a manner similar to that observed for constitutively recycling receptors.

To date, agonist-induced sequestration of several GPRs has been described. However, the mechanisms involved in mediating GPR sequestration remain largely undefined. The only apparent essential requirement appears to be occupancy of the receptor by agonist, with a direct correlation between β_2AR occupancy and sequestration having been observed (226). As mentioned, receptor coupling to G protein is not required (46, 59, 70, 147). Sequestration does not occur under conditions that specifically induce heterologous desensitization, suggesting that cAMP cannot induce sequestration. However, while several studies have suggested that βAR phosphorylation is not required for sequestration (35, 147, 350), recent studies by Ferguson et al. (98, 99) and Tsuga et al. (375) suggest that βARK-mediated phosphorylation may play a role in the sequestration of the β2AR and m2AChR, respectively. An even more critical role of nonvisual arrestins in mediating β2AR sequestration has been demonstrated in recent studies. Ferguson et al. (98) showed that overexpression of β-arrestin and arrestin3 in HEK cells rescued the agonist-dependent sequestration of sequestration-deficient β2AR mutants, while Goodman et al. (119b) identified nonvisual arrestins as clathrin-binding adaptor proteins that modulate endocytosis of wild-type β2AR. β-arrestin and arrestin3, but not visual arrestin, exhibited high-affinity binding to clathrin in vitro, and immunofluorescence microscopy of intact cells revealed an agonist-dependent co-localization of the β2AR with β-arrestin and clathrin. The sites of arrestin–clathrin interaction were subsequently localized to the C-terminus of β-arrestin and arrestin3 (119b, 194a) and residues 89–100 of the clathrin heavy chain N-terminal domain (119a).

As mentioned, multiple studies have demonstrated that functional uncoupling of the β2AR precedes its sequestration (147, 226, 304, 374, 387) and that inhibition of sequestration using either low temperature (64, 156, 373) or pretreatment with concanavalin A (277, 386, 387) does not effect rapid uncoupling or desensitization. What role, if any, does sequestration play in the regulation of the βAR? Perhaps βAR internalization plays a role in accelerating βAR down-regulation (the *loss* of receptors from the cell following prolonged exposure to agonist—see below) by increasing the rate of βAR degradation. Typically, membrane protein internalized to endosomes has two potential fates: it can be recycled back to the plasma membrane or directed to lysosomes. Some time-dependent signal linked to the duration of agonist exposure may determine the extent to which sequestered receptors are recycled or destroyed.

Although the role of sequestration in receptor desensitization remains elusive, recent studies suggest that sequestration may play an important role in the *resensitization* of the β2AR. Sibley et al. (330) had originally noted that sequestered receptors associated with the light vesicle fraction isolated from isoproterenol-desensitized erythrocytes were phosphorylated to a lesser degree (0.75 mol phosphate/mol receptor) than the total cellular pool of β2ARs (2.1 mol/mol). In addition, the light vesicle fraction was shown to contain a potent phosphatase activity capable of dephosphorylating adenylyl cyclases previously phosphorylated by βARK. Recently, Yu et al. (407) demonstrated that when β2AR sequestration was blocked via either su-

crose pretreatment of CHO cells or creation of a sequestration-defective β2AR, desensitized β2ARs failed to recover their capacity to stimulate adenylyl cyclase activity following removal of the pretreating agonist. Similar results were also obtained by Pippig et al. (277), who further demonstrated that resensitization and β2AR recycling were associated with dephosphorylation of the β2AR. In addition, inhibition of cellular serine/threonine protein phosphatases with calyculin A blocked β2AR resensitization. Thus, β2AR sequestration appears to play an important role in the dephosphorylation and resensitization of the desensitized β2AR.

Receptor Down-Regulation

Down-regulation, the loss of degradation of receptors from the cell, has been demonstrated for several GPRs. As opposed to the relatively rapid desensitization processes of receptor phosphorylation/uncoupling and sequestration, receptor down-regulation represents a chronic adaptation that occurs with prolonged (typically >1 h) exposure of the cell to agonist. While the molecular mechanisms underlying GPR down-regulation are not well understood, an increase in receptor degradation and/or a reduction in receptor synthesis are primarily implicated in the loss of cellular receptors. That receptors are degraded and not transiently sequestered is suggested by the associated prolonged recovery period from receptor down-regulation. Unlike the rapid recovery from short-term desensitization, full recovery from down-regulation can take days and requires new protein synthesis (89, 108, 237).

Down-regulation has been most extensively studied for the β2AR (interestingly, rhodopsin does not down-regulate). Despite numerous studies to date it is still difficult to say what exactly is required for and what facilitates βAR down-regulation. Down-regulation of the β2AR does not appear to require receptor phosphorylation since several studies have demonstrated that mutant β2ARs containing altered phosphorylation sites have normal patterns of down-regulation (61, 147, 350). Studies demonstrating normal down-regulation in both kin- s49 lymphoma cells (231, 321) and HC-1 hepatoma cells, which lack functional PKA (357), further suggest that PKA phosphorylation is not an obligatory event. A potential requirement for receptor–G protein coupling was suggested by the observation that s49 cyc- and unc- (defective in β2AR-G protein coupling) cells exhibited little or no agonist-induced down-regulation (231, 357). However, Bouvier et al. (34) demonstrated that down-regulation of wild-type β2ARs expressed in Chinese hamster fibroblasts could be induced by exposure of cells to cAMP analogs, forskolin, or phosphodiesterase inhibitors, although the rate of receptor loss was significantly slower than that observed for agonist-induced down-regulation. Mutagenesis of the PKA phosphorylation site of the β_2AR decreased the rate and extent of the agonist-induced down-regulation. Thus, although cAMP/PKA may not be required for down-regulation to occur, it may play a facilitatory role in the process in certain cell types.

Two different mechanisms by which the effects of cAMP/PKA are mediated have been proposed. Hadcock and Malbon (133) originally observed that chronic exposure of DDT$_1$MF-2 cells to isoproterenol, forskolin, or cholera toxin resulted in a time-dependent reduction in β_2AR mRNA levels. This reduction was ultimately determined to result from a decrease in β_2AR mRNA stability (75, 135) as opposed to a reduction in the rate of β_2AR gene transcription (75) [although down-regulation of other GPRs may be mediated in part by reduced transcription of the receptor gene (74)]. Thus, a reduction in β_2AR synthesis as a result of cAMP-mediated destablization of β_2AR mRNA appears to represent a principal mechanism of β_2AR down-regulation. However, an interesting observation by Bouvier et al. (34) suggests an additional PKA-mediated mechanism. The diminished down-regulation of the mutant β_2AR lacking PKA phosphorylation sites was accompanied by a loss of β_2AR mRNA equivalent to that observed in cells expressing the wild-type β_2AR. Therefore, enhanced degradation of the PKA-phosphorylated wild-type β_2AR is an attractive hypothesis explaining its greater down-regulation. Bouvier et al. (34) suggest that PKA-mediated phosphorylation of the β_2AR contributes to the initial loss of β_2ARs in down-regulation, whereas alterations in β_2AR mRNA levels mediate a latter stage of the down-regulation process.

The structural features of GPRs that confer a capacity for down-regulation are presently undetermined. Recent studies have suggested that the conserved cysteine in the C-terminal cytoplasmic tail of many GPRs close to the seventh TMD may play a role in down-regulation. This cysteine is palmitoylated in rhodopsin, the α_{2a}AR, and the β_2AR, and is important in β_2AR coupling and agonist-promoted desensitization (222). Mutation of this conserved cysteine in the human α_{2a}AR to a phenylalanine did not alter α_{2a}AR coupling or desensitization, but abolished agonist-induced down-regulation (90). Interestingly, the human α_{2b}AR lacks this cysteine and does not undergo down-regulation. However, certain GPRs known to possess the conserved cysteine are known not to down-regulate, leading Liggett and co-workers to propose that the presence of a palmitoylcysteine in the carboxy

tail of GPRs may be necessary, but not sufficient for agonist-promoted down-regulation (90).

While the initial rate of β_2AR down-regulation is dependent on the concentration of beta-agonist to which cells are exposed, several studies have also noted that chronic exposure of cells to very low concentrations of beta-agonists (that is, 3 nM epinephrine) (285) can promote desensitization and down-regulation. This observation raises some interesting questions regarding the potential effects of physiological concentrations of catecholamine on cells in vivo. Do circulating/local concentrations of catecholamines exert a constitutive suppression of β_2AR signaling in certain cells in vivo, and limit the potential range of responsiveness? Moreover, to what extent would rapid receptor phosphorylation/uncoupling, sequestration, and down-regulation exert an influence on such cells? With chronic exposure of cultured cells to moderate levels of beta-agonist, β_2AR levels can be reduced by 80%–90%. In addition, catecholamine-stimulated adenylyl cyclase activity may be abolished. Whether such complete ablation of β_2AR responsiveness ever occurs in vivo is unknown but appears unlikely; organ systems such as the lung and their β_2AR-containing cells appear to retain adequate responsiveness to beta-agonists following chronic beta-agonist exposure that produces significant β_2AR down-regulation. This has been demonstrated in studies of asthmatic patients in whom the bronchorelaxant effects of inhaled β-agonist appear minimally affected despite prior chronic use of high-dose beta-agonist inhalants (363). Moreover, airway epithelial cells harvested from normal (376) or asthmatic (274) subjects receiving chronic beta-agonist inhalant treatment displayed significant βAR down-regulation (35%–65% loss) and diminished, but present, isoproterenol-stimulated adenylyl cyclase activity. Thus, βAR down-regulation and the associated functional consequences may be somewhat limited by the in vivo condition.

Receptor Polymorphisms

Recent studies by Liggett and colleagues (125, 296, 377) have demonstrated multiple polymorphisms in the human β_2AR gene. Interestingly, two of the polymorphisms, arginine to glycine at amino acid 16 (Arg16u$\rightarrow$Gly) and glutamine to glutamic acid at amino acid 27 (Gln27$\rightarrow$Glu) encode receptors that, when expressed in Chinese hamster fibroblasts, exhibit enhancement of and resistance to, respectively, agonist-specific down-regulation (125). Additional studies from this group suggest that these polymorphisms have physiological consequences. Although it was determined that the frequency of β_2AR homozygous polymorphisms at amino acids 16 and 27 is no greater in asthmatics compared to nonasthmatics, the homozygous Arg16→Gly polymorphism is associated with a higher incidence of steroid dependency in asthmatics (296) and is overrepresented in nocturnal asthma (377). Thus, mutations of the β_2AR appear to impart distinct phenotypes of agonist-specific regulation and may contribute to the variability in responsiveness to beta-agonists observed in asthmatic populations. However, because the identified mutations lie outside of the putative principal functional and regulatory regions of the β_2AR, it is presently unclear how they mediate their effects.

Sensitization

Sensitization refers to the enhancement of receptor signaling via modification of the GPR pathway. Multiple mechanisms appear to exist through which sensitization can occur. One mechanism involves the up-regulation of receptor expression, which has been shown to occur for multiple GPRs following prolonged treatment with antagonists (29, 118, 398). In addition, glucocorticoids have been shown to up-regulate adenylyl cyclases through enhanced transcription of the adenylyl cyclase gene (76, 135). Moreover, glucocorticoids can mitigate the β-agonist induced down-regulation of adenylyl cyclases (135). This effect is appreciated in both cells and organ systems such as the lung following administration of drugs in vivo (232). However, the effects of glucocorticoids appear to be receptor-dependent; a recent study has determined that glucocorticoids down-regulate β_1AR expression while up-regulating adenylyl cyclase expression in C6 glioma cells (184).

As suggested above, PKC phosphorylation of G proteins and/or effectors represents another potential mechanism by which sensitization of GPR signaling occurs. $G_{\alpha i}$ is likely phosphorylated by phorbol esters in various cell types (171, 172, 290), while adenylyl cyclase appears to be a substrate in frog erythrocytes (406). However, the physiological significance of phorbol ester-induced effects of receptor regulation is unclear, since few hormones known to activate PKC can mimic the actions of phorbol esters on receptor responsiveness (172). Interestingly, sensitization of adenylyl cyclase in LM5 cells via P2 purinergic receptor stimulation could not be mimicked by m5AChR stimulation, despite the fact that carbachol (a muscarinic agonist) is a much more effective stimulator of PLC in LM5 cells than is ATP.

Several studies have also noted that chronic stimulation of various G_i-coupled receptors results in sensitization of agonist-or forskolin-stimulated adenylyl cyclase activity. For example, chronic pretreatment of NG108–

15 cells with carbachol (245) or opiates (210, 320, 395) led to increased basal and PGE$_1$-stimluated adenylyl cyclase activity. Prolonged treatment of opossum kidney cells with 5–HT1B receptor agonists resulted in enhanced forskolin-stimulated cAMP accumulation (281, 379). Chronic adenosine exposure of rat adipocytes expressing adenosine A1 receptors increased basal, isoproterenol-, NaF- and forskolin-stimulated adenylyl cyclase activity (270). While the responsible mechanisms are unclear, alterations in G_i levels or function (67, 270), G_s levels (270), or enhanced coupling between GPRs and G_s (4, 5) have been proposed to contribute.

Desensitization of Other GPR Pathways

The desensitization mechanisms of receptor phosphorylation/uncoupling, sequestration and down-regulation, while certainly not ubiquitous phenomena, appear to extend beyond the βAR to many other GPRs. Unfortunately, a comprehensive assessment of all GPRs whose regulation has been studied is beyond the scope of this review. Table 7.4 offers a summary of the modes of regulation evidenced in some of the more well-characterized GPRs. The receptors are loosely organized into groups based on actions on effectors (although many receptors clearly can regulate more than one effector). This summary is presented with the caveat that the presence and characteristics of modes of desensitization of certain receptors are cell-specific, for example, as has been clearly demonstrated for the 5–HT1A receptor (246).

The majority of receptors listed in Table 7.4 undergo agonist-induced phosphorylation/uncoupling, sequestration, and down-regulation. In several cases, receptor sequestration has not been examined. Of note, many receptors that couple to G_i and inhibit adenylyl cyclase (for example, adenosine A1, 5–HT1A, 5–HT1B, 5–HT1Dβ, and D2 dopamine receptors) appear to desensitize to a lesser degree and at a slower rate than G_s-coupled receptors. Frequently, desensitization is characterized by a small reduction in the potency of the receptor agonist with either no or a small reduction in the maximal inhibition of forskolin-stimulated adenylyl cyclase activity. Whether such a pattern of desensitization reflects receptor resistance to desensitization or a robustness of G_i-mediated signaling is unclear.

An interesting feature of the regulation of the majority of GPRs that activate PLC is the failure to demonstrate a role of PKC in agonist-induced desensitization. Homologous desensitization of the α_{1b}AR (212), m3AChR (369), H1 histamine (234) and thrombin receptor (165, 268) [as well as the agonist-induced attenuation of calcium mobilization through H1 hista-

TABLE 7.4. *Desensitization Features of G Protein–Coupled Receptors*

Receptor	Phosphorylation/ Uncoupling	Suspected Protein Kinases	Sequestration	Down-Regulation	References
Activators of cGMP Phosphodiesterase					
Rhodopsin	Rapid	GRK1	No	No	See text
Activators of Adenylyl Cylase					
β_1-adrenergic	Rapid	GRK2, 3, 5, PKA	Yes	Yes	(109, 124, 360, 378, 412)
β_2-adrenergic	Rapid	GRKs, PKA, PKC	Yes	Yes	See text
β_3-adrenergic *	No/minor, slow	— —	No —	No Minor	(47, 54, 221, 242) (55, 243, 244)
A2 adenosine	Rapid	GRKs	Yes	Yes	(58, 180, 265, 291)
D1 dopamine	Rapid	GRKs, PKA	Yes	Yes	(15, 30, 168, 251, 255)
IP prostanoid †	Unknown	—	—	Yes	(2, 183, 192, 193, 396)
H2 histamine	Rapid	—	No	No	(288, 310, 315)
Luteinizing hormone/ chorionic gonadotropin	Rapid	GRKs	Yes	Yes	(126, 216, 301, 309, 391, 413)
Follicle-stimulating hormone	Rapid	PKA	Yes	Yes	(120, 121, 216, 236, 308, 366)
Inhibitors of Adenylyl Cyclase					
m2 muscarinic	Rapid	GRK 2, 3	Yes	Yes	(81, 95, 117, 136, 158, 205– 207, 267, 300, 375, 393)
5-HT1A	Rapid	GRKs	—	No	(33, 127, 146, 246, 294, 381)
5-HT1B	Slow	PKC	—	Yes	(281, 379)
α_{2a}-adrenergic	Rapid	GRK2	Yes	Yes	(91–93, 107, 222)
α_{2b}-adrenergic	Rapid	—	Yes	Yes	(91–93, 169)
α_{2c}-adrenergic	No	—	No	No	(90–93)
A1 adenosine	Slow	—	Yes	Yes	(264, 270, 291)
A3 adenosine	Rapid	GRKs	Yes	Yes	(264, 266)
D2 dopamine	Slow	—	Yes	No ‡	(14, 16, 100, 411)
δ opioid	Rapid	GRKs	—	Yes	(213, 214, 271, 282, 410)
κ opioid	Moderate/ slow	GRK2	—	No	(295, 414)
μ opioid	Rapid		—	Yes	(57, 62, 282, 289, 409, 410)
Activators of Phospholipase C					
α_{1b} adrenergic	Rapid	GRK2, 3	Yes	Yes	(84, 102, 159, 212, 215)
m3 muscarinic	Rapid	GRK2, 3	Yes	Yes	(81, 158, 368, 369, 403)
Thrombin	Rapid	GRK3	Yes	—	(38, 39, 150, 165, 268)
H1 histamine	Rapid/intermediate	—	—	No	(40, 41, 83, 217, 234)
Cholecystokinin	Rapid	GRKs, PKC	Yes	Yes	(1, 112, 157, 259, 302, 382)

*Desensitization of the β_3-adrenergic has been reported in certain cell types.   †Agonist exposure results in rapid down-regulation of both $G_{s\alpha}$ and the IP receptor.   ‡The two isoforms of the D2 dopamine receptor may be differentially regulated, with the longer form (D2L) exhibiting agonist-induced up-regulation.

mine, bombesin, and ATP receptors (83, 390)] is not blocked by inhibitors of PKC or by depletion of PKC by chronic PMA pretreatment of cells. The absence of this direct feedback mechanism is unclear; it may reflect either the dominance of GRK-mediated desensitization or alternatively, the fact that multiple points of regulation (including dynamic regulation of IP_3 levels and IP_3 receptor responsiveness) exist along the pathway of receptor-mediated calcium release.

SUMMARY

In summary, the desensitization of GPR responsiveness involves multiple potential mechanisms that are invoked in a receptor- and cell-specific manner. While each component of the receptor– G protein– effector pathway may undergo acute modification or altered expression that affects signaling, alterations at the receptor locus appear to be the principal means by which both rapid and chronic desensitization occurs in many GPR signaling pathways. Three time-dependent mechanisms have been identified that can promote the desensitization that occurs with continuous exposure of a GPR to its specific agonist. Within seconds of agonist exposure, rapid *uncoupling* of the receptor from G protein is mediated by phosphorylation of the agonist-occupied receptor by GRKs, and the subsequent binding of arrestin proteins to the phosphorylated receptor. Within minutes of agonist exposure receptor *sequestration* may follow, whereby receptors are translocated from the plasma membrane to endosomes. Receptor internalization appears to represent a pathway for receptor dephosphorylation and resensitization, and potentially a mechanism for targeting receptors for lysosomal degradation. Chronic exposure (>1 h) to agonist can result in *down-regulation*, whereby a combination of increased receptor degradation and/or reduced receptor synthesis results in a net loss of receptors. Recovery from receptor down-regulation frequently takes days and requires new protein synthesis.

In addition, desensitization of a given GPR may also occur in the absence of its activation. In such instances activation of other signaling pathways can induce PKA or PKC phosphorylation of a GPR in an agonist-nonspecific manner, again resulting in the rapid uncoupling of the receptor from G protein. Alternatively, activation of other signaling pathways may also alter the responsiveness or expression of G proteins and effectors such that desensitization or *sensitization* of GPR pathways occurs.

It is important to re-emphasize that the modes and characteristics of regulation displayed by a given GPR

are both dependent on the receptor itself and the cell in which it is expressed. As noted, some receptors display but one mode of desensitization (for example, rhodopsin is rapidly uncoupled but does not sequester or down-regulate) while others (β_3AR, $\alpha_{2b}AR$) do not exhibit any appreciable desensitization. The cell-specific nature of GPR regulation is apparent in various studies of the 5–HT1A receptor. Agonist-induced desensitization of 5–HT1A receptor is not evident when the receptor is expressed in CHO cells (294). In contrast, rapid, agonist-induced uncoupling is observed of 5–HT1A receptors expressed in either HeLa or Sf9 cells (146, 246). However, 5–HT1A receptor uncoupling in HeLa cells appears to be mediated by PKC phosphorylation of the receptor, while in sf9 cells GRKs appear to play a dominant role. Further demonstration of the cell-specific nature of GPR regulation is suggested by Shih et al. (323). Using antisense oligodeoxynucleotides to mRNAs encoding βARK, PKA, or PKC, rapid agonist-induced desensitization of the adenylyl cyclase appears to be mediated predominately by βARK in DDT_1MF-2 and CHO cells, by PKA in rat osteosarcoma cells, and by both βARK and PKA in A431 cells.

Great strides in understanding the regulation of GPRs have been made in the last 20 years. Clearly, however, the road ahead is an exciting one, with many questions remaining to be answered. Clarification of the mechanisms by which GRKs and arrestins are regulated, as well as the delineation of the specificity of GRKs and arrestins for their receptor targets, represent important challenges. An increasing awareness of the effects of compartmentalization and membrane organization (249) suggests that more precise temporal and spatial analyses of second messenger flux are required for an accurate assessment of GPR regulation in certain cells. The wealth of information on GPR regulation provided to date through the use of in vitro assays, cell lines, and cell expression systems also needs to be supported by studies employing more physiologically relevant models. Toward this end, the development of in vivo models of desensitization and the use of genetically-engineered mice are encouraging. Ideally, such approaches will lead to the development of novel strategies for the management or cure of diseases through the manipulation of GPR signaling.

REFERENCES

1. Abdelmoumene, S., and J. D. Gardner. Cholecystokinin-induced desensitization of enzyme secretion in dispersed acini from guinea pig pancreas. *Am. J. Physiol.* 239(*Gastrointest. Liver Physiol.* 8): G272–G279, 1980.
2. Adie, E. J., I. Mullaney, F. R. McKenzie, and G. Milligan. Concurrent down-regulation of IP prostanoid receptors and

alpha-subunit of the stimulatory guanine-nucleotide-binding protein (Gs) during prolonged exposure of neuroblastoma × glioma cells to prostanoid agonist. Quantification and functional implications. *Biochem. J.* 285: 529–536, 1992.

3. Ambrose, C., M. James, G. Barnes, C. Lin, G. Bates, M. Altherr, M. Duyao, N. Groot, D. Church, J. J. Wasmuth, H. Lehrach, D. Housman, A. Buckler, J. F. Gusella, and M. E. MacDonald. A novel G protein-coupled receptor kinase gene cloned from 4p16.3. *Hum. Mol. Gene* 1: 697–703, 1992.

4. Ammer, H., and R. Schulz. Coupling of prostaglandin E1 receptors to the stimulatory GTP-binding protein Gs is enhanced in neuroblastoma × glioma (NG108–15) hybrid cells chronically exposed to an opioid. *Mol. Pharmacol.* 43: 556–563, 1993.

5. Ammer, H., and R. Schulz. Chronic activation of inhibitory delta-opioid receptors cross-regulates the stimulatory adenylate cyclase-coupled prostaglandin E1 receptor system in neuroblastoma x glioma (NG108–15) hybrid cells. *J. Neurochem.* 64: 2449–2457, 1995.

6. Anant, J. S., and B. K. Fung. In vivo farnesylation of rat rhodopsin kinase. *Biochem. Biophys. Res. Commun.* 183: 468–473, 1992.

7. Arriza, J. L., T. M. Dawson, R. B. Simerly, L. J. Martin, M. G. Caron, S. H. Snyder, and R. J. Lefkowitz. The G-protein-coupled receptor kinases βARK1 and βARK2 are widely distributed at synapses in rat brain. *J. Neurosci.* 12: 4045–4055, 1992.

8. Arshavsky, A., and M. D. Bownds. Regulation of the deactivation of photoreceptor G protein by its target enzyme and cGMP. *Nature* 357: 416–417, 1992.

9. Asano, T., T. Katada, A. G. Gilman, and E. M. Ross. Activation of the inhibitory GTP-binding protein of adenylate cyclase, Gi, by β-adrenergic receptors in reconstituted phospholipid vesicles. *J. Biol. Chem.* 259: 9351–9354, 1984.

10. Attramadal, H., J. L. Arriza, T. M. Dawson, J. Codina, M. M. Kwatra, S. H. Snyder, M. G. Caron, and R. J. Lefkowitz. β-arrestin2, a novel member of the arrestin/β-arrestin gene family. *J. Biol. Chem.* 267: 17882–17890, 1992.

11. Attramadal, H., F. Le Gac, T. Jahnsen, and V. Hansson. Beta-adrenergic regulation of Sertoli cell adenylyl cyclase: desensitization by homologous hormone. *Mol. Cell. Endocrinol.* 34: 1–6, 1984.

12. Barber, D. L., M. E. McGuire, and M. B. Ganz. Beta-adrenergic and somatostatin receptors regulate Na-H exchange independent of cAMP. *J. Biol. Chem.* 264: 21038–21042, 1989.

13. Barovsky, K., C. Pedone, and G. Brooker. Forskolin-stimulated cyclic AMP accumulation mediates protein synthesis-dependent refractoriness in C6–2B rat glioma cells. *J. Cyclic Nucleotide Protein Phosphor. Res.* 9: 181–189, 1983.

14. Barton, A. C., L. E. Black, and D. R. Sibley. Agonist-induced desensitization of D2 dopamine receptors in human Y-79 retinoblastoma cells. *Mol. Pharmacol.* 39: 650–658, 1991.

15. Bates, M. D., C. L. Olsen, B. N. Becker, A. F. J., J. P. Middleton, J. G. Mulheron, S. L. Jin, M. Conti, and J. R. Raymond. Elevation of cAMP is required for down-regulation, but not agonist-induced desensitization, of endogenous dopamine D1 receptors in opossum kidney cells. Studies in cells that stably express a rat cAMP phosphodiesterase (rPDE3) cDNA. *J. Biol. Chem.* 268: 14757–14763, 1993.

16. Bates, M. D., S. E. Senogles, J. R. Bunzow, S. B. Liggett, O. Civelli, and M. G. Caron. Regulation of responsiveness at D2 dopamine receptors by receptor desensitization and adenylyl cyclase sensitization. *Mol. Pharmacol.* 39: 55–63, 1991.

17. Benovic, J. L. Purification and characterization of the β-adrenergic receptor kinase. In: *Methods in Enzymology*, edited by T. Hunter and B. M. Sefton. New York: Academic Press, 1991, p. 351–362.

18. Benovic, J. L., A. De Blasi, W. C. Stone, M. G. Caron, and R. J. Lefkowitz. β-adrenergic receptor kinase: Primary structure delineates a multigene family. *Science* 246: 235–240, 1989.

19. Benovic, J. L., and J. Gomez. Molecular cloning and expression of GRK6: A new member of the G protein-coupled receptor kinase family. *J. Biol. Chem.* 268: 19521–19527, 1993.

20. Benovic, J. L., H. Kuhn, I. Weyand, J. Codina, M. G. Caron, and R. J. Lefkowitz. Functional desensitization of the isolated β-adrenergic receptor by the β-adrenergic receptor kinase: Potential role of an analog of the retinal protein arrestin (48 kDa protein). *Proc. Natl. Acad. Sci. USA* 84: 8879–8882, 1987.

21. Benovic, J. L., F. J. Mayor, C. Staniszewski, R. L. Lefkowitz, and M. G. Caron. Purification and characterization of the β-adrenergic receptor kinase. *J. Biol. Chem.* 262: 9026–9032, 1987.

22. Benovic, J. L., J. Onorato, M. J. Lohse, H. G. Dohlman, C. Staniszewski, M. G. Caron, and R. J. Lefkowitz. Synthetic peptides of the hamster β_2-adrenoceptor as substrates and inhibitors of the β-adrenoceptor kinase. *Br. J. Clin. Pharmacol.* 30: 3S–12S, 1990.

23. Benovic, J. L., J. J. Onorato, J. L. Arriza, W. C. Stone, M. Lohse, N. A. Jenkins, D. J. Gilbert, N. G. Copeland, M. G. Caron, and R. J. Lefkowitz. Cloning, expression, and chromosomal localization of β-adrenergic receptor kinase 2: A new member of the receptor kinase family. *J. Biol. Chem.* 266: 14939–14946, 1991.

24. Benovic, J. L., L. J. Pike, R. A. Cerione, C. Staniszewski, T. Yoshimasa, J. Codina, M. G. Caron, and R. J. Lefkowitz. Phosphorylation of the mammalian β-adrenergic receptor by cyclic AMP-dependent protein kinase. *J. Biol. Chem.* 260: 7094–7101, 1985.

25. Benovic, J. L., J. W. Regan, H. Matsui, F. J. Mayor, S. Cotecchia, L.M.F. Leeb-Lundberg, M. G. Caron, and R. J. Lefkowitz. Agonist-dependent phosphorylation of the α_2-adrenergic receptor by the β-adrenergic receptor kinase. *J. Biol. Chem.* 262: 17251–17253, 1987.

26. Benovic, J. L., W. C. Stone, K. Huebner, C. Croce, M. G. Caron, and R. J. Lefkowitz. cDNA cloning and chromosomal localization of the human β-adrenergic receptor kinase. *FEBS Lett.* 283: 122–126, 1991.

27. Benovic, J. L., R. H. Strasser, M. G. Caron, and R. J. Lefkowitz. β-Adrenergic receptor kinase: Identification of a novel protein kinase that phosphorylates the agonist-occupied form of the receptor. *Proc. Natl. Acad. Sci. USA* 83: 2797–2801, 1986.

28. Berstein, G., J. L. Blank, D. -Y. Jhon, J. H. Exton, S. G. Rhee, and E. M. Ross. Phospholipase C-β1 is a GTPase-activating protein for Gq/11, its physiological regulator. *Cell* 70: 411–418, 1992.

29. Bjornerheim, R., S. Golf, and V. Hansson. Effects of chronic pindolol treatment on human myocardial beta 1- and beta 2-adrenoceptor function. *Naunyn Schmiedebergs Arch. Pharmacol.* 342: 429–435, 1990.

30. Black, L. E., E. M. Smyk-Randall, and D. R. Sibley. Cyclic AMP-mediated desensitization of D1 dopamine receptor-coupled adenylyl cyclase in NS20Y neuroblastoma cells. *Mol. Cell. Neurosci.* 5: 567–575, 1994.

31. Blackshear, P. J., A. C. Nairn, and J. F. Kuo. Protein kinases 1988: a current perspective. *FASEB J.* 2: 2957–2969, 1988.

32. Blake, A. D., R. A. Mumford, H. V. Strout, E. . Slater, and C. D. Strader. Synthetic segments of the mammalian beta-adrenergic receptor are preferentially recognized by cAMP-dependent protein kinase and protein kinase C. *Biochem. Biophys. Res. Commun.* 147: 168–173, 1987.

33. Blier, P., and C. De Montigny. Modification of 5HT neuron properties by sustained administration of the 5HT1A agonist gepirone: Electrophysiological studies in the rat brain. *Synapse* 1: 470–480, 1987.

34. Bouvier, M., S. Collins, B. F. O'Dowd, P. T. Campbell, A. De Blasi, B. K. Kobilka, C. MacGregor, G. P. Irons, M. G. Caron, and R. J. Lefkowitz. Two distinct pathways for cAMP-mediated down-regulation of the β2–adrenergic receptor. Phosphorylation of the receptor and regulation of its mRNA level. *J. Biol. Chem.* 264: 16786–16792, 1989.

35. Bouvier, M., W. P. Hausdorff, A. De Blasi, B. F. O'Dowd, B. K. Kobilka, M. G. Caron, and R. J. Lefkowitz. Removal of phosphorylation sites from the β_2-adrenergic receptor delays onset of agonist-promoted desensitization. *Nature* 333: 370–373, 1988.

36. Bouvier, M., L. M. F. Leeb-Lundberg, J. L. Benovic, M. G. Caron, and R. J. Lefkowitz. Regulation of adrenergic receptor function by phosphorylation. II. Effects of agonist occupancy on phosphorylation of alpha 1- and beta 2-adrenergic receptors by protein kinase C and the cyclic AMP-dependent protein kinase. *J. Biol. Chem.* 262: 3106–3113, 1987.

37. Bownds, D., J. Dawes, J. Miller, and M. Stahlman. Phosphorylation of frog photoreceptor membranes induced by light. *Nature* 237: 125–127, 1972.

38. Brass, L. F. Homologous desensitization of HEL cell thrombin receptors. *J. Biol. Chem.* 267: 6044–6050, 1992.

39. Brass, L. F., M. Ahuja, E. Belmonte, S. Pizarro, A. Tarver, and J. A. Hoxie. The human platelet thrombin receptor. Turning it on and turning it off. *Ann. N. Y. Acad. Sci.* 714: 1–12, 1994.

40. Bristow, D. R., P. C. Banford, I. Bajusz, A. Vedat, and J. M. Young. Desensitization of histamine H1 receptor-mediated inositol phosphate accumulation in guinea pig cerebral cortex slices. *Br. J. Pharmacol.* 110: 269–274, 1993.

41. Bristow, D. R., and M. R. Zamani. Desensitization of histamine H1 receptor-mediated inositol phosphate production in HeLa cells. *Br. J. Pharmacol.* 109: 353–359, 1993.

42. Buczylko, J., C. Gutmann, and K. Palczewski. Regulation of rhodopsin kinase by autophosphorylation. *Proc. Natl. Acad. Sci. USA* 88: 2568–2572, 1991.

43. Bullrich, F., T. Druck, P. Kunapuli, J. Gomez, K. W. Gripp, B. Schlegelberger, J. Lasota, L. A. Cannizzaro, K. Huebner, and J. L. Benovic. Chromosomal mapping of the genes GPRK5 and GPRK6 encoding G protein-coupled receptor kinases GRK5 and GRK6. *Cytogenet. Cell Genet.* 70: 250–254, 1995.

44. Calabrese, G., M. Sallese, A. Stornaiuola, E. Morizio, G. Palka, and A. De Blasi. Assignment of the β-arrestin 1 gene (ARRB1) to human chromosone 11q13. *Genomics* 23: 168–171, 1994.

45. Calabrese, G., M. Sallese, A. Stornaiuola, L. Stuppia, G. Palka, and A. De Blasi. Chromosonal mapping of the human arrestin (SAG), β-arrestin2, (ARRB2), and the β-adrenergic receptor kinase 2 (ADRBK2) genes. *Genomics* 23: 286–288, 1994.

46. Campbell, P. T., M. Hnatowich, B. F. O'Dowd, M. G. Caron, R. J. Lefkowitz, and W. P. Hausdorff. Mutations of the human beta 2-adrenergic receptor that impairs coupling to Gs interfere with receptor down-regulation but not sequestration. *Mol. Pharmacol.* 39: 192–198, 1991.

47. Carpene, C., J. Galitzky, P. Collon, F. Esclapez, M. Dauzats, and M. Lafontan. Desensitization of beta-1, beta-2, but not beta-3, adrenoceptor-mediated lipolytic responses of adipo-cytes after long-term norepinephrine infusion. *J. Pharmacol. Exp. Ther.* 265: 237–247, 1993.

48. Cassel, D., H. Levkowitz, and D. Selinger. The regulatory GTPase cycle of turkey erythrocyte adenylate cyclase. *J. Cyclic Nucleotide Res.* 3: 393–406, 1977.

49. Cassel, D., and D. Selinger. Catecholamine-stimulated GTPase activity in turkey erythrocyte membranes. *Biochim. Biophys. Acta* 452: 537–551, 1976.

50. Cassel, D., and D. Selinger. Mechanism of adenylate cyclase activation by cholera toxin: Inhibition of GTPase hydrolysis at the regulatory site. *Proc. Natl. Acad. Sci. USA* 74: 3307–3311, 1977.

51. Cassill, J. A., M. Whitney, C.A.P. Joazeiro, A. Becker, and C. S. Zuker. Isolation of *Drosophila* genes encoding G protein-coupled receptor kinases. *Proc. Natl. Acad. Sci. USA* 88: 11067–11070, 1991.

52. Cerione, R. A., J. W. Regan, H. Nakata, J. Codina, J. L. Benovic, P. Gierschik, R. L. Somers, A. M. Spiegel, L. Birnbaumer, R. L. Lefkowitz, and M. G. Caron. Functional reconstitution of the α2–adrenergic receptor with guanine nucleotide regulatory proteins in phospholipid vesicles. *J. Biol. Chem.* 261: 3901–3909, 1986.

53. Cerione, R. A., C. Staniszewski, J. L. Benovic, R. J. Lefkowitz, and M. G. Caron. Specificity of the functional interactions of the β-adrenergic receptor and rhodopsin with guanine nucleotide regulatory proteins in phospholipid vesicles. *J. Biol. Chem.* 260: 1493–1500, 1985.

54. Chambers, J., J. Park, D. Cronk, C. Chapman, F. R. Kennedy, S. Wilson, and G. Milligan. Beta 3-adrenoceptor agonist-induced down-regulation of Gs alpha and functional desensitization in a Chinese hamster ovary cell line expressing a beta 3-adrenoceptor refractory to down-regulation. *Biochem. J.* 303: 973–978, 1994.

55. Chaudry, A., and J. G. Granneman. Influence of cell type upon the desensitization of the beta 3-adrenergic receptor. *J. Pharmacol. Exp. Ther.* 271: 1253–1258, 1994.

56. Chen, C. -Y., S. D. Dion, C. M. Kim, and J. L. Benovic. β-adrenergic receptor kinase: Agonist-dependent receptor binding promotes kinase activation. *J. Biol. Chem.* 268: 7825–7831, 1993.

57. Chen, Y., and L. Yu. Differential regulation of cAMP-dependent protein kinase and protein kinase C of the æ-opioid receptor coupling to a G protein-activated K^+ channel. *J. Biol. Chem.* 269: 7839–7842, 1994.

58. Chern, Y., H. -L. Lai, J. C. Fong, and Y. Liang. Multiple mechanisms for desensitization of A2a adenosine receptor-mediated cAMP elevation in rat pheochromocytoma PC12 cells. *Mol. Pharmacol.* 44: 950–958, 1993.

59. Cheung, A. H., R. A. Dixon, W. S. Hill, I. S. Sigal, and C. D. Strader. Separation of the structural requirements for agonist-promoted activation and sequestration of the β-adrenergic receptor. *Mol. Pharmacol.* 37: 775–779, 1990.

60. Cheung, A. H., R.R.C. Huang, M. P. Graziano, and C. D. Strader. Specific activation of Gs by synthetic peptides corresponding to an intracellular loop of the beta-adrenergic receptor. *FEBS Lett.* 279: 277–280, 1991.

61. Cheung, A. H., I. S. Sigal, R. A. Dixon, and C. D. Strader. Agonist-promoted sequestration of the beta 2-adrenergic receptor requires regions involved in functional coupling with Gs. *Mol. Pharmacol.* 35: 132–138, 1989.

62. Christie, M. J., J. T. Williams, and R. A. North. Cellular mechanisms of opioid tolerance: studies in single brain neurons. *Mol. Pharmacol.* 32: 633–638, 1987.

63. Chuang, D. -M., and E. Costa. Evidence for internalization of

the recognition site of β-adrenergic receptors during receptor subsensitivity induced by (-) isoproterenol. *Proc. Natl. Acad. Sci. USA* 76: 3024–3028, 1979.

63a. Chuang, T. T., H. LeVine III, and A. De Blasi. Phosphorylation and activation of beta-adrenergic receptor kinase by protein kinase C. *J. Biol. Chem.* 270: 1860–18665, 1995.

63b. Chuang, T. T., L. Paolucci, and A. De Blasi. Inhibition of G protein–coupled receptor kinase by Ca^{2+}/calmodulin. *J. Biol. Chem.* 271: 28691–28696, 1996.

64. Chuang, D. -M., W. J. Kinnier, L. Farber, and E. Costa. A biochemical study of receptor internalization during β-adrenergic receptor desensitization in frog erythrocytes. *Mol. Pharmacol.* 18: 348–355, 1980.

65. Chuang, T. T., M. Sallese, G. Ambrosini, G. Parruti, and A. De Blasi. High expression of β-adrenergic receptor kinase in human peripheral blood leukocytes: Isoproterenol and platelet activating factor can induce kinase translocation. *J. Biol. Chem.* 267: 6886–6892, 1992.

66. Clapham, D. E., and E. J. Neer. New roles for G-protein $\beta\gamma$-dimer in transmembrane signaling. *Nature* 365: 403–406, 1993.

67. Clark, R. B. Desensitization of hormonal stimuli coupled to regulation of cyclic AMP levels. In: *Advances in Cyclic Nucleotide and Protein Phosphorylation Research,* edited by P. Greengard and G. A. Robison. New York: Raven Press, 1986, p. 151–209.

68. Clark, R. B., J. Friedman, R. A. Dixon, and C. D. Strader. Identification of a specific site required for heterologous desensitization of the beta-adrenergic receptor by cAMP-dependent protein kinase. *Mol. Pharmacol.* 36: 343–348, 1989.

69. Clark, R. B., J. Friedman, J. A. Johnson, and M. W. Kunkel. Beta-adrenergic receptor desensitization of wild-type but not cyc- lymphoma cells unmasked by submillimolar Mg2+. *FASEB J.* 1: 289–297, 1987.

70. Clark, R. B., J. Friedman, N. Prashad, and A. E. Ruoho. Epinephrine-induced sequestration of the β-adrenergic receptor in cultured s49 wt and cyc- lymphoma cells. *J. Cyclic Nucleotide Res.* 10: 97–119, 1985.

71. Clark, R. B., M. W. Kunkel, J. Friedman, T. J. Goka, and J. A. Johnson. Activation of cAMP-dependent protein kinase for heterologous desensitization of adenylyl cyclase in s49 wild-type lymphoma cells. *Proc. Natl. Acad. Sci. USA* 85: 1442–1446, 1988.

72. Coleman, D. E., A. Berghuis, E. Lee, M. E. Linder, A. G. Gilman, and S. R. Sprang. Stuctures of the active confirmations of Giα1 and the mechanisms of GTP hydrolysis. *Science* 265: 1405–1412, 1994.

73. Coleman, D. E., E. Lee, M. B. Mixon, M. E. Linder, A. Berghuis, A. G. Gilman, and S. R. Sprang. Crystallization and preliminary crystallography studies of Giα1 and mutants of Giα1 in the GTP and GDP-bound states. *J. Mol. Biol.* 238: 630–638, 1994.

74. Collins, S. Recent perspectives on the molecular structure and regulation of the β2–adrenoceptor. *Life Sci.* 52: 2083–2091, 1993.

75. Collins, S., M. Bouvier, M. A. Bolanowski, M. G. Caron, and R. J. Lefkowitz. cAMP stimulates transcription of the β2–adrenergic receptor gene in response to short-term agonist exposure. *Proc. Natl. Acad. Sci. USA* 86: 4853–4857, 1989.

76. Collins, S., M. G. Caron, and R. J. Lefkowitz. β2–adrenergic receptors in hamster smooth muscle cells are transcriptionally regulated by glucocorticoids. *J. Biol. Chem.* 263: 9067–9070, 1988.

77. Craft, C. M., D. H. Whitmore, and A. F. Wiechmann. Cone arrestin identified by targeting expression of a functional family. *J. Biol. Chem.* 269: 4613–4619, 1994.

78. Crespo, P., N. Xu, W. F. Simonds, and J. S. Gutkind. Ras-dependent activation of MAP kinase pathway mediated by G-protein $\beta\gamma$ subunits. *Nature* 369: 418–420, 1994.

79. Dawson, T. M., J. L. Arriza, D. E. Jaworsky, F. F. Borisy, H. Attramadal, R. J. Lefkowitz, and G. V. Ronnett. β-Adrenergic receptor kinase-2 and β-arrestin2 as mediators of odorant-induced desensitization. *Science* 259: 825–829, 1993.

80. De Blasi, A., G. Parruti, and M. Sallese. Regulation of G protein-coupled receptor kinase subtypes in activated T lymphocytes. *J. Clin. Invest.* 95: 203–210, 1995.

81. DebBurman, S. K., P. Kunapuli, J. L. Benovic, and M. M. Hosey. Agonist-dependent phosphorylation of human muscarinic receptors in insect Sf9 cell membranes by G protein-coupled receptor kinases. *Mol. Pharmacol.* 47: 224–233, 1995.

82. DebBurman, S. K., J. Ptasienski, E. Boetticher, J. W. Lomasney, J. L. Benovic, and M. M. Hosey. Lipid-mediated regulation of G protein-coupled receptor kinases 2 and 3. *J. Biol. Chem.* 270: 5742–5747, 1995.

83. Dickenson, J. M., and S. J. Hill. Homologous and heterologous desensitization of histamine H1– and ATP-receptors in the smooth muscle cell line, DDT1MF-2: the role of protein kinase C. *Br. J. Pharmacol.* 110: 1449–1456, 1993.

84. Diviani, D., A. -L. Lattion, N. Larbi, P. Kunapuli, A. Pronin, J. L. Benovic, and S. Cotecchia. Effect of different G protein-coupled receptor kinases on phosphorylation and desensitization of the alpha1B-adrenergic receptor. *J. Biol. Chem.* 271: 5049–5058, 1996.

85. Dixon, B. S., R. Breckon, C. Burke, and R. J. Anderson. Phorbol esters inhibit adenylate cyclase activity in cultured collecting tubule cells. *Am. J. Physiol.* 254(*Cell Physiol.* 22): C183–C191, 1988.

86. Dixon, R.A.F., B. K. Kobilka, D. J. Strader, J. L. Benovic, H. G. Dohlman, T. Frielle, M. A. Bolanowski, C. D. Bennett, E. Rands, R. E. Diehl, R. A. Mumford, E. E. Slater, I. S. Sigal, M. G. Caron, R. J. Lefkowitz, and C. D. Strader. Cloning of the gene and cDNA for mammalian beta-adrenergic receptor and homology with rhodopsin. *Nature* 321: 75–79, 1986.

87. Dixon, R.A.F., I. S. Sigal, E. Rands, R. B. Register, M. R. Candelore, A. D. Blake, and C. D. Strader. Ligand binding to the β-adrenergic receptor involves its rhodopsin-like core. *Nature* 326: 73–77, 1987.

88. Dohlman, H. G., M. Bouvier, J. L. Benovic, M. G. Caron, and R. J. Lefkowitz. The multiple membrane spanning topography of the beta 2-adrenergic receptor. Localization of the sites of binding, glycosylation, and regulatory phosphorylation by limited proteolysis. *J. Biol. Chem.* 262: 14282–14288, 1987.

89. Doss, R. C., J. P. Perkins, and T. K. Harden. Recovery of β-adrenergic receptors following long term exposure of astrocytoma cells to catecholamines. *J. Biol. Chem.* 256: 12281–12286, 1981.

90. Eason, M. G., M. T. Jacinto, C. T. Theiss, and S. B. Liggett. The palmitoylated cysteine of the cytoplasmic tail of α2a-adrenergic receptors confers subtype-specific agonist-promoted downregulation. *Proc. Natl. Acad. Sci. USA* 91: 11178–11182, 1994.

91. Eason, M. G., H. Kurose, B. D. Holt, J. R. Raymond, and S. B. Liggett. Simultaneous coupling of alpha 2-adrenergic receptors to two G proteins with opposing effects. Subtype-selective coupling of alpha 2C10, alpha 2C4, and alpha 2C2 adrenergic receptors to Gi and Gs. *J. Biol. Chem.* 267: 15795–15801, 1992.

92. Eason, M. G., and S. B. Liggett. Subtype-selective desensitization of alpha 2-adrenergic receptors. Different mechanisms control short and long term agonist-promoted desensitization of alpha 2C10, alpha2C4, and alpha 2C2. *J. Biol. Chem.* 267: 25473–25479, 1992.

93. Eason, M. G., and S. B. Liggett. Functional alpha 2-adrenergic receptor-Gs coupling undergoes agonist-promoted desensitization in a subtype-selective manner. *Biochem. Biophys. Res. Commun.* 193: 318–323, 1993.

94. Eason, M. G., S. P. Moreira, and S. B. Liggett. Four consecutive serines in the third intracellular loop are the sites for beta-adrenergic receptor kinase-mediated phosphorylation and desensitization of the alpha 2A-adrenergic receptor. *J. Biol. Chem.* 270: 4681–4688, 1995.

95. El-Fakahany, E. E., B. E. Alger, W. S. Lai, T. A. Pitler, P. F. Worley, and J. M. Baraban. Neuronal muscarinic responses: role of protein kinase C. *FASEB J.* 2: 2575–2583, 1988.

96. Emorine, L. J., S. Marullo, M. M. Briend-Sutren, G. Patey, K. Tate, C. Delavier-Klutchko, and D. Strosberg. Molecular characterization of the human beta 3-adrenergic receptor. *Science* 245: 1118–1121, 1989.

97. Feng, D. F., and R. F. Doolittle. Progressive sequence alignment as a prerequisite to correct phylogenetic trees. *J. Mol. Evol.* 25: 351–360, 1987.

98. Ferguson, S.S.G., W.E.I. Downey, A.-M. Colapietro, L. S. Barak, L. Menard, and M. G. Caron. Role of β-arrestin in mediating agonist-promoted G protein-coupled receptor internalization. *Science* 271: 363–365, 1996.

99. Ferguson, S.S.G., L. Menard, L. S. Barak, W. J. Koch, A. Colapietro, and M. G. Caron. Role of phosphorylation in agonist-promoted β2–adrenergic receptor sequestration. *J. Biol. Chem.* 270: 24782–24789, 1995.

100. Filtz, T. M., R. P. Artymyshyn, W. Guan, and P. B. Molinoff. Paradoxical regulation of dopamine receptors in transfected 293 cells. *Mol. Pharmacol.* 44: 371–379, 1993.

101. Fishman, P., P. Mallorga, and J. F. Tallman. Catecholamine-induced desensitization of adenylate cyclase in rat glioma C6 cells: Evidence for a specific uncoupling of beta-adrenergic receptors from a functional regulatory component of adenylate cyclase. *Mol. Pharmacol.* 20: 310–318, 1981.

102. Fonseca, M. I., D. C. Button, and R. D. Brown. Agonist regulation of α1b-adrenergic receptor subcellular distribution and function. *J. Biol. Chem.* 270: 8902–8909, 1995.

103. Fowles, C., R. Sharma, and M. Akhtar. Mechanistic studies on the phosphorylation of photoexcited rhodopsin. *FEBS Lett.* 238: 56–60, 1988.

104. Frank, R. N., H. D. Cavanaugh, and K. R. Kenyon. Light-stimulated phosphorylation of bovine visual pigments by adenosine triphosphate. *J. Biol. Chem.* 248: 596–609, 1973.

105. Franke, R. R., T. P. Sakmar, R. M. Graham, and H. G. Khorana. Structure and function of rhodopsin: studies of the interaction between the rhodopsin cytoplasmic domain and transducin. *J. Biol. Chem.* 267: 14767–14774, 1992.

106. Franke, R. R., T. P. Sakmar, D. D. Oprian, and H. G. Khorana. A single amino acid substitution in rhodopsin (lysine 248 leucine) prevents activation of transducin. *J. Biol. Chem.* 263: 2119–2122, 1988.

107. Fraser, C. M., S. Arakawa, W. R. McCombie, and J. C. Venter. Cloning, sequence analysis, and permanent expression of a human alpha 2-adrenergic receptor in Chinese hamster ovary cells. Evidence for independent pathways of receptor coupling to adenylate cyclase attenuation and activation. *J. Biol. Chem.* 264: 11754–11761, 1989.

108. Frederich, R.C.J., G. L. Waldo, T. K. Harden, and J. P. Perkins. Characterization of agonist-induced beta-adrenergic receptor-specific desensitization in C62B glioma cells. *J. Cyclic Nucleotide Res.* 9: 103–118, 1983.

109. Freedman, N. J., S. B. Liggett, D. E. Drachman, G. Pei, M. G. Caron, and R. J. Lefkowitz. Phosphorylation and desensitization of the human β1–adrenergic receptor. *J. Biol. Chem.* 270: 17593–17961, 1995.

110. Fung, B. K., J. B. Hurley, and L. Stryer. Flow of information in the light-triggered cyclic nucleotide cascade of vision. *Proc. Natl. Acad. Sci. USA* 78: 151–156, 1981.

111. Gao, B., and A. G. Gilman. Cloning and expression of a widely distributed (type IV) adenylyl cyclase. *Proc. Natl. Acad. Sci. USA* 89: 10178–10182, 1991.

112. Gates, L. K., C. D. Ulrich, and L. J. Miller. Multiple kinases phosphorylate the pancreatic cholecystokiin receptor in an agonist-dependent manner. *Am. J. Physiol.* 264(*Gastrointest. Liver Physiol.* 33): G840–G847, 1993.

113. Gibbs, J. B. Ras C-terminal processing enzymes-new drug targets? *Cell* 65: 1–4, 1991.

114. Gibson, T. J., M. Hyvonen, A. Musacchio, and M. Saraste. PH domain: The first anniversary. *Trends Biochem. Sci.* 19: 349–353, 1994.

115. Gilman, A. G. G proteins: transducers of receptor-generated signals. *Annu. Rev. Biochem.* 56: 615–649, 1987.

116. Glass, D. B., and E. G. Krebs. Protein phosphorylation catalyzed by cyclic AMP-dependent and cyclic GMP-dependent protein kinases. *Annu. Rev. Pharmacol. Toxicol.* 20: 363–388, 1980.

117. Goldman, P. S., and N. M. Nathanson. Differential role of the carboxyl-terminal tyrosine in down-regulation and sequestration of the m2 muscarinic receptor. *J. Biol. Chem.* 269: 15640–15645, 1994.

118. Golf, S., and V. Hansson. Effects of beta blocking agents on the density of beta-adrenoceptors and adenylate cyclase response in human myocardium: intrinsic sympathomimetic activity favours receptor upregulation. *Cardiovasc. Res.* 20: 637–644, 1986.

119. Gomez, J., and J. L. Benovic. Molecular and regulatory properties of the adenylyl cyclase-coupled β-adrenergic receptors. In: *Molecular Biology of Receptors and Transporters: Receptors,* edited by M. Friedlander and M. Mueckler. New York: Academic Press, Inc., 1992, p. 1–34.

119a. Goodman, O. B. Jr., J. G. Krupnick, V. V. Gurevich, J. L. Benovic, and J. H. Keen. Arrestin/clathrin interaction: localization of the arrestin binding locus to the clathrin terminal domain. *J. Biol. Chem.* 272: 15017–15022, 1997.

119b. Goodman, O. B., J. G. Krupnick, F. Santini, V. V. Gurevich, R. B. Penn, A. Gagnon, J. H. Keen, and J. L. Benovic. β-Arrestin functions as a novel clathrin adaptor protein to promote agonist-specific G protein–coupled receptor internalization. *Nature* 383: 447–450, 1996.

120. Grasso, P., N. Leng, and L. E. Reichert. A synthetic peptide corresponding to the third cytoplasmic loop (residues 533–555) of the testicular follicle-stimulating hormone affects signal transduction in rat testis membranes and in intact cultures rat Sertoli cells. *Mol. Cell. Endocrinol.* 110: 35–41, 1995.

121. Grasso, P., T. A. Santa-Coloma, and L. E. Reichert. Correlation of the follicle-stimulating hormone (FSH) -receptor internalization with the sustained phase of FSH-induced calcium uptake by cultured rat Sertoli cells. *Endocrinology* 131: 2622–2628, 1992.

122. Green, D. A., and R. B. Clark. Adenylate cyclase coupling

proteins are not essential for agonist-specific desensitization of lymphoma cells. *J. Biol. Chem.* 256: 2105–2108, 1981.

123. Green, D. A., J. Friedman, and R. B. Clark. Epinephrine desensitization of adenylate cyclase from cyc- and s49 cultured lymphoma cells. *J. Cyclic Nucleotide Res.* 7: 161–172, 1981.

124. Green, S. A., and S. B. Liggett. A proline-rich region of the third intracellular loop imparts phenotypic β1– versus β2–adrenergic receptor coupling and sequestration. *J. Biol. Chem.* 269: 26215–26219, 1994.

125. Green, S. A., J. Turki, M. Innis, and S. B. Liggett. Amino-terminal polymorphisms in the human β2–adrenergic receptor impart distinct agonist-promoted regulatory properties. *Biochemistry* 33: 9414–9419, 1994.

126. Gudermann, T., M. Birnbaumer, and L. Birnbaumer. Homologous desensitization of the murine luteinizing hormone receptor expressed in L cells. *Mol. Cell. Endocrinol.* 110: 125–135, 1995.

127. Gulati, A., and H. N. Bhargava. Down-regulation of hypothalamic 5–HT1A receptors in morphine-abstinent rats. *Eur. J. Pharmacol.* 182: 253–259, 1990.

128. Gurevich, V. V., and J. L. Benovic. Cell-free expression of visual arrestin: Truncation mutagenesis identifies multiple domains involved in rhodopsin interaction. *J. Biol. Chem.* 267: 21919–21923, 1992.

129. Gurevich, V. V., and J. L. Benovic. Visual arrestin interaction with rhodopsin: Sequential multisite binding ensures strict selectivity toward light-activated phosphorylated rhodopsin. *J. Biol. Chem.* 268: 11628–11638, 1993.

130. Gurevich, V. V., and J. L. Benovic. Visual arrestin binding to rhodopsin. Diverse functional roles of positively charges residues within the phosphorylation-recognition region of arrestin. *J. Biol. Chem.* 270: 6010–6016, 1995.

131. Gurevich, V. V., S. B. Dion, J. J. Onorato, J. Ptasienski, C. M. Kim, R. Sterne-Marr, M. M. Hosey, and J. L. Benovic. Arrestin interactions with G protein-coupled receptors: Direct binding studies of wild-type, truncated, and chimeric arrestins with rhodopsin, β2-adrenergic, and m2 muscarinic cholinergic receptors. *J. Biol. Chem.* 270: 720–731, 1995.

132. Gurevich, V. V., R. M. Richardson, C. M. Kim, M. M. Hosey, and J. L. Benovic. Binding of wild type and chimeric arrestins to the m2 muscarinic cholinergic receptor. *J. Biol. Chem.* 268: 16879–16882, 1993.

133. Hadcock, J. R., and C. C. Malbon. Down-regulation of β-adrenergic receptors: Agonist-induced reduction in receptor mRNA levels. *Proc. Natl. Acad. Sci. USA* 85: 5021–5025, 1988.

134. Hadcock, J. R., J. D. Port, M. S. Gelman, and C. C. Malbon. Cross-talk between tyrosine kinase and G-protein-linked receptors. Phosphorylation of beta 2-adrenergic receptors in response to insulin. *J. Biol. Chem.* 267: 26017–26022, 1992.

135. Hadcock, J. R., H. Wang, and C. C. Malbon. Agonist-induced destabilization of β-adrenergic receptor mRNA. Attenuation of glucocorticoid-induced up-regulation of β-adrenergic receptors. *J. Biol. Chem.* 264: 19928–19933, 1989.

136. Haddad, E.-B., J. Rousell, J. C. W. Mak, and P. J. Barnes. Long-term carbachol treatment-induced down-regulation of muscarinic M2-receptors but not m2 receptor mRNA in a human lung cell line. *Br. J. Pharmacol.* 116: 2027–2032, 1995.

137. Haga, K., and T. Haga. Activation by G protein beta gamma subunits of agonist- or light-dependent phosphorylation of muscarinic acetylcholine receptors and rhodopsin. *J. Biol. Chem.* 267: 2222–2227, 1992.

138. Haga, K., K. Kameyama, and T. Haga. Synergistic activation of a G protein-coupled receptor kinase by G protein βγ subunits and mastoparan or related peptides. *J. Biol. Chem.* 269: 12594–12599, 1994.

139. Haga, T., K. Haga, and K. Kameyama. G protein-coupled receptor kinases. *J. Neurochem.* 63: 400–412, 1994.

140. Hanks, S. K., and A. M. Quinn. Protein kinase catalytic domain sequence database: Identification of conserved features of primary structure and classification of family members. *Meth. Enzymol.* 200: 38–81, 1991.

141. Harden, T. K. Agonist-induced desensitization of the β-adrenergic receptor-linked adenylate cyclase. *Pharmacol. Rev.* 35: 5–32, 1983.

142. Harden, T. K., C. U. Cotton, G. L. Waldo, J. K. Lutton, and J. P. Perkins. Catecholamine-induced alteration in sedimentation behavior of membrane bound β-adrenergic receptors. *Science* 210: 441–443, 1980.

143. Hargrave, P. A., and J. H. McDowell. Rhodopsin and phototransduction: A model system for G protein-linked receptors. *FASEB J.* 6: 2323–2331, 1992.

144. Hargrave, P. A., and J. H. McDowell. Rhodopsin and phototransuction. In: *Molelcular Biology of Receptors and Transporters: Receptors*, edited by M. Frielander and M. Mueckler. New York: Academic Press, 1992, p. 49–98.

145. Haribabu, B., and R. Snyderman. Identification of additional members of human G protein-coupled receptor kinase family. *Proc. Natl. Acad. Sci. USA* 90: 9398–9402, 1993.

146. Harrington, M. A., K. Shaw, P. Zhong, and R. D. Ciaranello. Agonist-induced desensitization and loss of high-affinity binding sites of stably expressed human 5–HT1A receptors. *J. Pharmacol. Exp. Ther.* 268: 1098–1106, 1994.

147. Hausdorff, W. P., M. Bouvier, B. F. O'Dowd, G. P. Irons, M. G. Caron, and R. J. Lefkowitz. Phosphorylation sites on two domains of the β2–adrenergic receptor are involved in distinct pathways of receptor desensitization. *J. Biol. Chem.* 264: 12657–12665, 1989.

148. Hawes, B. E., L. M. Luttrell, S. T. Exum, and R. J. Lefkowitz. Inhibition of G protein-coupled receptor signaling by expression of cytoplasmic domains of the receptor. *J. Biol. Chem.* 269: 15776–15785, 1994.

149. Hawes, B. E., T. van Biesen, W. J. Koch, L. M. Luttrell, and R. J. Lefkowitz. Distinct pathways of Gi- and Gq-mediated mitogen-activated protein kinase activation. *J. Biol. Chem.* 270: 17148–17153, 1995.

150. Hein, L., K. Ishii, S. R. Coughlin, and B. K. Kobilka. Intracellular targeting and trafficking of thrombin receptors. A novel mechanism for resensitization of a G protein-coupled receptor. *J. Biol. Chem.* 269: 27719–27726, 1994.

151. Henderson, R., J. M. Baldwin, T. A. Ceska, T. F. Zemlin, E. Beckman, and K. H. Downing. Model for the structure of bacteriorhodopsin based on high-resolution electron cryomicroscopy. *J. Mol. Biol.* 213: 899–929, 1990.

152. Hertel, C., S. J. Coulter, and J. P. Perkins. A comparison of catecholamine-induced internalization of beta-adrenergic receptors and receptor-mediated endocytosis of epidermal growth factor in human astrocytoma cells. Inhibition by phenylarsine oxide. *J. Biol. Chem* 260: 12547–12553, 1985.

153. Hertel, C., and J. P. Perkins. Receptor-specific mechanisms of desensitization of β-adrenergic receptor function. *Mol. Cell. Endocrinol.* 37: 245–256, 1984.

154. Hertel, C., M. Staehelin, and J. P. Perkins. Evidence for intravesicular β-adrenergic receptors in membrane fractions from desensitized cells: binding of the hydrophilic ligand CGP-12177

only in the presence of alamethicin. *J. Cyclic Nucleotide Res.* 9: 119–128, 1983.

155. Hogger, P., M. S. Shochkley, J. Lameh, and W. Sadee. Activating and inactivating mutations in N- and C-terminal i3 loop junctions of muscarinic acetylcholine hm1 receptors. *J. Biol. Chem.* 270: 7405–7410, 1995.

156. Homburger, V., M. Lucas, B. Cantau, J. Barabe, J. Penit, and J. Bockaert. Further evidence that desensitization of beta-adrenergic-sensitive adenylate cyclase proceeds in two steps. Modification of the coupling and loss of beta-adrenergic receptors. *J. Biol. Chem.* 255: 10436–10444, 1980.

157. Honda, T., H. Adachi, M. Noguchi, S. Sato, S. Onishi, E. Aoki, and K. Torizuka. Carbachol regulates cholecystokinin receptor on pancreatic acinar cells. *Am. J. Physiol.* 252(*Gastrointest. Liver Physiol.* 21): G77–G83, 1987.

158. Hosey, M. M., S. K. DebBurman, R. Pals-Rylaarsdam, R. M. Richardson, and J. L. Benovic. The role of G protein-coupled receptor kinases in the regulation of muscarinic cholinergic receptors. In: *Cholinergic Mechanisms: From Molecular Biology to Clinical Significance (Proceedings of the 9th International Symposium on Cholinergic Mechanisms*, edited by K. Loffelholz and J. Klein. New York: Elsevier, 1996, in press.

159. Hughes, R. J., and P. A. Insel. Agonist-mediated regulation of alpha 1- and beta 2-adrenergic receptor metabolism in a muscle cell line, BC3H-1. *Mol. Pharmacol.* 29: 521–530, 1986.

160. Hyde, D. R., K. L. Mecklenberg, J. A. Pollack, T. S. Vihtelic, and S. Benzer. Twenty *Drosophila* visual system cDNA clones: One is a homolog of human arrestin. *Proc. Natl. Acad. Sci. USA* 87: 1008–1112, 1990.

161. Inglese, J., N. J. Freedman, W. J. Koch, and R. J. Lefkowitz. Structure and mechanism of the G protein-coupled receptor kinases. *J. Biol. Chem.* 268: 23735–23738, 1993.

162. Inglese, J., J. F. Glickman, W. Lorenz, M. G. Caron, and R. J. Lefkowitz. Isoprenylation of a protein kinase: Requirement of farnesylation/α-carboxyl methylation for full enzymatic activity of rhodopsin kinase. *J. Biol. Chem.* 267: 1422–1425, 1992.

163. Inglese, J., W. J. Koch, M. G. Caron, and R. J. Lefkowitz. Isoprenylation in regulation of signal transduction by G-protein-coupled receptor kinases. *Nature* 359: 147–150, 1992.

164. Insel, P. A., L. C. Mahan, H. J. Motulsky, L. M. Stoolman, and A. M. Koachman. Time-dependent decreases in binding affinity of agonists for β-adrenergic receptors of intact s49 lymphoma cells. A mechanism of desensitization. *J. Biol. Chem.* 258: 13597–13605, 1983.

165. Ishii, K., J. Chen, M. Ishii, W. J. Koch, N. J. Freedman, R. J. Lefkowitz, and S. R. Coughlin. Inhibition of thrombin receptor signaling by a G-protein coupled receptor kinase: Functional specficity among G-protein coupled receptor kinases. *J. Biol. Chem.* 269: 1125–1130, 1994.

166. Iyengar, R., M. K. Baht, M. E. Riser, and L. Birnbaumer. Receptor-specific desensitization of the s49 lymphoma cell adenylyl cyclase: Unaltered behavior of the regulatory component. *J. Biol. Chem.* 256: 4810–4815, 1981.

166a. Jaber, M., W. J. Koch, H. Rockman, B. Smith, R. A. Bond, K. K. Sulik, J. Ross Jr., R. J. Lefkowitz, M. G. Caron, and B. Giros. Essential role of beta-adrenergic receptor kinase 1 in cardiac development and function. *Proc. Natl. Acad. Sci. USA* 93: 12974–12979, 1996.

167. Jelsema, C. L., and J. Axelrod. Stimulation of phospholipase A2 activity in bovine rod outer segments by the beta gamma subunits of transducin and its inhibition by the alpha subunit. *Proc. Natl. Acad. Sci. USA* 84: 3623–3627, 1987.

168. Jensen, A. A., U. B. Pedersen, A. Kiemer, N. Din, and P. H. Andersen. Functional importance of the carboxyl tail cysteine residues in the human D1 dopamine receptor. *J. Neurochem.* 65: 1325–1331, 1995.

169. Jewell-Moritz, E. A., and S. B. Liggett. The acidic motif within the intracellular loop of the alpha2C2 adrenergic receptor is required for agonist-promoted phosphorylation and desensitization. *Biochemistry* 34: 11946–11953, 1995.

170. Johnson, G. L., B. B. Wolfe, T. K. Harden, P. B. Molinoff, and J. P. Perkins. Role of β-adrenergic receptors in catecholamine-induced desensitization of adenylate cyclase in human astrocytoma cells. *J. Biol. Chem.* 252: 1472–1480, 1977.

171. Johnson, J. A., R. B. Clark, J. Friedman, R. A. Dixon, and C. D. Strader. Identification of a specific domain in the beta-adrenergic receptor required for phorbol ester-induced inhibition of catecholamine-stimulated adenylyl cyclase. *Mol. Pharmacol.* 38: 289–293, 1990.

172. Johnson, J. A., J. Friedman, R. D. Halligan, M. Birnbaumer, and R. B. Clark. Sensitization of adenylyl cyclase by P2 purinergic and m5 muscarinic receptor agonists in L cells. *Mol. Pharmacol.* 39: 539–546, 1991.

173. Johnson, J. A., T. J. Goka, and R. B. Clark. Phorbol ester-induced augmentation and inhibition of epinephrine-stimulated adenylate cyclase in S49 lymphoma cells. *J. Cyclic Nucleotide Protein Phosphor. Res.* 11: 199–216, 1986.

174. Jones, S.V.P., C. J. Heilman, and M. R. Brann. Functional responses of cloned muscarinic receptors expressed in CHO-K1 cells. *Mol. Pharmacol.* 40: 242–247, 1991.

175. Kakiuchi, S., and T. W. Rall. The influence of chemical agents on the accumulation of adenosine 3′, 5′-phosphate in slices of rabbit cerebellum. *Mol. Pharmacol.* 4: 367–378, 1968.

176. Karoor, V., K. Baltensperger, H. Paul, M. P. Czech, and C. C. Malbon. Phosphorylation of tyrosyl residues 350/354 of the β-adrenergic receptor is obligatory for counterregulatory effects of insulin. *J. Biol. Chem.* 270: 25305–25308, 1995.

177. Kassis, S., and P. H. Fishman. Functional alteration of the β-adrenergic receptor during desensitization of mammalian adenylate cyclase by β-agonists. *Proc. Natl. Acad. Sci. USA* 81: 6686–6690, 1984.

178. Kassis, S. M., M. Olasmaa, M. Sullivan, and P. H. Fishman. Desensitization of the β-adrenergic receptor-coupled adenylate cyclase in cultured mammalian cells: sequestration versus receptor function. *J. Biol. Chem.* 261: 12233–12337, 1986.

179. Katada, T., A. G. Gilman, Y. Watanabe, S. Bauer, and K. H. Jakobs. Protein kinase C phophorylates the inhibitory guanine-nucleotide protein and apparently suppresses its function in hormonal inhibition of adenylate cyclase. *Eur. J. Biochem.* 151: 431–437, 1985.

180. Keen, M., E. Kelly, P. Nobbs, and J. MacDermot. A selective binding site for 3H-NECA that is not an adenosine A2 receptor. *Biochem. Pharmacol.* 38: 3827–3833, 1989.

181. Kelleher, D. J., and G. L. Johnson. Characterization of rhodopsin kinase purified from bovine rod outer segments. *J. Biol. Chem.* 265: 2632–2639, 1990.

182. Kelleher, D. J., J. E. Pessin, A. E. Ruoho, and G. L. Johnson. Phorbol ester induces desensitization of adenylate cyclase and phopshorylation of the β-adrenergic receptor in turkey erythrocytes. *Proc. Natl. Acad. Sci. USA* 81: 4316–4320, 1984.

183. Kelly, E., M. Keen, P. Nobbs, and J. MacDermot. Segregation of discrete Gsα-mediated responses that accompany homologous or heterologous desensitization in two related somatic hybrids. *Br. J. Pharmacol.* 99: 309–316, 1990.

184. Kiely, J., J. R. Hadcock, S. W. Bahouth, and C. C. Malbon. Glucocorticoids down-regulate beta 1-adrenergic receptor ex-

presion by supressing transcription of the receptor gene. *Biochem. J.* 302: 397–403, 1994.

185. Kim, C. M., S. B. Dion, and J. L. Benovic. Mechanism of β-adrenergic receptor kinase activation by G proteins. *J. Biol. Chem.* 268: 15412–15418, 1993.

186. Kim, D., D. L. Lewis, L. Graziadei, E. J. Neer, D. Bar-Sagi, and D. E. Clapham. G-protein beta gamma-subunits activate the cardiac muscarinic K+-channel via phospholipase A2. *Nature* 337: 557–560, 1989.

187. Koch, W. J., J. Inglese, W. C. Stone, and R. J. Lefkowitz. The binding site for the βγ subunits of heterotrimeric G proteins on the β-adrenergic receptor kinase. *J. Biol. Chem.* 268: 8256–8260, 1993.

188. Koch, W. J., H. A. Rockman, P. Samama, R. Hamilton, R. A. Bond, C. Milano, and R. J. Lefkowitz. Cardiac function in mice overexpressing the β-adrenergic receptor kinase or a βARK inhibitor. *Science* 268: 1350–1353, 1995.

189. Kolakowsky, L. F. GCRDb: a G-protein-coupled receptor database. *Receptors Channels* 2: 1–7, 1994.

190. Kong, G., R. Penn, and J. L. Benovic. A β-adrenergic receptor kinase dominant negative mutant attenuates desensitization of the β₂-adrenergic receptor. *J. Biol. Chem.* 269: 13084–13087, 1994.

191. Koschel, K. A hormone-independent rise of adenosine 3′, 5′ -monophosphate desensitizes coupling of β-adrenergic receptors to adenylate cyclase in rat glioma C6–cells. *Eur. J. Biochem.* 108: 163–169, 1980.

192. Krane, A., J. MacDermot, and M. Keen. Desensitization of adenylate cyclase responses following exposure to IP prostanoid receptor agonists. Homologous and heterologous desensitization exhibit the same time course. *Biochem. Pharmacol.* 47: 953–959, 1994.

193. Krane, A., J. Malkhandi, L. Mercy, and M. Keen. The role of protein kinase A and protein kinase C in prostanoid IP receptor desensitization in NG108–15 cells. *Biochim. Biophys. Acta* 1206: 203–207, 1994.

194. Krebs, E. G., and J. A. Beavo. Phosphorylation-dephosphorylation of enzymes. *Annu. Rev. Biochem.* 48: 923–959, 1979.

194a. Krupnick, J. G., O. B. Goodman, Jr., J. H. Keen, and J. L. Benovic. Arrestin/clathrin interaction: localization of the clathrin binding domain of nonvisual arrestins to the C-terminus. *J. Biol. Chem.* 272: 15011–15016, 1997.

195. Kuhn, H. Light-dependent binding of rhodopsin kinase and other proteins to cattle photoreceptor membranes. *Biochemistry* 17: 4389–4395, 1978.

196. Kuhn, H., and W. J. Dreyer. Light dependent phosphorylation of rhodopsin by ATP. *FEBS Lett.* 20: 1–6, 1972.

197. Kuhn, H., S. W. Hall, and U. Wilden. Light-induced binding of 48-kDa protein to photoreceptor membranes is highly enhanced by phosphorylation of rhodopsin. *FEBS Lett.* 176: 473–478, 1984.

198. Kume, H., M. P. Graziano, and M. I. Kotlikoff. Stimulatory and inhibitory regulation of calcium-activated potassium channels by guanine nucleotide-binding proteins. *Proc. Natl. Acad. Sci. USA* 89: 11051–11055, 1992.

199. Kume, H., I. P. Hall, R. J. Washabau, K. Tagaki, and M. I. Kotlikoff. β-adrenergic agonists regulate KCa channels in airway smooth muscle by cAMP-dependent and -independent mechanisms. *J. Clin. Invest.* 93: 371–379, 1994.

200. Kunapuli, P., and J. L. Benovic. Cloning and expression of GRK5: A member of the G protein-coupled receptor kinase family. *Proc. Natl. Acad. Sci. USA* 90: 5588–5592, 1993.

201. Kunapuli, P., V. V. Gurevich, and J. L. Benovic. Phospholipid-stimulated autophosphorylation activates the G protein-coupled receptor kinase GRK5. *J. Biol. Chem.* 269: 10209–10212, 1994.

202. Kunkel, M. T., and E. G. Peralta. Charged amino acids required for signal transduction by the m3 muscarinic acetylcholine receptor. *EMBO J.* 12: 3809–3815, 1993.

203. Kunkel, M. W., J. Friedman, S. Shenolikar, and R. B. Clark. Cell-free heterologous desensitization of adenylyl cyclase in s49 lymphoma cell membranes mediated by cAMP-dependent protein kinase. *FASEB J.* 3: 2067–2074, 1989.

204. Kurz, J. B., and J. P. Perkins. Isoproterenol-initiated β-adrenergic receptor diacytosis in cultured cells. *Mol. Pharmacol.* 41: 375–381, 1992.

205. Kwatra, M. M., J. L. Benovic, M. G. Caron, R. J. Lefkowitz, and M. M. Hosey. Phosphorylation of chick heart muscarinic cholinergic receptors by the β-adrenergic receptor kinase. *Biochemistry* 28: 4543–4547, 1989.

206. Kwatra, M. M., E. Leung, A. C. Maan, K. K. McMahon, J. Ptasienski, R. Green, and M. M. Hosey. Correlation of agonist-induced phosphorylation of chick heart muscarinic receptors with receptor desensitization. *J. Biol. Chem.* 262: 16314–16321, 1987.

207. Kwatra, M. M., J. Ptasienski, and M. M. Hosey. The porcine heart m2 muscarinic receptor: agonist-induced phosphorylation and comparison of properties with chick heart receptor. *Mol. Pharmacol.* 35: 553–558, 1989.

208. Kwatra, M. M., D. A. Schwinn, J. Schreurs, J. L. Blank, C. M. Kim, J. L. Benovic, J. E. Krause, M. G. Caron, and R. J. Lefkowitz. The substance P receptor, which couples to Gq/11, is a substrate of β-adrenergic receptor kinases 1 and 2. *J. Biol. Chem.* 268: 9161–9164, 1993.

209. Lambright, D. G., J. P. Noel, H. E. Hamm, and P. B. Sigler. Structural determinants for activation of the α subunit of a heterotrimeric G protein. *Nature* 369: 621–628, 1994.

210. Lampert, A., M. Nirenberg, and W. A. Klee. Tolerance and dependence evoked by an endogenous opioid peptide. *Proc. Natl. Acad. Sci. USA* 73: 3165–3167, 1976.

211. Lands, A. M., A. Arnold, J. P. McAuliff, F. P. Luduena, and T.G.J. Brown. Differentiation of receptor systems activated by sympathomimetic amines. *Nature* 214: 597–598, 1967.

212. Lattion, A. -L., D. Diviani, and S. Cotecchia. Truncation of the receptor carboxyl terminus impairs agonist-dependent phosphorylation and desensitization of the α1b-adrenergic receptor. *J. Biol. Chem.* 269: 22887–22893, 1994.

213. Law, P. Y., D. S. Hom, and H. H. Loh. Loss of opiate receptor activity in neuroblastoma X glioma cells after chronic opiate treatment. A multi-step process. *Mol. Pharmacol.* 22: 1–4, 1982.

214. Law, P. Y., D. S. Hom, and H. H. Loh. Opiate receptor down-regulation and desensitization in neuroblastoma X glioma NG108–15 hybrid cells are two separate cellular adaptation processes. *Mol. Pharmacol.* 24: 413–424, 1983.

215. Leeb-Lundberg, L. M., S. Cotecchia, A. DeBlasi, M. G. Caron, and R. J. Lefkowitz. Regulation of adrenergic receptor function by phosphorylation. I. Agonist-promoted desensitization and phosphorylation of alpha 1-adrenergic receptors coupled to inositol phospholipid metabolism in DDT1 MF-2 smooth muscle cells. *J. Biol. Chem.* 262: 3098–3105, 1987.

216. Lerrant, Y., M. L. Kottler, F. Bergametti, M. Moumni, T. Blumberg-Tick, and R. Counis. Expression of gonadotropin-releasing hormone receptor gene is altered by GnRH agonist desensitization in a manner similar to that of gonadotropin

beta-subunit genes in normal and castrated rat pituitary. *Endocrinology* 136: 2803–2808, 1995.

217. Leurs, R., M. J. Smit, A. Bast, and H. Timmerman. Homologous histamine H1 receptor desensitization results in reduction of H1 receptor agonist efficacy. *Eur. J. Pharm.* 196: 319–322, 1991.

218. Liao, J. -F., and J. P. Perkins. Differential effects of antimycin A on endocytosis and exocytosis of transferrin also are observed for internalization and externalization of beta-adrenergic receptors. *Mol. Pharmacol.* 44: 364–370, 1993.

219. Liao, J. F. 1990. Characterization of agonist-induced internalization of β-adrenergic receptors and its down-regulation and desensitization. Yale University Ph.D. Thesis.

220. Liggett, S. B., M. Bouvier, W. P. Hausdorff, B. F. O'Dowd, M. G. Caron, and R. J. Lefkowitz. Altered patterns of agonist-stimulated cAMP accumulation in cells expressing mutant β2-adrenergic receptors lacking phosphorylation sites. *Mol. Pharmacol.* 36: 641–646, 1989.

221. Liggett, S. B., N. J. Freedman, D. A. Schwinn, and R. J. Lefkowitz. Structural basis for receptor subtype-specific regulation revealed by a chimeric β3/β2-adrenergic receptor. *Proc. Natl. Acad. Sci. USA* 90: 3665–3669, 1993.

222. Liggett, S. B., J. Ostrowski, L. C. Chesnut, H. Kurose, J. R. Raymond, M. G. Caron, and R. J. Lefkowitz. Sites of the third intracellular loop of the alpha 2A-adrenergic receptor confer short term agonist-promoted desensitization. Evidence for a receptor kinase-mediated mechanism. *J. Biol. Chem.* 267: 4740–4746, 1992.

223. Logothetis, D. E., Y. Karuchi, J. Galper, E. J. Neer, and D. E. Clapham. The βγ subunits of GTP-binding proteins activate the muscarinic K+ channel in heart. *Nature* 325: 321–326, 1987.

224. Lohse, M. J., S. Andexinger, J. Pitcher, S. Trukawinski, J. Codina, J. -P. Faure, M. G. Caron, and R. J. Lefkowitz. Receptor-specific desensitization with purified proteins: Kinase dependence and receptor specificity of β-arrestin and arrestin in the β2-adrenergic receptor and rhodopsin systems. *J. Biol. Chem.* 267: 8558–8564, 1992.

225. Lohse, M. J., J. L. Benovic, M. G. Caron, and R. J. Lefkowitz. β-Arrestin: A protein that regulates β-adrenergic receptor function. *Science* 248: 1547–1550, 1990.

226. Lohse, M. J., J. L. Benovic, M. G. Caron, and R. J. Lefkowitz. Multiple pathways of rapid β2-adrenergic receptor desensitization. Delineation with specific inhibitors. *J. Biol. Chem.* 265: 3202–3209, 1990.

227. Lorenz, W., J. Inglese, K. Palczewski, J. J. Onorato, M. G. Caron, and R. J. Lefkowitz. The receptor kinase family: Primary structure of rhodopsin kinase reveals similarities to the β-adrenergic receptor kinase. *Proc. Natl. Acad. Sci. USA* 88: 8715–8719, 1991.

228. Loudon, B., B. Perussia, and J. L. Benovic. Differentially regulated expression of the G protein-coupled receptor kinases, βARK and GRK6, during myelomonocytic cell development in vitro. *Blood* 88: 4547–4557, 1996.

229. Loudon, R. P., and J. L. Benovic. Expression, purification, and characterization of the G protein-coupled receptor kinase GRK6. *J. Biol. Chem.* 269: 22691–22697, 1994.

230. Luttrell, L. M., J. Ostrowski, S. Cotecchia, H. Kendell, and R. J. Lefkowitz. Antagonism of catecholamine receptor signalling by expression of cytoplasmic domains of the receptors. *Science* 259: 1453–1456, 1993.

231. Mahan, L. C., A. M. Koachman, and P. A. Insel. Do agonists promote rapid internalization of beta-adrenergic receptors? *Proc. Natl. Acad. Sci. USA* 82: 129–133, 1985.

232. Mak, J. K., M. Nishikawa, and P. J. Barnes. Glucocorticosteroids increase β2-adrenergic receptor transcription in human lung. *Am. J. Physiol.* 268: L41–L46, 1995.

233. Mayor, F. J., J. L. Benovic, M. G. Caron, and R. J. Lefkowitz. Somatostatin induces translocation of the β-adrenergic receptor kinase and desensitizes somatostatin receptors in S49 lymphoma cells. *J. Biol. Chem.* 262: 6468–6471, 1987.

234. McGreath, G., I. P. Hall, and S. J. Hill. Agonist-induced desensitization of histamine H1 receptor-mediated inositol phospholipid hydrolysis in human umbilical vein endothelial cells. *Br. J. Pharmacol.* 113: 823–830, 1994.

235. Mickey, J. V., R. Tate, D. Mullikan, and R. J. Lefkowitz. Regulation of adenylate cyclase-coupled β-adrenergic receptor binding sites by beta-adrenergic catecholamines in vitro. *Mol. Pharmacol.* 12: 409–419, 1975.

236. Minegishi, T., S. Igarashi, K. Nakamura, M. Nakamura, M. Tano, H. Shinozaki, K. Miyamoto, and Y. Ibuki. Functional expression of the recombinant human FSH receptor. *J. Endocrinol.* 141: 369–375, 1994.

237. Morishima, I., W. J. Thompson, G. A. Robinson, and S. J. Strada. Loss and restoration of sensitivity to epinephrine in cultured BHK cells: effect of inhibitors of RNA and protein synthesis. *Mol. Pharmacol.* 18: 370–378, 1980.

238. Mukherjee, C., M. G. Caron, and R. J. Lefkowitz. Catecholamine-induced subsensitivity of adenylate cyclase associated with a loss of β-adrenergic receptor binding sites. *Proc. Natl. Acad. Sci. USA* 72: 1945–1949, 1975.

239. Munshi, R., I. -H. Pang, P. C. Sternweis, and J. Linden. A1 adenosine receptors of bovine brain couple to guanine nucleotide-binding proteins Gi1, Gi2, and Go. *J. Biol. Chem.* 266: 22285–22289, 1991.

240. Murakami, A., T. Yajima, H. Sakuma, M. McLaren, and G. Inana. X-arrestin: a new retinal arrestin mapping to the X chromosome. *FEBS Lett.* 334: 203–209, 1993.

241. Musacchio, A., T. Gibson, P. Rice, J. Thompson, and M. Saraste. The PH domain: A common piece in the structural patchwork of signalling proteins. *Trends Biochem. Sci.* 18: 343–348, 1993.

242. Nantel, F., H. Bonin, L. J. Emorine, V. Zilberfarb, A. D. Strosberg, M. Bouvier, and S. Marullo. The human β3-adrenergic receptor is resistant to short term agonist-promoted desensitization. *Mol. Pharmacol.* 43: 548–555, 1993.

243. Nantel, F., M. Bouvier, D. Strosberg, and S. Marullo. Functional effects of long-term activation on human beta 2-adrenoceptor signalling. *Br. J. Pharmacol.* 114: 1045–1051, 1995.

244. Nantel, F., S. Marullo, S. Krief, A. D. Strosberg, and M. Bouvier. Cell-specific down-regulation of the beta 3-adrenergic receptor. *J. Biol. Chem.* 269: 13148–13155, 1994.

245. Nathanson, N. M., W. L. Klein, and M. Nirenberg. Regulation of adenylate cyclase activity mediated by muscarinic acetylcholine receptors. *Proc. Natl. Acad. Sci. USA* 75: 1788–7891, 1978.

246. Nebigil, C. G., M. N. Garnovskaya, S. J. Casanas, J. G. Mulheron, E. M. Parker, T. W. Gettys, and J. R. Raymond. Agonist-induced desensitization and phosphorylation of human 5-HT1A receptor expressed in sf9 insect cells. *Biochemistry* 34: 11954–11962, 1995.

247. Neer, E. J. G proteins: critical control points for transmembrane signals. *Protein Sci.* 3: 3–14, 1994.

248. Neer, E. J. Heterotrimeric G Proteins: Organizers of transmembrane signals. *Cell* 80: 249–257, 1995.

249. Neubig, R. R. Membrane organization in G-protein mechanisms. *FASEB J.* 8: 939–946, 1994.

250. Newman, K. B., J. R. Michael, and A. M. Feldman. Phorbol ester-induced inhibition of the beta-adrenergic system in pulmonary endothelium: Role of pertussis toxin-senstitive protein. *Am. J. Respir. Cell. Mol. Biol.* 1: 517–523, 1989.

251. Ng, G. Y., B. Mouillac, S. R. George, M. Caron, and M. Dennis. Desensitization, phosphorylation, and palmitoylation of the human D1 dopamine receptor. *Eur. J. Pharmacol.* 267: 7–19, 1994.

252. Noda, C., F. Shinjyo, A. Tomomura, S. Kato, T. Nakamura, and A. Ichihara. Mechanism of heterologous desensitization of the adenylate cyclase system by glucagon in primary cultures of adult rat hepatocytes. *J. Biol. Chem.* 259: 7747–7754, 1984.

253. Northup, J. K., M. D. Smigel, P. C. Sternweis, and A. G. Gilman. The subunits of the stimulatory regulatory components of adenylate cyclase. *J. Biol. Chem.* 258: 11369–11376, 1983.

254. O'Dowd, B. F., M. Hnatowich, J. W. Regan, W. M. Leader, M. G. Caron, and R. J. Lefkowitz. Site-directed mutagenesis of the cytoplasmic domains of the human β-adrenergic receptor. Localization of regions involved in G protein receptor coupling. *J. Biol. Chem.* 263: 15985–15992, 1988.

255. Ofori, S., O. Bugnon, and M. Schorderet. Agonist-induced desensitization of dopamine D-1 receptors in bovine retina and rat striatum. *J. Pharmacol. Exp. Ther.* 266: 350–357, 1993.

256. Okamoto, T., Y. Murayama, Y. Hayashi, M. Inagaki, E. Ogata, and I. Nishimoto. Identification of a Gs activator region of the β2–adrenergic receptor that is autoregulated via protein kinase A-dependent phosphorylation. *Cell* 67: 723–730, 1991.

257. Onorato, J. J., M. E. Gillis, Y. Liu, J. L. Benovic, and A. E. Ruoho. The β-adrenergic receptor kinase (GRK2) is regulated by phospholipids. *J. Biol. Chem.* 270: 21346–21353, 1995.

258. Onorato, J. J., K. Palczewski, J. Regan, M. Caron, R. J. Lefkowitz, and J. L. Benovic. Role of acidic amino acids in peptide substrates of the beta-adrenergic receptor kinase and rhodopsin kinase. *Biochemistry* 30: 5118–5125, 1991.

259. Ozcelebi, F., and L. J. Miller. Phosphopeptide mapping of cholecystokinin receptors on agonist-stimulated native pancreatic acinar cells. *J. Biol. Chem.* 270: 3435–3441, 1995.

260. Palczewski, K., A. Arendt, J. H. McDowell, and R. A. Hargrave. Substrate recognition determinants for rhodopsin kinase: Studies with synthetic peptides, polyanions, and polycations. *Biochemistry* 28: 8764–8770, 1989.

261. Palczewski, K., and J. L. Benovic. G-protein-coupled receptor kinases. *Trends Biochem. Sci.* 16: 387–391, 1991.

262. Palczewski, K., J. Buczylko, L. Lebioda, J. W. Crabb, and A. S. Polans. Identification of the N-terminal region in rhodopsin kinase involved in its interaction with rhodopsin. *J. Biol. Chem.* 268: 6004–6013, 1993.

263. Palczewski, K., J. H. McDowell., and P. A. Hargrave. Rhodopsin kinase: Substrate specificity and factors that influence activity. *Biochemistry* 27: 2306–2313, 1988.

264. Palmer, T. M., J. L. Benovic, and G. L. Stiles. Molecular basis for subtype-specific desensitization of inhibitory adenosine receptors: Analysis of a chimeric A1–A3 adenosine receptor. *J. Biol. Chem.* 271: 15272–15278, 1996.

265. Palmer, T. M., T. W. Gettys, K. A. Jacobson, and G. L. Stiles. Desensitization of the canine A2a adenosine receptor: Delineation of multiple processes. *Mol. Pharmacol.* 45: 21082–21094, 1994.

266. Palmer, T. M., T. W. Gettys, and G. L. Stiles. Differential interaction with and regulation of multiple G-proteins by the rat A3 adenosine receptor. *J. Biol. Chem.* 270: 16895–16902, 1995.

267. Pals-Rylaarsdam, R., Y. Xu, P. Witt-Enderby, J. L. Benovic, and M. M. Hosey. Desensitization and internalization of the m2 muscarinic acetylcholine receptor are directed by independent mechanisms. *J. Biol. Chem.* 270: 29004–29011, 1995.

268. Paris, S., I. Magnoldo, and J. Pouyssegar. Homologous desensitization of thrombin-induced phosphoinositide breakdown in hamster lung fibroblasts. *J. Biol. Chem.* 263: 11250–11256, 1988.

269. Parruti, G., F. Peracchia, M. Sallese, G. Ambrosini, M. Masini, D. Rotilio, and A. De Blasi. Molecular analysis of human β-arrestin-1: cloning, tissue distribution, and regulation of expression. Identification of two isoforms generated by alternative splicing. *J. Biol. Chem.* 268: 9753–9761, 1993.

270. Parsons, W. J., and G. L. Stiles. Heterologous desensitization of the inhibitory A1 adenosine receptor-adenylate cyclase system in rat adipocytes. Regulation of both Ns and Ni. *J. Biol. Chem* 262: 841–847, 1987.

271. Pei, G., B. L. Kieffer, R. J. Lefkowitz, and N. J. Freedman. Agonist-dependent phosphorylation of the mouse δ-opioid receptor: involvement of G protein-coupled receptor kinases but not protein kinase C. *Mol. Pharmacol.* 48: 173–177, 1995.

272. Penn, R. B., and J. L. Benovic. Structure of the human gene encoding the β-adrenergic receptor kinase. *J. Biol. Chem.* 269: 14924–14930, 1994.

273. Penn, R. B., S. G. Kelsen, and J. L. Benovic. Regulation of β-agonist- and prostaglandin E2-mediated adenylyl cyclase activity in human airway epithelial cells. *Am. J. Respir. Cell Mol. Biol.* 11: 496–505, 1994.

274. Penn, R. B., J. R. Shaver, J. G. Zangrilli, J. E. Fish, S. P. Peters, and J. L. Benovic. Effects of inflammation and acute beta-agonist inhalation on β2–adrenergic receptor signaling in human airways. *Am. J. Physiol. (Lung Cell. Mol. Physiol. 15)* L601–L608, 1996.

275. Pike, L. J., and R. J. Lefkowitz. Use of cell fusion techniques to probe the mechanism of catecholamine-induced desensitization of adenylate cyclase in frog erythrocytes. *Biochim. Biophys. Acta* 632: 354–365, 1980.

276. Pippig, S., S. Andexinger, K. Daniel, M. Puzicha, M. G. Caron, R. J. Lefkowitz, and M. J. Lohse. Overexpression of β-arrestin and β-adrenergic receptor kinase augment desensitization of β2-adrenergic receptor. *J. Biol. Chem.* 268: 3201–3298, 1993.

277. Pippig, S., S. Andexinger, and M. J. Lohse. Sequestration and recycling of beta 2-adrenergic receptors permit receptor resensitization. *Mol. Pharmacol.* 47: 666–676, 1995.

278. Pitcher, J. A., J. Inglese, J. B. Higgins, J. L. Arriza, P. J. Casey, C. Kim, J. L. Benovic, M. M. Kwatra, M. G. Caron, and R. J. Lefkowitz. Role of βγ subunits of G proteins in targeting the β-adrenergic receptor kinase to membrane-bound receptors. *Science* 257: 1264–1267, 1992.

279. Pitcher, J. A., K. Touhara, E. S. Payne, and R. J. Lefkowitz. Pleckstrin homology domain-mediated membrane association and activation of the β-adrenergic receptor kinase requires coordinate interaction with Gβγ subunits and lipid. *J. Biol. Chem.* 270: 11707–11710, 1995.

280. Pittman, R. N., and P. B. Molinoff. Interactions of agonists and antagonists with β-adrenergic receptors on intact L6 muscle cells. *J. Cyclic Nucleotide Res.* 6: 421–435, 1980.

281. Pleus, R. C., and D. B. Bylund. Desensitization and downregulation of the 5–hydroxytryptamine1B receptor in the opossum kidney cell line. *J. Pharmacol. Exp. Ther.* 261: 271–277, 1992.

281a. Post, S. R., O. Aguila-Buhain, and P. A. Insel. A key role for protein kinase A in homologous desensitization of the beta 2-adrenergic receptor pathway in S49 lymphoma cells. *J. Biol. Chem.* 271: 895–900, 1996.

282. Prather, P. L., A. W. Tsai, and P. Y. Law. Mu and delta opioid receptor desensitization in undifferentiated human neuroblastoma SHSY5Y cells. *Mol. Pharmacol.* 270: 177–184, 1994.

283. Premont, R. T., W. J. Koch, J. Inglese, and R. J. Lefkowitz. Identification, purification, and characterization of GRK5, a member of the family of G protein-coupled receptor kinases. *J. Biol. Chem.* 269: 6832–6841, 1994.

284. Premont, R. T., A. D. Macrae, R. H. Stoffel, N. Chung, J. A. Pitcher, C. Ambrose, J. Inglese, M. E. MacDonald, and R. J. Lefkowitz. Characterization of the G protein-coupled receptor kinase GRK4. Identification of four splice variants. *J. Biol. Chem.* 271: 6403–6410, 1996.

285. Proll, M. A., R. B. Clark, T. J. Goka, R. Barber, and R. W. Butcher. β-adrenergic receptor levels and function after growth of s49 lymphoma cells in low concentrations of epinephrine. *Mol. Pharmacol.* 42: 116–122, 1992.

286. Pronin, A. N., and J. L. Benovic. Regulation of the G protein–coupled receptor kinase GRK5 by protein kinase C *J. Biol. Chem.* 272: 3806–3812, 1997.

287. Pronin, A. N., and N. Gautam. Interaction between G-protein beta and gamma subunit types is selective. *Proc. Natl. Acad. Sci. USA* 89: 6220–6224, 1992.

287a. Pronin, A. N., D. K. Satpaev, V. Z. Slepak, and J. L. Benovic. Regulation of G protein–coupled receptor kinases by calmodulin and localization of calmodulin binding domain. In preparation.

288. Prost, A., S. Emami, and C. Gespach. Desensitization by histamine of H2 receptor-mediated adenylate cyclase activation in the human gastric cancer cell line HGT-1. *FEBS Lett.* 177: 227–230, 1984.

289. Puttfarcken, P. S., L. L. Werling, and B. M. Cox. Effects of chronic morphine exposure on opioid inhibition of adenylyl cyclase in 7315C cell membranes: a useful model for the study of tolerance at mu opioid receptors. *Mol. Pharmacol.* 33: 520–527, 1988.

290. Pyne, N. J., G. J. Murphy, G. Milligan, and M. D. Houslay. Treatment of intact hepatocytes with either the phorbol ester TPA or glucagon elicits the phosphorylation and functional inactivation of the inhibitory guanine nucleotide regulatory protein Gi. *FEBS Lett.* 243: 77–82, 1989.

291. Ramkumar, V., M. E. Olah, K. A. Jacobson, and G. L. Stiles. Distinct pathways of desensitization of A1– and A2–adenosine receptors in DDT1 MF-2 cells. *Mol. Pharmacol.* 40: 639–647, 1991.

292. Rapaport, B., K. D. Kaufman, and G. D. Chalzenbalk. Cloning of a member of the arrestin family from a human thyroid cDNA library. *Mol. Cell. Endocrinol.* 84: R39–R43, 1992.

293. Ray, K., C. Kunsch, L. M. Bonner, and J. D. Robishaw. Isolation of cDNA clones encoding eight different human G protein gamma subunits, including three novel forms designated the gamma 4, gamma 10, and gamma 11 subunits. *J. Biol. Chem.* 270: 21765–21771, 1995.

294. Raymond, J. R. Protein kinase C induces phosphorylation and desensitization of the human 5–HT1A receptor. *J. Biol. Chem.* 266: 14747–14753, 1991.

295. Raynor, K., H. Kong, J. Hines, G. Kong, J. Benovic, K. Yasuda, G. I. Bell, and T. Reisine. Molecular mechanisms of agonist-induced desensitization of the cloned mouse kappa opioid receptor. *J. Pharmacol. Exp. Ther.* 270: 1381–1386, 1994.

296. Reihsaus, M., M. Innis, N. MacIntyre, and S. B. Liggett. Mutations in the gene encoding the β2–adrenergic receptor in normal and asthmatic subjects. *Am. J. Respir. Cell. Mol. Biol.* 8: 334–339, 1993.

297. Reilly, T. M., and M. Blecher. On the mechanism of isoproterenol-induced desensitization of adenylate cyclase in cultured differentiated hepatocytes. *Biochim. Biophys. Acta* 720: 126–132, 1982.

298. Rens-Domiano, S., and H. E. Hamm. Structural and functional properties of heterotrimeric G-proteins. *FASEB J.* 9: 1059–1066, 1995.

299. Rich, K. A., J. Codina, G. Floyd, R. Sekura, J. D. Hildebrandt, and R. Iyengar. Glucagon-induced heterologous desensitization of the MDCK cell adenylyl cyclase. *J. Biol. Chem.* 259: 7893–7901, 1984.

300. Richardson, R. M., and M. M. Hosey. Agonist-induced phosphorylation and desensitization of human m2 muscarinic acetylcholine receptors in sf9 insect cells. *J. Biol. Chem.* 267: 22249–22255, 1992.

301. Rodriguez, M. C., Y. B. Xie, H. Wang, K. Collision, and D. L. Segaloff. Effects of truncations of the cytoplasmic tail of the luteinizing hormone/ chorionic gonadotropin receptor on receptor-mediated internalization. *Mol. Endocrinol.* 6: 327–336, 1992.

302. Roettger, B. F., R. U. Rentsch, D. Pinon, E. Holicky, E. Hadac, J. M. Larkin, and L. J. Miller. Dual pathways of internalization of the cholecystokinin receptor. *J. Cell Biol.* 128: 1029–1041, 1995.

303. Ross, E. M., A. C. Howlett, K. M. Ferguson, and A. G. Gilman. Reconstitution of hormone-sensitive adenylate cyclase activity with resolved components of the enzyme. *J. Biol. Chem.* 253: 6401–6412, 1978.

304. Roth, N. S., P. T. Campbell, M. G. Caron, R. J. Lefkowitz, and M. J. Lohse. Comparative rates of desensitization of β-adrenergic receptors by the β-adrenergic receptor kinase and the cyclic AMP-dependent protein kinase. *Proc. Natl. Acad. Sci. USA* 88: 6201–6204, 1991.

305. Rubenstein, R. R., M. E. Linder, and E. M. Ross. Selectivity of the β-adrenergic receptor among Gs, Gi's, and Go: Assay using recombinant α subunits in reconstituted phospholipid vesicles. *Biochemistry* 30: 10769–10777, 1991.

306. Sallese, M., M. S. Lombardi, and A. De Blasi. Two isoforms of G protein-coupled receptor kinase 4 identified by molecular cloning. *Biochem. Biophys. Res. Commun.* 199: 848–854, 1994.

307. Salomon, Y., C. Londos, and M. Rodbell. A highly sensitive adenylate cyclase assay. *Anal. Biochem.* 58: 541–548, 1974.

308. Sanchez-Yague, J., R. W. Hipkin, and M. Ascoli. Biochemical properties of the agonist-induced desensitization of the follicle-stimulating hormone and luteinizing hormone/chorionic gonadotropin-responsive adenylyl cyclase in cells expressing the recombinant gonadotropin receptors. *Endcrnology* 132: 1007–1016, 1993.

309. Sanchez-Yague, J., M. C. Rodriguez, D. L. Segaloff, and M. Ascoli. Truncation of the cytoplasmic tail of the lutropin/choriogonadotropin receptor prevents agonist-induced coupling. *J. Biol. Chem.* 267: 7217–7220, 1992.

310. Sawutz, D. G., K. Kalinyak, J. A. Whitsett, and C. L. Johnson. Histamine H2 receptor desensitization in HL-60 human promyelocytic leukemia cells. *J. Pharmacol. Exp. Ther.* 231: 1–7, 1984.

311. Schertler, G. F., C. Villa, and R. Henderson. Projection structure of rhodopsin. *Nature* 362: 770–772, 1993.

312. Schleicher, A., H. Kuhn, and K. P. Hofmann. Kinetics, binding constant, and activation energy of the 48-kDa protein-rhodopsin complex by extra-metarhodopsin II. *Biochemistry* 28: 1770–1775, 1989.

313. Schleicher, S., I. Boekhoff, J. Arriza, R. J. Lefkowitz, and H. Breer. A β-adrenergic kinase-like enzyme is involved in olfac-

tory signal termination. *Proc. Natl. Acad. Sci. USA* 90: 1420–1424, 1993.

314. Schmidt, C. J., T. C. Thomas, M. A. Levine, and E. J. Neer. Specificity of G protein β and γ subunit interactions. *J. Biol. Chem.* 267: 13807–13810, 1992.

315. Schreurs, J., M. O. Dailey, and H. Schulman. Pharmacological characterization of histamine H2 receptors on clonal cytolytic T lymphocytes. Evidence for histamine-induced desensitization. *Biochem. Pharmacol.* 33: 3375–3382, 1984.

316. Schubert, B., A. M. VanDongen, G. E. Kirsch, and A. M. Brown. Beta-adrenergic inhibition of cardiac sodium channels by dual G-protein pathways. *Science* 245: 516–519, 1989.

317. Schwarz, R. D., R. E. Davis, J. C. Jaen, C. J. Spencer, H. Tecle, and A. J. Thomas. Characterization of muscarinic receptors in recombinant cell lines. *Life Sci.* 52: 465–472, 1993.

318. Senogles, S. E., A. M. Spiegel, E. Padrell, R. Iyengar, and M. G. Caron. Specificity of receptor-G protein interactions. *J. Biol. Chem.* 265: 4507–4514, 1990.

319. Shapiro, R. A., and N. M. Nathanson. Deletion analysis of the mouse m1 muscarinic acetylcholine receptor: effects on phosphoinositide metabolism and down-regulation. *Biochemistry* 28: 8946–8950, 1989.

320. Sharma, S. K., W. A. Klee, and M. Nirenberg. Dual regulation of adenylate cyclase for narcotic dependence and tolerance. *Proc. Natl. Acad. Sci. USA* 72: 3092–3096, 1975.

321. Shear, M., P. A. Insel, K. L. Melmon, and P. Coffino. Agonist-specific refractoriness induced by isoproterenol. A study with mutant cells. *J. Biol. Chem.* 251: 7572–7576, 1976.

322. Shi, W., S. Osawa, C. D. Dickerson, and E. R. Weiss. Rhodopsin mutants discriminate sites important for the activation of rhodopsin kinase and Gt. *J. Biol. Chem.* 270: 2112–2119, 1995.

323. Shih, M., and C. C. Malbon. Oligodeoxynucleotides antisense to mRNA encoding protein kinase A, protein kinase C, and β-adrenergic receptor kinase reveal distinctive cell-type specific roles in agonist-induced desensitization. *Proc. Natl. Acad. Sci. USA* 91: 12193–12197, 1994.

324. Shinohara, T., B. Dietzschold, C. M. Craft, G. Wistow, J. J. Early, L. A. Donoso, J. Horwitz, and R. Tao. Primary and secondary structure of bovine retinal S antigen (48–kDa protein). *Proc. Natl. Acad. Sci. USA* 84: 6975–6979, 1987.

325. Shorr, R. G. L., R. J. Lefkowitz, and M. G. Caron. Purification of the beta-adrenergic receptor. Identification of the hormone binding subunit. *J. Biol. Chem.* 256: 5820–5826, 1981.

326. Shorr, R. G. L., M. W. Strohsacker, T. N. Lavin, R. J. Lefkowitz, and M. G. Caron. The beta 1-adrenergic receptor of the turkey erythrocyte. Molecular heterogeneity revealed by purification and photoaffinity labeling. *J. Biol. Chem.* 257: 12341–12350, 1982.

327. Sibley, D. R., D. Keifer, C. D. Strader, and R. J. Lefkowitz. Phosphorylation of the beta-adrenergic receptor in intact cells: relationship to heterologous and homologous mechanisms of adenylate cyclase desensitization. *Arch. Biochem. Biophys.* 258: 24–32, 1987.

328. Sibley, D. R., P. Nambi, J. R. Peters, and R. J. Lefkowitz. Phorbol diesters promote beta-adrenergic receptor phosphorylation and adenylate cyclase desensitization in duck erythrocytes. *Biochem. Biophys. Res. Commun.* 121: 973–979, 1984.

329. Sibley, D. R., J. R. Peters, P. Nambi, M. G. Caron, and R. J. Lefkowitz. Desensitization of the turkey erythrocyte adenylate cyclase. β-adrenergic receptor phosphorylation is correlated with attenuation of adenylate cyclase activity. *J. Biol. Chem.* 259: 9742–9749, 1984.

330. Sibley, D. R., R. H. Strasser, J. L. Benovic, K. Daniel, and R.

J. Lefkowitz. Phosphorylation/dephosphorylation of the β-adrenergic receptor regulates its functional coupling to adenylate cyclase and subcellular distribution. *Proc. Natl. Acad. Sci. USA* 83: 9408–9412, 1986.

331. Sibley, D. R., R. H. Strasser, M. G. Caron, and R. J. Lefkowitz. Homologous desensitization of adenylate cyclase is associated with phosphorylation of the β-adrenergic receptor. *J. Biol. Chem.* 260: 3883–3886, 1985.

332. Simon, M. I., M. P. Strathmann, and N. Gautam. Diversity of G proteins in signal transduction. *Science* 252: 802–808, 1991.

333. Simpson, A., and T. Pfeuffer. Functional desensitization of β-adrenergic receptors of avian erythrocytes by catecholamines and adenosine 3′, 5′ phosphate. *Eur. J. Biochem.* 111: 111–116, 1980.

334. Smith, D. P., B. H. Sheih, and C. S. Zuker. Isolation and structure of an arrestin gene from *Drosophila*. *Proc. Natl. Acad. Sci. USA* 87: 1003–1007, 1990.

335. Smith, W. C., A. H. Milam, D. Dugger, A. Arendt, P. A. Hargrave, and K. Palczewski. A splice variant of arrestin: Molecular cloning and localization in bovine retina. *J. Biol. Chem.* 269: 15407–15410, 1994.

336. Somers, R. L., and D. C. Klein. Rhodopsin kinase activity in the mammalian pineal and other tissues. *Science* 226: 182–184, 1984.

337. Sondek, J., D. G. Lambright, J. P. Noel, H. E. Hamm, and P. B. Sigler. GTPase mechanism of G proteins from the 1.7–A crystal structure of transducin alpha-GDPAlF-4. *Nature* 372: 276–279, 1994.

338. Stadel, J. M., A. De Lean, D. Mullikin-Kilpatrick, D. D. Sawyer, and R. J. Lefkowitz. Catecholamine-induced desensitization in turkey erythrocytes: cAMP mediated impairment of high affinity agonist binding without alteration in receptor number. *J. Cyclic Nucleotide Res.* 7: 37–47, 1981.

339. Stadel, J. M., P. Nambi, T. N. Lavin, S. L. Heald, M. G. Caron, and R. J. Lefkowitz. Catecholamine-induced desensitization of turkey erythrocyte adenylate cyclase. *J. Biol. Chem.* 257: 9242–9245, 1982.

340. Stadel, J. M., P. Nambi, R. G. L. Shorr, D. F. Sawyer, M. G. Caron, and R. J. Lefkowitz. Catecholamine-induced desensitization of turkey erythrocyte adenylate cyclase is associated with phosphorylation of the β-adrenergic receptor. *Proc. Natl. Acad. Sci. USA* 80: 3173–3177, 1983.

341. Stadel, J. M., B. Strulovici, P. Nambi, T. N. Lavin, M. M. Briggs, M. G. Caron, and R. J. Lefkowitz. Desensitization of the β-adrenergic receptor of frog erythrocytes. Recovery and characterization of the down-regulated receptors in sequestered vesicles. *J. Biol. Chem.* 258: 3032–3038, 1983.

342. Staehelin, M., and C. Hertel. [3H] CGP-12177, a beta-adrenergic ligand suitable for measuring cell surface receptors. *J. Recept. Res.* 3: 35–43, 1983.

343. Staehelin, M., P. Simons, J. K., and N. Wigger. CGP12177. A hydrophilic β-adrenergic receptor radioligand reveals high affinity binding of agonists to intact cells. *J. Biol. Chem.* 258: 3496–3502, 1983.

344. Sterne-Marr, R., Gurevich, V. V., Goldsmith, P., Bodine, R. C., Sanders, C., Donoso, L. A., and Benovic, J. L. Polypeptide variants of β-arrestin and arrestin3. *J. Biol. Chem.* 268: 15640–15648, 1993.

345. Sterne-Marr, R., and J. L. Benovic. Regulation of G protein-coupled receptors by receptor kinases and arrestins. In: *Vitamins and Hormones*, edited by G. Litwack. New York: Academic Press, 1995, p. 193–234.

346. Stoffel, R. H., R. R. Randall, R. T. Premont, R. J. Lefkowitz, and J. Inglese. Palmitoylation of G protein-coupled receptor

kinase, GRK6: Lipid modification diversity in the GRK family. *J. Biol. Chem.* 269: 27791–27794, 1994.

347. Strader, C. D., R. A. F. Dixon, A. H. Cheung, M. R. Candelore, A. D. Blake, and I. S. Sigal. Mutations that uncouple the β-adrenergic receptor from Gs and increase agonist affinity. *J. Biol. Chem.* 262: 16439–16443, 1987.

348. Strader, C. D., T. M. Fong, M. P. Graziano, and M. R. Tota. The family of G-protein-coupled receptors. *FASEB J.* 9: 745–754, 1995.

349. Strader, C. D., T. M. Fong, M. R. Tota, D. Underwood, and R. A. F. Dixon. Structure and function of G protein-coupled receptors. In: *Annual Review of Biochemistry,* edited by C. C. Richardson, J. N. Abelson, A. Meister and C. T. Walsh. Palo Alto, CA: Annual Reviews, Inc., 1994, p. 101–132.

350. Strader, C. D., I. S. Sigal, A. D. Blake, A. H. Cheung, R. B. Register, E. Rands, B. A. Zemcik, M. R. Candelore, and R. A. Dixon. The carboxyl terminus of the hamster beta-adrenergic receptor expresed in mouse L cells is not required for receptor sequestration. *Cell* 49: 855–863, 1987.

351. Strasser, R. H., J. L. Benovic, M. C. Caron, and R. J. Lefkowitz. β-Agonist- and prostaglandin E$_1$-induced translocation of the β-adrenergic receptor kinase: Evidence that the kinase may act on multiple adenylate cyclase-coupled receptors. *Proc. Natl. Acad. Sci. USA* 83: 6362–6366, 1986.

352. Strasser, R. H., D. R. Sibley, and R. J. Lefkowitz. A novel catecholamine-activated adenosine cyclic 3',5'-phosphate independent pathway for β-adrenergic receptor phosphorylation in wild-type and mutant s49 lymphoma cells: mechanism of homologous desensitization of adenylate cyclase. *Biochemistry* 25: 1371–1377, 1986.

353. Strasser, R. H., G. L. Stiles, and R. J. Lefkowitz. Translocation and uncoupling of the beta-adrenergic receptor in rat lung after catecholamine promoted desensitization in vivo. *Endocrinology* 115: 1392–1400, 1984.

354. Strosberg, A. D. Structure, function and regulation of the three β-adrenoceptor subtypes. *Obesity Res.* 3 (Suppl 4): 501S–505S, 1995.

355. Strulovici, B., J. M. Stadel, and R. J. Lefkowitz. Functional integrity of desensitized β-adrenergic receptors. Internalized receptors reconstitute catecholamine-stimulated adenylate cyclase activity. *J. Biol. Chem.* 258: 6410–6414, 1983.

356. Su, Y.-F., T. K. Harden, and J. P. Perkins. Isoproterenol-induced desensitization of adenylate cyclase in human astrocytoma cells. Relation of loss of hormonal responsiveness and decrement in β-adrenergic receptors. *J. Biol. Chem.* 254: 38–41, 1979.

357. Su, Y.-F., T. K. Harden, and J. P. Perkins. Catecholamine-specific desensitization of adenylate cyclase. Evidence for a multistep process. *J. Biol. Chem.* 255: 7410–7419, 1980.

358. Su, Y. F., L. Cubeddu-Ximenez, and J. P. Perkins. Regulation of adenosine 3':5'-monophosphate content of human astrocytoma cells: Desensitization to catecholamines and prostaglandins. *J. Cyclic Nucleotide Res.* 2: 257–270, 1976.

359. Su, Y. F., G. L. Johnson, L. Cubeddu-Ximenez, B. H. Leichtling, R. Ortmann, and J. P. Perkins. Regulation of adenosine 3':5'-monophosphate content of human astrocytoma cells: Mechanism of agonist-specific desensitization. *J. Cyclic Nucleotide Res.* 2: 271–285, 1976.

360. Suzuki, T., C. T. Nguyen, F. Nantel, H. Bonin, M. Valiquette, T. Frielle, and M. Bouvier. Distinct regulation of beta 1- and beta 2-adrenergic receptors in Chinese hamster fibroblasts. *Mol. Pharmacol.* 41: 542–548, 1992.

361. Tang, W.-J., and A. G. Gilman. Adenylyl cyclases. *Cell* 70: 869–872, 1991.

362. Tang, W.-J., and A. G. Gilman. Type-specific regulation of adenylyl cyclase by G protein βγ subunits. *Science* 254: 1500–1503, 1991.

363. Tattersfield, A. E. Effect of beta-agonists and anticholinergic drugs on bronchial reactivity. *Am. Rev. Respir. Dis.* 136: S64–S68, 1987.

364. Taussig, R., and A. G. Gilman. Mammalian membrane-bound adenylyl cyclases. *J. Biol. Chem.* 270: 1–4, 1995.

365. Teraski, W. L., G. Brooker, J. De Vellis, D. Inglish, C.-Y. Hsu, and R. D. Moylan. Involvement of cyclic AMP and protein synthesis in catecholamine refractoriness. *Adv. Cyclic Nucleotide Res.* 9: 33–52, 1978.

366. Themmen, A. P., L. J. Blok, M. Post, W. M. Baarends, J. W. Hoogerbrugge, M. Parmentier, G. Vassart, and J. A. Grootegoed. Follitropin receptor down-regulation involves a cAMP-dependent post-transcriptional decrease of receptor mRNA expression. *Mol. Cell. Endocrinol.* 78: R7–R13, 1991.

367. Thomason, P. A., S. R. James, P. J. Casey, and C. P. Downes. A G-protein βγ-subunit responsive phosphoinositide 3-kinase activity in human platelet cytosol. *J. Biol. Chem.* 269: 16525–16528, 1994.

368. Tobin, A. B., D. G. Lambert, and S. R. Nahorski. Rapid desensitization of muscarinic m3 receptor-stimulated polyphosphoinositide responses. *Mol. Pharmacol.* 42: 1042–1048, 1992.

369. Tobin, A. B., and S. R. Nahorski. Rapid agonist-mediated phosphorylation of m3–muscarinic receptors revealed by immunoprecipitation. *J. Biol. Chem.* 268: 9817–9823, 1993.

370. Toews, M. L., T. K. Harden, and J. P. Perkins. High-affinity binding of agonists to beta-adrenergic receptors on intact cells. *Proc. Natl. Acad. Sci. USA* 80: 3553–3557, 1983.

371. Toews, M. L., M. Liang, and J. P. Perkins. Agonists and phorbol esters desensitize β-adrenergic receptors by different mechanisms. *Mol. Pharmacol.* 32: 737–742, 1987.

372. Toews, M. L., and J. P. Perkins. Agonist-induced changes in beta-adrenergic receptors on intact cells. *J. Biol. Chem.* 259: 2227–2235, 1984.

373. Toews, M. L., and G. L. Waldo. Comparison of binding of 125I-iodopindolol to control and desensitized cells at 37 degrees and on ice. *J. Cyclic Nucleotide Res.* 11: 47–62, 1986.

374. Toews, M. L., G. L. Waldo, T. K. Harden, and J. P. Perkins. Relationship between an altered membrane form and a low affinity form of the beta-adrenergic receptor occuring during catecholamine-induced desensitization. Evidence for receptor internalization. *J. Biol. Chem.* 259: 11844–11850, 1984.

375. Tsuga, H., K. Kameyama, T. Haga, H. Kurose, and T. Nagao. Sequestration of muscarinic acetylcholine receptor m2 subtypes. Facilitation by G protein-coupled receptor kinase (GRK2) and attenuation by a dominant-negative mutant of GRK2. *J. Biol. Chem.* 269: 32522–32527, 1994.

376. Turki, J., S. A. Green, K. B. Newman, M. A. Meyers, and S. B. Liggett. Human lung cell β2–adrenergic receptors desensitize in response to in vivo administered β-agonist. *Am. J. Physiol.* 269: *(Lung Cell. Mol. Physiol.)* 13: L709–L714, 1995.

377. Turki, J., J. Pak, S. A. Green, R. J. Martin, and S. B. Liggett. Genetic polymorphisms of the β2–adrenergic receptor in nocturnal and nonnocturnal asthma. *J. Clin. Invest.* 95: 1635–1641, 1995.

378. Ungerer, M., G. Parruti, M. Bohm, A. Puzicha, A. DeBlasi, E. Erdman, and M. J. Lohse. Expression of beta-arrestins and beta-adrenergic receptor kinases in failing human heart. *Circ. Res.* 74: 206–213, 1994.

379. Unsworth, C. D., and P. B. Molinoff. Regulation of 5–hydroxy-

tryptamine1B receptor in opposum kidney cells after exposure to agonist. *Mol. Pharmacol.* 42: 464–470, 1992.

380. Valiquette, M., S. Parent, T. P. Loisel, and M. Bouvier. Mutation of tyrosine-141 inhibits insulin-promoted tyrosine phosphorylation and increased responsiveness of the human β_2-adrenergic receptor. *EMBO J.* 14: 5542–5549, 1995.

381. Varrault, A., V. Leviel, and J. Bockaert. 5HT1A-sensitive adenylyl cyclase of rodent hippocampal neurons: Effect of antidepressant treatments and chronic stimulation with agonists. *J. Pharmacol. Exp. Ther.* 257: 433–438, 1991.

382. Vinayek, R., M. Murakami, C. M. Sharp, R. T. Jensen, and J. D. Gardner. Carbachol desensitized pancreatic enzyme secretion by downregulation of receptors. *Am. J. Physiol.* 258 (*Gastrointest. Liver Physiol.* 27): G107–G121, 1990.

383. von Zastrow, M., and B. K. Kobilka. Ligand-regulated internalization and recycling of human beta 2-adrenergic receptors between the plasma membrane and endosomes containing transferrin receptors. *J. Biol. Chem.* 267: 3530–3538, 1992.

384. Wacker, W. B., L. A. Donoso, C. M. Kalsow, J. A. Yankeelov, and D. T. Organisciak. Experimental allergic uveitis: Isolation, characterization and localization of a soluble uveitopathogenic antigen from bovine tissue. *J. Immunol.* 119: 1949–1958, 1977.

385. Wade, S. M., H. K. Dalman, S.-Z. Yang, and R. R. Neubig. Multisite interactions of receptors and G proteins: enhanced potency of dimeric receptor peptides in modifying G protein function. *Mol. Pharmacol.* 45: 1191–1197, 1994.

386. Wakshull, E., C. Hertel, E. J. O'Keefe, and J. P. Perkins. Cellular redistribution of beta-adrenergic receptors in a human astrocytoma cell line: a comparison with the epidermal growth factor receptor in murine fibroblasts. *J. Cell. Biochem.* 29: 127–141, 1985.

387. Waldo, G. L., J. K. Northup, J. P. Perkins, and T. K. Harden. Characterization of an altered membrane form of the β-adrenergic receptor produced during agonist-induced desensitization. *J. Biol. Chem.* 258: 13900–13908, 1983.

388. Wall, M. A., D. E. Coleman, E. Lee, J. A. Ineguez-Lluhi, B. A. Posner, A. G. Gilman, and S. R. Sprang. The structure of the G protein heterotrimer Gi$\alpha_1\beta_1\gamma_2$. *Cell* 83: 1047–1058, 1995.

389. Walsh, D. A., and S. M. Van Patten. Multiple pathway signal transduction by the cAMP-dependent protein kinase. *FASEB J.* 8: 1227–1236, 1994.

390. Walsh, J. H., M. Bouzyk, and E. Rosengurt. Homologous desensitization of bombesin-induced increases in intracellular Ca2+ in quiescent Swiss 3T3 cells involves a protein kinase C-independent mechanism. *J. Cell. Physiol.* 156: 333–340, 1993.

391. Wang, H., D. L. Segaloff, and M. Ascoli. Lutropin/choriogonadotropin down-regulates its receptor by both receptor-mediated endocytosis and a cAMP-dependent reduction in receptor mRNA. *J. Biol. Chem.* 266: 780–785, 1991.

392. Wedegaertner, P. B., P. T. Wilson, and H. R. Bourne. Lipid modifications of trimeric G proteins. *J. Biol. Chem.* 270: 503–506, 1995.

393. Wei, H.-B., H. I. Yamamura, and W. R. Roeske. Downregulation and desensitization of the muscarinic M1 and M2 receptors in transfected fibroblast B82 cells. *Eur. J. Pharmacol.* 268: 381–391, 1994.

394. Wilden, U., S. W. Hall, and H. Kuhn. Phosphodiesterase activation by photoexcited rhodopsin is quenched when rhodopsin is phosphorylated and binds the intrinsic 48-kDa protein of rod outer segments. *Proc. Natl. Acad. Sci. USA* 83: 1174–1178, 1986.

395. Wilkening, D., and M. Nirenberg. Lipid requirement for long-lived morphine-dependent activations of adenylate cyclase of neuroblastoma x glioma hybrid cells. *J. Neurochem.* 34: 321–326, 1980.

396. Williams, R. J., and E. Kelly. Gs alpha-dependent and -independent desensitization of prostanoid IP receptor-activated adenylyl cyclase in NG108–15 cells. *Eur. J. Pharmacol.* 268: 177–186, 1994.

396a. Winstel, R., S. Freund, C. Krasel, E. Hoppe, and M. J. Lohse. Protein kinase cross-talk: membrane targeting of the beta-adrenergic receptor kinase by protein kinase C. *Proc. Natl. Acad. Sci. USA* 93: 2105–2109, 1996.

397. Wistow, G. J., A. Katial, C. Craft, and T. Shinohara. Sequence analysis of bovine retinal S-antigen: Relationships with α-transducin and G proteins. *FEBS Lett.* 196: 23–28, 1986.

398. Witt-Enderby, P. A., H. I. Yamamura, M. Halonen, J. Lai, J. D. Palmer, and J. Bloom. Regulation of airway muscarinic cholinergic receptor subtypes by chronic anticholinergic treatment. *Mol. Pharmacol.* 47: 485–490, 1995.

399. Wu, D., H. Jiang, and M. I. Simon. Different α_1–adrenergic receptor sequences required for activating different Gα subunits of Gq class of proteins. *J. Biol. Chem.* 270: 1995.

400. Yamada, T., Y. Takeuchi, N. Komori, H. Kobayashi, Y. Sakai, Y. Hotta, and H. Matsumoto. A 49-kilodalton phosphoprotein in the *Drosophila* photoreceptor is an arrestin homolog. *Science* 248: 483–486, 1990.

401. Yamaki, K., Y. Takahashi, S. Sakuragi, and K. Matsubara. Molecular cloning of the S-antigen cDNA from bovine retina. *Biochem. Biophys. Res. Commun.* 142: 904–910, 1987.

402. Yamaki, K., M. Tsuda, T. Kikuchi, K.-H. Chen, K.-P. Huang, and T. Shinohara. Structural organization of the human S-antigen gene. *J. Biol. Chem.* 265: 20757–20762, 1990.

403. Yang, J., C. D. Logsdon, T. E. Johansen, and J. A. Williams. Human m3 muscarinic acetylcholine receptor carboxy-terminal threonine residues are required for agonist-induced receptor down-regulation. *Mol. Pharmacol.* 44: 1158–1164, 1993.

404. Yarden, Y., H. Rodriguez, S. K. F. Wong, D. R. Brandt, D. C. May, J. Burnier, R. N. Harkins, E. Y. Chen, J. Ramachandran, A. Ullrich, and E. M. Ross. The avian beta-adrenergic receptor: primary structure and membrane topology. *Proc. Natl. Acad. Sci. USA* 83: 6795–6799, 1986.

405. Yatani, A., and A. M. Brown. Rapid beta-adrenergic modulation of cardiac calcium channel currents by a fast G protein pathway. *Science* 245: 71–74, 1989.

406. Yoshimasa, T., D. R. Sibley, M. Bouvier, R. J. Lefkowitz, and M. G. Caron. Cross-talk between cellular signalling pathways suggested by phorbol-ester-induced adenylate cyclase phosphorylation. *Nature* 327: 67–70, 1987.

407. Yu, S. S., and R. J. Lefkowitz. β-adrenergic receptor sequestration. A potential mechanism of receptor resensitization. *J. Biol. Chem.* 268: 337–341, 1993.

408. Yuan, N. Y., J. Friedman, B. S. Whaley, and R. B. Clark. cAMP-dependent protein kinase and protein kinase C consensus sites of the β-adrenergic receptor. *J. Biol. Chem.* 269: 23032–23038, 1994.

409. Zadina, J. E., S. L. Chang, L. J. Ge, and A. J. Kastin. Mu opiate receptor down-regulation by morphine and up-regulation by naloxone in SH-SY5Y human neuroblastoma cells. *J. Pharmacol. Exp. Ther.* 265: 254–262, 1993.

410. Zadina, J. E., L. M. Harrison, L. J. Ge, A. J. Kastin, and S. L. Chang. Differential regulation of mu and delta opiate receptors by morphine, selective agonists and antagonists and differentiating agents in SH-SY5Y human neuroblastoma cells. *J. Pharmacol. Exp. Ther.* 270: 1086–1096, 1994.

411. Zhang, L.-J., J. E. Lachowicz, and D. R. Sibley. The D$_{2S}$ and

D_{2L} dopamine receptor isoforms are differentially regulated in Chinese hamster ovary cells. *Mol. Pharmacol.* 45: 878–889, 1994.

412. Zhou, X. M., and P. H. Fishman. Desensitization of the human beta 1-adrenergic receptor. Involvement of the cyclic AMP-dependent kinase but not a receptor-specific protein kinase. *J. Biol. Chem.* 266: 7462–7268, 1991.

413. Zhu, X., T. Gudermann, M. Birnbaumer, and L. Birnbaumer. A luteinizing hormone receptor with a severely truncated cytoplasmic tail (LHR-ct628) desensitizes to the same degree as the full-length receptor. *J. Biol. Chem.* 268: 1723–1728, 1993.

414. Zukin, R. S., E. Pellirini-Giampietro, C. M. Knapp, and A. Tempel. Opioid receptor regulation. In: *Opioids*, edited by A. Herz. Berlin: Springer Verlag, 1994, p. 107–123.

8. Mammalian G$_s$-stimulated adenylyl cyclases

GEZHI WENG
YIBANG CHEN
RAVI IYENGAR

Department of Pharmacology, Mount Sinai School of Medicine of the City University of New York, New York, New York

CHAPTER CONTENTS

CELL SURFACE SIGNALING SYSTEMS are important cellular components used for information transfer into the cell. A large number of cell surface signaling systems use heterotrimeric G proteins as transducers. G protein–coupled systems recognize extracellular signals, such as hormones, neurotransmitters, and autocrine and paracrine factors, as well as sensory signals, such as light, odorants, and tastants. The receptors, upon receiving external signals, activate heterotrimeric G proteins. Activation of the G protein results in dissociation of the α-subunit from the $\beta\gamma$ complex. The guanosine triphosphate (GTP)–liganded Gα-subunit and the G$\beta\gamma$-subunits separately regulate effectors that are either ion channels or enzymes that synthesize or degrade intracellular messengers. The signal-transduction process mediated by heterotrimeric G proteins has been reviewed in detail (20, 42).

The multiplicity of receptors, G proteins, and effectors has been recognized for some time now. Well over 100 G protein–coupled receptors have been cloned and characterized. Twenty Gα-, five Gβ- and eleven Gγ-subunits have been identified as distinct molecular species. There is molecular and functional diversity at the level of direct effectors for heterotrimeric G proteins as well. The most extensively studied of the G protein effectors is the hormone-responsive adenylyl cyclase. In the past 6 years, nine mammalian adenylyl cyclases have been cloned. The isoforms of adenylyl cylase are different not only in their primary sequences but also in their signal recognition and integration capabilities. These different functional capabilities allow the cyclic adenosine monophosphate (cAMP) pathway to respond to a wide variety of external signals. In this chapter, we summarize the known properties of the various mammalian adenylyl cyclases and how these properties allow the cAMP pathway to play several important roles in cellular functions.

CLONING OF MAMMALIAN ISOFORMS

The first cloned mammalian adenylyl cyclase was Ca^{2+}/calmodulin (CaM)-stimulated brain enzyme from bovine brain membranes (36). Expression of the cDNA generated an adenylyl cyclase which was stimulated by Gα_s, forskolin, and Ca^{2+}/CaM (60). This enzyme is type 1 adenylyl cyclase (AC1).

Using this brain adenylyl cyclase sequence, cDNAs encoding eight additional mammalian adenylyl cyclase forms (types 2–9) have been identified. AC2 cDNA was cloned from rat brain (18) and AC4 cDNA from rat testes (19). A cDNA cloned from mouse S49 lymphoma cells encodes an adenylyl cyclase (AC7) related to AC2 (68). AC7 also has been cloned from human erythroleukemia cells (23). AC3 was cloned from the rat olfactory neuronal epithelial cDNA library (1). AC5 cDNAs have been cloned from dog heart cDNA library (25) and rat liver and kidney (46). AC6 cDNAs have been cloned from dog heart cDNA library (32), rat liver and kidney (46), mouse S49 lymphoma cells (49) and mouse NCB-20 cells (83). AC8 has been cloned from brain libraries of several species, including human and mouse (6, 16). AC9 has been cloned from a mouse brain library (49).

Comparison of the amino-acid sequences indicates that the overall similarity between the various mammalian adenylyl cyclases is about 50%. However, several individual sequences have considerably higher homology with each other. Such homology analysis indicates that there are at least five distinct families of mammalian adenylyl cyclase. Two of these families have multiple members: the type 2 family has three members, while the type 5 family has two members. The other isoforms (AC1, AC3, AC8, and AC9) are sufficiently divergent from each other and the multimember families that they are likely to be members of different subfamilies. The relationships between the different adenylyl cyclases are shown in Figure. 8.1.

In addition to nine separate gene products encoding the different adenylyl cyclases, multiple forms of adenylyl cyclase can arise from alternative splicing. Comparison of AC5 and AC6 cloned in our laboratory (46) with sequences reported by Ishikawa et al. (25) and Yoshimura and Cooper (83) suggested that there were N-terminal splice variants of AC5 and AC6. Krupinski and co-workers (5) have studied three splice variants of AC8. These were termed AC8-A, -B, and -C. In the case of AC8, the splice sites are spread throughout the protein. AC8-B lacks amino acids 802–831 of AC8-A and AC8-C lacks amino acids 666–682 of AC8-A. The

splice variants show different functional properties. For instance, AC8-C has a four- to fivefold lower affinity for adenosine triphosphate (ATP) than AC8–A, but a threefold higher affinity for Ca^{2+}/CaM. Thus, it appears that there are multiple molecular mechanisms by which different functional forms of adenylyl cyclases can be produced.

TISSUE DISTRIBUTION OF VARIOUS ADENYLYL CYCLASES

Almost all tissue-distribution studies of the cloned subtypes have been done on mRNAs and should be interpreted cautiously. AC1 mRNA appears to be present primarily in neuronal tissue (36, 77). AC2 enzyme mRNA has been detected only in brain and lung (18). Two other members of the AC2 family have varying distributions. AC4 enzyme mRNA appears to be widely distributed in trace amounts (19). AC7 enzyme mRNA has been found by Northern blotting in S49 lymphoma cells and in rat brain and heart (68). AC3 enzyme mRNA is abundant in olfactory tissue (1). However, it has been reported that AC3 mRNAs may be expressed at low levels in other tissues as well (76). mRNA detection by blotting, solution hybridization, and polymerase chain reaction (PCR) techniques indicates that AC5 and AC6 mRNAs are found at high levels in brain and heart, and at lower levels in several other tissues, including kidney, liver, lung, testes, adrenal glands, small intestine, and pancreas (45, 83). AC8 enzyme appears to be brain-specific (6, 16). In situ hybridization studies indicate that there are distinct patterns of distribution of types 1, 2, 5, and 8 enzymes in the brain. The AC5 enzyme appears to be localized primarily to the striatum (21). The AC9 enzyme is widely distributed. The highest amounts of AC9 mRNA are found in skeletal muscle, with significant expression in other tissues, such as brain, liver, kidney, heart, and lung. The tissue distributions for the mRNAs of various types of adenylyl cyclase are summarized in Table 8.1.

Little is known about the protein distribution of the various adenylyl cyclase isoforms. Antibodies specific to most types of adenylyl cyclase that can detect individual native proteins in tissues have not been obtained. The one exception is AC9, which has been identified in several tissues by immunoblotting (49). Subcellular distribution of adenylyl cyclase has been studied in brain regions using an antipeptide-antibody that recognizes all of the cloned mammalian adenylyl cyclases. Adenylyl cyclases are particularly concentrated at the postsynaptic density, a subcellular specialization in the postsynaptic region (41).

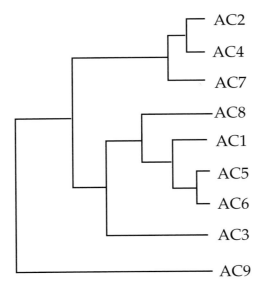

FIG. 8.1. Phylogenetic tree of adenylyl cyclases. Comparison was done according to the method of Sneath and Sokal (54) with the GCG program.

TABLE 8.1. *Tissue Distribution of the Various Adenylyl Cyclase mRNAs*

Adenylyl Cyclase Isoform	Tissues
1	Brain, neuronal tissue
2	Brain, lung
3	Abundant in olfactory neuroepithelia; found in brain and some other tissues
4	Widely distributed in trace amounts
5	Abundant in heart and striatum; widely distributed in trace amounts
6	Widely distributed in trace amounts
7	Heart, brain
8	Brain, neuronal tissue
9	Widely distributed

STRUCTURE AND CATALYTIC SITE

Adenylyl cyclases are integral membrane glycoproteins. The sizes of the native purified proteins are in the 110–180 kd range. From analysis of the deduced amino-acid sequences, all of the mammalian adenylyl cyclases are predicted to be transmembrane proteins with a complex topological structure similar to that of transporters and ion channels, with 12 transmembrane spans in two domains of six spans each. Sequence motifs in the predicted extracellular domain indicate that the protein has N-linked glycosylation. Both the N- and C-termini are predicted to be cytoplasmic. Two large cytoplasmic domains, a 350 amino-acid loop between the first and second sets of transmembrane domains and a 250–300 amino-acid tail following the second membrane domain, were predicted to contain the catalytic core of the enzyme, based on sequence similarity with cloned guanylyl cyclases. These two large intracellular domains share similarity with each other, and both are highly conserved among the known mammalian adenylyl cyclase sequences. The predicted topography of the mammalian adenylyl cyclases is shown in Figure 8.2. The conserved domains in the large cytoplasmic loop and tail are shown in solid black. These domains are similar to each other and to a single domain of cloned guanylyl cyclases (34). Cloned mammalian adenylyl cyclases do not have any obvious signature sequences for ATP binding, such as the P-loop. However, regions in both the central cytoplasmic loop and the C-terminal tail have homology with a single domain in cloned guanylyl cyclases, suggesting that these regions are involved in catalysis. Originally, data implicating these regions in catalytic activity comes from

studies on the *Drosophila* homolog of the bovine type 1 enzyme. This *Drosophila* type 1 adenylyl cyclase maps to the rutabaga genetic locus (38), which causes a defect in associative learning in flies and is correlated with a loss of CaM-stimulated adenylyl cyclase activity in the heads of affected flies (39). The loss of adenylyl cyclase activity results from a point mutation in the C-terminal cytoplasmic domain of *Drosophila* AC1. This mutation (Gly → Arg) changes a residue absolutely conserved among known G protein–regulated adenylyl cyclases (38). Point mutations that affect catalytic activity in both the central cytoplasmic loop and the C-terminal tail have been described (61). Point mutations of a conserved asparagine and arginine in the 1025–1030 region within the C-terminal domain of AC2 results in a very significant decrease catalytic activity. A second site suppressor for one of these mutants was also found close by (81). All of these observations have given rise to the notion that regions of the cytoplasmic tail are intimately involved in catalysis.

Expression of truncated forms of AC1 have shown that both the central cytoplasmic loop and the C-terminal tail are essential for catalytic activity. Expression of either half of the molecule does not yield a catalytically active enzyme. However, when the two halves are co-expressed, substantial catalytic activity is restored, and this activity can be regulated by a number of stimulators (61). That the two halves need to be co-expressed but do not need to be covalently linked to recover catalytic function suggests that interactions between the cytoplasmic domains of the two halves may be the primary requirement for catalysis. However, co-expression of the two halves does not result in full restoration of activity. Thus, one function of the transmembrane domains may be to optimize molecular interactions between the two cytoplasmic domains for efficient catalysis. The critical role of the central loop and C-terminal tail in adenylyl cyclase activity has been further established by the construction of a soluble adenylyl cyclase with the central loop of AC1 and the C-terminal tail of AC2. This soluble enzyme is stimulated by both Gα_s and forskolin (58). The two halves have been expressed individually and upon mixing shown to reconstitute a functional adenylyl cyclase in the presence of Gα_s and forskolin (73, 79). In the presence of Gα_s and forskolin, the affinity of the C-terminal tail for the central cytoplasmic loop is increased tenfold, suggesting that the function of Gα_s and forskolin is to promote interactions between the C-terminal tail and the central cytoplasmic loop. Further support for the idea that interaction between cytoplasmic domains results in a functional enzyme has come from studies on AC5. The expression of the two cytoplasmic domains of AC5 results in the Gα_s and

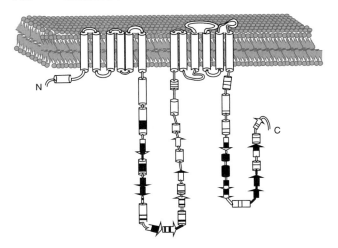

FIG. 8.2. Predicted topology and secondary structure of mammalian adenylyl cyclase. Secondary structure prediction was obtained by use of the PHD program (50). Cylinders represent helixes; wide arrows represent β-sheets; and the thin lines represent loops. Hydrophobic stretches, thought to be transmembrane regions, are depicted as being buried in the bilayer. Highly conserved regions are shown in solid black. The "N" and "C" indicate the N- and C-termini of the protein.

forskolin stimulated enzyme that is inhibited both by micromolar Ca^{2+} and $G\alpha_i$ (51).

The crystal structure of a truncated cytoplasmic tail of AC2 complexed with forskolin has been solved (86). The cytoplasmic tail exists as a dimer both in solution (73) as well as in crystal. The dimer has a wreath-like structure with a cleft in the center. Each dimeric structure contains two molecules of forskolin. Several residues that line the center of the ventral cavity have been shown by site-directed mutagenesis to bind either ATP or ATP analogs. Hence, the ventral cavity may contain the ATP binding site. Surprisingly, the forskolin binding site is close to the proposed ATP binding site. Forskolin binds to the two ends of the ventral cavity. As expected, the forskolin binding pockets are highly hydrophobic. This dimer of the cytoplasmic tail has been proposed as a model for the interaction between the central cytoplasmic loop and the C-terminal tail in the formation of an active enzyme. Further studies are required to determine the validity of this proposal. The cartoon in Figure 8.3 summarizes our current knowledge of structural features of the C-terminal tail of AC2. A surprising and perhaps disappointing aspect of this crystal structure is that even in the presence of forskolin, a clear outline of ATP binding pocket is not obvious. Perhaps, this will emerge as structures of the cytoplasmic loop–C-terminal tail complex are solved.

BASAL ACTIVITY

The different adenylyl cyclases have differing basal activities in the presence of Mg^{2+}. When we compared the basal activity of AC2 to AC6, we found that AC2 had nearly 25–fold greater activity than AC6. This, however, was not due to a difference in catalytic capacity since in the presence of Mn^{2+} and forskolin the difference in activity was only twofold (44). Thus, the Mg^{2+}-dependent basal activities of different adenylyl cyclases are likely to be very different. In addition to AC5 and AC6, AC3 is likely to be an isoform with low basal activity (1). In contrast, both AC1 and AC2 appear to have relatively higher basal activity in the presence of Mg^{2+} ions. The structural basis for this difference in basal activities is not known. It is possible that this may be caused in part by the differences in the catalytic site. It is also possible that the effect is due to allosteric regulation of adenylyl cyclase by divalent cations (55). Point mutations in AC1 that result in a selective decrease in Mg^{2+}-dependent basal activity without a corresponding decrease in Mn^{2+} plus forskolin (61) support the notion of divalent cation regulation of catalytic activity. Preliminary findings from the crystal structure (86) suggest that there may be a divalent cation binding site. The proposed location of this binding site at the interface between the two monomers suggests a mechanism by which divalent cations can allosterically regulate catalytic activity. The divalent cations may promote dimerization and thus stabilize the catalytic site. The structural features that result in the distinct basal activities of the different adenylyl cyclase need to be explored further.

REGULATION BY PROTEIN–PROTEIN INTERACTIONS

Ca^{2+}/Calmodulin

Calmodulin stimulation of brain adenylyl cyclases has been known for nearly two decades (4). Indeed, adenylyl cyclase was one of the first enzymes shown to be stimulated by CaM. There are three adenylyl cyclase isoforms stimulated by Ca^{2+}/CaM: AC1, AC3, and AC8. AC1 and AC8 are stimulated extensively by CaM (6, 59). AC3 is stimulated more modestly and in some situations requires co-stimulation by G protein subunits (13). Purified AC1 has been shown to be stimulated by Ca^{2+}/CaM (60). The half effective concentration (EC_{50}) for Ca^{2+}/CaM is around 25 nM. Vorherr et al. (66), using synthetic peptides have shown that amino acids 495–522 of AC1 are involved in Ca^{2+}/CaM stimulation. The importance of this region has been confirmed by Storm and colleagues (65) using site-directed mutagenesis. However, other regions may

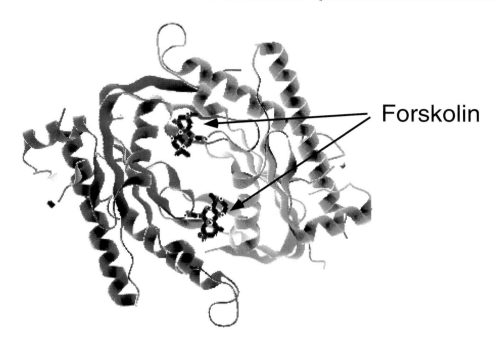

Forskolin

FIG. 8.3. A cartoon of the AC2 C-terminal dimer based on the solved x-ray structure. The dimer is formed by two monomers in close contact with each other. Two forskolin molecules are located at the interface of the monomers. The ribbons represent α-helixes and β-sheets. The thin lines represent disordered loops.

be involved as well. Tang et al. (61) have identified two amino acids, K350 and K923, which when mutated to Ala results in lacking of Ca^{2+}/CaM stimulation. The region, originally identified by Vorherr et al. is shown in Figure 8.4.

Homologous recombination techniques have been used to produce mice deficient in AC1. AC1–deficient mice show an approximately 50% decrease in CaM stimulation. Thus, it appears that AC8 also contributes substantially to the CaM-stimulated activity in neuronal cells. Mice lacking AC1 show a deficit in spatial learning. They also show a decrease in long-term potentiation of synaptic responses in the CA1 region of the hippocampus (75). Studies on the developmental expression of AC1 indicate progressively increasing expression in newborn mice for the first 16 days (65). This correlates well with the development of long-term potentiation in newborn mice.

G Protein Subunits

Gα_s. All nine mammalian adenylyl cyclases are stimulated by Gα_s. However, AC1 does not appear to be stimulated by receptors that activate G$_s$ (70). This may be because Gα_s stimulation is counterbalanced by inhibition by G$\beta\gamma$-subunits. This may be true for AC8

as well. All other adenylyl cyclases are stimulated by receptors that activate Gα_s.

Stimulation by Gα_s may involve multiple sites. Support for this notion comes largely from dose-response curves for Gα_s. Dose-response curves for GTPγS-stimulated Gα_s stimulation of AC2 stretch over three orders of magnitude (61). Using mutationally activated Gα_s, we found that there may be mechanistic differences in Gα_s-stimulation of the different adenylyl cyclases. Stimulation of AC1 appears to involve a single site but stimulation of AC2 and AC6 appears to involve multiple sites. For all three adenylyl cyclases, forskolin not only increases the affinity for Gα_s but also changes the profile of the curve such that stimulation by Gα_s appears to involve a single high affinity site (22). The locations of Gα_s sites on the various adenylyl cyclases are not fully understood. Scanning Ala mutation of AC1 has not proven very useful in locating Gα_s-binding regions since Tang and co-workers (61) find that the loss of Gα_s binding is almost always accompanied by the loss of basal and variously stimulated adenylyl cyclase activities. However, experiments suggest that the function of Gα_s is to stabilize the interactions between the two cytoplasmic domains (73, 79). Using this line of reasoning, mutations have been made in both cytoplasmic domains of the soluble adenylyl cyclase. Mutations in the region 880–990 of the cytoplasmic tail appear to decrease $G\alpha_s$ stimulation more than forskolin stimulation and hence have been postulated to be involved in $G\alpha_s$ binding (80). However this remains uncertain since basal or Mn^{2+}-stimulated activity cannot be measured in this system using the soluble enzyme. Recent studies in our laboratory have identified the region 660–682 of AC6 as being involved in $G\alpha_s$ interactions. However, this region appears to be involved only in stimulation of adenylyl cyclases by high concentrations of $G\alpha_s$ and may thus represent a "low-affinity" binding site for $G\alpha_s$. This region contains a motif conserved among the various adenylyl cyclases (9). It is not yet certain if this region within other adenylyl cyclases is involved in $G\alpha_s$ stimulation. The regions thought to be involved in $G\alpha_s$ interactions are depicted on a structural cartoon in Figure 8.4.

$G\alpha_i$. Inhibition of cAMP production by receptors that couple to pertussis toxin substrates has been known for the past fifteen years. However, extensive inhibition of adenylyl cyclase is seen only in some cells and tissues, while in others much more modest inhibition is observed. This confusing picture became clearer with the cloning of the various adenylyl cyclases. It was found that the different adenylyl cyclases were susceptible to differing extents of inhibition by activated $G\alpha_i$. AC6 was most extensively inhibited in intact cells (8) as well as in in vitro assays (62). AC5, which is very similar to AC6, also is extensively inhibited by $G\alpha_i$. Of the different adenylyl cyclases tested, AC2 was the least inhibitable in the intact cell (8). In in vitro assays, no inhibition of AC2 was observed (62). A unique feature of $G\alpha_i$ inhibition of AC2 in the intact cell is that activation of AC2 by protein kinase C results in abolishment of its capability to be regulated by $G\alpha_i$ (8). AC3 and AC1 also can be inhibited by $G\alpha_i$. Inhibition of adenylyl cyclase shows an interesting dichotomy: Ca^{2+}/CaM-stimulated activity of AC1 can be extensively inhibited, but activation by $G\alpha_s$ is far less susceptible to inhibition (62). All three G_i proteins are capable

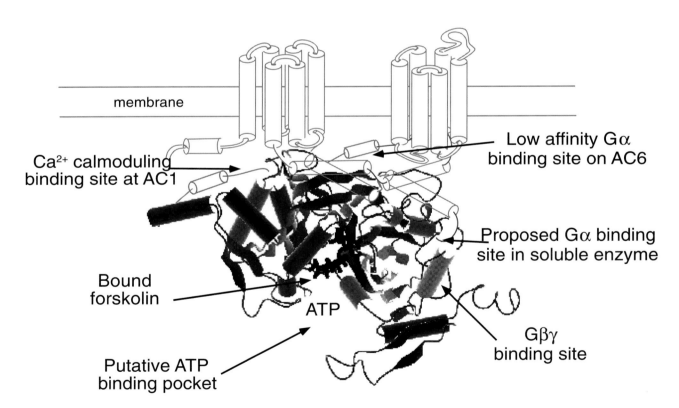

FIG. 8.4. A schematic drawing of the structure of adenylyl cyclases. The central region is the structure of central loop and C-terminus region based on the homology model using the C2 dimer as template. The secondary structure elements in gray are the regions not presented in the solved C2 dimer structure. The forskolin binding sites and putative ATP binding pocket are shown. Regions of adenylyl cyclase thought to be involved in interaction with G protein subunits and CaM are also labeled. The cylinders represent α-helixes and ribbons represent β-sheets. The thin lines represent disordered loops.

of inhibiting adenylyl cyclases both in the intact cell (74) and in vitro (64). Additionally, Bourne and co-workers (74) have shown that $G\alpha_z$, a G_i-related protein that is not pertussis toxin–sensitive, can inhibit adenylyl cyclases. This has been confirmed in in vitro assays (35).

The regions of adenylyl cyclases involved in $G\alpha_i$ interactions are unknown although the $G\alpha_i$ interaction sites are also within the cytoplasmic domains of AC5 (51). On the basis of kinetic analysis of the S49 cell adenylyl cyclase, Hildebrandt et al. (24) have proposed that there may be distinct sites of interaction for G_s and G_i. Gilman and co-workers (64) have come to a similar conclusion, based on the observation that $G\alpha_i$ stimulates AC2 in the presence of forskolin.

$G\beta\gamma$. Regulation of adenylyl cyclases by the $G\beta\gamma$-subunits is among the most complex phenomena studied in this system. AC2 and AC4 are stimulated conditionally by $G\beta\gamma$-subunits. For $G\beta\gamma$ stimulation, the enzymes need to be first stimulated by activated $G\alpha_s$ (57, 59). Since activated $G\alpha_s$ has low affinity for $G\beta\gamma$-subunits, it appears likely that $G\alpha_s$ and $G\beta\gamma$ bind to different sites on AC2. Purified AC2 is regulated by $G\alpha_s$- and $G\beta\gamma$-subunits (63); hence, regulation is likely to involve direct interaction between the G protein subunits and AC2. The notion that $G\alpha_s$ and $G\beta\gamma$ bind to different sites on AC2 gained further support with the identification of a region of AC2 involved in $G\beta\gamma$ signaling (7). Peptide encoding this region blocked stimulation by $G\beta\gamma$ but did not affect stimulation by $G\alpha_s$. The region encompassed by amino acids 956–982 of AC2 involved in $G\beta\gamma$ interactions is depicted in Figure 8.4. Studies using the yeast two-hybrid system have shown that the 956–982 region of AC2 directly interacts with $G\beta$- but not $G\gamma$-subunits (78). Within this region we had identified a motif QXXER, which is present in several other effectors regulated by $G\beta\gamma$ subunits. Studies on the presynaptic Ca^{2+} channels have shown that a region containing a similar motif is involved in $G\beta\gamma$ inhibition of the channels (67, 85).

In addition to stimulating AC2 and AC4, $G\beta\gamma$-subunits inhibit AC1 and AC8. $G\beta\gamma$ inhibition of CaM-stimulated adenylyl cyclase activity had been described previously but had ascribed the sequestration of CaM to $G\beta\gamma$ (31). Analysis with cloned AC1 showed that $G\beta\gamma$-subunits interacted directly with AC1 as well (63) and inhibited both $G\alpha_s$ and CaM stimulated adenylyl cyclase (63). However, the region in AC2 identified as being involved in $G\beta\gamma$ signaling is not conserved in AC1 or AC8. Hence, it is not known where on AC1 the $G\beta\gamma$ complex binds. The other adenylyl cyclases (AC3, AC5, AC6, and AC9) are not directly regulated by $G\beta\gamma$-subunits. AC7, which is closely related to AC2 and AC4, is likely to be stimulated by $G\beta\gamma$-subunits, though this has not been reported.

REGULATION BY SMALL MOLECULES

P-Site Ligands

Except for the unidentified adenylyl cyclase found in sperm, all mammalian adenylyl cyclases are inhibited by purine nucleotides. Inhibition is thought to occur due to direct interactions with a domain distinct from the catalytic site. This is called the P-site since inhibition is strictly dependent on the purine ring (30). All of the cloned mammalian adenylyl cyclases that have been tested are susceptible to P-site inhibition. The most potent inhibitors are dideoxy adenosine analogues (17). The stimulated activities of the enzyme, such as activity in the presence of Mn^{2+} or hormone-stimulated activity, are most susceptible to inhibition by the P-site ligand.

The exact location of the P-site is not known. However, it is possible that some P-site residues are also part of the catalytic site. Mutating Lys-923 to Ala in AC1 results in a greater than 90% inhibition of basal, G_s, and CaM-stimulated activities. The mutant enzyme has substantial (40% of wild-type) activity in the presence of Mn^{2+} and forskolin, but there is a 100–fold decrease in the sensitivity to inhibition by P-site ligands (61). This suggests that Lys-923 is important both for catalytic activity in the presence of Mg-ATP and for P-site ligands. Another implication of this observation is that the catalytic site may not be configured similarly for Mg-ATP and Mn-ATP.

Forskolin

The diterpene forskolin stimulates most mammalian adenylyl cyclases except the one expressed in sperm and testis. Forskolin interaction with the different adenylyl cyclases shows some interesting variations. Forskolin can stimulate adenylyl cyclase in the absence of $G\alpha_s$ (52). The extent of stimulation by forskolin in the absence of $G\alpha_s$ is highly variable. AC9 is the least stimulated, with only a twofold stimulation (49). In contrast, AC6 is highly stimulable, with maximal stimulations of up to 40–fold (44). AC2 and AC1 are in between, with five- to eightfold stimulation (44, 56). Although forskolin stimulates adenylyl cyclase in the absence of G_s, maximal activation by forskolin requires the presence of G_s (14). This synergistic effect is not observed in all adenylyl cyclases: for AC1, $G\alpha_s$, and forskolin, stimulations are additive, but for AC2, 5, and 6, these stimulations are synergistic (56). Binding of [^{3}H]-labeled forskolin to Sf9 cell membranes containing AC1 or AC2 indicates the presence of a single saturable binding site. The crystal structure of forskolin complex with the C-terminal cytoplasmic tail of AC2 has been solved. By itself the cytoplasmic tail dimerizes. There are two forskolin binding sites per dimer. The forskolin binding pockets are mostly hydrophobic, as expected. The forskolin binding sites are close to the interfaces between the monomers (86). This is pictorially depicted in Figure 8.3. If the dimer is reflective of the interactions between the central cytoplasmic loop and the C-terminal tail, then the function of forskolin as determined by the crystal structure would be to promote interactions between the two cytoplasmic domains. It is not certain, however, that there are two forskolin binding site per native adenylyl cyclase molecule.

Ca^{2+}

Cooper and Yoshimura (83) have reported that AC5 and AC6 are inhibited by micromolar amounts of Ca^{2+}. Elevation of Ca^{2+} specifically through capacitative Ca^{2+} entry is required for this inhibition (12). Inhibition of Ca^{2+} does not appear to involve CaM, though tight association of CaM with AC5 or 6 has not been rigorously tested. A soluble adenylyl cyclase derived from the cytoplasmic domains of AC5 is inhibited by low concentrations of Ca^{2+}, and this inhibition is relieved by the deletion of the 112 amino-acid carboxy-terminus region of the central cytoplasmic loop (51). Hence this region may be involved in Ca^{2+} inhibition. There are no well-characterized physiological effects associated with Ca^{2+} inhibition of adenylyl cyclases, but Cooper and co-workers (15) have proposed that the presence of Ca^{2+}-inhibitable adenylyl cyclases and cAMP-regulated Ca^{2+} channels can give rise to stable oscillations in both cAMP and Ca^{2+} levels. Such oscillations may encode some useful biological information.

REGULATION BY PROTEIN KINASES

Protein Kinase A

During studies on glucagon-induced desensitization in chick hepatocytes, one component of desensitization was cAMP-dependent. Reconstitution with G$_s$ did not restore full activity to membranes from cells treated with either glucagon or 8–Br-cAMP. Treatment of membranes from naive but not desensitized cells in vitro with protein kinase A resulted in decreased adenylyl cyclase activity (48). Studies on the kin$^-$ variant of S49 cells also indicate that protein kinase A treatment results in decreased forskolin-stimulated adenylyl cyclase activity (37, 48). Since G$_s$ is not a target for protein kinase A regulation (47), it appears that adenylyl cyclase is the most likely target for the protein kinase A–mediated phosphorylation. Analysis by PCR has shown that chick hepatocytes contain AC5 and AC6 (48). We also have cloned the mouse AC6 from S49 cells (48). Since chick hepatocytes and murine S49 cells have AC6 in common, we proposed that this may be one of the isoforms inhibited by protein kinase A–dependent phosphorylation (27), which we subsequently confirmed. Treatment of Sf9 cell membranes containing AC6 with protein kinase A results in decreased stimulation by Gα_s. There is a single predicted protein kinase A phosphorylation site in AC6. We have mutated the Ser at this site (Ser-674) to an Ala and tested to determine if effects of protein kinase A are lost. AC6 can be phosphorylated by protein kinase A; however, the S674A mutant AC6 is not phosphorylated by protein kinase A. Further, when S674A mutant AC6 is treated with protein kinase A, there is no effect on Gα_s stimulation. These observations indicate that protein kinase A regulates G$_s$ interactions with AC6 by phosphorylation at Ser-674 (9). Ishikawa and co-workers have shown that protein kinase A treatment of AC5 results in decreased activity as well (26). AC6 may be a locus of heterologous desensitization in several cell types. One recent study on PC12 cells shows that phosphorylation of AC6 may be responsible for A2a adenosine receptor–mediated desensitization of cAMP responses (11).

Protein Kinase C

Stimulation of adenylyl cyclase by activation of protein kinase C has been reported in many systems. Biochemical analysis has shown that adenylyl cyclase is a direct target for phosphorylation by protein kinase C (29, 53, 82). Such regulation represents physiologically relevant interactions between signaling pathways, since receptors that activate the protein kinase C pathway stimulate adenylyl cyclase (40); in one system protein kinase C–mediated elevation of cAMP is responsible for angiotensin II–stimulated steroidogenesis (2). Experiments in several laboratories show that AC2 is the enzyme most extensively stimulated by protein kinase C (28, 84). A noteworthy feature of the stimulation of AC2 by protein kinase C is the effect on basal activity. At low Mg^{2+} concentration, mimicking intracellular conditions, the basal activity of AC2 is stimulated five-to sixfold. Forskolin- and G$_s$-stimulated activities of AC2 are also increased, though not as extensively. When AC2 is expressed in Sf9 cells, it can be phosphorylated by phorbol ester activation of endogenous protein kinase C. This phosphorylation is accompanied by enhanced adenylyl cyclase activity (29). Zimmerman and Taussig (87) have shown that in vitro treatment of AC2 with protein kinase C results in activation of the enzyme. The other isoforms of adenylyl cyclase that have been tested (AC1, AC3, AC4, AC5, AC6) either are not stimulated by protein kinase C or are very modestly stimulated. AC5 shows an unusual response in that it is stimulated by protein kinase C in vitro (33) but not in the intact cell (28).

Calmodulin-Kinase

Storm and colleagues (69) have reported that elevation of Ca^{2+} suppresses activity of AC3 expressed in HEK-293 cells. An inhibitor of CaM-kinase relieves this suppression, suggesting that CaM-kinase may be involved. Co-expression of activated fragment of CaM-kinase also results in suppression of AC3 activity. In a recent study Storm and co-workers have shown that CaM-kinase II phosphorylates and inhibits AC3 in the intact cell (72). AC1 is also inhibited by CaM-kinase (71). Inhibition of about 50% results from suppression of maximal activity, rather than from a change in sensitivity to Ca^{2+}. This inhibition is specific for the isoforms of CaM-kinases. CaM-kinase IV inhibits AC1 while CaM-kinase II does not. Mutation of Ser-545 or Ser-552 in AC1 to Ala results in abolition of CaM-kinase–mediated inhibition of AC1. In contrast to AC1 and AC3, AC8 is not inhibited by either CaM-kinase II or IV. It is thought that such differential regulation could represent a mechanism of attenuation of receptor-regulated cAMP increases and could be a mechanism for connection between the cAMP and Ca^{2+} signaling pathways. It is also not known if other adenylyl cyclases are regulated by CaM-kinases.

Other Protein Kinases

AC9 can be activated by inhibition of the phosphatase calcineurin (43), suggesting that AC9 needs to be phosphorylated for it to be active. The identities of the protein kinases that can phosphorylate and activate AC9 remain unknown. Patel and co-workers (10) have reported that epidermal growth factor (EGF) stimulation of cAMP production is specifically observed when AC5 is expressed. It is not known if AC5 or other adenylyl cyclases are substrates for tyrosine kinases.

FUTURE DIRECTIONS

Cloning of the many mammalian adenylyl cyclases and characterization of the distinct regulatory features of the different adenylyl cyclases have led to the notion that the adenylyl cyclases can be loci of signal integration and sorting. Studies on long-term potentiation of synaptic responses in the CA1 region of the hippocampus have indicated that Ca^{2+}/CaM stimulation of adenylyl cyclase is important for long-term potentiation. However, the cAMP pathway, instead of communicating the signals that result in long-term potentiation, functions as a gate to regulate signal flow through other pathways (3). In addition to synaptic plasticity, the modulatory role of the cAMP pathway has been described in several biological processes, including cell differentiation, survival, and proliferation. Only in the case of synaptic plasticity has the role of Ca^{2+}/CaM-stimulated adenylyl cyclases been elucidated. In the other cases, the roles of individual adenylyl cyclases and their capability to receive and process signals from a variety of receptors remain to be determined.

Research in our laboratory is supported by NIH grants DK-38761 and GM-54508 and funds from the Aaron Diamond Foundation. G.W. is an Aaron Diamond Fellow.

REFERENCES

1. Bakalyar, H. A., and R. R. Reed. Identification of a specialized adenylyl cyclase that may mediate odorant detection. *Science* 250: 1403–1406, 1990.
2. Bird, I. A., J. I. Mason, K. Oka, and W. Rainey. Angiotensin-II stimulates an increase in cAMP and expression of 170c-hydroxylase cytochrome P450 in fetal bovine adrenocortical Cells. *Endocrinology* 132: 932–934, 1993.
3. Blitzer, R. D., T. Wong, R. Nouranifar, R. Iyengar, and E. M. Landau. Postsynaptic cAMP pathway gates early LTP in hippocampal CA1 region. *Neuron* 15: 1403–1414, 1995.
4. Brostrom, C. O., M. A. Brostrom, and D. J. Wolff. Calcium-dependent adenylate cyclase from rat cerebral cortex. Reversible activation by sodium fluoride. *J. Biol. Chem.* 252: 677–5685, 1977.
5. Cali, J. J., R. S. Parekh, and J. Krupinski. Splice variants of type VIII adenylyl cyclase. Differences in glycosylation and regulation by Ca^{2+}/calmodulin. *J. Biol. Chem.* 271: 1089–1095, 1996.
6. Cali, J. J., J. C. Zwaagstra, N. Mons, D. M. F. Cooper, and J. Krupinski. Type VIII adenylyl cyclase. A Ca^{2+}/calmodulin-stimulated enzyme expressed in discrete regions of rat brain. *J. Biol. Chem.* 269: 12190–12195, 1994.
7. Chen, J.-q., M. DeVivo, J. Dingus, A. Harry, J. Li, D. J. Carty, J. L. Blank, J. H. Exton, R. H. Stoffel, J. Inglese, R. J. Lefkowitz, D. E. Logothetis, J. D. Hildebrandt, and R. Iyengar. A region of adenylyl cyclase 2 critical for regulation by G protein $\beta\gamma$ subunits. *Science* 268: 1166–1169, 1995.
8. Chen, J.-q., and R. Iyengar. Inhibition of cloned adenylyl cyclases by mutant-activated Gi-alpha and specific suppression of

type 2 adenylyl cyclase inhibition by phorbol ester treatment. *J. Biol. Chem.* 268: 12253–12256, 1993.

9. Chen, Y., A. Harry, J. Li, M. J. Smit, X. Bai, R. Magnusson, J. Pieroni, G. Weng, and R. Iyengar. A Gα_s interaction region in adenylyl cyclase: selective involvement in protein kinase A regulaion of adenylyl cyclase 6. *Proc. Natl. Acad. Sci. U.S.A.*: accepted 1997.

10. Chen, Z., H. S. Nield, H. Sun, A. Barbier, and T. B. Patel. Expression of type V adenylyl cyclase is required for epidermal growth factor–mediated stimulation of cAMP accumulation. *J. Biol. Chem.* 270: 27525–27530, 1995.

11. Chern, Y., J. Y. Chiou, H. L. Lai, and M. H. Tsai. Regulation of adenylyl cyclase type VI activity during desensitization of the A2a adenosine receptor mediated cyclic AMP response: role for protein phosphatase 2A. *Mol. Pharmacol.* 48: 1–8, 1995.

12. Chiono, M., R. Mahey, G. Tate, and D. M. Cooper. Capacitative Ca^{2+} entry exclusively inhibits cAMP synthesis in C6–2B glioma cells. Evidence that physiologically evoked Ca^{2+} entry regulates Ca(2+)-inhibitable adenylyl cyclase in non-excitable cells. *J. Biol. Chem.* 270: 1149–1155, 1995.

13. Choi, E. J., Z. Xia, and D. R. Storm. Stimulation of the type III olfactory adenylyl cyclase by calcium and calmodulin. *Biochemistry* 31: 6492–6498, 1992.

14. Clark, R. B., T. J. Goka, D. A. Green, R. Barber, and R. W. Butcher. Differences in the forskolin activation of adenylate cyclases in wild-type and variant lymphoma cells. *Mol. Pharmacol.* 22: 609–613, 1982.

15. Cooper, D. M. F., N. Mons, and J. W. Karpen. Adenylyl cyclases and the interaction between calcium and cAMP signalling. *Nature* 374: 421–424, 1995.

16. Defer, N., O. Marinx, D. Stengel, A. Danisova, V. Iourgenko, I. Matsuoka, D. Caput, and J. Hanoune. Molecular cloning of the human type VIII adenylyl cyclase. *FEBS Lett.* 351: 109–113, 1994.

17. Desaubry, L., I. Shoshani, and R. A. Johnson. 2',5'-Dideoxyadenosine 3'-polyphosphates are potent inhibitors of adenylyl cyclases. *J. Biol. Chem.* 271: 2380–2382, 1996.

18. Feinstein, P. G., K. A. Schrader, H. A. Bakalyar, W.-J. Tang, J. Kuprinski, A. G. Gilman, and R. R. Reed. Molecular cloning and characterization of a Ca^{2+}/calmodulin-insensitive adenylyl cyclase from rat brain. *Proc. Natl. Acad. Sci. U.S.A.* 88: 10173–10177, 1991.

19. Gao, B., and A. G. Gilman. Cloning and expression of a widely distributed (type IV) adenylyl cyclase. *Proc. Natl. Acad. Sci. U.S.A.* 88: 10178–10182, 1991.

20. Gilman, A. G. G proteins: transducers of receptor-generated signals. *Annu. Rev. Biochem* 56: 651–693, 1987.

21. Glatt, C. E., and S. H. Snyder. Cloning and expression of an adenylyl cyclase localized to the corpus striatum. *Nature* 361: 536–538, 1993.

22. Harry, A., Y. Chen, R. Magnusson, R. Iyengar, and G. Weng. Differential regulation of adenylyl cyclase by Gα_s*. *J. Biol. Chem.* 272: 19017–19021, 1997.

23. Hellevuo, K., M. Yoshimura, M. Kao, P. L. Hoffman, D. M. Cooper, and B. Tabakoff. A novel adenylyl cyclase sequence cloned from the human erythroleukemia cell line. *Biochem. Biophys. Res. Commun.* 192: 311–318, 1993.

24. Hildebrandt, J. D., J. Hanoune, and L. Birnbaumer. Guanine nucleotide inhibition of cyc⁻ S49 mouse lymphoma cell membrane adenylyl cyclase. *J. Biol. Chem.* 257: 14723–14725, 1982.

25. Ishikawa, Y., S. Katsushika, L. Chen, N. J. Halnon, J. Kawabe, and C. J. Homcy. Isolation and characterization of a novel cardiac adenylyl cyclase cDNA. *J. Biol. Chem.* 267: 13553–13557, 1992.

26. Iwami, G., J. Kawabe, T. Ebina, P. J. Cannon, C. J. Homcy, and Y. Ishikawa. Regulation of adenylyl cyclase by protein kinase A. *J. Biol. Chem.* 270: 12481–12484, 1995.

27. Iyengar, R. Molecular and functional diversity of mammalian Gs-stimulated adenylyl cyclases. *FASEB J.* 7: 768–775, 1993.

28. Jacobowitz, O., J. Chen, R. T. Premont, and R. Iyengar. Stimulation of specific types of adenylyl cyclases by phorbol ester treatment. *J. Biol. Chem.* 268: 3829–3832, 1993.

29. Jacobowitz, O., and R. Iyengar. Phorbol ester-induced stimulation and phosphorylation of adenylyl cyclase 2. *Proc. Natl. Acad. Sci. U.S.A.* 91: 10630–10634, 1994.

30. Johnson, R. A., S. M. Yeung, D. Stubner, M. Bushfield, and I. Shoshani. Cation and structural requirements for P site-mediated inhibition of adenylate cyclase. *Mol. Pharmacol.* 35: 681–688, 1989.

31. Katada, T., K. Kasukabe, M. Oinuma, and M. Ui. A novel mechanism for the inhibition of adenylate cyclase via inhibitory GTP binding proteins. Calmodulin dependent inhibition of the cyclase catalyst by the βγ-subunits of GTP binding proteins. *J. Biol. Chem.* 262: 11897–11900, 1987.

32. Katsushika, S., L. Chen, J.-I. Kawabe, R. Nilakantan, N. J. Halnon, C. J. Homcy, and Y. Ishikawa. Cloning and characterization of a sixth adenylyl cyclase isoform: types V and VI constitute a subgroup within the mammalian adenylyl cyclase family. *Proc. Natl. Acad. Sci. U.S.A.* 89: 8774–8778, 1992.

33. Kawabe, J., G. Iwami, T. Ebina, S. Ohno, T. Katada, Y. Ueda, C. J. Homcy, and Y. Ishikawa. Differential activation of adenylyl cyclase by protein kinase C. *J. Biol. Chem.* 269: 16554–16558, 1994.

34. Koesling, D., E. Boheme, and G. Schultz. Guanylyl cyclases, a growing family of signal transducing enzymes. *FASEB J.* 5: 2785–2791, 1991.

35. Kozasa, T., J. R. Hepler, A. V. Smrcka, M. I. Simon, S. G. Rhee, P. C. Sternweis, and A. G. Gilman. Purification and characterization of recombinant G¹⁶ alpha from Sf9 cells: activation of purified phospholipase C isozymes by G-protein alpha subunits. *Proc. Natl. Acad. Sci. U.S.A.* 90: 9176–9180, 1993.

36. Krupinski, J., F. Coussen, H. A. Bakalyar, W.-J. Tang, P. G. Feinstein, K. Orth, C. Slaughter, R. R. Reed, and A. G. Gilman. Adenylyl cyclase amino acid sequence: possible channel- or transporter-like structure. *Science* 244: 1558–1564, 1989.

37. Kunkel, M. W., J. Friedman, S. Shenolikar, and R. B. Clark. Cell free heterologous desensitization of adenylyl cyclase in S49 cell membranes mediated by cAMP dependent kinase. *FASEB J.* 3: 2067–2074, 1989.

38. Levin, L. R., P.-Y. Han , P. M. Hwang, P. G. Feinstein, R. L. Davis, R. Randall, and R. R. Reed. The *Drosophila* learning and memory gene rutabaga encodes a Ca^{2+}/calmodulin responsive adenylyl cyclase. *Cell* 68: 479–489, 1992.

39. Livingstone, M. S., P. P. Sziber, and W. G. Quinn. Loss of calcium/calmodulin responsiveness in adenylate cyclase of rutabaga, a *Drosophila* learning mutant. *Cell* 37: 205–215, 1984.

40. Lustig, K. D., B. R. Conklin, P. Herzmark, R. Taussig, and H. R. Bourne. Type II adenylylcyclase integrates coincident signals from Gs, Gi, and Gq. *J. Biol. Chem.* 268: 13900–13905, 1993.

41. Mons, N., A. Harry, P. Dubourg, R. T. Premont, R. Iyengar, and D. M. Cooper. Immunohistochemical localization of adenylyl cyclase in rat brain indicates a highly selective concentration at synapses. *Proc. Natl. Acad. Sci. U.S.A.* 92: 8473–8477, 1995.

42. Neer, E. J. Heterotrimeric G proteins: organizers of transmembrane signals. *Cell* 80: 249–257, 1995.

43. Paterson, J. M., S. M. Smith, A. J. Harmar, and F. A. Antoni. Control of a novel adenylyl cyclase by calcineurin. *Biochem. Biophys. Res. Commun.* 214: 1000–1008, 1995.

44. Pieroni, J. P., A. Harry, J. Chen, O. Jacobowitz, R. P. Magnusson, and R. Iyengar. Distinct characteristics of the basal activities of adenylyl cyclases 2 and 6. *J. Biol. Chem.* 270: 21368–21373, 1995.

45. Pieroni, J. P., D. Miller, R. T. Premont, and R. Iyengar. Type 5 adenylyl cyclase distribution. *Nature* 363: 679, 1993.

46. Premont, R. T., J. Chen, H.-W. Ma, M. Ponnapalli, and R. Iyengar. Two members of a widely expressed subfamily of hormone stimulated adenylyl cyclases. *Proc. Natl. Acad. Sci. U.S.A.* 89: 9808–9813, 1992.

47. Premont, R. T., and R. Iyengar. Heterologous desensitization of the liver adenylyl cyclase: analysis of the role of G-proteins. *Endocrinology* 125: 1151–1160, 1989.

48. Premont, R. T., O. Jacobowitz, and R. Iyengar. Lowered responsiveness of the catalyst of adenylyl cyclase to stimulation by G$_s$ in heterologous desensitization: A role for cAMP dependent phosphorylation. *Endocrinology* 131: 2774–2783, 1992.

49. Premont, R. T., I. Matsuoka, M.-G. Mattei, Y. Pouille, N. Defer, and J. Hanoune. Identification and characterization of a widely expressed form of adenylyl cyclase. *J. Biol. Chem* 271: 13900–13907, 1996.

50. Rost, B., and C. Sander. Prediction of protein secondary structure at better than 70% accuracy. *J. Mol. Biol.* 232: 584–599, 1993.

51. Scholich, K., A. J. Barbier, J. B. Mullenix, and T. B. Patel. Characterization of soluble forms of nochimeric type V adenylyl cyclases. *Proc. Natl. Acad. Sci. U.S.A.* 94: 2915–2920, 1997.

52. Seamon, K. B. Forskolin and adenylate cyclase. *ISI Atlas of Science: Pharmacology* 1: 250–253, 1987.

53. Simmoteit, R. R., H. D. Schulzki, D. Palm, S. Mollner, and T. Pfeuffer. Chemical and functional analysis of components of adenylyl cyclase from human platelets treated with phorbol esters. *FEBS Lett.* 249: 189–194, 1991.

54. Sneath, P. H. A., and R. R. Sokal. *Numerical Taxonomy.* San Francisco: Freeman, 1973.

55. Somkuti, S. G., J. D. Hildebrandt, J. T. Herberg, and R. Iyengar. Divalent cation regulation of adenylyl cyclase. An allosteric site on the catalytic component. *J. Biol. Chem.* 257: 6387–6393, 1982.

56. Sutkowski, E. M., W.-J. Tang, C. W. Broome, J. D. Robbins, and K. B. Seamon. Regulation of forskolin interactions with type I, II, V, and VI adenylyl cyclases by G$_s$-α. *Biochemistry* 33: 12852–12859, 1994.

57. Tang, W.-J., and A. G. Gilman. Adenylyl cyclases. *Cell* 70: 869–872, 1992.

58. Tang, W.-J., and A. G. Gilman. Construction of a soluble adenylyl cyclase activated by G$_s$ alpha and forskolin. *Science* 268: 1769–1772, 1995.

59. Tang, W.-J., and A. G. Gilman. Type specific regulation of adenylyl cyclase by G protein $\beta\gamma$-subunits. *Science* 254: 1500–1503, 1991.

60. Tang, W.-J., J. Krupinski, and A. G. Gilman. Expression and characterization of calmodulin-activated (type I) adenylyl cyclase. *J. Biol. Chem.* 266: 8595–8603, 1991.

61. Tang, W.-J., M. Stanzel, and A. G. Gilman. Truncation and alanine-scanning mutants of type I adenylyl cyclase. *Biochemistry* 34: 14563–14572, 1995.

62. Taussig, R., J. A. Iniguez-Lluhi, and A. G. Gilman. Inhibition of adenylyl cyclase by G$_i$ alpha. *Science* 261: 218–221, 1993.

63. Taussig, R., L. M. Quarmby, and A. G. Gilman. Regulation of purified type I and II adenylyl cyclases by G protein $\beta\gamma$ subunits. *J. Biol. Chem.* 268: 9–12, 1993.

64. Taussig, R., W.-J. Tang, J. R. Hepler, and A. G. Gilman. Distinct patterns of bidirectional regulation of mammalian adenylyl cyclases. *J. Biol. Chem.* 269: 6093–6100, 1994.

65. Villacres, E. C., Z. Wu, W. Hua, M. D. Nielsen, J. J. Watters, C. Yan, J. Beavo, and D. R. Storm. Developmentally expressed Ca(2+)-sensitive adenylyl cyclase activity is disrupted in the brains of type I adenylyl cyclase mutant mice. *J. Biol. Chem.* 270: 14352–14357, 1995.

66. Vorherr, T., L. Knopfel, F. Hofmann, S. Mollner, T. Pfeuffer, and E. Carafoli. The calmodulin binding domain of nitric oxide synthase and adenylyl cyclase. *Biochemistry* 32: 6081–6088, 1993.

67. Waard, M. D., H. Liu, D. Walker, V. E. S. Scott, C. A. Gurnett, and K. P. Campbell. Direct binding of G-protein $\beta\gamma$ complex to voltage-dependent calcium channels. *Nature* 385: 446–450, 1997.

68. Watson, P. A., J. Krupinski, A. M. Kempinski, and C. D. Frankenfield. Molecular cloning and characterization of the type VII isoform of mammalian adenylyl cyclase expressed widely in mouse tissues and in S49 mouse lymphoma cells. *J. Biol. Chem.* 269: 28893–28898, 1994.

69. Wayman, G. A., S. Impey, and D. R. Storm. Ca^{2+} inhibition of type III adenylyl cyclase *in vivo*. *J. Biol. Chem.* 270: 21480–21486, 1995.

70. Wayman, G. A., S. Impey, Z. Wu, W. Kindsvogel, L. Prichard, and D. R. Storm. Synergistic activation of the type I adenylyl cyclase by Ca^{2+} and G$_s$-coupled receptors *in vivo*. *J. Biol. Chem.* 269: 25400–25405, 1994.

71. Wayman, G. A., J. Wei, S. Wong, and D. R. Storm. Regulation of type I adenylyl cyclase by calmodulin kinase IV in vivo. *Mol. Cell. Biol.* 16: 6075–6082, 1996.

72. Wei, J., G. Wayman, and D. R. Storm. Phosphorylation and inhibition of type III adenylyl cyclase by calmodulin-dependent protein kinase II in vivo. *J. Biol. Chem.* 271: 24231–24235, 1996.

73. Whisnant, R. E., A. G. Gilman, and C. W. Dessauer. Interaction of the two cytosolic domains of mammalian adenylyl cyclase. *Proc. Natl. Acad. Sci. U.S.A.* 93: 6621–6625, 1996.

74. Wong, Y. H., B. R. Conklin, and H. R. Bourne. G$_z$-mediated hormonal inhibition of cyclic AMP accumulation. *Science* 255: 339–342, 1992.

75. Wu, Z. L., S. A. Thomas, E. C. Villacres, Z. Xia, M. L. Simmons, C. Chavkin, R. D. Palmiter, and D. R. Storm. Altered behavior and long-term potentiation in type I adenylyl cyclase mutant mice. *Proc. Natl. Acad. Sci. U.S.A.* 92: 220–224, 1995.

76. Xia, Z., E. J. Choi, F. Wang, and D. R. Storm. The type III calcium/calmodulin-sensitive adenylyl cyclase is not specific to olfactory sensory neurons. *Neurosci. Lett.* 144: 169–173, 1992.

77. Xia, Z., C. Refsdal, K. M. Merchant, D. M. Dorsa, and D. R. Storm. Distribution of mRNA for the calmodulin-sensitive adenylate cyclase in rat brain: expression in areas associated with learning and memory. *Neuron* 6: 431–443, 1991.

78. Yan, K., and N. Gautam. A domain on the G protein β subunit interacts with both adenylyl cyclase 2 and the muscarinic atrial potassium channel. *J. Biol. Chem.* 271: 17597–17600, 1996.

79. Yan, S.-Z., D. Hahn, Z.-H. Huang, and W.-J. Tang. Two cytoplasmic domains of mammalian adenylyl cyclase form a G$_s\alpha$- and forskolin-activated enzyme *in vitro*. *J. Biol. Chem.* 271: 10941–10945, 1996.

80. Yan, S.-Z., Z.-H. Huang, V. D. Rao, J. H. Hurley, and W.-J. Tang. Three discrete regions of mammalian adenylyl cyclase from a site for G$_s\alpha$ activation. *J. Biol. Chem.* in press, 1997.

81. Yan, S.-Z., Z.-H. Huang, R. S. Shaw, and W.-J. Tang. The

conserved asparagine and arginine are essential for catalysis of mammalian adenylyl cyclase. *J. Biol. Chem.* 272: 12342–12349, 1997.

82. Yoshimasa, T., D. R. Sibley, M. Bouvier, R. J. Lefkowitz, and M. G. Caron. Cross-talk between cellular signalling pathways suggested by phorbol ester induced adenylate cyclase phosphorylation. *Nature* 327: 6770–6777, 1987.

83. Yoshimura, M., and D. M. F. Cooper. Cloning and expression of a Ca^{2+} inhibitable adenylyl cyclase from NCB-20 cells. *Proc. Natl. Acad. Sci. U.S.A.* 89: 6716–6720, 1992.

84. Yoshimura, M., and D. M. F. Cooper. Type Specifc stimulation of adenylyl cyclase by protein kinase C. *J. Biol. Chem.* 268: 4604–4607, 1993.

85. Zamponi, G. W., E. Bourinet, D. Nelson, J. Nargeot, and T. P. Snutch. Crosstalk between G proteins and protein kinase C mediated by the calcium channel α_1 subunit. *Nature* 385: 442–446, 1997.

86. Zhang, G., Y. Liu, A. E. Ruoho, and J. H. Hurley. Structure of the adenylyl cyclase catalytic core. *Nature* 386: 247–253, 1997.

87. Zimmerman, G. N., and R. Taussig. Protein kinase C alters the responses to G protein α and $\beta\gamma$ subunits. *J. Biol. Chem.* 271: 27161–27166, 1996.

9. Calcium signaling systems

STANKO S. STOJILKOVIC | *Endocrinology and Reproduction Research Branch, National Institute of Child Health and Human Development, National Institutes of Health, Bethesda, Maryland*

CHAPTER CONTENTS

TRANSDUCTION OF MANY NEUROTRANSMITTER AND HORMONAL STIMULI is mediated by an increase in the concentration of cytosolic calcium ion ($[Ca^{2+}]_i$). Such rises are critical for the control of many cellular functions, including membrane excitability, contraction, gene expression, hormone synthesis, and exocytosis (24, 362, 466). The dynamic relationships among extracellular, cytosolic, and intraorganelle calcium are diverse and essential for understanding the generation and control of Ca^{2+} signals. Calcium is differentially compartmentalized within the cell. The cytosol contains only a minor portion (10%–20%) of calcium, which is bound predominantly to soluble cytosolic proteins and membranes (359). The $[Ca^{2+}]_i$ in unstimulated cells is between 100 and 200 nM and can increase transiently to low-micromolar concentrations during agonist stimulation (26, 283, 354). The ratio between free and bound Ca^{2+} is about 1:100 (316, 464). The rest of the calcium is contained within the intracellular organelles, including the endoplasmic reticulum, sarcoplasmic reticulum, Golgi network, mitochondria, endosomes, lysosomes, and secretory vesicles. The total calcium in intracellular organelles is in a millimolar concentration range, and the level of free calcium is much higher than in the cytosol (359). Therefore, such membrane-bound compartments can serve as reservoirs for a transient increase in $[Ca^{2+}]_i$. The extracellular medium, with about 1 mM free calcium, represents an additional and practically unlimited reservoir of calcium for cells. For intracellular Ca^{2+} signaling, cells rely on the large electrochemical gradient of calcium across the plasma membrane (termed *"calcium entry"*) or on calcium release from intracellular stores (termed *"calcium mobilization"*).

Calcium homeostasis in body fluids is secured by two sources, diet and the bone matrix, avoiding any risk of calcium deprivation in the extracellular medium. In evolutionary terms, this favored the development of a system for intracellular Ca^{2+} signaling that depends exclusively on Ca^{2+} entry. The system is operative in excitable cells, which express a variety of voltage-gated plasma membrane calcium channels (VGCCs) (466). These and other plasma membrane channels in conjunction with plasma membrane (Na^+/K^+) adenosine triphosphatase (ATPase) and (Ca^{2+})ATPase are the essential elements of the *voltage-dependent calcium-signaling system* (234). Since the activation of VGCCs is associated with complex changes in plasma membrane potential (V_m), including activation and inactivation of several types of plasma membrane channel, we also refer to such Ca^{2+} entry as the "V_m *pathway.*"

Although the plasma membrane calcium gradients render a sufficient reservoir of calcium, intracellular reserves are highly advantageous for cells. They donate a different pattern of Ca^{2+} signaling within cells from that derived by the V_m-dependent pathway, which is potentially relevant for the selective control of cellular functions. Intracellular sources also provide a mechanism for the rapid attainment of equilibrium with the cytosol, which is important in the control of long-lasting excess of calcium in the cytosol. Such elevations of $[Ca^{2+}]_i$ occur in many nonexcitable and excitable cell types, including pancreatic acinar cells (138, 327), hepatocytes (188, 381), oocytes (89, 221), neurons (493), and pituitary cells (430, 461), and are mediated through calcium channels associated with intracellular organelles. These channels belong to two major classes: inositol(1,4,5)-trisphosphate (IP_3)-sensitive receptor (IP_3R) channels and ryanodine-sensitive calcium release (RyR) channels (103). These channels together with sarcoplasmic/endoplasmic reticulum calcium ATPase (SERCA)–type calcium pumps are the essential elements of the *calcium mobilization–dependent signaling system* (93, 232).

In general, a rapid and transient rise in $[Ca^{2+}]_i$ occurs spontaneously or (more frequently) in response to agonist stimulation. This increase is expressed commonly as prominent Ca^{2+} oscillations in single-cell studies. Both systems for Ca^{2+} signaling, voltage-dependent and calcium mobilization–dependent, can create oscillatory Ca^{2+} responses, the first being the *plasma membrane oscillator* and the second the *endoplasmic reticulum oscillator*. For some cellular functions, such as calcium-dependent excitability, the oscillatory nature of Ca^{2+} signals is essential. For others, periodic calcium release is not imperative (419) but provides additional features for the control of cellular functions. For example, the oscillatory nature of both Ca^{2+}-signaling systems leads to frequency coding of extracellular stimuli (169, 367, 381), which is an effi-

cient mechanism to inform the cell about the intensity of hormonal stimulation and, at the same time, to protect the cell from the toxic effects of high $[Ca^{2+}]_i$.

The role of plasma membrane receptors in the control of these two systems is critical. The V_m pathway is controlled predominantly by G_s- and G_i-coupled receptors (420). Control of calcium mobilization–dependent signaling systems is more diverse. The phospholipase C–controlled production of IP_3 is essential to initiate Ca^{2+} release through IP_3R channels, and this family of enzymes is activated by several G protein–coupled receptors, as well as by some tyrosine kinase receptors (24). These two classes of receptor are known as "*calcium-mobilizing receptors*" (see Chapter 11 by Exton in this *Handbook*). However, the importance of receptor regulation of Ca^{2+} release through RyR channels (if any) and the nature of these receptors are not known.

While the V_m-dependent pathway relies exclusively on extracellular Ca^{2+} entry, operation of the calcium-mobilizing system depends on both release of intracellular Ca^{2+} and Ca^{2+} entry. Calcium release predominates during the early phase of agonist stimulation, while Ca^{2+} entry is essential during sustained agonist stimulation (362). In this regard, the major difference between $[Ca^{2+}]_i$ responses of excitable and nonexcitable cells to calcium-mobilizing agonists is related to the Ca^{2+} entry that often follows Ca^{2+} mobilization from intracellular pools. In nonexcitable cells, the biochemical events that lead to Ca^{2+} mobilization commonly are accompanied by activation of a calcium-entry mechanism(s) other than VGCCs (362). In excitable cells, the VGCCs comprise the major calcium-delivery system during agonist stimulation (268, 420), though other systems, such as those operating in nonexcitable cells, may also participate in Ca^{2+} mobilization.

The spatial and temporal aspects of Ca^{2+} signals induced by voltage-gated calcium entry and mobilization of intracellular calcium vary depending on the receptor and cell type, the distribution of plasma membrane receptors and channels, and the intracellular distribution of calcium-release channels and endoplasmic reticulum (Ca^{2+})ATPase (354). In addition to the endoplasmic reticulum, the mitochondria (143) and nucleus (415) may participate in intracellular redistribution of calcium. Although other cytoplasmic organelles also are equipped with the mechanism for calcium influx and release, it is unlikely that they play an important role in a dynamic intracellular Ca^{2+} equilibrium (359).

Some cells express an additional system for self-potentiation of Ca^{2+} signaling and secretion. To be operative, this system requires loading of the secretory vesicles with ATP and its co-secretion with neurotransmitters or hormones, the expression of purinergic receptors or channels, and ecto-enzymes for rapid degradation of ATP (147, 171). The purinergic system may also participate in intercellular Ca^{2+} signaling in some tissues (326). In other cell types, gap junction channels provide the mechanism for intercellular calcium wave propagation (35, 413). Both systems are appropriate for an efficient synchronization of Ca^{2+} signals at the tissue level.

The complexity of the temporal and spatial organization of Ca^{2+} signals is in accord with the numerous intracellular functions of calcium ions. For example, Ca^{2+} signaling is required for many intracellular calcium storage compartment functions, including control of mitochondrial metabolism, "packaging" in the trans-Golgi network, exocytosis of secretory vesicles, and control of gene expression in the nucleus. The activity of several enzymes also depends on $[Ca^{2+}]_i$. These include calmodulin, protein kinase C, phospholipase C, and phospholipase D (119, 320, 450). In addition, cytosolic calcium is an active participant in the control of IP_3R and RyR channels (103, 189), and several plasma membrane potassium, sodium, chloride, and nonselective cationic channels (159). Calcium also has been implicated in the control of capacitive calcium entry (25) and cytoskeletal functions (42, 87, 348).

VOLTAGE-DEPENDENT CALCIUM-SIGNALING SYSTEM

Voltage-Gated Calcium Channels

The general feature of VGCCs is their sensitivity to depolarization. One group of these channels opens at more hyperpolarized potentials (low voltage–activated, LVA), and the other group requires large depolarizations to be activated (high voltage–activated, HVA). The LVA calcium channels usually show rapid and voltage-dependent inactivation. These channels are also named type I, low-threshold, fast, and slow deactivating. The HVA channels usually do not inactivate rapidly. These channels are also known as type II, high-threshold, slow inactivating, and fast deactivating (159). Functional studies in different cell types have revealed multiple types of LVA and HVA calcium channels, distinguished by ion selectivity, single channel conductance, pharmacology, metabolic regulation, and tissue localization. Based on such characterization, several types of VGCC were identified, including T-, L-, N-, P-, Q-, and R-type channels (484).

Molecular cloning has confirmed the great diversity among VGCCs (47, 53). This diversity is due to multiple genes for Ca^{2+} channel subunits and alternative splicing. A large single unit (200–260 kd) of VGCCs, called the "α_1-subunit," contains the voltage sensor, gating machinery, and a channel pore. The ancillary subunits, α_2/δ, β, and γ, modify the behavior of the α_1-subunit (484). In the mammalian brain, two major subfamilies of genes encode five different α_1-subunit classes (86, 98, 227, 302, 346, 386, 408, 412, 435, 445, 489). Class C, D, and S clones comprise the L-type superfamily of channels sensitive to dihydropyridines. The A, B, and E classes belong to another α_1 superfamily, with about 60% identity with each other and 45% with other members of the L-type superfamily. Class B clones encode N-type calcium channels, and information on the functional properties of the class A and class E α_1 subunits is more limited.

The co-existence of several types of VGCC in a single cell is common: T- and L-type channels are co-expressed frequently in several neurons (288) as well as other cell types, including pituitary gonadotrophs, lactotrophs, corticotrophs, somatotrophs, melanotrophs, and immortalized pituitary cells (37, 99, 190, 229, 256, 257, 404, 437, 462). In sensory neurons, T- and L-type channels are accompanied by N-type channels (322). Co-expression of several VGCC subtypes in the same cell is physiologically important to the control of transmitter release, spike initiation, and rhythmic action potential firing. For example, the characteristic properties of T-type channels are appropriate for the generation of action potentials (288). In this respect, hyperpolarization is necessary to remove the steady-state inactivation of T-type channels, and they inactivate rapidly (hence, "T" for transient). In contrast, L-type channels are opened by strong depolarizations and are noninactivating (hence, "L" for long-lasting). The slower activation and delayed inactivation kinetics of L-type channels are appropriate for mediating calcium influx during spontaneous electrical activity and agonist stimulation (298, 425). The T-type channels can be substituted by voltage-gated sodium channels, the activation of which depolarizes the cells to the level needed for activation of HVA channels (157).

Basal Pacemaker Activity

Repetitive spontaneous action potentials occur in many neuronal, neuroendocrine, endocrine, and smooth muscle cell types, including hypothalamic neurons (216), β pancreatic acinar cells (333), and pituitary cells (30, 101, 193). These action potentials occur as single spikes or as bursts of activity followed by quiescent periods. In some cell types, receptor activation leads to the initiation of firing or an increase in the frequency of spiking. Receptor activation also can lead to inhibition of spontaneous electrical activity. The ionic channel composition and duration of action potentials vary from cell to cell. The term "plasma membrane calcium oscillator" applies only to cells that drive action potentials associated with $[Ca^{2+}]_i$ spikes. In general, the duration of such action potentials is 50–500 ms, longer than typical sodium/potassium-driven action potentials (about 5 ms) (402).

In this chapter, the nature and receptor-dependent modulation of the plasma membrane oscillator are discussed using pituitary cells as examples. Within pituitary cells, spontaneous firing of action potentials is observed in gonadotrophs (210, 428), lactotrophs (229), somatotrophs (173, 229), and melanotrophs (467), as well as growth hormone and AtT-20 pituitary cell lines (30, 101, 193, 297). Sodium- and calcium-dependent action potentials have been reported in ovine gonadotrophs (157), GH_3 (growth hormone) lactosomatotrophs (30), and AtT-20 cells (4). Other cell studies have revealed only calcium-dependent activity, with no indication of a tetrodotoxin-sensitive sodium component (101, 193, 210). The action potential frequency in pituitary cells ranges from 0.1 to 1.5 Hz and is determined by the magnitude and duration of the afterhyperpolarization. Membrane depolarization by current injection increases the frequency of spontaneously occurring action potentials and induces electrical activity in silent cells (234). The ionic basis of action potentials and the mechanism of the pacemaker activity in pituitary cells have been reviewed elsewhere (99, 333).

Spontaneous action potential activity has been linked to the levels of $[Ca^{2+}]_i$ in unstimulated pituitary cells. This is typified by rat gonadotrophs, as shown in Figure 9.1. Spontaneous oscillatory patterns of $[Ca^{2+}]_i$ also occur in somatotrophs (161) and lactotrophs (255) and are responsible for the extracellular Ca^{2+}-dependent basal release of growth hormone and prolactin in vitro (426). Action potential–driven calcium transients also are observed in corticotrophs and the AtT-20 cell line (117, 204). In GH_3B_6 cells, an increase in the action potential frequency is followed by increases in the amplitude and duration of oscillations in $[Ca^{2+}]_i$ (394). During trains, basal $[Ca^{2+}]_i$ increases and rapidly reaches a steady state, fluctuating around a plateau level which depends linearly on action potential frequency in neurons (153). Both action potential activities and $[Ca^{2+}]_i$ fluctuations are abolished in the absence of extracellular calcium and in the presence of the L-type calcium channel blocker nifedipine (428). The spiking amplitude of spontaneous $[Ca^{2+}]_i$ fluctuations in cultured lactotrophs ranges from 60 to 260 nM (255), in somatotrophs from 50 to 450 nM (161), and in GH_3B_6 cells from 550 to 650 nM (394). In view of the differences in the amplitudes of the spontaneous Ca^{2+} spikes and the irregularity in their frequency,

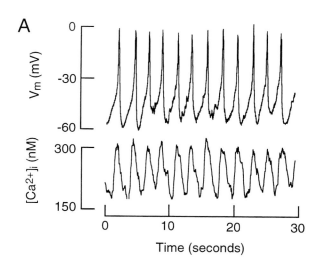

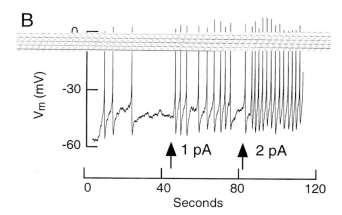

FIG. 9.1. Spontaneous plasma membrane oscillator activity in rat pituitary gonadotrophs. *A:* Simultaneous recording of membrane potential V_m and $[Ca^{2+}]_i$ during spontaneous firing of action potentials. *B:* Sensitivity of firing frequency to current injection. [From Li et al. (234) with permission.]

they are often termed "fluctuations" rather than "oscillations."

Agonist-Induced Modulation of Pacemaker Activity

Several hypothalamic neuropeptides, neurotransmitters, and peripheral hormones involved in the control of cell function operate by modulating the spontaneous activity of the pituitary membrane oscillator. Some of these factors show inhibitory action upon basal and agonist-activated membrane oscillators, while others operate through stimulation of the membrane oscillator. Negative control over the spontaneous activity of the membrane oscillator is exemplified by the action of somatostatin in somatotrophs, lactotrophs, and thyrotrophs; dopamine in lactotrophs and melanotrophs; and neuropeptide Y in gonadotrophs, lactotrophs, and melanotrophs. These agonists suppress electrical activity and the $[Ca^{2+}]_i$ fluctuations, leading to inhibition of hormone secretion (420). In contrast, growth hormone-releasing hormone (GHRH), corticotropin-releasing factor (CRF), and estradiol increase the activity of the membrane oscillatory system and hormone secretion in somatotrophs, corticotrophs, and lactotrophs, respectively (420).

Somatostatin. The inhibitory effect of somatostatin on electrical activity and $[Ca^{2+}]_i$ has been demonstrated in normal pituitary cells (161, 451). This action is accompanied by inhibition of growth hormone, prolactin, thyrotropin, and adrenocorticotropin release (344). Also, somatostatin suppresses spontaneous action potentials and associated $[Ca^{2+}]_i$ fluctuations in GH_3B_6 and AtT-20 immortalized pituitary cells (248). It has been suggested that somatostatin lowers $[Ca^{2+}]_i$ directly, through a blockade of VGCCs (230, 248, 250), and/or indirectly, by an increase in potassium conductance (200, 485, 495, 496). In pituitary tumor cells, somatostatin inhibits secretion through two distinct mechanisms: inhibition of adenylate cyclase (199) and a cAMP-independent mechanism that reduces Ca^{2+} influx (248, 394). Pretreatment of GH_3 cells with pertussis toxin abolishes somatostatin action (299, 494), suggesting that this agonist regulates the function of ionic channels through G_i and/or G_o proteins. A pertussis toxin–sensitive G protein also mediates the inhibition of voltage-gated calcium currents by somatostatin in AtT-20 cells (230). Experiments with selective blockers of different VGCCs in PC12 cells indicate that the effects of somatostatin on $[Ca^{2+}]_i$ are mediated by L-type calcium channels (458). The pertussis toxin-sensitive action of somatostatin on large-conductance Ca^{2+}-activated potassium channels (single-channel conductivity of 120 pS) may not involve direct effects of Ca^{2+}, cAMP, or G protein on the channels but may require protein dephosphorylation (485). In contrast, in growth hormone–secreting adenoma cells, somatostatin appears to activate potassium conductance by promoting the coupling of hormone receptors with channels through a G protein α-subunit. This action of somatostatin on membrane hyperpolarization is mediated through 55 pS potassium channels (496). However, the γ_3-subunit mediates the direct inhibitory action of pertussis toxin–sensitive G protein on VGCCs (198). Five subtypes of somatostatin receptors have been cloned, and all of them mediate inhibition of adenylyl cyclase, which is sensitive to pertussis toxin

(370). It also appears that somatostatin-2 and -5 mediate the endocrine actions of somatostatin by coupling to L-type calcium channels via G_i protein (127, 444).

Dopamine. Dopamine is a potent inhibitor of pituitary hormone secretion in mammals, amphibians, and some fish (219, 305, 349). In rat and frog melanotrophs (91, 137), rat lactotrophs (44, 104), and goldfish gonadotrophs (59), the inhibitory actions of dopamine are due to activation of dopamine D_2-like receptors. These receptors are negatively coupled to adenylate cyclase (85, 107), phospholipase C (48, 91), and phospholipase A_2 (44), as well as electrical membrane activity (176, 243, 446) and associated Ca^{2+} entry (255). The decrease in electrical membrane activity is linked to the modulation of several ionic channels, which ultimately lead, directly and/or indirectly, to reduced calcium entry through VGCCs. In rat lactotrophs (104), rat melanotrophs (490), and frog melanotrophs (468), dopamine induces membrane hyperpolarization by activating voltage-independent potassium channels, resulting in the suppression of action potential activity. Dopamine also reduces action potential duration by increasing the amplitude of voltage-dependent potassium currents (468). The dopamine-induced membrane hyperpolarizations and reduction in action potential duration by activation of voltage-dependent and -independent potassium channels indirectly leads to reduced calcium entry through VGCCs during action potential firing. In addition, in human prolactin-secreting adenoma cells (176), rat lactotrophs (137, 191, 242), rat and frog melanotrophs (191, 411, 468), and goldfish gonadotrophs (470), activation of dopamine D_2-like receptors directly inhibits Ca^{2+} entry through VGCCs. Dopamine also inhibits L-type VGCCs in GH_4C_1 pituitary cells expressing human D_2 and $D_{4.2}$, but not D_3, receptor cDNAs (396). Finally, the actions of dopamine are mediated by pertussis toxin–sensitive G proteins, which may be coupled directly and/or indirectly to potassium channels and VGCCs (104, 108, 240, 241, 243, 468). In rat lactotrophs, for example, the G_o subtype mediates the inhibitory actions of dopamine on VGCCs, while the G_i subtype mediates the activation of voltage-dependent potassium channels (240). Pertussis toxin–sensitive G proteins also are coupled to voltage-independent potassium channels in a cAMP- and Ca^{2+}-independent manner (50, 104).

Neuropeptide Y. In addition to somatostatin and dopamine, pituitary cell secretion is suppressed by hypothalamic neuropeptide Y. This effect is observed in rat gonadotrophs, lactotrophs, and melanotrophs (202,

393, 399, 480). In gonadotrophs, gonadotropin-releasing hormone (GnRH)-induced activation of VGCCs is suppressed by neuropeptide Y, through the enhancement of a hyperpolarizing potassium conductance. This effect is reduced markedly by treatment with pertussis toxin, suggesting the participation of a G protein in the activation of an inwardly rectifying potassium conductance (399). In lactotrophs, neuropeptide Y inhibits basal and thyrotropin-releasing hormone (TRH)-induced $[Ca^{2+}]_i$ response and prolactin secretion in a concentration- and extracellular calcium–dependent manner (480). In melanotrophs, neuropeptide Y inhibits spontaneous $[Ca^{2+}]_i$ fluctuations with a potency equal to its inhibition of secretion (393).

Growth Hormone–Releasing Hormone. In addition to somatostatin-induced inhibition of spontaneous fluctuations, somatotrophs possess a mechanism for increasing the activity of their membrane oscillator system. In these cells, GHRH increases $[Ca^{2+}]_i$ by promoting the influx of calcium through membrane ion channels, and this action is abolished in rat somatotrophs perifused with somatostatin (161). Also, GHRH increases calcium currents in ovine somatotrophs (63). These observations are consistent with the stimulatory actions of G_s proteins on L-type calcium channels (249). In addition, evidence suggests that depolarization of somatotrophs (64, 65), presumably due to activation of tetrodotoxin-insensitive sodium channels (187, 249), further facilitates calcium influx through L-type calcium channels. Increases in $[Ca^{2+}]_i$ induced by GHRH in somatotrophs appear to be mediated by AMP-dependent phosphorylation of sodium channels, leading to depolarization and activation of voltage-gated Ca^{2+} entry (313). In accord with this, both GHRH- and forskolin-induced rises in $[Ca^{2+}]_i$ are abolished by addition of calcium channel blockers such as cobalt and verapamil (160). Similar to forskolin treatment, phorbol ester–induced activation of protein kinase C in somatotrophs is followed by increased $[Ca^{2+}]_i$ due to an influx of extracellular calcium, which is suppressed by somatostatin (160, 249). These findings are comparable to those observed in growth hormone–secreting adenoma cells (102). Thus, interactions between the major second-messenger systems, calcium, cAMP, and protein kinase C may contribute to the coordinated regulation of the membrane oscillator in somatotrophs.

Corticotropin-Releasing Factor. In pituitary corticotrophs, CRF stimulates $[Ca^{2+}]_i$ oscillations, and this action is abolished in cells bathed in Ca^{2+}-deficient medium. CRF-induced Ca^{2+} oscillations can be mimicked by forskolin treatment in an extracellular Ca^{2+}-dependent manner (224). These data are consistent with the involvement of cAMP in the stimulation of corticotropin release by CRF (5) and the role of protein kinase A in the control of firing frequency in single corticotrophs (215). The protein kinase C activator phorbol myristate acetate (PMA) potentiates the effects of CRF on cAMP production in rat anterior pituitary cells (3), suggesting that the calcium-mobilizing receptors in these cells participate in CRF-stimulated adenylate cyclase activity. Also, CRF increases the frequency of action potentials and the subsequent $[Ca^{2+}]_i$ transients in cultured human corticotropic adenoma cells (142). In murine corticotropic adenoma (AtT-20) cells, CRF stimulates voltage-gated calcium influx. This action is mimicked by forskolin and 8-bromo-cAMP. In AtT-20, CRF- and cAMP-induced calcium influxes are attenuated by the dihydropyridine calcium channel blockers nifedipine and nisoldipine, as well as by verapamil (204, 247). Phorbol esters also stimulate calcium influx in AtT-20 cells but through a different intracellular site of action. While CRF activates cAMP-dependent protein kinase to stimulate calcium influx either by directly facilitating calcium conductance or by modifying the membrane potential, protein kinase C appears to act through a reduction in potassium current (369).

Estrogens. Estradiol-17β modulates Ca^{2+} signaling and secretion in pituitary cells, indirectly by activation of nuclear estrogen receptors and directly by nongenomic effects on plasma membrane channel conductivity. The genomic actions of estradiol include both Ca^{2+} mobilization and entry. Estradiol can have facilitatory or inhibitory effects, depending on its concentration, time of exposure, and interactions with progesterone (324, 325). In ovine gonadotrophs, estradiol enhances the current through L- and T-type calcium channels but not through sodium channels. In accordance with the genomic action of estradiol on these channels, no increase in the current occurs in cells with an inhibitor of protein synthesis, actinomycin (158). Pretreatment of female pituitary cell cultures with estradiol for 72 h also enhances Bay K 8644 (L-type calcium channel agonist)–induced luteinizing hormone and prolactin release but not growth hormone release (97).

Estradiol also increases spiking activity in lactotrophs immediately after its addition to the bathing solution. The increased spiking activity lasts for 3–30 min after application and is dependent on Ca^{2+} entry; subsequent exposure to estradiol is ineffective (101). This action is distinct from estradiol's long-term action on prolactin synthesis and release (152) and is consistent with a direct effect on the plasma membrane oscillator. This phenomenon also is observed in intestinal mucosal cells, in which estradiol directly stimulates calcium entry through L-type calcium channels (357). In contrast, estradiol inhibits VGCCs in neostriatal neurons (281) and vascular smooth muscle cells (309, 398, 500). However, very little is known about the molecular mechanism(s) of these nongenomic actions of estradiol on Ca^{2+} signaling.

CALCIUM MOBILIZATION–DEPENDENT SIGNALING SYSTEM

Inositol (1,4,5)-Triphosphate (IP₃) and IP₃ Receptor (IP₃R) Channels

The expression and operation of a voltage-dependent Ca^{2+} signaling system is typical for excitable cells. In nonexcitable cells, the mobilization of calcium from intracellular stores is the major source for Ca^{2+} signaling; however, this pathway is not unique to nonexcitable cells as calcium-release channels commonly are expressed in excitable cells as well (420). Calcium mobilization–dependent signaling systems are controlled by two classes of calcium-mobilizing receptor, seven-membrane-domain receptors coupled to G proteins and tyrosine kinase plasma membrane receptors. While receptors coupled to G_q, G_s, and G_i activate phospholipase C-β, tyrosine kinase C receptors activate phospholipase C-γ (see Chapter 11 by Exton in this *Handbook*). Both enzymes hydrolyze membrane-associated phosphatidylinositol-4,5-bisphosphate, leading to production of diacylglycerol and IP₃ (26, 320). Diacylglycerol remains in the plasma membrane, where it acts on protein kinase C. In contrast, IP₃ rapidly diffuses into the cytosol to release calcium from a fraction of the non-mitochondrial stores containing the specific intracellular receptors. Purification and functional reconstitution of the receptors have demonstrated that the binding sites for IP₃ and the calcium-release channels are the same molecular entity, the IP₃R channel (114).

The molecular structure of the IP₃R channel is similar to that of skeletal and cardiac muscle RyR channels (287). The IP₃R channels consist of four similar subunits, which are noncovalently associated (254, 286) to form a four-leaf clover–like structure (58), the center of which forms the calcium channel. The IP₃-binding sites are located within the first 788 residues of the N-terminus of each subunit (286, 293). Multiple IP₃R channel subtypes and splice variants exist (308), and different cellular and developmental expressions of these channels have been reported (293). Two inhibitors, heparin and decavanadate, competitively inhibit IP₃ binding to IP₃R channels (121, 122, 133); neither inhibitor is highly specific. A monoclonal antibody against the C-terminus of the IP₃R molecule also affects Ca^{2+} mobilization (294, 295).

The IP₃R channels are present in almost all cells, localized on the endoplasmic reticulum, nuclear membrane, and possibly the plasma membrane in some cell types. Functionally reconstituted purified IP₃R channels respond to IP₃ with an increase in the open probability due to a large conformational change. There are four conductance states of roughly 20 pS each, with a mean open time of about 10 ms (482). The relationship between saturation of the four binding sites and activation of the four conductance states is unclear, though it has been suggested that binding of one IP₃ molecule to the IP₃R is sufficient to fully activate the calcium channel (118, 482). The release of calcium is electrically compensated by an inward potassium flux (304).

The role of IP₃ in the spatial and temporal organization of Ca^{2+} signaling has been documented in a wide variety of cells. Injection of a fixed level of IP₃ or its non-metabolized forms into a single cell initiates oscillatory calcium responses in several cell types (429, 477). This indicates that fluctuations in IP₃ levels are not required for the oscillatory calcium response. Furthermore, an increase in IP₃ concentration leads to an increase in the oscillation frequency comparable to that observed in agonist-stimulated cells (429). As shown in Figure 9.2, IP₃ mimics the action of GnRH on spiking frequency in rat gonadotrophs. In addition to IP₃, several other factors modulate the activity of IP₃R channels, including cytosolic and luminal calcium (Fig. 9.3), protein kinase A (83), protein kinase C (113), calcium/calmodulin-dependent protein kinase II (146), adenine nucleotides (27), pH, and other intracellular factors (259). Thus, IP₃R channels not only are effectors in the Ca^{2+}-signaling pathway but also participate in signal transduction.

Cytosolic Calcium as a Co-agonist in the Control of IP₃R Channels. Early work on permeabilized fiber bundles from smooth muscle tissue suggested that cytosolic calcium was involved in the control of IP₃R channel gating. In the presence of stimulatory concentrations of IP₃, cytosolic calcium has a biphasic effect on Ca^{2+} release, activating it at low concentrations and inhibiting it at higher concentrations (170). This was confirmed by measuring the calcium dependence of the open probability of cerebellar Purkinje IP₃R channels incorporated into phospholipid bilayers (29). In *Xenopus laevis* oocytes, the inhibitory effect of calcium on IP₃-induced calcium release occurs on a much slower time scale than its activation (338). In synaptosomes, calcium triggers release in about 50 ms, while inactivation is delayed for nearly 0.5 s. Similarly, in pituitary gonadotrophs, activation time is 50–70 ms (211), and inactivation time is 1–1.2 s (472). A slight elevation in $[Ca^{2+}]_i$ converts IP₃R channels from a state of low

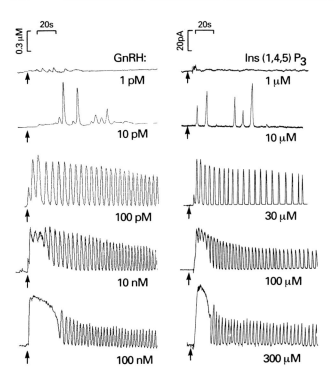

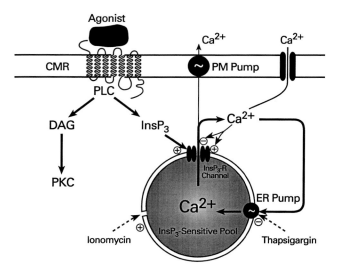

FIG. 9.3. Schematic representation of the endoplasmic reticulum *(ER)* oscillator. *CMR,* seven-membrane-domain calcium-mobilizing receptor; *PM,* plasma membrane; *PLC,* phospholipase C; *DAG,* diacyglycerol; *PKC,* protein kinase C; *InsP₃,* inositol(1,4,5)-trisphosphate.

FIG. 9.2. Comparison of effects of gonadotropin-releasing hormone *(GnRH) (left panels)* and inositol(1,4,5)-triphosphate *[Ins(1,4,5)P₃] (right panels)* on pattern of Ca^{2+} spiking in rat gonadotrophs: GnRH-induced $[Ca^{2+}]_i$ oscillations were measured in intact cells loaded with Indo 1-AM; IP₃-induced $[Ca^{2+}]_i$ oscillations were measured indirectly, by a calcium-controlled potassium current, and IP₃ was injected through the pipette. [From Stojilkovic et al. (429) with permission.]

affinity for IP₃ to a state of high affinity (358), which affects the ability of these channels to respond to IP₃ (260). Further elevation of $[Ca^{2+}]_i$ does not change the affinity of the receptor to IP₃ but decreases the conductance of the channel (258).

Endoplasmic Reticulum Calcium Excitability. Using an analogy to the Hodgkin-Huxley model for the electrical excitability of the plasma membrane (402), a simple mathematical model for pulsatile calcium release from the endoplasmic reticulum has been introduced (189, 232, 233). The first step in this model is IP₃ production and its binding to IP₃R channels, resulting in a small release of Ca^{2+} from the endoplasmic reticulum. Once released into the cytosol, Ca^{2+} initially exerts a positive feedback effect on the IP₃R channels, which augments Ca^{2+} release, leading to a large Ca^{2+} pulse or wave. *Endoplasmic reticulum calcium excitability* is the ability of such a small calcium increment to trigger a large

calcium pulse or wave. When $[Ca^{2+}]_i$ reaches a critical level, Ca^{2+} exerts a negative feedback effect on the IP₃R channel. During this refractory period, $[Ca^{2+}]_i$ undergoes a delicate distribution between the free and bound forms, which is influenced by endoplasmic reticulum (Ca^{2+})ATPase, the reuptake of calcium by mitochondria, and an exclusion of calcium from the cell by plasma membrane (Ca^{2+})ATPase and exchangers (Fig. 9.3). When the coordinate actions of these processes bring $[Ca^{2+}]_i$ to lower facilitatory levels, the process is repeated and another transient occurs.

The existence of the calcium concentration gradient across the endoplasmic reticulum membrane and the transient increase in calcium conductance through IP₃R channels is essential for the initiation of calcium excitability. Like plasma membrane potential, $[Ca^{2+}]_i$ represents the excitation variable in the calcium excitability of the endoplasmic reticulum membrane. The analogy between the two types of membrane-associated excitability goes beyond these general features. The positive and negative effects of calcium on IP₃R channels are analogous to voltage-gated activation and inactivation of the sodium channel, which is essential for the electrical excitability of neurons (159). This model broadens our understanding of agonist-induced Ca^{2+} oscillations in a general framework. When applied to a specific cell model, the pituitary gonadotroph, it reproduces the observed dynamics with remarkable agreement and helps to reveal properties specific to this cell type (189, 232, 233).

cADP Ribose and RyR Channels

RyR channels constitute a second class of intracellular calcium release channel. Although originally it was suggested that RyR channels are present only in skeletal muscle fibers and cardiac myocytes, we now know that they are expressed also in neurons, chromaffin cells, sea urchin eggs, and several nonexcitable cell types (409). They are named "RyR" since they were isolated based on their ability to bind ryanodine, a plant alkaloid (172, 174, 218). The RyR channel has three family members, R1–R3 (409). The skeletal R1 and cardiac R2 channels display a 66% identity, while the R3 channel is much shorter and is expressed in several non-muscle cell types (134, 329, 442, 506). Neuronal and sea urchin egg RyR channels resemble the cardiac R2 channel (273, 478). Like the IP_3R channels, RyR channels exist as tetramers, with a large N-terminal region forming heads and a C-terminal region forming the calcium channels (272). These channels are regulated by V_m, second messengers, and calcium (24).

Several lines of evidence implicate the cyclic adenosine 5′-diphosphate ribose (cADP-R) as a second messenger: (1) cADP-R activates ryanodine channels in a concentration range similar to that needed for IP_3 activation of IP_3R channels (222), (2) cADP-R is present in many cells and is generated from nicotinamide adenine dinucleotide (NAD) by two enzymes (73), and (3) intracellular cADP-R levels increase in response to agonist stimulation (223, 440). Calcium also activates RyR channels, resulting in Ca^{2+} release, a process known as "calcium-induced calcium release" (103, 409, 440). For example, a functional coupling between L-type calcium channels and RyR channels exists in cardiac myocytes, leading to release of Ca^{2+} from the sarcoplasmic reticulum, which in turn inactivates L-type channels (397). Furthermore, it is likely that cADP-R and calcium act as co-agonists in the control of Ca^{2+} release (130).

Calcium also inhibits RyR channels but in a millimolar concentration range, suggesting that such inhibition is not of physiological importance. In accord with the specificity of these channels, ryanodine, ruthenium red, and magnesium are blockers of RyR, but not IP_3R, channels (103). In the presence of Ca^{2+}, an inhibitor of IP_3R channels, heparin, activates RyR channels at physiological calcium concentrations, indicating that the RyR channels are quite specific (28). Such a dual pattern of regulation is sufficient to induce intracellular

calcium excitability for RyR channels as well. These channels are co-expressed frequently with IP_3R channels. However, the physiological importance of the co-expression of IP_3R and RyR release channels in the same cell types and their variable density within the cells are still largely unclear.

Calcium Pumps

Since cytosolic Ca^{2+} is in a nanomolar concentration range and intraluminal Ca^{2+} in a high-micromolar to low-millimolar concentration range, calcium uptake into intracellular organelles proceeds against its concentration gradient and, thus, requires energy to operate. Such transport occurs through two well-characterized pathways, $(Ca^{2+})ATPase$ and calcium electrogenic uniport. In all cells investigated, SERCA-type $(Ca^{2+})ATPases$ are expressed in both the sarcoplasmic reticulum and the endoplasmic reticulum (359). Calcium electrogenic uniport operates in mitochondria and utilizes mitochondrial membrane potential (see later under Intraorganelle calcium signaling).

Endoplasmic reticulum $(Ca^{2+})ATPases$ function as pumps in a manner comparable to the plasma membrane $(Ca^{2+})ATPases$, actively transporting calcium from the cytosol into internal stores. A variety of tissue-specialized isoforms of the SERCA pumps have been identified. All have a high affinity for calcium (0.1–0.4 μM) and transport it with a second-order, sigmoidal calcium dependence (251, 457). These characteristics are appropriate for maintaining low $[Ca^{2+}]_i$. There are several specific SERCA inhibitors, such as thapsigargin (387, 441, 449) and 2,5–di(tert-butyl)-1,4-benzohydroquinone (BHQ) (186, 301). Thapsigargin binds stoichiometrically to all SERCAs at the transmembrane segment M3 and causes an essentially irreversible inhibition of their activity by blocking the enzymes in the Ca^{2+}-free state (252, 321, 487). Thapsigargin shows high affinity (in a nanomolar concentration range) and high specificity for SERCA (without affecting the plasma membrane $[Ca^{2+}]ATPases$). The action of BHQ is similar to that of thapsigargin, but it has a significantly lower potency and reversible binding.

Inhibitors of SERCA exhibit complex effects on Ca^{2+} signaling in agonist-stimulated cells, depending on the concentration and time of exposure. For example, in gonadotrophs exposed briefly to thapsigargin and subsequently to GnRH, only one cycle of cytosolic Ca^{2+} oscillations occurs (169). After long-term thapsigargin treatment, the agonist is unable to induce any Ca^{2+} release due to a complete discharge of luminal calcium (169). In oscillating gonadotrophs, application of either thapsigargin or BHQ abolishes spiking (233, 428, 464), which is consistent with the conclusion that the endoplasmic reticulum calcium pump plays a major role in oscillation cycles. The importance of (Ca^{2+})-ATPases for the oscillatory response also is observed in other cell types (352). Overexpression of the SERCA1 pump in *X. laevis* oocytes leads to an increase in the frequency of Ca^{2+} spiking (45). In addition, thapsigargin itself can induce occasional spiking in pituitary gonadotrophs (169, 429, 434), lymphocytes (95), and pancreatic acinar cells (123, 124). Thus, although the role of the SERCA pumps is passive compared to the dynamic role of IP_3R channels in endoplasmic reticulum calcium excitability, it is of equal importance.

Intracellular Calcium Buffers

The diffusion rate of Ca^{2+} depends on cytosolic and endoplasmic reticulum calcium buffers. The concentration of buffer sites in cytosol is in the range 100–300 μM and in the millimolar range in the endoplasmic reticulum (283, 289). The cytosol contains slowly diffusible calcium-binding proteins which are capable of rapidly buffering cytosolic calcium. In addition, about 25% of cytosolic buffers are mobile (503). The ratio between free and bound calcium in cytosol is about 1:100 (153,316,464). It is possible that the effects of the buffers are significant near the calcium-release channels and that their saturation is required for the initiation of Ca^{2+} spikes and waves (352). In other words, the balance between the release of calcium from the endoplasmic reticulum and its binding to soluble proteins determines the spreading of localized Ca^{2+} signals.

Once Ca^{2+} is transported into the endoplasmic reticulum by (Ca^{2+})ATPase, a majority of it does not remain free. The mechanism that permits large quantities of calcium to be accumulated and quickly released is based on the binding of calcium to specific intraluminal proteins. Calsequestrin and calreticulin, calcium-binding proteins found in the reticular lumen, show the basic properties expected for a dynamic calcium-storage function: a high capacity and a low affinity for calcium (359). By buffering luminal free calcium concentrations, calsequestrin and calreticulin protect the accumulation of insoluble calcium phosphate precipitates. They also protect several endomembrane functions from the toxic effects of high luminal calcium concentrations (279). Calsequestrin and calreticulin are not single proteins but are expressed as multiple isoforms (120, 285). Overexpression of calreticulin inhibits repetitive IP_3-induced calcium waves. Deletion mutagenesis shows that calreticulin inhibition is mediated by the high-affinity–low-capacity calcium-binding do-main, which does not contribute significantly to calcium storage in the endoplasmic reticulum (46).

CALCIUM ENTRY CONTROLLED BY CALCIUM MOBILIZATION

It is generally accepted that activation of IP_3-dependent calcium mobilization is associated with depletion of the endoplasmic reticulum calcium pool and that Ca^{2+} entry is essential for sustaining agonist-induced Ca^{2+} spiking and refilling the intracellular calcium pools upon termination of receptor activation. The two phases of Ca^{2+} signaling during the sustained activation of phospholipase C–coupled receptors can be determined easily by comparing the responses of cell populations to a calcium-mobilizing agonist in the presence or absence of extracellular calcium (2, 7, 145, 177, 236, 433, 447). Receptor activation results in a transient increase in $[Ca^{2+}]_i$ in cells bathed in Ca^{2+}-deficient medium, while in a Ca^{2+}-containing medium the initial spike phase is accompanied by an additional plateau component (Fig. 9.4A). The sustained plateau phase can be further analyzed with specific blockers of plasma membrane calcium channels (Fig. 9.4B).

In general, several families of plasma membrane channels could be involved in such Ca^{2+} entry. So-called calcium release–activated calcium (CRAC) channels have received the most attention in this field (362). An additional class of plasma membrane channels that may participate in sustained Ca^{2+} entry is comprised of the nonselective cation channels (205). The structure of CRAC and nonselective calcium channels is unknown (25). Furthermore, in excitable cells, VGCCs mediate or participate in IP_3-induced Ca^{2+} entry (420). The truncated form of VGCCs also is expressed in both excitable and nonexcitable cells. The α_1-subunit of these channels lacks the first four transmembrane segments, but when it is co-expressed with the α_2- and β-subunits, it forms a functional and voltage-insensitive calcium channel (253). Another class of channels, the P_2 receptor channels, may participate in sustained Ca^{2+} entry in cells that secrete ATP in response to agonist stimulation (455).

Capacitative Calcium Entry

The idea of capacitative calcium entry, by analogy with a capacitor in an electrical circuit, implies that intracellular calcium stores prevent entry when they are charged but promote entry as soon as stored calcium is discharged (360). The similarities in the properties of this entry among different cell types suggest a common mechanism (361, 362). Capacitative calcium entry can

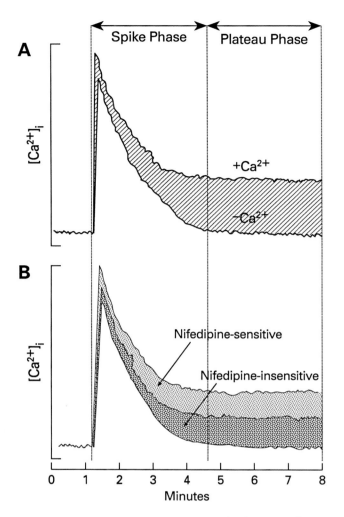

FIG. 9.4. Components of the agonist-induced calcium signal in an excitable cell. *A:* Spike and plateau phases of the $[Ca^{2+}]_i$ response to agonist stimulation can be resolved into a largely extracellular calcium–independent component and an influx-dependent component (dashed area). *B:* Extracellular calcium–dependent component in agonist-induced $[Ca^{2+}]_i$ response can be analyzed further by utilizing specific inhibitors of plasma membrane calcium channels.

Initially, it was suggested that capacitative entry is typical for nonexcitable cells and that such entry occurs through CRAC channels, in contrast to excitable cells, where VGCCs provide the pathway for calcium influx. However, the inositol phosphate system is also operative in excitable cells (362, 420) and in many instances is able to activate capacitative entry (61, 74, 106). Further investigations should clarify whether this entry is mediated solely through CRAC channels or if VGCCs or another class of calcium channels are regulated by the capacitative entry mechanism as well.

Calcium Release–Activated Calcium Channels. The structure of CRAC channels is still unknown. The low unitary cord conductance of Ca^{2+} entry (24 fS, in contrast to VGCCs, whose conductance is between 10 and 30 pS) is compatible with the role of a carrier in Ca^{2+} influx; however, results of noise analysis are more consistent with channel behavior (507). The absence of a potent and specific activating and inhibiting ligand for these channels makes it difficult to address their role in cellular calcium homeostasis. Channels are blocked by several trivalent and bivalent ions in the following order: $La^{3+} > Zn^{2+} > Cd^{2+} > Be^{2+} = Co^{2+} = Mn^{2+} > Ni^{2+} > Sr^{2+} > Ba^{2+}$ (163). Like VGCCs (88) and IP_3R channels (29), CRAC channels are sensitive to $[Ca^{2+}]_i$; both calcium-dependent inactivation and activation of these channels have been observed (350, 508–510). In contrast to VGCCs, CRAC channels are not activated by plasma membrane depolarization. Furthermore, recordings are made in hyperpolarized cells, resulting in an increase in the electrochemical gradient for calcium (271).

Initially, it was suggested that CRAC channels were IP_3R channels expressed in the plasma membrane. This hypothesis was supported by the presence of an immunospecific IP_3R channel expressed in the plasma membrane of T lymphocytes (192) and endothelial cells (129), as well as the ability of IP_3 and/or IP_4 to activate calcium channels on the cytoplasmic surface (303). Two findings, however, contradict this hypothesis: first, the single-cord conductivity of IP_3R channels is higher than that of CRAC channels; second, since Ca^{2+} entry into lymphocytes can be activated by thapsigargin (that is, without an increase in inositol phosphate production), these channels should be regulated by a mechanism other than IP_3 or IP_4 (95, 163, 262, 350). However, this could be explained by a dual regulation of CRAC channels by inositol phosphates and some other messenger(s) generated by the depletion of intracellular calcium pools.

The other proposal is that CRAC channels have a structure similar to the transient receptor potential (*trp*) protein from *Drosophila* mutants, whose photore-

be switched on by calcium-mobilizing agonists (74, 336, 350, 507), as well as by addition of IP_3 (31, 163, 336, 350), inhibition of (Ca^{2+})ATPase by thapsigargin (124, 262, 350, 441), discharge of the endoplasmic reticulum calcium content by the calcium ionophore ionomycin (95, 162, 163), or incubation of cells in Ca^{2+}-deficient conditions (162,350). Injection of heparin, an IP_3R channel inhibitor, completely blocks IP_3-induced Ca^{2+} mobilization and capacitative entry (31). All of these lines of evidence indicate that a decrease in endoplasmic reticulum calcium content is an effective signal for calcium influx.

ceptors are incapable of eliciting a sustained calcium response (148). The *trp* and related *trpl* gene products display significant amino-acid sequence similarity to the α-subunit of L-type VGCCs, but lack the specific basic residues in the S4 region which are responsible for the voltage sensitivity of VGCCs (355). In insects, photoreceptor signaling utilizes a phospholipase C–coupled system, implicating that the *trp* gene product may operate as a calcium channel activated by emptying intracellular calcium pools (290). In accord with this, when transfected in another cell type, the *trp* channel is sensitive to depletion of the endoplasmic reticulum. As with the IP_3R hypothesis, however, this explanation faces the problem of the difference in the conductances between the two channels (25).

Nonselective Cationic Channels. Several published observations support the view that the signal for capacitative calcium entry also can regulate calcium influx through calcium-conducting nonselective cation channels. Endothelial cells from human umbilical cord express a nonselective cation channel, with a K:Na:Ca permeation ratio of 1:0.9:0.2 and a single-channel conductance of about 27 pS (317). In these cells, application of histamine induced Ca^{2+} transients and an ionic current that reversed near 0 mV. The amplitude of this current closely correlates with the amplitude of the concomitant Ca^{2+} transients, suggesting that calcium influx through histamine-activated nonselective cation channels is responsible for Ca^{2+} spiking (318). A 50 pS nonselective cation channel is expressed in mast cells and contributes to the sustained increase in calcium following receptor activation. In contrast to CRAC channels, this form of Ca^{2+} entry is not blockable by dialyzing cells with the IP_3R channel inhibitor heparin (110). The depletion of intracellular calcium stores by thapsigargin also activates a calcium-conducting nonselective cation current in mouse pancreatic acinar cells, demonstrating more directly that capacitative calcium entry can be associated with channels other than CRAC (205).

Signals for Capacitative Calcium Entry. The mechanism of capacitative calcium entry is not only unclear but also a subject of debate (25, 362). The simplest way for IP_3 to regulate capacitative calcium influx is to activate directly IP_3R channels expressed in the plasma membrane. As discussed above, such a direct effect of IP_3 is inconsistent with several lines of evidence, pointing to an indirect action of this intracellular messenger. Two major hypotheses have been introduced to explain how information is transmitted from the endoplasmic reticulum to the plasma membrane calcium channels.

One is based on the importance of the topographical arrangement of the endoplasmic reticulum relative to the plasma membrane (conformational coupling models) and the other emphasizes the need for a diffusible messenger(s).

The conformational coupling models also presume the role of inositol phosphates in Ca^{2+} entry. These models propose the transfer of information directly from IP_3R channels to CRAC channels. The signal generated by the depletion of intracellular pools could be integrated by the large cytoplasmic head of the IP_3R channel, leading to a transmission of information to the CRAC channel through a protein–protein interaction (175). Since there are three separate isoforms of the IP_3R channel, which are expressed frequently in the same cell, it is possible that one of the isoforms is specifically responsible for such conformational coupling. This model also integrates the role of IP_4 and cytosolic calcium in the control of capacitative calcium entry. An IP_4-binding protein is a member of the family of guanosine triphosphatase (GTPase)-activating proteins (80), which have been implicated in the control of capacitative calcium entry. Thus, the proposed role of IP_4 in capacitative calcium entry (303) could be explained by an action on a G protein, which in turn participates in conformational coupling. The well-defined sensitivity of IP_3R channels to cytosolic calcium also could explain the bidirectional role of this cation on capacitative calcium entry (25).

An alternative protein–protein interaction model proposes a role for protein phosphorylation and dephosphorylation during information transfer. For example, activation of protein kinase C may lead to inhibition of capacitative entry (150, 300, 350, 351). A more complex role of protein kinase C in cellular calcium homeostasis includes a reduction in intracellular calcium-storage capacity and an augmentation of Ca^{2+} entry (374). In addition, several laboratories have suggested that phosphorylation of tyrosine residues may be important in the activation of capacitative entry. Thus, inhibition of tyrosine phosphorylation by tyrosine kinase inhibitors is associated with inhibition of receptor- and thapsigargin-induced capacitative entry. While the effects of these inhibitors on agonist-mediated Ca^{2+} entry may be due to inhibition of tyrosine kinase receptor–coupling with phospholipase C-γ, inhibition of thapsigargin-induced Ca^{2+} entry indicates a more direct role for tyrosine phosphorylation in capacitative entry (129, 392, 475).

The list of potential signals for capacitative calcium entry includes metabolites of cytochrome P-450 (12), cyclic guanosine monophosphate (cGMP) (335), and the novel diffusible messenger calcium influx factor

(CIF) (363), postulated to be a low-molecular-weight phosphorylated compound stored in the endoplasmic reticulum. Release of CIF into the cytosol is activated by Ca^{2+} released from the endoplasmic reticulum, which then diffuses to the plasma membrane and activates CRAC channels. It is notable that CIF also activates calcium influx when applied extracellularly (363). The low molecular weight of CIF may satisfy the need for a rapid diffusion of a soluble factor since the latency between Ca^{2+} release and entry in some cell types can be less than 100 ms (271). To be validated, this hypothesis should answer what this factor is and how it is generated.

Voltage-Gated Calcium Entry

Although excitable cells face the same problems as nonexcitable ones in reporting endoplasmic reticulum calcium content to the plasma membrane and activating Ca^{2+} entry, integration of the V_m pathway into endoplasmic reticulum–derived $[Ca^{2+}]_i$ oscillations has not received appropriate attention. An advance in this field was made using pituitary gonadotrophs, lactotrophs, and β-pancreatic cells as cell models (420). The following aspects of the interaction between IP_3-controlled calcium release and VGCC activity merit more detailed consideration: (1) kinetics of depletion and repletion of agonist-sensitive calcium pools; (2) synchronization of plasma membrane and endoplasmic reticulum oscillator activities; (3) control of voltage-gated calcium entry; and (4) the role of VGCCs in endoplasmic reticulum excitability.

Kinetics of Depletion and Repletion of the Endoplasmic Reticulum Calcium Pool.

Single gonadotrophs bathed in a Ca^{2+}-deficient medium show that agonist- and IP_3-stimulated cells oscillate for 3–10 min. Conversely, in the presence of calcium they oscillate for at least 60 min (428). In both Ca^{2+}-containing and Ca^{2+}-deficient media, the amplitudes of agonist-induced $[Ca^{2+}]_i$ transients decrease, albeit with different kinetics (211). These data indicate that gonadotrophs are very economical in terms of the reuptake of calcium but that extrusion mechanisms also are operative. Furthermore, these observations go against the argument that the I_{CRAC} influx pathway operates in agonist-stimulated gonadotrophs (211, 268) since hyperpolarization does not abolish Ca^{2+} influx through CRAC channels.

In general, the kinetics of changes in luminal calcium content in these cells reflect the pattern of Ca^{2+} spiking (Fig. 9.5) and can be summarized as follows: steady-state 1, before agonist application; transient 1, when Ca^{2+} entry is insufficient to compensate the extrusion

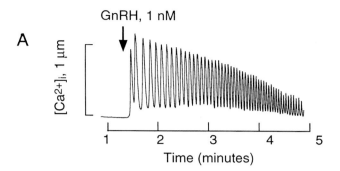

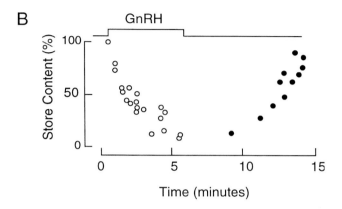

FIG. 9.5. Kinetics of depletion and repletion of agonist-sensitive calcium pool. *A:* Typical pattern of $[Ca^{2+}]_i$ oscillations in a single rat gonadotroph. *B:* Store calcium content is expressed as a percentage of prestimulus level. *Open circles,* endoplasmic reticulum calcium content during gonadotropin-releasing hormone *(GnRH)* stimulation. *Closed circles,* endoplasmic reticulum calcium content after withdrawal of GnRH. Estimation of intraluminal Ca^{2+} was done by ionomycin applied at different times after GnRH stimulation.

and intracellular redistribution of calcium, leading to a decrease in the amplitude of spiking; steady-state 2, when equilibrium is reached and the amplitude of spiking is stabilized; transient 2, upon the removal of the agonist, when Ca^{2+} entry dominates over extrusion; and back to steady-state 1, when the initial endoplasmic reticulum calcium content is reached (235). Thus, the V_m influx pathway is not sufficient to protect cells from depletion of the endoplasmic reticulum calcium pool but is essential for an equilibrium in calcium influx/efflux to be reached during sustained stimulation. Steady-state 2 equilibrium can provide long-lasting Ca^{2+} spiking, though the pool is almost completely depleted.

Synchronization of the Two Oscillators.

The association of changes in V_m with IP_3-controlled calcium release is a common feature in pituitary and other cell types regulated by calcium-mobilizing hormones. The level of integration of the two variables, $[Ca^{2+}]_i$ and V_m, varies according to the types of ion channel present in each cell type. For example, many nonexcitable cells operated by calcium-mobilizing receptors, exemplified by exocrine acinar cells (138, 327, 476), exhibit a simple association of V_m oscillations with $[Ca^{2+}]_i$. In these cells, agonist-induced $[Ca^{2+}]_i$ oscillations are highly synchronized with depolarizing transients. However, such V_m oscillations are dissociated from IP_3-induced Ca^{2+} entry since these cells do not possess VGCCs through which calcium can enter during operation of the cytoplasmic oscillator.

Pituitary cells exhibit a more complex pattern of synchronization of V_m and $[Ca^{2+}]_i$ oscillations due to their electrical excitability. In lactotrophs and growth hormone cell lines, TRH causes a biphasic $[Ca^{2+}]_i$ response that corresponds to the biphasic change in V_m (Fig. 9.6A). The spike phase of the $[Ca^{2+}]_i$ response

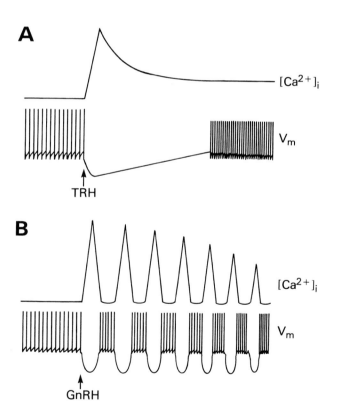

FIG. 9.6. Patterns of synchronization of $[Ca^{2+}]_i$ and membrane potentials in cells operated by calcium-mobilizing receptors. Schematic representation of thyroid-releasing hormone *(TRH)*-induced $[Ca^{2+}]_i$ and membrane potential *(V_m)* responses in lactotrophs *(A)* and gonadotropin-releasing hormone *(GnRH)*-induced $[Ca^{2+}]_i$ and V_m responses in gonadotrophs *(B)*. [From S. S. Stojilkovic and K. J. Catt. Calcium oscillations in anterior pituitary cells. *Endocr. Rev.* 13: 256–280, 1992, with permission. © The Endocrine Society.]

correlates temporally with the hyperpolarization phase, which is sufficient to abolish action potential firing. Transient hyperpolarization is followed by gradual depolarization, which ultimately leads to enhanced generation of action potentials for an extended period (6, 8, 173, 219, 332, 333). In accord with this, application of dihydropyridine calcium channel antagonists lowers the sustained rise in $[Ca^{2+}]_i$, confirming its dependence on an increase in the frequency of action potential (6, 333). A similar synchronization of electrical and biochemical events occurs in vasopressin-stimulated aortic cells (371).

The most complex interaction between $[Ca^{2+}]_i$ and V_m occurs in cells expressing both the plasma membrane and endoplasmic reticulum oscillators (Fig. 9.6B). For example, in gonadotrophs, the oscillatory rise in $[Ca^{2+}]_i$ in response to agonist stimulation switches the spontaneous firing of action potentials into a pattern composed of an immediate hyperpolarization followed by V_m oscillations with action potential firing at the peak of each spike (210, 428, 461) (Fig. 9.7). The participation of action potential–driven Ca^{2+} influx is minor during the initial phase of agonist stimulation and intracellular calcium mobilization but is important to the sustained operation of the cytoplasmic oscillator for maintenance of the endoplasmic reticulum calcium pool (211). In β-pancreatic cells, injection of IP_3 mimics the agonist (glucose) in activating oscillatory electrical activity similar to that observed in gonadotrophs (13). These observations support the view that there is a general scheme for the synchronization of electrical activity with operation of the cytoplasmic oscillator in cells in which both systems are operative. Furthermore, the coordinated and interdependent actions of the agonist-induced biochemical and electrical events maintain a long-lasting calcium signal during agonist stimulation.

Control of Voltage-Gated Calcium Entry. The VGCCs can be regulated by protein kinases C and A, G_i and G_o proteins, and cytosolic calcium (486). Since calcium-mobilizing receptors are coupled to the phospholipase C pathway, protein kinase C and cytosolic calcium represent the two major potential messengers involved in control of Ca^{2+} entry through VGCCs. Many calcium-mobilizing receptors are able to cross-couple to G proteins other than G_q/G_{11}, suggesting that the α- and β/γ-subunits of other G proteins, as well as cAMP protein kinase A, also may participate in the control of Ca^{2+} entry (for details, see Chapter 5, by Lledo et al., in this *Handbook*).

Several lines of evidence indicate that protein kinase C may affect VGCCs directly (414). Furthermore, in various cell types expressing VGCCs, the effects of the

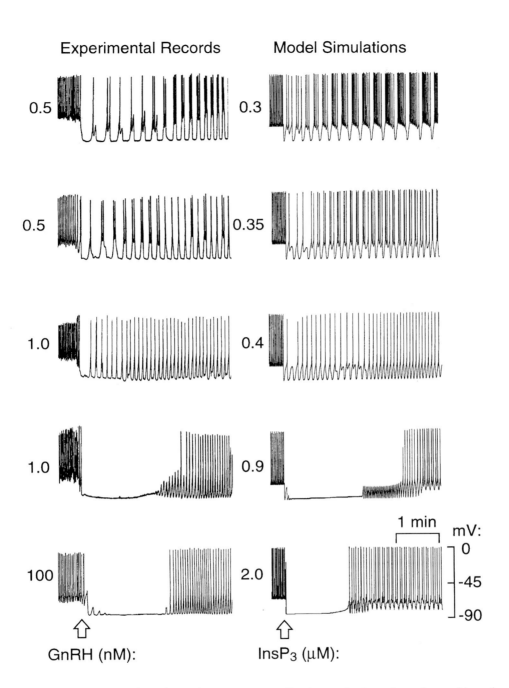

FIG. 9.7. Concentration-dependent voltage-response profiles in agonist (experimental records)- and inositol(1,4,5)-triphosphate *(InsP₃)* (model simulations) stimulated gonadotrophs. In experiments, increasing concentrations of gonadotropin-releasing hormone *(GnRH)* were applied at the *arrow*. In model simulations, increasing concentrations of InsP₃ were used. [From Li *et al.* (235) with permission.]

protein kinase C activator PMA on calcium homeostasis include both stimulation and inhibition of channel-mediated calcium influx (217, 364, 401). In pituitary gonadotrophs and growth hormone cells, Ca^{2+} entry also is stimulated by PMA and diacylglycerol (400, 421), and this response is predominantly dihydropyridine-sensitive (8, 178, 400, 421, 424). The existence of potential sites for phosphorylation in α_{1A}- and α_{1B}-subunits of VGCCs (414) is in accord with these observations. An alternative hypothesis proposes that the opening of calcium channels could be secondary to the closure of agonist-regulated potassium channels (20, 100) via activation of protein kinase C (8). While IP_3-mediated increases in $[Ca^{2+}]_i$ are responsible for activation of potassium currents, protein kinase C may phosphorylate potassium channels and suppress their activity. Ultimately, this action of protein kinase C would enhance the generation of action potentials and increase Ca^{2+} entry through VGCCs (333). Accordingly, phorbol esters mimic the TRH-induced sustained enhancement of spike generation in GH_3 cells (328). Activation of these channels in growth hormone cells is associated with phosphorylation by cAMP-dependent protein kinase, suggesting that both protein kinase A– and protein kinase C–dependent phosphorylations occur, depending on the second messenger produced during activation of specific types of receptor.

Cytosolic calcium negatively influences voltage-gated calcium entry. Such control involves two distinct regulatory mechanisms: calcium-controlled influx through calcium-activated potassium channels ($I_{K(Ca)}$) and VGCCs and calcium-controlled efflux through plasma membrane pumps and exchangers. The role of $I_{K(Ca)}$ in the control of calcium influx has been demonstrated in several pituitary cell types stimulated by TRH and GnRH (210, 376, 377, 461). An additional role of $[Ca^{2+}]_i$ on the direct inhibition of VGCCs should not be excluded since the conductivity of L-type calcium channels in gonadotrophs is sensitive to $[Ca^{2+}]_i$ (425, 432). Also, an essential calcium-binding motif for calcium-sensitive inactivation of L-type calcium channels has been described (88). Thus, it is possible that the conductivity of the L channels, in addition to their regulation by protein kinase C, is controlled by $[Ca^{2+}]_i$ and that such a dual control system is operative in several excitable cells, including gonadotrophs and lactotrophs.

A potential mechanism for communication between the endoplasmic reticulum and the plasma membrane in excitable cells, in which $[Ca^{2+}]_i$ itself is the messenger, has been suggested (235, 375). The mechanism of calcium-controlled calcium entry can be summarized as follows. In unstimulated cells with closed IP_3 chan-

nels, both plasma membrane and endoplasmic reticulum calcium influx and efflux are balanced, resulting in a basal $[Ca^{2+}]_i$. During agonist stimulation (transient 1 phase), this balance is broken at both membranes. At the endoplasmic reticulum membrane, Ca^{2+} release floods the cytosol with Ca^{2+}, activating $I_{K(Ca)}$ and reducing voltage-gated calcium entry. At steady-state 2, calcium fluxes across each membrane are again in balance, with $[Ca^{2+}]_i$ near basal levels. However, a balance is achieved with IP_3R channels that are more permeable to Ca^{2+} and with an almost completely depleted endoplasmic reticulum calcium content. Removal of the agonist again breaks the balance by reducing the calcium efflux through IP_3R channels, leading to a decrease in $[Ca^{2+}]_i$ due to activation of endoplasmic reticulum (Ca^{2+})ATPase. At the level of the plasma membrane, this decline causes an increase in net Ca^{2+} entry and a gradual refilling of the endoplasmic reticulum pool due to a reduction in Ca^{2+} extrusion and depolarization of the plasma membrane (235).

Role of Voltage-Gated Calcium Channels in Endoplasmic Reticulum Excitability.

In excitable cells, $InsP_3$ induces periodic Ca^{2+} mobilization at any membrane potential (209, 428). However, in cells held at hyperpolarized membrane potentials, at which VGCCs are not active, the oscillatory Ca^{2+} response occurs in a manner comparable to that observed in cells bathed in a Ca^{2+}-deficient medium (428). In both cases, Ca^{2+} response is associated with a progressive decrease in the frequency and amplitude of spiking, as well as the cessation of oscillations within 3–10 min. This is in contrast to the sustained rhythm achieved in nonclamped cells bathed in Ca^{2+}-containing medium (211), suggesting that, in addition to influencing the amplitude of the Ca^{2+} signal, Ca^{2+} entry through VGCCs influences the kinetics of intracellular calcium mobilization (209).

The frequency and duration of Ca^{2+} spiking are modulated by extracellular Ca^{2+} entry. For example, the decrease in the frequency and duration of Ca^{2+} spikes observed in hyperpolarized cells is reversed rapidly by membrane depolarization (Fig. 9.8). Several lines of evidence indicate that such depolarization effects are not related to the voltage and/or Ca^{2+} entry–dependent increase in IP_3 production. First, depolarization does not change the frequency of Ca^{2+} spiking in cells bathed in a Ca^{2+}-deficient medium. Second, an increase in $[Ca^{2+}]_i$ by addition of high concentrations of K^+, which induce membrane depolarization, or by addition of the VGCC activator Bay K 8644 is not associated with an increase in IP_3 production (434). This argues against calcium-dependent facilitation of phospholipase C activity. Third, depolarization-

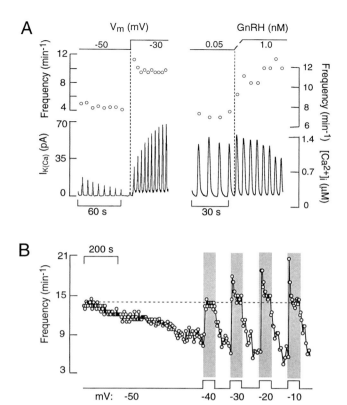

FIG. 9.8. Dependence of spiking frequency on agonist concentration and calcium influx. *A:* Modulation of Ca²⁺ spiking frequency by depolarization *(left panel)* and by increase in gonadotropin-releasing hormone *(GnRH)* concentration *(right panel)*. *B:* Membrane potential *(Vₘ)* dependence of depolarization on sustained GnRH-induced Ca²⁺ oscillations. Dashed horizontal line indicates maximum frequency response reached 150 s after initiation of oscillations at the holding potential of −50 mV. In a step-depolarization protocol, calcium-activated potassium current was employed as an indicator of cytosolic calcium concentration. [From Kukuljan et al. (211) with permission.]

IP₃R channels (29) and the hypothesis of endoplasmic reticulum excitability (189, 221), which suggests that IP₃ activates the IP₃R channels, sets the maximal rate of Ca²⁺ release, and makes the IP₃R channel sensitive to calcium (340). Thus, once the IP₃-induced liberation of calcium is initiated, the consequent rise in [Ca²⁺]ᵢ provides a positive feedback signal that leads to a progressive increase of its own release to the maximal rate determined by the IP₃ concentration (189). Furthermore, continuous depletion of the endoplasmic reticulum pool in hyperpolarized cells and the consequent reduction in the Ca²⁺ release gradient may be responsible for slowing down the response. The reduction in Ca²⁺ release subsequently can decrease the rate of activation of the receptor channel even for a constant high level of IP₃. In addition, at lower IP₃ concentrations, the excitability of the endoplasmic reticulum depends on action potential–driven calcium entry. In the absence of electrical activity, endoplasmic reticulum calcium excitability would decrease below the threshold required for an oscillatory pattern during sustained agonist stimulation (235).

These effects of depolarization-associated calcium entry explain why the pattern of the signal in gonadotrophs during sustained stimulation is so sensitive to the electrical activity of the plasma membrane (209, 211, 472). Action potential–driven calcium entry not only protects the cells from complete depletion of the endoplasmic reticulum calcium pool during sustained stimulation but also provides the extra calcium needed to reach the threshold level for a rapid increase in calcium efflux from the endoplasmic reticulum, such as occurs at the beginning of the rising phase of each spike. This establishes a highly regular periodic pattern of sustained spiking that can continue without alterations as long as IP₃ levels remain elevated and plasma membrane excitability is not modified.

TEMPORAL AND SPATIAL ORGANIZATION OF CALCIUM SIGNALS

Local and Global Calcium Spikes

A rise in [Ca²⁺]ᵢ can occur locally at a specific subcellular domain or globally when a calcium signal spreads throughout the cytoplasm. Both calcium influx and calcium mobilization can form local and global Ca²⁺ signals. An alternative or additional mechanism for localization of Ca²⁺ signals is Ca²⁺ accumulation in intracellular stores (417). In general, a local increase in calcium concentration occurs when there is no propagation of signal within the cell and calcium is buffered

induced modulation of sustained spiking also occurs in cells with "clamped" IP₃ levels (209, 211). These observations support the hypothesis that changes in [Ca²⁺]ᵢ, due to extracellular entry, modulate the oscillatory response by acting at the level of calcium liberation from the endoplasmic reticulum. Stimulation and inhibition of voltage-insensitive calcium entry in *Xenopus* oocytes also modulate the frequency of IP₃-induced Ca²⁺ spiking (136), indicating that the nature of channels involved in Ca²⁺ entry as well as changes in Vₘ are not essential for the observed effects.

The rapid effect of Ca²⁺ entry on sustained spiking is compatible with the activating role of this ion on and sequestered by cytosolic buffers and organelles, forming a steep spatial gradient (354). For example, depolarization-driven calcium entry produces two types of localized $[Ca^{2+}]_i$ increase close to the plasma membrane. At the mouth of an open calcium channel, $[Ca^{2+}]_i$ can reach hundreds of micromoles. These highly localized peaks are transient, with a time scale faster than that of calcium binding to its buffers, and relevant for co-localized processes (244). However, the equilibrated $[Ca^{2+}]_i$ in the layer close to the plasma membrane is about 1 μM (155, 391) and can exhibit a strong influence on the frequency and temporal profile of action potentials (234). In cells expressing RyR channels, voltage-gated calcium entry can spread to other areas due to calcium-induced calcium release. Thus, local increases in $[Ca^{2+}]_i$ can initiate a self-propagated signal in which calcium serves as a diffusible factor (24).

Calcium-mobilizing agonists also can lead to the formation of localized Ca^{2+} signals (calcium microgradients). As discussed in detail by Petersen et al. (354), such microgradients are the primary sites of a rise in $[Ca^{2+}]_i$ which spread or do not spread depending on agonist concentration and the distribution of IP3R channels. At subthreshold agonist concentrations, the two major factors for the generation of localized Ca^{2+} signals are the site of action of the primary stimulus and the density of calcium-mobilizing receptors on the plasma membrane. The focal and discrete injection of an agonist close to one region of the cell leads to a localized rise in $[Ca^{2+}]_i$ in a region of stimulation (493). Similarly, the initial rise of $[Ca^{2+}]_i$ in oocytes occurs at the point of sperm entry (295), and flash photolysis of caged IP3 induces a rise in $[Ca^{2+}]_i$ at certain spots or foci (221, 339). In pancreatic acinar cells, the IP3R channels are localized predominantly in a zone with secretory granules. Such a distribution provides localized Ca^{2+} signals independently of the regions of stimulation by agonist (354).

At higher agonist concentrations, Ca^{2+} signals spread from primary sites toward other cellular areas in a wave-like motion, suggesting that these spots serve as triggering zones (382). Calcium waves are markedly slower than electrical signals. Depending on the cell type, calcium propagates at 5–100 $\mu m/s$ (185, 282, 312, 452). The pattern of IP3R channel distribution is critical for wave propagation. For example, the density of IP3R channels in astrocytes varies within the cells, creating a nonlinear propagation of calcium waves, with several focal loci where the wave is amplified (493). Priming of cells with IP3 is required for wave propagation, but calcium serves as a positive feedback element (221). Thus, the same model used in the explanation of the oscilla-

tory response applies to wave propagation because these are manifestations of the same phenomenon, endoplasmic reticulum calcium excitability.

Cell Specificity of Calcium Signaling

Oscillatory Ca^{2+} signals are observed frequently in single-cell studies, following activation of phospholipase C pathways (115, 179, 283). However, not all cells operated by calcium-mobilizing receptors exhibit such oscillations; often, cells respond with nonoscillatory Ca^{2+} signals (126, 208, 280, 454). Figure 9.9 illustrates a case in which several cell types express the same calcium-mobilizing endothelin receptors and respond with nonoscillatory patterns of Ca^{2+} signaling. Similarly, in single Leydig cells and ovarian granulosa cells, GnRH induces a transient spike response, usually without a plateau phase (81, 454, 479). In two other cell types expressing GnRH and endothelin receptors, immortalized $\alpha T3–1$ gonadotrophs and GT1 neurons, agonists also induce nonoscillatory Ca^{2+} signals, but the pattern of this response is more complex than that observed in Leydig cells (206, 208, 269, 280, 427). As in the early Ca^{2+} measurements in cell suspensions, the calcium response in individual $\alpha T3–1$ and GT1–7 cells is composed of two phases: an early spike phase dependent on Ca^{2+} mobilization and a sustained plateau phase dependent on Ca^{2+} entry through VGCCs (269, 280). The most complex pattern of agonist-induced Ca^{2+} signaling is seen in pituitary gonadotrophs. Unlike other cells which express GnRH and endothelin receptors, gonadotrophs respond to physiological concentrations of agonists with base-line oscillatory spiking (169, 418, 423, 431).

Another difference in the Ca^{2+}-signaling responses of gonadotrophs and other cells operated by GnRH receptors is related to the mean duration of Ca^{2+} transients. In oscillating gonadotrophs, the duration of a single transient is 3–5 s (429), which is only one-tenth to one-fifteenth of that observed in Leydig cells (454). However, gonadotrophs also respond with a prolonged spike followed by a sustained plateau or spiking when stimulated with high GnRH concentrations (233). As shown in Figure 9.10, the duration of the spike response in gonadotrophs is comparable to that of Ca^{2+} spikes in Leydig cells. Also, there is no amplitude modulation of the Ca^{2+} response in gonadotrophs stimulated with GnRH in the 1 nM–1 μM concentration range. These observations raise the possibility that the spike phase of the biphasic calcium response in gonadotrophs and the single-spike calcium response in Leydig cells are driven by the same mechanism but that gonadotrophs express an additional sys-

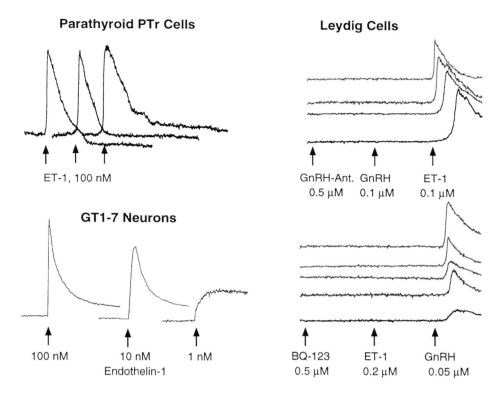

FIG. 9.9. Nonoscillatory calcium responses in single parathyroid cells, GT1-7 neurons, and Leydig cells. No obvious modulations of the amplitude of $[Ca^{2+}]_i$ response to increasing endothelin-1$(ET\text{-}1)$ concentrations were observed in parathyroid and Leydig cells. In GT1-7 cells, a consistent increase in the amplitude of $[Ca^{2+}]_i$ response to increasing concentrations of endothelin-1 was observed. *GnRH*, gonadotropin-releasing hormone; *GnRH-Ant.*, GnRh antagonist; *BQ-123*, ET_A receptor antagonist. [From M. Tomic, M. L. Dufau, K. K. Catt, and S. S. Stojilkovic. Calcium signaling in single rat Leydig cells. *Endocrinology* 136: 3422–3429, 1995. © The Endocrine Society.]

tem for Ca^{2+} signaling that operates at low agonist/IP_3 concentrations (454).

Receptor Specificity of Calcium Signaling

In general, activation of different calcium-mobilizing receptors expressed in the same cells should lead to similar patterns of spiking. This conclusion is enforced by the finding that non-metabolized IP_3 (429, 477) and the substances that facilitate IP_3R channel opening, such as thimerosal (36, 434), can induce Ca^{2+} oscillations similar to those induced by calcium-mobilizing agonists. Thus, the ligand–receptor and G protein–phospholipase C complexes are not directly involved in Ca^{2+} signaling, but the IP_3 concentration should translate their impact on the endoplasmic reticulum oscillator. In accord with this, the patterns of Ca^{2+} signals in gonadotrophs stimulated with GnRH, endothelin, and pituitary adenylate cyclase–activating polypeptide are highly comparable. Furthermore, injection of heparin inhibits the action of all three agonists,

confirming that IP_3 mediates the stimulatory action of these receptors through IP_3R channels (368, 434, 461). As shown in Figure 9.11, there are quantitative differences in the potencies of these agonists: GnRH is almost two and three orders of magnitude more potent than endothelin and pituitary adenylate cyclase–activating polypeptide, respectively.

Several factors other than IP_3 concentration can influence the pattern of Ca^{2+} spiking, including Ca^{2+} entry, (Ca^{2+})ATPase activity, and distribution of IP_3R channels. The different receptor-controlled calcium pump transport rates may underline the observed differences in the pattern of Ca^{2+} spiking in hepatocytes stimulated by two calcium-mobilizing agonists, vasopressin and phenylephrine. Vasopressin-induced spikes last longer, indicating a slower rate of recovery (381). In pancreatic acinar cells, acetylcholine and cholecystokinin induce distinct signaling patterns at low as well as high agonist concentrations: acetylcholine induces localized signals, while cholecystokinin induces global signals (353). These cells express both IP_3R and RyR chan-

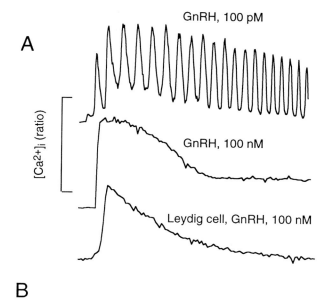

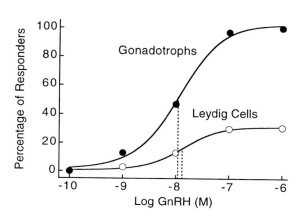

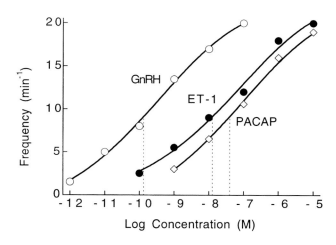

FIG. 9.11. Dependence of the frequency of Ca^{2+} spiking on agonist concentrations in rat gonadotrophs. Data for concentration responses for gonadotropin-releasing hormone *(GnRH)* and endothelin-1 *(ET-1)* were derived from Stojilkovic et al. (422) and those for pituitary adenylate cyclase–activating polypeptide *(PACAP)* from unpublished results.

FIG. 9.10. Comparison of the patterns of gonadotropin-releasing hormone *(GnRH)*-induced $[Ca^{2+}]_i$ responses in rat gonadotrophs and Leydig cells. *A:* Time dependence of the $[Ca^{2+}]_i$ response in the two cell types. Two *upper tracings* are from gonadotrophs and *bottom tracing* from a Leydig cell. *B:* Concentration-dependent effects of GnRH on the number of cells showing biphasic responses in gonadotrophs and Leydig cells. Dotted lines illustrate EC_{50} values.

nels but with different distributions within the cells. As discussed above, IP_3R channels are co-localized with secretory vesicles, which explains the localized Ca^{2+} signals in acinar cells. Cholecystokinin may activate an additional spreading factor which increases the sensitivity of IP_3R and/or RyR channels (354).

Concentration-Dependent Regulation

Transduction of signals by plasma membrane receptors ensures that changes in plasma hormone levels evoke appropriate changes in intracellular messenger concentrations. When calcium is the intracellular messenger, the pattern of transduction varies, depending on the cell type. For example, GnRH and endothelin induce a nonoscillatory calcium response in single Leydig cells and ovarian granulosa cells. Neither cell type shows modulation of the amplitude of the $[Ca^{2+}]_i$ response with increasing agonist concentrations, suggesting that the coupling of the inositol-phosphate pathway to Ca^{2+} signaling occurs in an "all-or-none" fashion. However, individual Leydig cells exhibit a high degree of the threshold concentration required for the initiation of Ca^{2+} signaling, and the concentration dependence of agonist action is related to an increase in the number of cells that respond to the agonist (Fig. 9.12). About 75% of granulosa cells and about 30% of purified Leydig cells respond to a supramaximal GnRH concentration with an increase in $[Ca^{2+}]_i$.

In two other cell types expressing GnRH receptors, immortalized αT3–1 gonadotrophs and GT1 neurons, GnRH also induces nonoscillatory, amplitude-modulated Ca^{2+} signals (208, 269, 280). In addition, a leftward shift in the EC_{50} for GnRH is evident in GT1 neurons (Fig. 9.12, central panels). These cells "sense" the changes in IP_3 concentration and respond by increases in the amplitude of the $[Ca^{2+}]_i$ response. The most complex pattern of GnRH-induced Ca^{2+} signaling is seen in pituitary gonadotrophs. As discussed above, these cells show an oscillatory pattern of Ca^{2+} signaling, with the frequency modulated by GnRH concentration. The EC_{50} for such frequency-modulated signaling

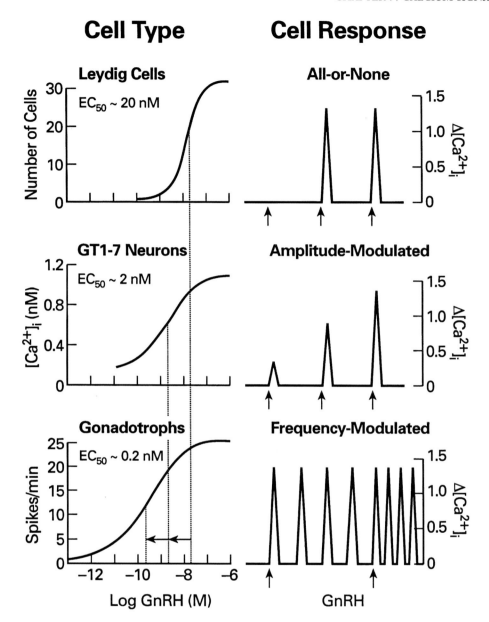

FIG. 9.12. Comparison of concentration dependence and $[Ca^{2+}]_i$ signaling patterns in Leydig cells, GT1-7 neurons, and pituitary gonadotrophs stimulated with gonadotropin-releasing hormone *(GnRH)*. *Left panels:* Data for concentration responses were derived from Iida et al. (169), Krsmanovic et al. (208), and Tomic et al. (453). *Right panels:* Schematic representation of the pattern of Ca^{2+} signals. [From M. Tomic, M. L. Dufau, K. J. Catt, and S. S. Stojikovic (454). Calcium signaling in single rat Leydig cells. *Endocrinology* 136: 3422–3429, 1995. © The Endocrine Society.]

is approximately ten times lower than that in GT1 neurons and about 100 times lower than that in Leydig cells (Fig. 9.12, bottom panels). The frequency of Ca^{2+} oscillations depends on agonist concentration in several other cell types, including hepatocytes (381), *Xenopus* oocytes (89), and endothelial cells (180). However, in some cells operated by calcium-mobilizing receptors, the mean amplitude of the response, rather than the frequency of spiking, increases with an increase in agonist concentration (138, 388, 499).

Intraorganelle Calcium Signaling

Propagation of Ca^{2+} signals within the cell is required for adequate regulation of cytosolic and membrane-associated cellular functions, such as control of the plasma membrane and endoplasmic reticulum channels' conductivities and enzyme activities. The requirement for calcium in the control of intracellular calcium storage compartment functions is also well established; however, the spreading of calcium signals into cytoplasmic organelles and the nucleus as well as the participation of these cellular compartments in a rapid cytosolic calcium response are not well characterized. In addition, the possibility that some of the compartments exhibit locally controlled Ca^{2+} signaling in response to receptor activation needs further clarification.

In general, a luminal calcium store may serve in a rapid Ca^{2+} response if the uptake, storage, and release of Ca^{2+} by an organelle is operative. Furthermore, a rapid rate of exchange between cytosolic and luminal calcium is required (111). The nucleus and all cytoplasmic organelles have the ability to uptake and release Ca^{2+}, no matter by which mechanism (359), but not all of the organelles are capable of rapid Ca^{2+} exchange across the membrane. For example, the exchange of Ca^{2+} between the secretory vesicles and cytosol is extremely low and slow (in hours) (111). The mechanism of Ca^{2+} loading and release by the Golgi complex and lysosomes is not well defined, but it is unlikely that these compartments play an important role in calcium signaling (359). Thus, although these structures presumably participate in intracellular calcium homeostasis, they are not essential for Ca^{2+} signaling.

Several reports indicate the participation of endosomes in the release of Ca^{2+} shortly after pinching off (94, 168). Caveolae, the small surface invaginations that eventually become vesicles, contain plasma membrane (Ca^{2+})ATPase and IP_3R channels (128, 129) and, thus, may participate in the control of intracellular Ca^{2+} signaling (Fig. 9.13). However, additional experiments are required to characterize the endocytotic mechanism for calcium signaling and its significance to oscillatory Ca^{2+} responses.

Nucleus. The nucleus is surrounded by a double membrane structure separating it from the cytoplasm. The perinuclear space is continuous with the endoplasmic reticulum (Fig. 9.13). Initial measurements of free calcium in the cytosol and nucleus showed a close parallelism in response (10, 237), suggesting that the Ca^{2+} level in the nucleus ($[Ca^{2+}]_n$) is not independently controlled. This suggestion is in accord with the old hypothesis that a passive diffusion of Ca^{2+} across nuclear pores leads to fast equilibration of $[Ca^{2+}]_i$ and $[Ca^{2+}]_n$. Thus, the nuclear envelope may serve only as a local reservoir for elevations of $[Ca^{2+}]_i$ and for its rapid diffusion from the cytosol into the nucleus.

However, this hypothesis is inconsistent with several lines of evidence. The nuclear membrane shares many features with the endoplasmic reticulum membrane, including expression of IP_3R channels, IP_4R, and (Ca^{2+})ATPase (203, 415). While IP_3R channels are expressed in the inner nuclear membrane, (Ca^{2+})ATPase and IP_4R are expressed in the outer membrane (166). The IP_3R channels in the nuclear membrane are sensitive to IP_3 and Ca^{2+}, are weakly regulated by ATP, and are mildly voltage-dependent (415). Also, the inositol lipid cycle takes place in the nucleus (261), implying that Ca^{2+} can be released from perinuclear stores directly to the nucleus. Indeed, such a release was reported by measuring $[Ca^{2+}]_n$ (131, 154). Furthermore, the presence of calcium-binding proteins in the nucleus (135) introduces another essential element for independent $[Ca^{2+}]_n$ regulation. Finally, diffusion across the nuclear pore is not as free as was previously assumed. The pore is not freely permeable to all ions (266), and its permeability can be regulated by the calcium content of the perinuclear store (347, 416) and ATP (267). These observations raise the possibility of an independently controlled nuclear calcium-signaling system. However, a direct comparison of $[Ca^{2+}]_i$ and $[Ca^{2+}]_n$ is still problematic due to experimental difficulties with calcium-sensitive dyes (11, 17, 77). Also, there seem to be cell-to-cell differences, suggesting a need for additional clarification (11, 201).

Mitochondria. The calcium efflux/influx system of the mitochondria differs from that of the endoplasmic reticulum and nucleus. Calcium influx occurs primarily via a calcium uniporter, which is very fast and does not require energy for its operation. Calcium efflux from the mitochondria requires ATP and occurs via Na^+-independent and -dependent mechanisms (79, 143) (Fig. 9.13). The operation of these two separate pathways permits a rapid exchange of Ca^{2+} across the inner mitochondrial membrane. In addition, the operation of large and nonspecific ion channels (mega channels) in the mitochondria has been proposed (245), but no information about the molecular nature of these channels is available.

The energy released by the passage of electrons along the respiratory chain of the mitochondria generates pH and voltage gradients across the inner membrane (291). The mitochondrial matrix is alkaline and negatively charged (-160 mV); thus, the membrane potential attracts any positive ion into the matrix and pushes OH^- ions out, which reinforces the effects of the pH gradient. The very low permeability of the inner

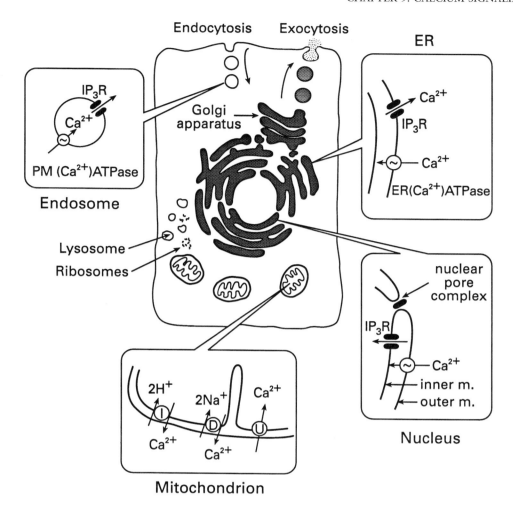

FIG. 9.13. Schematic representation of intracellular calcium releasable pools. *PM*, plasma membrane, *ER*, endoplasmic reticulum; *IP₃R*, inositol-(1,4,5)-triphosphate receptor; *m.*, membrane.

membrane to cations prevents massive Na^+ and K^+ fluxes. In contrast, Ca^{2+} entry is facilitated since the inner membrane contains a transport protein that efficiently moves calcium into the matrix using the voltage gradient as the driving force. Most of the calcium inside the mitochondrion precipitates as calcium phosphates, indicating that only a relatively small amount of energy is necessary to accumulate calcium (143). The enzyme ATP synthetase is stored in the inner membrane and synthesizes ATP in a reaction that is coupled with the inward flow of protons. At high calcium concentrations, ATP production in mitochondria is stopped and calcium is pumped into the cytosol (79).

Release of Ca^{2+} from the mitochondria is a highly complex process, and its physiological importance to $[Ca^{2+}]_i$ oscillations is disputable. The operation of two electroneutral antiporters, $2Na^+/Ca^{2+}$ and $2H^+/Ca^{2+}$,

has been implicated in experiments with ruthenium red and La^{3+} (79). Sodium-dependent transport dominates in muscle and neuronal tissues, and sodium-independent transport dominates in the liver and kidney (143). In activated cells, these antiporters catalyze the return of mitochondrial Ca^{2+} concentrations to the prestimulatory level. It also has been suggested that several VGCC inhibitors block the electroneutral antiporters but in a micromolar concentration range (79). Collapse of the mitochondrial membrane potential is associated with a rapid Ca^{2+} release, but it is unclear whether this process ever takes place under physiological conditions.

The importance of mitochondrial uptake and release of Ca^{2+} in V_m-controlled and calcium mobilization–dependent calcium signaling has been documented in several cell types. For example, in bullfrog sympathetic neurons, both depolarization-induced calcium entry and RyR channel–mediated calcium release are affected by the mitochondrial uncouplers (156). The dominant role of mitochondria over plasma membrane (Ca^{2+})ATPase and Na^+/Ca^{2+} exchange in $[Ca^{2+}]_i$ clearance is shown in depolarized chromaffin cells (125). In *Xenopus* oocytes, IP_3-induced Ca^{2+} wave activity is strengthened by oxidizable substrates that energize the mitochondria, as manifested by increases in the Ca^{2+} wave amplitude, velocity, and interwave period (183). In cultured oligodendrocytes, the characteristics of agonist-induced Ca^{2+} waves depend on mitochondrial localization and function (405). Some of the effects of the mitochondrial uncouplers should be interpreted with reservations since these compounds also affect nonmitochondrial stores (181).

AMPLIFICATION AND SYNCHRONIZATION OF CALCIUM SIGNALS

Initiation of Ca^{2+} signaling in a single cell by either the V_m-dependent or the calcium mobilization–dependent pathway can activate a mechanism for amplification of the initial signal in the same cell (positive autofeedback control) and/or to intercellular propagation of Ca^{2+} waves, leading to synchronization of Ca^{2+} signals at the tissue level. The functional implications of amplification and synchronization of Ca^{2+} signals are enormous. For example, an autofeedback mechanism in synaptic transmission may activate a local electrical circuit. Also, in the absence of cell-to-cell communication, the functional implications of oscillatory calcium signals would exist only at the cellular level. Such a local amplification and synchronization occur through autocrine/paracrine mechanisms or cell-to-cell contact. The purinergic system for Ca^{2+} signaling is suitable for both amplification of Ca^{2+} signals and spreading of Ca^{2+} signals to neighboring cells (147, 171, 326). Another common mechanism for communication by Ca^{2+} signaling between neighboring cells involves cell-to-cell transmission of ions and molecules through gap junction channels (213).

Purinergic Receptor Channels

Frequently, ATP is stored in secretory granules together with other neurotransmitters and hormones and is often co-secreted during agonist stimulation. Once released into the extracellular medium, ATP may bind to its plasma membrane receptors (P_2 purinergic receptors), leading to amplification of agonist-induced Ca^{2+} signals and the secretory response (43, 69, 147). Receptors for ATP belong to two major groups: G protein–coupled receptors (P_{2Y}), whose activation causes Ca^{2+} release from intracellular stores, and plasma membrane receptor channels (P_{2X}), whose activation promotes calcium influx (1, 82). As shown in Figure 9.14, the action of ATP during exocytosis may represent a positive feedback mechanism or the self-potentiation of Ca^{2+} signaling and secretion (autocrine regulation). In addition, ATP may diffuse and activate P_2 receptors in neighboring cells (paracrine regulation). However, it cannot act as a typical hormone since it is degraded rapidly by several ecto-ATPases (82).

Structure and Pharmacology. Purinergic P_2 receptor channels have been identified in both excitable and nonexcitable cells (22, 139, 385, 488). They are functionally heterogeneous, but in respect to ion selectivity and kinetic parameters of channel gating, they resemble acetylcholine- and serotonin-gated channels (21, 82). The overall transmembrane topology of these channels, however, resembles that of protein subunits from potassium channels, amiloride-sensitive sodium channels, and mechanosensitive ion channels (38). Seven channels from this family have been cloned and named P_{2X1}–P_{2X7}. Each P_{2X} receptor subunit appears to have intracellular N- and C-termini, two putative transmembrane domains (M1 and M2) with an intervening hydrophilic loop of abut 300 residues, and an adjacent hydrophobic segment (H5). There is 35%–50% identity and 50%–65% similarity between pairs of P_{2X} receptors (76). The expressed receptors differ among themselves with respect to the action of ATP analogs, the desensitization rate, and the effectiveness of antagonists (76).

The P_{2X1} and P_{2X3} ion channels are cation-selective, with relatively high calcium permeability (P_{Ca}/P_{Na} = 4). The proteins are composed of 399 and 397 amino acids, respectively. The pharmacology of P_{2X1} channels resembles that of classical P_{2X} channels in smooth muscle (469). However, the properties of P_{2X3} channels expressed in oocytes and HEK293 cells are comparable to those observed in rat sensory neurons and endogenous rat dorsal root ganglia, respectively (62, 228). The P_{2X3} mRNA is undetectable in RNA isolated from tissues other than dorsal root ganglion (62). The common characteristics of these two channels are their sensitivity to α,β-methylene-ATP and the P_2 channel antagonist suramin and their rapid desensitization to high agonist concentrations (62, 228, 469).

Another group of P_2 receptor channels is composed of P_{2X2}, P_{2X4}, P_{2X5}, and P_{2X6} channels. The members of this group do not respond to α,β-methylene-ATP and desensitize slowly compared to P_{2X1} and P_{2X3} channels. Similar to P_{2X1} and P_{2X3} channels, P_{2X2} and

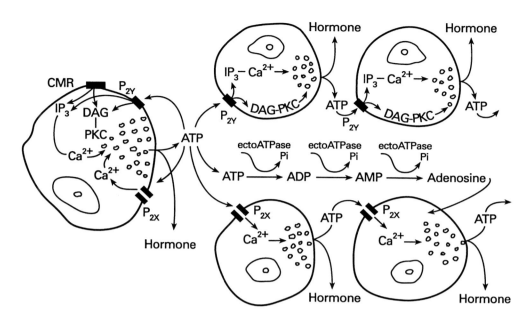

FIG. 9.14. Schematic representation of purinergic system for self-amplification of Ca^{2+} signals and secretion, as well as cell-to-cell spreading of Ca^{2+} signals. Co-secretion of ATP with hormone is essential for initiation of this signaling system. *CMR*, calcium-mobilizing receptors; *DAG*, diacylglycerol; *PKC*, protein kinase C; *IP$_3$*, inositol-(1,4,5)-triphosphate.

P_{2X5} channels are sensitive to suramin; however, P_{2X4} and P_{2X6} channels are not. The P_{2X2} channel is composed of 477 amino-acid proteins and contains two putative transmembrane domains with an intervening hydrophilic loop of abut 270 residues (38). The pharmacology of this receptor resembles that of native P_{2X} receptors on PC12 cells and some neurons (38). Northern blot analysis of a 2 kb transcript of P_{2X2} channels suggests its expression in the brain, spinal cord, intestine, and vas deferens. However, the most intense signal was observed with RNA from the pituitary (38, 139, 310, 373). Accordingly, P_{2X2}-like channels are expressed in pituitary gonadotrophs and several other unidentified anterior pituitary cell types (455). The P_{2X5} receptor contains 417 amino acids. The unique feature of this channel is a current with a small amplitude, only 5%–10% of that observed in other channels (76).

The P_{2X4} receptor RNA is expressed in spinal cord, lung, thymus, bladder, adrenal, testis, and brain, with a staining pattern that closely mirrors that of the P_{2X6} channel (34, 76). The predicted P_{2X6} channel protein has 379 amino acids, while the P_{2X4} channel has 388 amino acids (40, 76). In addition to tissue distribution, a common characteristic of these two channels is their insensitivity to suramin. The P_{2X7} channel shows low or no sensitivity to the P_{2X} channel antagonists suramin and pyridoxalphosphate-6–azophenyl-2',4'-disulfonic

acid and is insensitive to the P_{2X1} and P_{2X3} agonist α,β-methylene-ATP. The protein of this channel is the largest among P_{2X} proteins (599 amino acids). In contrast to other channels from this family, it represents a bifunctional molecule; it operates as a channel but also permeabilizes cells, forming large pores in the plasma membrane. Another distinguishing characteristic of P_{2X7} channels is their high sensitivity to BzATP (438). These and other characteristics of P_{2X7} channels are compatible with a pharmacological profile of the receptor previously termed P_{2Z} (139, 438, 448, 488).

Physiological Significance. In contrast to the well-characterized structure and pharmacology of P_2 channels, their physiological significance is not well understood. In general, calcium is the charge carrier through these channels, though the permeability of Ca^{2+} vs. Na^+ varies widely among cells (21). Thus, these can serve as calcium influx channels. Furthermore, since activation of ATP-controlled channels leads to plasma membrane depolarization, the $[Ca^{2+}]_i$ response to ATP could result from activation of VGCCs as well (21). Both of these actions are comparable to that observed in nonspecific cation and glutamate channels. For example, in pituitary gonadotrophs, P_2 receptor channels are not essential for spontaneous electrical activity, but their stimulation can activate the plasma membrane oscillator and modulate its activity (Fig. 9.15). In accord with this, depolarizing current initiates action firing of action potential in quiescent gonadotrophs and modulates the frequency pattern of firing in spontaneously active cells (234). These observations in gonadotrophs parallel those in noradrenergic neurons, where ATP analogs of increased enzymatic stability increase the action potential firing rate (460).

Also, ATP-gated calcium channels represent the potential calcium influx pathway that sustains IP_3-induced and endoplasmic reticulum–derived Ca^{2+} spiking (Fig. 9.16). In pituitary gonadotrophs, Ca^{2+}

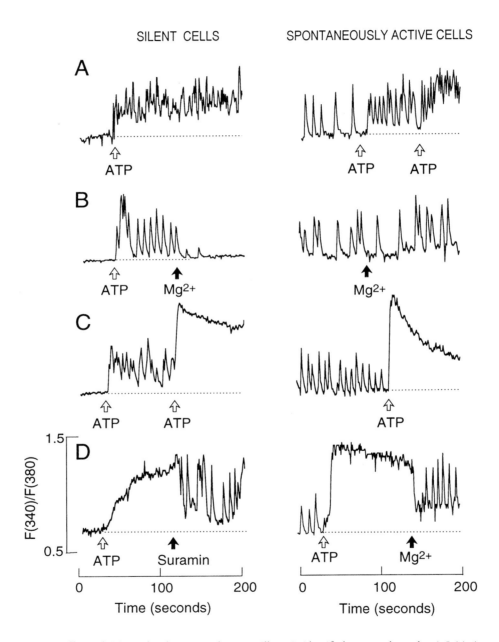

FIG. 9.15. Effects of ATP on the plasma membrane oscillator in identified rat gonadotrophs. *A:* Initiation of $[Ca^{2+}]_i$ spiking in silent cells by ATP *(left panel)* and modulation of spiking frequency in spontaneously active cells by increasing concentrations of ATP *(right panel)*. *B:* Effects of Mg^{2+} on ATP-induced spiking *(left panel)* and lack of effects of Mg^{2+} on spontaneously driven Ca^{2+} *(right panel)*. *C:* Addition of high (100 μM) ATP abolishes spontaneous and ATP-induced Ca^{2+} transients. *D:* In cells stimulated with high ATP, addition of P_2 receptor blocker suramin and Mg^{2+} reestablished the oscillatory pattern of $[Ca^{2+}]_i$ spiking. [From Tomic et al. (455) with permission.]

entry through P$_2$ receptor channels can modulate the frequency of IP$_3$-controlled Ca^{2+} spiking even at high and presumably nonphysiological concentrations of ATP (455). The best known co-agonist action of ATP is in synaptic transmission (109, 460, 505). This function of ATP has been studied in sympathetic nerves, where ATP acts as a co-transmitter with noradrenaline. In addition, the role of ATP has been implicated in parasympathetic, sensorimotor, and somatic neuromuscular transmissions (23, 43, 171). About 40% of hypothalamic cultured neurons respond to ATP by a rapid increase in [Ca^{2+}]$_i$ due to Ca^{2+} entry through P$_{2X}$ channels (68). The specific aspect of the paracrine action of ATP is cell-to-cell spread of Ca^{2+} signals in mast cells in the absence of gap-junctional communication (326) (Fig. 9.14).

In several cell types that secrete by an exocytotic mechanism, ATP-induced Ca^{2+} signals are sufficient to trigger hormone release. For example, in gonadotrophs (Fig. 9.16), chromaffin cells, β-pancreatic cells, and PC$_{12}$ cells, ATP induces an inward current and increases Ca^{2+} influx and hormone release (51, 171, 196, 310, 373, 455). In subpopulations of pituitary cells (49, 66, 67, 70, 84, 455), and of chromaffin and insulin-secreting cells (51, 132, 410), ATP also releases [Ca^{2+}]$_i$ from internal stores bathed in a Ca^{2+}-deficient medium. Finally, ATP is co-secreted during agonist- and depolarization-induced secretion of catecholamines and gonadotropins (54, 455). In the pineal gland, ATP potentiates the effect of noradrenaline in N'-acetyl-5–hydroxytryptamine production (112).

Secretion and Degradation of Adenosine Triphosphate. Adenosine triphosphate is co-stored with acetylcholine in a variety of peripheral and central synaptic vesicles and with noradrenaline in vesicles of sympathetic nerve terminals. It has been documented in synaptosomes from the mammalian brain and neuromuscular junction and the electric organ of the electric ray (116, 505). It is also co-secreted from chromaffin cells in a receptor-controlled and calcium-dependent manner (54). It is likely that ATP is co-secreted with neurotransmitters and hormones from many other cell types but that such secretion is masked by the activity of endogenous ectonucleotidases.

In many other cell types, the expression of ectonucleotidases and their participation in the dephosphorylation of ATP is well established (71, 92, 214, 238, 356, 456, 492, 498, 504). Ectonucleotidases are the set of plasma membrane–bound enzymes that dephosphorylate extracellular ATP, ADP, and AMP to adenosine in a sequential manner (345). Some of the cells express only ecto-ATPase, while in others ecto-ADPase and ecto-AMPase (5'-nucleotidase) are also operative (456, 498). It also has been reported that degradation of both ATP and ADP is controlled by the same enzyme, ATP-diphosphohydrolase (356, 492). The general characteristic of ecto-ATPase, ecto-ADPase, and ecto-AMPase is a dependence on extracellular Ca^{2+} and Mg^{2+} (345). Ecto-AMPase is inhibited specifically by α,β-methylene-ADP (92, 341). The operation of ectonucleotidase in a particular cell type is consistent with the hypothesis that ATP is co-secreted by target cells and that a mechanism for its degradation is needed to terminate the signal upon the removal of agonist.

Gap Junction Channels

More direct communication between cells is provided by gap junction channels. These channels differ from classical plasma membrane channels in that they exist between two cells, enabling the direct exchange of ions and small molecules, including cAMP and IP$_3$. Ion and

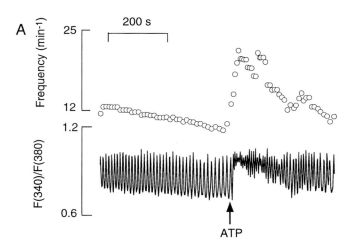
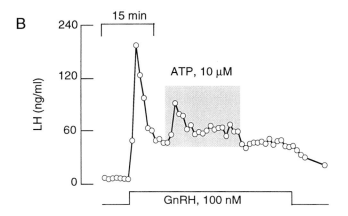

FIG. 9.16. Effects of extracellular ATP on gonadotropin-releasing hormone *(GnRH)*-induced [Ca^{2+}]$_i$ and secretory response. *A:* Effects of ATP on frequency of spiking during sustained GnRH stimulation. *B:* Effects of ATP on sustained GnRH-induced luteinizing hormone *(LH)* release in perifused pituitary cells. [From Tomic et al. (455) with permission.]

molecular movements occur by passive diffusion. Such permeability provides a mechanism for electrical and chemical communication between cells (213). These channels are expressed commonly in a variety of cell types from both vertebrates and invertebrates, as well as from plants. The role of gap junction channels is to maintain tissue homeostasis and to promote cell-to-cell signal transduction. For example, such coupling can ensure the spreading and synchronization of signals controlling secretion across large cell populations (413).

A multigene family of conserved proteins, connexins, is responsible for generating gap junctional channel oligomers between cells. Based on amino-acid sequences, this family can be categorized in two classes, α and β. Each molecule of connexin has four hydrophobic transmembrane domains, with N- and C-terminal tails located on the cytoplasmic membrane face. Six connexin subunits assemble into a hemichannel that spans the lipid bilayer. Two such structures from adjacent cells are connected by end-to-end interactions, forming a narrow extracellular gap (497). Since gap junction channels can be formed by a number of different connexins, they show different permeabilities. Single-channel conductances of these channels vary from tens to several hundred pico-Siemens (471). Signal transmission via gap junction channels is modulated by a variety of factors, including intercellular voltage, Ca^{2+}, pH, and the phosphorylation state of channels. The C-terminus is important in pH- and phosphorylation-mediated channel regulation. The voltage dependence of gap junction channels varies with the type of connexin. Several neurotransmitters and hormones, such as dopamine, acetylcholine, γ-aminobutyric acid, and estrogens, also affect signal transmission through these channels (497).

Gap-junctional coupling affects the electrophysiological characteristics and calcium signaling of interconnected cells. Both Ca^{2+} and K^+ can account for the electrical synchronization of cells. For example, in the pancreas, intercellular synchronization leads to an increase in the resting potential and its stabilization, which is critical in the promotion of β-cell responsiveness (278). In addition, agonist stimulation of islets and acini leads to intercellular propagation of Ca^{2+} waves (413). Coordination of Ca^{2+} signaling by gap junction channels also occurs in the intact liver. In this tissue, intracellular Ca^{2+} wave rates are constant but intercellular signal propagation increases with increases in agonist concentration (380). There are also indications that Ca^{2+} signals in glial cells can cause changes in $[Ca^{2+}]_i$ in surrounding neurons through gap junction channels (314). In GnRH neurons, gap junction channels may play an important role in the synchronization of electrical activity and pulsatile GnRH release (207,

263, 59b). Gap junction channels also are expressed by pituitary cells and play important roles in the modulation of cellular responses to external stimuli (see Chapter 18 by Denef in this *Handbook*).

In bovine aortic endothelial cell cultures, mechanical stimulation of a single cell increases $[Ca^{2+}]_i$ in the stimulated cell, which then spreads in the form of a wave to neighboring cells. In cells bathed in Ca^{2+}-deficient medium, there is no increase in $[Ca^{2+}]_i$ in stimulated cells, yet a Ca^{2+} wave occurs in adjacent cells, suggesting that Ca^{2+} per se is not a diffusible substance (90). Heparin inhibits propagation of intercellular Ca^{2+} waves, indicating that IP_3 moves through gap junctions to activate Ca^{2+} release in neighboring cells (35). However, a model simulation of these experimental data indicates that intercellular wave propagation cannot be explained by the simple diffusion of IP_3 since the required IP_3 concentration for diffusion is much higher than that reached by agonist stimulation (407). These experimental and theoretical observations suggest that a regenerative production of IP_3 is required for intercellular Ca^{2+} signaling and that Ca^{2+} is not a messenger for such a cycle of production. There are no experimental data on the mechanism of phospholipase C activation in neighboring cells by gap junction channels.

CELLULAR FUNCTIONS OF CALCIUM SIGNALS

Calcium signaling is critical for the control of many essential cellular responses. These include hormone synthesis and release, synaptic transmission, muscle contraction, gene expression and translation, protein synthesis and assembly, cell division and differentiation, apoptosis, and control of the activities of various enzymes and channels. A comprehensive review of such diverse cellular functions is beyond the scope of this chapter, which is focused primarily on calcium actions on the intracellular signaling pathways and the relevance of the pattern of calcium signals in controlling specific cellular processes. A review of the latter is limiting since little progress has been made in understanding the physiological significance of the complex spatial and temporal characteristics of agonist-induced Ca^{2+} signaling. This contrasts with the tremendous efforts, both experimental and computational, that have been devoted to the characterization of Ca^{2+} spiking and waves and the mechanisms underlying these phenomena.

Calcium-Controlled Enzymes

Calcium–Calmodulin-Dependent Enzymes. Cells contain a number of intracellular binding proteins. In all nonmuscle and smooth muscle cells, calmodulin (CaM) is the predominant Ca^{2+}-binding protein involved in the control of over 20 intracellular enzymes. Many of these enzymes are inhibited in an intramolecular manner, and the calcium–CaM complex releases this inhibition (277). A related calcium-binding protein, troponin C, dominates in skeletal muscle. Calmodulin is a single polypeptide chain of 148 amino acids and has been highly conserved during evolution. The sequence of troponin C is related to that of CaM, in accord with the view that it represents a specialized form of CaM. Both proteins have four high-affinity binding sites for Ca^{2+}, with a selectivity for Ca^{2+} over Mg^{2+}, and undergo a large conformational change when they bind Ca^{2+} (276). The CaM-binding domains of the target proteins are contained in 20-residue-long amino-acid sequences, which share no obvious amino-acid sequence homology (474). Still, the calcium–CaM complex can bind effectively to the CaM domains of all its target proteins (473).

Calmodulin mediates the calcium regulation of several intracellular functions, such as control of cyclic nucleotide and glycogen metabolism, secretion, motility, Ca^{2+} transport, and the cell cycle (246, 275). Activated CaM can bind directly to the effector protein and modulate its activity or indirectly through a family of calcium–CaM-dependent protein kinases and phosphatases (296, 307, 390). The kinase family includes myosin light chain kinase (MLCK), phosphorylase kinase, CaM kinase I, CaM kinase II, elongation factor (EF)-2 kinase (also known as CaM kinase III), and CaM kinase IV (307). Calmodulin kinase II is known as multifunctional Ca^{2+}/CaM-dependent protein kinase, while other members of this family are more specialized or dedicated to the regulation of a specific function (395).

The MLCKs belong to a heterogeneous group of enzymes broadly classified into invertebrate striated muscle and vertebrate smooth muscle/nonmuscle types (436). The inactive MLCK has a catalytic domain that is repressed by a substrate inhibitory domain. Activated CaM binds to MLCK, leading to a conformational change that depresses the catalytic site (274). In smooth muscle cells, the activated kinase phosphorylates a specific serine residue in the regulatory light chain that contributes to the control of myosin's interactions with actin. A decrease in $[Ca^{2+}]_i$ leads to dissociation of the kinase–CaM complex, as well as isomerization of the kinase to its inactive form (439). Additionally, MLCK may participate in the control of exocytosis. In rat basophilic cells, secretion is associated with diphosphorylation of myosin light chains by MLCK, as well as phosphorylation by protein kinase C. Selective inhibition of light chain phosphorylation by either kinase

suppresses exocytosis, indicating that the coordinate actions of MLCK and protein kinase C are required for agonist-induced secretion (72, 323). The participation of MLCK in exocytosis also has been implicated in studies with permeabilized chromaffin cells (212), insulin-secreting HIT-T15 cells (231), and GnRH-stimulated gonadotrophs (366).

Although the multifunctional CaM kinase II is widely distributed, it is highly concentrated in neuronal tissue and can be found in both soluble and particulate forms. The brain enzyme consists of three highly homologous subunits derived from two genes. The isolated enzyme exists as at least two isozymes (395). A rise in $[Ca^{2+}]_i$ leads to phosphorylation of CaM kinase II subunits as well as their substrates. Once the threshold is reached, however, the removal of $[Ca^{2+}]_i$ does not affect phosphorylation and the enzyme continues to phosphorylate at a high rate. This could be important for short- and/or long-term potentiation (39, 383, 395).

In neuronal tissue, CaM kinase II controls several other functions. For example, this enzyme phosphorylates tyrosine hydroxylase, the enzyme that catalyzes the hydroxylation of tyrosine to form dopa, which is converted subsequently to dopamine, noradrenaline, and adrenaline (39). These enzymes also are involved in the control of synaptic transmission. The effects of CaM kinase II on neurotransmitter release occur through phosphorylation of synapsin I, a protein associated with synaptic vesicles and actin. In the C-terminus of synapsin I, CaM kinase phosphorylates two specific sites, leading to a decrease in its binding to synaptic vesicles and actin filaments, which is essential for vesicular movement and fusion (140). In addition, CaM kinase II plays important roles in the cardiovascular system, epithelial cells, and liver (39, 395). The enzyme also has been implicated in the control of stimulus-transcription coupling (39); however, CaM kinase IV mediates the effects of calcium on gene expression (32). Finally, CaM kinase II is involved in regulation of the cell cycle by calcium (246, 443).

Among the other members of the calcium–CaM-dependent kinase family, phosphorylase kinase mediates glycogen breakdown in muscle cells. It is composed of four subunits, of which the β-subunit is activated by calcium–CaM (491). Although CaM kinase I exhibits a broad tissue distribution, its cellular functions are incompletely characterized (9). Phosphorylation and inactivation of eukaryotic EF-2, a protein that catalyzes the translocation of peptidyl tRNA on the ribosome, are mediated by CaM kinase III (292, 306). Activation of this enzyme correlates with $[Ca^{2+}]_i$ transients; phosphorylation of EF-2 occurs slightly after the Ca^{2+}

transient, followed by a rapid dephosphorylation shortly after $[Ca^{2+}]_i$ begins to decline (334). Expressed in neuronal, gonadal, and lymphoid tissues, CaM kinase IV regulates cAMP-responsive element-binding (CREB) protein–, cAMP-responsive element modulator τ (CREMτ)–, and serum response factor (SRF)–dependent gene expression (264). The protein exists in two monomeric forms, which are activated by calcium–CaM. The enzyme exhibits a unique three-step phosphorylation-dependent mechanism for its activation: binding of activated CaM, phosphorylation of the CaM-bound enzyme by a calcium–CaM-dependent kinase kinase, and autophosphorylation (60). The calcium–CaM complex also controls a serine-threonine protein phosphatase, calcineurin. This phosphatase is composed of a catalytic subunit, calcineurin A, and a regulatory subunit, calcineurin B. The catalytic subunit is activated by the binding of calcium–CaM (197).

Protein Kinase C. Protein kinase C initially was regarded as a single element in the cascade of phospholipase C–mediated cellular events, during which calcium and diacylglycerol were responsible for its integration into the signaling pathway (319). However, it is now known that mammalian cells express a family of several closely related protein kinase C isozymes (164, 165, 320). The classical group (A) consists of four isozymes, α, βI, βII, and γ, all single polypeptides containing four conserved (C_{1-4}) and five variable (V_{1-5}) regions. The C_2 region represents the calcium-binding domain. In addition to $[Ca^{2+}]_i$, protein kinase C enzymes are regulated by phosphatidylserine, diacylglycerol, and arachidonic acid and can be activated by phorbol esters (141). Another group (B) consists of four enzymes: δ, ϵ, η, and θ. This group lacks the C_2 region and thus does not require calcium for activation. The third group (C), composed of two atypical protein kinase C enzymes, ζ and λ, is also insensitive to cytosolic calcium (141, 165, 320).

Protein kinase C isozymes are involved in the control of a number of cellular processes, primarily at the membrane and nuclear levels. Membrane-controlled events include modulation of ion channels, control of phospholipases, and participation in exocytosis. At the nuclear level, protein kinase C is also essential in the control of gene expression, such as luteinizing hormone-β mRNA (14), prolactin (194), and early-response genes (57). As discussed below, all of these processes also are controlled by calcium independently of its action on protein kinase C activation, leading to complex interactions between these two messenger molecules.

Following recognition of the multiple subtypes and actions of protein kinase C, including four subtypes regulated by calcium, the specific roles of these individual isozymes in various effector functions have been analyzed. For example, two experiments indicate the role of protein kinase C-α in the control of phospholipase D. Overexpression of this subtype leads to up-regulation of phospholipase D activity in Swiss/3T3 cells (105). In Madin-Darby kidney cells, transfected with anti-sense protein kinase C-α, but not -β, phorbol ester–induced phospholipase D activity is attenuated (18). In RBL-2H3 cells, the α and ϵ isozymes of protein kinase C mediate feedback inhibition of phospholipase C and β and δ are stimulatory for exocytosis (330, 331). Another study, however, suggested that the α and β isozymes mediate the exocytotic response (311). Selective down-regulation of the ϵ isozyme demonstrates that this subtype is not necessary for exocytosis (195) but may participate in the regulation of prolactin gene transcription (194).

Phospholipases C, D, and A$_2$. For a detailed description of these enzymes and their regulation, including the role of calcium, see Chapter 11 by Exton in this *Handbook*. Here, three questions concerning the calcium dependence of the activity of these families of enzymes are discussed: Is the rise in $[Ca^{2+}]_i$ sufficient for their activation? Which pathway, calcium entry–dependent or calcium mobilization–dependent, is critical for the control of these enzymes? What are the modes of synchronization of protein kinase C and calcium actions on the activity of these enzymes?

In several neuronal cell types, depolarization-induced calcium entry leads to a modest increase in the activity of phospholipase C, as estimated by increases in IP$_3$ production (119). Such observations concur with in vitro studies of phospholipase C activity (372). However, the calcium dependence of IP$_3$ production is more complex than was proposed initially. In the majority of cells, including pituitary cells and hypothalamic neurons (434, 501), the rise in $[Ca^{2+}]_i$ is insufficient to activate phospholipase C; G protein–mediated activation of phospholipase C is a prerequisite for the development of sensitivity to calcium. Furthermore, the two calcium pathways activated by the G protein–phospholipase C complex show different efficiencies in the sensitization of IP$_3$ production. While the early calcium mobilization–dependent phase is relatively inefficient, the sustained calcium entry–dependent pathway is essential for the activity of the G protein–phospholipase C signaling system (19, 119, 167, 168). Thus, calcium may serve as a positive feedback element in the control of phospholipase C activity in agonist-activated cells.

Protein kinase C may negatively modulate phospholipase C, a feature sufficient to create an oscillatory Ca^{2+} response (151, 283). According to this model, calcium activates protein kinase C, which in turn generates an oscillatory Ca^{2+} signal through transient inhibition of phospholipase C; yet two lines of evidence argue against this hypothesis. First, in many cell types, injection of nonmetabolized IP_3 is sufficient to create an oscillatory Ca^{2+} response, demonstrating that oscillations in IP_3 are not required for oscillations in $[Ca^{2+}]_i$ (89, 221, 429, 477). Second, no obvious modulation of phospholipase C activity has been observed in several cell types, including gonadotrophs (502), treated with protein kinase C activators or in protein kinase C–depleted cells treated with agonists.

Protein kinase C stimulates phospholipase D activity in many cell types (see Chapter 11 by Exton in this *Handbook*). This action is facilitated by calcium entry through VGCCs. Depolarization-driven Ca^{2+} entry in both protein kinase C–replete and -depleted cells is sufficient to increase phospholipase D activity, as measured by the accumulation of phosphatidylethanol (501). Thus, calcium may facilitate phospholipase D independently of the protein kinase C pathway (450). Phospholipase A_2 shows a similar pattern of regulation by protein kinase C and calcium, a feature potentially important in understanding the cross-talk among multiple signal-activated phospholipases (16, 239, 406).

The calcium dependence of the adenylyl cyclase family of enzymes is discussed in detail in Chapter 8 by Weng et al. in this *Handbook*.

Calcium-Controlled Channels

The rise in $[Ca^{2+}]_i$ is an effective signal for the activation and/or inhibition of several plasma and endoplasmic reticulum membrane channels. The role of calcium in the control of IP_3R and RyR channels is discussed above under CALCIUM MOBILIZATION–DEPENDENT SIGNALING SYSTEM. In addition, the effects of calcium on L-type calcium channels and capacitative calcium entry are addressed above under *Voltage-Gated Calcium Entry* and *Signals for Capacitative Calcium Entry*, respectively. Several calcium-controlled potassium, chloride, and nonspecific channels also are expressed in the plasma membrane (159). Their characteristics are discussed briefly below.

The family of calcium-activated potassium channels is composed of at least three members: apamin-sensitive Ca^{2+}-activated K^+ (SK-K_{Ca}), apamin-resistant SK-K_{Ca}, and tetraethylammonium and carybdotoxin-sensitive BK-K_{Ca} channels. In agonist-stimulated gonadotrophs, the predominant mediators of the Ca^{2+}-dependent plasma membrane conductances are apamin-sensitive SK-K_{Ca} channels (210, 428, 461, 465). Expression of SK-K_{Ca} channels has been observed in other pituitary cell types, including corticotrophs (15,78), lactotrophs (481), thyrotrophs (384), immortalized GH_3 cells (220, 376), and other endocrine cells (315, 337). The SK-K_{Ca} channels show a higher sensitivity to Ca^{2+} than other calcium-activated potassium currents, rendering them appropriate for controlling the interspike interval by producing long hyperpolarizing pauses after action potentials, as well as spike frequency adaptation during depolarizing pulses (389). Consistent with this observation, an increase in the action potential spiking frequency follows addition of apamin to GH_3 pituitary cells (220). Also, increases in thyroid-stimulating hormone (TSH) and prolactin releases from cultured pituitary cells are observed after addition of apamin (15, 384, 481). Pituitary corticotrophs (15, 403) and GH_3 immortalized lactosomatotrophs (220) also express an apamin-insensitive, Ca^{2+}-activated current that is carried through BK-K_{Ca} channels. The intrinsic properties of BK-K_{Ca} channels are appropriate for regulation of action potential duration and the associated Ca^{2+} entry through VGCCs. In addition to BK-K_{Ca} channels, chromaffin cells and gonadotrophs express major apamin-sensitive and minor apamin-insensitive conductances (315, 337, 472b).

Calcium-activated chloride channels are present in many neurons and secretory cells. In addition to Cl^-, these channels are permeable to several other small anions. The opening of these channels is controlled by $[Ca^{2+}]_i$ and depolarization (159). In neurons, such channels may play a role similar to that of SK-K_{Ca} in pituitary cells (265). Because of its sensitivity to $[Ca^{2+}]_i$, the current through these channels is employed frequently in analyses of Ca^{2+} signaling in single cells (204, 327).

Calcium-activated nonselective (CAN) channels are expressed in many excitable and non-excitable cells. These channels are activated by an increase in $[Ca^{2+}]_i$ due to calcium influx and/or release from intracellular stores (343). They also provide a route for Ca^{2+} entry by two mechanisms. In a manner comparable to glutamate receptor channels and purinergic receptor channels, CAN channels depolarize cells, leading to activation of VGCCs and the subsequent influx of Ca^{2+}. These channels are permeable to Ca^{2+} and Ba^{2+} and, thus, can serve as calcium-permeant channels. They are voltage-insensitive and have a single-channel conductance of about 30 pS (342). The structure of these channels may relate to the *trpl* gene product of *Drosophila* (149) (see earlier under Capacitative Calcium Entry).

Calcium Signaling and Exocytosis

The cell biology of secretion and the role of calcium signals in exocytosis are discussed in Chapter 1 by Dannies in this *Handbook*. Here, the focus is on the pattern of Ca^{2+} signaling and its relationship to exocytosis. Two questions merit close attention: *(1)* oscillatory vs. nonoscillatory Ca^{2+} response and secretion and (2) frequency-coded signal and secretion.

The finding that in gonadotrophs GnRH induces oscillatory Ca^{2+} responses at low and intermediate concentrations and a biphasic response at high GnRH concentrations raised the question of which pattern is necessary for activation of secretion. Measurements of Ca^{2+} response and luteinizing hormone secretion in individual gonadotrophs, using a reverse hemolytic plaque assay, are consistent with the conclusion that individual secretory gonadotrophs respond with spike/plateau profiles, while nonsecretory gonadotrophs exhibit repetitive Ca^{2+} transients (225, 226). Contrasting these experiments, simultaneous measurements of luteinizing hormone release by capacitative measurements and Ca^{2+} signaling in a single cell suggest that each Ca^{2+} spike induces a burst of exocytosis (463). In accord with the extracellular Ca^{2+} independence of the initial phase of gonadotropin release in perifused pituitary cells (52, 387, 441, 449), exocytosis in single gonadotrophs is not abolished by a depletion of extracellular Ca^{2+} but is instead suppressed by the buffering of intracellular Ca^{2+}. Also, $[Ca^{2+}]_i$ elevations induced by photolysis of caged IP_3 trigger exocytosis (463). Finally, low GnRH concentrations induce baseline oscillatory Ca^{2+} responses in most individual gonadotrophs, though a significant increase in luteinizing hormone release occurs at the same temperature (453). Thus, the increase in $[Ca^{2+}]_i$, rather than the presence of the specific pattern of Ca^{2+} response, is essential for exocytosis.

The concentration-dependent regulation of secretion through frequency coding of Ca^{2+} signals is still not well defined. A reasonable correlation is found between the frequency of spiking and growth hormone release in spontaneously active somatotrophs (161). Also, several cell types show a complete concentration dependence of secretion by doses of agonists that induce frequency-controlled Ca^{2+} oscillations (179). However, the amplitude of Ca^{2+} spikes also may play an important role in secretion, as indicated in experiments with somatotrophs (161). In addition, exocytosis is not controlled exclusively by calcium (33, 41). Finally, the sensitivity of the secretory mechanism to calcium differs significantly between initial and sustained secretions (182). Thus, calcium is an essential element in the transduction of extracellular signals to exocytosis, but at the same time it represents only an intermediate step in such a transduction.

Mitochondrial Functions and Calcium Signals

Mitochondria do not serve only as sinks for calcium following agonist stimulation; calcium entry into these compartments is required for mitochondrial functions (79). Several mitochondrial dehydrogenase enzymes involved in oxidative ATP synthesis are regulated by calcium, such as pyruvate dehydrogenase, isocitrate dehydrogenase, and α-ketoglutaride dehydrogenase. These enzymes are regulated by calcium in the 0.2–2 μM concentration range (270).

It has been suggested that increases and decreases in $[Ca^{2+}]_i$ are translated into parallel changes in the concentration of mitochondrial Ca^{2+} ($[Ca^{2+}]_m$) (79). Accordingly, V_m-dependent and calcium mobilization–dependent $[Ca^{2+}]_m$ spiking occurs in intact hepatocytes (378, 379). Furthermore, each Ca^{2+} spike in hepatocytes is sufficient to cause a transient increase in $[Ca^{2+}]_m$ associated with a transient activation of Ca^{2+}-sensitive mitochondrial dehydrogenases. Such an action also triggers a sustained activation of mitochondrial metabolism if the spiking frequency is higher than 0.5/min. In contrast, sustained low-amplitude $[Ca^{2+}]_i$ responses and slow and partial elevations in $[Ca^{2+}]_i$ are ineffective at increasing $[Ca^{2+}]_m$ and dehydrogenase activities (144). These observations are supported by findings in chromaffin cells (156) and isolated mitochondria (359), where an increase in $[Ca^{2+}]_i$ to about 500 nM is required to activate calcium electrogenic uniport.

Nuclear Functions and Calcium Signals

A rise in $[Ca^{2+}]_i$ leads to the induction of several genes. Both calcium and cAMP are involved in the regulation of c-fos transcription (Fig. 9.17) via a well-characterized mechanism of calcium kinase– and cAMP-dependent phosphorylations of the dimeric transcription factor CREB (284, 365). Once phosphorylated, CREB stimulates induction of c-fos by binding to the CREB-responsive element located 60 base pairs upstream of the initiation site (Fig. 9.17). Protein kinase C is also involved in the control of c-fos expression, and this action is mediated by the serum-responsive factor, which binds to a serum-responsive element located 300 base pairs upstream of the mRNA initiation site (96, 459). Functional divergence between protein kinase C family members in the control of PMA-responsive transcriptional activation has been observed (184).

The relationship between the protein kinase C– and cAMP/Ca^{2+}-dependent initiations of transcription is still not well defined. Additionally, the role of oscillatory vs. nonoscillatory calcium signals has not been addressed. It is, however, interesting that Ca^{2+} exhibits a dual action on c-fos expression, stimulatory and inhibitory, depending on $[Ca^{2+}]_i$ (55, 56). Transcription of the c-fos gene in macrophages is modulated by

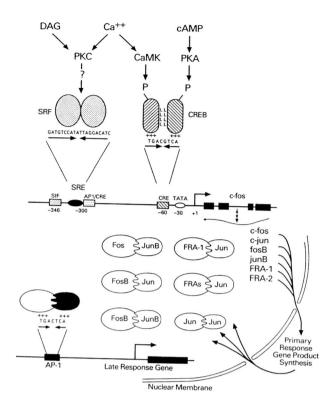

FIG. 9.17. Transcriptional regulation of *c-fos* by multiple intracellular messengers. *DAG*, diacylglycerol; *PKC*, protein kinase C; *CaMK*, calmodulin kinase; *PKA*, protein kinase A; *CREB*, cAMP-responsive element-binding protein; *SRF*, serum response factor. [From S. S. Stojilkovic, J. Reinhart, and K. J. Catt (431). GnRH receptors: structure and signal transduction pathways. *Endocr. Rev.* 15: 462–499, 1994, with permission. © The Endocrine Society.]

a calcium-dependent block to elongation (75). Also, transcriptional elongation of *c-fos* in HL-60 myeloid leukemia cells is extremely sensitive to $[Ca^{2+}]_i$. The $[Ca^{2+}]_i$ dose dependence of *c-fos* transcription and mRNA accumulation in these cells is bell-shaped, with facilitation at low and inhibition at high $[Ca^{2+}]_i$. In $\alpha T3-1$ cells, measurements of $[Ca^{2+}]_i$ in parallel with *c-fos* induction indicate that $[Ca^{2+}]_i$ elevations within the physiological range exert both stimulatory and inhibitory actions on gene expression (55). In HL-60 cells, the amplitude of the $[Ca^{2+}]_i$ response correlates with the fold induction of *c-fos* expression (483). Thus, the amplitude of the Ca^{2+} response may represent a signal for a dual action on transcriptional activity.

SUMMARY

Transduction of many hormonal and neurotransmitter stimuli through G protein–coupled receptors is medi-

ated by a rise in $[Ca^{2+}]_i$ due to activation of calcium-release channels within the endoplasmic reticulum membrane and/or activation of calcium-entry channels within the plasma membrane. In cells expressing calcium-mobilizing receptors, IP_3 mediates calcium discharge from endoplasmic reticulum by activating IP_3R channels, and this process is frequently followed by Ca^{2+} entry through plasma membrane calcium channels. In some excitable cells, activation of other subtypes of G protein–coupled receptor is associated with the stimulation or inhibition of calcium influx through plasma membrane calcium channels without affecting endoplasmic reticulum release channels. In other excitable cells, Ca^{2+} entry through plasma membrane channels leads to the activation of RyR channels by a process known as calcium-induced calcium release. Developments in the characterization of heterotrimeric G proteins have provided some insight into the question of how such diverse effects could be controlled by the same family of G protein–coupled receptors.

Single-cell measurements have shown that Ca^{2+} signaling can assume a variety of spatio-temporal patterns. For example, pituitary gonadotrophs and parotid acinar cells show a baseline oscillatory response to agonist stimulation with a frequency of 5–30 spikes/min. Hepatocytes, chondrocytes, glomerulosa cells, acinar cells, fibroblasts, and oocytes also respond to agonist stimulation with baseline oscillatory Ca^{2+} signaling but with a frequency of about 1 spike/min. In both cell types, modulation of the frequency of Ca^{2+} spiking by IP_3 concentration is the basis of the concentration dependence of agonist action. In contrast, many other cell types, including GT1 neurons, $\alpha T3-1$ gonadotrophs, lactotrophs, parathyroid PT-r cells, and testicular Leydig cells, respond to prolonged agonist stimulation with a single spike. Furthermore, no obvious threshold for activation of Ca^{2+} signaling is observed in some cells, a feature that leads to amplitude-modulated Ca^{2+} signaling in response to increasing agonist concentrations. In other cells, the amplitude of the $[Ca^{2+}]_i$ response to agonist stimulation is not altered by increasing agonist concentrations, but the number of responsive cells progressively increases. Such a variety in the patterns of Ca^{2+} signaling and encoding mechanisms raises several issues, including cell and receptor specificity of signaling pattern, phylogenic and ontogenic aspects of Ca^{2+} signaling, and modulation of the pattern of signaling in interconnected cells, which require further investigation.

It is not clear what endows some but not other cells operated by calcium-mobilizing receptors with the ability to oscillate, and this is one of the major topics of current investigations. The central dogma in the operation of the endoplasmic reticulum oscillator is that the co-agonist actions of IP$_3$ and calcium are required. Both stimulatory and inhibitory actions of calcium on IP$_3$-induced calcium response are believed to be essential for the oscillatory response. In the physiological concentration range, the effects of $[Ca^{2+}]_i$ are bidirectional; initially, increased $[Ca^{2+}]_i$ facilitates its own release, but this is followed by more slowly developing inhibition at higher concentrations. The opposing processes of fast activation and slow inactivation are reflected in the equilibrium open probability of the IP$_3$R channel, which exhibits a characteristic bell-shaped dependence on $[Ca^{2+}]_i$. The IP$_3$-sensitive intracellular pool also expresses a SERCA type of calcium pump, which is inhibited by thapsigargin and BHQ. It is likely that IP$_3$R channels and (Ca^{2+})ATPase function as an interacting pair of calcium regulators in the control of cytosolic and intra-luminal $[Ca^{2+}]$. Such an action implies that the regulatory role of IP$_3$ is permissive; that is, it potentiates opening of the channels by calcium.

The IP$_3$-controlled calcium release is highly synchronized with calcium influx. This is essential to sustain Ca^{2+} signaling and to prevent the possible remodulation of IP$_3$-induced Ca^{2+} spiking by calcium entry. In accord with this, voltage-gated and voltage-insensitive calcium entries are able to remodulate agonist and IP$_3$-induced Ca^{2+} spiking frequencies. Different calcium entry pathways can sustain IP$_3$-induced calcium mobilization, depending on the cell type. Most of the attention has been directed toward CRAC channels in non-excitable cells; however, the nature of these channels and the mechanism of their regulation are still not well defined. As opposed to nonexcitable cells, Ca^{2+} entry through VGCCs in excitable cells is essential for sustained agonist-induced Ca^{2+} spiking.

The plasma membrane oscillator *per se* and the physiological implications of its spontaneous and agonist-controlled activities are not well defined in excitable endocrine cells. While calcium release requires activation of G_q-coupled receptors in pituitary cells, Ca^{2+} entry through VGCCs is stimulated by both G_q and G_s-coupled receptors. However, activation of G_i- and G_o-coupled receptors is associated with inhibition of Ca^{2+} entry through VGCCs. In parallel to Ca^{2+} signaling, pituitary hormone secretion is stimulated by activation of G_q- and G_s-coupled receptors and inhibited by activation of G_i and G_o receptors. The ability of some G_q protein–coupled receptors to inhibit prolactin secretion after transient stimulation further suggests that a complex relationship exists between Ca^{2+} signaling and secretion in certain cells.

Interactions between calcium, CaM, and protein kinase C are essential in the control of signaling, secretion, and gene expression. Calmodulin and protein kinase C may control Ca^{2+} release and entry, the former by modulation of IP$_3$R channel function and the latter through control of VGCCs, sodium, potassium, and glutamate channels; or plasma membrane ATPases. Both calcium and protein kinase C also participate in the control of several enzymes involved in the cascade of intracellular signaling and secretion, including the exocytotic mechanism itself. Calcium is also involved in the stimulation of transcriptional activity in neuronal and endocrine cells. Both hormone release and gene transcription can be activated after the plasma membrane oscillator is rendered inoperative by the depletion of extracellular calcium, demonstrating that IP$_3$-induced Ca^{2+} release is sufficient to initiate such cellular responses.

I thank Melanija Tomic, Ann Katzur, and Fredrick Van Goor for their helpful discussions.

REFERENCES

1. Abbracchio, M. P., and G. Burnstock. Purinoreceptors: are there families of P2X and P2Y purinoreceotors? *Pharmacol. Ther.* 64: 445–475, 1994.
2. Abou-Samra, A. B., K. J. Catt, and G. Aguilera. Calcium-dependent control of corticotropin release in rat anterior pituitary cell cultures. *Endocrinology* 121: 965–971, 1987.
3. Abou-Samra, A.-B., J. P. Harwood, V. C. Manganiello, K. J. Catt, and G. Aguilera. Phorbol 12-myristate 13-acetate and vasopressin potentiate the effect of corticotropin-releasing factor on cyclic AMP production in rat anterior pituitary cells. *J. Biol. Chem.* 262: 1129–1136, 1987.
4. Adler, M., B. S. Wong, S. L. Sabol, N. Busin, M. B. Jackson, and F. F. Weight. Action potentials and membrane ion channels in clonal anterior pituitary cells. *Proc. Natl. Acad. Sci. U.S.A.* 80: 2086–2090, 1983.
5. Aguilera, G., J. P. Harwood, J. X. Wilson, J. Molrell, J. H. Brown, and K. J. Catt. Mechanisms of action of corticotropin-releasing factor and other regulators of corticotropin release in rat pituitary cells. *J. Biol. Chem.* 258: 8039–8045, 1983.
6. Albert, P. R., and A. H. Jr. Tashjian. Relationship of thyrotropin-releasing hormone-induced spike and plateau phases of cytosolic free Ca^{2+} concentrations to hormone secretion. Selective blockade using ionomycin and nifedipine. *J. Biol. Chem.* 259: 15350–15363, 1984.
7. Albert, P. R., and A. H. Jr. Tashjian. Thyrotropin-releasing hormone-induced spike and plateau in cytosolic free Ca^{2+} concentration in pituitary cells. Relation to prolactin release. *J. Biol. Chem.* 259: 5827–5832, 1984.
8. Albert, P. R., G. Wolfson, and A. H. Jr. Tashjian. Diacylglycerol increases cytosolic free Ca^{2+} concentration in rat pituitary cells. *J. Biol. Chem.* 262: 6577–6581, 1987.
9. Aletta, J. M., M. A. Selbert, A. C. Nairn, and A. M. Edelman. Activation of a calcium–calmodulin-dependent protein kinase I cascade in PC12 cells. *J. Biol. Chem.* 271: 20930–20934, 1996.
10. Allbritton, N. L., E. Oancea, M. A. Kuhn, and T. Meyer. Source of nuclear calcium signals. *Proc. Natl. Acad. Sci. U.S.A.* 91: 12458–12462, 1994.
11. Al-Mohanna, F. A., K.W.T. Caddy, and S. R. Bolsver. The

nucleus is insulated from large cytosolic calcium ion changes. *Nature* 367: 745–750, 1994.

12. Alvarez, J., M. Montero, and J. Garcia-Sancho. High affinity inhibition of Ca^{2+}-dependent K^+ channels by cytochrome P-450 inhibitors. *J. Biol. Chem.* 267: 11789–11793, 1992.

13. Ammala, C., O. Larsson, P. O. Berggern, K. Bokvist, L. J. Berggren, H. Kindmark, and P. Rorsman. Insoitol trisphosphate-dependent periodic activation of a Ca^{2+}-activated K^+ conductance in glucose-stimulated pancreatic β-cells. *Nature* 353: 849–852, 1991.

14. Andrews, W. V., R. A. Maurer, amd P. M. Conn. Stimulation of rat luteinizing hormone-beta messenger RNA levels by gonadotropin releasing hormone. Apparent role for protein kinase C. *J. Biol. Chem.* 263: 13755–13761, 1988.

15. Antoni, F. A., and G. Dayanithi. Blockade of K^+ channels reverses the inhibitory action of atriopeptin on secretagogue-stimulated ACTH release by perifused isolated rat anterior pituitary cells. *J. Endocrinol.* 126: 183–191, 1990.

16. Asaoka, Y., S.-I. Nakamura, K. Yoshida, and Y. Nishizuka. Protein kinase C, calcium and phospholipid degradation. *Trends Biochem. Sci.* 17: 414–417, 1992.

17. Badmintgon, M. N., A. K. Campbell, and C. M. Rembold. Differential regulation of nuclear and cytosolic Ca^{2+} in HeLa cells. *J. Biol. Chem.* 271: 31210–31214, 1996.

18. Balboa, M. A., B. L. Firestein, C. Godson, K. S. Bell, and P. A. Insel. Protein kinase Cα mediates phospholipase D activation by nucleotides and phorbol ester in Madin-Darby canine kidney cells. *J. Biol. Chem.* 269: 10511–10516, 1994.

19. Balla, T., S. Nakanishi, and K. J. Catt. Cation sensitivity of inositol 1,4,5-trisphosphate production and metabolism in agonist-stimulated adrenal glomerulosa cells. *J. Biol. Chem.* 269: 16101–16107, 1994.

20. Barros, F., G. M. Katz, G. J. Kaczorowski, and R. L. Vandlen. Calcium current in GH_3 cultured pituitary cells under whole-cell voltage clamp: inhibition by voltage-dependent potassium currents. *Proc. Natl. Acad. Sci. U.S.A.* 82: 1108–1112, 1985.

21. Bean, B. P. Pharmacology and electrophysiology of ATP-activated ion channels. *Trends Pharmacol. Sci.* 13: 87–90, 1992.

22. Benham, C. D., and R. W. Tsien. A novel receptor-operated Ca^{2+}-permeable channel activated by ATP in smooth muscle. *Nature* 328: 275–278, 1987.

23. Bennett, M. R., L. Farnell, W. G. Gibson, and S. Karunanithi. Quantal transmission at purinergic junctions: stochastic interaction between ATP and its receptors. *Biophys. J.* 68: 925–935, 1995.

24. Berridge, M. J. Inositol trisphosphate and calcium signaling. *Nature* 361: 315–325, 1993.

25. Berridge, M. J. Capacitative calcium entry. *Biochem. J.* 312: 1–11, 1995.

26. Berridge, M. J., and R. F. Irvine. Inositol phosphates and cell signalling. *Nature* 341: 197–205, 1989.

27. Bezprozvanny, I., and B. E. Ehrlich. ATP modulates the function of inositol 1,4,5-trisphosphate-gated channels at two sites. *Neuron* 10: 1175–1184, 1993.

28. Bezprozvanny, I. B., K. Ondrias, E. Kaftan, D. A. Stoyanovsky, and B. E. Ehrlich. Activation of the calcium release channel (ryanodine receptor) by heparin and other polyanions is calcium dependent. *Mol. Biol. Cell* 4: 347–352, 1993.

29. Bezprozvanny, I., J. Watras, and B. E. Ehrlich. Bell-shaped calcium-response curves of $Ins(1,4,5)P_3$- and calcium-gated channels from endoplasmic reticulum of cerebellum. *Nature* 351: 751–754, 1991.

30. Biales, B., M. A. Dicher, and A. Tischler. Sodium and calcium action potential in pituitary cells. *Nature* 267: 172–174, 1977.

31. Bird, S. J., M. F. Rossier, A. R. Hughes, S. B. Shears, D. L. Armstrong, and J. W. Putney. Activation of Ca^{2+} entry into acinar cells by a non-phosphorylatable inositol trisphosphate. *Nature* 352: 162–165, 1991.

32. Bito, H., K. Deisseroth, and R. W. Tsien. CREB phosphorylation and dephosphorylation: a Ca^{2+}- and stimulus duration-dependent switch for hippocampal gene expression. *Cell* 87: 1203–1214, 1996.

33. Blondel, O., G. I. Bell, and S. Seino. Inositol 1,4,5-trisphosphate receptors, secretory granules and secretion in endocrine and neuroendocrine cells. *Trends Neurosci.* 18: 157–161, 1995.

34. Bo, X., Y. Zhang, M. Nassar, G. Burnstock, and R. Schoepfer. A P2X purinoreceptor cDNA confering a novel pharmacological profile. *FEBS Lett.* 375: 129–133, 1995.

35. Boitano, S., E. R. Dirksen, and M. J. Sanderson. Intercellular propagation of calcium waves mediated by inositol trisphosphate. *Science* 258: 292–295, 1992.

36. Bootman, M. D., C. W. Taylor, and M. J. Berridge. The thiol reagent, thimerosal, evokes Ca^{2+} spikes in HeLa cells by sensitizing the inositol 1,4,5-trisphosphate receptor. *J. Biol. Chem.* 267: 25113–25119, 1992.

37. Bosma, M. M., and B. Hille. Electrophysiological properties of a cell line of the gonadotrope lineage. *Endocrinology* 130: 3411–3420, 1992.

38. Brake, A. J., M. J. Wagenbach, and D. Julius. New structural motif for ligand-gated ion channels defined by an ionotropic ATP receptor. *Nature* 371: 519–523, 1994.

39. Braun, A. P., and H. Schulman. The multifunctional calcium/calmodulin-dependent protein kinase: from form to function. *Annu. Rev. Physiol.* 57: 417–445, 1995.

40. Buell, G., C. Lewis, G. Collo, R. A. North, and A. Surprenant. An antagonist-insensitive P2X receptor expressed in epithelia and brain. *EMBO J.* 15: 55–62, 1996.

41. Burgoyne, R. D., and A. Morgan. Regulated exocytosis. *Biochem. J.* 293: 305–316, 1993.

42. Burgoyne, R. D., A. Morgan, and A. JH. O'Sullivan. The control of cytoskeletal actin and exocytosis in intact and permeabilized adrenal chromaffin cells: role of calcium and protein kinase C. *Cell. Signal.* 4: 323–334, 1989.

43. Burnstock, G. Physiological and pathological roles of purines: an update. *Drug Dev. Res.* 28: 195–206, 1993.

44. Caccavelli, L., D. Cussac, I. Pellegrini, V. Audinot, P. Jaquet, and A. Enjalbert. D_2 dopaminergic receptors: normal and abnormal transduction mechanisms. *Horm. Res.* 38: 78–83, 1992.

45. Camacho, P., and J. D. Lechleiter. Increased frequency of calcium waves in *Xenopus laevis* oocytes that express a calcium-ATPase. *Science* 260: 226–229, 1993.

46. Camacho, P., and J. D. Lechleiter. Calreticulin inhibits repetitive intracellular Ca^{2+} waves. *Cell* 82: 765–771, 1995.

47. Campbell, K. P., A. T. Leung, and A. H. Sharp. The biochemistry and molecular biology of the dihydropyridine-sensitive calcium channels. *Trends Neurosci.* 11: 425–430, 1988.

48. Canonico, P. L., C. A. Valdenergo, and R. M. Macleod. The inhibition of phosphatidylinositol turnover: a possible postreceptor mechanism for the prolactin secretion inhibiting effect of dopamine. *Endocrinology* 113: 7–14, 1990.

49. Carew, M. A., M.-L. Wu, G. J. Law, Y.-Z. Tseng, and W. T. Mason. Extracellular ATP activates calcium entry and mobilization via P_{2U}-purinoceptors in rat lactotrophs. *Cell Calcium* 16: 227–235, 1994.

50. Castelletti, L., M. Memo, C. Missale, P. F. Spano, and A. Valero. Potassium channels involved in the transduction mechanism of dopamine D_2 receptors in rat lactotrophs. *J. Physiol. (Lond.)* 410: 251–265, 1989.

51. Castro, E., J. Mateo, A. R. Tome, R. M. Barbosa, M. T. Miras-Portugal, and L. M. Rosario. Cell-specific purinergic receptors coupled to Ca^{2+} entry and Ca^{2+} release from internal stores in adrenal chromaffin cells. *J. Biol. Chem.* 270: 5098–5106, 1995.

52. Catt, K. J., and S. S. Stojilkovic. Calcium signaling and gonadotropin secretion. *Trends Endocrinol. Metab.* 1: 15–20, 1989.

53. Catterall, W. A. Structure and function of voltage-sensitive ion channels. *Science* 242: 50–61, 1988.

54. Cena, V., and E. Rojas. Kinetic characteristics of calcium-dependent, cholinergic receptor controlled ATP secretion from adrenal medullary chromaffin cells. *Biochim. Biophys. Acta* 1023: 213–222, 1990.

55. Cesnjaj, M., K. J. Catt, and S. S. Stojilkovic. Coordinate actions of calcium and protein kinase C in the expression of primary response genes in pituitary gonadotrophs. *Endocrinology* 135: 692–701, 1994.

56. Cesnjaj, M., L. Z. Krsmanovic, K. J. Catt, and S. S. Stojilkovic. Autocrine induction of c-fos expression in GT1 neuronal cells by gonadotropin-releasing hormone. *Endocrinology* 133: 3042–3045, 1993.

57. Cesnjaj, M., L. Zheng, K. J. Catt, and S. S. Stojilkovic. Dependence of stimulus-transcription coupling on phospholipase D in agonist-stimulated pituitary cells. *Mol. Biol. Cell* 9: 1037–1047, 1995.

58. Chadwick, C. C., A. Saito, and S. Fleischer. Isolation and characterization of the inositol trisphosphate receptor from smooth muscle. *Proc. Natl. Acad. Sci. U.S.A.* 87: 2132–2136, 1990.

59. Chang, J. P., K. L. Yu, A. O. Wong, and R. E. Peter. Differential actions of dopamine receptor subtypes on gonadotropin and growth hormone release *in vitro* in goldfish. *Neuroendocrinology* 51: 664–674, 1990.

59b. Charles, C. A., S. K. Kodali, and R. F. Tyndale. Intercellular calcium waves in neurons. *Mol. Cell. Neurosci.* 7: 337–353, 1996.

60. Chatila, T., K. A. Anderson, N. Ho, and A. R. Means. A unique phosphorylation-dependent mechanism for the activation of Ca^{2+}/calmodulin-dependent protein kinase type IV/GR. *J. Biol. Chem.* 271: 21542–21548, 1996.

61. Cheek, T. R., and O. Thastrup. Internal Ca^{2+} mobilization and secretion in bovine adrenal chromaffin cells. *Cell Calcium* 10: 213–221, 1989.

62. Chen, C.-C., A. N. Akoplan, L. Sivllott, D. Colquhoun, G. Burnstock, and J. N. Wood. A P2X purinoreceptor expressed by a subset of sensory neurons. *Nature* 377: 418–431, 1995.

63. Chen, C., and I. J. Clarke. Modulation of Ca^{2+} influx in the ovine somatotroph by growth hormone-releasing factor. *Am. J. Physiol.* 268(*Endocrinol. Metab.* 31): E204–EE212, 1995.

64. Chen, C., J. M. Israel, and J. D. Vincent. Electrophysiological responses of rat pituitary cells in somatotroph-enriched primary culture to human growth hormone releasing factor. *Neuroendocrinology* 50: 679–687, 1989.

65. Chen, C., J. Zhang, P. McNeill, M. Pullar, J. T. Cummins, and I. J. Clarke. Human growth hormone releasing factor (hGRF) modulates calcium currents in human growth hormone secreting adenoma cells. *Brain Res.* 604: 345–348, 1993.

66. Chen, Z.-P., M. Kratzmeier, A. Levy, C. A. McArdle, A. Poch, A. Day, A. K. Mukhopadhyay, and S. L. Lightman. Evidence for a role of pituitary ATP receptors in the regulation of pituitary function. *Proc. Natl. Acad. Sci. U.S.A.* 92: 5219–5223, 1995.

67. Chen, Z.-P., M. Kratzmeier, A. Poch, S. Xu, C. A. McArdle, A. Levy, A. K. Mukhopadhyay, and S. L. Lightman. Effects of extracellular nucleotides in the pituitary: adenosine trisphos-

68. phate receptor-mediated intracellular responses in gonadotrope-derived αT3–1 cells. *Endocrinology* 137: 248–256, 1996.

68. Chen, Z.-P., A. Levy, and S. L. Lightman. Activation of specific ATP receptors induces a rapid increase in intracellular calcium ions in rat hypothalamic neurons. *Brain Res.* 641: 249–256, 1994.

69. Chen, Z.-P., A. Levy, and S. L. Lightman. Nucleotides as extracellular signaling molecules. *J. Neuroendocrinol.* 7: 83–96, 1995.

70. Chen, Z.-P., A. Levy, C. A. McArdle, and S. L. Lightman. Pituitary ATP receptors: characterization and functional localization to gonadotropes. *Endocrinology* 135: 1280–1284, 1994.

71. Cheung, P. H., F. J. Dowd, J. E. Porter, and L. S. Li. A Ca^{2+}-ATPase from rat parotid gland plasma membranes has the characteristics of an ecto-ATPase. *Cell. Signal.* 4: 25–35, 1992.

72. Choi, O. H., R. S. Adelstein, and M. A. Beaven. Secretion from rat basophilic RBL-2H3 cells is associated with diphosphorylation of myosin light chains by myosin light chain kinase as well as phosphorylation by protein kinase C. *J. Biol. Chem.* 269: 536–541, 1994.

73. Clapper, D. L., T. F. Walseth, P. J. Dargoe, and H. C. Lee. Pyridine nucleotide metabolites stimulate calcium release from sea urchin egg microsomes desensitized to inositol trisphosphate. *J. Biol. Chem.* 262: 9561–9568, 1987.

74. Clementi, E., H. Scheer, D. Zavvhetti, C. Fasolato, T. Pozzan, and J. Meldolesi. Receptor-activated Ca^{2+} influx. *J. Biol. Chem.* 267: 2164–2172, 1992.

75. Collart, M. A., N. Tourkine, D. Belin, P. Vassalli, P. Jeanteur, and J.-M. Blanchard. c-fos gene transcription in murine macrophages is modulated by a calcium-dependent block to elongation in intron 1. *Mol. Cell. Biol.* 11: 2826–2831, 1991.

76. Collo, G., R. A. North, E. Kawashima, E. Merlo-Pich, S. Neidhart, A. Surprenant, and G. Buell. Cloning of P2X$_5$ and P2X$_6$ receptors and the distribution and properties of an extended family of ATP-gated ion channels. *J. Neurosci.* 16: 2495–2507, 1996.

77. Connor, J. A. Intracellular calcium mobilization by inositol 1,4,5-trisphosphate: intracellular movements and compartmentalization. *Cell Calcium* 14: 185–200, 1993.

78. Corcuff, J. B., N. C. Guerineau, P. Mariot, B. T. Lussier, and P. Mollard. Multiple cytosolic calcium signals and membrane electrical events evoked in single arginine vasopressin-stimulated corticotrophs. *J. Biol. Chem.* 268: 22313–22321, 1993.

79. Cox, D. A., and M. A. Matlib. Modulation of intramitochondrial free Ca^{2+} concentration by antagonists of Na^{+}-Ca^{2+} exchange. *Trends Pharmacol. Sci.* 14: 408–413, 1993.

80. Cullen, P. J., J. J. Hsuan, O. Truong, A. J. Letcher, T. R. Jackson, A. P. Dawson, and R. F. Irvine. Identification of a specific Ins(1,3,4,5)P$_4$-binding protein as a member of the GAP1 family. *Nature* 376: 527–530, 1995.

81. Currie, W. D., W. Li, K. G. Baimbridge, B. H. Yuen, and P.C.K. Leung. Cytosolic free calcium increased by prostaglandin F$_{2\alpha}$ (PGF$_{2\alpha}$), gonadotropin-releasing hormone, and angiotensin II in rat granulosa cells and PGF$_{2\alpha}$ in human granulosa cells. *Endocrinology* 130: 1837–1843, 1992.

82. Cusack, N. J. P$_2$ receptors: subclassification and structure-activity relationships. *Drug Dev. Res.* 28: 244–252, 1993.

83. Danoff, S. K., C. D. Ferris, C. Donath, G. A. Fischer, S. Munemitsu, A. Ullrich, S. H. Snyder, and C. A. Ross. Inositol 1,4,5-trisphosphate receptors: distinct neuronal and nonneuronal forms derived by alternative splicing differ in phosphorylation. *Proc. Natl. Acad. Sci. U.S.A.* 88: 2951–2955, 1991.

84. Davidson, J. S., I. K. Wakefield, U. Sohnius, P. A. van der

Merwe, and R. P. Millar. A novel extracellular nucleotide receptor coupled to phosphoinositidase-C in pituitary cells. *Endocrinology* 126: 80–87, 1990.

85. Decamilli, P., D. Marconi, and A. Spada. Dopamine inhibits adenylate cyclase in human prolactin secreting pituitary adenomas. *Nature* 278: 252–254, 1979.

86. de Jongh, K. S., C. Warner, A. A. Colvin, and W. A. Catterall. Characterization of the two size forms of the $\alpha 1$ subunit of skeletal muscle L-type calcium channels. *Proc. Natl. Acad. Sci. U.S.A.* 88: 10778–10782, 1991.

87. del Castillo, A. R., M. L. Vitale, and J.-M. Tfifaro. Ca^{2+} and pH determine the interaction of chromaffin cell scinderin with phosphatidylserine and phosphatidylinositol 4,5-biphosphate and its cellular distribution during nicotinic-receptor stimulation and protein kinase C activation. *J. Cell. Biol.* 119: 797–810, 1992.

88. de Leon, M., Y. Wang, L. Jones, E. Perez-Reyes, X. Wei, T. W. Soong, T. P. Snutch, and D. T. Yue. Essential Ca^{2+}-binding motif for Ca^{2+}-sensitive inactivation of L-type Ca^{2+} channels. *Science* 270: 1502–1506, 1995.

89. Delisle, S., K.-H. Krause, G. Denning, B.V.L. Potter, and M. J. Welsh. Effect of inositol trisphosphate and calcium on oscillating elevations of intracellular calcium in *Xenopus* oocytes. *J. Biol. Chem.* 265: 11726–11730, 1990.

90. Demer, L. L., C. M. Wortham, E. R. Dirksen, and M. J. Sanderson. Mechanical stimulation induces intercellular calcium signaling in bovine aortic endothelial cells. *Am. J. Physiol.* 264(*Heart Circ. Physiol.* 35): H2094–H2102, 1993.

91. Desrues, L., M. Lamacz, B. G. Jenks, H. Vaudry, and M. C. Tonon. Effect of dopamine on adenylate cyclase activity, polyphosphoinositide metabolism and cytosolic calcium concentrations in frog pituitary melanotrophs. *J. Endocrinol.* 136: 421–429, 1993.

92. Deussen, A., B. Bading, M. Kelm, and J. Schrader. Formation and salvage of adenosine by macrovascular endothelial cells. *Am. J. Physiol.* 264(*Heart Circ. Physiol.* 35): H692–H700, 1993.

93. de Young, G., and J. Keizer. A single pool IP$_3$-receptor based model for agonist stimulated Ca^{2+} oscillations. *Proc. Natl. Acad. Sci. U.S.A.* 89: 9895–9899, 1992.

94. Diaz, R., T. E. Wieleman, S. J. Anderson, and P. Stahl. The use of permeabilized cells to study the ion requirements of receptor-ligand dissociation in endosomes. *Biochem. J.* 260: 127–134, 1989.

95. Dolmetsch, R. E., and R. S. Lewis. Signalling between intracellular Ca^{2+} stores and depletion-activated Ca^{2+} channels generates $[Ca^{2+}]_i$ oscillations in T lymphocytes. *J. Gen. Physiol.* 103: 365–388, 1994.

96. Doucet, J. P., S. P. Squinto, and N. G. Bazan. Fos-jun and the primary genomic response in the nervous system. Possible physiological role and pathophysiological significance. *Mol. Neurobiol.* 4: 27–55, 1990.

97. Drouva, S. V., C. Bihoreau, E. Laplante, R. Rasolonjanahary, H. Clauser, and C. Kordon. Dihydropyridine-sensitive calcium channel activity related to prolactin, growth hormone, and luteinizing hormone release from anterior pituitary cells in culture: interactions with somatostatin, dopamine, and estrogens. *Endocrinology* 123: 2762–2773, 1988.

98. Dubel, S. J., T.V.B. Starr, J. Hell, M. K. Ahlijanian, J. J. Enyeart, W. A. Catterall, and T. P. Snutch. Molecular cloning of the α-1 subunit of an ω-conotoxin-sensitive calcium channel. *Proc. Natl. Acad. Sci. U.S.A.* 89: 5058–5062, 1992.

99. Dubinsky, J. M., and G. S. Oxford. Ionic currents in two strains of rat anterior pituitary tumor cells. *J. Gen. Physiol.* 83: 309–339, 1984.

100. Dubinsky, J. M., and G. S. Oxford. Dual modulation of K^+ channels by thyrotropin-releasing hormone in clonal pituitary cells. *Proc. Natl. Acad. Sci. U.S.A.* 82: 4282–4286, 1985.

101. Dufy, B., J. D. Vincent, H. Fleury, P. du Pasquier, D. Gourdji, and A. Toxoer-Vidal. Membrane effects of thyrotropin-releasing hormone and estrogen shown by intracellular recording from pituitary cells. *Science* 204: 309–311, 1979.

102. Dufy-Barbe, L., L. Bresson, P. Sartor, M.-F. Odessa, and B. Dufy. Calcium homeostasis in growth hormone (GH)-secreting adenoma cells: effect of GH-releasing factor. *Endocrinology* 131: 1436–1444, 1996.

103. Ehrlich, B. E., E. Kaftan, S. Bezprozvannaya, and I. Bezprozvanny. The pharmacology of intracellular Ca^{2+} release channels. *Trends Pharmacol. Sci.* 15: 145–149, 1994.

104. Einhorn, L. C., and G. S. Oxford. Guanine nucleotide binding proteins mediate D$_2$ dopamine receptor activation of a potassium channel in rat lactotrophs. *J. Physiol. (Lond.)* 462: 563–578, 1993.

105. Eldar, H., P. Ben-Av, U.-S. Schmidt, E. Livneh, and M. Liscovitch. Up-regulation of phospholipase D activity induced by overexpression of protein kinase C-α. *J. Biol. Chem.* 268: 12560–12564, 1993.

106. Ely, J. A., C. Ambroz, A. J. Baukal, S. B. Christensen, T. Balla, and K. J. Catt. Relationship between agonist- and thapsigargin-sensitive calcium pools in adrenal glomerulosa cells. *J. Biol. Chem.* 266: 18635–18641, 1991.

107. Enjalbert, A., and J. Backaert. Pharmacological characterization of the D$_2$ dopaminergic receptor negatively coupled with adenylate cyclase in rat anterior pituitary cells. *Mol. Pharmacol.* 23: 576–584, 1983.

108. Enjalbert, A., F. Musset, C. Chenard, M. Priam, C. Kordon, and S. Heisler. Dopamine inhibits prolactin secretion stimulated by the calcium channel agonist Bay-K-8644 through a pertussis toxin-sensitive G protein in anterior pituitary cells. *Endocrinology* 123: 406–412, 1988.

109. Evans, R. J., V. Derkach, and A. Surprenant. ATP mediates fast synaptic transmission in mammalian neurons. *Nature* 357: 503–505, 1992.

110. Fasolato, C., M. Hoth, G. Matthews, and R. Penner. Ca^{2+} and Mn^{2+} influx through receptor-mediated activation of nonspecific cation channels in mast cells. *Proc. Natl. Acad. Sci. U.S.A.* 90: 3068–3072, 1993.

111. Fasolato, C., M. Zottini, E. Clementi, D. Zaccetti, J. Meldolesi, and T. Pozzan. Intracellular Ca^{2+} pools in PC12 cells. Three intracellular pools are distinguished by their turnover and mechanisms of Ca^{2+} accumulation, storage, and release. *J. Biol. Chem.* 266: 20159–20167, 1991.

112. Ferreira, Z. S., N. J. Cipolla, and R. P. Markus. Presence of P2–purinoreceptors in the rat pineal gland. *Br. J. Pharmacol.* 112: 107–110, 1994.

113. Ferris, C. D., R. L. Huganir, D. S. Bredt, A. M. Cameron, and S. H. Snyder. Inositol trisphosphate receptor: phosphorylation by protein kinase C and calcium calmodulin-dependent protein kinases in reconstituted lipid vesicles. *Proc. Natl. Acad. Sci. U.S.A.* 88: 2232–2235, 1991.

114. Ferris, C. D., and S. H. Snyder. IP$_3$ receptor: ligand-activated calcium channels in multiple forms. *Adv. Second Messenger Phosphoprotein Res.* 26: 95–107, 1992.

115. Fewtrell, C. Ca^{2+} oscillations in non-excitable cells. *Annu. Rev. Physiol.* 55: 427–454, 1993.

116. Fielder, J. L., H. B. Pollard, and E. Rojas. Quantitative analysis

of depolarization-induced ATP release from mouse brain synaptosomes: external calcium dependent and independent processes. *J. Membr. Biol.* 127: 21–33, 1992.

117. Fiekers, J. F., and L. M. Konpoka. Spontaneous transients of $[Ca^{2+}]_i$ depend on external calcium and the activation of L-type voltage-gated calcium channels in a clonal pituitary cell line (AtT-20) of cultured mouse corticotropes. *Cell Calcium* 19: 327–336, 1996.

118. Finch, E. A., T. J. Turner, and S. M. Goldin. Calcium as a coagonist of inositol 1,4,5-trisphosphate-induced calcium release. *Science* 252: 443–446, 1991.

119. Fisher, S. K. Homologous and heterologous regulation of receptor-stimulated phosphoinositide hydrolysis. *Eur. J. Pharmacol.* 288: 231–250, 1995.

120. Fliegel, L., E. Leberer, N. M. Green, and D.H.S. MacLenan. The fast twitch muscle calsequesterin isoform predominates in rabbit slow-twich soleus muscle. *FEBS Lett.* 242: 297–300, 1989.

121. Fohr, K. J., J. Scott, G. A. Hilger, and M. Gratzl. Characterization of the inositol 1,4,5-trisphosphate-induced calcium release from permeabilized endocrine cells and its inhibition by decavanadate and *p*-hydroxymercuribenzoate. *Biochem. J.* 262: 83–89, 1989.

122. Fohr, K. J., Y. Wahl, R. Engline, T. P. Kemmer, and M. Gratzl. Decavanadate displaces inositol 1,4,5-trisphosphate (IP$_3$) from its receptor and inhibits IP$_3$ induced Ca^{2+} release in permeabilized pancreatic acinar cells. *Cell Calcium* 12: 735–742, 1991.

123. Foskett, J. K., C. M. Roifman, and D. Wong. Activation of calcium oscillations by thapsigargin in parotid acinar cells. *J. Biol. Chem.* 266: 2778–2782, 1991.

124. Foskett, J. K., and D.C.P. Wong. $[Ca^{2+}]_i$ inhibition of Ca^{2+} release-activated Ca^{2+} influx underlies agonist- and thapsigargin-induced $[Ca^{2+}]_i$ oscillations in salivary acinar cells. *J. Biol. Chem.* 269: 31525–31532, 1994.

125. Friel, D. D., and R. W. Tsien. An FCCP-sensitive Ca^{2+} store in bullfrog sympathetic neurons and its participation in stimulus-evoked changes in $[Ca^{2+}]_i$. *J. Neurosci.* 14: 4007–4024, 1994.

126. Fujii, Y., M. Tomic, S. S. Stojilkovic, T. Iida, M. L. Brandi, Y. Ogino, and K. Sakaguchi. Effects of endothelin-1 on Ca^{2+} signaling and secretion in parathyroid cells. *J. Bone Miner. Res.* 10: 716–725, 1995.

127. Fujii, Y., Y. Yamada, K. Chihara, N. Inagaki, and S. Seino. Somatostatin receptor subtype SSTR2 mediates the inhibition of high-voltage-activated calcium channels by somatostatin and its analogue SMS 201–995. *FEBS Lett.* 355: 117–120, 1994.

128. Fujimoto, T. Calcium pump of the plasma membrane is localized in caveolae. *J. Cell. Biol.* 120: 1147–1157, 1992.

129. Fujimoto, T., S. Nakade, A. Miyawaki, K. Mikoshiba, and K. Ogawa. Localization of inositol 1,4,5-trisphosphate receptor-like protein in plasmalemmal caveolae. *J. Cell. Biol.* 119: 1507–1513, 1992.

130. Galione, A., H. C. Lee, and W. B. Busa. Ca^{2+}-induced Ca^{2+} release in sea urchin egg homogenates: modulation by cyclic ADP-ribose. *Science* 253: 1143–1146, 1991.

131. Gerasimenko, O. V., J. V. Gerasimenko, A. V. Tepikin, and O. H. Petersen. ATP-dependent accumulation and inositol trisphosphate- or cyclic ADP-ribose-mediated release of Ca^{2+} from the nuclear envelope. *Cell* 80: 439–444, 1995.

132. Geschwind, J.-F., M. Hiriart, M. C. Glennon, H. Najafi, B. E. Corkey, F. M. Matschinsky, and M. Prentki. Selective activation of Ca^{2+} by extracellular ATP in a pancreatic β-cell line (HIT). *Biochim. Biophys. Acta* 1012: 107–115, 1989.

133. Ghosh, T. K., P. S. Eis, J. M. Mullaney, C. L. Ebert, and D. L. Gill. Competitive, reversible, and potent antagonism of inositol 1,4,5-trisphosphate-activated calcium release by heparin. *J. Biol. Chem.* 263: 11075–11079, 1988.

134. Giannini, G., E. Clementi, R. Ceci, G. Marziali, and V. Sorrentino. Expression of a ryanodine receptor-Ca^{2+} channel that is regulated by TGF-beta. *Science* 257: 91–94, 1992.

135. Gilchrist, J. S., M. P. Czubryt, and G. N. Pierce. Calcium and calcium-binding proteins in the nucleus. *Mol. Cell. Biochem.* 135: 79–88, 1994.

136. Girard, S., and D. Clapham. Acceleration of intracellular calcium waves in *Xenopus* oocytes by calcium influx. *Science* 260: 229–232, 1993.

137. Gomora, J. C., G. Avila, and G. Cota. Ca^{2+} current expression in pituitary melanotrophs of neonatal rats and its regulation by D$_2$ dopamine receptors. *J. Physiol. (Lond.)* 492: 763–737, 1996.

138. Gray, P.T.A. Oscillations of free cytosolic calcium evoked by cholinergc and catecholaminergic agonists in rat parotid acinar cells. *J. Physiol. (Lond.)* 406: 35–53, 1988.

139. Greenberg, S., F. di Virgilio, T. H. Steinberg, and S. C. Silvestein. Extracellular nucleotides mediate Ca^{2+} fluxes in J774 macrophages by two distinct mechanisms. *J. Biol. Chem.* 263: 10337–10343, 1988.

140. Greengard, P., F. Valtorta, A. J. Czernik, and F. Benfenati. Synaptic vesicle phosphoproteins and regulation of synaptic function. *Science* 259: 780–785, 1993.

141. Grunicke, H. H., and F. Uberall. Protein kinase C modulation. *Cancer Biol.* 3: 351–360, 1992.

142. Guerineau, N., J.-B. Corcuff, A. Tabarin, and P. Mollard. Spontaneous and corticotropin-releasing factor-induced cytosolic calcium transients in corticotrophs. *Endocrinology* 129: 409–420, 1991.

143. Gunter, T. E., K. K. Gunter, S.-S. Sheu, and C. E. Gavin. Mitochondrial calcium transport: physiological and pathological relevance. *Am. J. Physiol.* 267(*Cell Physiol.* 36): C313–C339, 1994.

144. Hajnoczky, G., L. D. Robb-Gaspers, M. B. Seitz, and A. P. Thomas. Decoding of cytosolic calcium oscillations in the mitochondria. *Cell* 82: 415–424, 1995.

145. Hansen, J. R., C. A. McArdle, and P. M. Conn. Relative roles of calcium derived from intra- and extracellular sources in dynamic luteinizing hormone release from perifused pituitary cells. *Mol. Endocrinol.* 1: 808–815, 1987.

146. Hanson, P. I., T. Meyer, L. Stryer, and H. Schulman. Dual role of calmodulin in autophosphorylation of multifunctional CaM kinase may underlie decoding of calcium signals. *Neuron* 12: 943–956, 1994.

147. Harden, T. K., J. L. Boyer, and R. A. Nicholas. P$_2$-purinergic receptors: subtype-associated signaling responses and structure. *Annu. Rev. Pharmacol. Toxicol.* 35: 541–579, 1995.

148. Hardie, R. C., and B. Minke. The trp gene is essential for a light-activated Ca^{2+} channel in *Drosophila* photoreceptors. *Neuron* 8: 643–651, 1992.

149. Hardie, R. C., and B. Minke. Novel Ca^{2+} channels underlying transduction in *Drosophila* photoreceptors: implications for phosphoinositide-mediated Ca^{2+} mobilization. *Trends Neurosci.* 16: 371–376, 1993.

150. Hardie, R. C., A. Peretz, E. Suss-Toby, A. Rom-Glas, S. A. Bishop, Z. Selinger, and B. Minke. Protein kinase C is required for light adaptation in *Drosophila* photoreceptor. *Nature* 363: 634–637, 1993.

151. Harootunian, A. T., J.P.Y. Kao, S. Paranjape, and R. Y. Tsien. Generation of calcium oscillations in fibroblasts by positive feedback between calcium and IP$_3$. *Science* 251: 75–78, 1991.

152. Haug, E., and K. M. Gautvik. Effects of sex steroids on

prolactin secreting rat pituitary cells in culture. *Endocrinology* 99: 1482–1489, 1976.

153. Helmchen, F., K. Imoto, and B. Sakmann. Ca^{2+} buffering and action potential-evoked Ca^{2+} signaling in dendrites of pyramidal neurons. *Biophys. J.* 70: 1069–1081, 1996.

154. Hennager, D. J., M. J. Welsh, and S. Delisle. Changes in either cytosolic or nucleoplasmic inositol 1,4,5-trisphosphate levels can control nuclear Ca^{2+} concentration. *J. Biol. Chem.* 270: 4959–4962, 1995.

155. Hernandez-Cruz, A., F. Sala, and P. R. Adams. Subcellular calcium transients visualized by confocal microscopy in a voltage-clamped vertebrate neurons. *Science* 247: 858–862, 1990.

156. Herrington, J., Y. B. Park, D. F. Babcook, and B. Hille. Dominant role of mitochondria in clearance of large Ca^{2+} loads from rat adrenal chromaffin cells. *Neuron* 16: 219–228, 1996.

157. Heyward, P. M., C. Chen, and I. J. Clarke. Inward membrane currents and electrophysiological responses to GnRH in ovine gonadotropes. *Neuroendocrinology* 61: 609–621, 1995.

158. Heyward, P. M., and I. J. Clarke. A transient effect of estrogen on calcium currents and electrophysiological responses to gonadotropin-releasing hormone in ovine gonadotropes. *Neuroendocrinology* 62: 543–552, 1995.

159. Hille, B. *Ionic Channels of Excitable Membranes.* Sunderland, MA: Sinauer, 1991.

160. Holl, R. W., M. O. Thorner, and D. A. Leong. Cytosolic free calcium in normal somatotropes: effects of forskolin and phorbol ester. *Am. J. Physiol.* 256(*Endocrinol. Metab.* 19): E373–E379, 1989.

161. Holl, R. W., M. O. Thorner, G. L. Mandell, J. A. Sullivan, Y. N. Sinha, and D. A. Leong. Spontaneous oscillations of intracellular calcium and growth hormone secretion. *J. Biol. Chem.* 263: 9682–9685, 1988.

162. Hoth, M., and R. Penner. Depletion of intracellular calcium stores activates a calcium current in mast cells. *Nature* 355: 353–355, 1992.

163. Hoth, M., and R. Penner. Calcium release-activated calcium current in rat mast cells. *J. Physiol. (Lond.)* 465: 359–386, 1993.

164. Huang, K.-P. The mechanism of protein kinase C activation. *Trends Neurosci.* 12: 425–432, 1989.

165. Huang, K.-P., and F. L. Huang. How is protein kinase C activated in CNS. *Neurochem. Int.* 22: 417–433, 1993.

166. Humbert, J. P., N. Matter, J. C. Artault, P. Koppler, and A. N. Malviya. Inositol 1,4,5-trisphosphate receptor is located in the inner buclear membrane vindicating regulation of nuclear calcium signaling by inositol 1,4,5-trisphosphate. Discrete distribution of inositol phosphate receptors to inner and outer nuclear membrane. *J. Biol. Chem.* 271: 478–485, 1996.

167. Hunyady, L., A. J. Baukal, M. Bor, J. A. Ely, and K. J. Catt. Regulation of 1,2-diacylglycerol production by angiotensin-II in bovine adrenal glomerulosa cells. *Endocrinology* 126: 1001–1008, 1990.

168. Hunyady, L., F. Merelli, A. J. Baukal, and K. J. Catt. Agonist-induced endocytosis and signal generation in adrenal glomerulosa cells. A potential mechanism for receptor-operated calcium entry. *J. Biol. Chem.* 266: 2783–2788, 1991.

169. Iida, T., S. S. Stojilkovic, S.-I. Izumi, and K. J. Catt. Spontaneous and agonist-induced calcium oscillations in pituitary gonadotrophs. *Mol. Endocrinol.* 5: 949–958, 1991.

170. Iino, M., and M. Endo. Calcium-dependent immediate feedback control of inositol 1,4,5-trisphosphate-induced Ca^{2+} release. *Nature* 360: 76–78, 1992.

171. Illes, P., and W. Norenberg. Neuronal ATP receptors and their mechanism of action. *Trends Pharmacol. Sci.* 14: 50–54, 1993.

172. Imagawi, T., J. S. Smith, R. Coronado, and K. J. Campbell. Purified ryanodine receptor from skeletal muscle sarcoplasmic reticulum is the Ca^{2+}-permeable pore of the calcium release channel. *J. Biol. Chem.* 262: 16636–16643, 1987.

173. Ingram, C. D., R. J. Bicknell, and W. T. Mason. Intracellular recordings from bovine anterior pituitary cells: modulation of spontaneous activity by regulators of prolactin secretion. *Endocrinology* 119: 2508–2515, 1986.

174. Inui, M., A. Saito, and S. Fleischer. Purification of the ryanodine receptor and identity with feet structures of junctional terminal cisternae of sarcoplasmic reticulum from fast skeletal muscle. *J. Biol. Chem.* 262: 1740–1747, 1987.

175. Irvine, R. F. "Qantal" Ca^{2+} release and the control of Ca^{2+} entry by inositol phosphates: a possible mechanism. *FEBS Lett.* 263: 5–9, 1990.

176. Israel, J.-M., P. Jaquet, and J.-D. Vincent. The electrical properties of isolated human prolactin-secreting adenoma cells and their modification by dopamine. *Endocrinology* 117: 1448–1455, 1985.

177. Izumi, S.-I., S. S. Stojilkovic, and K. J. Catt. Calcium mobilization and influx during the biphasic cytosolic calcium and secretory responses in agonist-stimulated pituitary gonadotrophs. *Arch. Biochem. Biophys.* 275: 410–428, 1989.

178. Izumi, S.-I., S. S. Stojilkovic, T. Iida, L. Z. Krsmanovic, R. J. Omeljaniuk, and K. J. Catt. Role of voltage-sensitive calcium channels in $[Ca^{2+}]_i$ and secretory responses to activators of protein kinase C in pituitary gonadotrophs. *Biochem. Biophys. Res. Commun.* 170: 359–367, 1990.

179. Jacob, R. Calcium oscillations in electrically non-excitable cells. *Biophysica Acta* 1052: 427–438, 1990.

180. Jacob, R. M., J. E. Merritt, T. J. Hallem, and T. J. Rink. Repetitive spikes in cytoplasmic calcium evoked by histamine in human endothelial cells. *Nature* 335: 40–45, 1988.

181. Jensen, J. R., and V. Rehder. FCCP releases Ca^{2+} from a non-mitochondrial store in an identified Helisoma neuron. *Brain Res.* 551: 311–314, 1991.

182. Jobin, R. M., M. Tomic, L. Zheng, S. S. Stojilkovic, and K. J. Catt. GnRH-induced potentiation of calcium-dependent exocytosis in pituitary gonadotrophs. *Endocrinology* 136: 3398–3405, 1995.

183. Jouaville, L. S., F. Ichas, E. L. Holmuhamedov, P. Camacho, and J. D. Lechleiter. Synchronization of calcium waves by mitochondrial substrates in *Xenopus laevis* oocytes. *Nature* 377: 438–441, 1995.

184. Karin, M., and T. Smeal. Control of transcriptional factors by signal transduction pathways: the beginning of the end. *Trends Biochem. Sci.* 17: 418–422, 1992.

185. Kasai, H., and G. J. Augustine. Cytosolic Ca^{2+} gradients triggering undirectional fluid secretion from exocrine pancreas. *Nature* 348: 735–738, 1990.

186. Kass, G. E., S. K. Duddy, G. A. Moore, and S. Orrenius. 2,5-Di(tert-butyl)1,4-benzohydroquinone rapidly elevates cytosolic Ca^{2+} concentration by mobilizing the inositol 1,4,5-trisphosphate-sensitive Ca^{2+} pool. *J. Biol. Chem.* 264: 15192–15198, 1989.

187. Kato, M., J. Hoyland, S. K. Sikdar, and W. T. Mason. Imaging of intracellular calcium in rat anterior pituitary cells in response to growth hormone releasing factor. *J. Physiol. (Lond.)* 447: 171–189, 1992.

188. Kawanishi, T., L. M. Blank, A. T. Harootunian, M. T. Smith, and R. Y. Tsien. Ca^{2+} oscillations induced by hormonal stimulation of individual fura-2-loaded hepatocytes. *J. Biol. Chem.* 264: 12859–12866, 1989.

189. Keizer, J., Y.-X. Li, S. S. Stojilkovic, and J. Rinzel. InsP$_3$-

induced Ca^{2+} excitability of the endoplasmic reticulum. *Mol. Biol. Cell* 6: 945–951, 1995.

190. Keja, J. A., and K. S. Kits. Single-channel properties of high- and low-voltage-activated calcium channels in rat pituitary melanotropic cells. *J. Neurophysiol.* 71: 840–855, 1994.

191. Keja, J. A., and K. S. Kits. Voltage dependence of G-protein-mediated inhibition of high-voltage-activated calcium channels in rat pituitary melanotropes. *Neuroscience* 62: 281–289, 1994.

192. Khan, A. A., J. P. Steiner, M. G. Klein, M. F. Schneider, and S. H. Snyder. IP_3 receptors: localization to plasma membrane of T cells and cocapping with the T cell receptor. *Science* 257: 815–818, 1992.

193. Kidokoro, Y. Spontaneous calcium action potentials in a clonal pituitary cell line and their relationship to prolactin secretion. *Nature* 258: 741–742, 1975.

194. Kiley, S. C., P. J. Parker, D. Fabbro, and S. Jaken. Differential regulation of protein kinase C isozymes by thyrotropin-releasing hormone in GH_4C_1 cells. *J. Biol. Chem.* 266: 23761–23768, 1991.

195. Kiley, S. C., P. J. Parker, D. Fabbro, and S. Jaken. Hormone- and phorbol ester-activated protein kinase C isozymes mediate a reorganization of the actin cytoskeleton associated with prolactin secretion in GH_4C_1 cells. *Mol. Endocrinol.* 6: 120–131, 1992.

196. Kim, K.-T., and W. Westhead. Cellular responses to Ca^{2+} from extracellular and intracellular sources are different as shown by simultaneous measurements of cytosolic Ca^{2+} and secretion from bovine chromaffin cells. *Proc. Natl. Acad. Sci. U.S.A.* 86: 9881–9885, 1989.

197. Klee, C. B., G. F. Draetta, and M. J. Hubbard. Calcineurin. *Adv. Enzymol. Relat. Areas Mol. Biol.* 61: 149–200, 1988.

198. Kleuss, C., H. Scherbul, J. Hescheler, G. Schultz, and B. Wittig. Selectivity in signal transduction determined by γ subunits of heterotrimeric G proteins. *Science* 259: 832–834, 1993.

199. Koch, B. D., and A. Schonbrunn. The somatostatin receptor is directly coupled to adenylate cyclase in GH_4C_1 pituitary cell membranes. *Endocrinology* 114: 1784–1790, 1984.

200. Koch, B. D., and A. Schonbrunn. Characterization of the cyclic AMP-independent actions of somatostatin in GH cells. *J. Biol. Chem.* 263: 226–234, 1988.

201. Kong, S. K., D. Tsang, K. N. Leung, and C. Y. Lee. Nuclear envelope acts as a calcium barrier in C6 glioma cells. *Biochem. Biophys. Res. Commun.* 218: 595–600, 1996.

202. Kongsamut, S., I. Shibuya, and W. W. Douglas. Melanotrophs of *Xenopus laevis* do respond directly to neuropeptide-Y as evidenced by reductions in secretion and cytosolic calcium pulsing in isolated cells. *Endocrinology* 133: 336–342, 1993.

203. Koppler, P., N. Matter, and A. N. Malviya. Evidence for stereospecific inositol 1,3,4,5-[^{3}H]tetrakisphosphate binding sites on rat liver nuclei. Delineating inositol 1,3,4,5-tetrakisphosphate interaction in nuclear calcium signaling process. *J. Biol. Chem.* 268: 26248–26252, 1993.

204. Korn, S. J., A. Bolden, and R. Horn. Control of action potentials and Ca^{2+} influx by the Ca^{2+}-dependent chloride current in mouse pituitary cells. *J. Physiol. (Lond.)* 439: 423–437, 1991.

205. Krause, E., F. Pfeiffer, A. Schmid, and I. Schulz. Depletion of intracellular calcium stores activates a calcium conducting nonselective cation current in mouse pancreatic acinar cells. *J. Biol. Chem.* 271: 32523–32528, 1996.

206. Krsmanovic, L. Z., S. S. Stojilkovic, T. Balla, S. Al-Damluji, R. I. Weiner, and K. J. Catt. Receptors and neurosecretory actions of endothelin in hypothalamic neurons. *Proc. Natl. Acad. Sci. U.S.A.* 88: 11124–11128, 1991.

207. Krsmanovic, L. Z., S. S. Stojilkovic, and K. J. Catt. Pulsatile gonadotropin-releasing hormone release and its regulation. *Trends Endocrinol. Metab.* 7: 56–59, 1996.

208. Krsmanovic, L. Z., S. S. Stojilkovic, L. M. Mertz, M. Tomic, and K. J. Catt. Expression of gonadotropin-releasing hormone receptors and autocrine regulation of neuropeptide release in immortalized hypothalamic neurons. *Proc. Natl. Acad. Sci. U.S.A.* 90: 3908–3912, 1993.

209. Kukuljan, M., E. Rojas, K. J. Catt, and S. S. Stojilkovic. Membrane potential regulates inositol 1,4,5-trisphosphate-controlled cytoplasmic Ca^{2+} oscillations in pituitary gonadotrophs. *J. Biol. Chem.* 269: 4860–4865, 1994.

210. Kukuljan, M., S. S. Stojilkovic, E. Rojas, and K. J. Catt. Apamin-sensitive potassium channels mediate agonist-induced oscillations of membrane potential in pituitary gonadotrophs. *FEBS Lett.* 301: 19–22, 1992.

211. Kukuljan, M., L. Vergara, and S. S. Stojilkovic. Modulation of the kinetics of inositol 1,4,5-trisphosphate-induced $[Ca^{2+}]_i$ oscillations by calcium entry in pituitary gonadotrophs. *Biophys. J.* 72: 698–707, 1997.

212. Kumakura, K., K. Sasaki, T. Sakuri, M. Ohara-Imaizumi, H. Misonou, S. Nakamura, Y. Matsuda, and Y. Nonomura. Essential role of myosin light chain kinase in the mechanism for MgATP-dependent priming of exocytosis in adrenal chromaffin cells. *J. Neurosci.* 14: 7695–7703, 1994.

213. Kumar, N. M., and N. B. Gilula. The gap junction communication channels. *Cell* 84: 381–388, 1996.

214. Kurihara, K., K. Hosoi, and T. Ueha. Characterization of ecto-nucleoside triphosphatase on A-431 human epidermoidal carcinoma cells. *Enzyme* 46: 213–220, 1992.

215. Kuryshev, Y. A., G. V. Childs, and A. K. Ritchie. Corticotropin-releasing hormone stimulation of Ca^{2+} entry in corticotropes is partially dependent on protein kinase A. *Endocrinology* 136: 3925–3935, 1995.

216. Kusano, K., S. Fueshko, H. Gainer, and S. Wray. Electrical and synaptic properties of embryonic luteinizing hormone–releasing hormone neurons in explant cultures. *Proc. Natl. Acad. Sci. U.S.A.* 92: 3918–3922, 1995.

217. Lacerda, A. E., D. Rampe, and A. M. Brown. Effects of protein kinase C activators on cardiac Ca^{2+} channels. *Nature* 335: 249–251, 1988.

218. Lai, F. A., H. P. Erickson, E. Rousseau, Q. Y. Liu, and G. Meissner. Purification and reconstitution of the calcium release channel. *Nature* 331: 315–319, 1988.

219. Lamberts, S.W.J., and R. M. MacLeod. Regulation of prolactin secretion at the level of the lactotrophs. *Endocr. Rev.* 7: 279–318, 1990.

220. Lang, D.G., and A. K. Ritchie. Tetraethylammonium blockade of apamin-sensitive and insensitive Ca^{2+}-activated K^+ channels in a pituitary cell line. *J. Physiol. (Lond.)* 425: 117–132, 1990.

221. Lechleiter, J. D., and D. E. Clapham. Molecular mechanisms of intracellular calcium excitability in *X. laevis* oocytes. *Cell* 69: 283–294, 1992.

222. Lee, H. C. Potentiation of calcium- and caffeine-induced calcium release by cyclic ADP-ribose. *J. Biol. Chem.* 268: 293–299, 1993.

223. Lee, H. C., R. Aarthus, and T. F. Walseth. Calcium mobilization by dual receptors during fertilization of sea urchin eggs. *Science* 261: 352–355, 1993.

224. Leong, D. A. A complex mechanism of facilitation in pituitary ACTH cells: recent single-cell studies. *J. Exp. Biol.* 139: 151–168, 1988.

225. Leong, D. A. A model for intracellular calcium signaling and

the coordinate regulation of hormone biosynthesis, receptors and secretion. *Cell Calcium* 12: 255–268, 1991.

226. Leong, D. A., and M. O. Thorner. A potential code of luteinizing hormone–releasing hormone-induced calcium ion responses in the regulation of luteinizing hormone secretion among individual gonadotropes. *J. Biol. Chem.* 266: 9016–9022, 1991.

227. Leung, A. T., T. Imagawa, and K. P. Campbell. Structural characterization of the 1,4-dihydropyridine receptor of the voltage-dependent Ca^{2+} channel from rabbit skeletal muscle. *J. Biol. Chem.* 262: 7943–7946, 1987.

228. Lewis, C., S. Neldhart, C. Holy, R. A. North, G. Buell, and A. Surprenant. Coexpression of P2X$_2$ and P2X$_3$ receptor subunits can account for ATP-gated currents in sensory neurons. *Nature* 377: 432–435, 1995.

229. Lewis, D. L., M. B. Goodman, P. A. St. John, and J. L. Barker. Calcium currents and fura-2 signals in fluorescence-activated cell sorted lactotrophs and somatotrophs of rat anterior pituitary. *Endocrinology* 123: 611–621, 1988.

230. Lewis, D. L., F. F. Weight, and A. Luini. A guanine nucleotide-binding protein mediates the inhibition of voltage-dependent calcium current by somatostatin in a pituitary cell line. *Proc. Natl. Acad. Sci. U.S.A.* 83: 9035–9039, 1986.

231. Li, G., E. Rungger-Brandle, I. Just, J.-C. Jonas, K. Aktories, and C. B. Wollheim. Effect of disruption of actin filaments by *Clostridium botulinum* C2 toxin on insulin secretion in HIT-T15 cells and pancreatic islets. *Mol. Biol. Cell* 4616: 1199–1213, 1994.

232. Li, Y.-X., J. Keizer, S. S. Stojilkovic, and J. Rinzel. Calcium excitability of the ER membrane: an explanation for IP$_3$-induced Ca^{2+} oscillations. *Am. J. Physiol.* 269(*Cell Physiol.* 32): C1079–C1092, 1995.

233. Li, Y.-X., J. Rinzel, J. Keizer, and S. S. Stojilkovic. Calcium oscillations in pituitary gonadotrophs: comparison of experiments and theory. *Proc. Natl. Acad. Sci. U.S.A.* 91: 58–62, 1994.

234. Li, Y.-X., J. Rinzel, L. Vergara, and S. S. Stojilkovic. Spontaneous electrical and calcium oscillations in pituitary gonadotrophs. *Biophys. J.* 69: 785–795, 1995.

235. Li, Y.-X., S. S. Stojilkovic, J. Keizer, and J. Rinzel. Sensing and refilling calcium stores in an excitable cell. *Biophys. J.* 72: 1080–1091, 1997.

236. Limor, R., D. Ayalon, A. M. Capponi, G. Childa, and Z. Naor. Cytosolic free calcium in cultured pituitary cells separated by centrifugal elutriation: effect of gonadotropin-releasing hormone. *Endocrinology* 120: 497–503, 1987.

237. Lin, C., G. Hajnoczky, and A. P. Thomas. Propagation of cytosolic calcium waves into the nuclei of hepatocytes. *Cell Calcium* 16: 247–258, 1994.

238. Lin, S. H., and W. E. Russell. Two Ca^{2+}-dependent ATPases in rat liver plasma membrane. The previously purified (Ca^{2+}-Mg^{2+})ATPase is not a Ca^{2+} pump but an ecto-ATPase. *J. Biol. Chem.* 263: 12253–12258, 1988.

239. Liscovitch, M. Crosstalk among multiple signal-activated phospholipases. *Trends Biochem. Sci.* 17: 393–399, 1992.

240. Lledo, P.-M., V. Homburger, J. Bockaert, and J. D. Vincent. Differential G protein-mediated coupling of D$_2$ dopamine receptors to K$^+$ and Ca^{2+} currents in rat anterior pituitary cells. *Neuron* 8: 455–463, 1992.

241. Lledo, P.-M., J.-M. Israel, and J.-D. Vincent. A guanine nucleotide-binding protein mediates the inhibition of voltage-dependent calcium currents by dopamine in rat lactotrophs. *Brain Res.* 528: 143–147, 1990.

242. Lledo, P.-M., P. Legendre, J.-M. Israel, and J.-D. Vincent. Dopamine inhibits two characterized voltage-dependent calcium currents in identified rat lactotroph cells. *Endocrinology* 127: 990–1001, 1990.

243. Lledo, P.-M., P. Legendre, J. Zhang, J.-M. Israel, and J.-D. Vincent. Effects of dopamine on voltage-dependent potassium currents in identified rat lactotroph cells. *Neuroendocrinology* 52: 545–555, 1990.

244. Llinas, R., M. Sugimori, and R. B. Silver. Microdomains of high calcium concentration in a presynaptic terminal. *Science* 256: 677–679, 1992.

245. Lohret, T. A., R. C. Murphy, T. Drgon, and K. W. Kinnally. Activity of the mitochondrial multiple conductance channel is independent of the adenine nucleotide translocator. *J. Biol. Chem.* 271: 4846–4849, 1996.

246. Lu, K. P., and A. R. Means. Regulation of the cell cycle by calcium and calmodulin. *Endocr. Rev.* 14: 40–58, 1993.

247. Luini, A., D. Lewis, S. Guild, D. Corda, and J. Axelrod. Hormone secretagogues increase cytosolic calcium by increasing cAMP in corticotropin-secreting cells. *Proc. Natl. Acad. Sci. U.S.A.* 82: 8034–8038, 1985.

248. Luini, A., D. Lewis, S. Guild, G. Schofield, and F. Weight. Somatostatin, an inhibitor of ACTH secretion, decreases cytosolic free calcium and voltage-dependent calcium current in a pituitary cell line. *J. Neurosci.* 6: 3128–3132, 1986.

249. Lussier, B. T., M. B. French, B. C. Moor, and J. Kraicer. Free intracellular Ca^{2+} concentration and growth hormone (GH) release from purified rat somatotrophs. III. Mechanism of action of GH-releasing factor and somatostatin. *Endocrinology* 128: 592–603, 1991.

250. Lussier, B. T., D. A. Wood, M. B. French, B. C. Moor, and J. Kraicer. Free intracellular Ca^{2+} concentration ([Ca^{2+}]$_i$) and growth hormone release from purified rat somatotrophs. II. Somatostatin lowers [Ca^{2+}]$_i$ by inhibiting Ca^{2+} influx. *Endocrinology* 128: 583–591, 1991.

251. Lytton, J., M. Westlin, S. E. Burk, G. E. Shull, and D. H. MacLennan. Functional comparisons between isoforms of the sarcoplasmic or endoplasmic reticulum family of calcium pumps. *J. Biol. Chem.* 267: 14483–14489, 1992.

252. Lytton, J., M. Westlin, and M. R. Hanley. Thapsigargin inhibits the sarcoplasmic or endoplasmic reticulum Ca-ATPase family of calcium pumps. *J. Biol. Chem.* 266: 17067–17071, 1991.

253. Ma, Y., E. Kobrinsky, and A. R. Mark. Cloning and expression of a novel truncated calcium channel from non-excitable cells. *J. Biol. Chem.* 270: 483–493, 1995.

254. Maeda, N., M. Niinobe, and K. Mikoshiba. A cerebellar Purkinje cell marker P$_{400}$ protein is an inositol 1,4,5-trisphosphate (InsP$_3$) receptor protein. Purification and characterization of InsP$_3$ receptor complex. *EMBO J.* 9: 61–67, 1990.

255. Malgaroli, A., L. Vallar, F. R. Elahi, T. Pozzan, A. Spada, and J. Meldolesi. Dopamine inhibits cytosolic Ca^{2+} increases in rat lactotroph cells. *J. Biol. Chem.* 262: 13920–13927, 1987.

256. Marchetti, C., G. V. Childs, and A. M. Brown. Membrane currents of identified isolated rat corticotropes and gonadotropes. *Am. J. Physiol.* 252(*Endocrinol. Metab.* 15): E340–E346, 1987.

257. Marchetti, C., G. V. Childs, and A. M. Brown. Voltage-dependent calcium currents in rat gonadotropes separated by centrifugal elutriation. *Am. J. Physiol.* 258(*Endocrinol. Metab.* 21): E589–E596, 1990.

258. Marshall, I.C.B., and C. W. Taylor. Biphasic effects of cytosolic Ca^{2+} on Ins(1,4,5)P$_3$-stimulated Ca^{2+} mobilization in hepatocytes. *J. Biol. Chem.* 268: 13214–13220, 1993.

259. Marshall, I.C.B., and C. W. Taylor. Regulation of inositol 1,4,5-trisphosphate receptors. *J. Exp. Biol.* 184: 161–182, 1993.

260. Marshall, I.C.B., and C. W. Taylor. Two calcium binding sites mediate the interconversion of liver inositol 1,4,5-trisphosphate receptors between three conformational states. *Biochem. J.* 301: 591–598, 1994.

261. Martelli, A. M., R. S. Gilmour, V. Bertagnolo, L. M. Neri, L. Manzoli, and L. Cocco. Nuclear localization and signaling activity of phosphoinositase C beta in Swiss 3T3 cells. *Nature* 358: 242–245, 1992.

262. Mason, M. J., M. P. Mahaut-Smith, and S. Grinstein. The role of intracellular Ca^{2+} in the regulation of the plasma membrane Ca^{2+} permeability of unstimulated rat lymphocytes. *J. Biol. Chem.* 266: 10872–10879, 1991.

263. Matesic, D. F., J. A. Germak, E. Dupont, and B. V. Madhukar. Immortalized hypothalamic luteinizing hormone–releasing hormone neurons express a connexin 26-like protein and display functional gap junction coupling assayed by fluorescence recovery after photobleaching. *Neuroendocrinology* 58: 485–492, 1993.

264. Matthews, R. P., C. R. Guthrie, L. M. Wailes, X. Zhao, A. R. Means, and G. S. McKnight. Calcium-calmodulin-dependent protein kinase types II and IV differentially regulate CREB-dependent gene expression. *Mol. Cell. Biol.* 14: 6107–6116, 1994.

265. Mayer, M. L. A calcium-activated chloride current generates the after-depolarization of rat sensory neurones in culture. *J. Physiol. (Lond.)* 364: 217–239, 1985.

266. Mazzanti, M., L. J. Defelice, J. Cohn, and H. Malter. Ion channels in the nuclear envelope. *Nature* 343: 764–767, 1990.

267. Mazzanti, M., B. Innocenti, and M. Rigatelli. ATP-dependent ionic permeability on nuclear envelope in *in situ* nuclei of *Xenopus* oocytes. *FASEB J.* 8: 231–236, 1994.

268. McArdle, C. A., W. Forrest-Owen, J. S. Davidson, R. Fowkes, R. Bunting, W. T. Mason, A. Poch, and M. Kratzmeier. Ca^{2+} entry in gonadotrophs and αT3-1 cells: does store-dependent Ca^{2+} influx mediate gonadotrophin-releasing hormone action? *J. Endocrinol.* 149: 155–169, 1996.

269. McArdle, C. A., R. Bunting, and W. T. Mason. Dynamic video imaging of cytosolic Ca^{2+} in the αT3-1, gonadotrope-derived cell line. *Mol. Cell. Endocrinol.* 3: 124–132, 1992.

270. McCormack, J. G., A. P. Halestrap, and R. M. Denton. Role of calcium ions in regulation of mammalian intramitochondrial metabolism. *Physiol. Rev.* 70: 391–425, 1990.

271. McDonald, T. V., B. A. Premack, and P. Gardner. Flash photolysis of caged inositol 1,4,5-trisphosphate activates plasma membrane calcium current in human T cells. *J. Biol. Chem.* 268: 3889–3896, 1993.

272. McPherson, P. S., and K. P. Campbell. The ryanodine receptor/ Ca^{2+} release channel. *J. Biol. Chem.* 268: 13765–13768, 1993.

273. McPherson, S. M., P. S. McPherson, L. Mathews, K. P. Campbell, and F. J. Longo. Cortical localization of a calcium release channel in sea urchin eggs. *J. Cell. Biol.* 116: 1111–1121, 1992.

274. Means, A. R., I. C. Bagchi, M. F. Vanberkum, and B. E. Kemp. Regulation of smooth muscle myosin light chain kinase by calmodulin. *Adv. Exp. Med. Biol.* 304: 11–24, 1991.

275. Means, A. R., and J. R. Dedman. Calmodulin—an intracellular calcium receptor. *Nature* 285: 73–77, 1980.

276. Means, A. R., and S. E. George. Calmodulin regulation of smooth myosin light-chain kinase. *J. Cardiovasc. Pharmacol.* 12: S25–S29, 1988.

277. Means, A. R., M. F. Vanberkum, I. Bagchi, K. P. Lu, and C. D. Rasmussen. Regulatory functions of calmodulin. *Pharmacol. Ther.* 50: 255–270, 1991.

278. Meda, P. The role of gap junction membrane channels in secretion and hormonal action. *J. Bioenerg. Biomembr.* 28: 369–377, 1996.

279. Meldolesi, J., A. Villa, P. Volpe, and T. Pozzan. Cellular sites of IP_3 action. *Adv. Second Messenger Phosphoprotein Res.* 26: 187–208, 1992.

280. Merelli, F., S. S. Stojilkovic, T. Iida, L. Z. Krsmanovic, L. Zheng, P. L. Mellon, and K. J. Catt. Gonadotropin-releasing hormone-induced calcium signaling in clonal pituitary gonadotrophs. *Endocrinology* 131: 925–932, 1992.

281. Mermelstein, P. G., J. B. Becker, and D. J. Surmeier. Estradiol reduces calcium currents in rat neostriatal neurons via a membrane receptor. *J. Neurosci.* 16: 595–604, 1996.

282. Meyer, T. Cell signaling by second messenger waves. *Cell* 64: 675–678, 1991.

283. Meyer, T., and L. Stryer. Calcium spiking. *Annu. Rev. Biophys. Chem.* 20: 153–174, 1991.

284. Meyer, T. E., and J. F. Habener. Cyclic adenosine 3′,5′-monophosphate response element binding protein (CREB) and related transcription-activating deoxyribonucleic acid-binding proteins. *Endocr. Rev.* 14: 269–290, 1993.

285. Michalak, M., R. E. Milner, K. Burns, and M. Opas. Calreticulin. *Biochem. J.* 285: 681–692, 1992.

286. Mignery, G. A., C. L. Newton, B. T. Archer, and T. C. Sudhof. Structure and expression of the rat inositol 1,4,5-trisphsophate receptor. *J. Biol. Chem.* 265: 12679–12685, 1990.

287. Mignery, G. A., T. C. Sudhof, K. Takei, and P. de Camilli. Putative receptor for inositol 1,4,5-trisphosphate similar to ryanodine receptor. *Nature* 342: 192–195, 1989.

288. Miller, R. J. Multiple calcium channels and neuronal function. *Science* 235: 46–52, 1987.

289. Milner, R. E., K. S. Famulski, and M. Michalak. Calcium binding proteins in the sarcoplasmic/endoplasmic reticulum of muscle and non-muscle cells. *Mol. Cell. Biochem.* 112: 1–13, 1992.

290. Minke, B., and Z. Selinger. Inositol lipid pathway in fly photoreceptors: excitation, calcium mobilization and retinal degradation. In: *Retinal Research,* edited by N. N. Osborne and G. J. Chader. New York: Pergamon, 1996, vol. 11, p. 99–124.

291. Mitchell, P. Coupling of phosphorylation to electron and hydrogen transfer by a chemiosmotic type of mechanism. *Nature* 191: 144–148, 1961.

292. Mitsui, K., M. Brady, H. C. Palfrey, and A. C. Nairn. Purification and characterization of calmodulin-dependent protein kinase III from rabbit reticulocytes and rat pancreas. *J. Biol. Chem.* 268: 13422–13433, 1993.

293. Miyawaki, A., T. Furuichi, Y. Ryou, S. Yoshikawa, T. Nakagawa, T. Saitoh, and K. Mikoshiba. Structure–function relationships of the mouse inositol 1,4,5-trisphosphate receptor. *Proc. Natl. Acad. Sci. U.S.A.* 88: 4911–4915, 1991.

294. Miyazaki, S., H. Shirakawa, K. Nakada, Y. Honda, M. Yuzaki, S. Nakade, and K. Mikoshiba. Antibody to the inositol trisphosphate receptor blocks thimerosal-enhanced Ca^{2+}-induced Ca^{2+} release and Ca^{2+} oscillations in hamster eggs. *FEBS Lett.* 309: 180–184, 1992.

295. Miyazaki, S., M. Yuzaki, K. Nakada, H. Shirakawa, S. Nakanishi, S. Nakade, and K. Mikoshiba. Block of Ca^{2+} wave and Ca^{2+} oscillation by antibody to the inositol 1,4,5-trisphosphate receptor in fertilized hamster eggs. *Science* 257: 251–255, 1992.

296. Molday, R. S. Calmodulin regulation of cyclic-nucleotide-gated channels. *Curr. Opin. Neurobiol.* 6: 445–52, 1996.

297. Mollard, P., N. Guerineau, C. Chiavaroli, W. Schlegel, and D. M. Cooper. Adenosine A1 receptor-induced inhibition of Ca^{2+} transients linked to action potentials in clonal pituitary cells. *Eur. J. Pharmacol.* 206: 271–277, 1991.

298. Mollard, P., J.-M. Theler, N. Guerineau, P. Vacher, C. Chiavaroli, and W. Schlegel. Cytosolic Ca^{2+} of excitable pituitary cells at resting potentials is controlled by steady state Ca^{2+} currents sensitive to dihydropyridines. *J. Biol. Chem.* 269: 25158–25164, 1994.

299. Mollard, P., P. Vacher, B. Dufy, and J. L. Barker. Somatostatin blocks Ca^{2+} action potential activity in prolactin-secreting pituitary tumor cells through coordinate actions of K$^+$ and Ca^{2+} conductances. *Endocrinology* 123: 721–732, 1988.

300. Montero, M., J. Garcia-Sancho, and J. Alvares. Transient inhibition by chemotactic peptide of a store-operated Ca^{2+} entry pathway in human neutrophils. *J. Biol. Chem.* 268: 13055–13061, 1993.

301. Moore, G. A., D. J. McConkey, G.E.N. Kass, P. J. O'Brien, and S. Orrenius. 2,5-Di(tert-butyl)-1,4-benzohydroquinone—a novel inhibitor of liver microsomal Ca^{2+} sequestration. *FEBS Lett.* 224: 331–336, 1987.

302. Mori, Y., T. Friedrich, M.-S. Kim, A. Mikami, J. Nakai, P. Ruth, E. Bosse, F. Hofmann, V. Flockerzi, and T. Furuichi. Primary structure and functional expression from complementary DNA of a brain calcium channel. *Nature* 350: 398–402, 1991.

303. Morris, A. P., D. V. Gallacher, R. F. Irvine, and O. H. Petersen. Synergism of inositol trisphosphate and tetrakisphosphate in activating Ca^{2+}-dependent K$^+$ channels. *Nature* 330: 653–655, 1987.

304. Muallem, S., M. Scheffield, S. Pandol, and G. Sachs. Inositol trisphosphate modification of ion transport in rough endoplasmic reticulum. *Proc. Natl. Acad. Sci. U.S.A.* 82: 4433–4437, 1985.

305. Musset, F., P. Bertrand, C. Kordon, and A. Enjalbert. Differential coupling with pertussis toxin-sensitive G proteins of dopamine and somatostatin receptors involved in regulation of adenohypophyseal secretion. *Mol. Cell. Endocrinol.* 73: 1–10, 1990.

306. Nairn, A. C., and H. C. Palfrey. Identification of the major Mr 100,000 substrate for calmodulin-dependent protein kinase III in mammalian cells as elongation factor-2. *J. Biol. Chem.* 262: 17299–17303, 1987.

307. Nairn, A. C., and M. R. Picciotto. Calcium/calmodulin-dependent protein kinases. *Semin. Cancer Biol.* 5: 295–303, 1994.

308. Nakagawa, T., H. Okano, T. Furuichi, J. Aruga, and K. Mikoshiba. The subtypes of the mouse inositol 1,4,5-trisphosphate receptor are expressed in a tissue specific and developmentally specific manner. *Proc. Natl. Acad. Sci. U.S.A.* 88: 6244–6248, 1991.

309. Nakajima, T., T. Lkitazawa, E. Hamada, H. Hazama, M. Omata, and Y. Kurachi. 17β-Estradiol inhibits the voltage-dependent L-type Ca^{2+} currents in aortic smooth muscle cells. *Eur. J. Pharmacol.* 294: 625–635, 1995.

310. Nakazawa, K., K. Fujimori, A. Takanaka, and K. Inoue. Comparison of adenosine triphosphate- and nicotine-activated inward currents in rat phaeochromocytoma cells. *J. Physiol.* 434: 647–660, 1991.

311. Naor, Z., H. D. Cohen, J. Hermon, and R. Limor. Induction of exocytosis in permeabilized pituitary cells by α- and β-type protein kinase C. *Proc. Natl. Acad. Sci. U.S.A.* 86: 4501–4504, 1989.

312. Nathanson, M. H., P. J. Padfield, A. J. O'Sullivan, A. D. Burghstahler, and J. D. Jamieson. Mechanism of Ca^{2+} wave propagation in pancreatic acinar cells. *J. Biol. Chem.* 267: 18118–18121, 1992.

313. Naumov, A. P., J. Herrington, and B. Hille. Actions of growth-hormone-releasing hormone on rat pituitary cells: intracellular calcium and ionic currents. *Pflugers Arch.* 427: 414–421, 1994.

314. Nedergaard, M. Direct signaling from astrocytes to neurons in cultures of mammalian brain cells. *Science* 263: 1768–1771, 1994.

315. Neely, A., and C. J. Lingle. Two components of calcium-activated potassium current in rat adrenal chromaffin cells. *J. Physiol. (Lond.)* 453: 97–131, 1992.

316. Neher, E., and G. J. Augustine. Calcium gradients and buffers in bovine chromaffin cells. *J. Physiol. (Lond.)* 450: 272–301, 1992.

317. Nilius, B. Permeation properties of a non-selective cation channel in human vascular endothelial cells. *Pflugers Arch.* 416: 609–611, 1990.

318. Nilius, B., G. Schwartz, M. Oike, and G. Droogmans. Histamine-activated, non-selective cation currents and Ca^{2+} transients in endothelial cells. *Pflugers Arch.* 424: 285–293, 1993.

319. Nishizuka, Y. Turnover of inositol phospholipids and signal transduction. *Science* 225: 1365–1369, 1984.

320. Nishizuka, Y. Intracellular signaling by hydrolysis of phospholipids and activation of protein kinase C. *Science* 258: 607–614, 1992.

321. Norregaard, A., B. Vilsen, and J. P. Andersen. Transmembrane segment M3 is essential to thapsigargin sensitivity of the sarcoplasmic reticulum Ca^{2+}-ATPase. *J. Biol. Chem.* 269: 26598–26601, 1994.

322. Nowycky, M. C., A. P. Fox, and R. W. Tsien. Three types of neuronal calcium channel with different calcium agonist sensitivity. *Nature* 316: 440–443, 1985.

323. Ohara-Imaizumi, M., T. Sakurai, S. Nakamura, S. Nakanishi, Y. Matsuda, S. Muramatsu, Y. Nonomura, and K. Kumakura. Inhibition of Ca^{2+}-dependent catecholamine release by myosin light chain kinase inhibitor, wortmannin, in adrenal chromaffin cells. *Biochem. Biophys. Res. Commun.* 185: 1016–1021, 1992.

324. Ortmann, O., F. Merelli, S. S. Stojilkovic, K. D. Schultz, G. Emons, and K. J. Catt. Modulation of calcium signaling and LH secretion by progesterone in pituitary gonadotrophs and clonal pituitary cells. *J. Steroid Biochem. Mol. Biol.* 48: 47–54, 1994.

325. Ortmann, O., S. S. Stojilkovic, M. Cesnjaj, G. Emons, and K. J. Catt. Modulation of cytoplasmic calcium signaling in rat pituitary gonadotrophs by estradiol and progesterone. *Endocrinology* 131: 1565–1568, 1992.

326. Osipchuk, Y., and M. Cahalan. Cell-to-cell spread of calcium signals mediated by ATP receptors in mast cells. *Nature* 359: 241–244, 1992.

327. Osipchuk, Y. V., M. Wakui, D. I. Yule, D. V. Gallacher, and O. H. Petersen. Cytoplasmic Ca^{2+} oscillations evoked by receptor stimulation, G-protein activation, internal application of inositol trisphosphate or Ca^{2+}: simultaneous microfluorimetry and Ca^{2+} dependent Cl$^-$ current recording in single pancreatic acinar cells. *EMBO J.* 9: 697–704, 1990.

328. Ostberg, B. C., O. Sand, T. Bjoro, and E. Haugh. The phorbol ester TPA induced hormone release and electrical activity in clonal rat pituitary cells. *Acta Physiol. Scand.* 126: 517–524, 1986.

329. Otsu, K., H. F. Willard, V. K. Khanna, F. Zorzato, N. M. Green, and D. H. MacLennan. Molecular cloning of cDNA encoding the Ca^{2+} release channel (ryanodine receptor) of rabbit cardiac muscle sarcoplasmic reticulum. *J. Biol. Chem.* 265: 13472–13483, 1990.

330. Ozawa, K., Z. Szallasi, M. G. Kazanietz, P. M. Blumberg, H.

Mischak, J. F. Mushinski, and M. A. Beaven. Ca^{2+}-dependent and Ca^{2+}-independent isozymes of protein kinase C mediate exocytosis in antigen-stimulated rat basophilic RBL-2H3 cells. *J. Biol. Chem.* 268: 1749–1756, 1993.

331. Ozawa, K., K. Yamada, M. G. Kazanietz, P. M. Blumberg, and M. A. Beaven. Different isozymes of protein kinase C mediate feedback inhibition of phospholipase C and stimulatory signals for exocytosis in rat RBL-2H3 Cells. *J. Biol. Chem.* 268: 2280–2283, 1993.

332. Ozawa, S., and N. Kimura. Membrane potential changes caused by thyrotropin-releasing hormone in the clonal GH_3 cell and their relationship to secretion of pituitary hormone. *Proc. Natl. Acad. Sci. U.S.A.* 76: 6017–6020, 1979.

333. Ozawa, S., and O. Sand. Electrophysiology of excitable endocrine cells. *Physiol. Rev.* 66: 887–952, 1986.

334. Palfrey, H. C., A. C. Nairn, L. L. Muldoon, and M. L. Villereal. Rapid activation of calmodulin-dependent protein kinase II in mitogen-stimulated human fibroblasts. Correlation with intracellular Ca^{2+} transients. *J. Biol. Chem.* 262: 9785–9792, 1987.

335. Pandol, S. J., and M. S. Schoeffield-Payne. Cyclic GMP mediates the agonist-stimulated increase in plasma membrane calcium entry in the pancreatic acinar cells. *J. Biol. Chem.* 265: 12846–12853, 1990.

336. Parekh, A. B., H. Terlau, and W. Stuhmer. Depletion of $InsP_3$ stores activates a Ca^{2+} and K^+ current by means of a phosphatase and a diffusible messenger. *Nature* 364: 814–818, 1993.

337. Park, Y. B. Ion selectivity and gating of small conductance Ca^{2+}-activated K^+ channels in cultured rat adrenal chromaffin cells. *J. Physiol. (Lond.)* 481: 555–570, 1994.

338. Parker, I., and I. Ivorra. Inhibition by Ca^{2+} of inositol trisphosphate-mediated Ca^{2+} liberation: a possible mechanism for oscillatory release of Ca^{2+}. *Proc. Natl. Acad. Sci. U.S.A.* 87: 260–264, 1990.

339. Parker, I., and I. Ivorra. Localized all-or-none calcium liberation by inositol trisphosphate. *Science* 250: 977–979, 1990.

340. Parker, I., Y. Yao, and V. Ilyin. Fast kinetics of calcium liberation induced in *Xenopus* oocytes by photoreleased inositol trisphosphate. *Biophys. J.* 70: 222–237, 1996.

341. Parker, K. E., and A. Scarpa. An ATP-activated nonselective cation channel in guinea pig ventricular myocytes. *Am. J. Physiol.* 269(*Heart Circ. Physiol.* 40): H789–H797, 1995.

342. Partridge, L. D., T. H. Muller, and D. Swandulla. Calcium-activated non-selective channels in the nervous system. *Brain Res. Rev.* 19: 319–325, 1994.

343. Partridge, L. D., and D. Swandulla. Calcium-activated non-specific cation channels. *Trends Neurosci.* 11: 69–72, 1988.

344. Patel, Y. C., and C. B. Srikant. Somatostatin mediation of adenohypophysial secretion. *Annu. Rev. Physiol.* 48: 551–567, 1986.

345. Pearson, J. D. Ectonucleotidases: measurement of activities and use of inhibitors. *Methods Pharmacol.* 6: 83–107, 1985.

346. Perez-Reyes, E., X. Wei, A. Castellano, and L. Birnbaumer. Molecular diversity of L-type calcium channels. *J. Biol. Chem.* 265: 20430–20436, 1990.

347. Perez-Tezic, C., J. Pyle, M. Jaconi, L. Stehno-Bittel, and D. E. Clapham. Conformational states of the nuclear pore complex induced by depletion of nuclear Ca^{2+} store. *Science* 273: 1875–1877, 1996.

348. Perrin, D., K. Moller, K. Hanke, and H.-D. Soling. cAMP and Ca^{2+}-mediated secretion in parotid acinar cells is associated with reversible changes in the organization of the cytoskeleton. *J. Cell. Biol.* 116: 127–134, 1992.

349. Peter, R. E., J. P. Chang, C. S. Nahorniak, R. J. Omeljaniuk, M. Sokolowska, S. H. Shih, and R. Billard. Interactions of catecholamines and GnRH in regulation of gonadotropin secretion in teleost fish. *Recent Prog. Horm. Res.* 42: 513–548, 1986.

350. Petersen, C. C., and M. J. Berridge. The regulation of capacitative calcium entry by calcium and protein kinase C in *Xenopus* oocytes. *J. Biol. Chem.* 269: 32246–32253, 1994.

351. Petersen, C. C., and M. J. Berridge. G-protein regulation of capacitative calcium entry may be mediated by protein kinases A and C in *Xenopus* oocytes. *Biochem. J.* 307: 663–668, 1995.

352. Petersen, C.C.H., O. H. Petersen, and M. J. Berridge. The role of endoplasmic reticulum calcium pumps during cytosolic calcium spiking in pancreatic acinar cells. *J. Biol. Chem.* 268: 22262–22264, 1993.

353. Petersen, C.C.H., E. C. Toescu, and O. H. Petersen. Different patterns of receptor-activated cytoplasmic oscillations in single pancreatic acinar cells: dependence on receptor type, agonist concentration and intracellular calcium buffering. *EMBO J.* 10: 527–533, 1991.

354. Petersen, O. H., C. H. Petersen, and H. Kasai. Calcium and hormone action. *Annu. Rev. Physiol.* 56: 297–319, 1994.

355. Phillips, A. M., A. Bull, and L. E. Kelly. Identification of a *Drosophila* gene encoding a calmodulin-binding protein with homology to the trp phototransduction gene. *Neuron* 8: 631–642, 1992.

356. Picher, M., J. Sevigny, P. D'Orleans-Juste, and A. R. Beaudoin. Hydrolysis of P_2-purinoreceptor agonists by a purified ecto-nucleotidase from the bovine aorta, the ATP-diphosphohydrolase. *Biochem. Pharmacol.* 51: 1453–1460, 1996.

357. Picotto, G., V. Massheimer, and R. Boland. Acute stimulation of intestinal cell calcium influx induced by 17 beta-estradiol via the cAMP messenger system. *Mol. Cell. Endocrinol.* 119: 129–134, 1996.

358. Pietri, F., M. Hilly, and J. P. Mauger. Calcium mediates the interconversion between two states of the liver inositol 1,4,5-trisphosphate receptor. *J. Biol. Chem.* 265: 17478–17485, 1990.

359. Pozzan, T., R. Rizzuto, P. Volpe, and J. Meldolesi. Molecular and cellular physiology of intracellular calcium stores. *Physiol. Rev.* 74: 596–636, 1994.

360. Putney, J. W., Jr. Capacitative calcium entry revisited. *Cell Calcium* 11: 611–624, 1990.

361. Putney, J. W., Jr. Inositol phosphates and calcium entry. *Adv. Second Messenger Phosphoprotein Res.* 26: 143–156, 1992.

362. Putney, J. W., Jr., and G.ST.J. Bird. The inositol phosphate-calcium signaling system in nonexcitable cells. *Endocr. Rev.* 14: 610–631, 1993.

363. Randriamampita, C., and R. Y. Tsien. Emptying of intracellular Ca^{2+} stores releases a novel small messenger that stimulates Ca^{2+} influx. *Nature* 364: 809–814, 1993.

364. Rane, S. G., and K. Dunlop. Kinase C activator 1–oleoyl-2–acetylglycerol attenuates voltage-dependent calcium current in sensory neurones. *Proc. Natl. Acad. Sci. U.S.A.* 83: 184–188, 1986.

365. Ransone, L. J., and I. M. Verma. Nuclear proto-oncogenes *fos* and *jun*. *Annu. Rev. Cell Biol.* 6: 539–557, 1990.

366. Rao, K., W.-Y. Paik, L. Zheng, R. M. Jobin, M. Tomic, H. Jiang, S. Nakanishi, and S. S. Stojilkovic. Wortmannin-sensitive and insensitive steps in calcium-controlled exocytosis in pituitary gonadotrophs. *Endocrinology*, 138: 1440–1449, 1997.

367. Rapp, P.E., and M. J. Berridge. The control of transepithelial potential oscillations in the salivary gland of *Calliphora erythrocephala*. *J. Exp. Biol.* 93: 119–132, 1981.

368. Rawlings, S. R., N. Demaurex, and W. Schlegel. Pituitary

adenylate cyclase-activating polypeptide increases $[Ca^{2+}]_i$ in rat gonadotrophs through an inositol trisphosphate-dependent mechanism. *J. Biol. Chem.* 269: 5680–5686, 1994.

369. Reisine, T. Phorbol esters and corticotropin-releasing factor stimulate calcium influx in the anterior pituitary tumor cell line, AtT-20, through different intracellular sites of action. *J. Pharmacol. Exp. Ther.* 248: 984–990, 1989.

370. Reisine, T., and G. I. Bell. Molecular biology of somatostatin receptors. *Endocr. Rev.* 16: 427–442, 1995.

371. Renterghen, C. V., G. Romey, and M. Lazdunski. Vasopressin modulates the spontaneous electrical activity in aortic cells (line A7r5) by acting on three different types of ionic channels. *Proc. Natl. Acad. Sci. U.S.A.* 85: 9365–9369, 1988.

372. Rhee, S. G., P.-G. Suh, S.-H. Ryu, and S. Y. Lee. Studies on inositol phospholipid-specific phospholipase C. *Science* 244: 546–550, 1989.

373. Rhoads, A. R., R. Parui, N.-D. Vu, R. Cadogan, and P. D. Wagner. ATP-induced secretion in PC12 cells and photoaffinity labeling of receptors. *J. Neurochem.* 61: 1657–1666, 1993.

374. Ribeiro, C.M.P., and J. W. Jr. PUTNEY. Differential effects of protein kinase C activation on calcium storage and capacitative calcium entry in NIH 3T3 cells. *J. Biol. Chem.* 271: 21522–21528, 1996.

375. Rinzel, J., J. Keizer, and Y.-X. Li. Modeling plasma membrane and endoplasmic reticulum excitability in pituitary cells. *Trends Endocrinol. Metab.* 7: 388–393, 1996.

376. Ritchie, A. K. Two distinct calcium-activated potassium currents in a rat anterior pituitary cell line. *J. Physiol. (Lond.)* 385: 591–609, 1987.

377. Ritchie, A. K. Thyrotropin-releasing hormone stimulates a calcium-activated potassium current in a rat anterior pituitary cell line. *J. Physiol. (Lond.)* 385: 611–625, 1987.

378. Rizzuto, R., M. Brini, M. Murgia, and T. Pozzan. Microdomains with high Ca^{2+} close to IP$_3$-sensitive channels are sensed by neighboring mitochondria. *Science* 262: 744–746, 1993.

379. Rizzuto, R., W. M. Simpson, M. Brini, and T. Pozzan. Rapid changes of mitochondrial Ca^{2+} revealed by specifically targeted recombinant aequorin. *Nature* 358: 325–327, 1992.

380. Robb-Gaspers, L. D., and A. P. Thomas. Coordination of Ca^{2+} signaling by intercellular propagation of Ca^{2+} waves in the intact liver. *J. Biol. Chem.* 270: 8102–8107, 1995.

381. Rooney, T. A., E. J. Sass, and A. P. Thomas. Characterization of cytosolic calcium oscillations induced by phenylaphrine and vasopressin in single fura-2-loaded hepatocytes. *J. Biol. Chem.* 264: 17131–17141, 1989.

382. Rooney, T. A., E. J. Sass, and A. P. Thomas. Agonist-induced cytosolic calcium oscillations originate from a specific locus in single hepatocytes. *J. Biol. Chem.* 265: 10792–10796, 1990.

383. Rotenberg, A., M. Mayford, R. D. Hawkins, E. R. Kandel, and R. U. Muller. Mice expressing activated CaMKII lack low frequency LTP and do not form stable place cells in the CA1 region of the hippocampus. *Cell* 87: 1351–1361, 1996.

384. Roussel, J. P., G. Mateu, and H. Astier. Blockade of potassium or calcium channels provokes modifications in TRH-induced TSH release from rat perifused pituitaries. *Endocr. Regul.* 26: 163–170, 1992.

385. Rozengurt, E., and L. A. Heppler. A specific effect of external ATP on the permeability of transformed 3T3 cells. *Biochem. Biophys. Res. Commun.* 67: 1581–1588, 1975.

386. Ruth, P., A. Rohrkasten, M. Biel, E. Bosse, S. Regulla, H. E. Meyer, V. Flockerzi, and F. Hofmann. Primary structure of the β subunit of the DHP-sensitive calcium channel from skeletal muscle. *Science* 245: 1115–1118, 1989.

387. Sagara, Y., F. F. Belda, L. Demeis, and G. Inesi. Characterization of the inhibition of intracellular Ca^{2+} transport ATPases by thapsigargin. *J. Biol. Chem.* 267: 12606–12613, 1992.

388. Sage, S. O., D. J. Adams, and C. van Breemen. Synchronized oscillations in cytoplasmic free calcium concentration in confluent bradykinin-stimulated bovine pulmonary artery endothelial cell monolayers. *J. Biol. Chem.* 264: 6–9, 1989.

389. Sah, P. Ca^{2+}-activated K^+ currents in neurones: types, physiological roles and modulation. *Trends Neurosci.* 19: 150–154, 1996.

390. Saimi, Y., and C. Kung. Ion channel regulation by calmodulin binding. *FEBS Lett.* 350: 155–158, 1994.

391. Sala, F., and A. Hernandez-Cruz. Calcium diffusion modeling in a spherical neuron. *Biophys. J.* 57: 313–324, 1990.

392. Sargeant, P., R. W. Farndale, and S. O. Sage. The tyrosine kinase inhibitors methyl 2,5-dihydroxynnamate and genistein reduce thrombin-evoked tyrosine phosphorylation and Ca^{2+} entry in human platelets. *FEBS Lett.* 315: 242–246, 1993.

393. Scheenen, W. J., H. G. Yntema, P. H. Willems, E. W. Roubos, J. R. Lieste, and B. G. Jenks. Neuropeptide Y inhibits Ca^{2+} oscillations, cyclic AMP, and secretion in melanotrope cells of *Xenopus laevis* via a Y1 receptor. *Peptides* 16: 889–895, 1995.

394. Schlegel, W., B. P. Winiger, P. Mollard, P. Vacher, F. Wuarin, G. R. Zahnd, C. B. Wollheim, and B. Dufy. Oscillations of cytosolic Ca^{2+} in pituitary cells due to action potentials. *Nature* 329: 719–721, 1987.

395. Schulman, H., and L. L. Lou. Multifunctional Ca^{2+}/calmodulin-dependent protein kinase: domain structure and regulation. *Trends Biochem. Sci.* 14: 62–66, 1989.

396. Seabrook, G. R., M. Knowles, N. Brown, J. Myers, H. Sinclair, S. Patel, S. B. Freedman, and G. McAllister. Pharmacology of high-threshold calcium currents in GH$_4$C$_1$ pituitary cells and their regulation by activation of human D$_2$ and D$_4$ dopamine receptors. *Br. J. Pharmacol.* 112: 728–734, 1994.

397. Sham, J.S.K., L. Cleemann, and M. Morad. Functional coupling of Ca^{2+} channels and ryanodine receptors in cardiac myocytes. *Proc. Natl. Acad. Sci. U.S.A.* 92: 121–125, 1995.

398. Shan, J., L. M. Resnick, Q. Y. Liu, X. C. Wu, M. Barbagallo, and P. K. Pang. Vascular effects of 17β-estradiol in male Sprague-Dawley rats. *Am. J. Physiol.* 266(*Heart Circ. Physiol.* 37): H967–H973, 1994.

399. Shangold, G. A., and R. J. Miller. Direct neuropeptide Y-induced modulation of gonadotrope intracellular calcium transients and gonadotropin secretion. *Endocrinology* 126: 2336–2342, 1990.

400. Shangold, G. A., S. N. Murphy, and R. J. Miller. Gonadotropin-releasing hormone-induced Ca^{2+} transients in single identified gonadotropes require both intracellular Ca^{2+} mobilization and Ca^{2+} influx. *Proc. Natl. Acad. Sci. U.S.A.* 85: 6566–6570, 1988.

401. Shearman, M. S., K. Sekiquchi, and Y. Nishizuka. Modulation of ion channel activity: a key function of the protein kinase C enzyme family. *Pharmacol. Rev.* 41: 211–237, 1989.

402. Shepherd, G. M. Neurobiology. New York: Oxford University Press, 1988.

403. Shipston, M. J., J. S. Kelly, and F. A. Antoni. Glucocorticoids block protein kinase A inhibition of calcium-activated potassium channels. *J. Biol. Chem.* 271: 9197–9200, 1996.

404. Simasko, S. M., G. A. Weiland, and R. E. Oswald. Pharmacological characterization of two calcium currents in GH$_3$ cells. *Am. J. Physiol.* 254(*Endocrinol. Metab.* 17): E328–E336, 1988.

405. Simpson, P. B., and J. T. Russell. Mitochondria support inositol 1,4,5-trisphosphate-mediated Ca^{2+} waves in cultured oligodendorocytes. *J. Biol. Chem.* 271: 33493–33501, 1996.

406. Slivka, S. R., and P. A. Insel. Phorbol ester and neomycin dissociate bradykinin receptor-mediated arachidonic acid release and polyphosphoinositide hydrolysis in Madin-Darby canine kidney cells. *J. Biol. Chem.* 263: 14640–14647, 1988.

407. Sneyd, J., A. C. Charles, and M. J. Sanderson. A model for the propagation of intercellular calcium waves. *Am. J. Physiol.* 266(*Cell Physiol.* 35): C293–C302, 1994.

408. Snutch, T. P., J. P. Leonard, M. M. Gilbert, H. A. Lester, and N. Davidson. Rat brain expresses a heterogeneous family of calcium channels. *Proc. Natl. Acad. Sci. U.S.A.* 87: 3391–3395, 1990.

409. Sorrentino, V., and P. Volpe. Ryanodine receptors: how many, where and why. *Trends Pharmacol. Sci.* 14: 98–103, 1993.

410. Squires, P. E., R.F.L. James, N.J.M. London, and M. J. Dunne. ATP-induced intracellular Ca^{2+} signals in isolated human insulin-secreting cells. *Pflugers Arch.* 427: 181–183, 1994.

411. Stack, J., and A. Surprenant. Dopamine actions on calcium currents, potassium currents and hormone release in rat melanotrophs. *J. Physiol. (Lond.)* 439: 37–58, 1991.

412. Starr, T.V.B., W. Prystay, and T. P. Snutch. Primary structure of a calcium channel that is highly expressed in the rat cerebellum. *Proc. Natl. Acad. Sci. U.S.A.* 88: 5621–5625, 1991.

413. Stauffer, P. L., H. Zhao, K. Luby-Phelps, R. L. Moss, R. A. Star, and S. Muallem. Gap junction communication modulates $[Ca^{2+}]_i$ oscillations and enzyme secretion in pancreatic acini. *J. Biol. Chem.* 268: 19769–19775, 1993.

414. Stea, A., T. W. Soong, and T. P. Snutch. Determinants of PKC-dependent modulation of a family of neuronal calcium channels. *Neuron* 15: 929–940, 1995.

415. Stehno-Bittel, L., A. Luckhoff, and D. E. Clapham. Calcium release from the nucleus by InsP$_3$ receptor channels. *Neuron* 14: 163–167, 1995.

416. Stehno-Bittel, L., C. Perez-Terzic, and D. E. Clapham. Diffusion across the nuclear envelope inhibited by depletion of the nuclear Ca^{2+} store. *Science* 270: 1835–1838, 1955.

417. Stendahl, O., K.-H. Krause, J. Krischer, P. Jerstrom, J.-M. Theler, R. A. Clark, J.-L. Carpentier, and D. P. Lew. Redistribution of intracellular Ca^{2+} stores during phagocytosis in human neutrophils. *Science* 265: 1439–1441, 1994.

418. Stojilkovic, S. S., T. Balla, S. Fukuda, M. Cesnjaj, F. Merelli, L. Z. Krsmanovic, and K. J. Catt. Endothelin ET_A receptors mediate the signaling and secretory actions of endothelins in pituitary gonadotrophs. *Endocrinology* 130: 465–474, 1992.

419. Stojilkovic, S. S., and K. J. Catt. Neuroendocrine actions of endothelins. *Trends Pharmacol. Sci.* 13: 385–391, 1992.

420. Stojilkovic, S. S., and K. J. Catt. Calcium oscillations in anterior pituitary cells. *Endocr. Rev.* 13: 256–280, 1992.

421. Stojilkovic, S. S., J. P. Chang, S.-I. Izumi, K. Tasaka, and K. J. Catt. Mechanisms of secretory responses to gonadotropin-releasing hormone and phorbol esters in cultured pituitary cells. *J. Biol. Chem.* 263: 17301–17306, 1988.

422. Stojilkovic, S. S., T. Iida, M. Cesnjaj, and K. J. Catt. Differential actions of endothelin and gonadotropin-releasing hormone in pituitary gonadotrophs. *Endocrinology* 131: 2821–2828, 1992.

423. Stojilkovic, S. S., T. Iida, F. Merelli, and K. J. Catt. Calcium signaling and secretory responses in endothelin-stimulated anterior pituitary cells. *Mol. Pharmacol.* 39: 762–770, 1991.

424. Stojilkovic, S. S., T. Iida, F. Merelli, A. Torsello, L. Z. Krsmanovic, and K. J. Catt. Interactions between calcium and protein kinase C in the control of signaling and secretion in pituitary gonadotrophs. *J. Biol. Chem.* 266: 10377–10384, 1991.

425. Stojilkovic, S. S., T. Iida, M. A. Virmani, S.-I. Izumi, E. Rojas, and K. J. Catt. Dependence of hormone secretion on activation–inactivation kinetics of voltage-sensitive Ca^{2+} channels in

426. Stojilkovic, S. S., S.-I. Izumi, and K. J. Catt. Participation of voltage-sensitive calcium channels in pituitary hormone secretion. *J. Biol. Chem.* 263: 13054–13061, 1988.

427. Stojilkovic, S. S., L. Z. Krsmanovic, D. J. Spergel, M. Tomic, and K. J. Catt. Calcium signaling and episodic secretory responses of GnRH neurons. *Methods Neurosci.* 20: 68–84, 1994.

428. Stojilkovic, S. S., M. Kukuljan, T. Iida, E. Rojas, and K. J. Catt. Integration of cytoplasmic calcium and membrane potential oscillations maintains calcium signaling in pituitary gonadotrophs. *Proc. Natl. Acad. Sci. USA* 89: 4081–4085, 1992.

429. Stojilkovic, S. S., M. Kukuljan, M. Tomic, E. Rojas, and K. J. Catt. Mechanism of agonist-induced $[Ca^{2+}]_i$ oscillations in pituitary gonadotrophs. *J. Biol. Chem.* 268: 7713–7720, 1993.

430. Stojilkovic, S. S., F. Merelli, T. Iida, L. Z. Krsmanovic, and K. J. Catt. Endothelin stimulation of cytosolic calcium and gonadotropin secretion in anterior pituitary cells. *Science* 248: 1663–1666, 1990.

431. Stojilkovic, S. S., J. Reinhart, and K. J. Catt. GnRH receptors: structure and signal transduction pathways. *Endocr. Rev.* 15: 462–499, 1994.

432. Stojilkovic, S. S., E. Rojas, A. Stutzin, S.-I. Izumi, and K. J. Catt. Desensitization of pituitary gonadotropin secretion by agonist-induced inactivation of voltage-sensitive calcium channels. *J. Biol. Chem.* 264: 10939–10942, 1989.

433. Stojilkovic, S. S., A. Stutzin, S.-I. Izumi, S. Dufour, A. Torsello, M. A. Virmani, E. Rojas, and K. J. Catt. Generation and amplification of the cytoplasmic calcium signal during secretory responses to gonadotropin-releasing hormone. *New Biol.* 3: 272–283, 1990.

434. Stojilkovic, S. S., M. Tomic, M. Kukuljan, and K. J. Catt. Control of calcium spiking frequency in pituitary gonadotrophs by a single-pool cytoplasmic oscillator. *Mol. Pharmacol.* 45: 1013–1021, 1994.

435. Striessnig, J., B. J. Murphy, and W. A. Catterall. Dihydropyridine receptor of L-type Ca^{2+} channels: identification of binding domains for [^{3}H](+)-PN200–110 and [^{3}H]azidopine within the α_1 subunit. *Proc. Natl. Acad. Sci. U.S.A.* 88: 10769–10773, 1991.

436. Stull, J. T., M. H. Nunnally, and C. H. Michnoff. Calmodulin-dependent protein kinases. In: *The Enzymes*, edited by E. G. Krebs and P. D. Boyer. Orlando, FL: Academic, 1986, p. 113–166.

437. Stutzin, A., S. S. Stojilkovic, K. J. Catt, and E. Rojas. Characteristics of two types of calcium channels in rat pituitary gonadotrophs. *Am. J. Physiol.* 257(*Cell Physiol.* 26): C865–C874, 1989.

438. Surprenant, A., F. Rassendren, E. Kawashima, R. A. North, and G. Buell. The cytosolic P_{2Z} receptor for extracellular ATP identified as a P_{2X} receptor (P2X$_7$). *Science* 272: 735–738, 1996.

439. Sweeney, H. L., B. F. Bowman, and J. T. Stull. Myosin light chain phosphorylation in vertebrate striated muscle: regulation and function. *Am. J. Physiol.* 264(*Cell Physiol.* 33): C1085–C1095, 1993.

440. Takasawa, S., K. Nata, H. Yonekura, and H. Okamoto. Cyclic ADP-ribose in insulin secretion from pancreatic β cells. *Science* 259: 370–373, 1993.

441. Takemura, H., A. R. Hughes, O. Thastrup, and J. W. Putney. Activation of calcium entry by the tumor promoter thapsigargin in parotid acinar cells. *J. Biol. Chem.* 264: 12266–12271, 1989.

442. Takeshima, H., S. Nishimura, T. Matsumoto, H. Ishida, K. Kangawa, N. Manamino, H. Matsuo, M. Ueda, M. Hanaoka, and T. Hirose. Primary structure and expression from complementary DNA of sceletal muscle ryanodine receptor. *Nature* 339: 439–445, 1989.

443. Takuwa, N., W. Zhou, and Y. Takuwa. Calcium, calmodulin and cell cycle progression. *Cell. Signal.* 7: 93–104, 1995.

444. Tallent, M., G. Liapakis, A. M. O'Carroll, S. J. Lolait, M. Dichter, and T. Reisine. Somatostatin receptor subtypes SSTR2 and SSTR5 couple negatively to an L-type Ca^{2+} current in the pituitary cell line AtT-20. *Neuroscience* 71: 1073–1081, 1996.

445. Tanabe, T., H. Takeshima, A. Mikami, V. Flockerzi, H. Takahashi, K. Kangawa, M. Kojima, H. Matsuo, T. Hirose, and S. Numa. Primary structure of the receptor for calcium channel blockers from skeletal muscle. *Nature* 328: 313–318, 1987.

446. Taraskevich, P. S., and W. W. Douglas. Catecholamines of supposed inhibitory hypophysiotrophic function suppress action potentials in prolactin cells. *Nature* 276: 832–834, 1978.

447. Tasaka, K., S. S. Stojilkovic, S.-I. Izumi, and K. J. Catt. Biphasic activation of cytosolic free calcium and LH responses by gonadotropin-releasing hormone. *Biochem. Biophys. Res. Commun.* 154: 398–403, 1988.

448. Tatham, P.E.R., and M. Lindau. ATP-induced pore formation in the plasma membrane of rat peritoneal mast cells. *J. Gen. Physiol.* 95: 459–476, 1990.

449. Thastrup, O., P. J. Cullen, B. K. Drobak, M. R. Hanley, and A. P. Dawson. Thapsigargin, a tumor promoter, discharges intracellular Ca^{2+} stores by specific inhibition of the endoplasmic reticulum Ca^{2+}-ATPase. *Proc. Natl. Acad. Sci. U.S.A.* 87: 2466–2470, 1990.

450. Thompson, N. T., R. W. Bonser, and L. G. Garland. Receptor-coupled phospholipase D and its inhibition. *Trends Pharmacol. Sci.* 12: 404–408, 1991.

451. Thorner, M. O., R. W. Holl, and D. A. Leong. The somatotrope: an endocrine cell with functional calcium transients. *J. Exp. Biol.* 139: 169–179, 1988.

452. Toescu, E. C., A. M. Lawrie, O. H. Petersen, and D. V. Gallacher. Spatial and temporal distribution of agonist-evoked cytoplasmic Ca^{2+} signals in exocrine acinar cells analyzed by digital image microscopy. *EMBO J.* 11: 1623–1629, 1992.

453. Tomic, M., M. Cesnjaj, K. J. Catt, and S. S. Stojilkovic. Developmental and physiological aspects of Ca^{2+} signaling in agonist-stimulated pituitary gonadotrophs. *Endocrinology* 135: 1762–1771, 1994.

454. Tomic, M., M. L. Dufau, K. J. Catt, and S. S. Stojilkovic. Calcium signaling in single rat Leydig cells. *Endocrinology* 136: 3422–3429, 1995.

455. Tomic, M., R. M. Jobin, L. A. Vergara, and S. S. Stojilkovic. Expression of purinergic receptor channels in their role in calcium signaling and hormone release in pituitary gonadotrophs. *J. Biol. Chem.* 271: 21200–21208, 1996.

456. Torres, M., J. Pintor, and M. T. Miras-Portugal. Presence of ectonucleotidases in cultured chromaffin cells: hydrolysis of extracellular adenine nucleotides. *Arch. Biochem. Biophys.* 279: 37–44, 1990.

457. Toyofuku, T., K. Kurzydlowski, J. Lytton, and D. H. MacLennan. The nuclear binding/hinge domain plays a crucial role in determining isoform-specific Ca^{2+} dependence of organellar Ca^{2+}-ATPases. *J. Biol. Chem.* 267: 14490–14496, 1992.

458. Traina, G., S. Cannistraro, and P. Bagnoli. Effects of somatostatin on intracellular calcium concentration in PC12 cells. *J. Neurochem.* 66: 485–492, 1996.

459. Treisman, R. The serum responsive element. *Trends Biochem. Sci.* 17: 423–426, 1992.

460. Tschopl, M., L. Harms, W. Norenberg, and P. Illes. Excitatory effects of adenosine 5′-trisphosphate on rat locus coeruleus neurones. *Eur. J. Pharmacol.* 213: 71–77, 1992.

461. Tse, A., and B. Hille. GnRH-induced Ca^{2+} oscillations and rhythmic hyperpolarizations of pituitary gonadotropes. *Science* 255: 462–464, 1992.

462. Tse, A., and B. Hille. Role of voltage-gated Na^+ and Ca^{2+} channels in gonadotropin-releasing hormone-induced membrane potential changes in identified rat gonadotropes. *Endocrinology* 132: 1475–1481, 1993.

463. Tse, A., F. W. Tse, W. Almers, and B. Hille. Rhythmic exocytosis stimulated by GnRH-induced calcium oscillations in rat gonadotropes. *Science* 260: 82–84, 1993.

464. Tse, A., F. W. Tse, and B. Hille. Calcium homeostasis in identified rat gonadotrophs. *J. Physiol. (Lond.)* 477: 511–525, 1994.

465. Tse, A., F. W. Tse, and B. Hille. Modulation of Ca^{2+} oscillation and apamin-sensitive, Ca^{2+}-activated K^+ current in rat gonadotropes. *Pflugers Arch.* 430: 645–652, 1995.

466. Tsien, R. W., and R. Y. Tsien. Calcium channels, stores, and oscillations. *Annu. Rev. Cell Biol.* 6: 715–760, 1990.

467. Valentijn, J. A., E. Louiset, H. Vaudry, and L. Cazin. Dopamine-induced inhibition of action potentials in cultured frog pituitary melanotrophs is mediated through activation of potassium channels and inhibition of calcium and sodium channels. *Neuroscience* 42: 29–39, 1991.

468. Valentijn, J. A., H. Vaudry, and L. Cazin. Multiple control of calcium channel gating by dopamine D_2 receptors in frog pituitary melanotrophs. *Ann. N. Y. Acad. Sci.* 680: 211–228, 1993.

469. Valera, S., N. Hussy, R. J. Evans, N. Adami, A. Surprenant, and G. Buell. A new class of ligand-gated ion channel defoined by P2X receptor for extracellular ATP. *Nature* 371: 516–519, 1994.

470. van Goor, F., J. I. Goldberg, and J. P. Chang. Dopamine actions on calcium current in identified goldfish (*Carassius aureatus*) gonadotropin cells. In: *Reproductive Physiology of Fish*, edited by F. Goetz and P. Thomas. 1995, p. 61–63.

471. Veenstra, R. D. Size and selectivity of gap junction channels formed from different connexins. *J. Bioenerg. Biomembr.* 28: 327–337, 1996.

472. Vergara, L. A., S. S. Stojilkovic, and E. Rojas. GnRH induced cytosolic calcium oscillations in pituitary gonadotrophs: phase resetting by membrane depolarization. *Biophys. J.* 69: 1606–1614, 1995.

472b. Vergara, L., E. Rojas, and S. S. Stojilkovic. A novel calcium-activated apamin-insensitive potassium current in pituitary gonadotrophs. *Endocrinology* 138 (in press), 1997.

473. Vogel, H. J. Calmodulin: a versatile calcium mediator protein. *Biochem. Cell. Biol.* 72: 357–376, 1994.

474. Vogel, H. J., and M. Zhang. Protein engineering and NMR studies of calmodulin. *Mol. Cell. Biochem.* 149/150: 3–15, 1995.

475. Vostal, J. C., W. L. Jackson, and N. R. Shulman. Cytosolic and stored calcium antagonistically control tyrosine phosphorylation of specific platelet proteins. *J. Biol. Chem.* 266: 16911–16916, 1991.

476. Wakui, M., Y. V. Osipchuk, and O. H. Petersen. Receptor-activated cytoplasmic Ca^{2+} spiking mediated by inositol trisphosphate is due to Ca^{2+}-induced Ca^{2+} release. *Cell* 63: 1025–1032, 1990.

477. Wakui, M., B.V.L. Potter, and O. H. Petersen. Pulsatile intracellular calcium release does not depend on fluctuations in inositol trisphosphate concentration. *Nature* 339: 317–320, 1989.

478. Walton, P. D., J. A. Airey, J. L. Sutko, C. F. Beck, G. A. Mignery, T. C. Sudhof, T. J. Bdeerinck, and M. H. Ellisman. Ryanodine and inositol trisphosphate receptors coexist in avian cerebellar Purkinje neurons. *J. Cell. Biol.* 113: 1145–1157, 1991.

479. Wang, J., K. G. Baimbridge, and P.C.K. Leung. Changes in cytosolic free calcium ion concentrations in individual rat granulosa cells: effect of luteinizing hormone–releasing hormone. *Endocrinology* 124: 1912–1917, 1989.

480. Wang, J., P. Ciofi, and W. R. Crowley. Neuropeptide Y suppresses prolactin secretion from rat anterior pituitary cells: evidence for interactions with dopamine through inhibitory coupling to calcium entry. *Endocrinology* 137: 587–594, 1996.

481. Wang, X., T. Inukai, M. A. Greer, and S. E. Greer. Evidence that Ca^{2+}-activated K^+ channels participate in the regulation of pituitary prolactin secretion. *Brain Res.* 662: 83–87, 1994.

482. Watras, J., I. Bezprozvanny, and B. E. Ehrlich. Inositol 1,4,5-trisphosphate-gated channels in cerebellum: presence of multiple conductance states. *J. Neurosci.* 11: 3239–3245, 1991.

483. Werlen, G., D. Belin, B. Conne, E. Roche, D. P. Lew, and M. Prentki. Intracellular Ca^{2+} and the regulation of early response gene expression in HL-60 myeloid leukemia cells. *J. Biol. Chem.* 268: 16596–16601, 1993.

484. Wheeler, D. B., A. Randall, W. A. Sather, and R. W. Tsien. Neuronal calcium channels encoded by the α_{1A} subunit and their contribution to excitatory synaptic transmission in the CNS. *Prog. Brain Res.* 105: 65–78, 1995.

485. White, R. E., A. Schonbrunn, and D. L. Armstrong. Somatostatin stimulates Ca^+ activated K^+ channels through protein dephosphorylation. *Nature* 351: 570–573, 1991.

486. Wickman, K., and D. E. Clapham. Ion channel regulation by G proteins. *Physiol. Rev.* 75: 865–885, 1995.

487. Wictome, M., I. Henderson, A. G. Lee, and J. M. East. Mechanism of inhibition of the calcium pump of sarcoplasmic reticulum by thapsigargin. *Biochem. J.* 283: 525–529, 1992.

488. Wiley, J. S., R. Chen, and G. P. Jamieson. The ATP^{4-} receptor-operated channel (P_2Z class) of human lymphocytes allows Ba^{2+} and ethidium$^+$ uptake: inhibition of fluxes by suramin. *Arch. Biochem. Biophys.* 305: 54–60, 1993.

489. Williams, M. E., P. F. Brust, D. H. Feldman, S. Patthi, S. Simerson, A. Maroufi, A. F. McCue, G. Velicelebi, S. B. Ellis, and M. M. Harpold. Structure and functional expression of an ω-conotoxin-sensitive human N-type calcium channel. *Science* 257: 389–395, 1992.

490. Williams, P. J., B. A. MacVicar, and Q. J. Pittman. A dopaminergic inhibitory postsynaptic potential mediated by an increased potassium conductance. *Neuroscience* 31: 673–681, 1989.

491. Xu, Y. H., D. A. Wilkinson, and G. M. Carlson. Divalent cations but not other activators enhance phosphorylase kinase's affinity for glycogen phosphorylase. *Biochemistry* 35: 5014–5021, 1996.

492. Yagi, K., M. Shinbo, M. Hashizume, L. S. Shimba, S. Kurimura, and Y. Miura. ATP diphosphohydrolase is responsible for ecto-ATPase and ecto-ADPase activites in bovine aorta endothelial and smooth muscle cells. *Biochem. Biophys. Res. Commun.* 180: 1200–1206, 1991.

493. Yagodin, S. V., L. Holtzclaw, C. A. Sheppard, and J. T. Russell. Nonlinear propagation of agonist-induced cytoplasmic calcium waves in single astrocytes. *J. Neurobiol.* 25: 265–280, 1994.

494. Yamashita, N., I. Kojima, N. Shibuya, and E. Ogata. Pertussis

toxin inhibits somatostatin-induced K^+ conductance in human pituitary tumor cells. *Am. J. Physiol.* 253(*Endocrinol. Metab.* 16): E28–E32, 1987.

495. Yamashita, N., N. Shibuya, and E. Ogata. Hyperpolarization of the membrane potential caused by somatostatin in dissociated human pituitary adenoma cells that secrete growth hormone. *Proc. Natl. Acad. Sci. U.S.A.* 83: 6198–6202, 1986.

496. Yatani, A., J. Codina, R. D. Sekura, L. Birnbaumer, and A. M. Brown. Reconstitution of somatostatin and muscarinic receptor mediated stimulation of K^+ channels by isolated G_K protein in clonal rat anterior pituitary cell membranes. *Mol. Endocrinol.* 1: 283–289, 1987.

497. Yeager, M., and B. J. Nicholson. Structure of gap junction intercellular channels. *Cur. Opin. Struct. Biol.* 6: 183–192, 1996.

498. Yoshimura, Y., M. Nishida, and J. Kawada. An ecto-ATPase of thyroidal cell membrane. *Endocrinol. Jpn.* 30: 769–775, 1983.

499. Yule, D. I., and D. V. Gallacher. Oscillations in cytosolic calcium in single pancreatic acinar cells stimulated by acetylcholine. *FEBS Lett.* 239: 358–362, 1988.

500. Zhang, F., J. L. Ram, P. R. Standley, and J. R. Sowers. 17β-Estradiol attenuates voltage-dependent Ca^{2+} currents in A7r5 vascular smooth muscle cell line. *Am. J. Physiol.* 266(*Cell Physiol.* 35): C975–C980, 1994.

501. Zheng, L., L. Z. Krsmanovic, L. A. Vergara, K. J. Catt, and S. S. Stojilkovic. Dependence of intracellular signaling and neurosecretion on phospholipase D activation in immortalized gonadotropin-releasing hormone neurons. *Proc. Natl. Acad. Sci. U.S.A.* 94: 1573–1578, 1997.

502. Zheng, L., S. S. Stojilkovic, L. Hunyady, L. Z. Krsmanovic, and K. J. Catt. Sequential activation of phospholipase C and phospholipase D in agonist-stimulated gonadotrophs. *Endocrinology* 134: 1446–1454, 1994.

503. Zhou, Z., and E. Neher. Mobile and immobile calcium buffers in bovine chromaffin cells. *J. Physiol. (Lond.)* 469: 245–273, 1993.

504. Ziganshin, A. U., L. E. Ziganshin, B. E. King, and G. Burnstock. Characteristics of ecto-ATPase of *Xenopus* oocytes and the inhibitory actions of suramin on ATP breakdown. *Pflugers Arch.* 429: 412–418, 1995.

505. Zimmermann, H. Signaling via ATP in the nervous system. *Trends Neurosci.* 17: 420–426, 1994.

506. Zorzato, F., J. Fuji, K. Otsu, M. Philips, N. M. Green, F. A. Lai, G. Meissner, and D. H. MacLennan. Molecular cloning of cDNA encoding human and rabbit forms of the Ca^{2+} release channel (ryanodine receptor) of skeletal muscle sarcoplasmic reticulum. *J. Biol. Chem.* 265: 2244–2256, 1990.

507. Zweifach, A., and R. S. Lewis. Mitogen-regulated Ca^{2+} current of T lymphocytes is activated by depletion of intracellular Ca^{2+} stores. *Proc. Natl. Acad. Sci. U.S.A.* 90: 6295–6299, 1993.

508. Zweifach, A., and R. S. Lewis. Rapid inactivation of depletion-activated calcium current (I_{CRAC}) due to local calcium feedback. *J. Gen. Physiol.* 105: 209–226, 1995.

509. Zweifach, A., and R. S. Lewis. Slow calcium-dependent inactivation of depletion-activated calcium current. Store-dependent and -independent mechanisms. *J. Biol. Chem.* 270: 14445–14451, 1995.

510. Zweifach, A., and R. S. Lewis. Calcium-dependent potentiation of store-operated calcium channels. *J. Gen. Physiol.* 107: 597–610, 1996.

10. Protein kinases and phosphatases in cellular signaling

KAREN L. LEACH | *Cell Biology and Inflammation Research, Pharmacia & Upjohn, Inc., Kalamazoo, Michigan*

CHAPTER CONTENTS

PROTEIN PHOSPHORYLATION is an important cellular switch that plays a key role in all aspects of regulation, including carbohydrate, amino-acid, and lipid metabolism (70). Historically, the discovery of protein phosphorylation is attributed in part to the work of Carl and Gertrude Cori, who, in the 1930s, identified active and inactive forms of glycogen phosphorylase. The mechanism accounting for these forms was demonstrated in the 1950s through the work of Edwin Krebs and Edmond Fischer. These researchers demonstrated a requirement for adenosine triphosphate (ATP) for the interconversion of the two forms of phosphorylase, leading to the establishment of phosphorylation/dephosphorylation as the regulatory mechanism (178).

These initial efforts led the way for a variety of studies demonstrating the involvement of phosphorylation and dephosphorylation reactions in many cellular processes. Most important was the identification of stimulated protein phosphorylation and dephosphorylation in response to cellular activation by a number of agents, including hormones, growth factors, and neurotransmitters. The change in phosphorylation state of a protein acts as a switch, triggering conformational changes. These changes lead to altered protein function, resulting in an observable physiological response to an agonist. These experiments firmly established that protein phosphorylation/dephosphorylation serves as a means of coupling extracellular signals to intracellular events, making this covalent modification a primary component of signal transduction.

Protein phosphorylation offers a number of advantages for cellular regulation (70). Phosphorylation/dephosphorylation reactions are mediated by highly specific regulatory enzymes. As discussed below, many of the enzymes involved have unique substrate specificities and/or regulatory protein requirements for activity. Therefore, in contrast to allosteric regulation, phosphorylation/dephosphorylation reactions offer the ability to affect a single biochemical step.

Another advantage afforded by these reactions is the high degree of signal amplification that can be achieved. Many of the proteins which become phosphorylated and/or dephosphorylated are part of a signal cascade; for example, the original signal of growth factor binding to its membrane receptor is markedly increased. Thus, a very small amount of extracellular agent can result in a large intracellular signal. Finally, phosphorylation/dephosphorylation reactions have multiple functions; that is, the same enzyme can act on proteins from a variety of different cellular pathways, thereby linking distinct metabolic processes.

PROTEIN KINASE AND PHOSPHATASE CLASSIFICATION

Protein kinases and phosphatases are classified according to their amino-acid substrate specificity. These include serine/threonine, tyrosine, dual specificity (serine/threonine/tyrosine), histidine, and cysteine. Relatively little is known concerning the last two subtypes, and most of the kinases and phosphatases involved in cellular signal-transduction pathways are of the first three types. Serine/threonine kinases and phosphatases catalyze phosphate transfer to and from an alcohol group; thus, these enzymes utilize either serine or threonine residues as substrates. In contrast, tyrosine kinases and phosphatases specify phosphate transfer to and from phenolic groups. The most recent addition to the kinase and phosphatase families is the group of dual-specificity enzymes, which phosphorylate/dephosphorylate serine, threonine, and tyrosine residues equally.

PROTEIN KINASE STRUCTURE

Despite these differences in amino-acid substrate specificity, there are a number of conserved features in all kinases (105, 128, 307). Sequence alignment of over 100 kinase proteins has identified a conserved catalytic core of approximately 270 residues that is shared among all kinases. Hanks and Quinn (104) further identified 12 major conserved subdomains within the catalytic core, which were predicted to be important for catalytic function. Each of the subdomains contains a number of highly conserved amino acids, interspersed with variable regions. The N-terminus is characterized by a Gly-X-Gly-X-X-Gly consensus sequence, followed by an invariant Lys 15–20 residue downstream, both of which form part of the ATP-binding site. Subdomains VI–IX contain additional conserved residues that are involved in nucleotide binding, while region VIII contains the triplet Ala-Pro-Glu, which is important for catalytic activity. The conserved sequence Asp-Leu-Lys-Pro-Glu-Asn in domain VI is highly characteristic of serine/threonine kinases, while the sequence Asp-Leu-Ala-Ala-Arg-Asn or Asp-Leu-Arg-Ala-Ala-Asn is

specific for tyrosine kinases. Finally, the C-terminus of the catalytic domain is characterized by the presence of an invariant arginine.

These signature sequences, characteristic of protein kinases, have allowed the identification of new family members based on homology cloning. Overall, it has been predicted that as many as 2000 protein kinases exist (127). In addition, many of the known kinases exist as isoforms, which further increases the total number of kinases. Clearly, the greatest challenge is to identify the regulation and function of all of these proteins.

Serine/Threonine Kinases

The kinase catalytic core, containing the consensus sequences described above, resides in the C-terminus, and the N-terminus usually acts as a regulatory site. For a wide variety of serine/threonine kinases, kinase activity is regulated via specific binding of agents to the N-terminus. These include cyclic nucleotides, calmodulin, and diacylglycerol, to name a few. Increases in the cellular concentration of these regulators result in their binding to their respective kinases and kinase activation. Thus, stimulation of kinase activity is intimately linked to the concentration of specific second messengers.

Tyrosine Kinases

In the case of tyrosine kinases, both cytosolic and growth factor receptor kinases exist (1, 252, 314). For receptor tyrosine kinases, the regulatory domain is the site of extracellular binding of the receptor ligand, while the tyrosine kinase region is located intracellularly. In general, growth factor binding to its cognate receptor results in receptor dimerization and autophosphorylation, which activates the tyrosine kinase activity of the receptor. Growth factors such as platelet-derived growth factor (PDGF), epidermal growth factor (EGF), fibroblast growth factor (FGF), and insulin utilize this signaling pathway. Activation of tyrosine kinase on the receptor results in phosphorylation of intracellular substrates. In addition, the autophosphorylated tyrosine residues of the kinase serve as a docking site for proteins that contain SH2 domains, which further serves as a switch for downstream signaling pathways.

Dual-Specificity Kinases

There are relatively fewer members of the dual-specificity kinase family, due to their recent discovery

(195). The best characterized member is mitogen-activated protein (MAP) kinase kinase, which is activated via phosphorylation by MAP kinase kinase kinase as part of a signaling cascade. Activated MAP kinase kinase then phosphorylates MAP kinase on both Tyr and Thr in the sequence Tyr-Glu-Thr, leading to its activation (231, 275, 332, 333). Less than 20 members of the dual-specificity kinase family have been identified, and some of these have yet to be identified in mammalian cells.

PROTEIN PHOSPHATASE STRUCTURE

Conserved sequences that are common to both serine/threonine and tyrosine kinases have been identified. However, this is not true for the phosphatases; serine/threonine phosphatases share no structural homology with the tyrosine phosphatases (38). Thus, homology cloning of new phosphatases has lagged behind that of the kinases. In addition, biochemical analysis of phosphatases is more difficult than that of kinases since substrate specificity often is not known. Furthermore, phosphatase assays are more difficult since prior phosphorylation of the substrate is required. Overall, this has resulted in the identification of fewer phosphatases than kinases.

Serine/Threonine Phosphatases

Despite these limitations, considerable information is known about phosphatase family members. Four major serine/threonine phosphatases are known: protein phosphatase (PP) 1, PP2A, PP2B (also known as calcineurin), and PP2C (130, 284). Calcineurin, PP1, and PP2A are approximately 40%–50% homologous in their catalytic domains, while PP2C is structurally distinct (38). The crystal structure of PP1 has been published, and comparison between conserved residues of PP1, PP2A, and calcineurin predicts that the tertiary structures of these enzymes are very similar (88). Calcineurin and PP2C require calcium/calmodulin and Mg^{2+}, respectively, while PP1 and PP2A have no cation requirements, though the crystal structure of PP1 demonstrates that two metal ions are bound near the active site.

Tyrosine Phosphatases

Tyrosine phosphatases exist as both intracellular and receptor-like transmembrane enzymes. Protein tyrosine phosphatase (PTP) 1B, an intracellular enzyme, was the first tyrosine phosphatase discovered (150, 309).

Overall, at least 40 different tyrosine phosphatases have been identified (71, 321). Sequence analysis has shown that all tyrosine phosphatases share a conserved catalytic domain of approximately 230 amino acids. Within this domain is an 11-residue stretch that contains Cys and Arg residues essential for catalysis. Several of the intracellular phosphatases also contain domains that direct enzyme localization within cells (321). For example, truncation of residues C-terminal to the catalytic domain of PTP 1B results in cytoplasmic localization compared to the membrane localization of the wild-type form. Another phosphatase, PTP 1C, contains two SH2 domains upstream from the catalytic domain, which direct its coupling to tyrosine-phosphorylated proteins.

In general, the transmembrane enzymes have an extracellular domain often containing fibronectin or immunoglobulin repeats, indicative of a ligand-binding domain (71, 321). However, for the majority of transmembrane phosphatases, the ligand(s) to which they bind is not known. These phosphatases also contain a transmembrane region and an intracellular region which usually consists of two catalytic domains. The role of the two catalytic domains is not understood; mutation of the first domain often abolishes catalytic activity, while similar mutations in the second domain are without effect. Additional studies have suggested that the second domain may regulate the substrate specificity of the enzyme.

Dual-Specificity Phosphatases

A phosphatase from vaccinia virus, VH1, was the first dual-specificity phosphatase to be identified (47, 48, 343). Subsequently, other family members were identified, including MKP1 and PAC1, which dephosphorylate mitogen-activated kinases (28, 300, 322); KAP, which dephosphorylates cyclin-dependent kinase 2 (cdk2) (262); and cdc25. The dual-specificity phosphatases share the active site conserved sequence (HCXXGXXR) found in all tyrosine phosphatases. Outside this catalytic region, however, the sequences are dissimilar.

KINASE AND PHOSPHATASE REGULATION

Regulation of enzymatic activity is an important and multifaceted step. Historically, considerable attention has been directed toward kinase regulation. However, it is important to remember that the net state of phosphorylation of a protein is the result of a dynamic equilibrium between protein kinases and phosphatases

(37, 301). Previously it was thought that phosphatase activity was constitutive, but it is now clear that dephosphorylation reactions are subject to many levels of regulation.

Localization

As outlined above, second messengers and receptor ligands play a major role in activating specific kinases and phosphatases. In addition, localization of kinases and phosphatases within cells serves as a means of regulating enzyme activity. Substrates and/or binding proteins appear to play a role in directing the subcellular localization of enzymes. The phosphatase PP1 associates with glycogen via a glycogen-binding, or G-, subunit (284). Cyclic adenosine monophosphate (cAMP)–dependent protein kinase A (PKA) is localized to subcellular sites via binding of the PKA regulatory subunit to A kinase anchor proteins (AKAPs) (36, 272). Protein kinase A and AKAP 79 co-localize to hippocampal neurons, and binding of PKA to AKAP 79 is inhibited by preincubation with a peptide derived from the conserved amphipathic helix region of AKAPs (272). This targeting of enzymes may restrict phosphorylation/dephosphorylation to select substrates, which in turn would regulate kinase/phosphatase involvement in distinct physiological pathways.

Phosphorylation

Phosphorylation/dephosphorylation also is important in modulating kinase and phosphatase activity (269); that is, the enzymes that mediate these events are themselves subject to similar modifications. In T cells, the CD45 tyrosine phosphatase is phosphorylated by the tyrosine kinase $p56^{lck}$, thus activating CD45–mediated dephosphorylation (29). The activation cascade for MAP kinase is mediated by sequential phosphorylation and activation of the various MAP kinase members (7, 32, 333). The cell-cycle kinases and phosphatases also are sensitive to control by phosphorylation, as described in detail later under Regulation via Phosphorylation.

Regulation via Autoinhibitory Domains

Another means of enzyme regulation is through intrasteric control mediated by autoinhibitory domains contained within the protein (107, 156, 157, 290, 291). Some enzymes, such as PKA, protein kinase C (PKC), cyclic guanosine monophosphate (cGMP)-dependent protein kinase, calmodulin-dependent protein kinase, calcineurin, and phosphatase 1, are maintained in an inhibited state by their autoinhibitory domains. These domains are thought to act by folding back on the active site within the protein, thereby masking the active site. Binding of activating ligand (cAMP in the case of PKA, calcium and calmodulin for calcineurin) relieves this inhibition, resulting in activation of the enzyme.

The inhibitory domains for PKA share sequence homology with the substrate sequence of the kinase, except that they lack the phosphorylatable serine or threonine. This same pseudosubstrate motif holds true for the other enzyme autoinhibitory domains. Thus, this stretch of amino acids acts as a "pseudosubstrate" that binds to the catalytic site.

Synthetic peptides based on these sequences are useful as pharmacological probes of enzyme function. Pseudosubstrate peptides competitively inhibit enzymatic activity in vitro. These peptides are highly specific and potent inhibitors for the enzyme from which they are derived. They have been used as inhibitors in intact cells, by microinjection, or in permeabilized cells (65). In addition, Grove et al. (95, 96) transfected cells with a gene encoding the PKA pseudosubstrate region and demonstrated inhibition of cAMP-stimulated gene expression.

Substrate Specificity

Consensus substrate sites generally have not been identified for tyrosine kinases. However, consensus motifs have been identified for a variety of serine/threonine kinases (for review see refs. 104, 158). Many of these motifs are similar, requiring a Lys or Arg N-terminal and/or C-terminal to the phosphorylated Ser or Thr. In fact, a number of proteins serve as in vitro substrates for multiple kinases, suggesting that phosphorylation of a protein by a particular kinase may be determined in large part via co-localization of substrate and kinase, rather than by strict kinase/substrate requirements.

Dual-specificity kinases are unique in that their consensus substrate sequence is Ser/Thr followed by a Pro. Accordingly, these kinases appear to have a narrow substrate specificity. For example, the dual-specificity MAP kinase kinase utilizes only MAP kinase as a substrate.

Much less is known about phosphatase substrate specificities. In general, the serine/threonine phosphatases, with the exception of calcineurin (see later under CALCINEURIN), are considered to have broad substrate specificities, and no consensus sequences for dephosphorylation have been identified.

Like their kinase counterparts, the dual-specificity phosphatases have a narrow substrate specificity. They utilize a number of substrates in vitro, but their physiological substrates are specific. For example, PAC1 dephosphorylates only MAP kinase, while the only known physiological substrates for cdc25 are the cyclin-dependent kinases (130).

PROTEIN KINASE C

Protein kinase C plays a major role in the signal-transduction pathway of a variety of ligands. Molecular cloning studies have established that PKC exists as a family of closely related proteins. The PKC isoforms are highly homologous within their amino-acid sequences, and all possess serine/threonine kinase activity. Based on their co-factor requirements, the PKC isoforms have been classified into three groups. The first group, called conventional PKCs (α, β_I, β_{II}, and γ) require calcium, phospholipid, and diacylglycerol (DAG) or phorbol ester for full activity, while the novel PKCs (δ, ϵ, η, and θ) require only DAG or phorbol ester. The third group of atypical PKCs (ζ, ι, and λ) do not require either calcium or DAG for enzymatic activity (for review, see refs. 17, 232, 294).

Structure

The C-terminal region of the PKCs contains a catalytic domain. The N-terminal region is the regulatory domain, which contains a pseudosubstrate inhibitory domain and two highly conserved constant regions, C1 and C2 (Fig. 10.1). The C2 region is responsible for calcium binding, and the PKC isozymes which lack the C2 domain (the novel and atypical isoforms) are insensitive to calcium for enzymatic activity (294, 295). The importance of this region for binding calcium was demonstrated in deletion experiments, showing that C2 deletion mutants no longer require calcium for either kinase or phorbol ester binding (242).

The C1 region contains the phospholipid and DAG/phorbol ester–binding sites (17, 242). This region contains a zinc finger structure, consisting of two conserved cysteine-rich regions, cys1 and cys2, each of which binds two zinc ions. Both cysteine-rich regions are required for DAG (or phorbol ester) binding, and the atypical PKCs, which contain only one cysteine-rich region, do not bind DAGs (154, 155, 242, 264, 283, 295). The early observation by Nishizuka and co-workers (24) that phorbol esters specifically activate PKC has been useful for studying the role of PKC in cellular pathways. However, several proteins unrelated to PKC, including the guanosine triphosphatase (GTPase)–activating protein n-chimaerin and the nematode protein unc-13, have been shown to contain the same zinc finger structure as PKC, and these proteins also bind phorbol esters (5, 14, 206). These results suggest that treatment of cells with phorbol esters may activate proteins other than just PKC and that caution must be used in interpreting the results of such experiments.

The nuclear magnetic resonance (NMR) solution structure as well as the crystal structure of cys2 have been determined (122, 340). The upper third of this three-dimensional structure is highly hydrophobic and contains the phorbol ester/DAG–binding groove, while the area below is composed primarily of positively charged amino acids. Binding of phorbol ester covers the polar interior and allows insertion of the hydrophobic binding domain into the membrane. Thus, phorbol esters change the protein surface, stabilizing the membrane-inserted state of the cys2 region, without

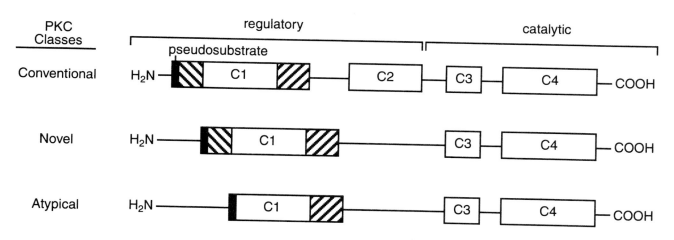

FIG. 10.1. Structure of protein kinase C *(PKC)* enzymes. Conserved *(C1–4)* regions are indicated. *C1* contains two cysteine-rich regions and binds phorbol ester/diacyglycerol (DAG). Atypical PKCs contain only one cysteine-rich region and do not bind DAG/phorbol ester. *C2* is responsible for calcium-binding activity, and the ATP-binding site is in *C3*.

causing a marked conformational change. Comparisons between phorbol esters and the physiological activator DAG demonstrate that the C20-hydroxyl of the phorbol ester, which hydrogen-bonds to the cys2 domain, is analogous to the 3-hydroxyl of DAG. These results explain the ability of the phorbol esters to functionally mimic DAGs in binding to and activating PKC.

Activation by Lipid Second Messengers.

It has been demonstrated that PKC is activated by DAGs, generated in response to cellular stimulation with agonists that hydrolyze phosphatidylinositol 4,5-bisphosphate (PIP_2) (233, 295). These DAGs are rapidly produced and degraded, resulting in rapid PKC activation (187). Originally, PIP_2-derived DAGs were thought to be the sole source of lipid PKC activators, but accumulating evidence has demonstrated that other lipid second messengers also stimulate PKC. For example, PKC is activated by phosphatidylcholine-derived DAGs (86, 219). Phosphatidylcholine hydrolysis is stimulated by some agonists, including vasopressin and angiotensin II in hepatocytes; interleukin-1 in T cells; and PDGF, α-thrombin, and EGF in IIC9 fibroblasts (22, 138, 187, 256, 273). The exact mechanism leading to phosphatidylcholine breakdown is unknown, but both phospholipase C and D activities may be involved. In many cells, phosphatidycholine-derived DAGs can be distinguished from PIP_2-derived DAGs based on differences in fatty acid composition (256). In addition, the magnitude and time course of DAG accumulation from PIP_2 vs. phosphatidylcholine varies; in general, PIP_2 hydrolysis yields DAGs that accumulate more rapidly than DAGs generated from phosphatidylcholine breakdown (16, 330). The phosphatidylcholine-derived DAGs may lead to a sustained activation of PKC since the kinetics of DAG accumulation are more prolonged compared with PIP_2-generated DAGs (62, 225, 331).

Other lipids also stimulate PKC activity (225, 233). For example, stimulation of phospholipase A_2 results in an increase in free fatty acids. Free fatty acids, such as oleic, linoleic, and arachidonic acids, stimulate PKC activity in vitro, while saturated fatty acids are without effect (184, 289, 338). Phospholipase A_2 activation also leads to the generation of lysophosphatidylcholine, which has been shown to potentiate cellular responses such as proliferation. For example, addition of lysophosphatidylcholine potentiates the ability of DAG plus ionomycin to activate T lymphocytes (15).

Lipid second messengers also may serve as a means of selective PKC isozyme activation (225). For example, cholesterol sulfate activates PKC η but not PKC α or δ (137); PKC ζ is not activated by either calcium or DAG/phorbol esters, but addition of phosphatidylinositol 3,4,5-trisphosphate (PIP_3) selectively activates this isozyme (226). Taken together, these results suggest that a number of different lipid-signaling pathways may converge on PKC activation and that the PKC isoforms vary in sensitivity to these activators.

Isozyme Specificity

The use of phorbol esters as PKC activators has suggested a role for PKC in many cellular pathways, including neurotransmitter release, inflammatory responses, and growth and differentiation. The question of how one enzyme can be involved in so many different cellular functions has been answered in part by the demonstration of PKC isoforms. Results from a wide variety of studies indicate that the individual PKC isozymes may be differentially involved in cellular signaling (46). There are several areas in which isozyme selectivity is displayed. As discussed above, differential activation of isozymes by lipid second messengers has been demonstrated. In addition, isozyme expression levels vary in different tissue and cell types. Other areas of isozyme selectivity include substrate specificity, down-regulation, and localization.

Substrate Specificity.

Relatively little is known concerning the physiological substrates of PKC, and most of the available information concerning substrate specificity is the result of in vitro experiments. In most examples, differences between the isozymes are small, and Michaelis-Menten constant (K_m) and maximal velocity (V_{max}) values for most substrates do not differ by more than threefold (153, 204, 205, 288). However, some specificity has been demonstrated. For example, histone IIIS is a good substrate for most of the isozymes, though it is not phosphorylated by PKC ϵ, η, or δ (239, 240, 281, 282). The EGF receptor is phosphorylated more readily by PKC α than PKC β (135), while PKC β, but not PKC α or γ, phosphorylates the vitamin D receptor (125). Also, PKC α, β_I, and γ phosphorylate glycogen synthase kinase-3β (GSK-3β) with approximately equal potency, while PKC ϵ phosphorylates GSK-3β poorly, if at all (46, 90). These results indicate that substrate specificities do exist, though studies utilizing physiological substrates are required to further define the basis of isozyme selectivity.

Expression.

Heterogeneity in PKC isozyme expression has been demonstrated (327). For example, PKC α is widely expressed in almost all cells and tissues, while PKC γ is present only in the brain and spinal cord (232). Compared to PKC α, the β isoforms are more restricted in their expression; PKC ζ and λ are found in many tissues, but PKC η is expressed predominantly in the lung and skin (10, 243). In most cell types, only a subset of all of the PKC isoforms are expressed, suggesting that the various isoforms are functionally distinct (18, 26, 244).

Down-Regulation. Degradation of PKC is involved in its regulation. Prolonged treatment of cells with phorbol esters results in a loss or down-regulation of PKC activity and immunoreactivity. Young et al. (339) demonstrated that phorbol ester treatment of cells results in an increased rate of degradation of the PKC protein with no effect on the rate of synthesis. In FRSK cells, treatment with the protease inhibitors N-tosyl-phenylalanine chloromethyl ketone (TPCK) or leupeptin prevents the down-regulation of PKC, suggesting the involvement of a serine protease in the degradation pathway (31).

The PKC isozymes display differential sensitivity to down-regulation. Treatment of Swiss 3T3 cells with bombesin results in the selective down-regulation of PKC δ and ϵ protein levels, while PKC ζ levels are unchanged (241). Similarly, in GH$_4$C$_1$ cells, thyrotropin-releasing hormone (TRH) decreases PKC ϵ levels with no effect on PKC α or β (11, 162, 164). The mechanism by which certain isozymes resist this activator-induced degradation is not known. However, this down-regulation protocol produces cells that are functionally deficient in selective PKC isozymes; thus, it is a useful tool to study the role of PKC isozymes in various cellular pathways.

Localization. Early experiments by a number of investigators demonstrated that treatment of cells with PKC activators results in a translocation of PKC from the soluble fraction to the particulate fraction (plasma membrane) (63, 177, 228, 329). Subsequent studies showed that various PKC isozymes are differentially localized to other subcellular locations, including the nucleus, cytoskeleton, and Golgi (118, 163, 186, 189, 215). The mechanism(s) of this isozyme-selective localization is not known, but PKC structure may be a determinant. Mochly-Rosen and co-workers have identified PKC-binding proteins, termed "RACKs" (receptor for activated C kinase), that specifically and saturably bind PKC (214, 215, 270). The RACK1-binding site was mapped to the C2 region of PKC β, and peptides from this region inhibit PKC β translocation and function in *Xenopus* oocytes (271). These results suggest that specific regions of the PKC isoforms play a role in directing their location within cells. This isozyme-selective localization may serve as a means for selective substrate phosphorylation and, thus, as a basis for isozyme-selective functions in vivo.

Using immunological and biochemical analyses, a number of laboratories have demonstrated the presence of PKC in the nucleus of liver (207) HL-60 cells (118), 3T3 cells, and IIC9 cells (52, 68, 185, 186, 308). In some systems, PKC appears to be constitutively expressed in the nucleus. For example, in liver, PKC β is present in nuclei from unstimulated tissues (207). Likewise, PKC ζ was detected by immunofluorescence in nuclei from resting Purkinje cells (102). In contrast, in a number of other cell models, such as 3T3, IIC9, and HL-60 cells, PKC is present in nuclei prepared from stimulated, but not unstimulated, cells. Stimuli resulting in PKC nuclear localization include phorbol myristate acetate (PMA), bryostatin, insulin-like growth factor-1, and α-thrombin (52, 67, 68, 185, 186, 308).

The mechanism(s) leading to PKC nuclear localization is not known. Bryostatin and PMA may be able to directly activate PKC, while mitogens such as α-thrombin may act by altering nuclear DAG levels. Treatment of IIC9 cells with α-thrombin results in increased nuclear DAG levels, as well as a specific increase in nuclear PKC α levels (186). Analysis of molecular species profiles of induced DAGs indicates that phosphatidylcholine hydrolysis is the predominant, if not exclusive, source of the α-thrombin-induced nuclear DAGs (147, 265). Similarly, insulin-like growth factor-1 treatment of 3T3 cells results in increased nuclear DAG levels and decreased mass levels of intranuclear phosphoinositides (52). The time course of DAG elevation is quite rapid and is accompanied by a rise in nuclear PKC. Taken together, the results of the IIC9 cell and 3T3 cell studies are consistent with the hypothesis that changes in nuclear DAG levels may be a determinant of PKC nuclear localization.

The mechanism(s) leading to isozyme-selective nuclear localization has been investigated in several studies. The hinge region separates the regulatory and catalytic domains of PKC, and deletion mutants of PKC α indicate that this region contains nuclear localization sequences that are masked by regulatory domain components in wild-type PKC (146). Fields and co-workers (117, 118) have demonstrated selective nuclear localization of β_{II}, but not α, PKC in K-562 erythroleukemia cells following bryostatin treatment. The increased nuclear PKC is accompanied by increased lamin B phosphorylation and nuclear envelope breakdown, supporting the hypothesis that lamin B is a physiological nuclear substrate for PKC. Studies with chimeras, in which the regulatory and catalytic domains of α and β_{II} PKC were exchanged, indicated that the catalytic domains contain important determinants for isoform localization and function since only chimeras containing the β_{II} catalytic domain localized to the nucleus

(319). Additional delineation of the enzyme regions responsible for specific subcellular localization should help in further investigations of the structural basis for isozyme-specific functions.

Activation of PKC causes rapid changes in the cytoskeleton, including actin polymerization and cell ruffling (326). In Y-1 cells, PKC is associated with the cytoskeletal fraction (248). A number of cytoskeletal proteins have been identified as PKC substrates, including caldesmon, adducin, and microtubule-associated protein 2 (124, 305, 323). Jaken and co-workers (161, 163) have demonstrated that treatment of GH_4C_1 cells with either phorbol esters or the physiological agonist TRH results in PKC α association with the detergent-insoluble cytoskeletal fraction. They used a blot overlay assay to identify PKC-binding proteins, including the cytoskeletal proteins vinculin, talin, and MARCKS (myristoylated alanine-rich C kinase substrate) (27, 134). These proteins are also PKC substrates, and phosphorylation of MARCKS and annexin II by PKC has been shown to regulate their properties (2, 3, 227, 280). Mapping experiments indicate that more than one PKC domain is involved in binding to the cytoskeletal proteins, including the PKC substrate-binding site and the N-terminal autoinhibitory (pseudosubstrate) domain, suggesting that protein secondary structure plays an important role in directing PKC isozymes to discrete subcellular locations (194).

Isozymes in Cellular Function

As discussed above, PKC isozymes are involved in many different cellular responses. As for all kinase and phosphatase families, determining the role of individual isozymes is difficult since the available kinase inhibitors lack specificity. However, several different approaches have been used successfully to address this issue. Overexpression of eight PKC isozymes in NIH 3T3 cells was used to characterize the subcellular distribution of the isoforms (91). In a similar experiment, the effect of each overexpressed isozyme on cell growth was examined (213): PKC δ caused cells to grow more slowly, while overexpression of PKC ϵ resulted in increased growth rates and higher cell densities than in wild-type cells. In addition, PKC ϵ-overexpressing cells grew in soft agar and formed tumors in nude mice. These results suggest that PKC ϵ, but not PKC δ, is involved in neoplastic transformation.

A similar approach has been used in T cells, where overexpression of constitutively active PKC isozymes demonstrated that PKC ϵ, but not PKC ζ, stimulated nuclear factor kappa B (NF-κB) and nuclear factor of activated T cells activity (80). Transfection of kinase-

defective mutants results in a "dominant negative" phenotype, which proved useful in demonstrating that PKC ζ is required for NF-kB activation (51, 200). Overall, the advantage of these systems is that all of the isoforms are expressed often in one cell type, simplifying comparisons. In addition, the functional effects of an individual isoform can be examined directly. However, a major disadvantage of overexpression studies is that the normal pathways of activation and regulation have been circumvented, and the overexpressed phenotype may bear little resemblance to the physiological phenotype and function.

Antisense experiments also have been used to define isotype-specific functions (4, 43, 201). In kidney cells stably transfected with antisense PKC α, phorbol ester–stimulated arachidonic acid release was inhibited, while antisense PKC β had no effect (87). Phorbol ester–stimulated induction of the adhesion molecule ICAM-1 was inhibited 60%–70% in human lung carcinoma cells following treatment with PKC α antisense oligonucleotides (44). Introduction of antisense PKC α into glioblastoma cells resulted in no change in the protein levels of PKC β, γ, ϵ, and ζ as detected by Western blot analysis, while expression of PKC α was completely undetectable (6). These cells displayed an increase in doubling time with reduced serum-dependent growth, suggesting that PKC α plays an important role in growth control in these cells. Taken together, the results of antisense experiments demonstrate the specificity of the antisense probes and suggest that this approach is useful for determining the roles of the individual isozymes in cellular signaling pathways.

CALCINEURIN

Enzyme Structure

Calcineurin (CaN) is a serine/threonine phosphatase which is highly expressed in brain tissue, and accumulating evidence suggests that it is involved in neuronal function (169, 172). However, CaN has gained significant interest because it also plays a key role in T-cell activation and is the molecular target of the immunosuppressive drugs FK506 and cyclosporin A (CsA) (196, 267). Thus, CaN serves as a good example of the role of a phosphatase in signal-transduction pathways.

First identified in 1978 as a calmodulin-binding protein in bovine brain (173), CaN was subsequently further purified and shown to contain intrinsic phosphatase activity that is dependent on both calcium and calmodulin (297). Thus, it is unique among the serine/threonine phosphatases in that its enzymatic activity is sensitive to levels of a second messenger, calcium. In addition, although it shares considerable homology with the catalytic region of the serine/threonine phosphatases PP1 and PP2A (40%–50% amino-acid identity), CaN differs significantly in composition from these phosphatases since it is a heterodimer (139, 320). The CaN A-subunit (61 kd) contains the catalytic site as well as a calmodulin-binding site, while the B-subunit (19 kd) is the regulatory subunit which binds calcium. The two subunits co-purify under mild conditions, and cross-linking experiments have demonstrated that they exist in a 1:1 stoichiometry (170, 173).

The B-subunit was purified to homogeneity, and its amino-acid sequence indicated that it contains four "EF" hand high-affinity calcium-binding sites, as found in other calcium-binding proteins, such as troponin C and calmodulin (9, 170). Overall, CaN B shows 35% sequence homology with calmodulin, but several lines of evidence demonstrate that the two proteins are not functionally interchangeable. Calmodulin cannot substitute for CaN B in supporting phosphatase activity from reconstituted A- plus B-subunits, and conversely, CaN B cannot replace calmodulin in the activation of CaN A (171, 174, 210). The N-terminus of CaN B is myristoylated, which may serve as a determinant in the localization of the enzyme, especially to membrane compartments (8, 175).

The A-subunit is composed of several distinct domains: a catalytic site, a CaN B–binding region, a calmodulin-binding site, and an autoinhibitory domain (Fig. 10.2). Enzymatic activity is regulated by binding of both the B-subunit and calmodulin (296, 304). The A-subunit has very low phosphatase activity on its own, but activity is increased approximately 200-fold in the presence of calmodulin and the B-subunit (254). Calcium binding to the B-subunit lowers the K_m for substrates with a small effect on V_{max}, while calmodulin increases V_{max} with little or no effect on K_m (254, 255, 296).

Calmodulin binds with high affinity to the A-subunit in the presence, but not in the absence, of calcium. Cross-linking experiments and gel filtration studies have demonstrated that CaN A and calmodulin form a 1:1 complex (170, 303). Molecular cloning of CaN A has identified a 24-amino-acid calmodulin-binding domain based on sequence homology to other known calmodulin-binding proteins (139, 167).

Limited proteolysis experiments have been useful in defining the functional domains of CaN A (126, 203). Treatment of CaN with trypsin results in a 43 kd protein fragment which binds CaN B and retains phosphatase activity. However, the trypsinized enzyme is insensitive to calmodulin and can no longer bind to immobilized calmodulin, thus demonstrating that the CaN B–binding site on the A-subunit is separate from the calmodulin-binding site. Watanabe et al. (325) demonstrated that a fusion protein containing residues 328–390 of the A-subunit binds the B-subunit. Mutagenesis of four hydrophobic amino acids in this region totally prevented binding of the B-subunit to CaN A, though calmodulin binding was unaffected. These results suggest that hydrophobic interactions are essential for the association of the A- and B-subunits. Crystallization of CaN has demonstrated that CaN B consists of two globular calcium-binding domains, each containing two EF hand motifs, flanked by a β strand (93). These globular domains form a hydrophobic groove which binds to the α-helical B-subunit-binding site on the A-subunit.

The autoinhibitory domain of the A-subunit also was elucidated by proteolysis experiments. Treatment with clostipain cleaves CaN to produce a 57 kd protein which binds calmodulin, but its phosphatase activity is independent of calcium and calmodulin (126). These results are analogous to those obtained with the calmodulin-dependent proteins calmodulin-dependent kinase and myosin light chain kinase, both of which contain autoinhibitory domains. For these enzymes, as well as for CaN, the autoinhibitory domains bind to and inhibit the catalytic sites. Binding of calcium and calmodulin causes a conformational change which disrupts the autoinhibitory domain binding, thereby relieving the inhibition of the enzyme. Hashimoto et al. (109) synthesized peptides corresponding to the

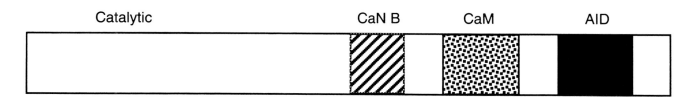

FIG. 10.2. Schematic of calcineurin A-subunit, showing the catalytic domain, *(CaN B)*–binding domain, calmodulin *(CaM)*-binding domain, and autoinhibitory domain *(AID)*

COOH-terminal residues of CaN and demonstrated that a peptide corresponding to residues 457–482 inhibited CaN activity in vitro. Using [^{32}P]myosin light chain as a substrate and intact CaN, an IC$_{50}$ of approximately 10 μM was obtained (109).

Isoforms

Molecular cloning of both the CaN A- and B-subunits has demonstrated that isoforms exist (98, 99, 139, 166, 221). There are three isoforms of CaN A (α, β, and γ), which are highly conserved across species (84, 114, 311). Isoforms Aα and Aβ are highly expressed in brain tissue, and the human α gene is 84% identical to the β gene (222). Despite this high homology, the two genes are found on different chromosomes, indicating that they are not physically linked (83). The β form contains a proline-rich amino-terminus which is not present in the α form, and the two isoforms also differ in their C-terminal amino acids (99). In addition, splicing variants of both isoforms have been identified. The third CaN isoform, γ, was identified as a nonneural isoform that appears to be expressed specifically in testis. It is 70%–80% identical to the α and β isoforms and differs predominantly in several regions in the C-terminus of the protein (221). Additional, uncharacterized CaN isoforms may exist, as suggested by the observation of a unique polymerase chain reaction (PCR) product identified in PC12 cells (317).

As with the A-subunit, the B-subunit has both isoforms and splice variants (25). The α isoform was cloned from a brain library, while the β isoform, which contains an additional nine amino acids, is testis-specific (220). Overall, these two isoforms show approximately 80% amino-acid identity. The amino-acid sequences of the human and bovine CaN Bα isoforms are identical, and the β isoforms also are highly conserved across species, indicating the functional conservation of this protein (100, 229, 312).

Ubiquitously expressed in all tissues, the highest levels of CaN are found in brain, where CaN represents approximately 1% of total brain protein. The levels in brain are at least 20 times higher than those in any other tissue, and detection of CaN protein levels in tissues other than brain is difficult (169, 172, 320). Within the brain, radioimmunoassay experiments demonstrate high levels in neural tissue, predominantly in the cerebrum, olfactory bulb, and cerebellum. As shown by subcellular fractionation studies, CaN is found in both the soluble and particulate fractions (302). In immunostaining experiments in rat brain, CaN reactivity was found in the cell bodies of neurons, both as diffuse cytoplasmic staining and as punctate staining, suggestive of membrane association (165, 328).

Substrate Specificity

Calcineurin can dephosphorylate a variety of proteins phosphorylated at serine or threonine residues, as well as several nonprotein molecules, such as para-nitrophenyl phosphate and 4-methylumbelliferyl phosphate (12, 192, 247). Although the K$_m$ for the nonprotein phosphocompounds is typically very high (in the millimolar range), these substrates have proved useful for characterizing the enzymatic reaction. Based on the observation that CaN binds to type II cAMP-dependent protein kinase through the RII-subunit (110), Blumenthal et al. (21) demonstrated that CaN dephosphorylates the RII-subunit. Proteolytic fragments of the RII-subunit were used to identify the exact site of dephosphorylation. A 19-amino-acid synthetic peptide of this region is dephosphorylated by CaN with a K$_m$ of 26 μM, similar to that of the RII protein (21).

Overall, CaN has a narrower substrate specificity than does PP1 or PP2A (172, 304). However, no overall consensus substrate sequence for CaN has been identified. Synthetic phosphopeptides have been used to define substrate requirements for CaN (21, 53). Peptides that are optimally dephosphorylated by CaN contain basic residues on the N-terminal side of the phosphoserine or phosphothreonine, with a basic residue at the -3 position being particularly important. In addition, acidic residues adjacent to the C-terminal side of the phosphoamino acid are negative regulators of dephosphorylation. Examination of peptides of various lengths showed that amino-acid additions N-terminal to the phosphorylated residue markedly improve dephosphorylation, though no optimal sequence was demonstrated. Taken together, the results of these studies indicate that the specificity of CaN is determined by higher-order structural features, rather than by a specific consensus sequence.

Endogenous Substrates

The search for endogenous substrates of CaN has centered on brain proteins, due to the high level of expression of CaN in brain. Calcineurin dephosphorylates synapsin I, DARPP-32, GAP-43 (neuromodulin), and protein K.-F with similar K$_m$ values; however, comparison of the catalytic efficiencies (kcat/K$_m$) indicates that dephosphorylation of only DARPP-32, GAP-43, and protein K.-F occur at significant rates in vitro (168, 199).

Evidence for these phosphoproteins serving as endogenous CaN substrates in cells or tissues is accumulating, especially for DARPP-32. Highly expressed in the neostriatum, DARPP-32 is a dopamine-regulated, 32 kd protein substrate for cAMP-dependent kinase

(111). It inhibits PP1 at nanomolar concentrations in vitro; however, DARPP-32 is active as an inhibitor only when it is phosphorylated on Thr34. At this same site, CaN dephosphorylates DARPP-32, thus regulating its activity. In intact neurons, dopamine binding to D_1 receptors activates PKA, resulting in DARPP-32 phosphorylation. Activation of CaN occurs as a result of glutamate binding to its receptors and a subsequent rise in calcium levels. In addition, DARPP-32 is phosphorylated by casein kinase II on Ser137, which in turn inhibits CaN dephosphorylation of Thr34 (50). Thus, the regulation of DARPP-32 activity exemplifies the complex interrelationships between cellular kinases and phosphatases which modulate signal-transduction pathways.

It has been suggested that CaN plays a role in axonal elongation and that the cytoskeletal protein tau serves as a substrate. During initial outgrowth of neurites, CaN reactivity is localized to the growth cones. Tau is maintained in a phosphorylated state during this time, as demonstrated by immunoreactivity with an antibody that specifically recognizes the phosphorylated, but not the dephosphorylated, form of the protein (66). Treatment of cultures from embryonic rat cerebellum with a peptide inhibitor of CaN prevents axonal elongation and inhibits tau reactivity with the phosphorylation-dependent antibody.

Hyperphosphorylated tau is found in the paired helical filaments associated with Alzheimer's disease, and the abnormal phosphorylation sites on the protein have been mapped. Gong et al. (89) demonstrated that dephosphorylation of all six of these sites in vitro occurred preferentially with CaN, while PP1 and PP2A had little or no effect. Overall, these results, as well as those from the neurite extension experiments summarized above, suggest that CaN plays a role in modulating tau function, thereby affecting normal neuronal development, as well as Alzheimer's disease pathology.

T-Cell Activation

Calcineurin may have important biological roles in addition to its involvement in neuronal function. These additional roles have been elucidated as a result of experiments aimed at defining the mechanism of action of the immunosuppressant drugs CsA and FK506.

These drugs inhibit the early steps of antigen-stimulated T-cell activation and have a very similar profile of cellular activity (42, 182, 196, 266, 267, 313). For example, both drugs inhibit T-cell activation induced by mitogenic lectins, as well as activation resulting from treatment of cells with the combination of PMA and a calcium ionophore. In contrast, neither drug inhibits T-cell activation induced by CD28 liga-

tion. Both CsA and FK506 prevent activation of a variety of cytokine genes, including interleukin (IL)-2, granulocyte-macrophage colony-stimulating factor, IL-4, and tumor necrosis factor (TNF)α. The drugs bind with high affinity to intracellular proteins, termed "immunophilins." The immunophilin for CsA is cyclophilin, while that for FK506 is FKBP-12. Structurally, these two immunophilins share no homology, yet they both contain peptidyl-prolyl isomerase activity. This enzymatic activity catalyzes the cis–trans interconversion of peptidyl-prolyl bonds, which is involved in protein folding in cells. Binding of the drugs to their respective immunophilins inhibits the isomerase activity of the proteins.

Because of the overlapping spectrum of biological activity of CsA and FK506 and since both drugs, acting through unrelated proteins, inhibit isomerase activity, it was originally hypothesized that inhibition of this enzymatic activity was responsible for the action of the drugs. That hypothesis subsequently was proved incorrect. First, rapamycin, another immunosuppressant, also binds to FKBP-12 and inhibits its isomerase activity. However, rapamycin does not inhibit antigen-stimulated T-cell activation or cytokine gene transcription; rather, it inhibits IL-2–dependent T-cell proliferation (19, 56). Thus, the biological activity of rapamycin does not correlate with isomerase inhibition. Second, a number of nonimmunosuppressive analogs of FK506 and CsA were synthesized and tested. Despite a lack of biological activity, these compounds bind with high affinity to their respective immunophilins and inhibit isomerase activity (20). Taken together, these results indicate that isomerase inhibition is not sufficient to explain the mechanism of action of CsA and FK506.

The mechanism was discovered by Liu et al. (198), who immobilized either FK506–FKBP-12 or CsA–cyclophilin and demonstrated specific binding of CaN to the complexes. Importantly, binding of the complexes to CaN inhibits the phosphatase activity of the enzyme in vitro. Additional evidence supports the hypothesis that CaN is the molecular target of the immunosuppressants. First, the ability of a number of FK506 and CsA analogs to inhibit the phosphatase activity of CaN in vitro correlates with their ability to inhibit T-cell activation (197). Second, treatment of cells with FK506 or CsA inhibits the cellular activity of CaN (73). Third, overexpression of a constitutively active form of CaN in T cells renders the cells more resistant to the effects of the drugs (34, 235).

The interaction of the FKBP-12–FK506 complex with CaN has been studied using a variety of approaches (101, 133, 152, 211). Chemical cross-linking studies demonstrated binding of the drug–immunophilin complexes to CaN B but only in the presence of

CaN A (133). Deletion mutants of the CaN A-subunit were used to show that the calmodulin-binding and autoinhibitory domains were not required for the binding of CaN to FKBP-12–FK506, though the CaN B-subunit was necessary, but not sufficient, for complex formation (35). Mutations in CaN B that prevent binding of FKBP-12–FK506 to the CaN complex were identified; these same mutations also inhibited activation of the phosphatase activity of CaN A. These results are consistent with those obtained from the X-ray structure of the ternary complex of CaN A, CaN B, and FKBP-12–FK506 (93). The principal site of interaction between FKBP-12–FK506 and CaN is a hydrophobic cleft located at the interface of CaN B and the CaN B-binding domain on CaN A; FKBP-12–FK506 makes contact with CaN B as well as with CaN A. In the ternary complex, FK506 is located 25 Å from the active site of CaN. Thus, the drug–immunophilin complex does not directly inhibit phosphatase activity, but rather, inhibition is mediated by FKBP-12–FK506 physically blocking access of the substrate to CaN. Crystal structure results demonstrate that only the FK506–FKBP-12 complex can bind to the CaN A–CaN B surface; neither the drug nor the immunophilin alone forms the required surface for interaction. Taken together, these results elucidate the mechanism of FK506–FKBP-12 binding and inhibition of CaN, and they raise the possibility of designing specific inhibitors that mimic the drug–immunophilin complex.

Evidence suggests that CaN is not just involved in mediating the actions of FK506 and CsA but that it plays a role in the physiological pathway of T-cell activation. O'Keefe et al. (235) demonstrated that, in cells transfected with CaN, PMA, and ionophore-stimulated IL-2N driven gene expression was increased approximately twofold. Furthermore, in cells overexpressing a constitutively active form of CaN, IL-2-driven gene expression was stimulated approximately 150-fold in the presence of PMA alone, indicating that active CaN can replace the usual requirement for ionophore. Similar results were obtained by Clipstone and Crabtree (34), who demonstrated reporter gene activity in CaN-transfected cells at suboptimal concentrations of ionomycin that elicited little or no activity in control cells. Taken together, these results demonstrate that CaN overexpression augments T-cell activation resulting from both calcium and PKC stimulation and suggest that CaN plays a key role in this process.

Nuclear Factor of Activated T Cells as a Substrate

As stated above, CsA and FK506 regulate cytokine gene, including IL-2 gene, transcription. Interleukin 2 plays a key role in controlling T-cell proliferation,

and consequently, numerous studies have focused on understanding IL-2 gene proliferation. Results of these studies have demonstrated that transcriptional activation requires nuclear factor of activated T cells (NFAT), a DNA-binding protein which binds to specific sites on the regulatory regions of the cytokine genes (42, 266, 313).

Molecular cloning and biochemical studies have provided insights into the actions of NFAT. The approximately 120 kd NFAT is a member of a gene family whose members contain a rel homology domain which is important for DNA-binding activity (208, 234). In addition, a serine/proline repeat region, of unknown function, is present in each of the family members (193). The original NFAT members were termed "NFAT$_c$" and "NFAT$_p$," and the newest member to be identified is NFAT$_c$3, which is highly expressed in the thymus (116). In unactivated T cells, NFAT DNA-binding activity is localized primarily in the cytosol, and following T-cell activation, activity is detected in the nucleus. Nuclear NFAT forms a complex with fos and jun, and mutations in NFAT that inhibit binding to these proteins eliminate NFAT-mediated gene transcription (143–145). Furthermore, treatment of cells with either CsA or FK506 inhibits the appearance of NFAT-binding activity in the nucleus (60, 72).

The results with CsA and FK506 suggest that NFAT is a CaN substrate, either direct or indirect, in T cells (208, 209). Treatment of NFAT$_p$ immunoprecipitated from murine HT-2 cells with CaN in vitro results in its dephosphorylation demonstrating that NFAT$_p$ is an in vitro substrate for CaN (276). Treatment of NFAT$_p$ immunoprecipitated from ^{32}P-labeled HT-2 cells results in its migration as an approximately 120 kd protein that is localized to the cytosol of cells. Treatment of cells with ionomycin results in a decrease in the molecular weight of NFAT$_p$ and a loss of ^{32}P, demonstrating NFAT$_p$ dephosphorylation. Dephosphorylation is accompanied by localization of the protein to the nuclear fraction. Dephosphorylation and nuclear localization are completely blocked by preincubation of cells with FK506, consistent with the hypothesis that NFAT$_p$ is a CaN substrate.

These results suggest the scheme shown in Figure 10.3. T-cell activation causes a rise in intracellular calcium levels, which can activate CaN, either directly or indirectly, resulting in the dephosphorylation of NFAT and allowing nuclear localization and subsequent gene activation. By inhibiting CaN, FK506 and CsA inhibit NFAT dephosphorylation, thus preventing nuclear localization and transcriptional activation. A putative nuclear localization sequence has been identified in the carboxyl terminal region of the NFAT rel domain (193). Phosphorylation of this sequence may

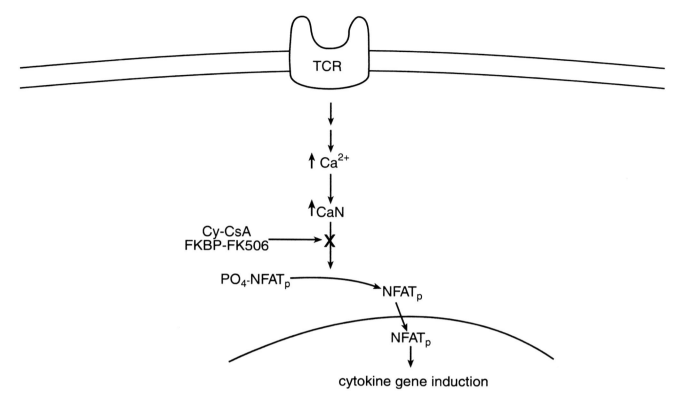

FIG. 10.3. Schematic of T-cell calcineurin *(CaN)* activation pathway. Antigen stimulation of the T-cell receptor *(TCR)* results in increased cytosolic calcium levels, resulting in CaN activation. CaN dephosphorylates (either directly or indirectly) the nuclear factor of activated T cells *(NFAT)*. Dephosphorylated NFAT translocates to the nucleus, where it regulates induction of several cytokine genes, including interleukin 2 and tumor necrosis factor-α.

be an important determinant of NFAT localization. Experimental results support this overall scheme, though it is important to note that it is not known whether NFAT is a direct substrate for CaN in cells. Based on cross-talk between kinases and phosphatases, which occurs in many systems, it is possible that CaN regulates another phosphatase that in turn acts directly on NFAT. ^{32}P peptide mapping of NFAT isolated from cells and identification of phosphorylated residues is an important next step that should help answer this question.

Additional mechanisms of regulation may exist for NFAT. For example, Park et al. (249) demonstrated that the human homolog of $NFAT_p$ is constitutively present in the nucleus of human B (Raji) and T (Jurkat) cells. Dephosphorylation of $NFAT_p$ is blocked by pretreatment of cells with FK506, as is DNA-binding activity. Calcineurin dephosphorylates $NFAT_p$ in vitro, suggesting that, as for the other NFAT family members, it is an endogenous substrate. Since $NFAT_p$ is constitutively localized to the nucleus in these cells, these results suggest that CaN is also localized to the nucleus, either constitutively or as a result of cellular activation.

FK506 and Cyclosporin A as Probes of Calcineurin Action

The identification of FK506 and CsA, when bound to their immunophilins, as specific CaN inhibitors has been useful for investigating a potential role for CaN in various pathways. Prior to the discovery of the mechanism of these drugs, few specific CaN inhibitors were available. Calmodulin inhibitors, which inhibit all calmodulin-dependent proteins, or phosphatase inhibitors, such as okadaic acid, which also inhibit PP1 and PP2A, were the primary pharmacological tools available. The autoinhibitory peptide inhibitor is a specific and selective inhibitor of CaN but cannot be used in intact cell studies since it does not readily penetrate the membrane.

The use of FK506 and/or CsA has suggested a role for CaN in several different signal pathways. For example, both drugs inhibit calcium-mediated amylase secretion in pancreatic acinar cells (94), Na$^+$/K$^+$-ATPase activity in rat nephrons (183), degranulation of cytotoxic T lymphocytes (58), and neutrophil migration on vitronectin (112). In AtT20 pituitary cells, treatment with FK506 stimulates adrenocorticotropic hormone release, suggesting that CaN normally plays an inhibitory role in the signal-transduction pathway of hormone secretion (13). In most of these systems, a potential role for CaN is consistent with a previously characterized calcium-dependent requirement for the biological effect.

A role for CaN in apoptosis also has been proposed (103, 337, 341). Treatment of T-cell hybridomas with anti-CD3 antibody induces programmed cell death, which is inhibited by co-incubation with either FK506 or CsA (74). Calcineurin activity in cellular lysates was inhibited under these conditions, with an IC_{50} of 0.6 nM for FK506, which correlated closely with the IC_{50} value for inhibition of apoptosis. A similar inhibitory effect of CsA was observed in studies examining immunoglobulin M (IgM)–mediated apoptosis in B cells (23). Further work obviously is required to define the role(s) for CaN in these various signal-transduction pathways, but the use of FK506 and CsA provides the first step in that process.

ROLE OF CDC25 IN CELL-CYCLE PROGRESSION

Progression through the cell cycle is regulated at two major checkpoints: the transitions from G_1 to S and from G_2 to M. Much of our knowledge of the regulation of these steps in mammalian cells has come from studies in fission yeast, *Drosophila*, and frogs, where it has been demonstrated that there are common mechanisms for progression through the cell cycle involving the sequential activation of cyclin-dependent kinases. Regulation of these kinases occurs at several levels; thus, they serve as an interesting example of the complex role played by kinases and phosphatases in signal transduction.

Overview of Cell-Cycle Proteins

Cyclin-Dependent Kinases and Cyclins. The cyclin-dependent kinases (cdks), as their name implies, require binding to a cyclin protein for enzymatic activity (121, 258). There are multiple cdk family members, named "cdk1–cdk7," as well as multiple cyclin proteins, termed "cyclins A– H." Additional homologs of both families are likely to be identified as PCR cloning techniques are applied to various tissues and cell types. All cdks share a high degree of homology at the amino-acid level (40% identity). In particular, the sequence EGVPSTAIRESLLKE (amino acids 42–55) of cdk1, commonly called the "PSTAIR region," is highly conserved among the cdks. The various cdks display different specificities with respect to cyclin binding: for ex-

ample, cdk4 binds only cyclin D, while cdk2 binds both cyclins E and A.

Binding of the various cyclins to their cdk partners results in an increase in cdk activity and progression through the cell cycle (287). The cyclins display less homology with each other, except for a conserved domain of approximately 100–150 amino acids, called the "cyclin box," which is responsible for both binding to and activation of cdk (286). Cyclins are required for kinase activity, but they also confer substrate specificity. Cyclins A and B form complexes with cdk2, yet only the cyclin A–cdk2 complex phosphorylates the retinoblastoma (Rb)-related p107 protein in vitro (253). It has been demonstrated that cdk1 (cdc2) can be substituted for cdk2 without affecting substrate phosphorylation, further supporting the model in which the cyclin subunit plays a dual role in cell-cycle control (253).

The cyclins have been divided into two groups, depending on the portion of the cell cycle in which they are expressed. Cyclins C, D, and E are referred to as the "G_1 cyclins" because they control passage through G_1. They were originally identified in budding yeast as proteins encoded by CLN genes that enable passage through a G_1 restriction point, termed "START" (285, 286). Cyclin D expression is maximal in early to mid-G_1 phase, whereas cyclin E levels are highest at the G_1/S transition. Overexpression of cyclin E in fibroblasts shortens the G_1 phase and results in a decrease in cell size (237). In addition, microinjection of anti-cyclin E antibodies blocks the entry of cells into S phase, demonstrating that cyclin E is essential for the G_1/S phase transition (238).

In contrast, cyclins A and B are referred to as the "mitotic cyclins" because they control progression into mitosis. Microinjection of either cyclin A or B into *Xenopus* oocytes induces maturation (259). Inactivation of cyclin A in fibroblasts during the G_1 phase, by either specific antibodies or antisense RNAs, results in the inhibition of DNA synthesis (81, 245). Cyclin B controls the G_2/M transition, and prevention of cyclin B degradation arrests cells in mitosis (132).

Although there are at least seven cdk members, most information is known about cdk1, also called cdc2, and cdk2 (217, 315). Many of the other cdk isoforms have been identified, primarily through homology cloning, but their biological roles are not well defined. All of the cdks are serine/threonine kinases, with a molecular weight of 35–40 kd (223). They possess an unusual substrate specificity in that they phosphorylate the consensus sequence (S/T)PX(K/R) (230). Because of this requirement for a proline adjacent to the phosphorylated residue, they are often referred to as "proline-directed kinases," as described above.

An increase in cdk activity resulting from binding of cyclin to cdk causes cellular progression. In general, cdk levels are constant throughout the cell cycle, but cyclin levels vary (217). The G_1 cyclins (C, D, and E) contain Pro-Glu-Ser-Thr (PEST) sequences within their C-terminus, which are important recognition motifs for rapid proteolysis. In contrast, a 40-amino-acid region in the N-terminus of cyclins A and B, termed the "destruction box," is responsible for proteolysis. Proteolysis of these cyclins occurs via a ubiquitin-dependent pathway (30, 85). N-terminal truncation mutants of cyclin B are resistant to proteolysis, and *Xenopus* extracts expressing this mutant are unable to exit mitosis (224). The exact signal initiating cyclin destruction is not known, and it has been suggested that a cyclin-dependent enzyme is involved in conjugating ubiquitin to cyclin (85). Hershko et al. (113) isolated a fraction from clam oocytes that is activated by cdc2 and promotes cyclin degradation.

Cyclin-Dependent Kinase Inhibitors. While cyclins activate cdk activity, another group of proteins, cyclin-dependent kinase inhibitors (CKIs), act as inhibitors of cyclin–cdk complexes (129, 217). As with the other cell-cycle proteins, the inhibitors exist as a large family, of which there are at least seven members. The inhibitors fall into two classes, based on the cdks that they inhibit. In mammalian cells, p21 and p27 form one class, binding to and inhibiting cdk2– and cdk4–cyclin complexes, while p15 and p16 show specificity for cdk4– and cdk6–cyclin complexes. These inhibitors bind directly to the cyclin–cdk complex and inhibit kinase activity with high affinity (129, 217, 287).

Regulation of the cdk inhibitors is not completely understood, but they appear to respond to different cellular signals. For example, p21 levels are increased at the transcriptional level by p53, a transcriptional regulator that mediates cell-cycle arrest following DNA damage (55, 59). Stimulation of T cells with IL-2 induces a decrease in p27 levels, while transforming growth factor (TGF)-β increases p27 levels by inducing release of p27 from a heat-labile cellular compartment (49, 69, 260). In contrast, TGF-β treatment increases p15 protein levels approximately 30-fold in human keratinocytes (106), resulting in a drop in the activities of cdk4 and cdk6.

Overexpression of p27 and p21 arrests cells in G_1, consistent with the hypothesis that the CKIs are negative regulators of cell-cycle progression (257, 261, 310, 336). Transfection of p21 into malignant cells suppresses cell growth (336). In addition, introduction of p21 directly into established tumors inhibits tumor growth, suggesting that gene transfer of the CKIs serves as a potential therapeutic in the treatment of cancer.

Cdc2

The kinase that plays a pivotal role in cell-cycle progression by directing the cell to enter mitosis was identified first in yeast as maturation-promoting factor (MPF), a dimeric protein consisting of cdc2 kinase and cyclin B. Activation of cdc2–cyclin B is the rate-limiting step for cells to enter mitosis and occurs primarily as a result of regulated phosphorylation/dephosphorylation of the cdc2 molecule. The cdc2 protein kinase acts by phosphorylating a wide variety of mitotic substrates, such as histones, nuclear lamins, and microtubule-associated proteins (30, 54, 191). Phosphorylation of these substrates results in the cellular changes associated with mitosis, such as nuclear envelope breakdown. The remainder of this section discusses this regulation in more detail, focusing on the action of the phosphatase cdc25.

Cdc2 contains three major sites of phosphorylation, which have been demonstrated to control its function (39, 92, 179). These sites are Thr14, Tyr15, and Thr161 in the human cdc2 protein (Fig. 10.4). Similar sites have been identified on other cdk isoforms and are thought to play similar roles in regulating kinase activity.

Regulation via Phosphorylation. Phosphorylation of Thr161 is required for the kinase activity of cdc2–cyclin B, and mutations at this residue result in cdc2 that is devoid of histone kinase activity (293). A separate protein kinase, CAK (cdk-activating kinase), is responsible for Thr161 phosphorylation. Also called "cdk7," CAK requires cyclin H for activity (190, 202, 263, 292, 335) and has been shown to be a component of TFIIH, which is responsible for phosphorylating RNA polymerase II during transcription (64, 274) and is required for nucleotide excision repair, suggesting that cell-cycle components are also involved in DNA repair.

The crystal structure of cdk2, both free and bound to cyclin A, has been reported, and this has advanced our understanding of the important regulatory sites on these proteins (45, 148, 218). Because of the high homology among the cdk proteins, the information gained from cdk2 is applicable to the other kinase family members, including cdc2. Overall, the cdk structure is similar to that of cAMP-dependent kinase in that it consists of two lobes, with the ATP- and substrate-binding sites located between the lobes. The Thr161 phosphorylation site is contained within the "T-loop" of cdk, residues 152–170. This loop blocks access to the substrate-binding site, effectively acting as an autoinhibitor of cdk. Phosphorylation of Thr161 is thought to induce a conformational change in the loop, exposing the substrate-binding site.

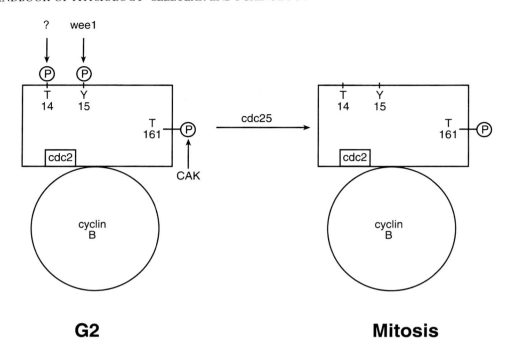

FIG. 10.4. Schematic of cdc2 kinase regulation. Cyclin B binds to cdc2, which is phosphorylated on Thr14, Tyr15 (by wee1), and Thr161 (by cdk-activating kinase *[CAK]*). The cdc25 phosphatase induces mitosis by dephosphorylating Thr14 and Tyr15. Exit from mitosis is regulated by cyclin degradation and Thr161 dephosphorylation.

While Thr161 phosphorylation plays an activating role in cdk regulation, phosphorylations at Thr14 and Tyr15 are inhibitory. In the cdk2 crystal structure, both of these residues are located in a glycine-rich loop located above the phosphates of ATP. Phosphorylation of these sites is believed to alter ATP orientation, or the general conformation of the active site (148).

Tyr15 is phosphorylated by a kinase called "wee1," and this phosphorylation inhibits the kinase activity of cdc2 (136, 188, 250, 324). In humans, wee1 is not able to phosphorylate Thr14, and a separate Thr14 kinase activity has been identified, but not yet purified, in both *Xenopus* and human cells (176). Wee1 activity is regulated throughout the cell cycle, with the lowest level of activity during mitosis (61). In fission yeast, this drop in wee1 activity is the result of C-terminal phosphorylation of wee1 by the protein kinase Nim1 (40, 251, 334). Whether this same regulatory mechanism exists in mammalian cells is not known since a human homolog of Nim1 has not been identified. However, *Xenopus* extracts contain a kinase activity that inactivates wee1, suggesting that a similar regulatory control exists (306).

A kinase called myt1 that phosphorylates cdc2 on both Thr14 and Tyr15 was cloned from *Xenopus* (219a). Sequence analysis demonstrates that myt1 is

most similar to members of the wee1 family, with 39% identity to *Xenopus* wee1. An interesting aspect of myt1 is the presence of a putative transmembrane segment located C-terminal to the kinase domain. Fractionation experiments indicated that the 55 kDa myt1 protein is localized predominantly to the membrane fraction. The human form of myt1, cloned from a HeLa cDNA library, shares 46% sequence identity with the *Xenopus* form (195a). Northern analysis of myt1 mRNA levels demonstrated expression in HaLa and Jurkat cells, but not in primary peripheral blood lymphocytes. Golgi and ER staining of HeLa cells was observed using a human myt1 peptide antibody. Deletion of the myt1 transmembrane region resulted in a nuclear staining pattern.

Cdc25

As stated above, phosphorylations of cdc2 on Thr14 and Tyr15 inhibit its kinase activity, and dephosphorylation of these sites is required to activate the enzyme. This dephosphorylation is catalyzed by cdc25. This phosphatase was identified first in fission yeast as a gene required to initiate mitosis. Yeast mutants that lack cdc25 accumulate the phosphorylated form of cdc2 (92). Similarly, immunodepletion of cdc25 from

Xenopus extracts prevents entry into M phase (181). Furthermore, overproduction of cdc25 protein in yeast results in the inappropriate initiation of mitosis before completion of S phase. These early experiments established that cdc25 is a rate-limiting mitotic inducer and suggested that cdc25 and wee1 act in opposition to each other (121, 277).

The cdc25 gene was identified and cloned by rescue of a fission yeast cdc25 temperature-sensitive mutant, and the human homolog was then cloned via PCR. The cloned human 55–60 kd protein is about 40% identical to the yeast protein and was shown to rescue the same yeast cdc25 temperature-sensitive mutant, demonstrating functional conservation of the protein (212, 278).

In PCR cloning experiments, it has been demonstrated that cdc25 isoforms exist. These isoforms, cdc25A, cdc25B, and cdc25C, share about 40% identity in the catalytic C-terminal region (76, 278). All of them contain the "cdc25 box" of highly conserved amino acids required for phosphatase activity and can rescue yeast lacking a cdc25 gene, further demonstrating the conservation of function in all of the isoforms. Cdc25 is a dual-specificity phosphatase. Although initial sequence analysis of the cdc25 protein did not demonstrate any obvious similarities to protein phosphatases, cdc25 was shown subsequently to share sequence homology with the VH1 phosphatase from vaccinia virus (47, 48, 97). VH1 phosphatase is a member of the family of dual-specificity phosphatases which dephosphorylate both tyrosine and threonine residues. The sequence I/VFHCEXXXXR, which is localized to the catalytic domain near the COOH terminus of cdc25, is conserved in all protein tyrosine phosphatases and is required for catalytic activity (76, 79).

The phosphatase activity of cdc25 was confirmed using para-nitrophenylphosphate (57, 180, 299, 316). Phosphatase activity co-purifies with the cdc25 protein, and a mutant protein lacking the critical cysteine from the I/VFHCEXXXXR motif lacks enzymatic activity. Activity is highly dependent on the presence of dithiothreitol (DTT), and vanadate, but not ethylenediaminetetraacetic acid (EDTA), inhibits dephosphorylation (57).

Cdc25 is a highly selective phosphatase that utilizes nonprotein substrates poorly. For example, the K_m for dephosphorylation of para-nitrophenylphosphate is 50 mM (57). However, cdc25 readily dephosphorylates cdc2 (180, 299, 316), and the sites of dephosphorylation are Thr14 and Tyr15, the residues shown to be important in regulating cdc2 activity (123). Cdc25 immunoprecipitated from HeLa cells dephosphorylates immunoprecipitated cdc2, and phosphatase activity is highest in mitotic cells (316). Addition of the bacterially

expressed protein to oocyte extracts dephosphorylates the cdc2–cyclin B complex, resulting in an increase in its histone kinase activity (79, 149, 180, 299). Furthermore, mutations in the active site of cdc25 which block enzymatic activity also block activation of cdc2–cyclin B and entry of cells into mitosis (79). These results demonstrate the functional coupling between dephosphorylation and mitotic induction, highlighting the key role of this phosphatase in cellular proliferation.

Phosphorylation Regulates Activity. Like cdc2, the level of cdc25 protein remains fairly constant throughout the cell cycle (82). Thus, regulation of cdc25 activity is not the result of a rise and fall in the protein but, rather, occurs primarily through changes in the cdc25 phosphorylation state. These changes have been demonstrated for cdc25B and cdc25C, though it is now clear that cdc25A also is regulated via phosphorylation (see later under *Isoforms*). The cdc25B and C proteins are phosphorylated extensively at the entry of cells into M phase, which is accompanied by a shift in molecular weight from approximately 70 kd to 98 kd. Concomitant with the phosphorylation is a marked increase in phosphatase activity (140, 142, 181). Treatment of oocyte extracts with okadaic acid, a phosphatase inhibitor, prevents the dephosphorylation of cdc25 and accelerates progression of the cell cycle (181). Izumi et al. (142) demonstrated that treatment of purified cdc25 with either PP1 or PP2A dephosphorylates the protein and inhibits its ability to activate cdc2.

A number of studies have focused on identifying the kinase(s) responsible for phosphorylating cdc25. ^{32}P-labeling experiments have identified the sites of phosphorylation in the N-terminal portion of cdc25. Both serine and threonine, but not tyrosine, are phosphorylated. Cdc2–cyclin A and cdc2–cyclin B phosphorylate cdc25 in vitro and result in a mobility shift similar to that in intact cells. Furthermore, the amino-acid residues phosphorylated by cdc2–cyclin B in vitro are identical to those phosphorylated in intact cells (119, 298). Cdc25 phosphorylated by cdc2–cyclin B becomes activated, as shown by an increase in phosphatase activity (119, 140, 181). Mitotic HeLa cell extracts depleted of cdc2 or cyclin B lose their ability to phosphorylate cdc25, while depletion of cdk2 has no effect (119). In contrast, other kinases, such as MAP kinase and cAMP-dependent protein kinase, also phosphorylate purified cdc25 in vitro, but these kinases do not cause a mobility shift in the protein or stimulate its phosphatase activity (140).

Regulation of cdc25 phosphorylation has been investigated in mutational studies. Ser/Pro or Thr/Pro, usually with a basic residue nearby, are minimal consensus sequences for the cyclin-dependent kinases. *Xenopus* cdc25 contains 14 of these sites, with 13 of them located in the N-terminus. Of the 13, five are conserved between the *Xenopus* and human cdc25 proteins (140). Various combinations of these sites were mutated and tested for phosphorylation-induced mobility shifts following incubation with cdc2–cyclin B. Only when all five sites were mutated was the mobility shift completely inhibited, indicating that the shift accompanying entry into M phase is the result of multiple phosphorylation events. Mutation of these sites decreases the activation of cdc25 by cdc2 in vitro by approximately 90%, and the mutant cdc25 proteins are unable to activate cdc2 kinase activity, further demonstrating the link between cdc25 phosphorylation and enzymatic activity (140).

These results suggest a positive feedback system between cdc25 and cdc2, whereby phosphorylation of cdc25 by cdc2 increases its phosphatase activity toward cdc2. However, this model also raises the question of how the initial activation of cdc2–cyclin B occurs (39). It has been suggested that phosphorylation of cdc25 is catalyzed by cdc2–cyclin A before entry into mitosis since cdc2–cyclin A has been shown to be active in late G_2 (33, 318). However, activation of cdc2–cyclin B by cdc25 can occur in oocyte extracts depleted of cyclin A (318), suggesting that other kinases besides cdc2–cyclin A phosphorylate and activate cdc25. Alternatively, nonphosphorylated cdc25 has a low level of phosphatase activity, which may be sufficient to trigger the initial dephosphorylation and activation of cdc2–cyclin B. Cdc25 is dephosphorylated by both PP1 and PP2A, and inhibition of either of these phosphatases produces the net effect of activating cdc25.

In fact, several groups have identified kinases other than cdc2–cyclin A or cdc2–cyclin B that phosphorylate cdc25. Treatment of *Xenopus* extracts depleted of cdc2, cdk2, and the cyclins with the phosphatase inhibitor microcystin results in the phosphorylation and activation of cdc25 (141). Furthermore, addition of microcystin to these broken cell preparations results in chromosome condensation and nuclear envelope breakdown, similar to control M phase extracts, though nuclear lamin phosphorylation does not occur in microcystin-treated extracts. Calmodulin-dependent kinase phosphorylates and activates cdc25 in vitro, though the amino-acid residues phosphorylated are distinct from those phosphorylated by cdc2 (141). However, microcystin-induced cdc25 activation occurs in the presence of ethyleneglycoltetraacetic acid (EGTA), which presumably prevents calmodulin-dependent kinase activation. These results suggest that cdc25 is not a physiological substrate for calmodulin-dependent kinase; however, the microcystin results indicate the presence of other kinases which can activate cdc25.

Ogg et al. (236) identified a kinase in HeLa cell extracts based on its binding to immobilized cdc25. The site of cdc25 phosphorylation was identified as Ser216, which is distinct from those phosphorylated by cdc2–cyclin B (298). The kinase activity was purified from rat liver cytosol and co-eluted with two proteins of approximately 36–38 kd. Whether Ser216 phosphorylation results in an increase in cdc25 phosphatase activity is not known, but the results of such experiments will help to distinguish whether this kinase plays an important regulatory role in cdc25 function.

Isoforms. As stated above, cdc25 exists as a gene family, all of the members of which have phosphatase activity. However, differences among the isoforms have been identified. For example, addition of cyclin B, but not cyclin A or D, to cdc25A directly stimulates phosphatase activity approximately threefold, while cdc25B activity is less sensitive to addition of the cyclin (76). This activation by cyclin B occurs in the absence of cdc2 and suggests that cyclin B has an additional role besides binding to and activating cdc2. The interaction of cyclin B with cdc2 and the activation of cdc25 depend on the presence of the "P-box," a region of the cyclin sequence that shares homology with certain tyrosine phosphatases (342). Taken together, these results demonstrate differential activation of the cdc25 isoforms and identify an important functional domain of cyclin B.

The most pronounced differences among the isoforms are observed with cdc25A since this isoform regulates entry into S phase, while cdc25B and C regulate entry into M. As with cdc25B and -C, cdc25A enzymatic activity is regulated by phosphorylation. Cdc25A is phosphorylated during S phase, and phosphorylation appears to be mediated by cdk2–cyclin E since immunodepletion of either cdk2 or cyclin E prevents the phosphorylation of cdc25A (120). In addition, cdc25A is stably associated with both cdk2 and cyclin E in co-immunoprecipitation experiments. Injection of cdc25A antibodies into normal rat kidney cells blocks entry of cells from the G_1 phase of the cycle into S (120, 151, 212). While it has been demonstrated that cdc2–cyclin B is a substrate for cdc25B and cdc25C, the physiological substrate for cdc25A is not known. Taken together, the results of these experiments suggest that the cdc25 isoforms regulate events in different parts of the cell cycle and that the regulation of isoform phosphatase activity is differentially regulated by cdk–cyclin partners.

Interaction With Cellular Proteins. Protein–protein interactions are important determinants in subcellular localization and substrate specificity for a wide variety of enzymes. Raf-1 co-precipitates with cdc25 in HeLa cells, and the interaction is not dependent on the kinase activity of raf-1 since a kinase-defective mutant binds cdc25 (77). Raf-1 preferentially associates with cdc25A, compared to cdc25B, and interaction of raf-1 with cdc25C is barely detectable, indicating differential binding to cdc25 isoforms. Furthermore, cdc25 is phosphorylated by raf-1, with a concomitant increase in phosphatase activity. These results support the hypothesis that raf-1 interaction with cdc25 may play a role in activation of the cell cycle in response to mitogens (77).

The two-hybrid yeast system was utilized to identify proteins from HeLa cells that interact with cdc25 (41). Two members of the 14–3–3 protein family bind specifically to cdc25 in vitro, and cdc25 and 14–3–3 co-precipitate from intact HeLa cells. Binding of 14–3–3 to cdc25 does not affect phosphatase activity; thus, the functional significance of this interaction is not known. However, 14–3–3 proteins have been shown to associate with a number of signal-transduction proteins, including raf-1 (75), Bcr-Abl (268), and middle T antigen (246), suggesting that cdc25 interaction with 14–3–3 proteins plays a role in directing the subcellular localization and activity of cdc25.

Role in Cancer. Aberrations in cell-cycle proteins are implicated in cancer (108, 115, 131, 216, 279). Cyclin D1 expression levels were increased in approximately one-third of 50 esophageal cancers examined, as well as in about 15% of breast cancers. Overexpression of cyclins A, B, and E was observed in a number of different tumor lines, with overexpression of cyclin E in ten of ten lines (160). Furthermore, the cyclin E gene was amplified, and several cyclin E variant proteins were present, suggesting that cyclin E acts as an oncogene. In breast cancer, alterations in cyclin E expression worsen with increasing stage of the tumor (159). Increased cyclin RNA stability also may contribute to cell-cycle deregulation since in normal cells cyclin degradation acts as a switch to limit cdk activity (160).

Cdc25 may also play a role in oncogenesis (78). As shown by in situ hybridization, cdc25B was overexpressed in 32% of neoplastic breast tissue samples examined, and patients with high levels of cdc25B expression in tumor cells had a recurrence rate at 10 years of approximately 40% compared to 29% of those who expressed low levels of cdc25B. Cdc25A and cdc25B, but not cdc25C, cooperate with ras to cause focus formation in normal mouse fibroblasts, and injection of the ras-cdc25 co-transfected cells into nude mice results in tumor formation. In fibroblasts lacking the tumor-suppressor protein Rb, transfection of the cdc25A gene alone causes cellular transforma-

tion, further supporting the idea that cdc25 isoforms can act as oncogenes (78).

Regulation of the cell cycle is a complex process, involving many different proteins and a cascade of phosphorylation/dephosphorylation events. The cell cycle has far-reaching effects since it controls growth and differentiation, as well as apoptosis. Thus, cell-cycle regulation has important therapeutic implications in areas such as cancer, inflammation, and degenerative diseases. Although it is clear that many of the major protein players have been identified, it is also highly likely that additional proteins, with as yet uncharacterized activities, exist and further regulate this process.

CONCLUSIONS

The complete biochemical details of the function and regulation of both the new and established enzymes are not known; however, a number of common themes have emerged.

First, the enzymes exist as isozyme families. In general, the isoforms are highly homologous, yet close examination demonstrates that structural differences exist. These differences play an important role in the differential activation of the various isozymes. In the case of the PKC family, the presence or absence of the C2 domain regulates activation by DAG. Although more than one isozyme may be present in a given cell, each isozyme may carry out a specific cellular function.

Second, the targeting and localization of the various isozymes is an important determinant of function. For example, PKA is localized to specific cellular compartments through association with AKAP proteins. In hippocampal neurons, disruption of PKA–AKAP binding disrupts PKA-dependent regulation (and presumably phosphorylation) of α-amino-3-hydroxy-5methyl-4-isoxazole propionic acid (AMPA)/kainate currents. Compartmentalization of kinases and phosphatases appears to be a key regulatory event, dictating the intracellular substrates and, thus, the involvement of the enzymes in specific cellular pathways.

Third, both kinases and phosphatases are part of an interconnecting signaling network in which extensive cross-talk between the various members occurs. Although they are often diagrammed as linear pathways, it is clear that the signal-transduction pathways are complex. As exemplified by the cell-cycle cdc2 kinase, many of the enzymes are themselves regulated via phosphorylation; thus, activation of ancillary kinases and phosphatases may have far-reaching cellular effects.

Defining the roles of kinases and phosphatases in signal-transduction pathways is an exciting area of research that promises to lead to new discoveries about cellular regulation.

I thank the colleagues in my laboratory for their critical comments and discussion.

REFERENCES

1. Aaronson, S. A. Growth factors and cancer. *Science* 254: 1146–1150, 1991.

2. Aderem, A. Signal transduction and the actin cytoskeleton: the roles of MARCKS and profilin. *Trends. Biol. Sci.* 17: 438–443, 1992.

3. Aderem, A. The MARCKS brothers: a family of protein kinase C substrates. *Cell* 71: 713–716, 1992.

4. Ahmad, S., and R. I. Glazer. Expression of the antisense cDNA for protein kinase Cα attenuates resistance in doxorubicin-resistant MCF-7 breast carcinoma cells. *Mol. Pharmacol.* 43: 858–862, 1993.

5. Ahmed, S., I. N. Maruyama, R. Kozma, J. Lee, S. Brenner, and L. Lim. The *Caenorhabditis elegans unc*-13 gene product is a phospholipid-dependent high-affinity phorbol ester receptor. *Biochem. J.* 287: 995–999, 1992.

6. Ahmad, S., T. Mineta, R. L. Martuza, and R. I. Glazer. Antisense expression of protein kinase Cα inhibits the growth and tumorigenicity of human glioblastoma cells. *Neurosurgery* 35: 904–909, 1994.

7. Ahn, N. G. The MAP kinase cascade. Discovery of a new signal transduction pathway. *Mol. Cell. Biochem.* 127: 201–209, 1993.

8. Aitken, A., P. Cohen, S. Santikarn, D. H. Williams, A. G. Calder, A. Smith, and C. B. Klee. Identification of the NH$_2$-terminal blocking group of calcineurin B as myristic acid. *FEBS Lett.* 150: 314–318, 1982.

9. Aitken, A., C. B. Klee, and P. Cohen. The structure of subunit B of calcineurin. *Eur. J. Biochem.* 139: 663–671, 1984.

10. Akimoto, K., K. Mizuno, S. Osada, S. Hirai, S. Tanuma, K. Suzuki, and S. Ohno. A new member of the third class in the protein kinase C family, PKC lambda, expressed dominantly in an undifferentiated mouse embryonal carcinoma cell line and also in many tissues and cells. *J. Biol. Chem.* 269: 12677–12683, 1994.

11. Akita, Y., S. Ohno, Y. Yajima, and K. Suzuki. Possible role of Ca^{2+}-independent protein kinase C isozyme, nPKCϵ, in thyrotropin-releasing hormone-stimulated signal transduction: differential downregulation in GH$_4$C$_1$ cells. *Biochem. Biophys. Res. Commun.* 172: 184–189, 1990.

12. Anthony, F. A., D. L. Merat, and W. Y. Cheung. A spectrofluorimetric assay of calmodulin-dependent protein phosphatase using 4-methylumbelliferyl phosphate. *Anal. Biochem.* 155: 103–108, 1986.

13. Antoni, F. A., M. J. Shipston, and S. M. Smith. Inhibitory role for calcineurin in stimulus-secretion coupling revealed by FK506 and cyclosporin A in pituitary corticotrope tumor cells. *Biochem. Biophys. Res. Commun.* 194: 226–233, 1993.

14. Areces, L. B., M. G. Kazanietz, and P. M. Blumberg. Close similarity of baculovirus-expressed n-chimaerin and protein kinase Cα as phorbol ester receptors. *J. Biol. Chem.* 269: 19553–19558, 1994.

15. Asaoka, Y., M. Oka, K. Yoshida, Y. Sasaki, and Y. Nishizuka. Role of lysophosphatidylcholine in T-lymphocyte activation: involvement of phospholipase A$_2$ in signal transduction through protein kinase C. *Proc. Natl. Acad. Sci. U.S.A.* 1992.

16. Augert, G., P. F. Blackmore, and J. H. Exton. Changes in the concentration and fatty acid composition of phosphoinositides induced by hormones in hepatocytes. *J. Biol. Chem.* 264: 2574–2580, 1989.

17. Azzi, A., D. Boscoboinik, and C. Hensey. The protein kinase C family. *Eur. J. Biochem.* 208: 547–557, 1992.

18. Baier, G., D. Telford, L. Giampa, K. M. Coggeshall, G. Baier-Bitterlick, N. Isakov, and A. Altman. Molecular cloning and characterization of PKCΦ, a novel member of the protein kinase C (PKC) gene family expressed predominantly in hematopoietic cells. *J. Biol. Chem.* 268: 4997–5004, 1993.

19. Bierer, B. E., P. S. Mattila, R. F. Standaert, L. A. Herzenberg, S. J. Burakoff, G. Crabtree, and S. L. Schreiber. Two distinct signal transmission pathways in T lymphocytes are inhibited by complexes formed between an immunophilin and either FK506 or rapamycin. *Proc. Natl. Acad. Sci. U.S.A.* 87: 9231–9235, 1990.

20. Bierer, B. E., P. K. Somers, T. J. Wandless, S. J. Burakoff, and S. L. Schreiber. Probing immunosuppressant action with a nonnatural immunophilin ligand. *Science* 250: 556–558, 1990.

21. Blumenthal, D. K., K. Takio, R. S. Hansen, and E. G. Krebs. Dephosphorylation of cAMP-dependent protein kinase regulatory subunit (type II) by calmodulin-dependent protein phosphatase. *J. Biol. Chem.* 261: 8140–8145, 1986.

22. Bocckino, S. B., P. F. Blackmore, and J. H. Exton. Stimulation of 1,2-diacylglycerol accumulation in hepatocytes by vasopressin, epinephrine, and angiotensin II. *J. Biol. Chem.* 260: 14201–14207, 1985.

23. Bonnefoy-Berard, N., L. Genestier, M. Flacher, and J. P. Revillard. The phosphoprotein phosphatase calcineurin controls calcium-dependent apoptosis in B cell lines. *Eur. J. Immunol.* 24: 325–329, 1994.

24. Castagna, M., Y. Takai, K. Kaibuchi, K. Sano, U. Kikkawa, and Y. Nishizuka. Direct activation of calcium-activated, phospholipid-dependent protein kinase by tumor-promoting phorbol esters. *J. Biol. Chem.* 257: 7847–7851, 1982.

25. Chang, C. D., H. Mukai, T. Kuno, and C. Tanaka. cDNA cloning of an alternatively spliced isoform of the regulatory subunit of Ca^{2+}/calmodulin-dependent protein phosphatase (calcineurin Bα2). *Biochim. Biophys. Acta* 1217: 174–180, 1994.

26. Chang, J. D., Y. Xu, M. K. Raychowdhury, and J. A. Ware. Molecular cloning and expression of a cDNA encoding a novel isoenzyme of protein kinase C (nPKC). *J. Biol. Chem.* 268: 14208–14214, 1993.

27. Chapline, C., K. Ramsay, T. Klauck, and S. Jaken. Interaction cloning of protein kinase C substrates. *J. Biol. Chem.* 268: 6858–6861, 1993.

28. Charbonneau, H., and N. K. Tonks. 1002 protein phosphatases? *Annu. Rev. Cell Biol.* 8: 463–493, 1992.

29. Charbonneau, H., N. K. Tonks, K. A. Walsh, and E. H. Fischer. The leukocyte common antigen (CD45): a putative receptor-linked protein tyrosine phosphatase. *Proc. Natl. Acad. Sci. U.S.A.* 85: 7182–7186, 1988.

30. Charollais, R. H., S. Tiwari, and N.S.B. Thomas. Into and out of G1: the control of cell proliferation. *Biochimie* 76: 887–894, 1994.

31. Chida, K., N. Kato, and T. Kuroki. Down regulation of phorbol diester receptors by proteolytic degradation of protein kinase C in a cultured cell line of fetal rat skin keratinocytes. *J. Biol. Chem.* 261: 13013–13018, 1986.

32. Clarke, P. R. Switching off MAP kinases. *Curr. Biol.* 4: 647–650, 1994.

33. Clarke, P. R., D. Leiss, M. Pagano, and E. Karsenti. Cyclin A-

and cylin B-dependent kinases are regulated by different mechanisms in *Xenopus* egg extracts. *EMBO J.* 11: 1751–1761, 1992.

34. Clipstone, N. A., and G. R. Crabtree. Identification of calcineurin as a key signalling enzyme in T-lymphocyte activation. *Nature* 357: 695–697, 1992.

35. Clipstone, N. A., D. F. Fiorentino, and G. R. Crabtree. Molecular analysis of the interaction of calcineurin with drug-immunophilin complexes. *J. Biol. Chem.* 269: 26431–26437, 1994.

36. Coghlan, V. M., B. A. Perrino, M. Howard, L. K. Langeberg, J. B. Hicks, W. M. Gallatin, and J. D. Scott. Association of protein kinase A and protein phosphatase 2B with a common anchoring protein. *Science* 267: 108–112, 1995.

37. Cohen, P. Signal integration at the level of protein kinases, protein phosphatases and their substrates. *Trends Biol. Sci.* 17: 408–413, 1992.

38. Cohen, P., and P.T.W. Cohen. Protein phosphatases come of age. *J. Biol. Chem.* 264: 21435–21438, 1989.

39. Coleman, T. R., and W. G. Dunphy. Cdc2 regulatory factors. *Curr. Biol.* 6: 877–882, 1994.

40. Coleman, T. R., Z. Tang, and W. G. Dunphy. Negative regulation of the Wee1 protein kinase by direct action of the nim1/cdr1 mitotic inducer. *Cell* 72: 919–929, 1993.

41. Conklin, D. S., K. Galaktionov, and D. Beach. 14–3–3 proteins associate with cdc25 phosphatases. *Proc. Natl. Acad. Sci. U.S.A.* 92: 7892–7896, 1995.

42. Crabtree, G. R., and N. A. Clipstone. Signal transmission between the plasma membrane and nucleus of T lymphocytes. *Annu. Rev. Biochem.* 63: 1045–1083, 1993.

43. Dean, N. M., and R. McKay. Inhibition of protein kinase C-α expression in mice after systemic administration of phosphorothioate antisense oligodeoxynucleotides. *Proc. Natl. Acad. Sci. U.S.A.* 91: 11762–11766, 1994.

44. Dean, N. M., R. McKay, T. P. Condon, and C. F. Bennett. Inhibition of protein kinase C-α expression in human A549 cells by antisense oligonucleotides inhibits induction of intracellular adhesion molecule 1 (ICAM-1) mRNA by phorbol esters. *J. Biol. Chem.* 269: 16416–16424, 1994.

45. DeBondt, H. L., J. Rosenblatt, J. Jancarik, H. D. Jones, D. O. Morgan, and S. Kim. Crystal structure of cyclin-dependent kinase 2. *Nature* 363: 595–602, 1993.

46. Dekker, L. V., and P. J. Parker. Protein kinase C—a question of specificity. *Trends Biol. Sci.* 19: 73–77, 1994.

47. Denu, J. M., and J. E. Dixon. A catalytic mechanism for the dual-specific phosphatases. *Proc. Natl. Acad. Sci. U.S.A.* 92: 5910–5914, 1995.

48. Denu, J. M., G. Zhou, L. Wu, R. Zhao, J. Yuvaniyama, M. A. Saper, and J. E. Dixon. The purification and characterization of a human dual-specific protein tyrosine phosphatase. *J. Biol. Chem.* 270: 3796–3803, 1995.

49. Desai, D., H. C. Wessling, R. P. Fisher, and D. O. Morgan. Effects of phosphorylation by CAK on cyclin binding by CDC2 and CDK2. *Mol. Cell. Biol.* 15: 345–350, 1995.

50. Desdoutis, F., J. C. Siciliano, P. Greengard, and J. Girault. Dopamine- and cAMP-regulated phosphoprotein DARPP-32: phosphorylation of ser-137 by casein kinase I inhibits dephosphorylation of thr-34 by calcineurin. *Proc. Natl. Acad. Sci. U.S.A.* 92: 2682–2685, 1995.

51. Diaz-Meco, M. T., E. Berra, M. A. Munico, L. Sanz, J. Lozano, I. Dominguez, V. Diaz-Golpe, M. T. Lain de Lera, J. Alcami, C. V. Paya, F. Arenzana-Seisdedos, J. Virelizier, and J. Moscat. A dominant negative protein kinase C zeta subspecies blocks NF-kB activation. *Mol. Cell. Biol.* 13: 4770–4775, 1993.

52. Divecha, N., H. Banfic, and R. F. Irvine. The phosphoinositide cycle exists in the nuclei of Swiss 3T3 cells under the control of

a receptor (for IGF-1) in the plasma membrane, and stimulation of the cycle increases nuclear diacylglycerol and apparently induces translocation of protein kinase C to the nucleus. *EMBO J.* 10: 3207–3214, 1991.

53. Donella-Dean, A., M. H. Krinks, M. Ruzzene, C. B. Klee, and L. A. Pinna. Dephosphorylation of phosphopeptides by calcineurin (protein phosphatase 2B). *Eur. J. Biochem.* 219: 109–117, 1994.

54. Draetta, G. Cell cycle control in eukaryotes: molecular mechanisms of cdc2 activation. *Trends. Biol. Sci.* 15: 379–383, 1990.

55. Dulic, V., W. K. Kaufmann, S. J. Wilson, T. D. Tisty, E. Lees, J. W. Harper, S. J. Elledge, and S. I. Reed. p53–dependent inhibition of cyclin-dependent kinase activities in human fibroblasts during radiation-induced G1 arrest. *Cell* 76: 1013–1023, 1994.

56. Dumont, F. J., M. J. Staruch, S. K. Koprak, M. R. Melino, and N. H. Sigal. Distinct mechanisms of suppression of murine T cell activation by the related macrolides FK506 and rapamycin. *J. Immunol.* 144: 251–258, 1990.

57. Dunphy, W. G., and A. Kumagai. The cdc25 protein contains an intrinsic phosphatase activity. *Cell* 67: 189–196, 1991.

58. Dutz, J. P., D. A. Fruman, S. J. Burakoff, and B. E. Bierer. A role for calcineurin in degranulation of murine cytotoxic T lymphocytes. *J. Immunol.* 150: 2591–2598, 1993.

59. El-Deiry, W. S., J. W. Harper, P. M. O'Connor, V. E. Velculescu, C. E. Canman, J. Jackman, J. A. Pietenpol, M. Burrell, D. E. Hill, Y. Wang, K. G. Wiman, W. E. Mercer, M. B. Kastan, K. W. Kohn, S. J. Elledge, K. W. Kinzler, and B. Vogelstein. WAF1/CIP1 is induced in p53–mediated G1 arrest and apoptosis. *Cancer Res.* 54: 1169–1174, 1994.

60. Emmel, E. A., C. L. Verweij, D. B. Durand, K. M. Higgins, E. Lacy, and G. R. Crabtree. Cyclosporin A specifically inhibits function of nuclear proteins involved in T cell activation. *Science* 246: 1617–1619, 1989.

61. Enoch, T., and P. Nurse. Mutation of fission yeast cell cycle control genes abolishes dependence of mitosis on DNA replication. *Cell* 60: 665–673, 1990.

62. Exton, J. H. Signaling through phosphatidylcholine breakdown. *J. Biol. Chem.* 265: 1–4, 1990.

63. Farrar, W. L., T. P. Thomas, and W. B. Anderson. Altered cytosol/membrane enzyme redistribution on interleukin-3 activation of protein kinase C. *Nature* 315: 235–237, 1985.

64. Feaver, W., J. Q. Svejstrup, N. L. Henry, and R. D. Kornberg. Relationship of cdk-activating kinase and RNA polymerase II CTD kinase TFIIH/TFIIK. *Cell* 79: 1103–1109, 1994.

65. Fernandez, A., J. Mery, M. Vandromme, M. Basset, J. Cavadore, and N.J.C. Lamb. Effective intracellular inhibition of the cAMP-dependent protein kinase by microinjection of a modified form of the specific inhibitor peptide PKI in living fibroblasts. *Exp. Cell Res.* 195: 468–477, 1991.

66. Ferreira, A., R. L. Kincaid, and K. S. Kosik. Calcineurin is associated with the cytoskeleton of cultured neurons and has a role in the acquisition of polarity. *Mol. Biol. Cell* 4: 1225–1238, 1993.

67. Fields, A. P., S. M. Pincus, A. S. Kraft, and W. S. May. Interleukin-3 and bryostatin 1 mediate rapid nuclear envelope protein phosphorylation in growth factor-dependent FDC-P1 hematopoietic cells. A possible role for nuclear protein kinase C. *J. Biol. Chem.* 264: 21896–21901, 1989.

68. Fields, A. P., G. Tyler, A. S. Kraft, and W. S. May. Role of nuclear protein kinase C in the mitogenic response to platelet-derived growth factor. *J. Cell Sci.* 96: 107–114, 1990.

69. Firpo, E. J., A. Koff, M. J. Solomon, and J. M. Roberts. Inactivation of a cdk2 inhibitor during interleukin 2-induced

proliferation of human T lymphocytes. *Mol. Cell. Biol.* 14: 4889–4901, 1994.

70. Fischer, E. H. Protein phosphorylation: a historical overview. In: *Signal Transduction and Protein Phosphorylation*, edited by L.M.G. Heilmeyer. New York: Plenum Press, 1987, p. 3–10.

71. Fischer, E. H., H. Charbonneau, and N. K. Tonks. Protein tyrosine phosphatases: a diverse family of intracellular and transmembrane enzymes. *Science* 253: 401–406, 1991.

72. Flanagan, W. M., B. Corthesy, R. J. Bram, and G. R. Crabtree. Nuclear association of a T-cell transcription factor blocked by FK-506 and cyclosporin A. *Nature* 352: 803–807, 1991.

73. Fruman, D. A., C. B. Klee, B. E. Bierer, and B. E. Burakoff. Calcineurin phosphatase activity in T lymphocytes is inhibited by FK506 and cyclosporin A. *Proc. Natl. Acad. Sci. U.S.A.* 89: 3686–3690, 1992.

74. Fruman, D. A., P. E. Mather, S. J. Burakoff, and B. E. Bierer. Correlation of calcineurin phosphatase activity and programmed cell death in murine T cell hybridomas. *Eur. J. Immunol.* 22: 2513–2517, 1992.

75. Fu, H., K. Xia, D. C. Pallas, C. Cui, K. Conroy, R. P. Narsimhan, H. Mamon, R. J. Collier, and T. M. Roberts. Interaction of the protein kinase Raf-1 with 14–3–3 proteins. *Science* 266: 126–129, 1994.

76. Galaktionov, K., and D. Beach. Specific activation of cdc25 tyrosine phosphatases by B-type cyclins: evidence for multiple roles of mitotic cyclins. *Cell* 67: 1181–1194, 1991.

77. Galaktionov, K., C. Jessus, and D. Beach. Raf1 interaction with cdc25 phosphatase ties mitogenic signal transduction to cell cycle activation. *Genes Dev.* 9: 1046–1058, 1995.

78. Galaktionov, K., A. K. Lee, J. Eckstein, G. Draetta, J. Meckler, M. Loda, and D. Beach. cdc25 phosphatases as potential human oncogenes. *Science* 269: 1575–1578, 1995.

79. Gautier, J., M. J. Solomon, R. N. Booher, J. F. Bazan, and M. W. Kirschner. cdc25 is a specific tyrosine phosphatase that directly activates p34^cdc2^. *Cell* 67: 197–211, 1991.

80. Genot, E. M., P. J. Parker, and D. A. Cantrell. Analysis of the role of protein kinase C-α, -ϵ, and -zeta in T cell activation. *J. Biol. Chem.* 270: 9833–9839, 1995.

81. Gerard, F., U. Strausfeld, A. Fernandez, and N. J. Lamb. Cyclin A is required for the onset of DNA replication in mammalian fibroblasts. *Cell* 67: 1169–1172, 1991.

82. Girard, F., U. Strausfield, J. Cavadore, P. Russell, A. Fernandez, and N.J.C. Lamb. cdc25 is a nuclear protein expressed constitutively throughout the cell cycle in nontransformed mammalian cells. *J. Cell. Biol.* 118: 785–794, 1992.

83. Giri, P. R., S. Higuchi, and R. L. Kincaid. Chromosomal mapping of the human genes for the calmodulin-dependent protein phosphatase (calcineurin) catalytic subunit. *Biochem. Biophys. Res. Commun.* 181: 252–258, 1991.

84. Giri, P. R., C. A. Marietta, S. Higuchi, and R. L. Kincaid. Molecular and phylogenetic analysis of calmodulin-dependent protein phosphatase (calcineurin) catalytic subunit genes. *DNA Cell Biol.* 11: 415–424, 1992.

85. Glotzer, M., A. W. Murray, and M. W. Kirschner. Cyclin is degraded by the ubiquitin pathway. *Nature* 349: 132–136, 1991.

86. Go, M., K. Sekiguchi, H. Nomura, U. Kikkawa, and Y. Nishizuka. Further studies on the specificity of diacylglycerol for protein kinase C activation. *Biochem. Biophys. Res. Commun.* 144: 598–605, 1987.

87. Godson, C., K. S. Bell, and P. A. Insel. Inhibition of expression of protein kinase C α by antisense cDNA inhibits phorbol ester–mediated arachidonate release. *J. Biol. Chem.* 268: 11946–11950, 1993.

88. Goldberg, J., H. Huang, Y. Kwon, P. Greengard, A. C. Nairn, and J. Kuriyan. Three-dimensional structure of the catalytic subunit of protein serine/threonine phosphatase-1. *Nature* 376: 745–752, 1995.

89. Gong, C. X., T. J. Singh, I. Grundke-Iqbal, and K. Iqbal. Alzheimer's disease abnormally phosphorylated τ is dephosphorylated by protein phosphatase 2B (calcineurin). *J. Neurochem.* 62: 803–806, 1994.

90. Goode, N., K. Hughes, J. R. Woodgett, and P. J. Parker. Differential regulation of glycogen synthase kinase-3β by protein kinase C isotypes. *J. Biol. Chem.* 267: 16878–16882, 1992.

91. Goodnight, J., H. Mischak, W. Kolch, and J. F. Mushinski. Immunocytochemical localization of eight protein kinase C isozymes overexpressed in NIH 3T3 cells. *J. Biol. Chem.* 270: 9991–10001, 1995.

92. Gould, K. L., and P. Nurse. Tyrosine phosphorylation of the fission yeast cdc2^+^ protein kinase regulates entry into mitosis. *Nature* 342: 39–45, 1989.

93. Griffith, J. P., J. L. Kim, E. E. Kim, M. D. Sintchak, J. A. Thomson, M. J. Fitzgibbon, M. A. Fleming, P. R. Caron, K. Hsiao, and M. A. Navia. X-ray structure of calcineurin inhibited by the immunophilin-immunosuppressant FKBP12–FK506 complex. *Cell* 82: 507–522, 1995.

94. Groblewski, G. E., A. C. C. Wagner, and J. A. Williams. Cyclosporin A inhibits Ca^{2+}/calmodulin-dependent protein phosphatase and secretion in pancreatic acinar cells. *J. Biol. Chem.* 269: 15111–15117, 1994.

95. Grove, J. R., P. J. Deutsch, D. J. Price, J. F. Habener, and J. Avruch. Plasmids encoding PKI (1–31), a specific inhibitor of cAMP-stimulated gene expression, inhibit the basal transcriptional activity of some but not all cAMP-regulated DNA response elements in JEG-3 cells. *J. Biol. Chem.* 19506–19513, 1989.

96. Grove, J. R., D. J. Price, H. M. Goodman, and J. Avruch. Recombinant fragment of protein kinase inhibitor blocks cyclic AMP-dependent gene transcription. *Science* 238: 530–533, 1987.

97. Guan, K., S. S. Broyles, and J. E. Dixon. A tyr/ser phosphatase encoded by vaccinia virus. *Nature* 350: 359–361, 1991.

98. Guerini, D., M. J. Hubbard, M. H. Krinks, and C. B. Klee. Multiple forms of calcineurin, a brain isozyme of the calmodulin-stimulated protein phosphatase. In: *The Biology and Medicine of Signal Transduction*, edited by Y. Nishizuka. New York: Raven, 1990, p. 242–250.

99. Guerini, D., and C. B. Klee. Cloning of human calcineurin A: evidence for two isozymes and identification of a polyproline structural domain. *Proc. Natl. Acad. Sci. U.S.A.* 86: 9183–9187, 1989.

100. Guerini, D., M. H. Krinks, J. M. Sikela, W. E. Hahn, and C. B. Klee. Isolation and sequence of a cDNA clone for human calcineurin B, the calcium-binding subunit of the calcium/calmodulin stimulated protein phosphatase. *DNA* 8: 675–682, 1989.

101. Haddy, A., S. K. Swanson, T. L. Born, and F. Rusnak. Inhibition of calcineurin by cyclosporin A-cyclophilin requires calcineurin B. *FEBS Lett.* 314: 37–40, 1992.

102. Hagiwara, M., C. Uchida, N. Usuda, T. Nagata, and H. Kidaka. Zeta-related protein kinase C in nuclei of nerve cells. *Biochem. Biophys. Res. Commun.* 168: 161–168, 1990.

103. Haldar, S., N. Jena, and C. M. Croce. Inactivation of bcl-2 by phosphorylation. *Proc. Natl. Acad. Sci. U.S.A.* 92: 4507–4511, 1995.

104. Hanks, S. K., and A. M. Quinn. Protein kinase catalytic domain sequence database: identification of conserved features of pri-

mary structure and classification of family members. *Methods Enzymol.* 200: 38–77, 1991.

105. Hanks, S. K., A. M. Quinn, and T. Hunter. The protein kinase family: conserved features and deduced phylogeny of the catalytic domains. *Science* 241: 42–52, 1988.

106. Hannon, G. J., and D. Beach. p15^INK4B is a potential effector of TGF-β-induced cell cycle arrest. *Nature* 371: 257–260, 1994.

107. Hardie, G. Pseudosubstrates turn off protein kinases. *Nature* 335: 592–593, 1988.

108. Hartwell, L. H. and M. B. Kastan. Cell cycle control and cancer. *Science* 266: 1821–1828, 1994.

109. Hashimoto, Y., B. A. Perrino, and T. R. Soderling. Identification of an autoinhibitory domain in calcineurin. *J. Biol. Chem.* 265: 1924–1927, 1990.

110. Hathaway, D. R., R. S. Adelstein, and C. B. Klee. Interaction of calmodulin with myosin light chain kinase and cAMP-dependent protein kinase in bovine brain. *J. Biol. Chem.* 256: 8183–8189, 1981.

111. Hemmings, H. C., S. I. Walaas, C. C. Ouimet, and P. Greengard. Dopaminergic regulation of protein phosphorylation in the striatum: DARPP-32. *Trends Neurosci.* 10: 377–383, 1987.

112. Hendley, B., C. B. Klee, and F. R. Maxfield. Inhibition of neutrophil chemokinesis on vitronectin by inhibitors of calcineurin. *Science* 258: 296–299, 1992.

113. Hershko, A., D. Ganoth, V. Sudakin, A. Dahan, L. H. Cohen, F. C. Luca, J. V. Ruderman, and E. Eytan. Components of a system that ligates cyclin to ubiquitin and their regulation by the protein kinase cdc2. *J. Biol. Chem.* 269: 4940–4946, 1994.

114. Higuchi, S., J. Tamura, P. R. Giri, J. W. Polli, and R. L. Kincaid. Calmodulin-dependent protein phosphatase from *Neurospora crassa*. *J. Biol. Chem.* 266: 18104–18112, 1991.

115. Hirama, T., and H. P. Koeffler. Role of the cyclin-dependent kinase inhibitors in the development of cancer. *Blood* 86: 841–854, 1995.

116. Ho, S. N., D. J. Thomas, L. A. Timmerman, X. Li, U. Francke, and G. R. Crabtree. NFATc3, a lymphoid-specific NFATc family member that is calcium-regulated and exhibits distinct DNA binding specificity. *J. Biol. Chem.* 270: 19898–19907, 1995.

117. Hocevar, B. A., D. J. Burns, and A. P. Fields. Identification of protein kinase C (PKC) phosphorylation sites on human lamin B. *J. Biol. Chem.* 268: 7545–7552, 1993.

118. Hocevar, B. A., and A. P. Fields. Selective translocation of β_II-protein kinase C to the nucleus of human promyelocytic (HL60) leukemia cells. *J. Biol. Chem.* 266: 28–33, 1991.

119. Hoffmann, I., P. R. Clarke, M. J. Marcote, E. Karsenti, and G. Draetta. Phosphorylation and activation of human cdc25-C by cdc2–cyclin B and its involvement in the self-amplification of MPF at mitosis. *EMBO J.* 12: 53–63, 1993.

120. Hoffmann, I., G. Draetta, and E. Karsenti. Activation of the phosphatase activity of human cdc25A by a cdk2–cyclin E dependent phosphorylation at the G_1/S transition. *EMBO J.* 13: 4302–4310, 1994.

121. Hoffmann, I., and E. Karsenti. The role of cdc25 in checkpoints and feedback controls in the eukaryotic cell cycle. *J. Cell Sci.* 18: 75–79, 1994.

122. Hommel, U., M. Zurini, and M. Luyten. Solution structure of a cysteine rich domain of rat protein kinase C. *Nature Struct. Biol.* 1: 383–387, 1994.

123. Honda, R., Y. Ohba, A. Nagata, H. Okayama, and H. Yasuda. Dephosphorylation of human p34^cdc2 kinase on both Thr-14 and Tyr-15 by human cdc25B phosphatase. *FEBS Lett.* 318: 331–334, 1993.

124. Hoshi, M., T. Akiyama, Y. Shinohara, Y. Mitata, H. Ogawara, E. Nishida, and H. Sakai. Protein kinase C-catalyzed phosphorylation of the microtubule-binding domain of microtubule-associated protein 2 inhibits its ability to induce tubulin polymerization. *Eur. J. Biochem.* 174: 225–230, 1988.

125. Hsieh, J., P. W. Jurutka, M. A. Galligan, C. M. Terpening, C. A. Haussler, D. S. Samuels, Y. Shimizu, N. Shimizu, and M. R. Haussler. Human vitamin D receptor is selectively phosphorylated by protein kinase C on serine 51, a residue crucial to its trans-activation function. *Proc. Natl. Acad. Sci. U.S.A.* 88: 9315–9319, 1991.

126. Hubbard, M. J.. and C. B. Klee. Functional domain structure of calcineurin A: mapping by limited proteolysis. *Biochemistry* 28: 1868–1874, 1989.

127. Hunter, T. A thousand and one protein kinases. *Cell* 50: 823–829, 1987.

128. Hunter, T. Protein kinase classification. *Methods Enzymol.* 200: 3–37, 1991.

129. Hunter, T. Braking the cycle. *Cell* 75: 839–841, 1993.

130. Hunter, T. Protein kinases and phosphatases: the yin and yang of protein phosphorylation and signaling. *Cell* 80: 225–236, 1995.

131. Hunter, T., and J. Pines. Cyclins and cancer. *Cell* 66: 1071–1074, 1991.

132. Hunter, T., and J. Pines. Cyclins and cancer II: cyclin D and cdk inhibitors come of age. *Cell* 79: 573–582, 1994.

133. Husi, H., M. A. Luyten, and M. G. M. Zurini. Mapping of the immunophilin-immunosuppressant site of interaction on calcineurin. *J. Biol. Chem.* 269: 14199–14204, 1994.

134. Hyatt, S. L., L. Liao, C. Chapline, and S. Jaken. Identification and characterization of α-protein kinase C binding proteins in normal and transformed REF52 cells. *Biochemistry* 33: 1223–1228, 1994.

135. Ido, M., K. Sekiguchi, U. Kikkawa, and Y. Nishizuka. Phosphorylation of the EGF receptor from A431 epidermoid carcinoma cells by three distinct types of protein kinase C. *FEBS Lett.* 219: 215–218, 1987.

136. Igarishi, M., A. Nagata, S. Jinno, K. Suto, and H. Okayama. Wee1^+-like gene in human cells. *Nature* 353: 80–82, 1991.

137. Ikuta, T., K. Chida, O. Tajima, Y. Matsuura, M. Iwamori, Y. Ueda, K. Mizuno, S. Ohno, and T. Kuroki. Cholesterol sulfate, a novel activator for the eta isoform of protein kinase C. *Cell Growth Differ.* 5: 943–947, 1994.

138. Irving, H. R., and J. H. Exton. Phosphatidylcholine breakdown in rat liver plasma membranes. Roles of guanine nucleotides and P2-purigenic agonists. *J. Biol. Chem.* 262: 3440–3443, 1987.

139. Ito, A., T. Hashimoto, M. Hirai, T. Takeda, H. Shuntoh, T. Kuno, and C. Tanaka. The complete primary structure of calcineurin A, a calmodulin binding protein homologous with protein phosphatases 1 and 2A. *Biochem. Biophys. Res. Commun.* 163: 1492–1497, 1989.

140. Izumi, T., and J. L. Maller. Elimination of cdc2 phosphorylation sites in the cdc25 phosphatase blocks initiation of M-phase. *Mol. Biol. Cell* 4: 1337–1350, 1993.

141. Izumi, T., and J. L. Maller. Phosphorylation and activation of the *Xenopus* cdc25 phosphatase in the absence of cdc2 and cdk2 kinase activity. *Mol. Biol. Cell* 6: 215–226, 1995.

142. Izumi, T., D. M. Walker, and J. L. Maller. Periodic changes in phosphorylation of the *Xenopus* cdc25 phosphatase regulate its activity. *Mol. Biol. Cell* 3: 927–939, 1992.

143. Jain, J., P. G. McCaffrey, Z. Miner, T. K. Kerppola, J. N. Lambert, G. L. Verdine, T. Curran, and A. Rao. The T-cell transcription factor NFATp is a substrate for calcineurin and interacts with Fos and Jun. *Nature* 365: 352–355, 1993.

144. Jain, J., P. G. McCaffrey, V. E. Valge-Archer, and A. Rao. Nuclear factor of activated T cells contains Fos and Jun. *Nature* 356: 801–804, 1992.

145. Jain, J., Z. Miner, and A. Rao. Analysis of the preexisting and nuclear forms of nuclear factor of activated T cells. *J. Immunol.* 151: 837–848, 1993.

146. James, G., and E. N. Olson. Deletion of the regulatory domain of protein kinase C α exposes regions in the hinge and catalytic domains that mediate nuclear targeting. *J. Cell Biol.* 116: 863–874, 1992.

147. Jarpe, M. B., K. L. Leach, and D. M. Raben. α-Thrombin-induced nuclear sn-1,2-diacylglycerols are derived from phosphatidylcholine hydrolysis in cultured fibroblasts. *Biochemistry* 33: 526–534, 1994.

148. Jeffrey, P. D., A. A. Russo, K. Polyak, E. Gibbs, J. Hurwitz, J. Massague, and N. P. Pavletich. Mechanism of CDK activation revealed by the structure of a cyclin A-CDK2 complex. *Nature* 376: 313–320, 1995.

149. Jessus, C., and D. Beach. Oscillation of MPF is accompanied by periodic association between cdc25 and cdc2–cyclin B. *Cell* 68: 323–332, 1992.

150. Jia, Z., D. Barford, A. J. Flint, and N. K. Tonks. Structural basis for phosphotyrosine peptide recognition by protein tyrosine phosphatase 1B. *Science* 268: 1754–1758, 1995.

151. Jinno, S., K. Suto, A. Nagata, M. Igarashi, Y. Kanaoka, H. Nojima, and H. Okayama. Cdc25A is a novel phosphatase functioning early in the cell cycle. *EMBO J.* 13: 1549–1556, 1994.

152. Kawamura, A., and M. S. Su. Interaction of FKBP12–FK506 with calcineurin A at the B subunit-binding site. *J. Biol. Chem.* 270: 15463–15466, 1995.

153. Kazanietz, M. G., L. B. Areces, A. Bahador, H. Mischak, J. Goodnight, J. F. Mushinski, and P. M. Blumberg. Characterization of ligand and substrate specificity for the calcium-dependent and calcium-independent protein kinase C isozymes. *Mol. Pharmacol.* 44: 298–307, 1993.

154. Kazanietz, M. G., X. R. Bustelo, M. Barbacid, W. Kolch, H. Mischak, G. Wong, G. R. Pettit, J. D. Bruns, and P. M. Blumberg. Zinc finger domains and phorbol ester pharmacophore. *J. Biol. Chem.* 269: 11590–11594, 1994.

155. Kazanietz, M. G., S. Wang, G. W. A. Milne, N. E. Lewin, H. L. Liu, and P. M. Blumberg. Residues in the second cysteine-rich region of protein kinase C δ relevant to phorbol ester binding as revealed by site-directed mutagenesis. *J. Biol. Chem.* 270: 21852–21859, 1995.

156. Kemp, B. E., and R. B. Pearson. Intrasteric regulation of protein kinases and phosphatases. *Biochim. Biophys. Acta* 1094: 67–76, 1991.

157. Kemp, B. E., R. B. Pearson, C. House, P. J. Robinson, and A. R. Means. Regulation of protein kinases by pseudosubstrate prototopes. *Cell. Signal.* 1: 303–311, 1989.

158. Kennelly, P. J., and E. G. Krebs. Consensus sequences as substrate specificity determinants for protein kinases and protein phosphatases. *J. Biol. Chem.* 266: 15555–15558, 1991.

159. Keyomarsi, K., N. O'Leary, G. Molnar, E. Lees, H. J. Finger, and A. B. Pardee. Cyclin E, a potential prognostic marker for breast cancer. *Cancer Res.* 380–385, 1994.

160. Keyomarsi, K., and A. B. Pardee. Redundant cyclin overexpression and gene amplification in breast cancer cells. *Proc. Natl. Acad. Sci. U.S.A.* 90: 1112–1116, 1993.

161. Kiley, S. C., and S. Jaken. Protein kinase C: interactions and consequences. *Trends Cell Biol.* 4: 223–227, 1994.

162. Kiley, S. C., P. J. Parker, D. Fabbro, and S. Jaken. Differential regulation of protein kinase C isozymes by thyrotropin-releasing hormone in GH$_4$C$_1$ cells. *J. Biol. Chem.* 266: 23761–23768, 1991.

163. Kiley, S. C., P. J. Parker, D. Fabbro, and S. Jaken. Hormone- and phorbol ester-activated protein kinase C isozymes mediate a reorganization of the actin cytoskeleton associated with prolactin secretion in GH$_4$C$_1$ cells. *Mol. Endocrinol.* 6: 120–131, 1992.

164. Kiley, S. C., D. Schaap, P. J. Parker, L.-L. Hsieh, and S. Jaken. Protein kinase C heterogeneity in GH$_4$C$_1$ rat pituitary cells. Characterization of a calcium-independent phorbol ester receptor. *J. Biol. Chem.* 265: 15704–15712, 1990.

165. Kincaid, R. L., C. D. Balaban, and M. L. Billingsley. Differential localization of calmodulin-dependent enzymes in rat brain: evidence for selective expression of cyclic nucleotide phosphodiesterase in specific neurons. *Proc. Natl. Acad. Sci. U.S.A.* 84: 1118–1122, 1987.

166. Kincaid, R. L., P. R. Giri, S. Higuchi, J. Tamura, S. C. Dixon, C. A. Marietta, D. A. Amorese, and B. M. Martin. Cloning and characterization of molecular isoforms of the catalytic subunit of calcineurin using nonisotopic methods. *J. Biol. Chem.* 265: 11312–11319, 1990.

167. Kincaid, R. L., M. S. Nightingale, and B. M. Martin. Characterization of a cDNA clone encoding the calmodulin-binding domain of mouse brain calcineurin. *Proc. Natl. Acad. Sci. U.S.A.* 85: 8983–8987, 1988.

168. King, M. M., C. Y. Huang, P. B. Chock, A. C. Nairn, H. C. Hemmings, K. J. Chan, and P. Greengard. Mammalian brain phosphoproteins as substrates for calcineurin. *J. Biol. Chem.* 259: 8080–8083, 1984.

169. Klee, C. B., and P. Cohen. The calmodulin-regulated protein phosphatase. *Mol. Aspects Cell Regul.* 5: 225–248, 1988.

170. Klee, C. B., T. H. Crouch, and M. H. Krinks. Calcineurin: a calcium and calmodulin-binding protein of the nervous system. *Proc. Natl. Acad. Sci. U.S.A.* 76: 6270–6273, 1979.

172. Klee, C. B., G. F. Draetta, and M. J. Hubbard. Calcineurin. *Adv. Enzymol. Relat. Areas Mol. Biol.* 61: 149–200, 1988.

173. Klee, C. B., and M. H. Krinks. Purification of cyclic 3′,5′-nucleotide phosphodiesterase inhibitory protein by affinity chromatography on activator protein coupled to sepharose. *Biochemistry* 17: 120–128, 1978.

174. Klee, C. B., M. H. Krinks, A. J. Manalan, G. F. Draetta, and D. L. Newton. In: *Advances in Protein Phosphatases 1*, edited by W. Merlevede and J. DiSalvo. Belgium: Leuven University Press, 1985, p. 135–146.

175. Klee, C. B., and T. C. Vanaman. Calmodulin. *Adv. Prot. Chem.* 35: 213–321, 1982.

176. Kornbluth, S., B. Sebastian, T. Hunter, and J. Newport. Membrane localization of the kinase which phosphorylates p34^{cdc2} on threonine 14. *Mol. Biol. Cell* 5: 273–282, 1994.

177. Kraft, A. S., and W. B. Anderson. Phorbol esters increase the amount of Ca^{2+}, phospholipid-dependent protein kinase associated with plasma membrane. *Nature* 301: 621–623, 1983.

178. Krebs, E. G. The growth of research on protein phosphorylation. *Trends Biochem. Sci.* 19: 439, 1994.

179. Krek, W., and E. A. Nigg. Differential phosphorylation of vertebrate p34^{cdc2} kinase at the G1/S and G2/M transitions of the cell cycle: identification of major phosphorylation sites. *EMBO J.* 10: 305–316, 1991.

180. Kumagai, A., and W. G. Dunphy. The cdc25 protein controls tyrosine dephosphorylation of the cdc2 protein in a cell-free system. *Cell* 64: 903–914, 1991.

181. Kumagai, A., and W. G. Dunphy. Regulation of the cdc25

protein during the cell cycle in *Xenopus* extracts. *Cell* 70: 139–151, 1992.

182. Kunz, J., and M. N. Hall. Cyclosporin A, FK506 and rapamycin: more than just immunosuppression. *Trends Biochem. Sci.* 18: 334–338, 1993.

183. Lea, J. P., J. M. Sands, S. J. McMahon, and J. A. Tumlin. Evidence that the inhibition of Na$^+$/K$^+$-ATPase activity by FK506 involves calcineurin. *Kidney Int.* 46: 647–652, 1994.

184. Leach, K. L., and P. M. Blumberg. Modulation of protein kinase C activity and [^{3}H]phorbol 12,13-dibutyrate binding by various tumor promoters in mouse brain cytosol. *Cancer Res.* 45: 1958–1963, 1985.

185. Leach, K. L., E. A. Powers, V. A. Ruff, S. Jaken, and S. Kaufmann. Type 3 protein kinase C localization to the nuclear envelope of phorbol ester-treated NIH 3T3 cells. *J. Cell Biol.* 109: 685–695, 1989.

186. Leach, K. L., V. A. Ruff, M. B. Jarpe, L. D. Adams, D. Fabbro, and D. M. Raben. α-Thrombin stimulates nuclear diglyceride levels and differential nuclear localization of protein kinase C isozymes in IIC9 cells. *J. Biol. Chem.* 267: 21816–21822, 1992.

187. Leach, K. L., V. A. Ruff, T. M. Wright, M. S. Pessin, and D. M. Raben. Dissociation of protein kinase C activation and sn-1,2-diacylglycerol formation. *J. Biol. Chem.* 266: 3215–3221, 1991.

188. Lee, M. S., T. Enoch, and H. Piwnica-Worms. *mik1$^+$* encodes a tyrosine kinase that phosphorylates p34^{cdc2} on tyrosine 15. *J. Biol. Chem.* 269: 30530–30537, 1994.

189. Lehel, C., Z. Olah, G. Jakab, and W. B. Anderson. Protein kinase C✓ is localized to the Golgi via its zinc-finger domain and modulates Golgi function. *Proc. Natl. Acad. Sci. U.S.A.* 92: 1406–1410, 1995.

190. Levedakou, E. N., M. He, E. W. Baptist, R. J. Craven, W. G. Cance, P. L. Welcsh, A. Simmons, S. L. Naylor, R. J. Leach, T. B. Lewis, A. Bowcock, and E. T. Liu. Two novel human serine/threonine kinase with homologies to the cell cycle regulating *Xenopus* MO15, and NIMA kinases: cloning and characterization of their expression pattern. *Oncogene* 9: 1977–1988, 1994.

191. Lewin, B. Driving the cell cycle: M phase kinase, its partners, and substrates. *Cell* 64: 748–752, 1990.

192. Li, H.-C. Activation of brain calcineurin phosphatase towards nonprotein phosphoesters by Ca^{2+}, calmodulin, and Mg^{2+}. *J. Biol. Chem.* 265: 8801–8807, 1984.

193. Li, X., S. N. Ho, J. Luna, J. Giacalone, D. J. Thomas, L. A. Timmerman, G. R. Crabtree, and U. Francke. Cloning and chromosomal localization of the human and murine genes for the T-cell transcription factors NFATc and NFATp. *Cytogenet. Cell Genet.* 68: 185–191, 1995.

194. Liao, L., S. L. Hyatt, C. Chapline, and S. Jaken. Protein kinase C domains involved in interactions with other proteins. *Biochemistry* 33: 1229–1233, 1994.

195. Lindberg, R. A., M. A. Quinn, and T. Hunter. Dual-specificity protein kinases: will any hydroxyl do? *Trends Biochem. Sci.* 17: 114–119, 1992.

195a. Liu, F., J. J. Stanton, Z. Wu, and H. Piwnica-Worms. The human myt1 kinase preferentially phosphorylates cdc2 on threonine 14 and localizes to the endoplasmic reticulum and Golgi complex. *Mol. Cell Biol.* 17: 571–583. 1997.

196. Liu, J. FK506 and cyclosporin, molecular probes for studying intracellular signal transduction. *Immunol. Today* 14: 290–295, 1993.

197. Liu, J., M. W. Albers, T. J. Wandless, S. Luan, D. G. Alberg,

P. J. Belshaw, P. Cohen, C. MacKintosh, C. B. Klee, and S. L. Schreiber. Inhibition of T cell signaling by immunophilin–ligand complexes correlates with loss of calcineurin phosphatase activity. *Biochemistry* 31: 3896–3901, 1992.

198. Liu, J., J. D. Farmer, W. S. Lane, J. Friedman, I. Weissman, and S. L. Schreiber. Calcineurin is a common target of cyclophilin-cyclosporin A and FKBP-FK506 complexes. *Cell* 66: 807–815, 1991.

199. Liu, Y., and D. R. Storm. Dephosphorylation of neuromodulin by calcineurin. *J. Biol. Chem.* 264: 12800–12804, 1989.

200. Lozano, J., E. Berra, M. M. Munico, M. T. Diaz-Meco, I. Dominguez, L. Sanz, and J. Moscat. Protein kinase C zeta isoform is critical for kappa B-dependent promoter activation by sphingomyelinase. *J. Biol. Chem.* 269: 19200–19202, 1994.

201. Maier, J.A.M., and G. Ragnotti. An oligomer targeted against protein kinase Cα prevents interleukin-1α induction of cyclooxygenase expression in human endothelial cells. *Exp. Cell Res.* 205: 52–58, 1993.

202. Makela, T. P., J. Tassan, E. A. Nigg, S. Frutiger, G. J. Hughes, and R. A. Weinberg. A cyclin associated with the CDK-activating kinase MO15. *Nature* 371: 254–257, 1994.

203. Manalan, A. S., and C. B. Klee. Activation of calcineurin by limited proteolysis. *Proc. Natl. Acad. Sci. U.S.A.* 80: 4291–4295, 1983.

204. Marais, R. M., O. Nguyen, J. R. Woodgett, and P. J. Parker. Studies on the primary sequence requirements for PKC-α, -β$_1$ and -γ peptide substrates. *FEBS Lett.* 277: 151–155, 1990.

205. Marais, R. M., and P. J. Parker. Purification and characterization of bovine brain protein kinase C isotypes α, β and gamma. *Eur. J. Biochem.* 182: 129–137, 1989.

206. Maruyama, I. N., and S. Brenner. A phorbol ester/diacylglycerol-binding protein encoded by the *unc-13* gene of *Caenorhabditis elegans*. *Proc. Natl. Acad. Sci. U.S.A.* 88: 5729–5733, 1991.

207. Masmoudi, A., G. Labourdette, M. Mersel, F. L. Huang, K. Huang, G. Vincendon, and A. N. Malviya. Protein kinase C located in rat liver nuclei. Partial purification and biochemical and immunocytochemical characterization. *J. Biol. Chem.* 264: 1172–1179, 1989.

208. McCaffrey, P. G., C. Luo, T. K. Kerppola, J. Jain, T. M. Badalian, A. M. Ho, E. Burgeon, W. S. Lane, J. N. Lambert, T. Curran, G. L. Verdine, A. Rao, and P. G. Hogan. Isolation of the cyclosporin-sensitive T cell transcription factor NFATp. *Science* 262: 750–754, 1993.

209. McCaffrey, P. G., B. A. Perrino, T. R. Soderling, and A. Rao. NFATp, a T lymphocyte DNA-binding protein that is a target of calcineurin and immunosuppressive drugs. *J. Biol. Chem.* 268: 3747–3752, 1993.

210. Merat, D. L., Z. Y. Hu, T. E. Carter, and W. Y. Cheung. Bovine brain calmodulin-dependent protein phosphatase. *J. Biol. Chem.* 260: 11053–11059, 1985.

211. Milan, D., J. Griffith, M. Su, E. R. Price, and F. McKeon. The latch region of calcineurin B is involved in both immunosuppressant–immunophilin complex docking and phosphatase activation. *Cell* 79: 437–447, 1994.

212. Millar, J. B., J. Blevitt, L. Gerace, S. Sadhu, C. Featherstone, and P. Russell. p55^{cdc25} is a nuclear protein required for the initiation of mitosis in human cells. *Proc. Natl. Acad. Sci. U.S.A.* 10500–10504, 1991.

213. Mischak, H., J. Goodnight, W. Kolch, G. Martiny-Baron, C. Schaechtle, M. G. Kazanietz, P. M. Blumberg, J. H. Pierce, and J. F. Mushinski. Overexpression of protein kinase C-δ and -ε in NIH 3T3 cells induced opposite effects on growth,

morphology, anchorage dependence, and tumorigenicity. *J. Biol. Chem.* 268: 6090–6096, 1993.

214. Mochly-Rosen, D., H. Khaner, and J. Lopez. Identification of intracellular receptor proteins for activated protein kinase C. *Proc. Natl. Acad. Sci. U.S.A.* 88: 3997–4000, 1991.

215. Mochly-Rosen, D., H. Khaner, J. Lopez, and B. L. Smith. Intracellular receptors for activated protein kinase C. *J. Biol. Chem.* 266: 14866–14868, 1991.

216. Morgan, D. O. Cell cycle control in normal and neoplastic cells. *Curr. Opin. Genet. Dev.* 2: 33–37, 1992.

217. Morgan, D. O. Principles of cdk regulation. *Nature* 374: 131–134, 1995.

218. Morgan, D. O., and H. L. De Bondt. Protein kinase regulation: insights from crystal structure analysis. *Curr. Opin. Cell Biol.* 6: 239–246, 1994.

219. Mori, T., Y. Takai, B. Yu, J. Takahashi, Y. Nishizuka, and T. Fujikura. Specificity of the fatty acyl moieties of diacylglycerol for the activation of calcium-activated, phospholipid-dependent protein kinase. *J. Biochem. (Tokyo)* 91: 427–431, 1982.

219a. Mueller, P. R., T. R. Coleman, A. Kumagai, and W. G. Dunphy. Myt1: a membrane-associated inhibitory kinase that phosphorylates cdc2 on both threonine-14 and tyrosine-15. *Science* 270: 86–90, 1995.

220. Mukai, H., C. D. Change, H. Tanaka, A. Ito, T. Kuno, and C. Tanaka. cDNA cloning of a novel testis-specific calcineurin B-like protein. *Biochem. Biophys. Res. Commun.* 179: 1325–1330, 1991.

221. Muramatsu, T., P. R. Giri, S. Higuchi, and R. L. Kincaid. Molecular cloning of a calmodulin-dependent phosphatase from murine testis: identification of a developmentally expressed nonneural enzyme. *Proc. Natl. Acad. Sci. U.S.A.* 89: 529–533, 1992.

222. Muramatsu, T., and R. L. Kincaid. Molecular cloning of a full-length cDNA encoding the catalytic subunit of human calmodulin-dependent protein phosphatase (calcineurin Aα). *Biochim. Biophys. Acta* 1178: 117–120, 1993.

223. Murray, A. W. Cyclin-dependent kinases: regulators of the cell cycle and more. *Curr. Biol.* 1: 191–195, 1994.

224. Murray, A. W., M. J. Solomon, and M. W. Kirschner. The role of cyclin synthesis and degradation in the control of maturation promoting factor activity. *Nature* 339: 280–286, 1989.

225. Nakamura, S., and Y. Nishizuka. Lipid mediators and protein kinase C activation for the intracellular signaling network. *J. Biochem. (Tokyo)* 115: 1029–1034, 1994.

226. Nakanishi, H., K. A. Brewer, and J. H. Exton. Activation of the zeta isozyme of protein kinase C by phosphatidylinositol 3,4,5-trisphosphate. *J. Biol. Chem.* 268: 13–16, 1993.

227. Nakaoka, T., N. Kojima, T. Ogita, and S. Tsuji. Characterization of the phosphatidylserine-binding region of rat MARCKS (myristoylated, alanine-rich protein kinase C substrate). *J. Biol. Chem.* 270: 12147–12151, 1995.

228. Naor, Z., J. Zer, H. Zakut, and J. Hermon. Characterization of pituitary calcium-activated, phospholipid-dependent protein kinase: redistribution by gonadotropin-releasing hormone. *Proc. Natl. Acad. Sci. U.S.A.* 82: 8203–8207, 1985.

229. Nargang, C. E., D. A. Bottorff, and K. Adachi. Isolation and characterization of a cDNA clone coding for the calcium-binding subunit of calcineurin from bovine brain: an identical amino acid sequence to the human protein. *DNA Seq.* 4: 313–318, 1994.

230. Nigg, E. A. Targets of cyclin-dependent protein kinases. *Curr. Opin. Cell Biol.* 5: 187–193, 1993.

231. Nishida, E., and Y. Gotoh. The MAP kinase cascade is essential for diverse signal transduction pathways. *Trends. Biochem. Sci.* 18: 128–132, 1993.

232. Nishizuka, Y. The molecular heterogeneity of protein kinase C and its implications for cellular regulation. *Nature* 334: 661–665, 1988.

233. Nishizuka, Y. Membrane phospholipid degradation and protein kinase C for cell signalling. *Neurosci. Res.* 15: 3–5, 1992.

234. Northrup, J. P., S. N. Ho, L. Chen, D. J. Thomas, L. A. Timmerman, G. P. Nolan, A. Admon, and G. R. Crabtree. NF-AT components define a family of transcription factors targeted in T-cell activation. *Nature* 369: 497–502, 1994.

235. O'Keefe, S. J., J. Tamura, R. L. Kincaid, M. J. Tocci, and E. A. O'Neill. FK506 and CsA-sensitive activation of the interleukin-2 promoter by calcineurin. *Nature* 357: 692–695, 1992.

236. Ogg, S., B. Gabrielli, and H. Piwnica-Worms. Purification of a serine kinase that associates with and phosphorylates human cdc25C on serine 216. *J. Biol. Chem.* 269: 30461–30469, 1994.

237. Ohtsubo, M., and J. M. Roberts. Cyclin-dependent regulation of G_1 in mammalian fibroblasts. *Science* 259: 1908–1912, 1993.

238. Ohtsubo, M., A. M. Theodoras, J. Schumacker, J. M. Roberts, and M. Pagano. Human cyclin E, a nuclear protein essential for the G_1-to-S phase transition. *Mol. Cell. Biol.* 15: 2612–2624, 1995.

239. Olivier, A. R., S. C. Kiley, C. Pears, D. Schaap, S. Jaken, and P. J. Parker. Protein kinase C-delta and -epsilon: a functional appraisal. *Biochem. Soc. Trans.* 20: 603–607, 1992.

240. Olivier, A. R., and P. J. Parker. Expression and characterization of protein kinase C-δ. *Eur. J. Biochem.* 200: 805–810, 1991.

241. Olivier, A. R., and P. J. Parker. Bombesin, platelet-derived growth factor, and diacylglycerol induce selective membrane association and down-regulation of protein kinase C isotypes in Swiss 3T3 cells. *J. Biol. Chem.* 269: 2758–2763, 1994.

242. Ono, Y., T. Fujii, K. Igarashi, T. Kuno, C. Tanaka, U. Kikkawa, and Y. Nishizuka. Phorbol ester binding to protein kinase C requires a cysteine-rich zinc-finger-like sequence. *Proc. Natl. Acad. Sci. U.S.A.* 86: 4868–4871, 1989.

243. Osada, S., K. Mizuno, T. C. Saido, Y. Akita, K. Suzuki, T. Kuroki, and S. Ohno. A phorbol ester receptor/protein kinase, nPKC, a new member of the protein kinase C family predominantly expressed in lung and skin. *J. Biol. Chem.* 265: 22434–22440, 1990.

244. Osada, S., K. Mizuno, T. C. Saido, K. Suzuki, T. Kuroki, and S. Ohno. A new member of the protein kinase C family, nPKCΦ, predominantly expressed in skeletal muscle. *Mol. Cell. Biol.* 12: 3930–3938, 1992.

245. Pagano, M., R. Pepperkok, F. Verde, W. Ansorge, and G. Draetta. Cyclin A is required at two points in the human cell cycle. *EMBO J.* 11: 961–971, 1992.

246. Pallas, D. C., H. Fu, L. D. Cripe, R. J. Collier, and T. M. Roberts. Association of the polyoma virus middle tumor antigen with 14–3–3 proteins. *Science* 265: 535–537, 1994.

247. Pallen, C. J., and J. H. Wang. Calmodulin-stimulated dephosphorylation of p-nitrophenylphosphate and free phosphotyrosine by calcineurin. *J. Biol. Chem.* 258: 8550–8553, 1983.

248. Papadopoulos, V. P., and P. F. Hall. Isolation and characterization of protein kinase C from Y-1 adrenal cell cytoskeleton. *J. Cell Biol.* 108: 553–567, 1989.

249. Park, J., N. R. Yaseen, P. G. Hogan, A. Rao, and S. Sharma. Phosphorylation of the transcription factor NFATp inhibits

its DNA binding activity in cyclosporin A-treated human B and T cells. *J. Biol. Chem.* 270: 20653–20659, 1995.

250. Parker, L. L., and H. Piwnica-Worms. Inactivation of the p34^{cdc2}–cyclin B complex by the human WEE1 tyrosine kinase. *Science* 257: 1955–1957, 1992.

251. Parker, L. L., S. A. Walter, P. G. Young, and H. Piwnica-Worms. Phosphorylation and inactivation of the mitotic inhibitor Wee1 by the nim1/cdr1 kinase. *Nature* 363: 736–738, 1993.

252. Pazin, M. J., and L. T. Williams. Triggering signaling cascades by receptor tyrosine kinases. *Trends Biochem. Sci.* 17: 374–378, 1992.

253. Peeper, D. S., L. L. Parker, M. E. Ewen, M. Toebes, F. L. Hall, M. Xu, A. Zantema, A. J. van der Eb, and H. Piwnica-Worms. A- and B-type cyclins differentially modulate substrate specificity of cyclin–cdk complexes. *EMBO J.* 12: 1947–1954, 1993.

254. Perrino, B. A., Y. Fong, D. A. Brickey, Y. Saitoh, Y. Ushio, K. Fukunaga, E. Miyamoto, and T. R. Soderling. Characterization of the phosphatase activity of a baculovirus-expressed calcineurin A isoform. *J. Biol. Chem.* 267: 15965–15969, 1992.

255. Perrino, B. A., L. Y. Ng, and T. R. Soderling. Calcium regulation of calcineurin phosphatase activity by its B subunit and calmodulin. *J. Biol. Chem.* 270: 340–346, 1995.

256. Pessin, M. S., and D. M. Raben. Molecular species analysis of 1,2-diacylglycerides stimulated by alpha-thrombin in cultured fibroblasts. *J. Biol. Chem.* 264: 8729–8738, 1989.

257. Peter, M., and I. Herskowitz. Joining the complex: cyclin-dependent kinase inhibitory proteins and the cell cycle. *Cell* 79: 181–184, 1994.

258. Pines, J. Cyclins and cyclin-dependent kinases: take your partners. *Trends Biochem. Sci.* 18: 195–197, 1993.

259. Pines, J., and T. Hunt. Molecular cloning and characterization of the mRNA for cyclin from sea urchin eggs. *EMBO J.* 6: 2987–2995, 1987.

260. Polyak, K., J. Kato, M. J. Solomon, C. J. Scherr, J. Massague, J. M. Roberts, and A. Koff. p27^{KIP1}, a cyclin-Cdk inhibitor, links transforming growth factor-β and contact inhibition to cell cycle arrest. *Genes Dev.* 8: 9–22, 1994.

261. Polyak, K., M. Lee, H. Erdjument-Bromage, A. Koff, J. M. Roberts, P. Tempst, and J. Massague. Cloning of p27^{Kip1}, a cyclin-dependent kinase inhibitor and a potential mediator of extracellular antimitogenic signals. *Cell* 78: 59–66, 1994.

262. Poon, R.Y.C., and T. Hunter. Dephosphorylation of cdk2 Thr^{160} by the cyclin-dependent kinase interacting phosphatase KAP in the absence of cyclin. *Science* 270: 90–93, 1995.

263. Poon, Y.C.R., K. Yamahita, J. P. Adamczewski, T. Hunt, and J. Shuttleworth. The cdc2–related protein p40^{MO15} is the catalytic subunit of a protein kinase that can activate p33^{cdk2} and p34^{cdc2}. *EMBO J.* 12: 3123–3132, 1993.

264. Quest, A.F.G., E.S.G. Bardes, and R. M. Bell. A phorbol ester binding domain of protein kinase C. *J. Biol. Chem.* 269: 2953–2960, 1994.

265. Raben, D. M., M. B. Jarpe, and K. L. Leach. Nuclear lipid metabolism in NEST: nuclear envelope signal transduction. *J. Membr. Biol.* 142: 1–7, 1994.

266. Rao, A. NFATp: a transcription factor required for the coordinate induction of several cytokine genes. *Immunol. Today* 15: 274–281, 1994.

267. Rao, A. NFATp, a cyclosporin-sensitive transcription factor implicated in cytokine gene induction. *J. Leukocyte Biol.* 57: 536–542, 1995.

268. Reuther, G. W., H. Fu, L. D. Cripe, R. J. Collier, and A. M. Pendergast. Association of the protein kinases c-Bcr and Bcr-Abl with proteins of the 14–3–3 family. *Science* 266: 129–133, 1994.

269. Roach, P. Multisite and hierarchal protein phosphorylation. *J. Biol. Chem.* 266: 14139–14142, 1991.

270. Ron, D., C. Chen, J. Caldwell, L. Jamieson, E. Orr, and D. Mochly-Rosen. Cloning of an intracellular receptor for protein kinase C: a homolog of the β subunit of G proteins. *Proc. Natl. Acad. Sci. U.S.A.* 91: 839–843, 1994.

271. Ron, D., J. Luo, and D. Mochly-Rosen. C2 region-derived peptides inhibit translocation and function of β protein kinase C *in vivo*. *J. Biol. Chem.* 270: 24180–24187, 1995.

272. Rosenmund, C., D. W. Carr, S. E. Bergeson, G. Nilaver, J. D. Scott, and G. L. Westbrook. Anchoring of protein kinase A is required for modulation of AMPA/kainate receptors on hippocampal neurons. *Nature* 368: 853–855, 1994.

273. Rosoff, P. M., N. Savage, and C. A. Dinarello. Interleukin-1 stimulates diacylglycerol production in T lymphocytes by a novel mechanism. *Cell* 54: 73–81, 1988.

274. Roy, R., J. P. Adamczewski, T. Seroz, W. Vermeulen, J. Tassan, L. Schaeffer, E. A. Nigg, J.H.J. Hoeijmakers, and J. Egly. The MO15 cell cycle kinase is associated with the TFIIH transcription-DNA repair factor. *Cell* 79: 1093–1101, 1994.

275. Ruderman, J. V. MAP kinase and the activation of quiescent cells. *Curr. Biol.* 5: 207–213, 1993.

276. Ruff, V. A., and K. L. Leach. Direct demonstration of NFAT$_p$ dephosphorylation and nuclear localization in activated HT-2 cells using a specific NFAT$_p$ polyclonal antibody. *J. Biol. Chem.* 270: 22602–22607, 1995.

277. Russell, P., and P. Nurse. cdc25$^+$ functions as an inducer in the mitotic control of fission yeast. *Cell* 45: 145–153, 1986.

278. Sadhu, K., S. I. Reed, H. Richardson, and P. Russell. Human homolog of fission yeast cdc25 mitotic inducer is predominantly expressed in G$_2$. *Proc. Natl. Acad. Sci. U.S.A.* 87: 5139–5143, 1990.

279. Said, T. K., and D. Medina. Cell cyclins and cyclin-dependent kinase activities in mouse mammary tumor development. *Carcinogenesis* 16: 823–830, 1995.

280. Sarafian, T., L. Pradel, J. Henry, D. Aunis, and M. Bader. The participation of annexin II (calpactin I) in calcium-evoked exocytosis requires protein kinase C. *J. Cell Biol.* 114: 1135–1147, 1991.

281. Schaap, D., and P. J. Parker. Expression, purification, and characterization of protein kinase C-ε. *J. Biol. Chem.* 265: 7310–7307, 1990.

282. Schaap, D., P. J. Parker, A. Bristol, R. Kriz, and J. Knopf. Unique substrate specificity and regulatory properties of PKC-ε: a rationale for diversity. *FEBS Lett.* 243: 351–357, 1989.

283. Selbie, L. A., C. Schmitz-Peiffer, Y. Sheng, and T. J. Biden. Molecular cloning and characterization of PKC iota, an atypical isoform of protein kinase C derived from insulin-secreting cells. *J. Biol. Chem.* 268: 24296–24302, 1993.

284. Shenolikar, S. Protein serine/threonine phosphatases—new avenues for cell regulation. *Annu. Rev. Cell Biol.* 10: 55–86, 1994.

285. Sherr, C. J. Mammalian G$_1$ cyclins. *Cell* 73: 1059–1065, 1993.

286. Sherr, C. J. Growth factor-regulated G$_1$ cyclins. *Stem Cells* 12: 47–57, 1994.

287. Sherr, C. J. G1 phase progression: cycling on cue. *Cell* 79: 551–555, 1994.

288. Sheu, F., R. M. Marais, P. J. Parker, N. G. Bazan, and A. Routtenberg. Neuron-specific protein F1/GAP-43 shows substrate specificity for the beta subtype of protein kinase C. *Biochem. Biophys. Res. Commun.* 171: 1236–1243, 1990.

289. Shinomura, T., Y. Asaoka, M. Oka, K. Yoshida, and Y. Nishizuka. Synergistic action of diacylglycerol and unsaturated fatty acid for protein kinase C activation: its possible implications. *Proc. Natl. Acad. Sci. U.S.A.* 88: 5149–5153, 1991.

290. Soderling, T. R. Protein kinases. *J. Biol. Chem.* 265: 1823–1826, 1990.

291. Soderling, T. R. Protein kinases and phosphatases: regulation by autoinhibitory domains. *Biotechnol. Appl. Biochem.* 18: 185–200, 1993.

292. Solomon, M. J., J. W. Harper, and J. Shuttleworth. CAK, the p34^cdc2 activating kinase, contains a protein identical or closely related to p40. *EMBO J.* 12: 3133–3142, 1993.

293. Solomon, M. J., T. Lee, and M. W. Kirschner. Role of phosphorylation in p34^cdc2 activation: identification of an activating kinase. *Mol. Biol. Cell* 3: 13–27, 1992.

294. Stabel, S. Protein kinase C—an enzyme and its relatives. *Semin. Cancer Biol.* 5: 277–284, 1994.

295. Stabel, S., and P. J. Parker. Protein kinase C. *Pharmacol. Ther.* 51: 71–95, 1991.

296. Stemmer, P. M., and C. B. Klee. Dual calcium ion regulation of calcineurin by calmodulin and calcineurin B. *Biochemistry* 33: 6859–6866, 1994.

297. Stewart, A. A., T. S. Ingebritsen, A. Manalan, C. B. Klee, and P. Cohen. Discovery of a Ca^{2+}- and calmodulin-dependent protein phosphatase. *FEBS Lett.* 137: 80–84, 1982.

298. Strausfield, U., A. Fernandez, J. Capony, F. Girard, N. Lautredou, J. Derancourt, J. Labbe, and N.J.C. Lamb. Activation of p34^cdc2 protein kinase by microinjection of human cdc25c into mammalian cells. *J. Biol. Chem.* 269: 5989–6000, 1994.

299. Strausfeld, U., J. C. Labbe, D. Fesquet, J. C. Cavadore, A. Picard, K. Sadhu, P. Russell, and M. Doree. Dephosphorylation and activation of a p34^cdc2/cyclin B complex *in vitro* by human cdc25 protein. *Nature* 351: 242–245, 1991.

300. Sun, H., C. H. Charles, L. F. Lau, and N. K. Tonks. MKP-1 (3CH134), an immediate early gene product, is a dual specificity phosphatase that dephosphorylates MAP kinase in vivo. *Cell* 75: 487–493, 1993.

301. Sun, H., and N. K. Tonks. The coordinated action of protein tyrosine phosphatases and kinases in cell signaling. *Trends Biochem. Sci.* 19: 480–484, 1994.

302. Tallant, E. A., and W. Y. Cheung. Calmodulin-dependent protein phosphatase: a developmental study. *Biochemistry* 22: 3630–3635, 1983.

303. Tallant, E. A., and W. Y. Cheung. Characterization of bovine brain calmodulin-dependent protein phosphatase. *Arch. Biochem. Biophys.* 232: 269–279, 1984.

304. Tallant, E. A., and W. Y. Cheung. Calmodulin-dependent protein phosphatase. In: *Calcium and Cell Function,* edited by W. Y. Cheung. Orlando, FL: Academic, 1986, p. 71–111.

305. Tanaka, T., H. Ohta, K. Kanda, H. Hidaka, and K. Sobue. Phosphorylation of high M_r caldesmon by protein kinase-C modulates the regulatory function of this protein on the interaction between actin and myosin. *Eur. J. Biochem.* 188: 495–500, 1990.

306. Tang, Z., T. R. Coleman, and W. G. Dunphy. Two distinct mechanisms for negative regulation of the Wee1 protein kinase. *EMBO J.* 12: 3427–3436, 1993.

307. Taylor, S. S., D. R. Knighton, J. Zheng, J. M. Sowadski, C. S. Gibbs, and M. J. Zoller. A template for the protein kinase family. *Trends Biochem. Sci.* 18: 84–89, 1993.

308. Thomas, T. P., H. S. Talwar, and W. B. Anderson. Phorbol ester-mediated association of protein kinase C to the nuclear

309. Tonks, N. K., C. D. Diltz, and E. H. Fischer. Purification of the major protein-tyrosine-phosphatase of human placenta. *J. Biol. Chem.* 263: 6722–6730, 1988.

310. Toyoshima, H., and T. Hunter. p27, a novel inhibitor of G1 cyclin-cdk protein kinase activity, is related to p21. *Cell* 78: 67–74, 1994.

311. Ueki, K., and R. L. Kincaid. Interchangeable associations of calcineurin regulatory subunit isoforms with mammalian and fungal catalytic subunits. *J. Biol. Chem.* 268: 6554–6559, 1993.

312. Ueki, K., T. Muramatsu, and R. L. Kincaid. Structure and expression of two isoforms of the murine calmodulin-dependent protein phosphatase regulatory subunit (calcineurin B). *Biochem. Biophys. Res. Commun.* 187: 537–543, 1992.

313. Ullman, K. S., J. P. Northrup, C. L. Verweij, and G. R. Crabtree. Transmission of signals from the T lymphocyte antigen receptor to the genes responsible for cell proliferation and immune function: the missing link. *Annu. Rev. Immunol.* 8: 421–452, 1990.

314. Ullrich, A., and J. Schlessinger. Signal transduction by receptors with tyrosine kinase activity. *Cell* 61: 203–212, 1990.

315. van den Heuvel, S., and E. Harlow. Distinct roles for cyclin-dependent kinases in cell cycle control. *Science* 262: 2050–2054, 1993.

316. Villa-Moruzzi, E. Activation of the cdc25c phosphatase in mitotic HeLa cells. *Biochem. Biophys. Res. Commun.* 196: 1248–1254, 1993.

317. Wadzinski, B. E., L. E. Heasley, and G. L. Johnson. Multiplicity of protein serine-threonine phosphatases in PC12 pheochromocytoma and FTO-2B hepatoma cells. *J. Biol. Chem.* 265: 21504–21508, 1990.

318. Walker, D. H., and J. L. Maller. Role of cyclin A in the dependence of mitosis on completion of DNA replication. *Nature* 354: 314–317, 1991.

319. Walker, D. H., N. R. Murray, D. J. Burns, and A. P. Fields. Protein kinase C chimeras: catalytic domains of α and β_{II} protein kinase C contain determinants for isotype-specific function. *Proc. Natl. Acad. Sci. U.S.A.* 92: 9156–9160, 1995.

320. Wallace, R. W., E. A. Tallant, and W. Y. Cheung. High levels of a heat-labile calmodulin-binding protein (CaM-BP$_{80}$) in bovine neostriatum. *Biochemistry* 19: 1831–1837, 1980.

321. Walton, K. M., and J. E. Dixon. Protein tyrosine phosphatases. *Annu. Rev. Biochem.* 62: 101–120, 1993.

322. Ward, Y., S. Gupta, P. Jensen, M. Wartmann, R. J. Davis, and K. Kelly. Control of MAP kinase activation by the mitogen-induced threonine/tyrosine phosphatase PAC1. *Nature* 367: 651–654, 1994.

323. Waseem, A., and H. C. Palfrey. Identification and protein kinase C-dependent phosphorylation of α-adducin in human fibroblasts. *J. Cell Sci.* 96: 93–98, 1990.

324. Watanabe, N., M. Broome, and T. Hunter. Regulation of the human WEE1Hu cdk tyrosine 15-kinase during the cell cycle. *EMBO J.* 14: 1878–1891, 1995.

325. Watanabe, Y., B. A. Perrino, B. H. Chang, and T. R. Soderling. Identification in the calcineurin A subunit of the domain that binds the regulatory B subunit. *J. Biol. Chem.* 270: 456–460, 1995.

326. Weinstein, I. B., P. B. Fisher, A. Mufson, and H. Yamasaki. Action of phorbol esters in cell culture: mimicry of transformation, altered differentiation, and effects on cell membranes. *J. Supramol. Struct.* 12: 195–208, 1979.

fraction in NIH 3T3 cells. *Cancer Res.* 48: 1910–1919, 1988.

327. Wetsel, W. C., W. A. Khan, I. Merchenthaler, H. Rivera, A. E. Halpern, H. M. Phung, A. Negro-Vilar, and Y. A. Hannun. Tissue and cellular distribution of the extended family of protein kinase C isoenzymes. *J. Cell Biol.* 117: 121–133, 1992.

328. Wood, J. G., R. W. Wallace, J. N. Whitaker, and W. Y. Cheung. Immunocytochemical localization of calmodulin and a heat-labile calmodulin-binding protein (CaM-BP$_{80}$) in basal ganglia of mouse brain. *J. Cell. Biol.* 84: 66–76, 1980.

329. Wooten, M. W., and R. W. Wrenn. Phorbol ester induces intracellular translocation of phospholipid/Ca^{2+}-dependent protein kinase and stimulates amylase secretion in isolated pancreatic acini. *FEBS Lett.* 171: 183–186, 1984.

330. Wright, T. M., L. A. Rangan, H. S. Shin, and D. M. Raben. Kinetic analysis of 1,2-diacylglycerol mass levels in cultured fibroblasts. Comparison of stimulation by alpha-thrombin and epidermal growth factor. *J. Biol. Chem.* 263: 9374–9380, 1988.

331. Wright, T. M., H. S. Shin, and D. M. Raben. Sustained increase in 1,2-diacylglycerol precedes DNA synthesis in epidermal-growth-factor-stimulated fibroblasts. Evidence for stimulated phosphatidylcholine hydrolysis. *Biochem. J.* 267: 501–507, 1990.

332. Wu, J., J. K. Harrison, L. A. Vincent, C. Haystead, T.A.J. Haystead, H. Michel, D. F. Hunt, K. R. Lynch, and T. W. Sturgill. Molecular structure of a protein-tyrosine/threonine kinase activating p42 mitogen-activated protein (MAP) kinase: MAP kinase kinase. *Proc. Natl. Acad. Sci. U.S.A.* 90: 173–177, 1993.

333. Wu, J., H. Michel, P. Dent, T. Haystead, D. F. Hunt, and T. W. Sturgill. Activation of MAP kinase by a dual specificity tyr/thr kinase. *Adv. Second Messenger Phosphoprotein Res.* 28: 219–225, 1993.

334. Wu, L., and P. Russell. Nim1 kinase promotes mitosis by inactivating Wee1 tyrosine kinase. *Nature* 363: 738–741, 1993.

335. Wu, L., A. Yee, L. Liu, D. Carbonaro-Hall, N. Venkatesan, V. T. Tolo, and F. L. Hall. Molecular cloning of the human CAK1 gene encoding a cyclin-dependent kinase-activating kinase. *Oncogene* 9: 2089–2096, 1994.

336. Yang, Z., N. D. Perkins, T. Ohno, E. Nabel, and G. J. Nabel. The p21 cyclin-dependent kinase inhibitor suppresses tumorigenicity *in vivo*. *Nature Med.* 1: 1052–1056, 1995.

337. Yazdanbakhsh, K., J. Choi, Y. Li, L. F. Lau, and Y. Choi. Cyclosporin A blocks apoptosis by inhibiting the DNA binding activity of the transcription factor Nur77. *Proc. Natl. Acad. Sci. U.S.A.* 92: 437–441, 1995.

338. Yoshida, K., Y. Asaoka, and Y. Nishizuka. Platelet activation by simultaneous actions of diacylglycerol and free unsaturated fatty acids. *Proc. Natl. Acad. Sci. U.S.A.* 89: 6443–6446, 1992.

339. Young, S., P. J. Parker, A. Ullrich, and S. Stabel. Down-regulation of protein kinase C is due to an increased rate of degradation. *Biochem. J.* 244: 775–779, 1987.

340. Zhang, G., M. G. Kazanietz, P. M. Blumberg, and J. H. Hurley. Crystal structure of the Cys2 activator-binding domain of protein kinase Cδ in complex with phorbol ester. *Cell* 81: 917–924, 1995.

341. Zhao, Y., Y. Tozawa, R. Iseki, M. Mukai, and M. Iwata. Calcineurin activation protects T cells from glucocorticoid-induced apoptosis. *J. Immunol.* 154: 6346–6354, 1995.

342. Zheng, X., and J. V. Ruderman. Functional analysis of the P box, a domain in cyclin B required for the activation of cdc25. *Cell* 75: 155–164, 1993.

343. Zhou, G., J. M. Denu, L. Wu, and J. E. Dixon. The catalytic role of Cys^{124} in the dual specificity phosphatase VHR. *J. Biol. Chem.* 269: 28084–28090, 1994.

11. Phospholipid-derived second messengers

JOHN H. EXTON | *Howard Hughes Medical Institute and Department of Molecular Physiology and Biophysics, Vanderbilt University School of Medicine, Nashville, Tennessee*

CHAPTER CONTENTS

THE INITIAL DISCOVERY by Hokin and Hokin (119, 120) that cholinergic agents induce the turnover of inositol phospholipids in pancreas and brain led to a vast new area of biological research. In a classic review, Michell (223) demonstrated the widespread nature of the phenomenon and proposed that it was intimately involved in the mechanism of action of many agonists. Later work (14) showed that the inositol phospholipid that is initially hydrolyzed is not phosphatidylinositol (PI), but phosphatidylinositol 4,5-bisphosphate (PIP_2). This led to the demonstration that the product of phospholipase C (PLC) action on PIP_2, namely, inositol 1,4,5-trisphosphate (IP_3), is a major intracellular signal that mobilizes Ca^{2+} from nonmitochondrial stores (13, 14, 327).

In parallel studies, Nishizuka (239) discovered protein kinase C (PKC) and found that it depends on phospholipids, especially phosphatidylserine, for activity and is regulated by Ca^{2+} and 1,2-diacylglycerol (DAG). Protein kinase C was found to exist in many isoforms, many of which were widely distributed, and the enzyme was proposed to play an important role in cell signaling. Since DAG is the other product of PLC action on PIP_2, it became apparent that PIP_2 hydrolysis is bifunctional in that it generates two intracellular signals (14). Studies of the molecular mechanism by which agonists activate PIP_2-specific PLC subsequently showed that there are two major systems, one involving growth factors and the tyrosine kinase activity of their receptors and one involving heterotrimeric G proteins that are either sensitive or insensitive to pertussis toxin (87, 284).

Measurements of the changes in the level and chemical composition of DAG in cells stimulated with agonists revealed that another phospholipid was being hydrolyzed, and this was identified as phosphatidylcholine (PC) (19, 85). Surprisingly, the phospholipase responsible for the hydrolysis of PC in most cells was found to be phospholipase D (PLD) (19, 85). The product of PLD action, phosphatidic acid (PA), is rapidly converted to DAG by phosphatidate phosphohydrolase (PAP), accounting for the second phase of DAG accumulation observed in many stimulated cells (19, 85, 86). Agonist activation of PLD was found to occur through receptors linked to heterotrimeric G proteins and receptors with tyrosine kinase activity, but the molecular mechanisms involved are still unclear (86). Phosphatidic acid is generally considered to be an intracellular signal, but its physiological targets have not been rigorously defined.

Hydrolysis of PC and phosphatidylethanolamine by phospholipase A_2 (PLA_2) has long been known to be a major source of the arachidonic acid (AA) that accumulates in many stimulated cells (69, 70). This is subsequently converted to a variety of eicosanoids, depending on the cell type. As in the case of PLD, the molecular mechanisms by which agonists activate PLA_2 are incompletely defined (69, 86).

Another phospholipid involved in cell signaling is sphingomyelin, (SM) which is hydrolyzed by sphingomyelinase (SMase) in response to certain cytokines (70, 112, 165). The hydrolysis releases P-choline and ceramide, and the latter acts as an intracellular signal, apparently by controlling certain protein kinases and phosphatases (112, 165). Although important physiological effects have been attributed to the activation of SMase, the mechanisms involved in the generation of these effects are largely undefined.

INOSITOL PHOSPHOLIPID HYDROLYSIS

Functional Significance

Inositol Trisphosphate and Ca^{2+} Mobilization. As alluded to above, PIP_2 hydrolysis is a widespread cellular response to many hormones, neurotransmitters, growth factors, and related agonists. Activation of PLC isozymes that are specific for inositol-containing phospholipids (designated "PI-PLC isozymes") leads to rapid hydrolysis of PIP_2 in the plasma membrane and a prompt increase of IP_3 in the cytosol (14, 87) (Fig. 11.1). This promotes the release of Ca^{2+} from components of the endoplasmic reticulum by binding to IP_3 receptors. These receptors exist in several isoforms, which have a membrane-spanning domain in the C-terminus and a large N-terminal domain ending in the IP_3-binding site (94, 222). Four of the receptors combine to form an IP_3-sensitive Ca^{2+} channel. The heterogeneity of the receptors comes from the existence of separate genes and from alternative splicing in the IP_3-binding domain (222). They show partial homology with ryanodine receptors, which also form Ca^{2+} channels in the endoplasmic reticulum and are part of the T-tubule foot structures of the sarcoplasmic reticulum (201). Ryanodine opens the channels at nanomolar concentrations but closes them at higher concentrations. Caffeine also can open ryanodine channels, which are present in many different cell types. The putative intracellular signal cyclic adenosine diphosphate ribose (cADPR) (184) also activates ryanodine channels in some cell types (317).

Studies of the effects of Ca^{2+}-mobilizing agonists on single cells have revealed that the increase in Ca^{2+} first occurs in a localized region and spreads as a wave throughout the cell (15, 17). The Ca^{2+} stores at the initiation site appear to be more sensitive to IP_3 (17), and the released Ca^{2+} triggers a regenerative response that propagates outward. A key factor in wave propagation is Ca^{2+}-induced Ca^{2+} release, whereby the Ca^{2+} released from the initiation site diffuses out to cause the release of Ca^{2+} from other stores, which then provide Ca^{2+} to propagate the wave further (15). Both IP_3- and cADPR-sensitive Ca^{2+} stores display Ca^{2+}-induced Ca^{2+} release, and both compounds enhance the sensitivity of their receptors to the stimulatory action of Ca^{2+} (17). Most studies show that Ca^{2+} is stimulatory at low concentrations but becomes inhibitory at high concentrations, and the latter effect may terminate the release of Ca^{2+} (27).

Calcium release may be localized in the form of a "spark" or "puff," or it may lead to regenerating waves that are reflected in the oscillations in cytosolic Ca^{2+} observed in many cells (17, 27). Several models have been advanced to explain periodic Ca^{2+} spike initiation and wave propagation (15, 17, 27, 48). Groups of cells also may show synchronized oscillations, and the diffusible signal may be IP_3, which crosses gap junctions (17).

Mobilization of intracellular Ca^{2+} by agonists is typically followed by an influx of extracellular Ca^{2+}, which sustains the elevation of cytosolic Ca^{2+} (15, 264). Studies of the entry of Ca^{2+} have shown that it is due to the opening of specific plasma membrane channels, termed "Ca^{2+} release–activated Ca^{2+} channels," that are regulated by the Ca^{2+} content of the intracellular stores (16, 17, 48, 264, 276) (Fig. 11.1). The channels are formed by subunits corresponding to the Trp proteins of the *Drosophila* photoreceptor, which form light-activated Ca^{2+} channels (20a). Evidence for the existence of a factor released from the stores that controls the channels has been presented

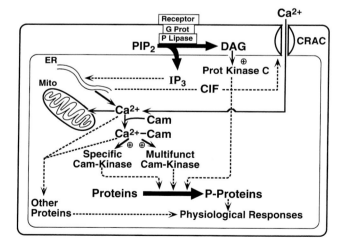

FIG. 11.1. Mechanisms involved in physiological responses mediated by receptors linked through G proteins to phosphoinositide phospholipase C. *G Prot*, G protein; *P Lipase*, phospholipase C; *PIP₂*, phosphatidylinositol 4,5–P₂; *IP₃*, inositol 1,4,5–P₃; *DAG*, 1,2–diacylglycerol; *CIF*, putative Ca^{2+} influx factor; *CRAC*, Ca^{2+}-release-activated Ca^{2+} channel; *ER*, endoplasmic reticulum; *Mito*, mitochondrion; *Cam*, calmodulin.

(281, 335), but its chemical nature has not been defined. An alternative hypothesis is that the cytoplasmic head of the IP$_3$ receptor is apposed to the Ca^{2+} channel and regulates it through a protein–protein interaction (16).

Consistent with its function as a dynamic intracellular signal, IP$_3$ is rapidly metabolized by a 5-phosphatase and a 3-kinase to generate inositol 1,4-bisphosphate and inositol 1,3,4,5-tetrakisphosphate, respectively (312). These phosphate esters are further degraded by specific phosphatases (312). Inositol 1,4-bisphosphate has no known biological activity, whereas the role of inositol 1,3,4,5-tetrakisphosphate remains unclear (366).

Diacylglycerol and Protein Kinase C Activation.
Hydrolysis of PIP$_2$ produces DAG, and this can activate all of the isozymes of PKC except the ζ and λ (ι) atypical forms (241) (Fig. 11.1). Like tumor-promoting phorbol esters, DAG interacts with the C1 domain of the typical (conventional and new) PKC isoforms to activate them in a phosphatidylserine-dependent manner (240). In the case of the Ca^{2+}-dependent (conventional) α, β_1, β_2, and γ isoforms, DAG also lowers the concentration of Ca^{2+} required to activate the enzyme (239). The accumulation of DAG in the plasma membrane due to activation of PI-PLC is associated with translocation of PKC isozymes from the cytosol to this site. Reversal of the activation of PKC occurs as a result of the metabolism of DAG. This occurs principally by conversion of DAG to monoacylglycerol by DAG lipase, but there is also formation of PA by DAG kinase. These lipids are metabolized further in the plasma membrane or the endoplasmic reticulum.

The physiological substrates of PKC isozymes have not been fully defined, but a substrate in most cells is MARCKS (myristoylated alanine-rich C-kinase substrate), which is thought to be involved in chemotaxis and other processes involving changes in cell shape and mobility (22). Another common substrate is pleckstrin, which becomes phosphorylated during platelet activation (116, 130). Also, PKC phosphorylates certain growth factor receptors, α_1-adrenergic receptors, Na$^+$/H$^+$ antiporter isoforms, and certain types of ion channel (86). In many cases, phosphorylation of these proteins is associated with activity changes. In addition to MARCKS, neurogranin and neuromodulin are prominent PKC substrates in brain, and functional changes have been attributed to their phosphorylation (308). Several nuclear substrates of PKC have been identified, and some PKC isozymes have been identified in the nucleus (34). There is evidence of the presence of PI-PLC in the nucleus (7, 87). α-Thrombin increases nuclear DAG in fibroblasts (138, 182), but the mechanisms by which this occurs are unknown. Some of the in vivo nuclear substrates of PKC are lamin B, a constituent of the nuclear lamina, and DNA topoisomerase I and myogenin, two proteins that interact with DNA (34).

Accumulation of DAG in response to agonists is biphasic in most cell types (85, 86). The first, transient peak is associated with release of IP$_3$ and is enriched in arachidonic and stearic acids, which are the major fatty acids in inositol phospholipids. The second, prolonged component has a different fatty acid composition and is accompanied by release of choline, consistent with its origin from PC and perhaps other phospholipids (85, 86). Some agonists, for example, interleukin-1, cause the accumulation of ether-linked species (alkyl acylglycerol and alkenyl acylglycerol), which arise from ethanolamine plasmalogens (364). These species inhibit activation of PKC by ester-linked DAG species derived from other phospholipids (64, 231).

Although PKC is the major target of agonist-derived DAG in cells, other proteins are potentially influenced by this lipid. These include n-chimaerin, which contains a cysteine-rich region homologous to those in PKC and a sequence homologous to Bcr, a guanosine triphosphatase (GTPase)–activating protein (GAP) for the small M_r protein Rho (3). DAG kinase, which contains cysteine-rich motifs similar to PKC, undergoes membrane translocation in response to DAG (208). GTP:phosphocholine cytidyltransferase, which catalyzes the rate-limiting step in PC synthesis, also has a motif that resembles the cysteine-rich regions of PKC and undergoes translocation and activation when cellular levels of DAG increase (137, 148). Another possible target of DAG is acidic sphingomyelinase, which is implicated in the production of ceramide from sphingomyelin (304).

Phosphoinositide Phospholipases as Targets of Hormones and Growth Factors

Mechanisms of Activation Involving G Proteins.
Early studies of the effects of GTP analogs on PI hydrolysis in plasma membranes and permeabilized cells indicated the involvement of heterotrimeric G proteins in the regulation of PI-PLC (87). Work with pertussis toxin showed that both toxin-sensitive and -insensitive G proteins were involved, depending on the agonist and cell type (220). It is now known that the toxin-insensitive G proteins that mediate agonist control of PI-PLC are members of the G$_q$ family of G proteins, which include G$_q$, G$_{11}$, G$_{14}$, G$_{15}$, and G$_{16}$, whereas the toxin-sensitive G proteins are subtypes of G$_i$ (G$_{i1-3}$) and of G$_o$ (G$_{o1,2}$) (87) (Fig. 11.2). Stimulation of PI-PLC by the G$_q$ family

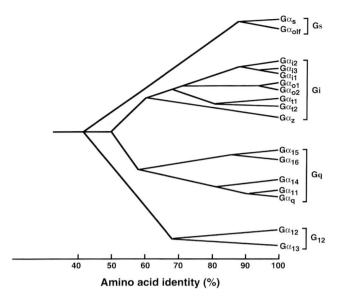

FIG. 11.2. Heterotrimeric G protein families. The four families of G protein α-subunits are displayed in terms of their amino-acid identity. [Reproduced from Simon et al. (314a), with permission.]

is considered to be mediated by their α-subunits and that of G_i and G_o by their βγ complexes. However, this may not always be the case (322).

The many isoforms of PI-PLC are divided into three families (β, γ, δ isozymes) (186, 284) (Fig. 11.3). All of the isozymes have two regions (X and Y) of high sequence similarity that are believed to represent the catalytic domain, and there is a pleckstrin homology domain in the N-terminus (186). All of the isozymes are Ca^{2+}-dependent and contain Ca^{2+} lipid–binding (CaLB) domains. There are four mammalian β isozymes, which have long C-terminal sequences; two γ isozymes, which have Src homology (SH2 and SH3) domains and PH domains between the X and Y regions; and three δ isozymes, which have short C-terminal sequences and are of lower M_r than the other forms (186) (Fig. 11.3).

All four PI-PLC β isozymes are regulated by G_q α-subunits, though the β1 isozyme shows the largest activation and the β2 isozyme the least (87). The β1 and β3 isozymes are widely distributed, whereas the β2 isozyme is confined to cells of hematopoietic origin

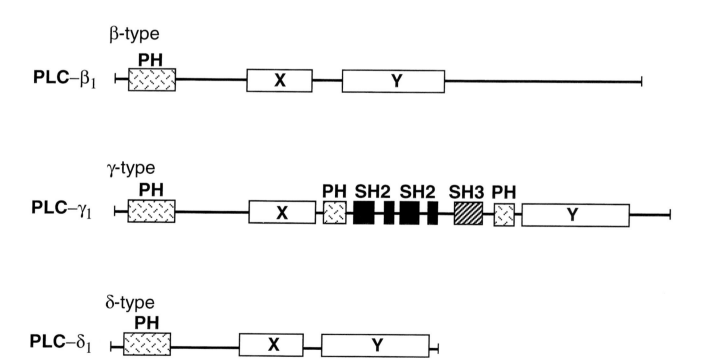

FIG. 11.3. Structural features of the β, γ, and δ isotypes of phosphoinositide phospholipase C. The conserved X and Y domains are believed to be involved in catalysis. *PH*, pleckstrin homology domain; *SH2* and *SH3*, Src homology domains.

and the $\beta 4$ isozyme is found mainly in the retina (183). The most widespread members of the G_q family are G_q and G_{11}, though tissue differences occur; G_{15} and G_{16} are mouse/human homologs and are restricted to hematopoietic cells; and G_{14} has a wider distribution but is found mainly in kidney, lung, spleen, and testis (87).

A very large number of agonists acting through specific receptor subtypes utilize pertussis toxin–insensitive G proteins (presumably G_q family members) to activate PI-PLC (220). These include epinephrine and norepinephrine (α_1-adrenergic receptors), vasopressin (V1 receptors), acetylcholine (M1, M3, and M5 receptors), angiotensin II (AT$_1$ receptors), serotonin (5HT$_2$ receptors), adenosine triphosphate (ATP) (P$_{2Y}$ purinergic receptors), thromboxane A$_2$, histamine (H1 receptors), bombesin (BB$_1$ and BB$_2$ receptors), bradykinin (B$_1$ and B$_2$ receptors), cholecystokinin and gastrin, endothelin (ET$_A$ and ET$_B$ receptors), neurotensin receptor (NTR), and tachykinins (NK receptors).

Like other receptors that couple to G proteins, the receptors that interact with G_q have seven transmembrane helices (Fig. 11.4) that are arranged ring-like to form a helical bundle (9a, 29a, 363a). They also have N-terminal extracellular and C-terminal cytoplasmic tails of variable length and three extracellular and three cytoplasmic loops (300). Most studies have identified sequences in the third cytoplasmic loop, which is of variable length, as critical for selective interaction with G proteins, with the second loop and the C-terminal tail contributing some determinants of specificity (9a, 87, 300, 363a). In most cases, ligands bind to residues in certain transmembrane helices, and this causes a separation of the helices and the postulated opening of a crevice in the intracellular surface of the receptor for the binding/activation of specific G proteins (9a, 29a, 300, 363a). This leads to the release of guanosine diphosphate (GDP) from the guanine nucleotide–binding cleft of the G protein α-subunit and its replace-

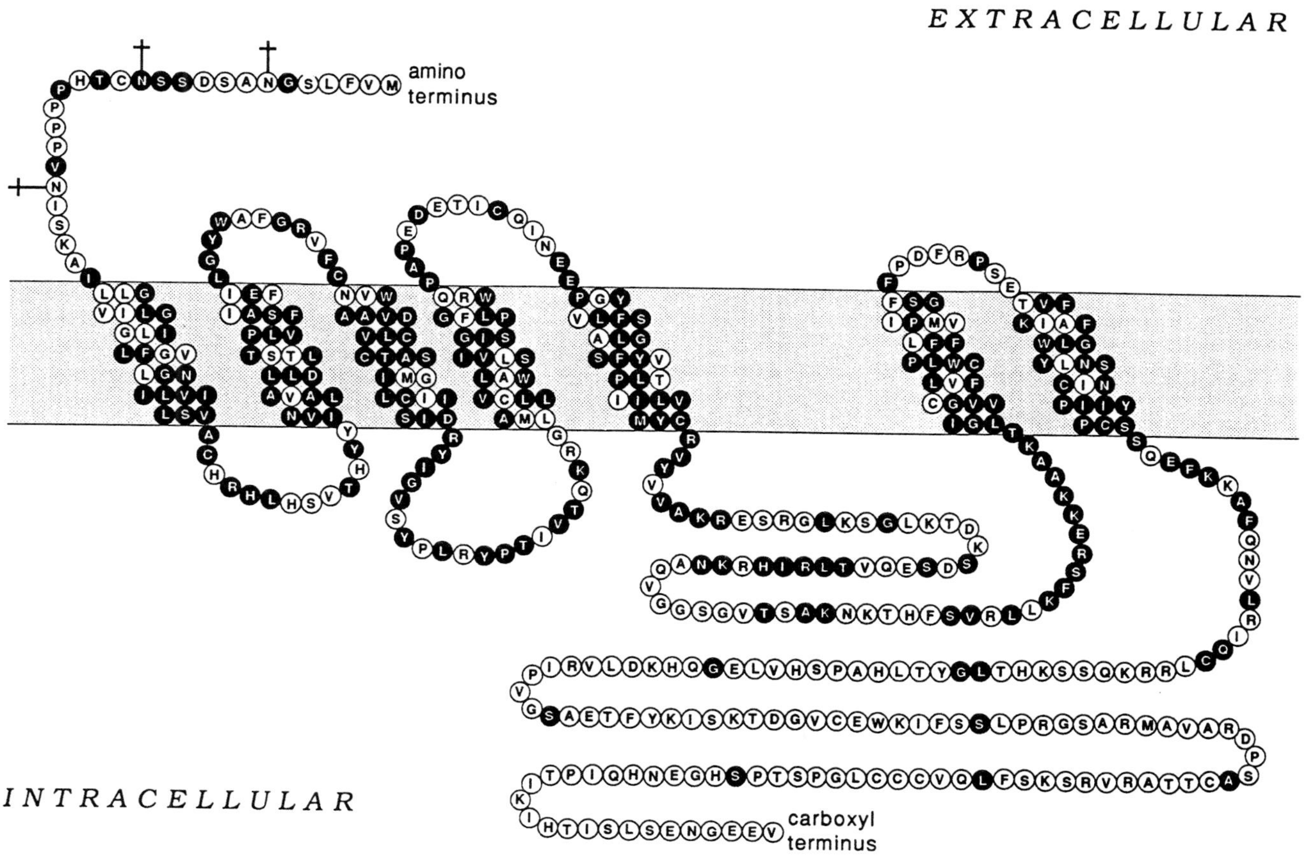

FIG. 11.4. Transmembrane-spanning model of the bovine α_{1A}-adrenergic receptor. The seven transmembrane helices are defined on the basis of hydropathic analysis. Black residues are those common to the hamster α_{1B}-adrenergic receptor. Presumed glycosylation sites are marked with crosses. [Reproduced from Schwinn et al. (304a), with permission.]

ment by GTP (58, 178) (Fig. 11.5). Other changes subsequent to GTP binding occur, including activation of the α-subunit and its dissociation from the receptor and the $\beta\gamma$ complex. The activated α-subunit interacts with a specific effector(s), but the change in the activity of the effector is transient because the α-subunit possesses an intrinsic GTPase activity which hydrolyzes the bound GTP to GDP, leading to inactivation of the α-subunit and reformation of the heterotrimeric G-protein complex (58). In the persistent presence of agonist, continuing generation of GTP-liganded α-subunits occurs and the activation (or inactivation) of the effector is maintained unless the system becomes desensitized. Additional proteins regulate the interaction of receptors with G proteins. These include a recently discovered family of proteins termed RGSs (regulators of G protein–dependent signaling), which act as negative regulators by stimulating the hydrolysis of GTP bound to G protein α-subunits (79a).

The α-subunits of the G_q family have a low intrinsic GTP/GDP exchange activity, and stimulation of this activity by agonist-bound receptor produces a rapid and large increase in PIP$_2$ hydrolysis (87). The subunits also possess low GTPase activity, but this is activated by PI-PLCβ isozymes (87) and certain RGS proteins (118b), leading to a rapid turnoff of IP$_3$ production when an agonist is withdrawn. The α-subunits interact

with a defined domain in the C-terminal region of the PI-PLCβ isozymes (87, 186), and the domain on the α-subunit involved in this interaction contains residues in the third α-helix and an adjacent sequence in the GTPase component of the molecule (6, 87, 178, 355). It is of particular interest that the sequences involved in interaction with PI-PLCβ are close to a switch region whose conformation changes when the α-subunit is activated (178, 355). In contrast, a major region of the α-subunit involved in receptor interaction is the C-terminal tail (58, 87, 178). The molecular mechanisms by which receptors activate G proteins and by which G proteins alter the activity of effectors remain to be defined.

The pertussis toxin–sensitive mechanism of agonist activation of PIP$_2$ hydrolysis (220) involves subtypes of G_i and G_o proteins. A surprising feature of the system is that the activating component of the G proteins is not the α-subunit but the $\beta\gamma$ complex (87, 186, 325) (Fig. 11.6). The PI-PLC isozymes that are targets of the $\beta\gamma$ complex are members of the PI-PLCβ family, with the exception of the β_4 isozyme. In contrast to the case with G_q α-subunits, the β_3 isozyme shows the greatest response to $\beta\gamma$ and the β_1 isozyme shows the least (87, 186, 325). The $\beta\gamma$ complex can regulate other effectors, including certain adenylate cyclase isoforms, the muscarinic-regulated cardiac K$^+$ channel, a

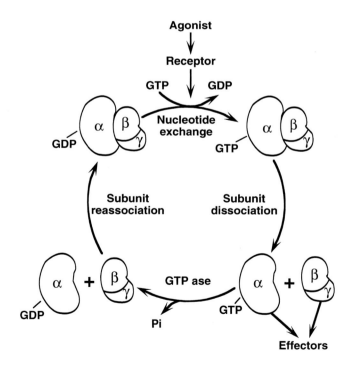

FIG. 11.5. Mechanisms involved in activation/deactivation of heterotrimeric G proteins.

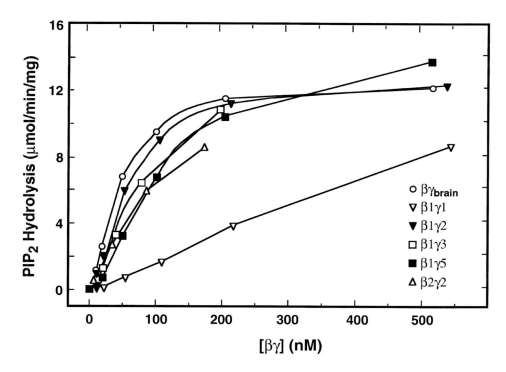

FIG. 11.6. Stimulation of phosphoinositide phospholipase $\beta3$ by G protein $\beta\gamma$-subunits. Experimental conditions were as described in Blank et al. (22a). $\beta\gamma$-subunits were prepared from bovine brain or produced by recombinant means in Sf9 cells. [From unpublished studies by J. L. Blank, J. A. Iniguez-Luihi, N. Ueda, A. G. Gilman, and J. H. Exton.]

PI 3-kinase isoenzyme, and β-adrenergic receptor kinases (49, 87, 325).

The domain at on PI-PLCβ_2 at which the $\beta\gamma$ complex interacts has been narrowed to a 60 amino acid sequence in the X region (170b). Thus, the domains for binding of α_q and $\beta\gamma$ are well separated, and the enzymes are activated by these subunits in an additive manner (186). Five different subtypes of G protein β-subunit and 12 subtypes of γ-subunit have been identified. In contrast to the high effector specificity observed for different G protein α-subunits, little effector selectivity has been reported for β- and γ-subunits, apart from a low potency for the $\beta_1\gamma_1$ complex in activating PI-PLC and adenylyl cyclase isoforms (Fig. 11.6) (87, 325).

Signaling through G_i and G_o provides the possibility of bifunctional control of effectors through α-subunits and $\beta\gamma$ complexes. Thus, receptor activation of G_i could release α_i, which would inhibit adenylyl cyclase, and $\beta\gamma$, which could activate PI-PLC. Such bifunctional signaling has been shown in Chinese hamster ovary (CHO) cells expressing M2 muscarinic receptors and a pertussis toxin–resistant mutant of α_{i2} (129). Although the concentrations of $\beta\gamma$ required to activate

effectors in vitro are high relative to the effective concentrations of α-subunits (87, 325), G_i and G_o are more abundant than most other G proteins, and studies in intact cells have shown that control of PI-PLC and adenylyl cyclase through the $\beta\gamma$ complex does occur (164).

The agonists and receptors linked to G_i include epinephrine and norepinephrine (α_2-adrenergic receptors), acetylcholine (M2 and M4 receptors), glutamate (mGluR receptors), serotonin ($5HT_1$ receptors), adenosine (A_1 and A_3 receptors), bradykinin, thrombin, fMet-Leu-Phe, and somatostatin. Although activation of these receptors is associated with a decrease in cyclic adenosine monophosphate (cAMP), changes in PIP_2 hydrolysis are not always apparent. This may be due to the fact that high concentrations of $\beta\gamma$ are required to activate PI-PLC (87, 325). Alternatively, it might reflect differences in the tissue distribution of PI-PLC and adenylyl cyclase isozymes (325) and/or differences in the subtypes of $\beta\gamma$ released.

Mechanisms of Activation Involving Tyrosine Kinases.
Many growth factors activate PI-PLCγ1. Examples are

epidermal growth factor (EGF), platelet-derived growth factor (PDGF), basic fibroblast growth factor (bFGF), hepatocyte growth factor (HGF), and nerve growth factor (NGF) (186). Binding of these growth factors to their receptors results in dimerization of the receptors and activation of their intrinsic tyrosine kinase activity (Fig. 11.7). This induces phosphorylation of the receptor itself (autophosphorylation) and other cellular proteins. Autophosphorylation occurs on specific tyrosine residues in the cytoplasmic segment of the receptors (Fig. 11.7) (118, 262). The phosphorylated tyrosines and surrounding residues provide high-affinity binding sites for cytoplasmic proteins. These include PI-PLCγ1; the 85 kd regulatory subunit of PI 3-kinase; Ras GAP; SH2–containing adaptor proteins such as Grb2, Shc, Crk, and Nck; the soluble tyrosine kinase Src; and the tyrosine phosphatase Syp (118, 262).

Association of these proteins to specific receptor sequences containing phosphotyrosine (P-Tyr) involves their SH2 domains in most cases and results in functional changes. These include changes in their enzymatic activity or their ability to bind to proline-rich sequences in other proteins through their SH3 domains (262). The P-Tyr residues to which PI-PLCγ1 specifically associates have been identified in the PDGF β receptor (47, 118, 186), the NGF receptor (246), and the FGF receptor (225, 270). However, identification of a binding site(s) for the enzyme is less precise for the EGF receptor (318).

Association of PI-PLCγ1 with the EGF, FGF, and PDGF receptors is accompanied by its phosphorylation on three tyrosine residues (Tyr771, 783, and 1254) (158). Phosphorylation of Tyr783 is required for the enzyme to be activated by PDGF (156) but not for its association with the PDGF receptor. However, it has been difficult to show that phosphorylation of the enzyme results in an increase in activity in vitro. Tyrosine phosphorylation of PI-PLCγ1 by growth factors and other agonists also promotes its association with actin components of the cytoskeleton (106, 186). Targeting the enzyme to the plasma membrane probably plays a role in its activation (186).

Nonreceptor protein tyrosine kinases also can phosphorylate and activate PI-PLCγ isozymes in response to activation of certain cell-surface receptors. Examples of such receptors are the T-cell antigen receptor, the immunoglobulin E (IgE) receptor (FcεRI), the IgG receptors (Fcγ-Rs), membrane-bound immunoglobulin (mIgM), and certain cytokine receptors (for interleukin 6, erythropoietin, oncostatin M, ciliary neurotrophic factor, leukemia inhibitory factor) (186, 284). These receptors have no intrinsic tyrosine kinase activity but can activate cytosolic tyrosine kinases (members of the Src, Csk, Tec, Jak, and Syk families) (280a, 332). Some of these kinases associate with and phosphorylate PI-PLCγ isozymes (234). Activation of certain receptors linked to G_i or G_q also is associated with tyrosine phosphorylation of PI-PLCγ and other cell proteins (87, 106, 107, 209, 210, 333, 339). The mechanisms by which these receptors promote this tyrosine phosphorylation is unclear, but they could involve a Ca^{2+}-

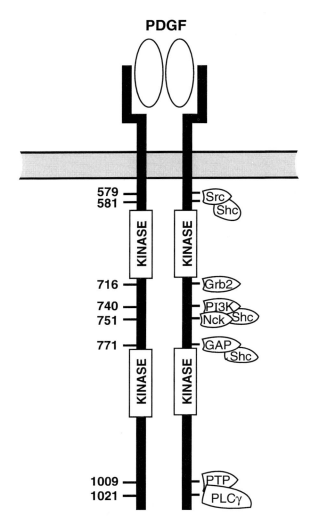

FIG. 11.7. Structure of the β receptor for platelet-derived growth factor (PDGF). The figure presents schematically the binding domain for PDGF, the tyrosine kinase domains, the numbered phosphorylatable tyrosine residues, and the proteins that associate with these. *Src*, Src family members; *Grb2, Shc*, and *Nck*, adapter proteins with SH2 and SH3 domains; *PI3K*, the regulatory subunit of phosphatidylinositol 3-kinase; *GAP*, the GTPase-activating protein of Ras; *PTP*, a protein tyrosine phosphatase variously designated PTP1D, Syp, SHPTP2, or PTP2C; *PLCγ*, the γ isozyme of phosphoinositide phospholipase C.

regulated tyrosine kinase(s) (386a). Activation of PI-PLC by collagen and antibodies to β_2 integrins acting through membrane receptors and a tyrosine phosphorylation–dependent pathway has been shown (50).

Activation of PI-PLCγ by growth factors results in increases in IP$_3$ and Ca^{2+} that are of slower onset and generally of smaller magnitude than those induced by G protein–linked agonist activation of PI-PLCβ (115, 142, 236, 385). The role of PI-PLC activation in the mitogenic action of growth factors has been explored by examining the effects of mutations in their receptors that abolish coupling to this enzyme. These studies have shown that PI-PLC activation is not required for stimulation of DNA synthesis by FGF (127, 225, 270). Mutant FGF receptors that are unable to activate PI-PLCγ and to stimulate PI hydrolysis show reduced activation of Raf-1 and microtubule-associated protein (MAP) kinase but a normal proliferative response to acidic FGF (aFGF) (127). Studies with PDGF (68a, 154, 290, 306, 346) have not given clearcut results, but suggest roles for both PI-PLC and PI 3-kinase in the growth response. Mice with disruption of the gene for PI-PLCγ1 show embryonic lethality, indicating a critical role for the enzyme in mammalian growth and development (280b).

PHOSPHATIDYLINOSITOL 3,4,5-TRISPHOSPHATE SYNTHESIS

Phosphatidylinositol 3-Kinases as Targets of Hormones and Growth Factors

To replenish PIP$_2$ broken down in response to agonist stimulation, PI is phosphorylated by PI 4-kinase to form PI 4-P (PIP), which is then converted to PIP$_2$ by PIP 5-kinase (Fig. 11.8) (14). In addition to these lipid kinases, cells possess 3-kinases that phosphorylate PI, PIP and PIP$_2$ on position 3 of the *myo*inositol ring (96, 324) (Fig. 11.8). The products are PI 3-P, PI 3,4-P$_2$, and PI 3,4,5-P$_3$ (PIP$_3$), but there is much evidence that the physiologically important compound is PIP$_3$ (324). Unlike PIP$_2$, which is hydrolyzed by PI-PLC to produce two intracellular signals, PIP$_3$ is not a substrate for known phospholipases and does not appear to produce signaling molecules (324). Many growth factors and G protein–linked agonists activate PI 3-kinase in their target cells. The G protein–linked agonists include thrombin, f-Met-Leu-Phe, platelet-activating factor, and ATP (96, 324). The response is inhibited by pertussis toxin (324), implying the involvement of G$_i$ subtypes. The probable mediator is the G protein $\beta\gamma$ complex since this has been shown to activate directly

and indirectly a PI 3-kinase isozyme (96, 323, 336, 392). The small M_r G proteins Ras, Rho, and Rac also have been implicated in the control of PI 3-kinase (171, 260, 288, 288a, 391, 396), and there is evidence that Rac is regulated via this PI kinase (41, 117, 242).

The growth factors that activate PI 3-kinase include PDGF, EGF, FGF, NGF, HGF, and colony-stimulating factor 1 (CSF-1) (96, 261, 324). The enzyme also is activated by insulin and insulin-like growth factor 1 (IGF-1) (96, 261, 324). In addition, activation of the T-cell antigen receptor and receptors for other cytokines (interleukins 2, 3, and 4 and granulocyte-macrophage colony-stimulating factor) activate the enzyme via soluble tyrosine kinases of the Src family (324).

There are several mammalian isoforms of PI 3-kinase, most of which consist of a regulatory 85 kd α- or β-subunit associated with a 110 kd α-, β-, γ-, or δ-catalytic subunit (261, 353b). An exception is the PI 3-kinase that is the target of the subunits of heterotrimeric G proteins. This isozyme consists of a 110 kd catalytic subunit (p110γ) which does not have a binding site for a 85 k subunit (326), but has a pleckstrin homology domain that binds G protein $\beta\gamma$ subunits (1). Interestingly, the p110α catalytic subunit exhibits a protein serine kinase activity that phosphorylates the regulatory subunit, resulting in a loss of PI 3-kinase activity (73, 176). The physiological relevance of this protein kinase activity is unknown.

As described above for the activation of PI-PLCγ, growth factors induce autophosphorylation of their receptors, providing specific docking sites for the SH2 domains of the 85 kd subunit of PI 3-kinase (36, 96, 247, 261, 271, 324, 353) (Fig. 11.6). The 85 kd subunit also can associate with the adapter protein Grb2. In the case of insulin and IGF-1, there is minimal association of this subunit with the receptor itself. Instead, it binds to the insulin receptor substrate (IRS)-1 when this becomes associated with the activated receptor and phosphorylated on specific tyrosine residues (96). In some cells, EGF activates PI 3-kinase without promoting association of the enzyme with the EGF receptor (320). Activation of the enzyme may be mediated by an adapter protein (p120^{cbl}), which is phosphorylated by the EGF receptor (319). Activation also may occur through heterodimerization and tyrosine phosphorylation of erbB3, a protein related to the EGF receptor (157). Plasma membrane localization of PI 3-kinase is a critical component of signaling through this enzyme. Its substrate (PIP$_2$) is in the membrane, and it activates its downstream effectors at this site (74a, 161b).

The association of PI 3-kinase with polyoma middle T antigen was one of the first indications that this enzyme played a role in cell signaling (151). In cells

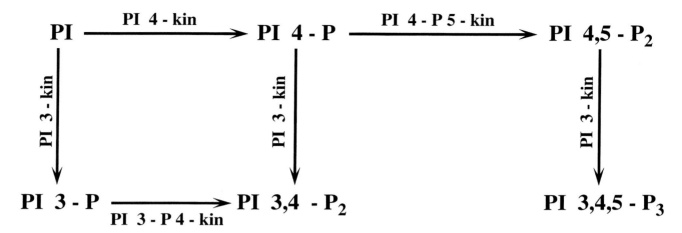

FIG. 11.8. Pathways of synthesis of 3-phosphorylated phosphoinositides. *PI 3-kin*, phosphatidylinositol 3-kinase; *PI 4-kin*, phosphatidylinositol 4-kinase; *PI 3-P 4-kin*, phosphatidylinositol 3-P 4-kinase; *PI 4-P 5-kin*; phosphatidylinositol 4-P 5-kinase.

transformed by polyoma virus, middle T antigen forms a complex with c-Src, which then phosphorylates middle T antigen on several tyrosines residues, including Tyr315. The 85 kd subunit of PI 3-kinase then associates with Tyr315 and surrounding amino acids through its SH2 domains (96, 324). As noted above, soluble tyrosine kinases, including members of the Src family, can associate with and activate PI 3-kinase, but the relative extent to which SH2 and SH3 domains are involved in the associations is unclear (324).

The mechanisms by which association of the regulatory subunit of PI 3-kinase with tyrosine-phosphorylated domains leads to an increase in the activity of the 110 kd catalytic subunit are undefined. A change in the conformation of the 85 kd subunit upon binding of appropriate phosphopeptides has been observed (324), and this is presumably transmitted to the 110 kd subunit. The sites of interaction between the subunits have been localized to a region between the two SH2 domains of the regulatory subunit and a small region in the N-terminus of the catalytic subunit (124, 161).

Role of Phosphatidylinositol 3-Kinase in Cell Function

Although many agonists have been shown to activate PI 3-kinase or to promote its association with their receptors, an increase in PIP_3 has not been demonstrated always because the lipid is present at low levels and its measurement is not easy. Thus, few correlations have been made between changes in the level of PIP_3 and the cellular events that it has been proposed to mediate. Compared with PI 3-P and PI 3,4-P_2, PIP_3 increases most rapidly and to the greatest fold extent

after agonist stimulation, consistent with it being the physiologically significant product of activated PI 3-kinase (324). However, many of the cellular changes that PI 3-kinase is supposed to mediate occur on a slower time scale, suggesting the involvement of a signaling cascade(s). In the case of PDGF, the role of PI 3-kinase has been explored by mutating the tyrosine residues in the PDGF β receptor with which the 85 kd regulatory subunit associates (Fig. 11.7) (89, 153, 154, 238, 347, 363). Mutation of these residues to phenylalanine results in a loss of activation of PI 3-kinase and an impairment of the mitogenic or proliferative effect of the growth factor (68a, 89, 154, 347). Although the adapter protein Nck also binds to the sequence around one of the phosphorylated tyrosines with which p85 associates (Fig. 11.7) (238), other data support a role for PI 3-kinase in mitogenesis (96). However, in some studies, the mutant receptors still mediate a significant mitogenic response (154, 347), indicating the involvement of other factors.

The idea that an additional signal is involved in the stimulation of DNA synthesis is supported by the observation that the G protein–linked agonists f-Met-Leu-Phe and thrombin are not mitogenic, though they produce large increases in PIP_3 (96, 324). It is also consistent with the finding that microinjection of antibodies specific for the 110 kd subunit of PI 3-kinase into fibroblasts inhibited DNA synthesis induced by PDGF or EGF but not that induced by CSF-1, bombesin, or lysophosphatidic acid (287).

Mutant PDGF receptors also have been used to implicate PI 3-kinase in membrane ruffling, which is due to the polymerization of actin at the inner surface of the plasma membrane (363), and in the translocation of the insulin-stimulable glucose transporter GLUT4 (149), though the latter probably requires additional signaling pathways (131). A role for PI 3-kinase in the stimulation of Na^+/H^+ exchange by PDGF also has been indicated (196), but the data additionally implicate PI-PLCγ. Another approach has involved the microinjection of a phosphorylated peptide corresponding to the binding site for the 85 kd subunit, and the data suggest that the enzyme is involved in membrane ruffling (168). Injection of a similar peptide into *Xenopus* oocytes stimulates glucose transport (194), in agreement with other evidence for a role of the enzyme in regulating this process as noted below.

Mutations of the regulatory or catalytic subunits of PI 3-kinase have been employed to define its cellular role. A mutant 85 kd subunit to which the catalytic subunit cannot bind has been overexpressed in cells and found to inhibit membrane ruffling induced by PDGF (363), insulin, IGF1, or V12Ras (168, 288a). This mutant regulatory subunit also blocked glucose transport and translocation of GLUT1 in response to insulin in CHO cells (114). A constitutively active form of the catalytic subunit expressed in adipocytes promotes GLUT4 translocation (212a, 332a) and membrane ruffling (212a). Expression of this mutant catalytic subunit in NIH 3T3 fibroblasts induces transcription from the promoter for *c-fos* (125). The latter activity is potentiated by c-Ras and inhibited by dominant negative forms of Ras or Raf-1. In addition, expression of the catalytic subunit of PI 3-kinase in *Xenopus* oocytes increases the amount of Ras·GTP (125). Expression of the 85 kd subunit inhibits insulin stimulation of the transcription of *c-fos* in CHO cells presumably by inhibiting the activation of endogenous PI 3-kinase (380). As NIH 3T3 cells, there is evidence in these cells that activation of the *c-fos* serum response element involves Ras and Raf-1 (380). Overexpression of wild-type and mutant forms of the 85 kd subunit strongly inhibits cellular transformation induced by constitutively active V12Ras, but not by vSrc (288a), implying a role for PI 3-kinase in addition to the Raf/MAP kinase pathway in Ras-induced transformation.

Monocyte colony-stimulating factor has been shown to promote the interaction of the 85 kd subunit of PI 3-kinase with the adapter protein Grb2 and with Sos, a guanine nucleotide exchange factor for Ras (298). Formation of the complex would explain the interaction between PI 3-kinase and Ras. However, other pathways that are not dependent on PI 3-kinase activation can activate the Ras/MAP kinase pathway (38, 55, 91, 114, 211).

As indicated above, there is evidence that in some cells, PI 3-kinase may be involved in activation of the Ras/Raf-1/MAP kinase pathway. The enzyme is involved in agonist activation of pp70^{S6K}, a protein serine kinase that phosphorylates the S6 ribosomal protein (38, 45, 362, 368a). In many cells, pp70^{S6K} is important for G1 cell-cycle transition, and inhibition of its activation by rapamycin leads to a failure of cells to enter S phase (46).

The immediate intracellular targets of PIP$_3$ are various protein kinases. Early reports indicated that certain isozymes of PKC could be activated by PIP$_3$ in vitro (232, 259, 341), and there is evidence that the atypical isozymes ζ and λ are activated in vivo (3a, 118c). Another target of the products of PI 3-kinase is Akt, a serine/threonine kinase that is also called PKB. This is regulated by PI 3,4-bisphosphate through its pleckstrin homology domain (64a, 94b–94e). In addition, it can be phosphorylated and activated by another protein kinase (PDK1), which itself is potently activated by PIP$_3$ (4a). Insulin and growth factors rapidly activate Akt in cells via PI 3-kinase (34a, 62b, 64a, 74a, 94d, 161b, 164b). Glycogen synthase kinase-3 has been identified as a substrate for Akt (62a), but other physiological substrates are likely. Akt has been implicated in the stimulation of glucose uptake and glucose transporter translocation and expression by insulin in adipocytes (164c). Other targets of PIP$_3$ have recently been identified. One (GRP1) has a region of high sequence similarity to the yeast Sec7 protein (160a). A related protein (cytohesin 1), which also binds PIP$_3$, regulates integrin B2 and stimulates guanine nucleotide exchange on the small G protein ARF (160a, 164d). These proteins may be involved in the regulation of protein sorting and membrane trafficking by PIP$_3$. Another target is the protein AP-3, which is involved in synaptic vesicle formation and recycling (113a).

The fungal metabolite wortmannin has been shown to be a potent inhibitor of PI 3-kinase in intact cells and in vitro (5, 251, 382) and has been used extensively to explore the role of the enzyme in cell responses. Another inhibitor that has been used is the quercetin analog LY294002 (358). Many studies have demonstrated that wortmannin at nanomolar concentrations or LY294002 at micromolar concentrations inhibits the effect of insulin or IGF-1 on glucose transport or glucose transporters (38, 54, 104, 250). Inhibition of neutrophil activation by f-Met-Leu-Phe also has been reported (5, 72, 75, 251). Other effects of wortmannin and LY294002 include inhibition of the following processes: histamine release mediated by the IgE receptor in basophilic cells (382); membrane ruffling induced by insulin, IGF-1, or PDGF (168, 363); glycogen synthase activation by insulin (297, 376); activation of Na^+/H^+ exchange (196) and of pp70^{S6K} activity (45) by PDGF; and prevention of apoptosis by PDGF and other growth factors in PC12 cells (104).

The observation that wortmannin inhibits membrane ruffling (168, 242, 288a, 363, 372) implies that PI 3-kinase is involved in actin polymerization. This is supported by the induction of membrane ruffling in cells expressing constitutively active PI 3-kinase (212a). Associations between PI 3-kinase and focal adhesion kinase (40, 41) and α-actin (313) have been observed. The small M_r G protein Rac has been implicated in the membrane ruffling induced by growth factors and insulin (167, 286), and there is evidence that PI 3-kinase lies upstream to Rac in the induction of the response (117, 167, 242). Association of PI 3-kinase with GTP-Rac has been observed in cell lysates and in vivo (342, 396), but the interaction may not be direct (288, 342, 396).

A role for PI 3-kinase in the internalization and degradation of the PDGF receptor is indicated by studies of mutations of the receptor (143, 144) and of the association of the receptor with PI 3-kinase in clathrin-coated vesicles (150). Studies with wortmannin also have indicated a role for the enzyme in endocytosis (214a, 313b). Further work has indicated that the enzyme is required for the diversion of the receptor to a degradative pathway (143). The gene for the inherited disease ataxia telangiectasia encodes a protein similar to the catalytic subunit of PI 3-kinase (301). The disease is characterized by cerebellar degeneration, dilated conjunctival blood vessels, and severe deficiencies in immune responses. There is much evidence that PI 3-kinase is involved in the suppression of programed cell death (apoptosis) and that Akt mediates the effect (94a, 118a). The ability of NGF to prevent apoptosis in neuronal (PC-12) cells was inhibited by wortmannin, and PDGF failed to prevent apoptosis in cells expressing mutant receptors that cannot activate PI 3-kinase (384). Overexpression of Akt in cerebellar neurons also prevented apoptosis, and dominant negative forms of the kinase interfered with the ability of growth factors to prevent the phenomenon (82a). Additional evidence for roles of PI 3-kinase and Akt, but not $pp70^{S6K}$, in cell survival has been obtained (94a, 152a, 384a), but the mechanisms remain obscure.

PHOSPHATIDYLCHOLINE HYDROLYSIS

Many agonists cause the breakdown of phosphatidylcholine (PC) in a variety of cells (19, 24). The phospholipase activities involved are of the A_2, C, and D varieties. In contrast to phospholipase A_2, which acts on several phospholipids, PLD is specific for PC in most cell types (86). Phosphatidylcholine-phospholipase C (PC-PLC) activity has been much less studied, and it is not certain that PC-PLC exists as a separate enzyme in mammalian cells. The number of cell types in which PC hydrolysis by PLD has been shown is very large, and this is also true for the agonists that elicit the response (19, 24). Activation of receptors linked to heterotrimeric G proteins and those linked to or containing tyrosine kinase activity stimulates PC-PLD, and tumor-promoting phorbol esters elicit this response in most cell types.

Phosphatidylcholine Hydrolysis by Phospholipase D and Its Functional Significance

The products of PC-PLD activity are choline and phosphatidic acid (PA), which are further metabolized. Choline is phosphorylated by choline kinase to phosphocholine, which is then reincorporated into PC after conversion to cytidine diphosphate-choline. Because of the high resting levels of choline and phosphocholine (0.1–0.3 mM and 0.2–2 mM, respectively) in most cells (263), these compounds are not considered to be signaling molecules. However, activation of PC-PLD in many cells can increase PA levels two- or three-fold, and this lipid is considered to be an intracellular signal (86). In addition, PA is rapidly converted to DAG, which is an activator of many PKC isozymes (86).

Although the generation of signaling molecules may be an important component of PC-PLD activation, it is also possible that the decrease in PC and/or the increase in PA and DAG in the membranes where the enzyme is activated may lead to physical changes that may facilitate membrane fusion and other changes. Such a possibility has been suggested for the PC-PLD present in Golgi membranes (170, 229).

Phosphatidic acid has been reported to have many effects in vitro, including stimulatory effects on PKC, β-adrenergic receptor kinase (in the presence of G protein $\beta\gamma$-subunits) and other protein kinases (25, 86, 98, 155, 185, 189, 200, 233, 272), a tyrosine phosphatase (343, 395), PI-PLCγ (132, 145), and PI 4P-kinase (228). Inhibition of Ras GAP (344), disruption of the interaction of Rac with RhoGDI (44), and activation of n-chimaerin (3), an activator of Rac GAP, also have been described. Early reports showed inhibition of adenylyl cyclase and stimulation of Ca^{2+} influx (86) and a later report, binding of PA to Raf-1 kinase (98). However, the physiological relevance of these in vitro observations has not been established. There is better evidence that PA plays a role in the respiratory burst observed in neutrophils stimulated by chemotactic peptides, though other factors are involved (12, 86, 200, 280, 293).

In studies with intact cells, addition of PA promotes PIP_2 hydrolysis, Ca^{2+} mobilization, and PLA_2 activation, with resulting secondary changes (86, 299). PA and bacterial PLD also have been reported to be mitogenic (86, 166) and to stimulate stress fiber formation (86). In some studies, these effects can be attributed to lysophosphatidic acid (LPA) contamination (92, 135, 348), but dose-response studies indicate a separate role for PA in some cases (349). Whereas many cells have surface receptors for LPA (226, 227a, 338, 350), evidence that these exist for PA is lacking. If PA enters cells, this may involve a dephosphorylation/rephosphorylation cycle in which the molecule actually traversing the plasma membrane is DAG (257, 267).

Major roles have been proposed for PLD and PA in vesicle transport from the endoplasmic reticulum to the Golgi complex as well as within the Golgi stacks (17a, 41a, 147, 170, 170a, 229). Golgi-enriched membranes contain PLD activity that is stimulated by ARF (41a, 170, 275), and it has been proposed that the PLD activity plays a role in the action of ARF to form coated vesicles from Golgi membranes (41a, 170a). For example, in Golgi from cells with high constitutive PLD activity, formation of coated vesicles does not require ARF (170a), and addition of bacterial or mammalian PLD stimulates vesicle budding (41a) or coatomer binding (170a). Furthermore, ethanol and butanol, which decrease PA formation by PLD, inhibit the formation or release of coated vesicles (41a, 170a). Transport from the endoplasmic reticulum to the Golgi complex in CHO cells has also been shown to be inhibited by primary alcohols, and the inhibition is reversed by exogenous PA (17a).

The major metabolic fate of PA generated by PC-PLD activation is its conversion to DAG by PAP. This enzyme exists in at least two isozymic forms, and the plasma membrane-associated form (PAP2) (65, 136) is presumably responsible for the hydrolysis of agonist-generated PA. The other form (PAP1) is associated with the cytosol and endoplasmic reticulum and is involved in the conversion of PA to DAG that occurs during triacylglycerol and phospholipid synthesis. Some of the PA produced in the plasma membrane may be transported to the endoplasmic reticulum for this lipid synthesis.

Another fate of PA is hydrolysis by a specific PLA$_2$ to produce LPA (337). This reaction is prominent in platelets (226), but it is not known to what extent it occurs in other cells. LPA is recognized to be an important intercellular messenger (227a). It produces many effects in cells that are mediated by a G protein–linked plasma membrane receptor(s) (134, 226). The G proteins are probably members of both the G$_i$, G$_{12}$ and G$_q$ families since some effects are inhibited by pertussis toxin, whereas others are not (226, 227a). The cellular effects of LPA include hydrolysis of PIP$_2$ with consequent Ca^{2+} mobilization and PKC activation (133, 226, 227). There is also liberation of arachidonic acid due to Ca^{2+}-independent activation of PLA$_2$ (93) and activation of PLD by a PKC-dependent mechanism (110, 226, 227, 352). A reduction in cAMP occurs in fibroblasts, presumably due to activation of G$_i$ (226). There also has been a report that LPA increases cAMP in myeloma cells (340).

One of the important effects of LPA is its stimulation of growth (134), and there is evidence that much of the growth-stimulatory action of serum is due to LPA. Although LPA stimulates DNA synthesis and cell division in most cell types, it inhibits the growth of myeloma cells (340) and suppresses the differentiation of neuroblastoma cells (134). Since the mitogenic action of LPA is inhibited by pertussis toxin, it probably involves G$_i$, and there is much evidence that it involves the Ras/MAP kinase signaling pathway (121, 123, 134, 172, 173, 226). The probable mediator of Ras activation is the $\beta\gamma$-subunit of G$_i$, and a non-receptor tyrosine kinase may be involved (226, 227, 227a). Also, LPA activates PI 3-kinase. This activation may be mediated by the $\beta\gamma$-subunit (96, 336, 392) or may be secondary to Ras or Rho activation (171, 288). The molecular interactions between G protein $\beta\gamma$-subunits, tyrosine kinases, and PI 3-kinase in regulation of the Ras/MAP kinase pathway in vivo are still poorly defined (227a).

Another prominent effect of LPA is the induction of stress fiber formation in fibroblasts due to actin polymerization (285). Like other G$_q$- and G$_i$-linked agonists, LPA induces tyrosine phosphorylation of cellular proteins, including focal adhesion kinase and paxillin (121, 172, 173, 226, 227, 309). This is accompanied by recruitment of these and other proteins to focal adhesion sites in the cell, the initiation of focal adhesions, and the assembly of actin stress fibers (226, 227). A critical component of the tyrosine phosphorylation and actin polymerization mechanism is the small G protein Rho (134, 226, 227, 282, 285, 288). Treatment of cells with the *Clostridium botulinum* C3 exozyme, which ADP-ribosylates and inactivates Rho, blocks stress fiber formation, and also tyrosine phosphorylation of focal adhesion kinase and paxillin induced by LPA and other G protein–linked agonists (134, 226, 227, 282, 285, 288). The effect of Rho on actin polymerization may be mediated by Rho-associated kinase (Rho kinase), which phosphorylates and inactivates myosin light chain phosphatase (159a). Although there is evidence that LPA and Rho family members control PC-PLD (30, 110, 204, 314, 352), the role of this enzyme in actin polymerization remains uncertain (109, 110, 227).

As indicated above, there is much evidence that the effects of LPA are mediated by a cell surface receptor (134, 226, 227, 338, 350), but it is unclear whether the 40 kd protein identified by cross-linking to an LPA derivative (350) is the functional receptor. Although there have been two reports of the cloning of the LPA receptor (106a, 117a), neither is entirely convincing (227a). There have been few studies of the metabolism of extracellular LPA in cells, but in fibroblasts, it is principally converted to monoacylglycerol, which is then converted to triacylglycerol (351). PA and DAG appear to be minor products.

Phospholipase D as a Target of Hormones and Growth Factors

Although initial reports of PC hydrolysis in cells stimulated by phorbol esters, growth factors, and other agonists concluded that the hydrolysis occurred by a PLC mechanism, later work showed that the enzyme activated was PLD in most cases (19, 85, 86). The evidence for this came from time-course measurements of PA and choline in addition to DAG and P-choline. However, the recognition that PLD specifically catalyzed a transphosphatidylation reaction, whereby the phosphatidyl group of PC is transferred to primary alcohols, such as ethanol, propanol, and butanol, allowed the use of this reaction to demonstrate that a large number of agonists stimulated PC-PLD in a large variety of cells and tissues (19, 85, 86). Because of the activity of PAP, much of the DAG accumulating in agonist-treated cells is derived from PC via PA, and this is particularly true for the second phase of DAG formation (19, 85, 86).

Properties of Phospholipase D. Until recently, information on the properties and regulation of PC-PLD has been severely limited by the absence of purified or cloned forms of the mammalian enzyme. Although there have been several descriptions of partially purified PLD (32, 86, 215, 330, 357), there has been only one report of a fully purified PC-PLD (252). The purified enzyme was obtained from porcine lung microsomes (252) and has an M_r of 190,000. It is specific for PC and carries out the transphosphatidylation reaction. It has a pH optimum of 6.6 and is stimulated by 1–2 mM Ca^{2+} and Mg^{2+} and by unsaturated fatty acids in the presence of Mg^{2+}·

Two alternatively spliced forms of a human PLD that is stimulated by the small G protein ADP ribosylation factor (ARF) have been cloned (111a, 111b). Its molecular mass is 120 kd, and it has several sequences that are conserved in PLDs from yeast and plant species. Activity is selective for PC, and the enzyme catalyzes the transphosphatidylation reaction. It is stimulated by PIP$_2$ and PIP$_3$ but inhibited by oleate. ARF

strongly activates the enzyme expressed in either Sf9 insect cells or COS-7 cells, and the homogeneous enzyme purified from Sf9 cells responds directly to ARF, Rho and PKC-α (111a, 111b). Interestingly, the stimulatory effect of PKC-α does not require ATP, implying a non-phosphorylation mechanism. Synergism between the effects of ARF, Rho and PKC-α is observed, and the Rho family members Rac and Cdc42 have some stimulatory activity (111b). A PC-PLD corresponding to the shorter form of human PLD (hPLD1b) also has been cloned from rat brain (259a). Its properties strongly resemble those of hPLD1b, except that synergism between the small G proteins and PKCα is not evident. Another PC-PLD termed PLD2 has been cloned from mouse embryo (57a) and rat brain (164c). This has a high basal activity and is inhibited by oleate. It responds to PIP$_2$, but not to small G proteins or PKC.

Studies of PC-PLD have been enhanced by the observation that the activity of the enzyme is greatly increased by PIP$_2$ (33, 193) and that the enzyme from neutrophils, HL-60 cells, and most mammalian tissues is markedly stimulated by ARF in the presence of GTPγS (32, 33, 57, 275). These findings led to the partial purification of a PC-PLD from porcine brain membranes (32), which was shown by hydrodynamic analysis to have an M_r of 95,000 (32). This enzyme is activated by ARF plus GTPγS but only if a cytosolic factor(s) is present (32, 315), as previously noted for neutrophils and HL60 cells by other workers (29, 177). Recent studies with expressed cloned PC-PLD (hPLD1) purified from Sf9 cells have demonstrated that PIP$_2$ and PIP$_3$ directly activate the enzyme and that it interacts directly with ARF and Rho family proteins (111b).

Biochemical and cloning studies show that different isozymes of PC-PLD exist. For example, an ARF-responsive enzyme, partially purified from rat brain, is different from another PLD isolated from this source; it depends on oleate for activity and is not stimulated by ARF or PIP$_2$ (215). Membranes from rat liver and HL60 cells also contain a PC-PLD that is activated predominantly by members of the Rho family of small G proteins (30, 204, 314). As described above, two PLD isozymes with very different properties (hPLD1 and PLD2) have been cloned (57a, 111a, 111b, 164a).

In addition to factors that stimulate PLD, cells also contain several inhibitors of the enzyme (46a, 111c, 157a, 182a, 195a). Some of these have been defined, namely synaptojanin, which is a phosphatase that acts by hydrolyzing PIP$_2$, (46a, 157a), fodrin, a nonerythroid form of spectrin that binds actin (195a), and AP3, a synapse-specific clathrin assembly protein that interacts directly with PLD (182a). It is unclear whether these inhibitors play a role in the physiological control of PLD.

Role of Protein Kinase C in Phospholipase D Regulation.

The fact that agonists whose receptors are linked to heterotrimeric G proteins or that exhibit intrinsic tyrosine kinase activity activate PLD (19, 85, 86) indicates that signals initiated by G protein activation or by receptor autophosphorylation and possible tyrosine phosphorylation of cytosolic proteins are capable of influencing the activity of the enzyme. Although the possibility exists that heterotrimeric G proteins and receptor tyrosine kinases can directly activate PC-PLD in a manner analogous to the β and γ isozymes of PI-PLC, no evidence exists for such mechanisms. It is more likely that PKC and/or other signaling proteins are involved.

Early work demonstrating that PC hydrolysis could be activated by phorbol esters in many cell types pointed to a role of PKC in the regulation of PC-PLD (19, 85). In some cases, agonist stimulation of PC hydrolysis was totally or largely inhibited by PKC inhibitors or down-regulation of the enzyme, implying that PKC plays a major role in the mechanism of regulation of the enzyme (86) (Fig. 11.9). However, in other cases, agonist stimulation of PC-PLD was decreased little, if at all, by these treatments, indicating the involvement of other mechanisms (86, 329). Because of the lack of specificity of some of the PKC inhibitors, that is, the possibility that they affect other protein kinases, and because they may have effects on PLD and other enzymes of lipid metabolism (86, 266), the use of these inhibitors to define a role for PKC may be questioned (86). Likewise, down-regulation of PKC by prolonged treatment with phorbol esters could have secondary effects. For these reasons, studies using multiple approaches to the role of PKC in PLD activation by agonists (9, 86, 108, 187, 329, 385, 386) are more valid.

More direct evidence for a role of PKC in PLD regulation has come from cell studies in which α and β isozymes of PKC were overexpressed (84, 256, 258), depleted by antisense methods (9), or added directly to isolated membranes (59, 60). Other examples are experiments with cells that overexpress PI-PLCγ or cells that express mutant PDGF receptors (187, 386). Cells with higher PI-PLC activity showed an enhanced PLD response to PDGF, which was completely blocked by PKC down-regulation (187), and cells expressing mutant PDGF receptors that could not couple to PI-PLCγ or activate PKC exhibited a complete loss of PLD activation by the growth factor (386).

There have been studies of the regulation of PLD by PKC in vitro (59, 60, 186a, 194, 248, 249, 259a, 316) including experiments with purified cloned enzymes

(111b). Although one of these studies supported a phosphorylation-dependent mechanism (194), the others, surprisingly, did not. In particular, one study showed that activation of PLD in fibroblast membranes occurred in the demonstrated absence of ATP and was dissociated from the phosphorylation of PKC substrates (59). The PKC isozymes involved in the phosphorylation-independent effect required phorbol ester and Ca^{2+} for full activity, and it was later shown that only the α and β isozymes were effective (60, 249). Studies with cloned expressed hPLD1 purified from Sf9 cells have shown clearly that PKCα can activate the enzyme in the absence of ATP (111b). Phorbol ester–dependent association of PLD with PKCα has been shown in vitro and in immunoprecipitates from NIH3T3 fibroblasts treated with phorbol ester (186a). These data sug-

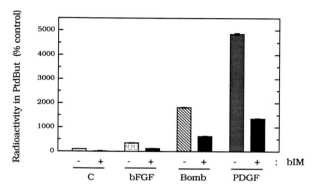

A. **bis-Indolylmaleimide**

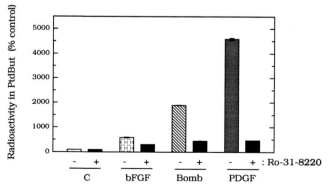

B. **Ro-31-8220**

FIG. 11.9. Effects of protein kinase C inhibitors (bis-indolylmaleimide and Ro-31–8220) on stimulation of phospholipase D by basic fibroblast growth factor (*bFGF*), bombesin (*Bomb*), and platelet-derived growth factor (*PDGF*) in Swiss 3T3 cells. Phospholipase D activity was measured by the formation of radioactive phosphatidylbutanol (*PtdBut*) in cells previously labeled with [³H] myristic acid. [Reproduced from Yeo and Exton (385), with permission.]

gest that the two proteins can interact directly in vitro and in vivo. Large synergistic interactions between PKCα and ARF or Rho in the activation of PLD have been observed (111b, 249, 316). The molecular bases for these interesting effects are unknown, but they could be of physiological significance.

In summary, although different cell types show a variable dependence of agonist-stimulated PLD activation on PKC, the consensus of the evidence is that it is an important regulatory factor. Although there is much evidence that PKC can control the enzyme by a nonphosphorylation mechanism in vitro, it is probable that additional mechanisms operate in vivo. This is because the stimulation of the enzyme by phorbol ester in intact cells is much greater than that observed with isolated membranes (for example, 259a). If a phosphorylation mechanism is involved, it is not known if PKC directly phosphorylates and activates the enzyme or controls it through a regulatory cascade.

Role of Small G Proteins in Phospholipase D Regulation.

Small G proteins of the ARF and Rho families have been implicated in the regulation of PC-PLD. Large in vitro effects of activated ARF proteins have been demonstrated for homogeneous hPLD1 (111b) and also the enzyme in neutrophils, HL60 cells, and brain (Fig. 11.10) (32, 33, 57, 315); these include mammalian ARFs 1, 3, 4, 5, and 6, with the nonmyristoylated forms being very much less potent (32, 33). Stimulation of HL60 cells with f-Met-Leu-Phe or phorbol ester potentiates the effect of GTPγS on PLD in the membrane fraction (122). This treatment also causes translocation of ARF to the membranes, as shown by Western blotting.

In studies utilizing HEK cells stably expressing M3 muscarinic receptors, activation of PLD by carbachol is inhibited by brefeldin A (294). Since this is an inhibitor of the activation of ARF by GTP/GDP exchange, these data imply a role for ARF in the activation of PLD by certain agonists. This was supported by the observation that carbachol promoted translocation of ARF from cytosol to membranes (294). These data point to a role for ARF in the regulation of the enzyme in intact cells. However, it has not been shown that agonists activate ARF, that is, increase its GTP/GDP ratio in cells.

The effect of ARF on the enzyme is amplified by a 50–55 kd cytosolic protein (29, 32, 122, 164, 177, 315), but its nature remains to be determined. The domain in ARF responsible for the activation of PLD is different from that which interacts with cholera toxin (387). The stimulatory effect of ARF and GTP analogues on PLD activity is observed not only in plasma membranes but also in Golgi-enriched mem-

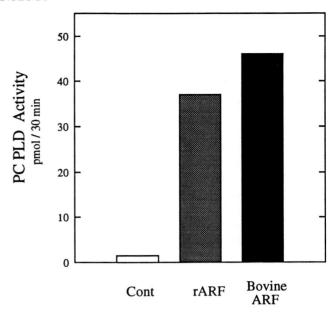

FIG. 11.10. Stimulation of HL60 phospholipase D by recombinant ADP-ribosylation factor (ARF) (*rARF*) and ARF purified from bovine brain. Phospholipase D partially purified from HL60 membranes was assayed in the presence of GTPγS and the ARF forms. [Data replotted from Brown et al. (33), with permission.]

branes, nuclei, and cytosol (10a, 170, 275, 314). Activation of PLD in the Golgi complex is sensitive to brefeldin A. Some investigators have suggested that activation of PLD by ARF in the Golgi complex could produce the membrane lipid changes required for vesicular transport (147, 170a, 229).

Phospholipase D is regulated also by Rho family proteins in membranes from liver, brain, and HL60 cells (30, 174, 204, 275, 314). A specific inhibitor of Rho activation, Rho GDP dissociation inhibitor (Rho-GDI), inhibits PLD activation by GTP analogues in membranes from liver and HL60 cells (30, 204, 248, 314) (Fig. 11.11). Moreover, the response is restored by readdition of RhoA and Rac1 (204, 314). A partially purified preparation of PLD from rat brain membranes has been shown to be activated by RhoA (174) and this has been demonstrated for two cloned enzymes (111b, 259a). However, a PLD that responds only to Rho family proteins has not been purified or cloned. Synergistic interactions between RhoA and ARF and/or PKC in the regulation of PLD have been observed with membrane preparations and purified enzymes (111b, 174, 314, 315, 316). These suggest that the regulation of PLD in vivo may be very complex. As described below, there is evidence that Rho family members activate tyrosine and serine/threonine kinases and that these could be involved in the activation of PLD.

Studies in fibroblasts overexpressing wild-type, constitutively active, and dominant negative forms of Rac1 have provided evidence for a role of this small G protein in the control of PLD by EGF (118d). The mechanisms by which growth factor receptors activate Rho family members are unknown, though the specific association of a Rho family member with the activated human and murine PDGFβ receptors has been reported in studies with fibroblasts (397). In addition, it has been suggested that activation of Rac is dependent upon Grb2 since antibodies to this adapter protein block Rac, but not Rho, activation (219). There is evidence for another coupling between the Ras and Rho signaling pathways. This is because expression of the N-terminal domain of Ras-GAP produces a complex with p190 Rho-GAP and leads to cellular changes consistent with reduced Rho activity (197). There is also evidence that Rho proteins play a role in the regulation of PLD by agonists that activate heterotrimeric G proteins (203). For example, scrape loading the C3 exoenzyme from *C. botulinum* into fibroblasts greatly inhibits the activation of PC-PLD by LPA, endothelin 1, and phorbol ester (Fig. 11.12) (203). Since this toxin ADP-ribosylates and inactivates Rho much more efficiently than Rac and CDC42, these data impli-

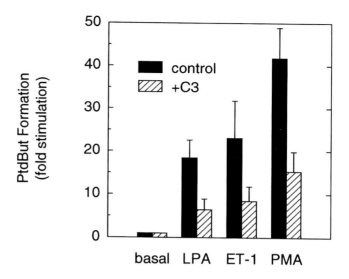

FIG. 11.12. Effects of C3 exoenzyme of *Clostridium botulinum* on the stimulation of phospholipase D in Rat1 fibroblasts by lysophosphatidic acid (*LPA*), endothelin-1 (*ET-1*), and phorbol myristate acetate (*PMA*). The exoenzyme was introduced into cells by scrape-loading 24 h prior to labeling with [^{3}H]myristic acid and 48 h prior to assay of phospholipase D by measurement of [^{3}H]phosphatidylbutanol (*PtdBut*) formation. [Reproduced from Malcolm et al. (203), with permission.]

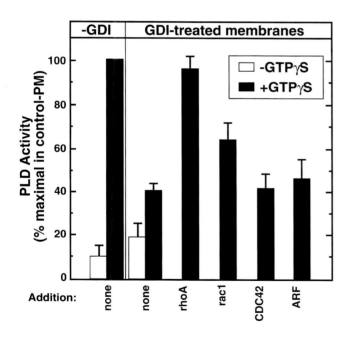

FIG. 11.11. Effects of Rho GDP dissociation inhibitor (*GDI*) and Rho family members on activation of phospholipase D (*PLD*) by GTPγS in rat liver plasma membranes. Membranes were treated with GDI and then washed and incubated with or without GTPγS in the absence or presence of RhoA, Rac1, Cdc42, or ARF. Phospholipase D was assayed by transphosphatidylation with ethanol. [Reproduced from Malcolm et al. (204), with permission.]

cate a Rho protein in the action of these agonists on PC-PLD. Selective translocation of Rho family proteins from cytosol to membranes has been observed in fibroblasts treated with PDGF and LPA (94a). LPA and endothelin 1 promote translocation of RhoA and Cdc42 to a low-speed membrane fraction, whereas PDG causes relocalization of Racl to a high-speed fraction. Since membrane association of the Rho proteins is determined by the ratio of bound GTP to GDP, these findings imply that PDGF activates Rac and that the other agonists activate Rho and Cdc42 (94a).

Role of Ca^{2+} Ions in Phospholipase D Regulation. Agonist-stimulated PC hydrolysis is partly dependent upon extracellular and/or intracellular Ca^{2+} (95, 96, 329). In addition, activation of PC breakdown by Ca^{2+} ionophores has been observed in many cell types (86, 95, 329). The role of Ca^{2+} could be attributed to the involvement of Ca^{2+}-dependent PKC isozymes, but other mechanisms are possible. Purified or partially purified forms of PC-PLD are not dependent upon Ca^{2+} ions for activity, though they may show activation by submillimolar concentrations of these ions (32, 111b, 252, 314, 330). Higher Ca^{2+} concentrations are generally inhibitory. It is uncertain if physiological changes in Ca^{2+} play a role in the regulation of the enzyme.

Role of Cytosolic Tyrosine Kinases and Serine/Threonine Kinases in Phospholipase D Regulation. Most growth factors whose receptors possess intrinsic tyrosine kinase activity are capable of activating PC-PLD (19, 85, 86). In addition, there is evidence, based on the effects of vanadate and tyrosine kinase inhibitors, that a soluble tyrosine kinase(s) is involved in the activation of the enzyme by agonists linked to heterotrimeric G proteins (31, 131a, 214, 303, 329a, 345, 359, 367). Furthermore, in permeabilized cells, vanadate, whose actions include inhibition of tyrosine phosphatases, enhances the stimulation of PLD by GTPγS (28, 82, 175), whereas tyrosine kinase inhibitors decrease the response (28, 82, 175, 214). Tyrosine phosphorylation of PLD in response to H_2O_2 has recently been demonstrated in PC12 pheochromocytoma cells (131b). The phosphorylation induced by H_2O_2 or carbachol is Ca^{2+}-dependent, implying the involvement of PYK2 or another Ca^{2+}-dependent protein tyrosine kinase (131a, 131b).

Studies of the action of Rho as a mediator of stress fiber formation indicate the involvement of tyrosine kinases upstream and downstream from Rho (242, 285). In addition, treatment of fibroblasts with C. botulinum C3 exoenzyme to inactivate Rho causes a decrease in tyrosine phosphorylation of multiple proteins in response to GTPγS in vitro (305) and to bombesin and endothelin in intact cells (282). There has been a report of a novel hippocampal tyrosine kinase (p120[ACK]) that binds to the GTP-bound form of the Rho family member CDC42 (205).

In addition to tyrosine kinases, serine/threonine kinases have been reported to be targets of Rho family proteins (8, 162, 173, 206, 212, 393). The kinases that are activated by Rac and Cdc42 have been designated "p21–activated protein kinases" (PAKs) and are related to the STE 20 kinase that is involved in pheromone action and is a target of G protein $\beta\gamma$-subunits in Saccharomyces cerevisiae (212). The PAKs have been implicated in the pathway(s) by which Rac and Cdc42 activate the stress-activated protein kinase (SAPK)/Jun N-terminal kinase (JNK) pathway (106b, 188a, 243). In addition, Rho has specific protein kinase targets (for example, ROKα, ROKβ, p160[ROCK], and PKN (188a, 188b, 243). Although Rho can interact directly with PLD (111b), it may exert additional effects through these kinases.

Agonist-Stimulated Phosphatidylcholine Hydrolysis by Phospholipase C

Compared with the multitude of reports on the cellular role of PC-PLD, there have been few studies of PC-PLC. Because of the metabolic interconversion of DAG and PA and of P-choline and choline, it is unclear to what extent this enzyme plays a role in PC hydrolysis in mammalian cells. The enzyme has been purified from bacterial and plant sources, but although there have been reports of its activity in mammalian tissues (19, 85, 86), the enzyme has not been purified from an animal source. In some studies, evidence has been presented that agonist-stimulated PC hydrolysis in cells occurs by PLC in addition to PLD. This has included time-course studies of the changes in P-choline, choline, DAG, and PA and of the use of ethanol to suppress PA formation by PLD and of propranolol to inhibit DAG formation from PA in cells in which PC is predominantly, but not exclusively, labeled (11, 97, 128, 199, 213, 277, 289). However, the results of these experiments are not conclusive, and other studies have found that PLC plays little, if any, role in DAG formation from PC (2, 20, 37, 61, 76, 88, 273, 328). An analysis of three cell types has shown considerable differences in the formation of DAG by PC-PLD vs. PC-PLC (126).

Activation of PC-PLC directly produces DAG for activation of PKC, as well as P-choline, which has been proposed to be required for the mitogenic actions of PDGF, EGF, and FGF (63, 140). The enzyme also has been implicated in the action of transforming growth factor (TGF) β (74, 111). Moscat and co-workers have provided evidence that PLC-mediated hydrolysis of PC is required for the mitogenic action of PDGF in fibroblasts (179) and that PC-PLC is regulated by Ras (35, 80, 195). Furthermore, cells expressing bacterial PC-PLC show a transformed phenotype (141), and Xenopus oocytes microinjected with this enzyme undergo maturation (68). In fibroblasts in which PKC is downregulated, PDGF does not activate PLD, but still induces increases in DAG and phosphocholine, implying activation of PL-PLC (353a). Treatment of the cells with bacterial PC-PLC increases DAG and mimics the activation of the MAP kinase-signaling pathway by PDGF (353a). These findings support a role for PC-sPLC in growth factor signaling through MAP kinase. Other studies have employed D609 as an inhibitor of PC-PLC, but its specificity is questionable (353a). It is not clear how these findings can be integrated into the generally accepted pathways of transcriptional control by growth factors and Ras.

Agonist-Stimulated Phosphatidylcholine Hydrolysis by Phospholipase A_2

Stimulation of many cell types leads to the release of arachidonic acid, which is subsequently converted to a variety of potent extracellular eicosanoid mediators, including prostaglandins, leukotrienes, and thromboxanes. Arachidonic acid is released from PC, phosphatidylethanolamine, (PE) and PI due mainly to PLA$_2$ activity, and this is generally accepted to be the rate-limiting reaction for eicosanoid biosynthesis. Alternative pathways for arachidonic acid formation are its release from DAG due to DAG lipase activity (10, 21, 274) and its release from phospholipids due to sequential PLA$_1$ and lysophospholipase activity (268, 269). The extent to which these pathways are involved in agonist-stimulated arachidonic acid formation is unknown. It is generally assumed that they are minor, but this may not be the case (269). Also, PLA$_2$ is involved in the formation of platelet-activating factor from phospholipids, with an alkyl ether linkage at the sn-1 position.

Phospholipases of the A$_2$ type are classified into four groups and are either secretory or cytosolic (69). The secretory forms are of low mass (10–20 kd) and have five to seven disulfide pairs. They are found in the pancreas and secretory granules of neutrophils and platelets and in snake and bee venoms (69). The cytosolic forms are of higher molecular mass (90–110 kd) and show no homology with the secretory forms. There is evidence that they are the forms regulated by agonists (52, 53, 169, 187a, 190, 292). Although the relative rates differ depending on the isoforms and assay conditions, PC, PE, and PI are hydrolyzed by PLA$_2$ (53). Arachidonic acid is the preferred fatty acid in the sn-2 position (53), but other polyunsaturated acids can be released from this site. The enzyme can hydrolyze both alkylether and acyl forms of the phospholipids, but different isoforms vary in their relative rates of hydrolysis of these types of phospholipid.

Some forms of cytosolic PLA$_2$ are Ca^{2+}-independent (1a), whereas others are activated by physiological concentrations of Ca^{2+} (52, 105, 169), and activation is associated with translocation to membranes (51) (Fig. 11.13). Binding of Ca^{2+} is to a Ca^{2+} lipid binding domain in the N-terminal sequence of the enzyme (51, 53, 311). This domain also mediates membrane association of the enzyme (53, 235). Cytosolic PLA$_2$ is phosphorylated by MAP kinase on a specific residue (Ser505) and this is associated with activation of the enzyme (53, 191, 237) (Fig. 11.13). There is evidence that this phosphorylation occurs in intact cells in response to certain agonists (83, 279, 296, 375). However, PKC also has been implicated in the regulation of PLA$_2$ in some cells (53) (Fig. 11.13). Thus, phorbol myristate acetate can stimulate arachidonic acid release and induce phosphorylation and activation of cytosolic PLA$_2$ (100, 278, 279, 331, 365, 373, 374), and PKC down-regulation frequently impairs the effects of agonists on PLA$_2$ phos-

phorylation and arachidonic acid release (42, 100, 283, 331, 369). Since MAP kinase activation by agonists can occur by both PKC-dependent and -independent mechanisms (55, 202), it is possible that some of the effects of PKC on PLA$_2$ are mediated by MAP kinase (Fig. 11.13) (187a). The PKC isozyme specificity for activation of PLA$_2$ has not been explored in detail, but indirect evidence indicates a role for PKCα (100). Recently, cytosolic PLA$_2$ has been shown to be phosphorylated by p38 kinase (169a), a member of the MAP kinase family. The phospholipase is also a physiological target of p38 kinase in thrombin-stimulated receptors, although the phosphorylation is not required for PLA$_2$ activation (169a).

Many agonists whose receptors are linked to G$_i$ and G$_q$ activate PLA$_2$, and there is much evidence that the enzyme is controlled by G proteins (53, 56, 86). However, efforts to demonstrate direct regulation of PLA$_2$ by G protein subunits have been unsuccessful, and it is generally believed that the control is indirect. Agonists that activate G$_i$ and G$_q$ have been shown to activate MAP kinase (4, 23, 26, 62, 76, 121, 123, 134, 163, 173, 202, 226, 361, 371) and are known to stimulate PKC via PI-PLC (9) (Fig. 11.13). Because MAP kinase and PKC are able to induce the phosphorylation of cytosolic PLA$_2$ and stimulate arachidonic acid release, as described above, these would seem to be the mechanisms by which the G proteins activate PLA$_2$. The PKC-independent regulation of MAP kinase by G$_i$ appears to involve the $\beta\gamma$-subunit of the G protein (62, 90, 163) and a phosphorylation cascade involving Ras (4, 163, 371) (Fig.

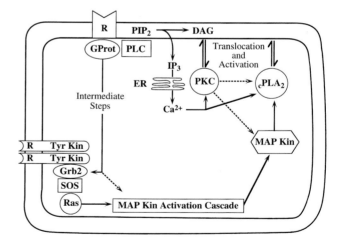

FIG. 11.13. Mechanisms of regulation of cytosolic phospholipase A$_2$ ($cPLA_2$) by growth factors and agonists linked to G proteins (GProt). $Tyr Kin$ tyrosine kinase; SOS, nucleotide exchange factor (GDP-dissociation stimulator) for Ras; DAG, 1,2-diacylglycerol; ER, endoplasmic reticulum; PLC, phospholipase C; PKC, protein kinase C; PIP_2, phosphatidylinositol 4,5-P$_2$; IP_3, inositol 1,4,5-P$_3$.

11.13). Regulation of the kinase by agonists that activate G_q also involves Ras (26, 361) and probably the α-subunit of the G protein.

Arachidonic acid release also can be stimulated by EGF, PDGF, bFGF, CSF-1, and TGFα in several cell types (42, 86, 101, 152, 295, 296, 321, 360, 375). The ability of these growth factors to induce arachidonic acid release is probably the result of their activation of MAP kinase, which occurs through a Ras-mediated pathway (55, 296, 307, 369, 375) (Fig. 11.13). The major kinase that phosphorylates and activates PLA$_2$, MAP kinase, may be involved in the transcriptional control of the enzyme that is also observed (53). In addition to activating PLA$_2$ when added to cells alone, some growth factors enhance the activation induced by G protein–linked agonists (83, 207). This may be due to simultaneous increases in MAP kinase activity and cytosolic Ca^{2+}, which enhance the translocation of cytosolic PLA$_2$ to the membranes (83).

Interleukin-1β (IL-1β), transforming growth factor-β (TFG-B), and tumor necrosis factor (TNFα) also enhance PLA$_2$ activity in fibroblasts and mesangial cells (53, 302) by mechanisms involving increased transcription. In an interesting development, Rac has been found to be essential for EGF-induced arachidonic acid production in fibroblasts (265). Thus, a dominant negative mutant of Rac (RacN17) inhibits EGF-dependent arachidonic acid release and leukotriene formation, and cells expressing a constitutively active Rac mutant (RacV12) exhibit enhanced leukotriene synthesis (265). Studies of the activation of Rac by growth factors in cells suggest the involvement of PI 3-kinase (167, 242).

SPHINGOMYELIN HYDROLYSIS AND ITS FUNCTIONAL SIGNIFICANCE

A rapidly developing concept in the study of lipid-based cell signaling is the sphingomyelin pathway (112, 165, 224, 265, 394) (Fig. 11.14). It is now recognized that TNFα, interferon γ (IFNγ), 1, 25–dihydroxyvitamin D$_3$ (vitamin D$_3$), IL-1β, NGF, and other neurotrophins stimulate the hydrolysis of SM by sphingomyelinase. The products are ceramide and P-choline (Fig. 11.14). Basal P-choline levels in most cells are very high and it seems unlikely that this compound acts as an intracellular signal. However, SM levels decline and ceramide levels increase significantly in several cell types in response to the agents listed above (81, 159, 217, 253, 254, 304). Activation of sphingomyelinase is rapid with TNFα, IL-1β, and neurotrophins, that is, detectable within a few minutes (78, 81, 159, 217, 304), whereas that with vitamin D$_3$ and IFNγ is slower,

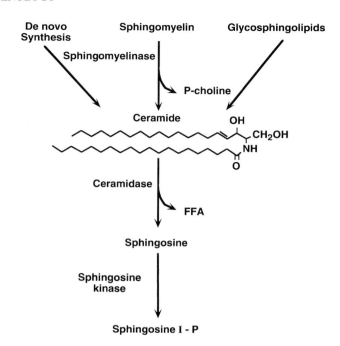

FIG. 11.14 Pathways of formation and breakdown of ceramide.

that is, maximal at 1.5–2 h (159, 253, 254). The mechanisms by which the receptors for these agents are coupled to the sphingomyelinase are unknown.

Ceramide has been proposed as an important intracellular signal because of its effects on cell growth, differentiation, and viability (112, 165, 224, 265, 394), which are similar to those induced by vitamin D$_3$, TNFα, and IFNγ. Thus, exogenous ceramides mimic the effects of these agents to induce differentiation of HL60 cells (18, 159, 253, 254). Low concentrations of C$_2$-ceramide and its analogs are also antiproliferative in several malignant and other cell lines (265). Ceramide induces a G_o/G_1 arrest in cell-cycle progression (139) and promotes dephosphorylation of the retinoblastoma gene product Rb, which has been implicated as an inhibitor of the cell cycle (67).

Tumor necrosis factor is a potent inducer of the nuclear transcription factor NF-κB, and many of its transcriptional effects appear to be mediated by this factor (356). Kolesnick and associates (165, 381) and Kronke and associates (198, 304) have provided evidence that activation of NF-κB by TNF is mediated by sphingomyelinase. However, the role of ceramide in the activation of NF-κB is unclear (66, 112a, 198, 304).

Initial studies indicated that ceramide was cytotoxic, but further work has shown that it plays a role in cellular senescence (354a), induces programmed cell death (apoptosis) (112a) and mediates the effects of radiation, TNFα, and the Fas/APO-1 cell surface antigen on apoptosis (245, 298a, 334). Ceramide also has been implicated in the regulation of protein trafficking (39, 192, 291). The specificity of action of ceramide has been shown in several studies by comparing the effects of its analogs and isomers (265).

Some intracellular targets for ceramide have been identified, namely, proteases of the interleukin converting enzyme (ICE) family (112a). The lipid also activates a ceramide-activated protein kinase (81, 216, 217) and a ceramide-activated protein phosphatase (77, 79, 370). The kinase is a proline-directed serine/threonine kinase that is membrane-associated (216). The phosphatase is a member of the phosphatase 2A class and is potently inhibited by okadaic acid (79). However, the physiological targets of these enzymes have not been defined, though the ceramide-activated kinase has been reported to phosphorylate Raf-1, a protein kinase that is a target of activated Ras (383). Raf-1 may be directly activated by ceramide (129a). In HL60 cells, TNFα has been reported to activate the SAPK/JNK pathway, leading to stimulation of AP-1-dependent gene transcription and translocation of NF-κB to the nucleus, resulting in stimulation of NFκB-dependent gene transcription (364). Treatment of cells with sphingomyelinase or ceramide also induced activation of these protein kinases and induction of c-*jun* (364), consistent with the view that ceramide acts as a second messenger for TNFα (165, 304, 381). There has also been a report that ceramide initiates apoptosis through the SAPK/JNK pathway (355a) and that the lipid activates SAPK/JNK through a protein kinase termed TAK1 (313a).

A role for ceramide in the activation of PKC and PLD is indicated by the observation that treatment of skin fibroblasts or epidermal cells with sphingomyelinase or C$_2$-ceramide blocks translocation of PKCα, but not PKCϵ, and inhibits the activation of PLD induced by bradykinin or exogenous DAG (146). Another soluble analog of ceramide, C$_6$-ceramide, also inhibits PLD activation in young fibroblasts treated with serum or phorbol ester (354). Senescent WI-38 fibroblasts, which have elevated endogenous ceramide, do not show a PLD response to serum (354), indicating a possible role for this lipid in cell senescense. Inhibitory effects of C$_2$- and C$_6$-ceramide and sphingomyelinase on PLD activation by LPA, phorbol myristate acetate, thrombin, and serum in rat fibroblasts also have been reported (102).

Sphingosine is another metabolite of sphingomyelin, which is produced by removal of the fatty acyl group from ceramide (Fig. 11.14). It can be converted to sphingosine 1-phosphate (SPP) by a specific kinase. Sphingosine was recognized to be an inhibitor of PKC (113, 221, 368) and PAP (181, 230) and can produce dramatic cytoskeletal changes in association with tyrosine phosphorylation of multiple substrates (310). In cells, SPP has a number of in vitro and in vivo effects and has been proposed as an intracellular signal (71, 99, 103, 255, 388, 390). It mobilizes intracellular Ca^{2+} (99, 390) by an IP$_3$-independent mechanism (218) and increases PA by activating PLD (71, 160, 180, 389). Activation of sphingosine kinase by PDGF and serum has been observed in fibroblasts, and it has been proposed that the resulting formation of SPP may be involved in the stimulation of DNA synthesis (255). The signaling pathways involved in the mitogenic action of SPP are largely unknown. However, inhibition of the response by pertussis toxin (103) suggests that it is mediated by a receptor coupled to a G protein of the G$_i$/G$_o$ family. Sphingosine 1-phosphate is normally present in plasma and serum (384b), and it interacts with a high affinity receptor in atrial myocytes (34a).

SUMMARY

Phospholipid-derived second messengers are now recognized to play major roles in the control of cellular functions and in the communication between cells. The first recognized cell-signaling system involving phospholipids was the agonist-induced hydrolysis of inositol phospholipids (PIP$_2$). The function and mechanism of action of the released IP$_3$ as a mediator of Ca^{2+} mobilization is now clear, but the mechanisms involved in the generation of the complex changes in cell Ca^{2+} (sparks and waves) and in the stimulation of Ca^{2+} influx are still obscure. Protein kinase C remains the major target of the DAG produced by PIP$_2$ breakdown, but the specific functions of the various PKC isozymes are unclear. The β and γ isozymes of PI-PLC play roles in the regulation of PIP$_2$ hydrolysis by G protein–linked agonists and growth factors, respectively, but the function(s) of the δ isozyme is unknown. G protein regulation of PI-PLC involves either α-subunits of the G$_q$ family or $\beta\gamma$-subunits of the G$_i$ family, and the molecular details of their interactions are being defined. The major mechanism by which growth factor receptors activate PI-PLCγ is through recruitment to specific phosphorylated tyrosine residues in their cytoplasmic domains, but it is not clear how this leads to activation.

Both PIP$_3$ and the PI 3-kinase isozymes that generate it from PIP$_2$ are now recognized to be involved in agonist control of many important cellular processes, including mitogenesis and regulation of the cell cycle, actin polymerization and the resulting morphological changes, glucose transport, and exocytosis. Growth factors activate PI 3-kinase through a mechanism similar to that for PI-PLCγ except that different autophosphorylation sites are involved. Agonists linked to G_i also activate the enzyme through a mechanism involving βγ-subunits. Several small G proteins (Ras, Rho, and Rac) have been implicated in both upstream and downstream events involving PI 3-kinase, but the pathways are poorly defined.

Hydrolysis of PC by PLD is a very widespread response to many agonists. Regulation of PLD appears to be complex, with evidence for roles of PKC and other serine/threonine kinases, Ca^{2+}, Rho, ARF, and soluble tyrosine kinases. With the cloning of PLD isozymes, the mechanisms involved in the regulation of PLD should become clearer. The initial product of PLD is PA and several cellular effects have been ascribed to this lipid. However, it is largely converted to DAG in most cells and to LPA in platelets and other cells. Diacylglycerol derived from PC via PLD activates Ca^{2+}-independent isozymes of PKC, whereas LPA released from platelets is now recognized as a major intercellular messenger, acting on a receptor(s) coupled to G_q or G_i to mobilize Ca^{2+}, stimulating growth via the Ras/MAP kinase pathway, and inducing actin polymerization and tyrosine phosphorylation to form stress fibers and focal adhesions via Rho proteins.

Phospholipase A_2 has long been recognized as the major cellular enzyme producing arachidonic acid for the production of various eicosanoids. This function is probably subserved by the cytosolic form of the enzyme, whereas the lower M_r secretory forms perform other functions. Many agonists activate PLA_2 and the mechanisms involve MAP kinase, PKC, and Ca^{2+}, though their roles are not clear.

Sphingomyelin hydrolysis by sphingomyelinase to yield ceramide is a major physiological response to TNFα, IFNγ, IL-1, and certain other agonists. Ceramide activates a protein kinase and phosphatase and has important effects on cell growth, differentiation, and viability, including the induction of apoptosis. It regulates the cell cycle and stimulates NF-κB-dependent gene transcription. Another product of sphingomyelin metabolism is SPP, which can mobilize Ca^{2+} and induce mitogenesis.

The concept that cells utilize their membrane lipids to generate intracellular and extracellular signaling molecules has progressed far beyond the early reports of cell phospholipids being utilized as a source of eicosanoids and platelet-activating factor and of inositol phospholipid hydrolysis being linked to changes in cell Ca^{2+}. The most exciting new developments are the widespread occurrence of PC hydrolysis by PLD and the recognition of PIP_3, PI 3-kinase, ceramide, and sphingomyelinase as mediating important signaling pathways in the control of many cellular events, including growth and apoptosis.

I thank Judy Childs for the major role she played in the preparation of this chapter.

REFERENCES

1. Abram, C. S., J. Zhang, C. P. Downes, X-w. Tang, W. Zhao, and S. E. Rittenhouse. Phosphopleckstrin inhibits Gβγ-activable platelet phosphatidylinositol-4,5-bisphosphate 3-kinase. *J. Biol. Chem.* 271: 25192–25197, 1996.

1a. Ackerman, E. J., E. S. Kempner, and E. A. Dennis. Ca^{2+}-independent cytosolic phospholpase A_2 from macrophage-like P388D21 cells. Isolation and characterization. *J. Biol. Chem.* 269: 9227–9233, 1994.

2. Ahmed, A., R. Plevin, M. H. Shoaibi, S. A. Fountain, R. A. Ferriani, and S. K. Smith. Basic FGF activates phospholipase D in endothelial cells in the absence of inositol-lipid hydrolysis. *Am. J. Physiol.* 266 (*Cell Physiol.*) 35): C206–C212, 1994.

3. Ahmed, S., J. Lee, R. Kozma, A. Best, C. Monfries, and L. Lim. A novel functional target for tumor-promoting phorbol esters and lysophosphatidic acid. The p21*rac*-GTPase activating protein *n*-chimaerin. *J. Biol. Chem.* 268: 10709–10712, 1993.

3a. Akimoto, K., R. Takahashi, S. Moriya, N. Nishioka, J. Takayanagi, K. Kimura, Y. Fukui, S-i. Osada, K. Mizuno, S-i. Hirai, A. Kazlauskas, and S. Ohno. EGF or PDGF receptors activate atypical PKCλ through phosphatidylinositol 3-kinase. *EMBO J.* 15: 788–798, 1996.

4. Alblas, J., E. J. van Corven, P. L. Hordijk, G. Milligan, and W. H. Moolenaar. G_i-mediated activation of the p21^{ras}-mitogen-activated protein kinase pathway by α2-adrenergic receptors expressed in fibroblasts. *J. Biol. Chem.* 268: 22235–22238, 1993.

4a. Alessi, D. R., S. R. James, C. P. Downes, A. B. Holmes, P.R.J. Gaffney, C. B. Reese, and P. Cohen. Characterization of a 3-phosphoinositide-dependent protein kinase which phosphorylates and activates protein kinase Bα. *Curr. Biol.* 7: 261–269, 1997.

5. Arcaro, A., and M. P. Wymann. Wortmannin is a potent phosphatidylinositol 3-kinase inhibitor: the role of phosphatidylinositol 3,4,5-trisphosphate in neutrophil responses. *Biochem. J.* 296: 297–301, 1993.

6. Arkinstall, S., C. Chabert, K. Maundrell, and M. Peitsch. Mapping regions of $G_{αq}$ interacting with PLCβ1 using multiple overlapping synthetic peptides. *FEBS Lett.* 364: 45–50, 1995.

7. Asano, M., K. Tamiya-Koizumi, Y. Homma, T. Takenawa, Y. Nimura, K. Kojima, and S. Yoshida. Purification and characterization of nuclear phospholipase C specific for phosphoinositides. *J. Biol. Chem.* 269: 12360–12366, 1994.

8. Bagrodia, S., S. J. Taylor, C. L. Creasy, J. Chernoff, and R. A. Cerione. Identification of a mouse p21$^{Cdc42/Rac}$ activated kinase. *J. Biol. Chem.* 270: 22731–22737, 1995.

9. Balboa, M. A., B. L. Firestein, C. Godson, K. S. Bell, and P. A. Insel. Protein kinase $C_α$ mediates phospholipase D activation by nucleotides and phorbol ester in Madin-Darby canine kidney cells. Stimulation of phospholipase D is independent of activation of polyphosphoinositide-specific phospholipase C and phospholipase A_2. *J. Biol. Chem.* 269: 10511–10516, 1994.

9a. Baldwin, J. M. Structure and function of receptors coupled to G proteins. *Curr. Opin. Cell Biol.* 6: 180–190, 1994.

10. Balsinde, J., E. Diez, and F. Mollinedo. Arachidonic acid release from diacylglycerol in human neutrophils. Translocation of diacylglycerol-deacylating enzyme activities from an intracellular pool to plasma membrane upon cell activation. *J. Biol. Chem.* 266: 15638–15643, 1991.

10a. Banno, Y., K. Tamiya-Koizumi, H. Oshima, A. Morikawa, S. Yoshida, and Y. Nozawa. Nuclear ADP-ribosylation factor (ARF)- and oleate-dependent phospholipase D (PLD) in rat liver cells. Increases of ARF-dependent PLD activity in regenerating liver cells. *J. Biol. Chem.* 272: 5208–5213, 1997.

11. Barnett, R. L., L. Ruffini, L. Ramsammy, R. Pasmantier, M. M. Friedlaender, and E. P. Nord. Angiotensin-mediated phosphatidylcholine hydrolysis and protein kinase C activation in mesangial cells. *Am. J. Physiol.* 265 (*Cell Physiol.* 34): C1100–C1108, 1993.

12. Bauldry, S. A., D. A. Bass, S. L. Cousart, and C. E. McCall. Tumor necrosis factor α priming of phospholipase D in human neutrophils. Correlation between phosphatidic acid production and superoxide generation. *J. Biol. Chem.* 266: 4173–4179, 1991.

13. Berridge, M. J. Rapid accumulation of inositol trisphosphate reveals that agonists hydrolyse polyphosphoinositides instead of phosphatidylinositol. *Biochem. J.* 212: 849–858, 1983.

14. Berridge, M. J. Inositol trisphosphate and diacylglycerol as second messengers. *Biochem. J.* 220: 345–360, 1984.

15. Berridge, M. J. Inositol trisphosphate and calcium signalling. *Nature* 361: 315–325, 1993.

16. Berridge, M. J. Capacitative calcium entry. *Biochem. J.* 312: 1–11, 1995.

17. Berridge, M. J., and G. Dupont. Spatial and temporal signalling by calcium. *Curr. Opin. Cell Biol.* 6: 267–274, 1994.

17a. Bi, K., M. G. Roth, and N. T. Ktistakis. Phosphatidic acid formation by phospholipase D is required for transport from the endoplasmic reticulum to the Golgi complex. *Curr. Biol.* 7:301–307, 1997.

18. Bielawska, A., C. M. Linardic, and Y. A. Hannun. Ceramide-mediated biology. Determination of structural and stereospecific requirements through the use of *N*-acyl-phenylaminoalcohol analogs. *J. Biol. Chem.* 267: 18493–18497, 1992.

19. Billah, M. M., and J. C. Anthes. The regulation and cellular functions of phosphatidylcholine hydrolysis. *Biochem. J.* 269: 281–291, 1990.

20. Billah, M. M., S. Eckel, T. J. Mullmann, R. W. Egan, and M. I. Siegel. Phosphatidylcholine hydrolysis by phospholipase D determines phosphatidate and diglyceride levels in chemotactic peptide-stimulated human neutrophils. Involvement of phosphatidate phosphohydrolase in signal transduction. *J. Biol. Chem.* 264: 17069–17077, 1989.

20a. Birnbaumer, L., X. Zhu, M. Jiang, G. Boulay, M. Peyton, B. Vannier, D. Brown, D. Platano, H. Sadeghi, E. Stefani, and M. Birnbaumer. On the molecular basis and regulation of cellular capacitative calcium entry: Roles for Trp proteins. *Proc. Natl. Acad. Sci. U.S.A.* 93: 15195–15202, 1996.

21. Bishop, W. R., and R. M. Bell. Attenuation of *sn*-1,2-diacylglycerol second messengers. Metabolism of exogenous diacylglycerols by human platelets. *J. Biol. Chem.* 261: 12513–12519, 1986.

22. Blackshear, P. J. The MARCKS family of cellular protein kinase substrates. *J. Biol. Chem.* 268: 1501–1504, 1993.

22a. Blank, J. L., K. A. Brattain, and J. H. Exton. Activation of cytosolic phosphoinositide phospholipase C by G-protein βγ subunits. *J. Biol. Chem.* 267: 23069–23075, 1992.

23. Blumer, K. J., and G. L. Johnson. Diversity in function and regulation of MAP kinase pathways. *Trends Biochem. Sci.* 19: 236–240, 1994.

24. Bocckino, S. B., and J. H. Exton. Phosphatidic acid. In: *Handbook of Lipid Research,* edited by R. M. Bell, S. M. Prescott, and J. H. Exton. New York: Plenum, 1996, p. 75–124.

25. Bocckino, S. B., P. B. Wilson, and J. H. Exton. Phosphatidate-dependent protein phosphorylation. *Proc. Natl. Acad. Sci. U.S.A.* 88: 6210–6213, 1991.

26. Bogoyevitch, M. A., P. E. Glennon, M. B. Andersson, A. Clerk, A. Lazou, C. J. Marshall, P. J. Parker, and P. H. Sugden. Endothelin-1 and fibroblast growth factors stimulate the mitogen-activated protein kinase signaling cascade in cardiac myocytes. The potential role of the cascade in the integration of two signaling pathways leading to myocyte hypertrophy. *J. Biol. Chem.* 269: 1110–1119, 1994.

27. Bootman, M. D., and M. J. Berridge. The elemental principles of calcium signalling. *Cell* 83: 675–678, 1995.

28. Bourgoin, S., and S. Grinstein. Peroxides of vanadate induce activation of phospholipase D in HL-60 cells. Role of tyrosine phosphorylation. *J. Biol. Chem.* 267: 11908–11916, 1992.

29. Bourgoin, S., D. Harbour, Y. Desmarais, Y. Takai, and A. Beaulier. Low molecular weight GTP-binding proteins in HL-60 granulocytes. Assessment of the role of ARF and of a 50-kDa cytosolic protein in phospholipase D activation. *J. Biol. Chem.* 270: 3172–3178, 1995.

29a. Bourne, H. R. How receptors talk to trimeric G proteins. *Curr. Opin. Cell Biol.* 9: 134–142, 1997.

30. Bowman, E. P., D. J. Uhlinger, and J. D. Lambeth. Neutrophil phospholipase D is activated by a membrane-associated Rho family small molecular weight GTP-binding protein. *J. Biol. Chem.* 268: 21509–21512, 1993.

31. Briscoe, C. P., A. Martin, M. Cross, and M.J.O. Wakelam. The roles of multiple pathways in regulating bombesin-stimulated phospholipase D activity in Swiss 3T3 fibroblasts. *Biochem. J.* 306: 115–122, 1995.

32. Brown, H. A., S. Gutowski, R. A. Kahn, and P. C. Sternweis. Partial purification and characterization of Arf-sensitive phospholipase D from porcine brain. *J. Biol. Chem.* 270: 14935–14943, 1995.

33. Brown, H. A., S. Gutowski, C. R. Moomaw, C. Slaughter, and P. C. Sternweis. ADP-ribosylation factor, a small GTP-dependent regulatory protein, stimulates phospholipase D activity. *Cell* 75: 1137–1144, 1993.

34. Buchner, K. Protein kinase C in the transduction of signals toward and within the cell nucleus. *Eur. J. Biochem.* 228: 211–221, 1995.

34a. Bünemann, M., K. Liliom, B. K. Brandts, L. Pott, J-L. Tseng, D. M. Desiderio, G. Sun, D. Miller, and G. Tigyi. A novel membrane receptor with high affinity for lysosphingomyelin and sphingosine 1-phosphate in atrial myocytes. *EMBO J.* 15:5527–5534, 1996.

34b. Burgering, B.M.T., and P. J. Coffer. Protein kinase B (c-Akt) in phosphatidylinositol-3-OH kinase signal transduction. *Nature* 376: 599–602, 1995.

35. Cai, H., P. Erhardt, J. Szeberenyi, M. T. Diaz-Meco, T. Johansen, J. Moscat, and G. M. Cooper. Hydrolysis of phosphatidylcholine is stimulated by Ras proteins during mitogenic signal transduction. *Mol. Cell. Biol.* 12: 5329–5335, 1992.

36. Carpenter, C. L., K. R. Auger, M. Chanudhur, M. Yoakim, B. Schaffhausen, S. Shoelson, and L. C. Cantley. Phosphoinositide 3-kinase is activated by phosphopeptides that bind to the SH2 domains of the 85-kDa subunit. *J. Biol. Chem.* 268: 9478–9483, 1993.

37. Chabot, M. C., L. C. McPhail, R. L. Wykle, D. A. Kennerly, and C. E. McCall. Comparison of diglyceride production from

choline-containing phosphoglycerides in human neutrophils stimulated with N-formylmethionyl-leucylphenylalanine, ionophore A23187 or phorbol 12-myristate 13–acetate. *Biochem. J.* 286: 693–699, 1992.

38. Cheatham, B., C. J. Vlahos, L. Cheatham, L. Wang, J. Blenis, and C. R. Kahn. Phosphatidylinositol 3-kinase activation is required for insulin stimulation of pp70 S6 kinase, DNA synthesis, and glucose transporter translocation. *Mol. Cell. Biol.* 14: 4902–4911, 1994.

39. Chen, C.-S., A. G. Rosenwald, and R. E. Pagano. Ceramide as a modulator of endocytosis. *J. Biol. Chem.* 270: 13291–13297, 1995.

40. Chen, H.-C., and J.-L. Guan. Association of focal adhesion kinase with its potential substrate phosphatidylinositol 3-kinase. *Proc. Natl. Acad. Sci. U.S.A.* 91: 10148–10152, 1994.

41. Chen, H.-C., and J.-L. Guan. Stimulation of phosphatidylinositol 3'-kinase association with focal adhesion kinase by platelet-derived growth factor. *J. Biol. Chem.* 269: 31229–31233, 1994.

41a. Chen, Y-G., A. Siddhanta, C. D. Austin, S. M. Hammond, T-C. Sung, M. A. Frohman, A. J. Morris, and D. Shields. Phospholipase D stimulates release of nascent secretory vesicles from the *trans*-Golgi network. *J. Cell Biol.* 138:495–504, 1997.

42. Chow, S. C., and G. Powis. Mechanisms of platelet-derived growth factor–induced arachidonic acid release in Swiss 3T3 fibroblasts: the role of a localized increase in free Ca^{2+} concentration beneath the plasma membrane and the activation of protein kinase C. *Biochim. Biophys. Acta* 1179: 81–88, 1993.

44. Chuang, T.-H., B. B. Bohl, and G. M. Bokoch. Biologically active lipids are regulators of Rac GDO complexation. *J. Biol. Chem.* 268: 26206–26211, 1993.

45. Chung, J., T. C. Grammer, K. P. Lemon, A. Kazlauskas, and J. Blenis. PDGF-and insulin-dependent pp70^{S6K} activation mediated by phosphatidylinositol-3–OH kinase. *Nature* 370: 71–75, 1994.

46. Chung, J., C. J. Kuo, G. R. Crabtree, and J. Blenis. Rapamycin-FKBP specifically blocks growth-dependent activation of and signalling by the 70 kDa S6 protein kinase. *Cell* 79: 1229–1236, 1992.

46a. Chung, J-K., F. Sekiya, H-S. Kang, C. Lee, J-S. Han, S. R. Kim, Y. S. Bae, A. J. Morris, and S. G. Rhee. Synaptojanin inhibition of phospholipase D activity by hydrolysis of phosphatidylinositol 4,5-bisphosphate. *J. Biol. Chem.* 272:15980–15985, 1997.

47. Claesson-Welsh, L. Platelet-derived growth factor receptor signals. *J. Biol. Chem.* 269: 32023–32026, 1994.

48. Clapham, D. E. Calcium signalling. *Cell* 80: 259–268, 1995.

49. Clapham, D. E., and E. J. Neer. New roles for G-protein βγ-dimers in transmembrane signalling. *Nature* 365: 403–406, 1993.

50. Clark, E. A., and J. S. Brugge. Integrins and signal transduction pathways: the road taken. *Science* 268: 233–239, 1995.

51. Clark, J. D., L.-L. Lin, R. W. Kriz, C. S. Ramesha, L. A. Sultzman, A. Y. Lin, N. Milona, and J. L. Knopf. A novel arachidonic acid–selective cytosolic PLA$_2$ contains a Ca^{2+}-dependent translocation domain with homology to PKC and GAP. *Cell* 65: 1043–1051, 1991.

52. Clark, J. D., N. Milona, and J. L. Knopf. Purification of a 110-kilodalton cytosolic phospholipase A$_2$ from the human monocytic cell line U937. *Proc. Natl. Acad. Sci. U.S.A.* 87: 7708–7712, 1990.

53. Clark, J. D., A. R. Schievella, E. A. Nalefski, and L.-L. Lin. Cytosolic phospholipase A$_2$. *J. Lipid Mediat. Cell Signal.* 12: 83–117, 1995.

54. Clarke, J. F., P. W. Young, K. Yonezawa, M. Kasuga, and G. D. Holman. Inhibition of the translocation of GLUT1 and GLUT4 in 3T3–L1 cells by the phosphatidylinositol 3-kinase inhibitor, wortmannin. *Biochem. J.* 300: 631–635, 1994.

55. Cobb, M. H., and E. J. Goldsmith. How MAP kinases are regulated. *J. Biol. Chem.* 270: 14843–14846, 1995.

56. Cockcroft, S. G-protein-regulated phospholipases C, D and A$_2$-mediated signalling in neutrophils. *Biochim. Biophys. Acta* 1113: 135–160, 1992.

57. Cockcroft, S., G.M.H. Thomas, A. Fensome, B. Geny, E. Cunningham, I. Gout, I. Hiles, N. F. Totty, O.Truong, and J. J. Hsuan. Phospholipase D: a downstream effector of ARF in granulocytes. *Science* 263: 523–526, 1994.

57a. Colley, W. C., T-C Sung, R. Roll, J. Jenco, S. M. Hammond, Y. Altshuller, D. Bar-Sagi, A. J. Morris, and M. A. Frohman. Phospholipase D2, a distinct phospholipase D isoform with novel regulatory properties that provokes cytoskeletal reorganization. *Curr. Biol.* 7: 191–201, 1997.

58. Conklin, B. R., and H. R. Bourne. Structural elements of Gα subunits that interact with Gβγ, receptors, and effectors. *Cell* 73: 631–641, 1993.

59. Conricode, K. M., K. A. Brewer, and J. H. Exton. Activation of phospholipase D by protein kinase C. Evidence for a phosphorylation-independent mechanism. *J. Biol. Chem.* 267: 7199–7202, 1992.

60. Conricode, K. M., J. L. Smith, D. J. Burns, and J. H. Exton. Phospholipase D activation in fibroblast membranes by the α and β isoforms of protein kinase C. *FEBS Lett.* 342: 149–153, 1994.

61. Cook, S. J., and M.J.O. Wakelam. Analysis of the water-soluble products of phosphatidylcholine breakdown by ion-exchange chromatography. Bombesin and TPA (12–O–tetradecanoylphorbol 13-acetate) stimulate choline generation in Swiss 3T3 cells by a common mechanism. *Biochem. J.* 263: 581–587, 1989.

62. Crespo, P., N. Xu, W. F. Simonds, and J. S. Gutkind. Ras-dependent activation of MAP kinase pathway mediated by G-protein βγ subunits. *Nature* 369: 418–420, 1994.

62a. Cross, D.A.E., D. R. Alessi, P. Cohen, M. Andjelkovich, and B. A. Hemmings. Inhibition of glycogen synthase kinase-3 by insulin mediated by protein kinase B. *Nature* 378: 785–789, 1995.

62b. Cross, D.A.E., P. W. Watt, M. Shaw, J. van der Kaay, C. P. Downes, J. C. Holder, and P. Cohen. Insulin activates protein kinase B, inhibits glycogen synthase kinase-3 and activates glycogen synthase by rapamycin-insensitive pathways in skeletal muscle and adipose tissue. *FEBS Lett.* 406:211–215, 1997.

63. Cuadrado, A., A. Carnero, F. Dolfi, B. Jimenez, and J. C. Lacal. Phosphorylcholine: a novel second messenger essential for mitogenic activity of growth factors. *Oncogene* 8: 2959–2968, 1993.

64. Daniel, L. W., G. W. Small, and J. D. Schmitt. Alkyl-linked diglycerides inhibit protein kinase C activation by diacylglycerols. *Biochem. Biophys. Res. Commun.* 151: 291–297, 1988.

64a. Datta, K., A. Bellacosa, T. O. Chan, and P. N. Tsichlis. Akt is a direct target of the phosphatidylinositol 3-kinase. Activation by growth factors, v-src and v-Ha-ras, in Sf9 and mammalian cells. *J. Biol. Chem.* 271: 30835–30839, 1996.

65. Day, C. P., and S. J. Yeaman. Physical evidence for the presence of two forms of phosphatidate phosphohydrolase in rat liver. *Biochim. Biophys. Acta* 1127: 87–94, 1992.

66. Dbaibo, G. S., L. M. Obeid, and Y. A. Hannun. Tumor necrosis factor-α (TNF-α) signal transduction through ceramide. Dissociation of growth inhibitory effects of TNF-α from activation of nuclear factor-k. *J. Biol. Chem.* 268: 17762–17766, 1993.

67. Dbaibo, G. S., M. Y. Pushkareva, S. Jayadev, J. K. Schwarz, J. M. Horowitz, L. M. Obeid, and Y. A. Hannun. Retinoblastoma gene product as a downstream target for a ceramide-dependent pathway of growth arrest. *Proc. Natl. Acad. Sci. U.S.A.* 92: 1347–1351, 1995.

68. de Herreros, A. G., I. Dominguez, M. T. Diaz-Meco, G. Graziani, M. E. Cornet, P. H. Guddal, T. Johansen, and J. Moscat. Requirement of phospholipase C-catalyzed hydrolysis of phosphatidylcholine for maturation of *Xenopus laevis* oocytes in response to insulin and *ras* p21. *J. Biol. Chem.* 266: 6825–6829, 1991.

68a. DeMali, K. A., C. C. Whiteford, E. T. Ulug, and A. Kazlauskas. Platelet-derived growth factor-dependent cellular transformation requires either phospholipase Cγ or phosphatidylinositol 3 kinase. *J. Biol. Chem.* 272: 9011–9018, 1997.

69. Dennis, E. A. Diversity of group types, regulation, and function of phospholipase A₂. *J. Biol. Chem.* 269: 13057–13060, 1994.

70. Dennis, E. A., S. G. Rhee, M. M. Billah, and Y. A. Hannun. Role of phospholipases in generating lipid second messengers in signal transduction. *FASEB J.* 5: 2068–2077, 1991.

71. Desai, N., H. Zhang, A. Olivera, M. E. Mattie, and S. Spiegel. Sphingosine-1–phosphate, a metabolite of sphingosine, increases phosphatidic acid levels by phospholipase D activation. *J. Biol. Chem.* 267: 23122–23128, 1992.

72. Dewald, B., M. Thelen, and M. Baggiolini. Two transduction sequences are necessary for neutrophil activation by receptor agonists. *J. Biol. Chem.* 263: 16179–16184, 1988.

73. Dhand, R., I. Hiles, G. Panayotou, S. Roche, M. J. Fry, I. Gout, N. F. Totty, O. Truong, P. Vicendo, K. Yonezasa, M. Kasuga, S. A. Courtneidge, and M. D. Waterfield. PI 3-kinase is a dual specificity enzyme: autoregulation by an intrinsic protein-serine kinase activity. *EMBO J.* 13: 522–533, 1994.

74. Diaz-Meco, M. T., I. Dominguez, L. Sanz, M. M. Municio, E. Berra, M. E. Cornet, A. G. de Herreros, T. Johansen, and J. Moscat. Phospholipase C-mediated hydrolysis of phosphatidylcholine is a target of transforming growth factor β1 inhibitory signals. *Mol. Cell. Biol.* 12: 302–308, 1992.

74a. Didichenko, S. A., B. Tilton, B. A. Hemmings, K. Ballmer-Hofer, and M. Thelen. Constitutive activation of protein kinase B and phosphorylation of p47^phox by a membrane-targeted phosphoinositide 3-kinase. *Curr. Biol.* 6: 1271–1278, 1996.

75. Ding, J., C. J. Vlahos, R. Liu, R. F. Brown, and J. A. Badwey. Antagonists of phosphtidylinositol 3-kinase block activation of several novel protein kinases in neutrophils. *J. Biol. Chem.* 270: 11684–11691, 1995.

76. Dinh, T. T., and D. A. Kennerly. Assessment of receptor-dependent activation of phosphatidylcholine hydrolysis by both phospholipase D and phospholipase C. *Cell Regul.* 2: 229–309, 1991.

77. Dobrowsky, R. T., and Y. A. Hannun. Ceramide stimulates a cytosolic protein phosphatase. *J. Biol. Chem.* 267: 5048–5051, 1992.

78. Dobrowsky, R. T., G. M. Jenkins, and Y. A. Hannun. Neurotrophins induce sphingomyelin hydrolysis. Modulation by co-expression of p75^NTR with Trk receptors. *J. Biol. Chem.* 270: 22135–22142, 1995.

79. Dobrowsky, R. T., C. Kamibayashi, M. C. Mumby, and Y. A. Hannun. Ceramide activates heterotrimeric protein phosphatase 2A. *J. Biol. Chem.* 268: 15523–15530, 1993.

79a. Dohlman, H. G., and J. Thorner. RGS proteins and signaling by heterotrimeric G proteins. *J. Biol. Chem.* 272: 3871–3874, 1997.

80. Dominguez, K., M. S. Marshall, J. B. Gibbs, A. G. de Herreros, M. E. Cornet, G. Graziani, M. T. Diaz-Meco, T. Johansen, F. McCormick, and J. Moscat. Role of GTPase activating protein in mitogenic signalling through phosphatidylcholine-hydrolysing phospholipase C. *EMBO J.* 10: 3215–3220, 1991.

81. Dressler, K. A., S. Mathias, and R. N. Kolesnick. Tumor necrosis factor-α activates the sphingomyelin signal transduction pathway in a cell-free system. *Science* 255: 1715–1718, 1992.

82. Dubyak, G. R., S. J. Schomisch, D. J. Kusner, and M. Xie. Phospholipase D activity in phagocytic leucocytes is synergistically regulated by G-protein- and tyrosine kinase-based mechanisms. *Biochem. J.* 292: 121–128, 1993.

82a. Dudek, H., S. R. Datta, T. F. Franke, M. J. Birnbaum, R. Yao, G. M. Cooper, R. A. Segal, D. R. Kaplan, and M. E. Greenberg. Regulation of neuronal survival by the serine-threonine protein kinase Akt. *Science* 275: 661–665, 1997.

83. Durstin, M., S. Durstin, T.F.P. Molski, E. L. Becker, and R. I. Sha'afi. Cytoplasmic phospholipase A₂ translocates to membrane fraction in human neutrophils activated by stimuli that phosphorylate mitogen-activated protein kinase. *Proc. Natl. Acad. Sci. U.S.A.* 91: 3142–3146, 1994.

84. Eldar, H., P. Ben-Av, U.-S. Schmidt, E. Livneh, and M. Liscovitch. Up-regulation of phospholipase D activity induced by over-expression of protein kinase C-α. Studies in intact Swiss/3T3 cells and in detergent-solubilized membranes in vitro. *J. Biol. Chem.* 268: 12560–12564, 1993.

85. Exton, J. H. Signalling through phosphatidylcholine breakdown. *J. Biol. Chem.* 265: 1–4, 1990.

86. Exton, J. H. Phosphatidylcholine breakdown and signal transduction. *Biochim. Biophys. Acta* 1212: 26–42, 1994.

87. Exton, J. H. Regulation of phosphoinositide phospholipases by hormones, neurotransmitters and other agonists linked to G-proteins. *Annu. Rev. Pharmacol. Toxicol.* 36: 481–509, 1996.

88. Fallman, M., M. Gullberg, C. Hellberg, and T. Andersson. Complement receptor-mediated phagocytosis is associated with accumulation of phosphatidylcholine-derived diglyceride in human neutrophils. Involvement of phospholipase D and direct evidence for a positive feedback signal of protein kinase C. *J. Biol. Chem.* 267: 2656–2663, 1992.

89. Fantl, W. J., J. A. Escobedo, G. A. Martin, C. W. Turck, M. del Rasario, F. McCormick, and L. T. Williams. Distinct phosphotyrosines on a growth factor receptor bind to specific molecules that mediate different signaling pathways. *Cell* 69: 413–423, 1992.

90. Faure, M., T. A. Voyno-Yasenetskaya, and H. R. Bourne. cAMP and βγ subunits of heterotrimeric G proteins stimulate the mitogen-activated protein kinase pathway in COS-7 cells. *J. Biol. Chem.* 269: 7851–7854, 1994.

91. Feig, L. A. Guanine-nucleotide exchange factors: a family of positive regulators of Ras and related GTPases. *Curr. Opin. Cell Biol.* 6: 204–211, 1994.

92. Ferguson, J. E., and M. R. Hanley. Phosphatidic acid and lysophosphatidic acid stimulate receptor-regulated membrane currents in the *Xenopus laevis* oocyte. *Arch. Biochem. Biophys.* 297: 388–392, 1992.

93. Fernandez, B., M. A. Balboa, J. A. Solis-Herruzo, and J. Balsinde. Phosphatidate-induced arachidonic acid mobilization in mouse peritoneal macrophages. *J. Biol. Chem.* 269: 26711–26716, 1994.

94. Ferris, C. D., and S. H. Snyder. Inositol 1,4,5-trisphosphate-activated calcium channels. *Annu. Rev. Physiol.* 54: 469–488, 1992.

94a. Fleming, I. N., C. M. Elliott, and J. H. Exton. Differential translocation of Rho family GTPases by lysophosphatidic acid, endothelin-1, and platelet-derived growth factor. *J. Biol. Chem.* 271: 33067–33073, 1996.

94b. Franke, T. F., D. R. Kalan, and L. C. Cantley. P13K: Downstream AKTion blocks apoptosis. *Cell* 88: 435–437, 1997.

94c. Franke, T. F., D. R. Kaplan, L. C. Cantley, and A. Toker. Direct regulation of the Akt proto-oncogene product by phosphatidylinositol-3,4-bisphosphate. *Science* 275: 665–668, 1997.

94d. Franke, T. F., S-I. Yang, T. O. Chan, K. Datta, A. Kazlauskas, D. K. Morrison, D. R. Kaplan, and P. N. Tsichlis. The protein kinase encoded by the Akt proto-oncogene is a target of the PDGF-activated phosphatidylinositol 3-kinase. *Cell* 81: 727–736, 1995.

94e. Frech, M., M. Andjelkovic, E. Ingley, K. K. Reddy, J. R. Falck, and B. A. Hemmings. High affinity binding of inositol phosphates and phosphoinositides to the pleckstrin homology domain of RAC/protein kinase B and their influence on kinase activity. *J. Biol. Chem.* 272: 8474–8481, 1997.

95. Freeman, E. J., G. M. Chisolm, and E. A. Tallant. Role of calcium and protein kinase C in the activation of phospholipase D by angiotensin II in vascular smooth muscle cells. *Arch. Biochem. Biophys.* 319: 84–92, 1995.

96. Fry, M. J. Structure, regulation and function of phosphoinositide 3-kinases. *Biochim. Biophys. Acta* 1226: 237–268, 1994.

97. Fu, T., Y. Okano, and Y. Nozawa. Differential pathways (phospholipase C and phospholipase D) of bradykinin-induced biphasic 1,2-diacylglycerol formation in non-transformed and K-*ras*-transformed NIH-3T3 fibroblasts. Involvement of intracellular Ca^{2+} oscillations in phosphatidylcholine breakdown. *Biochem. J.* 283: 347–354, 1992.

98. Ghosh, S., J. C. Strum, V. A. Sciorra, L. Daniel, and R. M. Bell. Raf-1 kinase possesses distinct binding domains for PS and PA: phosphatidic acid regulates the translocation of Raf-1 in TPA stimulated MDCK cells. *J. Biol. Chem.* 271: 8472–8480, 1996.

99. Ghosh, T. K., J. Bian, and D. L. Gill. Intracellular calcium release mediated by sphingosine derivatives generated in cells. *Science* 248: 1653–1656, 1990.

100. Godson, C., B. A. Weiss, and P. A. Insel. Differential activation of protein kinase C α is associated with arachidonate release in Madin-Darby canine kidney cells. *J. Biol. Chem.* 265: 8369–8372, 1990.

101. Goldberg, H. J., M. M. Viegas, B. L. Margolis, J. Schlessinger, and K. L. Skorecki. The tyrosine kinase activity of the epidermal-growth-factor receptor is necessary for phospholipase A_2 activation. *Biochem. J.* 267: 461–465, 1990.

102. Gomez-Munoz, A., A. Martin, L. O'Brien, and D. N. Brindley. Cell-permeable ceramides inhibit the stimulation of DNA synthesis and phospholipase D activity by phosphatidate and lysophosphatidate in rat fibroblasts. *J. Biol. Chem.* 269: 8937–8943, 1994.

103. Goodemote, K. A., M. E. Mattie, A. Berger, and S. Spiegel. Involvement of a pertussis toxin–sensitive G protein in the mitogenic signaling pathways of sphingosine 1-phosphate. *J. Biol. Chem.* 270: 10272–10277, 1995.

104. Gould, G. W., T. J. Jess, G. C. Andrews, J. J. Herbst, R. J. Plevin, and E. M. Gibbs. Evidence for a role of phosphatidylinositol 3-kinase in the regulation of glucose transport in *Xenopus* oocytes. *J. Biol. Chem.* 269: 26622–26625, 1994.

105. Gronich, J. H., J. V. Bonventre, and R. A. Nemenoff. Purification of a high-molecular-mass form of phospholipase A_2 from rat kidney activated at physiological calcium concentrations. *Biochem. J.* 271: 37–43, 1990.

106. Guinebault, C., B. Payrastre, G. Mauco, M. Breton, M. Plantavid, and H. Chap. Rapid and transient translocation of PLC-γ1 to the cytoskeleton of thrombin-stimulated platelets. Evidence for a role of tyrosine kinases. *Cell. Mol. Biol. (Noisy-le-grand)* 40: 687–693, 1994.

106a. Guo, Z., K. Liliom, D. J. Fischer, I. C. Bathurst, L. D. Tomei, M. C. Kiefer, and G. Tigyi. Molecular cloning of a high-affinity receptor for the growth factor-like lipid mediator lysophosphatidic acid from *Xenopus* oocytes. *Proc. Natl. Acad. Sci. U.S.A.* 93: 14367–14372, 1996.

106b. Gutkind, J. S., and L. Vitale-Cross. The pathway linking small GTP-binding proteins of the Rho family to cytoskeletal

components and novel signaling kinase cascades. *Cell Dev. Biol.* 7: 683–690, 1996.

107. Gusovsky, F., J. E. Lueders, E. C. Kohn, and C. C. Felder. Muscarinic receptor-mediated tyrosine phosphorylation of phospholipase C-γ. An alternative mechanism for cholinergic-induced phosphoinositide breakdown. *J. Biol. Chem.* 268: 7768–7772, 1993.

108. Gustavsson, L., G. Moehren, M. E. Torres-Marquez, C. Benistant, R. Rubin, and J. B. Hoek. The role of cytosolic Ca^{2+}, protein kinase C, and protein kinase A in hormonal stimulation of phospholipase D in rat hepatocytes. *J. Biol. Chem.* 269: 849–859, 1994.

109. Ha, K.-S., and J. H. Exton. Activation of actin polymerization by phosphatidic acid derived from phosphatidylcholine in IIC9 fibroblasts. *J. Cell Biol.* 123: 1789–1796, 1993.

110. Ha, K.-S., E.-J. Yeo, and J. H. Exton. Lysophosphatidic acid activation of phosphatidylcholine-hydrolysing phospholipase D and actin polymerization by a pertussis toxin–sensitive mechanism. *Biochem. J.* 303: 55–59, 1994.

111. Halstead, J., K. Kemp, and R. A. Ignotz. Evidence for involvement of phosphatidylcholine-phospholipase C and protein kinase C in transforming growth factor-β signaling. *J. Biol. Chem.* 270: 13600–13603, 1995.

111a. Hammond, S. M., Y. M. Altshuller, T-C. Sung, S. A. Rudge, K. Rose, J. Engebrecht, A. J. Morris, and M. A. Frohman. Human ADP-ribosylation factor-activated phosphatidylcholine-specific phospholipase D defines a new and highly conserved gene family. *J. Biol. Chem.* 270: 29640–29643, 1995.

111b. Hammond, S. M., J. M. Jenco, S. Nakashima, K. Cadwallader, Q-m. Gu, S. Cook, Y. Nozawa, G. D. Prestwich, M. A. Frohman, and A. J. Morris. Characterization of two alternately spliced forms of phospholipase D1. Activation of the purified enzymes by phosphatidylinositol 4,5-bisphospate, ADP-ribosylation factor, and Rho family monomeric GTP-binding proteins and protein kinase C-α. *J. Biol. Chem.* 272: 3860–3868, 1997.

111c. Han, J-S., J-K. Chung, H-S. Kang, J. Donaldson, Y. S. Bae, and S. G. Rhee. Multiple forms of phospholipase D inhibitor from rat brain cytosol. Purification and characterization of heat-labile form. *J. Biol. Chem.* 271:11163–11169, 1996.

112. Hannun, Y. A. The sphingomyelin cycle and the second messenger function of ceramide. *J. Biol. Chem.* 269: 3125–3128, 1994.

112a. Hannun, Y. A. Functions of ceramide in coordinating cellular responses to stress. *Science* 274: 1855–1859, 1996.

113. Hannun, Y. A., C. R. Loomis, A. H. Merill, Jr., and R.M. Bell. Sphingosine inhibition of protein kinase C activity and of phorbol dibutyrate binding in vitro and in human platelets. *J. Biol. Chem.* 261: 12604–12609, 1986.

113a. Hao, W., Z. Tan, K. Prasad, K. K. Reddy, J. Chen, G. D. Prestwich, J. R. Falck, S. B. Shears, and E. M. Lafer. Regulation of AP-3 function by inositides. Identification of phosphatidylinositol 3,4,5-trisphosphate as a potent ligand. *J. Biol. Chem.* 272: 6393–6398, 1997.

114. Hara, K., K. Yonezawa, H. Sakaue, A. Ando, K. Kotani, T. Kitamura, Y. Kitamura, H. Ueda, L. Stephens, T. R. Jackson, P. T. Hawkins, R. Dhand, A. E. Clark, G. D. Holman, M. D. Waterfield, and M. Kasuga. 1-Phosphatidylinositol 3-kinase activity is required for insulin-stimulated glucose transport but not for RAS activation in CHO cells. *Proc. Natl. Acad. Sci. U.S.A.* 91: 7415–7419, 1994.

115. Hasegawa-Sasaki, H., F. Lutz, and T. Sasaki. Pathway of phospholipase C activation initiated with platelet-derived growth factor is different from that initiated with vasopressin and bombesin. *J. Biol. Chem.* 263: 12970–12976, 1988.

116. Haslam, R. J., J. A. Lynham, and J.E.B. Fox. Effects of collagen,

ionophore A23187 and prostaglandin E$_1$ on the phosphorylation of specific proteins in blood platelets. *Biochem. J.* 178: 397–406, 1979.

117. Hawkins, P. T., A. Eguinoa, R.-G. Qiu, D. Stokoe, F. T. Cooke, R. Walters, S. Wennstrom, L. Claesson-Welsh, T. Evans, M. Symons, and L. Stephens. PDGF stimulates an increase in GTP-Rac via activation of phosphoinositide 3-kinase. *Curr. Biol.* 5: 393–403, 1995.

117a. Hecht, J. H., J. A. Weiner, S. R. Post, and J. Chun. *Ventricular Zone Gene-1* (VZG-1) encodes a lysophosphatidic acid receptor expressed in neurogenic regions of the developing cerebral cortex. *J. Cell Biol.* 135:1071–1083, 1996.

118. Heldin, C.-H. Dimerization of cell surface receptors in signal transduction. *Cell* 80: 213–223, 1995.

118a. Hemmings, B. A. Akt signaling: Linking membrane events to life and death decisions. *Science* 275: 628–630, 1997.

118b. Hepler, J. R., D. M. Berman, A. G. Gilman, and T. Kozasa. RGS4 and GAIP are GTPase-activating proteins for G$_{q\alpha}$. and block activation of phospholipase Cβ by γ-thio-GTP-G$_{q\alpha}$. *Proc. Natl. Acad. Sci. U.S.A.* 94: 428–432, 1997.

118c. Herrera-Velit, P., K. L. Knutson, and N. E. Reiner. Phosphatidylinositol 3-kinase-dependent activation of protein kinase C-ζ in bacterial lipopolysaccharide-treated human monocytes. *J. Biol. Chem.* 272:16445–16452, 1997.

118d. Hess, J. A., A. H. Ross, R-G. Qiu, M. Symons, and J. H. Exton. Role of Rho family proteins in phospholipase D activation by growth factors. *J. Biol. Chem.* 272: 1615–1620, 1997.

119. Hokin, L. E., and M. R. Hokin. Effects of acetylcholine on the turnover of phosphoryl units in individual phospholipids of pancreas slices and brain cortex slices. *Biochim. Biophys. Acta* 18: 102–110, 1955.

120. Hokin, M. R., and L. E. Hokin. Enzyme secretion and the incorporation of P^{32} into phospholipids of pancreas slices. *J. Biol. Chem.* 203: 967–977, 1953.

121. Hordijk, P. L., I. Verlaan, E. J. van Corven, and W. H. Moolenaar. Protein tyrosine phosphorylation induced by lysophosphatidic acid in rat-1 fibroblasts. Evidence that phosphorylation of MAP kinase is mediated by the G$_i$-p21^{ras} pathway. *J. Biol. Chem.* 269: 645–651, 1994.

122. Houle, M. G., R. A. Kahn, P. H. Naccache, and S. Bouirgoin. ADP-ribosylation factor translocation correlates with potentiation of GTPγS-stimulated phospholipase D activity in membrane fractions of HL-60 cells. *J. Biol. Chem.* 270: 22795–22800, 1995.

123. Howe, L. R., and C. J. Marshall. Lysophosphatidic acid stimulates mitogen-activated protein kinase activation via a G-protein-coupled pathway requiring p21^{ras} and p74^{raf-1}. *J. Biol. Chem.* 268: 20717–20720, 1993.

124. Hu, P., and J. Schlessinger. Direct association of p110β phosphatidylinosiol 3-kinase with p85 is mediated by an N-terminal fragment of p110β. *Mol. Cell. Biol.* 14: 2577–2583, 1994.

125. Hu, Q., A. Klippel, A. J. Muslin, W. J. Fantl, and L. T. Williams. Ras-dependent induction of cellular responses by constitutively active phosphatidylinositol-3 kinase. *Science* 268: 100–102, 1995.

126. Huang, C., and M. C. Cabot. Phorbol diesters stimulate the accumulation of phosphatidate, phosphatidylethanol, and diacylglycerol in three cell types. Evidence for the indirect formation of phosphatidylcholine-derived diacylglycerol by a phospholipase D pathway and direct formation of diacylglycerol by a phospholipase C pathway. *J. Biol. Chem.* 265: 14858–14863, 1990.

127. Huang, J., M. Mohammadi, G. A. Rodrigues, and J. Schlessinger. Reduced activation of RAF-1 and MAP kinase by a fibroblast growth factor receptor mutant deficient in stimula-

tion of phosphatidylinositol hydrolysis. *J. Biol. Chem.* 270: 5065–5072, 1995.

128. Huang, R., G. L. Kucera, and S. E. Rittenhouse. Elevated cytosolic Ca^{2+} activates phospholipase D in human platelets. *J. Biol. Chem.* 266: 1652–1655, 1991.

129. Hunt, T. W., R. C. Carroll, and E. G. Peralta. Heterotrimeric G proteins containing G$_{\alpha i3}$ regulate multiple effector enzymes in the same cell. Activation of phospholipase C and A$_2$ and inhibition of adenylyl cyclase. *J. Biol. Chem.* 269: 29565–29570, 1994.

129a. Huwiler, A., J. Brunner, R. Hummel, M. Vervoordeldonk, S. Stabel, H. van den Bosch, and J. Pfeilschifter. Ceramide-binding and activation defines protein kinase c-Raf as a ceramide-activated protein kinase. *Proc. Natl. Acad. Sci. U.S.A.* 93: 6959–6963, 1996.

130. Imaoka, T., J. A. Lynham, and R. J. Haslam. Purification and characterization of the 47,000-dalton protein phosphorylated during degranulation of human platelets. *J. Biol. Chem.* 258: 11404–11414, 1983.

131. Isakoff, S. J., C. Taha, E. Rose, J. Marcusohn, A. Klip, and E. Y. Skolnik. The inability of phosphatidylinositol 3-kinase activation to stimulate GLUT4 translocation indicates additional signaling pathways are required for insulin-stimulated glucose uptake. *Proc. Natl. Acad. Sci. U.S.A.* 92: 10247–10251, 1995.

131a. Ito, Y., S. Nakashima, H. Kanoh, annd Y. Nozawa. Implication of Ca^{2+}-dependent protein tyrosine phosphorylation in carbachol-induced phospholipase D activation in rat pheochromocytoma PC12 cells. *J. Neurochem.* 68:419–425, 1997.

131b. Ito, Y., S. Nakashima, and Y. Nozawa. Hydrogen peroxide-induced phospholipase D activation in rat pheochromocytoma PC12 cells: Possible involvement of Ca^{2+}-dependent protein tyrosine kinase. *J. Neurochem.* 69:729–736, 1997.

132. Jackowski, S., and C. O. Rock. Stimulation of phosphtidylinositol 4,5-bisphosphate phospholipase C activity by phosphatidic acid. *Arch. Bichem. Biophys.* 268: 516–524, 1989.

133. Jalink, K., T. Hengeveld, S. Mulder, F. R. Postma, M.-F. Simon, H. Chap, G. A. van der Marel, J. H. van Boom, W. J. van Blitterswijk, and W. H. Moolenaar. Lysophosphatidic acid-induced Ca^{2+} mobilization in human A431 cells: structure–activity analysis. *Biochem. J.* 307: 609–616, 1995.

134. Jalink, K., P. L. Hordijk, and W. H. Moolenaar. Growth factor-like effects of lysophosphatidic acid, a novel lipid mediator. *Biochim. Biophys. Acta* 1198: 185–196, 1994.

135. Jalink, K., E. J. van Corven, and W.H. Moolenaar. Lysophosphatidic acid, but not phosphatidic acid, is a potent Ca^{2+}-mobilizing stimulus for fibroblasts. Evidence for an extracellular site of action. *J. Biol. Chem.* 265: 12232–12239, 1990.

136. Jamal, Z., A. Martin, A. Gomez-Munoz, and D. N. Brindley. Plasma membrane fractions from rat liver contain a phosphatidate phosphohydrolase distinct from that in the endoplasmic reticulum and cytosol. *J. Biol. Chem.* 266: 2988–2996, 1991.

137. Jamil, H., A. K. Uital, and D. E. Vance. Evidence that cyclic AMP-induced inhibition of phosphatidylcholine biosynthesis is caused by a decrease in cellular diacylglycerol levels in cultured rat hepatocytes. *J. Biol. Chem.* 267: 1752–1760, 1992.

138. Jarpe, M. B., K. L. Leach, and D. M. Raben. α-Thrombin-induced nuclear *sn*-1,2-diacylglycerols are derived from phosphatidylcholine hydrolysis in cultured fibroblasts. *Biochemistry* 33: 526–534, 1994.

139. Jayadev, S., B. Liu, A. E. Bielawska, J. Y. Lee, F. Nazaire, M. Y. Pushkareva, L. M. Obeid, and Y. A. Hannun. Role for ceramide in cell cycle arrest. *J. Biol. Chem.* 270: 2047–2052, 1995.

140. Jimenez, B., L. del Peso, S. Montaner, P. Esteve, and J. C. Lacal. Generation of phosphorylcholine as an essential event in the activation of Raf-1 and MAP-kinases in growth factor-induced mitogenic stimulation. *J. Cell. Biochem.* 57: 141–149, 1995.

141. Johansen, T., G. Bjorkoy, A. Overvatn, M. T. Diaz-Meco, T. Traavik, and J. Moscat. NIH 3T3 cells stably transfected with the gene encoding phosphatidylcholine-hydrolyzing phospholipase C from *Bacillus cereus* acquire a transformed phenotype. *Mol. Cell. Biol.* 14: 646–654, 1994.

142. Johnson, R. M., and J. C. Garrison. Epidermal growth factor and angiotensin II stimulate formation of inositol 1,4,5- and inositol 1,3,4-trisphosphate in hepatocytes. Differential inhibition by pertussis toxin and phorbol 12-myristate 13-acetate. *J. Biol. Chem.* 262: 17285–17293, 1987.

143. Joly, M., A. Kazlauskas, and S. Corvera. Phosphatidylinositol 3-kinase activity is required at a postendocytic step in platelet-derived growth factor receptor trafficking. *J. Biol. Chem.* 270: 13225–13230, 1995.

144. Joly, M., A. Kazlauskas, F. S. Fay, and S. Corvera. Disruption of PDGF receptor trafficking by mutation of its PI-3 kinase binding sites. *Science* 263: 684–687, 1994.

145. Jones, G. A., and G. Carpenter. The regulation of phospholipase C-γ1 by phosphatidic acid. Assessment of kinetic parameters. *J. Biol. Chem.* 268: 20845–20850, 1993.

146. Jones, M. J., and A. W. Murray. Evidence that ceramide selectively inhibits protein kinase C-α translocation and modulates bradykinin activation of phospholipase D. *J. Biol. Chem.* 270: 5007–5013, 1995.

147. Kahn, R. A., J. K. Yucei, and V. Malhotra. ARF signaling: a potential role for phospholipase D in membrane traffic. *Cell* 75: 1045–1048, 1993.

148. Kalmar, G. B., R. J. Kay, A. Lachance, R. Aebersold, and R. B. Cornell. Cloning and expression of rat liver CTP:phosphocholine cytidylyltransferase: an amphipathic protein that controls phosphatidylcholine synthesis. *Proc. Natl. Acad. Sci. U.S.A.* 87: 6029–6033, 1990.

149. Kamohara, S., H. Hayashi, M. Todaka, F. Kanai, K. Ishii, T. Imanaka, J. A. Escobedo, L. T. Williams, and Y. Ebina. Platelet-derived growth factor triggers translocation of the insulin-regulatable glucose transporter (type 4) predominantly through phosphatidylinositol 3-kinase binding sites on the receptor. *Proc. Natl. Acad. Sci. U.S.A.* 92: 1077–1081, 1995.

150. Kapeller, R., R. Chakrabarti, L. Cantley, F. Fay, and S. Corvera. Internalization of activated platelet-derived growth factor receptor-phosphatidylinositol-3′ kinase complexes: potential interactions with the microtubule cytoskeleton. *Mol. Cell. Biol.* 13: 6052–6063, 1993.

151. Kaplan, D. R., D. C. Pallas, W. Morgan, B. Schaffhausen, and T. M. Roberts. Mechanisms of transformation by polyoma virus middle T antigen. *Biochim. Biophys. Acta* 948: 345–364, 1988.

152. Kast, R., G. Furstenberger, and F. Marks. Activation of cytosolic phospholipase A₂ by transforming growth factor-α in HEL-30 keratinocytes. *J. Biol. Chem.* 268: 16795–16802, 1993.

152a. Kauffman-Zeh, A., P. Rodriguez-Viciana, E. Ulrich, C. Gilbert, P. Coffer, J. Downward, and G. Evan. Suppression of a c-Myc-induced apoptosis by Ras signaling through PI(3)K and PKB. *Nature* 385: 544–548, 1997.

153. Kazlauskas, A., and J. A. Cooper. Autophosphorylation of the PDGF receptor in the kinase insert region regulates interactions with cell proteins. *Cell* 58: 1121–1133, 1989.

154. Kazlauskas, A., A. Kashishian, J. A. Cooper, and M. Valius.

155. Khan, W. A., G. C. Blobe, A. L. Richards, and Y. A. Hannun. Identification, partial purification, and characterization of a novel phospholipid-dependent and fatty acid–activated protein kinase from human platelets. *J. Biol. Chem.* 269: 9729–9735, 1994.

156. Kim, H. K., J. W. Kim, A. Zilberstein, B. Margolis, J. G. Kim, J. Schlessinger, and S. G. Rhee. PDGF stimulation of inositol phospholipid hydrolysis requires PLC-γ1 phosphorylation on tyrosine residues 783 and 1254. *Cell* 65: 435–441, 1991.

157. Kim, H. H., S. L. Sierke, and J. G. Koland. Epidermal growth factor–dependent association of phosphatidylinositol 3-kinase with the erbB3 gene product. *J. Biol. Chem.* 269: 24747–24755, 1994.

157a. Kim, J. H., Y. J. Suh, T. G. Lee, Y. Kim, S. S. Bae, M. J. Kim, J. D. Lambeth, P-G. Suh, and S. H. Ryu. Inhibition of phospholipase D by a protein factor from bovine brain cytosol. Partial purification and characterization of the inhibition mechanism. *J. Biol. Chem.* 271:25213–25219, 1996.

158. Kim, J. W., S. S. Sim, U.-H. Kim, S. Nishibe, M. I. Wahl, G. Carpenter, and S. G. Rhee. Tyrosine residues in bovine phospholipase C-γ phosphorylated by the epidermal growth factor receptor in vitro. *J. Biol. Chem.* 265: 3940–3943, 1990.

159. Kim, M.-Y., C. Linardic, L. Obeid, and Y. Hannun. Identification of sphingomyelin turnover as an effector mechanism for the action of tumor necrosis factor α and γ-interferon. Specific role in cell differentiation. *J. Biol. Chem.* 266: 484–489, 1991.

159a. Kimura, K., M. Ito, M. Amano, K. Chihara, Y. Fukata, M. Nakafuku, B. Yamamori, J. Feng, T. Nakano, K. Okawa, A. Iwamatsu, and K. Kaibuchi. Regulation of myosin phosphatase by Rho and Rho-associated kinase (Rho-kinase). *Science* 273: 245–248, 1996.

160. Kiss, Z., and W. B. Anderson. ATP stimulates the hydrolysis of phosphatidylethanolamine in NIH 3T3 cells. Potentiating effects of guanosine triphosphates and sphingosine. *J. Biol. Chem.* 265: 7345–7350, 1990.

160a. Klarlund, J. K., A Guilherme, J. J. Holik, J. V. Virbasius, A. Chawla, and M. P. Czech. Signaling by phosphoinositide-3,4,5-trisphosphate through proteins containing pleckstrin and Sec7 homology domains. *Science* 275: 1927–1930, 1997.

161. Klippel, A., J. A. Escobedo, M. Hirano, and L. T. Williams. The interaction of small domains between the subunits of phosphatidylinositol 3-kinase determines enzyme activity. *Mol. Cell. Biol.* 14: 2675–2685, 1994.

161a. Klippel A., W. M. Kavanaugh, D. Pot, and L. T. Williams. A specific product of phosphatidylinositol 3-kinase directly activates the protein kinase Akt through its pleckstrin homology domain. *Mol. Cell. Biol.* 17: 338–344, 1997.

161b. Klippel, A., C. Reinhard, W. M. Kavanaugh, G. Apell, M-A. Escobedo, and L. T. Williams. Membrane localization of phosphatidylinositol 3-kinase is sufficient to activate multiple signal-transducing kinase pathways. *Mol. Cell. Biol.* 16: 4117–4127, 1996.

162. Knaus, U. G., S. Morris, H.-J. Dong, J. Chernoff, and G. M. Bokoch. Regulation of human leukocyte p21–activated kinases through G protein-coupled receptors. *Science* 269: 221–223, 1995.

163. Koch, W. J., B. E. Hawes, L. F. Allen, and R. J. Lefkowitz. Direct evidence that Gᵢ-coupled receptor stimulation of mitogen-activated protein kinase is mediated by Gβγ activation of p21ras. *Proc. Natl. Acad. Sci. U.S.A.* 91: 12706–12710, 1994.

GTPase-activating protein and phosphatidylinositol 3-kinase bind to distinct regions of the platelet-derived growth factor receptor β subunit. *Mol. Cell. Biol.* 12: 2534–2544, 1992.

164. Koch, W. J., B. E. Hawes, J. Inglese, L. M. Luttrell, and R. J. Lefkowitz. Cellular expression of the carboxyl terminus of a G protein-coupled receptor kinase attenuates $G_{\beta\gamma}$-mediated signaling. *J. Biol. Chem.* 269: 6193–6197, 1994.

164a. Kodaki, T., and S. Yamashita. Cloning, expression, and characterization of a novel phospholipase D complementary DNA from rat brain. *J. Biol. Chem.* 272: 11408–11413, 1997.

164b. Kohn, A. D., K. S. Kovacina, and R. A. Roth. Insulin stimulates the kinase activity of RAC-PK, a pleckstrin homology domain containing ser/thr kinase. *EMBO J.* 14: 4288–4295, 1995.

164c. Kohn, A. D., Summers, S. A., M. J. Birnbaum, and R. A. Roth. Expression of a constitutively active Akt Ser/Thr kinase in 3T3-L1 adipocytes stimulates glucose uptake and glucose transporter 4 translocation. *J. Biol. Chem.* 271: 31372–31378, 1996.

164d. Kolanus, W., W. Nagel, B. Schiller, L. Zeitlmann, S. Godar, H. Stockinger, and B. Seed. $\alpha L\beta 2$ integrin/LFA-1 binding to ICAM-1 induced by cytohesin-1, a cytoplasmic regulatory molecule. *Cell* 86: 233–242, 1996.

165. Kolesnick, R., and D. W. Golde. The sphingomyelin pathway in tumor necrosis factor and interleukin-1 signaling. *Cell* 77: 325–328, 1994.

166. Kondo, T., H. Inui, F. Konishi, and T. Inagami. Phospholipase D mimics platelet-derived growth factor as a competence factor in vascular smooth muscle cells. *J. Biol. Chem.* 267: 23609–23616, 1992.

167. Kotani, K., K. Hara, K. Kotani, K. Yonezawa, and M. Kasuga. Phosphoinositide 3-kinase as an upstream regulator of the small GTP-binding protein Rac in the insulin signaling of membrane ruffling. *Biochem. Biophys. Res. Commun.* 208: 985–990, 1995.

168. Kotani, K., K. Yonezawa, K. Hara, H. Ueda, Y. Kitamura, H. Sakaue, A. Ando, A. Chavanieu, B. Calas, F. Grigorescu, M. Nishiyama, M. D. Waterfield, and M. Kasuga. Involvement of phosphoinositide 3-kinase in insulin- or IGF-1–induced membrane ruffling. *EMBO J.* 13: 2313–2321, 1994.

169. Kramer, R. M., E. F. Roberts, J. Manetta, and J. E. Putnam. The Ca^{2+}-sensitive cytosolic phospholipase A_2 is a 100 kDa protein in human monoblast U937 cells. *J. Biol. Chem.* 266: 5268–5272, 1991.

169a. Kramer, R. M., E. F. Roberts, S. L. Um, A. G. Borsch-Haubold, S. P. Watson, M. J. Fisher, and J. A. Jakubowski. p38 mitogen-activated protein kinase phosphorylates cytosolic phospholipase A_2 (cPLA$_2$) in thrombin-stimulated platelets. Evidence that proline-directed phosphorylation is not required for mobilization of arachidonic acid by cPLA$_2$. *J. Biol. Chem.* 271: 27723–27729, 1996.

170. Ktistakis, N. T., H. A. Brown, P. C. Sternweis, and M. G. Roth. Phospholipase D is present on Golgi-enriched membranes and its activation by ADP ribosylation factor is sensitive to brefeldin A. *Proc. Natl. Acad. Sci. U.S.A.* 92: 4952–4956, 1995.

170a. Ktistakis, N. T., H. A. Brown, M. G. Waters, P. C. Sternweis, and M. G. Roth. Evidence that phospholipase D mediates ADP ribosylation factor-dependent formation of Golgi coated vesicles. *J. Cell Biol.* 134: 295–306, 1996.

170b. Kuang, Y., Y. Wu, A. Smrcka, H. Jiang, and D. Wu. Identification of a phyospholipase C β_2 region that interacts with $G\beta\gamma$. *Proc. Natl. Acad. Sci. U.S.A.* 93: 2964–2968, 1996.

171. Kumagai, N., N. Morri, K. Fujisawa, Y. Nemoto, and S. Narumiya. ADP-ribosylation of rho p21 inhibits lysophosphatidic acid–induced protein tyrosine phosphorylation and phosphatidylinositol 3-kinase activation in cultured Swiss 3T3 cells. *J. Biol. Chem.* 268: 24535–24538, 1993.

172. Kumagai, N., N. Morii, K. Fujisawa, T. Yoshimasa, K. Nakao, and S. Narumiya. Lysophosphatidic acid induces tyrosine phosphorylation and activation of MAP-kinase and focal adhesion kinase in cultured Swiss 3T3 cells. *FEBS Lett.* 329: 273–276, 1993.

173. Kumagai, N., N. Morii, T. Ishizaki, N. Watanabe, K. Fukisawa, Y. Saito, and S. Narumiya. Lysophosphatidic acid–induced activation of protein Ser/Thr kinases in cultured rat 3Y1 fibroblasts. Possible involvement in rho p21–mediated signalling. *FEBS Lett.* 366: 11–16, 1995.

174. Kuribara, H., K. Tago, T. Yokozeki, T. Sasaki, Y. Takai, N. Morii, S. Narumiya, T. Katada, and Y. Kanaho. Synergistic activation of rat brain phospholipase D by ADP-ribosylation factor and *rho*A p21, and its inhibition by *Clostridium botulinum* C3 exoenzyme. *J. Biol. Chem.* 270: 25667–25671, 1995.

175. Kusner, D. J., S. J. Schomisch, and G. R. Dubyak. ATP-induced potentiation of G-protein-dependent phospholipase D activity in a cell-free system from U937 promonocytic leukocytes. *J. Biol. Chem.* 268: 19973–19982, 1993.

176. Lam, K., C. L. Carpenter, N. B. Ruderman, J. C. Friel, and K. L. Kelly. The phosphatidylinositol 3-kinase serine kinase phosphorylates IRS-1. Stimulation by insulin and inhibition by wortmannin. *J. Biol. Chem.* 269: 20648–20652, 1994.

177. Lambeth, J. D., J.-Y. Kwak, E. P. Bowman, D. Perry, D. J. Uhlinger, and I. Lopez. ADP-ribosylation factor functions synergistically with a 50-kDa cytosolic factor in cell-free activation of human neutrophil phospholipase D. *J. Biol. Chem.* 270: 2431–2434, 1995.

178. Lambright, D. G., J. P. Noel, H. E. Hamm, and P. B. Sigler. Structural determinants for activation of the α-subunit of a heterotrimeric G protein. *Nature* 369: 621–628, 1994.

179. Larrodera, P., M. E. Cornet, M. T. Diaz-Meco, M. Lopez-Barahona, I. Diaz-Laviada, P. H. Guddal, T. Johansen, and J. Moscat. Phospholipase C–mediated hydrolysis of phosphatidylcholine is an important step in PDGF-stimulated DNA synthesis. *Cell* 61: 1113–1120, 1990.

180. Lavie, Y., and M. Liscovitch. Activation of phospholipase D by sphingoid bases in NG108–15 neural-derived cells. *J. Biol. Chem.* 265: 3868–3872, 1990.

181. Lavie, Y., O. Piterman, and M. Liscovitch. Inhibition of phosphatidic acid phosphohydrolase activity by sphingosine. Dual action of sphingosine in diacylglycerol signal termination. *FEBS Lett.* 277: 7–10, 1990.

182. Leach, K. L., V. A. Ruff, M. B. Jarpe, L. D. Adams, D. Fabbro, and D. M. Raben. α-Thrombin stimulates nuclear diglyceride levels and differential localization of protein kinase C isozymes in IIC9 cells. *J. Biol. Chem.* 267: 21816–21822, 1992.

182a. Lee, C., H-S. Kang, J-K. Chung, F. Sekiya, J-R. Kim, J-S. Han, S. R. Kim, Y. S. Bae, A. J. Morris, and S. G. Rhee. Inhibition of phospholipase D by clathrin assembly protein 3 (AP3). *J. Biol. Chem.* 272:15986–15992, 1997.

183. Lee, C.-W., D. J. Park, K.-H. Lee, C. G. Kim, and S. G. Rhee. Purification, molecular cloning, and sequencing of phospholipase C-$\beta 4$. *J. Biol. Chem.* 268: 21318–21327, 1993.

184. Lee, H. C. Cyclic ADP-ribose: a new member of a super family of signalling cyclic nucleotides. *Cell. Signal.* 6: 591–600, 1994.

185. Lee, M.-H., and R. M. Bell. Supplementation of the phosphatidyl-L-serine requirement of protein kinase C with nonactivating phospholipids. *Biochemistry* 31: 5176–5182, 1992.

186. Lee, S. B., and S. G. Rhee. Significance of PIP$_2$ hydrolysis and regulation of phospholipase C isozymes. *Curr. Opin. Cell Biol.* 7: 183–189, 1995.

186a. Lee, T. G., J. B. Park, S. D. Lee, S. Hong, J. H. Kim, Y. Kim, K. S. Yi, S. Bae, Y. A. Hannun, L. M. Obeid, P-G. Suh, and S. H. Ryu. Phorbol myristate acetate-dependent association of protein kinase Cα with phospholipase D1 in intact cells. *Biochim. Biophys. Acta* 1347:199–204, 1997.

187. Lee, Y. H., H. S. Kim, J.-K. Pai, S. H. Ryu, and P.-G. Suh. Activation of phospholipase D induced by platelet-derived growth factor is dependent upon the level of phospholipase C-γ1. *J. Biol. Chem.* 269: 26842–26847, 1994.

187a. Leslie, C. C. Properties and regulation of cytosolic phospholipase A₂. *J. Biol. Chem.* 272:16709–16712, 1997.

188. Leung, T., E. Manser, L. Tan, and L. Lim. A novel serine/threonine kinase binding the ras-related RhoA GTPase which translocates the kinase to peripheral membranes. *J. Biol. Chem.* 270: 29051–29054, 1995.

188a. Lim, L., E. Manser, T. Leung, and C. Hall. Regulation of phosphorylation pathways by p21 GTPases. *Eur. J. Biochem.* 242: 171–185, 1996.

188b. Lim, L., C. Hall, and C. Monfries. Regulation of actin cytoskeleton by Rho-family GTPases and their associated proteins. *Cell Dev. Biol.* 7: 699–706, 1996.

189. Limatola, C., D. Schaap, W. H. Moolenaar, and W. J. van Blitterswijk. Phosphatidic acid activation of protein kinase C-ζ overexpressed in COS cells: comparison with other protein kinase C isotypes and other acidic lipids. *Biochem. J.* 394: 1001–1008, 1994.

190. Lin, L.-L., A. Y. Lin, and J. L. Knopf. Cytosolic phospholipase A₂ is coupled to hormonally regulated release of arachidonic acid. *Proc. Natl. Acad. Sci. U.S.A.* 89: 6147–6151, 1992.

191. Lin, L.-L., M. Wartmann, A. Y. Lin, J. L. Knopf, A. Seth, and R. J. Davis. cPLA₂ is phosphorylated and activated by MAP kinase. *Cell* 72: 269–278, 1993.

192. Linardic, C. M., S. Jayadev, and Y. A. Hannun. Brefeldin A promotes hydrolysis of sphingomyelin. *J. Biol. Chem.* 267: 14909–14911, 1992.

193. Liscovitch, M., V. Chalifa, P. Pertile, C.-S. Chen, and L. C. Cantley. Novel function of phosphatidylinositol 4,5-bisphosphate as a cofactor for brain membrane phospholipase D. *J. Biol. Chem.* 269: 21403–21406, 1994.

194. Lopez, I., D. J. Burns, and J. D. Lambeth. Regulation of phospholipase D by protein kinase C in human neutrophils. Conventional isoforms of protein kinase C phosphorylate a phospholipase D-related component in the plasma membrane. *J. Biol. Chem.* 270: 19465–19472, 1995.

195. Lopez-Barahona, M., P. L. Kaplan, M. E. Cornet, M. T. Diaz-Meco, P. Larrodera, I. Diaz-Laviada, A. M. Municio, and J. Moscat. Kinetic evidence of a rapid activation of phosphatidylcholine hydrolysis by Ki-*ras* oncogene. Possible involvement in late steps of the mitogenic cascade. *J. Biol. Chem.* 265: 9022–9026, 1990.

195a. Lukowski, S., M-C. Lecomte, J-P. Mira, P. Marin, H. Gautero, F. Russo-Marie, and B. Geny. Inhibition of phospholipase D activity by fodrin. An active role for the cytoskeleton. *J. Biol. Chem.* 271:24164–24171, 1996.

196. Ma, Y.-H., H. P. Reusch, E. Wilson, J. A. Escobedo, W. J. Fantzl, L. T. Williams, and H. E. Ives. Activation of Na⁺/H⁺ exchange by platelet-derived growth factor involves phosphatidylinositol 3'-kinase and phospholipase Cγ. *J. Biol. Chem.* 269: 30734–30739, 1994.

197. McGlade, J., B. Brunkhorst, D. Anderson, G. Mbamalu, J. Settleman, S. Dedhar, M. Rozakis-Adcock, L. B. Chen, and T. Pawson. The N-terminal region of GAP regulates cytoskeletal structure and cell adhesion. *EMBO J.* 12: 3073–3081, 1993.

198. Machleidt, T., K. Wiegmann, T. Henkel, S. Schutze, P. Baeuerle, and M. Kronke. Sphingomyelinase activates proteolytic IκB-α

degradation in a cell-free system. *J. Biol. Chem.* 269: 13760–13765, 1994.

199. McKenzie, F. R., K. Seuwen, and J. Pouyssegur. Stimulation of phosphatidylcholine breakdown by thrombin and carbachol but not by tyrosine kinase receptor ligands in cells transfected with M1 muscarinic receptors. Rapid desensitization of phosphocholine-specific (PC) phospholipase D but sustained activity of PC-phospholipase C. *J. Biol. Chem.* 267: 22759–22769, 1992.

200. McPhail, L. C., D. Qualliotine-Mann, and K. A. Waite. Cell-free activation of neutrophil NADPH oxidase by a phosphatidic acid–regulated protein kinase. *Proc. Natl. Acad. Sci. USA* 92: 7931–7935, 1995.

201. McPherson, P. S., and K. P. Campbell. The ryanodine receptor/Ca²⁺ release channel. *J. Biol. Chem.* 268: 13765–13768, 1993.

202. Malarkey, K., C. M. Belham, A. Paul, A. Graham, A. McLess, P. H. Scott, and R. Plevin. The regulation of tyrosine kinase signalling pathways by growth factor and G-protein-coupled receptors. *Biochem. J.* 309: 361–375, 1995.

203. Malcolm, K. C., C. M. Elliott, and J. H. Exton. Evidence for RhoA-mediated agonist stimulation of phospholipase D in rat 1 fibroblasts. Effects of *Clostridium botulinum* C3 exoenzyme. *J. Biol. Chem.* 271: 13135–13139, 1996.

204. Malcolm, K. C., A. H. Ross, R.-G. Qie, M. Symons, and J. H. Exton. Activation of rat liver phosphoplipase D by the small GTP-binding protein RhoA. *J. Biol. Chem.* 269: 25951–25954, 1994.

205. Manser, E., T. Leung, H. Salihuddin, L. Tan, and L. Lim. A non-receptor tyrosine kinase that inhibits the GTPase activity of p21ᶜᵈᶜ⁴². *Nature* 363: 364–367, 1993.

206. Manser, E., T. Leung, H. Salihuddin, Z.-s. Zhao, and L. Lim. A brain serine-threonine protein kinase activated by Cdc42 and Rac1. *Nature* 367: 40–46, 1994.

207. Margolis, B. L., B. J. Holub, D. A. Troyer, and K. L. Skorecki. Epidermal growth factor stimulates phospholipase A₂ in vasopressin-treated rat glomerular mesangial cells. *Biochem. J.* 256: 469–474, 1988.

208. Maroney, A. C., and I. G. Macara. Phorbol ester-induced translocation of diacylglycerol kinase from cytosol to the membrane in Swiss 3T3 fibroblasts. *J. Biol. Chem.* 264: 2537–2544, 1989.

209. Marrero, M. B., W. G. Paxton, J. L. Duff, B. C. Berk, and K. E. Bernstein. Angiotensin II stimulates tyrosine phosphorylation of phospholipase C-γ1in vascular smooth muscle cells. *J. Biol. Chem.* 269: 10935–10939, 1994.

210. Marrero, M. B., B. Schieffer, W. G. Paxton, E. Schieffer, and K. E. Bernstein. Electroporation of pp60ᶜ⁻ˢʳᶜ antibodies inhibits the angiotensin II activation of phospholipase C-γ1 in rat aortic smooth muscle cells. *J. Biol. Chem.* 270: 15734–15738, 1995.

211. Marshall, C. J. Specificity of receptor tyrosine kinase signaling: transient versus sustained extracellular signal-regulated kinase activation. *Cell* 80: 179–185, 1995.

212. Martin, G. A., G. Bollag, F. McCormick, and A. Abo. A novel serine kinase activated by rac1/CDC42Hs-dependent autophosphorylation is related to PAK65 and STE20. *EMBO J.* 14: 1970–1978, 1995.

212a. Martin, S. S., T. Haruta, A. J. Morris, A. Klippel, L. T. Williams, and J. M. Olefsky. Activated phosphatidylinositol 3-kinase is sufficient to mediate actin rearrangement and GLUT4 translocation in 3T3-L1 adipocytes. *J. Biol. Chem.* 271: 17605–17608, 1996.

213. Martinson, E. A., D. Goldstein, and J. H. Brown. Muscarinic receptor activation of phosphatidylcholine hydrolysis. Relationship to phosphoinositide hydrolysis and diacylglycerol metabolism. *J. Biol. Chem.* 264: 14748–14754, 1989.

214. Martinson, E. A., S. Scheible, and P. Presek. Inhibition of phospholipase D of human platelets by protein tyrosine kinase inhibitors. *Cell. Mol. Biol.* (*Noisy-le-grand*) 40: 627–634, 1994.

214a. Martys, J. L., C. Wjasow, D. M. Gangi, M. C. Kielian, T. E. McGraw, and J. M. Backer. Wortmannin-sensitive trafficking pathways in Chinese hamster ovary cells. Differential effects on endocytosis and lysosomal sorting. *J. Biol. Chem.* 271: 10953–10962, 1996.

215. Massenburg, D., J.-S. Han, M. Liyanage, W. A. Patton, S. G. Rhee, J. Moss, and M. Vaughan. Activation of rat brain phospholipase D by ADP-ribosylation factors 1,5, and 6: separation of ADP-ribosylation factor–dependent and oleate-dependent enzymes. *Proc. Natl. Acad. Sci. U.S.A.* 91: 11718–11722, 1994.

216. Mathias, S., K. A. Dressler, and R. N. Lolesnick. Characterization of a ceramide-activated protein kinase: stimulation by tumor necrosis factor α. *Proc. Natl. Acad. Sci. U.S.A.* 88: 10009–10013, 1991.

217. Mathias, S., A. Younes, C.-C. Kan, I. Orlow, C. Joseph, and R. N. Kolesnick. Activation of the sphingomyelin-signaling pathway in intact EL4 cells and in a cell-free system by IL-1β. *Science* 259: 519–522, 1993.

218. Mattie, M., G. Brooker, and S. Spiegel. Sphingosine-1–phosphate, a putative second messenger, mobilizes calcium from internal stores via an inositol trisphosphate-independent pathway. *J. Biol. Chem.* 269: 3181–3188, 1994.

219. Matuoka, L., F. Shibasaki, M. Shibata, and T. Takenawa. Ash/Grb-2, a SH2/SH3–containing protein, couples to signaling for mitogenesis and cytoskeletal reorganization by EGF and PDGF. *EMBO J.* 12: 3467–3473, 1993.

220. Meldrum, E., P. J. Parker, and A. Carozzi. The PtdIns-PLC superfamily and signal transduction. *Biochim. Biophys. Acta* 1092: 49–71, 1991.

221. Merrill, Jr., A. H., A. M. Sereni, V. L. Stevens, Y. A. Hannun, R. M. Bell, and J. M. Kinkade, Jr. Inhibition of phorbol ester–dependent differentiation of human promyelocytic leukemic (HL-60) cells by sphinganine and other long-chain bases. *J. Biol. Chem.* 261: 12610–12615, 1986.

222. Mikoshiba, K. Inositol 1,4,5-trisphosphate receptor. *Trends Pharmacol. Sci.* 14: 86–89, 1993.

223. Mitchell, R. H. Inositol phospholipids and cell surface receptor function. *Biochim. Biophys. Acta* 415: 81–147, 1975.

224. Mitchell, R. H., and M. J. O. Wakelam. Sphingolipid signalling. *Cur. Biol.* 4: 370–373, 1994.

225. Mohammadi, M., C. A. Dionne, W. Li, N. Li, T. Spivak, A. M. Honegger, M. Jaye, and J. Schlessinger. Point mutation in FGF receptor eliminates phosphatidylinositol hydrolysis without affecting mitogenesis. *Nature* 358: 681–684, 1992.

226. Moolenaar, W. H. Lysophosphatidic acid, a multifunctional phospholipid messenger. *J. Biol. Chem.* 270: 12949–12952, 1995.

227. Moolenaar, W. H. Lysophosphatidic acid signaling. *Curr. Opin. Cell Biol.* 7: 203–210, 1995.

227a. Moolenaar, W. H., O. Kranenburg, F. R. Postma, and G.C.M. Zondag. Lysophosphatidic acid: G-protein signalling and cellular responses. *Curr. Opin. Cell. Biol.* 9: 168–173, 1997.

228. Moritz, A., P. N. E. DeGraan, W. H. Gispen, and K.W.A. Wirtz. Phosphatidic acid is a specific activator of phosphatidylinositol-4–phosphate kinase. *J. Biol. Chem.* 267: 7207–7210, 1992.

229. Moss, J., and M. Vaughan. Structure and function of ARF proteins: activators of cholera toxin and critical components of intracellular vesicular transport processes. *J. Biol. Chem.* 270: 12327–12330, 1995.

230. Mullman, T. J., M. I. Siegel, R. W. Egan, and M. M. Billah. Sphingosine inhibits phosphatidate phosphohydrolase in human neutrophils by a protein kinase C–independent mechanism. *J. Biol. Chem.* 266: 2013–2016, 1991.

231. Musial, A., A. Mandal, E. Coroneos, and M. Kester. Interleukin-1 and endothelin stimulate distinct species of diglycerides that differentially regulate protein kinase C in mesangial cells. *J. Biol. Chem.* 270: 21632–21638, 1995.

232. Nakanishi, H., K. A. Brewer, and J. H. Exton. Activation of the ζ isozyme of protein kinase C by phosphatidylinositol 3,4,5-trisphosphate. *J. Biol. Chem.* 268: 13–16, 1993.

233. Nakanishi, H., and J. H. Exton. Purification and characterization of the ζ isoform of protein kinase C from bovine kidney. *J. Biol. Chem.* 267: 16347–16354, 1992.

234. Nakanishi, O., F. Shibasaki, M. Hidaka, Y. Monna, and T. Takenawa. Phospholipase C-γ₁ associates with viral and cellular *src* kinases. *J. Biol. Chem.* 268: 10754–10759, 1993.

235. Nalefski, E. A., L. A. Sultzman, D. M. Martin, R. W. Kriz, P. S. Towler, J. L. Knopf, and J. D. Clark. Delineation of two functionally distinct domains of cytosolic phospholipase A_2, a regulatory Ca^{2+}-dependent lipid-binding domain and a Ca^{2+}-independent catalytic domain. *J. Biol. Chem.* 269: 18239–18249, 1994.

236. Nanberg, E., and E. Rozengurt. Temporal relationship between inositol polyphosphate formation and increases in cytosolic Ca^{2+} in quiescent 3T3 cells stimulated by platelet-derived growth factor, bombesin and vasopressin. *EMBO J.* 7: 2741–2747, 1988.

237. Nemenoff, R. A., S. Winitz, N.-X. Qian, V. V. Putten, G. L. Johnson, and L. E. Heasley. Phosphorylation and activation of a high molecular weight form of phospholipase A_2 by p42 microtubule-associated protein 2 kinase and protein kinase C. *J. Biol. Chem.* 268: 1960–1964, 1993.

238. Nishimura, R., W. Li, A. Kashishian, A. Mondino, M. Zhou, J. Cooper, and J. Schlessinger. Two signaling molecules share a phosphotyrosine-containing binding site in the platelet-derived growth factor receptor. *Mol. Cell. Biol.* 13: 6889–6896, 1993.

239. Nishizuka, Y. The role of protein kinase C in cell surface signal transduction and tumour promotion. *Nature* 308: 693–698, 1984.

240. Nishizuka, Y. Intracellular signaling by hydrolysis of phospholipids and activation of protein kinase C. *Science* 258: 607–612, 1992.

241. Nishizuka, Y. Protein kinase C and lipid signaling for sustained cellular responses. *FASEB J.* 9: 484–496, 1995.

242. Nobes, C. D., P. Hawkins, L. Stephens, and A. Hall. Activation of the small GTP-binding proteins rho and rac by growth factor receptors. *J. Cell Sci.* 108: 225–233, 1995.

243. Narumiya, S. The small GTPase Rho: Cellular functions and signal transduction. *J. Biochem.* 120: 215–228, 1996.

245. Obeid, L. M., C. M. Linardic, L. A. Karolak, and Y. A. Hannun. Programmed cell death induced by ceramide. *Science* 259: 1769–1771, 1993.

246. Obermeier, A., H. Halfter, K.-H. Wiesmuller, G. Jung, J. Schlessinger, and A. Ullrich. Tyrosine 785 is a major determinant of Trk–substrate interaction. *EMBO J.* 12: 933–941, 1993.

247. Obermeier, A., R. Lammers, K.-H. Wiesmuller, G. Jung, J. Schlessinger, and A. Ullrich. Identification of Trk binding sites for SHC and phosphatidylinositol 3′-kinase and formation of a multimeric signaling complex. *J. Biol. Chem.* 268: 22963–22966, 1993.

248. Ohguchi, K., Y. Banno, S. Nakashima, and Y. Nozawa. Activation of membrane-bound phospholipase D by protein kinase C in HL60 cells: synergistic action of a small GTP-binding

protein RhoA. *Biochem. Biophys. Res. Commun.* 211: 306–311, 1995.

249. Ohguchi, K., Y. Banno, S. Nakashima, and Y. Nozawa. Regulation of membrane-bound phospholipase D by protein kinase C in HL60 cells. Synergistic action of small GTP-binding protein RhoA. *J. Biol. Chem.* 271: 4366–4372, 1996.

250. Okada, T., Y. Kawano, T. Sakakibara, O. Hazeki, and M. Ui. Essential role of phosphatidylinositol 3-kinase in insulin-induced glucose transport and antilipolysis in rat adipocytes. Studies with a selective inhibitor wortmannin. *J. Biol. Chem.* 269: 3568–3573, 1994.

251. Okada, T., L. Sakuma, Y. Fukui, O. Hazeki, and M. Ui. Blockage of chemotactic peptide-induced stimulation of neutrophils by wortmannin as a result of selective inhibition of phosphatidylinositol 3-kinase. *J. Biol. Chem.* 269: 3563–3567, 1994.

252. Okamura, S.-I., and S. Yamashita. Purification and characterization of phosphatidylcholine phospholipase D from pig lung. *J. Biol. Chem.* 269: 31207–31213, 1994.

253. Okazaki, T., R. M. Bell, and Y. A. Hannun. Sphingomyelin turnover induced by vitamin D_3 in HL-60 cells. Role in cell differentiation. *J. Biol. Chem.* 264: 19076–19080, 1989.

254. Okazaki, T., A. Bielawska, R. M. Bell, and Y. A. Hannun. Role of ceramide as a lipid mediator of $1\alpha,25$-dihydroxyvitamin D_3-induced HL-60 cell differentiation. *J. Biol. Chem.* 265: 15823–15831, 1990.

255. Olivera, A., and S. Spiegel. Sphingosine-1–phosphate as second messenger in cell proliferation induced by PDGF and FCS mitogens. *Nature* 365: 557–560, 1993.

256. Pachter, J. A., J.-K. Pai, R. Mayer-Ezell, J. M. Petrin, E. Dobek, and W. R. Bishop. Differential regulation of phosphoinositide and phosphatidylcholine hydrolysis by protein kinase C-β1 overexpression. Effects on stimulation by α-thrombin, guanosine 5'-O-(thiotriphosphate), and calcium. *J. Biol. Chem.* 267: 9826–9830, 1992.

257. Pagano, R. E., and K. J. Longmuir. Phosphorylation, transbilayer movement, and facilitated intracellular transport of diacylglycerol are involved in the uptake of a fluorescent analog of phosphatidic acid by cultured fibroblasts. *J. Biol. Chem.* 260: 1909–1916, 1985.

258. Pai, J.-K., E. A. Dobek, and W. R. Bishop. Endothelin-1 activates phospholipase D and thymidine incorporation in fibroblasts overexpressing protein kinase C_1. *Cell Regul.* 2: 897–903, 1991.

259. Palmer, R. H., L. V. Dekker, R. Woscholski, J. A. Le Good, R. Gigg, and P. J. Parker. Activation of PRK1 by phosphatidylinositol 4,5-bisphosphate and phosphatidylinositol 3,4,5-trisphosphate. A comparison with protein kinase C isotypes. *J. Biol. Chem.* 270: 22412–22416, 1995.

259a. Park, S-K., J. J. Provost, C. D. Bae, W-T. Ho, and J. H. Exton. Cloning and characterization of phospholipase D from rat brain. *J. Biol. Chem.* In press.

260. Parker, P. J. PI 3-kinase puts GTP on the Rac. *Curr. Biol.* 5: 577–579, 1995.

261. Parker, P. J., and M. D. Waterfield. Phosphatidylinositol 3-kinase: a novel effector. *Cell Growth Differ.* 3: 747–752, 1992.

262. Pawson, T. Protein modules and signalling networks. *Nature* 373: 573–580, 1995.

263. Pelech, S. L., and D. E. Vance. Regulation of phosphatidylcholine biosynthesis. *Biochim. Biophys. Acta* 779: 217–251, 1984.

264. Penner, R., C. Fasolato, and M. Hoth. Calcium influx and its control by calcium release. *Curr. Opin. Neurobiol.* 3: 368–374, 1993.

265. Peppelenbosch, M. P., R.-G. Qiu, A.M.M. de Vries-Smits,

L.G.J. Tertoolen, S. W. de Laat, F. McCormick, A. Hall, M. H. Symons, and J. L. Bos. Rac mediates growth factor–induced arachidonic acid release. *Cell* 81: 849–856, 1995.

266. Perianin, A., C. Combadiere, E. Pedruzzi, B. Djerdjouri, and J. Hakim. Staurosporine stimulates phospholipase D activation in human polymorphonuclear leukocytes. *FEBS Lett.* 315: 33–37, 1993.

267. Perry, D. K., V. L. Stevens, T. S. Widlanski, and J. D. Lambeth. A novel *ecto*-phosphatidic acid phosphohydrolase activity mediates activation of neutrophil superoxide generation by exogenous phosphatidic acid. *J. Biol. Chem.* 268: 25302–25310, 1993.

268. Pete, M. J., and J. H. Exton. Purification of a lysophospholipase from bovine brain that selectively deacylates arachidonoyl-substituted lysophosphatidylcholine. *J. Biol. Chem.* 271: 18114–18121, 1996.

269. Pete, M. J., D. W. Wu, and J. H. Exton. Subcellular fractions of bovine brain degrade phosphatidylcholine by sequential deacylation of the *sn-1* and *sn-2* positions. *Biochim. Biophys. Acata* 1299: 325–332, 1996.

270. Peters, K. G., J. Marie, E. Wilson, H. E. Ives, J. Escobedo, M. Del Rosario, D. Merda, and L. T. Williams. Point mutation of an FGF receptor abolishes phosphatidylinositol turnover and Ca^{2+} flux but not mitogenesis. *Nature* 358: 678–681, 1992.

271. Piccione, E., R. D. Chase, S. M. Domchek, P. Hu, M. Chaudhuri, J. M. Backer, J. Schlessinger, and S. E. Shoelson. Phosphatidylinositol 3-kinase p85 SH2 domain specificity defined by direct phosphopeptide/SH2 domain binding. *Biochemistry* 32: 3197–3202, 1993.

272. Pitcher, J. A., K. Touhara, E. S. Payne, and R. J. Lefkowitz. Pleckstrin homology domain–mediated membrane association and activation of the β-adrenergic receptor kinase requires coordinate interaction with $G_{\beta\gamma}$ subunits and lipid. *J. Biol. Chem.* 270: 11707–11710, 1995.

273. Plevin, R., and M. J. O. Wakelam. Rapid desensitization of vasopressin-stimulated phosphatidylinositol 4,5-bisphosphate and phosphatidylcholine hydrolysis questions the role of these pathways in sustained diacylglycerol formation in A10 vascular smooth-muscle cells. *Biochem. J.* 285: 759–766, 1992.

274. Prescott, S. M., and P. W. Majerus. Characterization of 1,2-diacylglycerol hydrolysis in human platelets. Demonstration of an arachidonoyl-monacylglycerol intermediate. *J. Biol. Chem.* 258: 764–769, 1983.

275. Provost, J. J., J. Fudge, S. Israelit, A. R. Siddiqi, and J. H. Exton. Tissue specific distribution and subcellular distribution of phospholipase D in rat. Evidence for distinct RhoA- and ARF-regulated isozymes. *Biochem. J.* 319: 285–291, 1996.

276. Putney, J. W., Jr., and G. S. J. Bird. The signal for capacitative calcium entry. *Cell* 75: 199–201, 1993.

277. Pyne, S., and N. J. Pyne. Bradykinin-stimulated phosphatidate and 1,2-diacylglycerol accumulation in guinea-pig airway smooth muscle: evidence for regulation "down-stream" of phospholipases. *Cell. Signal.* 6: 269–277, 1994.

278. Qiu, Z.-H., M. S. de Carvalho, and C. C. Leslie. Regulation of phospholipase A_2 activation by phosphorylation in mouse peritoneal macrophages. *J. Biol. Chem.* 268: 24506–24513, 1993.

279. Qiu, Z.-H., and C. C. Leslie. Protein kinase C–dependent and –independent pathways of mitogen-activated protein kinase activation in macrophages by stimuli that activate phospholipase A_2. *J. Biol. Chem.* 269: 19480–19487, 1994.

280. Qualliotine-Mann, D., D. E. Agwu, M. D. Ellenburg, C. E. McCall, and L. C. McPhail. Phosphatidic acid and diacylglycerol synergize in a cell-free system for activation of NADPH

oxidase from human neutrophils. *J. Biol. Chem.* 268: 23843–23849, 1993.

280a. Qian, D., and A. Weiss. T cell antigen receptor signal transduction. *Curr. Opin. Cell Biol.* 9: 205–212, 1997.

280b. Ji, Q.-S., G. E. winnier, K. D. Niswender, D. Horstman, R. Wisdom, M. A. Magnuson, and G. Carpenter. Essential role of the tyrosine kinase substrate phospholipase C-γ1 in mammalian growth and development. *Proc. Natl. Acad. Sci. U.S.A.* 94: 2999–3003, 1997.

281. Randriamampita, C., and R. Y. Tsien. Emptying of intracellular Ca^{2+} stores releases a novel small messenger that stimulates C influx. *Nature* 364: 809–814, 1993.

282. Rankin, S., N. Morii, S. Narumiya, and E. Rozengurt. Botulinum C3 exoenzyme blocks the tyrosine phosphorylation of p125^{FAK} and paxillin induced by bombesin and endothelin. *FEBS Lett.* 354: 315–319, 1994.

283. Rao, G. N., B. Lassegue, R. W. Alexander, and K. K. Griendling. Angiotensin II stimulates phosphorylation of high-molecular-mass cytosolic phospholipase A$_2$ in vascular smooth-muscle cells. *Biochem. J.* 299: 197–201, 1994.

284. Rhee, S. G., and K. D. Choi. Regulation of inositol phospholipid-specific phospholipase C isozymes. *J. Biol. Chem.* 267: 12393–12396, 1992.

285. Ridley, A. J., and A. Hall. The small GTP-binding protein rho regulates the assembly of focal adhesions and actin stress fibers in response to growth factors. *Cell* 70: 389–399, 1992.

286. Ridley, A. J., H. F. Paterson, C. L. Johnston, D. Diekmann, and A. Hall. The small GTP-binding protein rac regulates growth factor–induced membrane ruffling. *Cell* 70: 401–410, 1992.

287. Roche, S., M. Koegl, and S. A. Courtneidge. The phosphatidylinositol 3-kinase α is required for DNA synthesis induced by some, but not all, growth factors. *Proc. Natl. Acad. Sci. U.S.A.* 91: 9185–9189, 1994.

288. Rodriguez-Viciana, P., P. H. Warne, R. Dhand, B. Vanhaesebroeck, I. Gout, M. J. Fry, M. D. Waterfield, and J. Downward. Phosphatidylinositol-3–OH kinase as a direct target of Ras. *Nature* 370: 527–532, 1994.

288a. Rodriguez-Viciana, P., P. H. Warne, A. Khwaja, B. M. Marte, D. Pappin, P. Das, M. D. Waterfield, A. Ridley, and J. Downward. Role of phosphoinositide 3-OH kinase in cell transformation and control of the actin cytoskeleton by ras. *Cell* 89:457–467, 1997.

289. Roldan, E. R. S., and T. Murase. Polyphosphoinositide-derived diacylglycerol stimulates the hydrolysis of phosphatidylcholine by phospholipase C during exocytosis of the ram sperm acrosome. Effect is not mediated by protein kinase C. *J. Biol. Chem.* 269: 23583–23589, 1994.

290. Ronnstrand, L., S. Mori, A.-K. Arridsson, A. Eriksson, C. Wernstedt, U. Hellman, L. Claesson-Welsh, and C.-H. Heldin. Identification of two C-terminal autophosphorylation sites in the PDGF β-receptor: involvement in the interaction with phospholipase C-γ. *EMBO J.* 11: 3911–3919, 1992.

291. Rosenwald, A. G., and R. E. Pagano. Inhibition of glycoprotein traffic through the secretory pathway by ceramide. *J. Biol. Chem.* 268: 4577–4579, 1993.

292. Roshak, A., G. Sathe, and L. A. Marshall. Suppression of monocyte 85-kDa phospholipase A$_2$ by antisense and effects on endotoxin-induced prostaglandin biosynthesis. *J. Biol. Chem.* 269: 25999–26005, 1994.

293. Rossi, F., M. Grzeskowiak, V. D. Bianca, F. Calzetti, and G. Gandini. Phosphatidic acid and not diacylglycerol generated by phospholipase D is functionally linked to the activation of the NADPH oxidase by FMLP in human neutrophils. *Biochem. Biophys. Res. Commun.* 168: 320–327, 1990.

294. Rumenapp, U., M. Geiszt, F. Wahn, M. Schmidt, and K. H. Jakobs. Evidence for ADP-ribosylation-factor-mediated activation of phospholipase D by m3 muscarinic acetylcholine receptor. *Eur. J. Biochem.* 234: 240–244, 1995.

295. Sa, G., and P. L. Fox. Basic fibroblast growth factor–stimulated endothelial cell movement is mediated by a pertussis toxin–sensitive pathway regulation phospholipase A$_2$ activity. *J. Biol. Chem.* 269: 3219–3225, 1994.

296. Sa, G., G. Murugesan, M. Jaye, Y. Ivashchenko, and P. L. Fox. Activation of cytosolic phospholipase A$_2$ by basic fibroblast growth factor via p42 mitogen-activated protein kinase–dependent phosphorylation pathway in endothelial cells. *J. Biol. Chem.* 270: 2360–2366, 1995.

297. Sakaue, H., K. Hara, T. Noguchi, T. Matozaki, K. Kotani, W. Ogawa, K. Yonezawa, M. D. Waterfield, and M. Kasuga. Ras-independent and wortmannin-sensitive activation of glycogen synthase by insulin in Chinese hamster ovary cells. *J. Biol. Chem.* 270: 11304–11309, 1995.

298. Saleem, A., S. Kharbanda, Z.-M. Yuan, and D. Kufe. Monocyte colony-stimulating factor stimulates binding of phosphatidyl-inositol 3-kinase to Grb2.Sos complexes in human monocytes. *J. Biol. Chem.* 270: 10380–10383, 1995.

298a. Santana, P., L. A. Pena, A. Haimovitz-Friedman, S. Martin, D. Green, M. McLoughlin, C. Cordon-Cardo, E. H. Schuchman, Z. Fuks, and R. Kolesnick. Acid sphingomyelinase-deficient human lymphoblasts and mice are defective in radiation-induced apoptosis. *Cell* 86: 189–199, 1996.

299. Sato, T., T. Ishimot, S. Akiba, and T. Fujii. Enhancement of phospholipase A$_2$ activation by phosphatidic acid endogenously formed through phospholipase D action in rat peritoneal mast cell. *FEBS Lett.* 323: 23–26, 1993.

300. Savarese, T. M., and C. M. Fraser. In vitro mutagenesis and the search for structure–function relationships among G protein-coupled receptors. *Biochem. J.* 283: 1–19, 1992.

301. Savitsky, K., A. Bar-Shira, S. Gilad, G. Rotman, Y. Ziv, L. Vanagaite, D. A. Tagle, S. Smith, T. Uziel, S. Sfez, M. Ashkenazi, I. Pecker, M. Frydman, R. Harnik, S. R. Patanjali, A. Simmons, G. A. Clines, A. Sartiel, R. A. Gatti, L. Chessa, O. Sanai, M. F. Lavin, N. G. J. Jaspers, A.M.R. Taylor, C. F. Arlett, T. Miki, S. M. Weissman, M. Lovett, F. S. Collins, and Y. Shiloh. A single ataxia telangiectasia gene with a product similar to PI-3 kinase. *Science* 268: 1749–1753, 1995.

302. Schalkwijk, C. G., E. de Vet, J. Pfeilschifter, and H. van den Bosch. Interleukin-1β and transforming growth factor-β$_2$ enhance cytosolic high-molecular-mass phospholipase A$_2$ activity and induce prostaglandin E$_2$ formation in rat mesangial cells. *Eur. J. Biochem.* 210: 169–176, 1992.

303. Schmidt, M., S. M. Huwe, B. Fasselt, D. Homann, U. Rumenapp, J. Sandmann, and K. H. Jakobs. Mechanisms of phospholipase D stimulation by m3 muscarinic acetylcholine receptors. Evidence for involvement of tyrosine phosphorylation. *Eur. J. Biochem.* 225: 667–675, 1994.

304. Schutze, S., K. Potthoff, T. Machleidt, D. Berkovic, K. Wiegmann, and M. Kronke. TNF activates NF-kB by phosphatidylcholine-specific phospholipase C–induced "acidic" sphingomyelin breakdown. *Cell* 71: 765–776, 1992.

304a. Schwinn, D. A., J. W. Lomasney, W. Lorenz, P. J. Szklut, R. T. Fremeau, Jr., T. L. Yang-Feng, M. G. Caron, R. J. Lefkowitz, and S. Cotecchia. Molecular cloning and expression of the cDNA for a novel α$_1$-adrenergic receptor subtype. *J. Biol. Chem.* 265: 8183–8189, 1990.

305. Seckl, M. J., N. Morii, S. Narumiya, and E. Rozengurt. Guanosine 5'-3-O-(Thio)triphosphate stimulates tyrosine phosphory-

lation of p125^{FAK} and paxillin in permeabilized Swiss 3T3 cells. Role of p21^{rho}. *J. Biol. Chem.* 270: 6984–6990, 1995.

306. Seedorf, K., B. Millauer, G. Kostka, J. Schlessinger, and A. Ullrich. Differential effects of carboxyl-terminal sequence deletions on platelet-derived growth factor receptor signaling activities and interactions with cellular substrates. *Mol. Cell. Biol.* 12: 4347–4356, 1992.

307. Seger, R., and E. G. Krebs. The MAPK signaling cascade. *FASEB J.* 9: 726–735, 1995.

308. Seki, K., H.-C, Chen, and K.-P, Huang. Dephosphorylation of protein kinase C substrates, neurogranin, neuromodulin, and MARCKS, by calcineurin and protein phosphatases 1 and 2A. *Arch. Biochem. Biophys.* 316: 673–679, 1995.

309. Seufferlelin, T., and E. Rozengurt. Lysophosphatidic acid stimulates tyrosine phosphorylation of focal adhesion kinase, paxillin, and p130. Signaling pathways and cross-talk with platelet-derived growth factor. *J. Biol. Chem.* 269: 9345–9351, 1994.

310. Seufferlelin, T., and E. Rozengurt. Sphingosine induces p125^{FAK} and paxillin tyrosine phosphorylation, actin stress fiber formation, and focal contact assembly in Swiss 3T3 cells. *J. Biol. Chem.* 269: 27610–27617, 1994.

311. Sharp, J. D., D. L. White, X. G. Chiou, T. Goodson, G. C. Gamboa, D. McClure, S. Burgett, J. Hoskins, P. L. Skatrud, J. R. Sportsman, G. W. Becker, L. H. Kang, E. F. Roberts, and R. M. Kramer. Molecular cloning and expression of human Ca^{2+}-sensitive cytosolic phospholipse A$_2$. *J. Biol. Chem.* 266: 14850–14853, 1991.

312. Shears, S. B. Metabolism of inositol phosphates. *Adv. Second Messenger and Phosphoprotein Res.* 26: 63–92, 1992.

313. Shibasaki, F., K. Fukami, Y. Fukui, and T. Takenawa. Phosphatidylinositol 3-kinase binds to α-actinin through the p85 subunit. *Biochem. J.* 302: 551–557, 1994.

313a. Shirakabe, K., K. Yamaguchi, H. Shibuya, K. Irie, S. Matsuda, T. Moriguchi, Y. Gotoh, K. Matsumoto, and E. Nishida. TAK1 mediates the ceramide signaling to stress-activated protein kinase/c-Jun N-terminal kinase. *J. Biol. Chem.* 272: 8141–8144, 1997.

313b. Shpetner, H., M. Joly, D. Hartley, and S. Corvera. Potential sites of PI-3 kinase function in the endocytic pathway revealed by the PI-3 kinase inhibitor, wortmannin. *J. Cell. Biol.* 132: 595–605, 1996.

314. Siddiqi, A. R., J. L. Smith, A. H. Ross, R.-G. Qiu, M. Symons, and J. H. Exton. Regulation of phospholipase D in HL60 cells. Evidence for a cytosolic phospholipase D. *J. Biol. Chem.* 270: 8466–8473, 1995.

314a. Simon, M. I., M. P. Strathmann, and N. Gautam. Diversity of G proteins in signal transduction. *Science* 252: 802–808, 1991.

315. Singer, W. D., H. A. Brown, G. M. Bokoch, and P. C. Sternweis. Resolved phospholipase D activity is modulated by cytosolic factors other than Arf. *J. Biol. Chem.* 270: 14944–14950, 1995.

316. Singer, W. D., H. A. Brown, X. Jiang, and P. C. Sternweis. Regulation of phospholipase D by protein kinase C is synergistic with ADP-ribosylation factor and independent of protein kinase activity. *J. Biol. Chem.* 271: 4504–4510, 1996.

317. Sitsapesan, R., S. J. McGarry, and A. J. Williams. Cyclic ADP-ribose, the ryanodine receptor and Ca^{2+} release. *Trends Pharmacol. Sci.* 16: 386–391, 1995.

318. Soler, C., L. Beguinot, and G. Carpenter. Individual epidermal growth factor receptor autophosphorylation sites do not stringently define association motifs for several SH2–containing proteins. *J. Biol. Chem.* 269: 12320–12324, 1994.

319. Soltoff, S., and L. C. Cantley. p120^{cbl} is a cytosolic adapter protein that associates with phosphoinositide 3-kinase in re-

sponse to epidermal growth factor in PC12 and other cells. *J. Biol. Chem.* 271: 563–567, 1996.

320. Soltoff, S. P., K. L. Carraway III, S. A. Prigent, W. G. Gullick, and L. C. Cantley. ErbB3 is involved in activation of phosphatidylinositol 3-kinase by epidermal growth factor. *Mol. Cell. Biol.* 14: 3550–3558, 1994.

321. Spaargaren, M., S. Wissink, L.H.K. Defize, S. W. de Laat, and J. Boonstsra. Characterization and identification of an epidermal-growth-factor-activated phospholipase A$_2$. *Biochem. J.* 287: 37–43, 1992.

322. Stehno-Bittle, L., G. Krapivinsky, L. Krapivinsky, C. Perez-Terzie, and D. E. Clapham. The G protein $\beta\gamma$ subunit transduces the muscarinic receptor signal for Ca^{2+} release in *Xenopus* oocytes. *J. Biol. Chem.* 270: 30068–30074, 1995.

323. Stephens, L., A. Smrcka, F. T. Cooke, T. R. Jackson, P. C. Sternweis, and P. T. Hawkins. A novel phosphoinositide 3 kinase activity in myeloid-derived cells is activated by G protein $\beta\gamma$ subunits. *Cell* 77: 83–93, 1994.

324. Stephens, L. R., T. R. Jackson, and P. T. Hawkins. Agonist-stimulated synthesis of phosphatidylinositol (3,4,5)-trisphosphate: a new intracellular signalling system? *Biochim. Biophys. Acta* 1179: 27–75, 1993.

325. Sternweis, P. C. The active role of $\beta\gamma$ in signal transduction. *Curr. Opin. Cell Biol.* 6: 198–203, 1994.

326. Stoyanov, B., S. Volinia, T. Hanck, I. Rubio, M. Loubtchenkov, D. Malek, S. Stoyanova, B. Banhaesebroeck, R. Dhand, B. Nurnberg, P. Gierschik, K. Seedorf, J. J. Hsuan, M. D. Waterfield, and R. Wetzker. Cloning and characterization of a G protein-activated human phosphoinositide-3 kinase. *Science* 269: 690–693, 1995.

327. Streb, H., R. F. Irvine, M. J. Berridge, and I. Schulz. Release of Ca^{2+} from a nonmitochondrial intracellular store in pancreatic acinar cells by inositol-1,4,5-trisphosphate. *Nature* 306: 67–69, 1983.

328. Strum, J. C., A. B. Nixon, L. W. Daniel, and R. L. Wykle. Evaluation of phospholipase C and D activity in stimulated human neutrophils using a phosphono analog of choline phosphoglyceride. *Biochim. Biophys. Acta* 1169: 25–29, 1993.

329. Sugiyama, T., T. Sakai, Y. Nozawa, and N. Oka. Prostaglandin F$_{2\alpha}$-stimulated phospholipase D activation in osteoblast-like MC3t#-E1 cells: involvement in sustained 1,2-diacylglycerol production. *Biochem. J.* 298: 479–484, 1994.

329a. Suzuki, A., J. Shinoda, Y. Oiso, and O. Kozawa. Tyrosine kinase is involved in angiotensin II-stimulated phospholipase D activation in aortic smooth muscle cells: Function of Ca^{2+} influx. *Atherosclerosis* 121:119–127, 1996.

330. Taki, T., and J. N. Kanfer. Partial purification and properties of a rat brain phospholipase D. *J. Biol. Chem.* 254: 9761–9765, 1979.

331. Takuwa, N., M. Kumada, K. Yamashita, and Y. Takuwa. Mechanisms of bombesin-induced arachidonate mobilization in Swiss 3T3 fibroblasts. *J. Biol. Chem.* 266: 14237–14243, 1991.

332. Taniguchi, T. Cytokine signaling through nonreceptor protein tyrosine kinases. *Science* 268: 251–255, 1995.

332a. Tanti, J-F., T. Gremeaux, S. Grillo, V. Calleja, A. Klippel, L. T. Williams, E. Van Obberghen, and Y. Le Marchand-Brustel. Overexpression of a constitutively active form of phosphatidylinositol 3-kinase is sufficient to promote Glut 4 translocation in adipocytes. *J. Biol. Chem.* 271: 25227–25232, 1996.

333. Tate, B. F., and S. E. Rittenhouse. Thrombin activation of human platelets causes tyrosine phosphorylation of PLC-γ_2. *Biochim. Biophys. Acta* 1178: 281–285, 1993.

334. Tepper, C. G., S. Jayadev, B. Liu, A. Bielawska, R. Wolff, S. Yonehara, Y. A. Hannun, and M. F. Seldin. Role for ceramide

as an endogenous mediator of Fas-induced cytotoxicity. *Proc. Natl. Acad. Sci. U.S.A.* 92: 8443–8447, 1995.

335. Thomas, D., and M. R. Hanley. Evaluation of calcium influx factors from stimulated jurkat T-lymphocytes by microinjection into *Xenopus* oocytes. *J. Biol. Chem.* 270: 6429–6432, 1995.

336. Thomason, P. A., S. R. James, P. J. Casey, and C. P. Downes. A G-protein $\beta\gamma$-subunit-responsive phosphoinositide 3-kinase activity in human platelet cytosol. *J. Biol. Chem.* 269: 16525–16528, 1994.

337. Thomson, F. J., and M. A. Clark. Purification of a phosphatidic-acid-hydrolysing phospholipase A_2 from rat brain. *Biochem. J.* 306: 305–309, 1995.

338. Thomson, F. J., L. Perkins, D. Ahern, and M. Clark. Identification and characterization of a lysophosphatidic acid receptor. *Mol. Pharmacol.* 45: 718–723, 1994.

339. Thurston, A. W., Jr., S. G. Rhee, and S. D. Shukla. Role of guanine nucleotide-binding protein and tyrosine kinase in platelet-activating factor activation of phospholipase C in A431 cells: proposal for dual mechanisms. *J. Pharmacol. Exp. Ther.* 266: 1106–1112, 1993.

340. Tigyi, G., D. L. Dyer, and R. Miledi. Lysophosphatidic acid possesses dual action in cell proliferation. *Proc. Natl. Acad. Sci. U.S.A.* 91: 1908–1912, 1994.

341. Toker, A., M. Meyer, K. K. Reddy, J. R. Falck, R. Aneja, S. Aneja, A. Parra, D. J. Burns, L. M. Ballas, and L. C. Cantley. Activation of protein kinase C family members by the novel polyphosphoinositides PtdIns-3,4,-P_2 and PtdIns-3,4,5-P_3. *J. Biol. Chem.* 269: 32358–32367, 1994.

342. Tolias, K. F., L. C. Cantley, and C. L. Carpenter. Rho family GTPases bind to phosphoinositide kinases. *J. Biol. Chem.* 270: 17656–17659, 1995.

343. Tomic, S., U. Greiser, R. Lammers, A. Kharitonenkov, E. Imyanitov, A. Ullrich, and F.D. Bohmer. Association of SH2 domain protein tyrosine phosphatases with the epidermal growth factor receptor in human tumor cells. Phosphatidic acid activates receptor dephosphorylation by PTP1C. *J. Biol. Chem.* 270: 21277–21284, 1995.

344. Tsai, M.-H., C.-L, Yu, F.-S. Wie, and D. W. Stacy. The effect of GTPase activating protein upon Ras is inhibited by mitogenically responsive lipids. *Science* 243: 522–526, 1989.

345. Uings, I. J., N. T. Thompson, R. W. Randall, G. D. Spacey, R. W. Bonser, A. T. Hudson, and L. G. Garland. Tyrosine phosphorylation is involved in receptor coupling to phospholipase D but not phospholipase C in the human neutrophil. *Biochem. J.* 281: 597–600, 1992.

346. Valius, M., C. Bazenet, and A. Kazlauskas. Tyrosines 1021 and 1009 are phosphorylation sites in the carboxyl terminus of the platelet-derived growth factor receptor β subunit and are required for binding of phospholipase Cγ and a 64-kilodalton protein, respectively. *Mol. Cell. Biol.* 13: 133–143, 1993.

347. Valius, M., and A. Kazlauskas. Phospholipase C-γ1 and phosphatidylinositol 3 kinase are the downstream mediators of the PDGF receptor's mitogenic signal. *Cell* 73: 321–334, 1993.

348. van Corven, E.J., A. Groenink, K. Jalink, T. Eichholtz, and W.H. Moolenaar. Lysophosphatidate-induced cell proliferation: identification and dissection of signaling pathways mediated by G proteins. *Cell* 59: 45–54, 1989.

349. van Corven, E. J., A. Van Rijswijk, K. Jalink, R. L. van der Bend, W. J. van Blitterswijk, and W. H. Moolenaar. Mitogenic action of lysophosphatidic acid and phosphatidic acid on fibroblasts. Dependence on acyl-chain length and inhibition by suramin. *Biochem. J.* 281: 163–169, 1992.

350. van der Bend, R. L., J. Brunner, K. Jalink, E. J. van Corven, W. H. Moolenaar, and W. J. van Blitterswijk. Identification of a putative membrane receptor for the bioactive phospholipid, lysophosphatidic acid. *EMBO J.* 11: 2495–2501, 1992.

351. van der Bend, R. L., J. De Widt, E. J. van Corven, W. H. Moolenaar, and W. J. van Blitterswijk. Metabolic conversion of the biologically active phospholipid, lysophosphatidic acid, in fibroblasts. *Biochim. Biophys. Acta* 1125: 110–112, 1992.

352. van der Bend, R. L., J. De Widt, E. J. Van Corven, W. H. Moolenaar, and W. J. Van Blitterswijk. The biologically active phospholipid, lysophosphatidic acid, induces phosphatidylcholine breakdown in fibroblasts via activation of phospholipase D. Comparison with the response to endothelin. *Biochem. J.* 285: 235–240, 1992.

353. van der Geer, P., and T. Hunter. Mutation of Tyr697, a GRB2–binding site, and Tyr721, a PI 3-kinase binding site, abrogates signal transduction by the murine CSF-1 receptor expressed in rat-2 fibroblasts. *EMBO J.* 12: 5161–5172, 1993.

353a. van Dijk, M.C.M., F J.G. Muriana, J. de Widt, H. Hilkmann, and W. J. van Blitterswijk. Involvement of phosphatidylocholine-specific phospholipase C in platelet-derived growth factor-induced activation of the mitogen-activated protein kinase pathway in rat-1 fibroblasts. *J. Biol. Chem.* 272: 11011–11016, 1997.

353b. Vanmhaesebroeck, B.M.J. Welham, K. Kotani, R. Stein, P. H. Warne, M. J. Zvelebil, K. Higashi, S. Volinia, J. Downward, and M. D. Waterfield. p110δ, a novel phosphoinositide 3-kinase in leukocytes. *Proc. Natl. Acad. Sci. U.S.A.* 94: 4330–4335, 1997.

354. Venable, M. E., G. C. Blobe, and L. M. Obeid. Identification of a defect in the phospholipase D/diacylglycerol pathway in cellular senescence. *J. Biol. Chem.* 269: 26040–26044, 1994.

354a. Venable, M. E., J. Y. Lee, M. J. Smyth, A. Bielawska, and L. M. Obeid. Role of ceramide in cellular senescence. *J. Biol. Chem.* 270: 30701–30708, 1995.

355. Venkatakrishnan, G., and J. H. Exton. Identification of determinants in the α subunit of G_q required for phospholipase C activation. *J. Biol. Chem.* 271: 5066–5074, 1996.

355a. Verheij, M., R. Bose, X. H. Lin, B. Yao, W. D. Jarvis, S. Grant, M. J. Birrer, E. Szabo, L. I. Zon, J. M. Kyriakis, A. Halmovitz-Friedman, Z. Fuks, and R. N. Kolesnick. Requirement for ceramide-initiated SAPK/JNK signalling in stress-induced apoptosis. *Nature* 380: 75–79, 1996.

356. Vilcek, J., and T. H. Lee. Tumor necrosis factor. New insights into the molecular mechanisms of its multiple actions. *J. Biol. Chem.* 266: 7313–7316, 1991.

357. Vinggaard, A. M., and H. S. Hansen. Characterization and partial purification of phospholipase D from human placenta. *Biochim. Biophys. Acta* 1258: 169–176, 1995.

358. Vlahos, C. J., W. F. Matter, K. Y. Hui, and R. F. Brown. A specific inhibitor of phosphatidylinositol 3-kinase, 2-(4-morpholinyl)-8-phenyl-4H-1-benzopyran-4-one (LY294002). *J. Biol. Chem.* 269: 5241–5248, 1994.

359. Ward, D. T., J. Ohanian, A. M. Heagerty, and V. Ohanian. Phospholipase D–induced phosphatidate production in intact small arteries during noradrenaline stimulation: involvement of both G-protein and tyrosine-phosphorylation-linked pathways. *Biochem. J.* 307: 451–456, 1995.

360. Warner, L. C., N. Hack, S. E. Egan, H. J. Goldberg, R. A. Weinberg, and K. L. Skorecki. RAS is required for epidermal growth factor–stimulated arachidonic acid release in rat-1 fibroblasts. *Oncogene* 8: 3249–3255, 1993.

361. Watanabe, T., I. Waga, Z.-i. Honda, K. Kurokawa, and T. Shimizu. Prostaglandin $F_{2\alpha}$ stimulates formation of p21^{ras}–GTP complex and mitogen-activated protein kinase in NIH-

3T3 cells via G_q-protein-coupled pathway. *J. Biol. Chem.* 270: 8984–8990, 1995.

362. Weng, Q.-P., K. Andrabi, A. Klippel, M. T. Kozlowski, L. T. Williams, and J. Avruch. Phosphatidylinositol 3-kinase signals activation of p70 S6 kinase in situ through site-specific p70 phosphorylation. *Proc. Natl. Acad. Sci. USA* 92: 5744–5748, 1995.

363. Wennstrom, S., P. Hawkins, F. Cooke, K. Hara, K. Yonezawa, M. Kasuga, T. Jackson, L. Claesson-Welsh, and L. Stephens. Activation of phosphoinositide 3-kinase is required for PDGF-stimulated membrane ruffling. *Curr. Biol.* 4: 385–393, 1994.

363a. Wess, J. G-protein-coupled receptors: molecular mechanisms involved in receptor activation and selectivity of G-protein regulation. *FASEB J.* 11: 346–354, 1997.

364. Westwick, J. K., A. E. Bielawska, G. Dhaibo, Y. A. Hannun, and D. A. Brenner. Ceramide activates the stress-activated protein kinases. *J. Biol. Chem.* 270: 22689–22692, 1995.

365. Wijkander, J., and R. Sundler. Regulation of arachidonate-mobilizing phospholipase A_2 by phosphorylation via protein kinase C in macrophages. *FEBS Lett.* 311: 299–301, 1992.

366. Wilcox, R. A., and S. R. Nahorski. Does Ins(1,3,4,5)P_4 play a role in Ca^{2+} signaling? In: *Signal-Activated Phospholipases*, edited by M. Liscovitch. R. G. Landes, 1994, p. 189–212.

367. Wilkes, L. C., V. Patel, J. R. Purkiss, and M. R. Boarder. Endothelin-1 stimulated phospholipase D in A10 vascular smooth muscle derived cells is dependent on tyrosine kinase. *FEBS Lett.* 322: 147–150, 1993.

368. Wilson, E., M. C. Olcott, R. M. Bell, A. H. Merrill, Jr., and J. D. Lambeth. Inhibition of the oxidative burst in human neutrophils by sphingoid long-chain bases. Role of protein kinase C in activation of the burst. *J. Biol. Chem.* 261: 12616–12623, 1986.

368a. Wilson, M., A. R. Burt, G. Milligan, and N. G. Anderson. Wortmannin-sensitive activation of p70^s6k by endogenous and heterologously expressed G_i-coupled receptors. *J. Biol. Chem.* 271: 8537–8540, 1996.

369. Winitz, S., S. K. Gupta, N.-X. Qian, L. E. Heasley, R. A. Nemenoff, and G. L. Johnson. Expression of a mutant G_{i2} α subunit inhibits ATP and thrombin stimulation of cytoplasmic phospholipase A_2-mediated arachidonic acid release independent of Ca^{2+} and mitogen-activated protein kinase regulation. *J. Biol. Chem.* 269: 1889–1895, 1994.

370. Wolff, R. A., R. T. Dobrowsky, A. Bielawska, L. M. Obeid, and Y. A. Hannun. Role of ceramide-activated protein phosphatase in ceramide-mediated signal transduction. *J. Biol. Chem.* 269: 19605–19609, 1994.

371. Worthen, G. S., N. Avdi, A. M. Buhl, N. Suzuki, and G. L. Johnson. FMLP activates Ras and Raf in human neutrophils. Potential role in activation of MAP kinase. *J. Clin. Invest.* 94: 815–823, 1994.

372. Wymann, M., and A. Arcaro. Platelet-derived growth factor–induced phosphatidylinositol 3-kinase activation mediates actin rearrangements in fibroblasts. *Biochem. J.* 298: 617–620, 1994.

373. Xing, M., and R. Mattera. Phosphorylation-dependent regulation of phospholipase A_2 by G-proteins and Ca^{2+} in HL60 granulocytes. *J. Biol. Chem.* 267: 25966–25975, 1992.

374. Xing, M., P. L. Wilkins, B. K. McConnell, and R. Mattera. Regulation of phospholipase A_2 activity in undifferentiated and neutrophil-like HL60 cells. Lineage between impaired responses to agonists and absence of protein kinase C–dependent phosphorylation of cytosolic phospholipase A_2. *J. Biol. Chem.* 269: 3117–3124, 1994.

375. Xu, X.-X., C. O. Rock, Z.-H Qiu, C. C. Leslie, and S. Jackow-ski. Regulation of cytosolic phospholipase A_2 phosphorylation and eicosanoid production by colony-stimulating factor 1. *J. Biol. Chem.* 269: 31693–31700, 1994.

376. Yamamoto-Hondo, R., K. Tobe, Y. Kaburagi, K. Ueki, S. Asai, M. Yachi, M. Shirouzu, J. Yodoi, Y. Akanuma, S. Yokoyama, Y. Yazaki, and T. Kadowski. Upstream mechanisms of glycogen synthase activation by insulin and insulin-like growth factor-I. Glycogen synthase activation is antagonized by wortmannin or ly204–2 but not by rapamycin or by inhibiting p21^ras. *J. Biol. Chem.* 270: 2729–2734, 1995.

380. Yamauchi, K., K. Holt, and J.E. Pessin. Phosphatidylinositol 3-kinase functions upstream of Ras and Raf in mediating insulin stimulation of *c-fos* transcription. *J. Biol. Chem.* 268: 14597–14600, 1993.

381. Yang, Z., M. Costanzo, D. W. Golde, and R. N. Kolesnick. Tumor necrosis factor activation of the sphingomyelin pathway signals nuclear factor kB translocation in intact HL-60 cells. *J. Biol. Chem.* 268: 20520–20523, 1993.

382. Yano, H., S. Nakanishi, K. Kimura, N. Hanai, Y. Saitoh, Y. Fukui, Y. Nonomura, and Y. Matsuda. Inhibition of histamine secretin by wortmannin through the blockade of phosphatidyl-inositol 3-kinase in RBL-2H3 cells. *J. Biol. Chem.* 268: 25846–25856, 1993.

383. Yao, B., Y. Zhang, S. Delilkat, S. Mathias, S. Basu, and R. Kolesnick. Phosphorylation of Raf by ceramide-activated protein kinase. *Nature* 378: 307–310, 1995.

384. Yao, R., and G. M. Cooper. Requirement for phosphatidylinositol-3 kinase in the prevention of apoptosis by nerve growth factor. *Science* 267: 2003–2006, 1995.

384a. Yao, R., and G. M. Cooper. Growth factor-dependent survival of rodent fibroblasts requires phosphatidylinositol 3-kinase but is independent of pp70^S6K activity. *Oncogene* 13: 343–351, 1996.

384b. Yatomi, Y., Y. Igarashi, L. Yang, N. Hisano, R. Qi, N. Asazuma, K. Satoh, Y. Ozaki, and S. Kume. Sphingosine 1-phosphate, a bioactive sphingolipid abundantly stored in platelets, is a normal constituent of human plasma and serum. *J. Biochem.* 121:969–973, 1997.

385. Yeo, E.-J., and J. H. Exton. Stimulation of phospholipase D by epidermal growth factor requires protein kinase C activation in Swiss 3T3 cells. *J. Biol. Chem.* 270: 3980–3988, 1995.

386. Yeo, E.-J., A. Kazlauskas, and J. H. Exton. Activation of phospholipase C-γ is necessary for stimulation of phospholipase D by platelet-derived growth factor. *J. Biol. Chem.* 269: 27823–27826, 1994.

386a. Yu, H., X. Li, G. S. Marchetto, R. Dy, D. Hunter, B. Calvo, T. L. Dawson, M. Wilm, R. J. Anderegg, L. M. Graves, and H. S. Earp. Activation of a novel calcium-dependent protein-tyrosine kinase. Correlation with c-Jun N-terminal kinase but not mitogen-activated protein kinase activation. *J. Biol. Chem.* 271: 29993–29998, 1996.

387. Zhang, G.-F., W. A. Patton, F.-J. S. Lee, M. Liyanage, J.-S. Han, S. G. Rhee, J. Moss, and M. Vaughan. Different ARF domains are required for the activation of cholera toxin and phospholipase D. *J. Biol. Chem.* 270: 21–24, 1995.

388. Zhang, H., N. E. Buckley, K. Gibson, and S. Spiegel. Sphingosine stimulates cellular proliferation via a protein kinase C–independent pathway. *J. Biol. Chem.* 265: 76–81, 1990.

389. Zhang, H., N. N. Desai, J. M. Murphey, and S. Spiegel. Increases in phosphatidic acid levels accompany sphingosine-stimulated proliferation of quiescent Swiss 3T3 cells. *J. Biol. Chem.* 265: 21309–21316, 1990.

390. Zhang, H., N. N. Desai, A. Olivera, T. Seki, G. Brooker, and S. Spiegel. Sphingosine-1–phosphate, a novel lipid, involved in cellular proliferation. *J. Cell. Biol.* 114: 155–167, 1991.

391. Zhang, J., W. G. King, S. Dillon, A. Hall, L. Feig, and S. E. Rittenhouse. Activation of platelet phosphatidylinositide 3-kinase requires the small GTP-binding protein Rho. *J. Biol. Chem.* 268: 22251–22254, 1993.

392. Zhang, J., J. Zhang, J. L. Benovic, M. Sugai, R. Wetzker, I. Gout, and S. E. Rittenhouse. Sequestration of a G-protein $\beta\gamma$ subunit or ADP-ribosylation of Rho can inhibit thrombin-induced activation of platelet phosphoinositide 3-kinases. *J. Biol. Chem.* 270: 6589–6594, 1995.

393. Zhang, S., J. Han, M. A. Sells, J. Chernoff, U. G. Knaus, R. J. Ulevitch, and G. M. Bokoch. Rho family GTPases regulate p38 mitogen-activated protein kinase through the downstream mediator Pak1. *J. Biol. Chem.* 270: 23934–23936, 1995.

394. Zhang, Y., and R. Kolesnick. Signaling through the sphingomyelin pathway. *Endocrinology* 136: 4157–4160, 1995.

395. Zhao, Z., S.-H. Shen, and E. H. Fischer. Stimulation by phospholipids of a protein-tyrosine-phosphatase containing two *src* homology 2 domains. *Proc. Natl. Acad. Sci. U.S.A.* 90: 4251–4255, 1993.

396. Zheng, Y., S. Bagrodia, and R. A. Cerione. Activation of phosphoinositide 3-kinase activity by Cdc42Hs binding to p85. *J. Biol. Chem.* 269: 18727–18730, 1994.

397. Zubiaur, M., J. Sancho, C. Terhorst, and D. V. Faller. A small GTP-binding protein, Rho, associates with the platelet-derived growth factor type-β receptor upon ligand binding. *J. Biol. Chem.* 270: 17221–17228, 1995.

12. Membrane receptor–linked disease states

V. NEBES
J. WALL | *The Thyroid Eye Disease Research Laboratory, Department of Ophthalmology, Allegheny General Hospital, Pittsburgh, Pennsylvania*

DISORDERS OF ENDOCRINE RECEPTORS and of their effector molecules are associated with clearly defined disease states. We focus in this chapter on *(1)* genetic disorders of receptors, *(2)* guanosine triphosphate disorders of the (GTP)-binding proteins (G proteins) that are closely linked with receptor activation, and *(3)* disorders in which the receptor is the target of autoantibodies, whether or not other features of an autoimmune reaction are present.

GENETIC DISORDERS OF RECEPTOR AND EFFECTOR MOLECULES

Types of Receptor

There are three main families of endocrine receptors, defined according to the number of transmembrane segments of the molecule and their signal-transduction system(s). The seven transmembrane receptors are the most common and include luteinizing hormone (LH), follicle-stimulating hormone (FSH), thyroid-stimulating hormone (TSH), somatostatin, and vasopressin receptors. These receptors are closely linked to the G proteins, which modulate their interaction with effector molecules, and can be subdivided into three classes: rhodopsin-like receptors, glucagon and calcitonin receptors, and glutamate metabotrophic receptors. Among disorders of the seven transmembrane receptors are both genetic and acquired abnormalities, including some of the most common clinical syndromes such as Graves' disease, precocious puberty, retinitis pigmentosa, and nephrogenic diabetes insipidus. A much less common receptor is the four-transmembrane-segment receptor, or ligand-gated ion channel family, which includes gamma-aminobutyric acid (GABA), glycine, 5-hydroxytryptamine, adenosine triphosphate (ATP), and acetylcholine (Ach) receptors. This latter group may be activated extracellularly or intracellularly. Genetic disorders of these receptors are uncommon, though antibodies against the Ach receptor are associated with a classical and fairly common organ-specific autoimmune disorder. The third type of receptor has a single-transmembrane segment and includes receptors for growth hormone and other peptide hormones, insulin, cytokines, and growth factors. More than 50 members of this family have been identified. These receptors have a large extracellular domain and show similarities with the immunoglobulin G (IgG) molecule. They also can be divided into several families: the protein tyrosine kinase, guanylate cyclase, serine/threonine kinase, multisubunit, tumor necrosis factor (TNF), nerve growth factor (NGF), phosphotyrosine phosphate, and plasma protein receptor families. Abnormalities of these receptors are associated with relatively common and well-defined clinical syndromes (reviewed in ref. 66).

Clinical Disorders

Receptor disorders may be classified as sporadic (tumors, adenomas, multinodular goiters), genetic, or autoimmune (Graves' disease, myasthenia gravis, and some cases of hypothyroidism, insulin resistance, and asthma). While some are common, such as Graves' disease, which affects about 1% of the adult population, and others fairly common, most are quite rare. Receptor abnormalities and the resulting buildup of hormone and resistance to hormonal action were predicted following the revolution in molecular biology and were identified from their often profound clinical effects. Clinical disorders result from mutations of the receptor or effector molecules, abnormal receptor regu-

lation, antibodies to receptors, receptor-specific cross-over disease, and receptor oncogenes. These disorders affect the three main signal-transduction pathways: G protein–coupled, non-G protein–coupled, and tyrosine kinase or protein kinase ligand–gated ion channels. Mixed polygenic/sporadic disorders are much less common. There is overlap since disorders of receptors may be (1) endocrine or nonendocrine, (2) sporadic or congenital, and (3) G protein–linked or not. Most disorders of hormone receptors lead to hormone resistance and deficiency (rather than excess), though one of the most common, Graves' disease, is caused by the stimulating action of an antibody reactive with the TSH receptor.

G Proteins

The G proteins are a subfamily of the GTP–binding protein superfamily, comprising the G proteins, which are the most common; *ras* (a GTPase) and *ras*-like proteins (oncogenes); and various elongation and initiation factors of ribosomal protein synthesis. These latter proteins are less well defined. More than 16 G proteins have been identified. Their function is to transduce information across the cell membrane by coupling various and diverse receptors to their effector proteins. The "on" and "off" states are regulated by factors such as hormones, neurotransmitters, and sensory stimuli, acting as exchange factors which allow guanosine diphosphate (GDP) to be released and GTP to be bound. The G proteins, which bind tightly to the cytoplasmic surface of plasma membranes, are associated with seven transmembrane domain receptors but not with the other two families of receptors. Agonist binding to these receptors leads to a conformational change in intracellular loops that promotes binding to a G protein. A living cell contains a variety of receptors, G proteins, and effector proteins. Receptor–effector coupling by G proteins is not usually totally specific or promiscuous; that is, G proteins bind to many receptors in the same cell (reviewed in ref. 204).

G Protein Alterations in Disease States. There are many different ways in which the G proteins may be abnormal, including (1) mutations in genes encoding G protein subunits, Albright hereditary osteodystrophy (AHO), McCune-Albright syndrome, some somatotroph adenomas, thyroid tumors, and adrenal cortical and ovarian tumors; (2) changes in expression of G protein subunit mRNA and/or function and some cases of non-insulin-dependent diabetes mellitus (NIDDM), dilated cardiomyopathy, and alcoholism; (3) posttranslational modifications of G proteins by the bacterial exotoxins *Vibrio cholerae* (CTX) and *Bordetella per-*

tussis (PTX) on intestinal epithelial cells and islet cells; and *(4)* some other, less well-defined abnormalities of the effector proteins. In this chapter, we discuss several of these disorders, focusing on those most representative of a certain abnormality or associated with classical endocrine syndromes.

Immunodeficiency. Pertussis toxin–sensitive G proteins play a critical role in transducing signals in polymorphonuclear neutrophils and lymphocytes, and defects in migration and activation of these cells have been identified in human disease. As a result, PTX infection may cause severe lymphocytosis. In addition, PTX blocks the normal trafficking of T lymphocytes from the thymus in a transgenic mouse model. Although few disorders of the immune system involving receptors or proteins linked with receptor activation have been recognized, it seems likely that this will be a subject of great interest in the future.

Receptors and Oncogenes

There are many genes whose products are involved in the regulation of normal cell growth. Oncogenes, of which there are more than 50, are capable of transforming prototypes. Protooncogenes, defined as the normal cellular counterparts of the oncogenes, play a role in normal growth control and differentiation and encode important components of the receptor signal-transduction pathway. These include membrane-associated GTP-binding proteins, receptors with tyrosine kinase activity, and nuclear proteins, some of which may have transcriptional activity. The relationship between protooncogenes and receptor diseases is discussed in this chapter, focusing on those protooncogenes which serve as receptors, such as the epidermal growth factor (EGF) receptor.

Antibodies Against Receptors and Autoimmune Disorders

Some fairly common disorders are associated with antibodies to hormone or other receptors. In some cases, these antibodies play a role in the development of clinical syndromes, while in others they are secondary to some other process but may be useful diagnostic markers. The best model of a receptor antibody–induced disease is Graves' hyperthyroidism, in which anti-TSH receptor antibodies are almost certainly directly responsible for thyroid cell hyperactivity and the clinical features of thyrotoxicosis. Another classical disorder caused by receptor antibodies is myasthenia gravis, in which antibodies against the Ach receptor cause chronic muscle weakness and fatigability. In some

other cases, the role of the antibodies, such as those reactive with the β-adrenergic receptor, is unclear. While it is possible to produce experimental polyclonal or monoclonal antibodies against other receptors, no corresponding clinical syndromes have been recognized and the significance of these antibodies is unclear. The role of receptor antibodies in the pathogenesis of human autoimmune disorders is discussed in detail in this chapter.

SEVEN-TRANSMEMBRANE-RECEPTOR/G PROTEIN–COUPLED DISORDERS

The largest family of hormone membrane receptors is comprised of the seven-transmembrane-segment receptors that bind heterotrimeric G proteins. More than 100 members of this family, which includes receptors for numerous hormones, neurotransmitters, and paracrine substances, as well as light, gustatory, and olfactory signals, have been identified. These receptors are composed of an extracellular amino-terminal domain of varying length, seven hydrophobic transmembrane domains connected by three extracellular and three intracellular hydrophilic loops, and a cytoplasmic C-terminal domain that contains potential phosphorylation sites involved in regulation of receptor activity. For small ligands, the transmembrane helices are involved in binding, whereas for larger ligands, such as the glycoprotein hormones, the N-terminal domain also may be important for binding. The intracellular parts of these receptors form a G protein–coupling site. The receptors remain in inactive conformations until ligand binds, thereby changing the receptor conformation to an active form that can bind heterotrimeric G proteins (reviewed in ref. 66).

Thyroid-Stimulating Hormone Receptor/Toxic Thyroid Hyperplasia/Thyroid-Stimulating Hormone Resistance

Most G protein–coupled receptors contain a short N-terminal extracellular domain. In contrast, the thyrotropin, or TSH, receptor has a large glycosylated extracellular domain (398 amino acids), which is involved in hormone binding. Receptors for TSH, LH, and FSH form a subgroup of glycoprotein hormone receptors within the family of GTP-binding, protein-coupled receptors due to their similar large glycosylated extracellular domains. Binding of TSH to the receptor activates adenyl cyclase via the stimulating heterotrimeric G protein $G\alpha_s$. At high concentrations of TSH, the phospholipase C/diacylglycerol/inositol phosphate pathway is activated (70). The TSH receptor gene, which has ten exons, has been mapped to chromosome 14q31

(128, 183). The TSH receptor cDNA encodes a 764-amino-acid sequence (127, 152). Structure–function relationships of the TSH receptor have been reviewed (153).

Toxic Thyroid Hyperplasia.

The molecular structure of the TSH receptor is well known and will be discussed in more detail later in this chapter. Toxic thyroid hyperplasia (TTH) is a rare autosomal dominant disorder caused by germ-line mutations that encode constitutively activated TSH receptor (49). Patients are clinically and biologically hyperthyroid and have a goiter but no features of autoimmunity or extrathyroidal signs of Graves' disease such as ophthalmopathy or dermopathy. Both of the TSH receptor gene mutations linked to TTH occur in exon 10, which encodes the seven transmembrane domains and the cytoplasmic tail region. V509A alters a codon expressed in the third and C672Y alters a codon expressed in the seventh transmembrane domain. In vitro expression studies show that both mutations constitutively activate adenyl cyclase (49). In addition, point mutations are found in about 50% of toxic adenomas. This leads to activation of adenyl cyclase (via G_s), increased cyclic adenosine monophosphate cyclic adenosine monophosphate (cAMP) production, and clonal expansion of the mutated cell and adenoma, which manifests clinically as a thyroid nodule (5) and, in some cases, hyperthyroidism (36). While the most common abnormality is a single-amino-acid change in the third intracellular loop, large insertions and deletions also have been described. Some cases of simple goiter or nodule are associated with genetic abnormalities, although their significance has not been determined.

Resistance to Thyroid-Stimulating Hormone.

Resistance to TSH has been reported to be an autosomal recessive condition linked to mutations in the TSH receptor (206). Patients were euthyroid and had normal serum concentrations of thyroid hormone but high concentrations of TSH. The TSH receptor nucleotide sequence has been analyzed in three patients with congenital primary hypothyroidism associated with TSH unresponsiveness (208) and found to be the same as the normal TSH receptor sequence in two patients, while a heterozygous polymorphism in codon 601 was found in one patient, indicating absence of structural abnormalities (208). Mutations were found in exon 6, which encodes part of the extracellular domain. In vitro studies showed that receptors encoded with the P162A mutation did not stimulate adenyl cyclase in response to hormone, whereas cells with the I167N mutation required 20-fold higher levels of TSH for maximal stimulation of cAMP (206).

Luteinizing Hormone Receptor/Precocious Puberty/ Leydig Cell Hypoplasia

The lutropin, or luteinizing hormone receptor is a single polypeptide of 674 amino acids with a predicted molecular mass of 75 ka and an apparent mass of 93 kd due to posttranslational modifications, primarily glycosylation. The extracellular domain has 14 copies of an imperfectly repeated leucine-rich sequence of about 25 amino acids, similar to that found in a family of leucine-rich glycoproteins. This diverse family of leucine-rich glycoproteins includes a collagen-binding proteoglycan, PG40, the alpha-2 serum glycoprotein, the *Drosophila* Toll gene product, the yeast adenylyl cyclase, the α-chain of human platelet protein 1b, and the acid-labile subunit of the insulin-like growth factor (IGF)–binding protein complex. The extracellular domain of the LH receptor binds to LH with similar affinity as the full-length receptor when expressed in COS cells (reviewed in ref. 194). The transmembrane domain is very similar in sequence to other members of the seven-transmembrane superfamily of receptors. The cDNA for the human LH receptor was identified and characterized in 1990 (145). The LH receptor gene has been localized to the short arm of human chromosome 2 (2p21) (146a).

Familial Male-Limited Precocious Puberty.

The syndrome of familial male-limited precocious puberty (FMPP), also called testotoxicosis, has been linked to LH receptor gene mutations (reviewed in refs. 63, 196). Mutant receptors stimulate cAMP production in the absence of hormone, inducing primary hyperplasia of Leydig cells and excess testicular androgen production. Signs of puberty usually appear by 2–3 years of age, followed by rapid virilization and advanced skeletal maturation. The mode of inheritance is autosomal dominant or sporadic. The syndrome is diagnosed from the history, evidence of pubertal development on physical examination, pubertal levels of serum testosterone (greater than 20 nmol/l, normal prepubertal levels being less than 0.1 nmol/l), prepubertal gonadotropin values, and a negative response to the gonadotropin-releasing hormone (GnRH) stimulation test. It also may be associated with pseudohypoparathyroidism.

Mutations in the Luteinizing Hormone Receptor Gene.

Mutations in the LH receptor gene that co-segregate with FMPP have been identified in regions that encode the second (M398T), fifth (1542L), and sixth transmembrane segments (M5711, T577I, D578G, and C581R) and in the third extracellular domain (A568V, D564G) (112, 114, 117, 199, 238). A heterozygous autosomal dominant mutation encoding substitution of Asp578 with gly in transmembrane helix 6 of the LH receptor was found in nine American FMPP families by Kosugi et al. (112). In vitro expression of these mutants in COS cells revealed constitutively activated receptors, manifested as increased basal cAMP production, whereas basal inositol phosphate production and hormone-binding affinity were comparable to those of the wild-type receptor (94). This result is clinically significant since the D578G mutation occurs in 78% of patients with FMPP (123). The location of the amino-acid substitutions near the third intracellular loop is similar to those found in some mutant α1B-adrenergic receptors, which release receptors from inactive conformation. Mutations in a region of the LH receptor gene that encode the second transmembrane segment also cause constitutive elevation of cAMP, but hormone-induced cAMP production was low (198). The A568V mutation also was shown to cause constitutive activation of the receptor in COS cells, yielding fourfold increases in intracellular cAMP levels. The mutation did not alter ligand binding. Mutations of the homologous alanine residue in the α1-adrenergic, FSH, and TSH receptors also resulted in constitutive adenyl cyclase activation, suggesting that this alanine residue is crucial for signal transduction and a potential site for oncogenic mutations in G protein-coupled receptors (122). All except one of the constitutively activating mutations in the LH receptor characterized to date encode changes in the region 542–581. This region encodes part of the fifth transmembrane segment, the third cytoplasmic loop, and the sixth transmembrane segment encoded by a 120 bp region of exon 11, which may contain hot spots for receptor activation (122). In sum, these studies strongly suggest that autonomous Leydig cell activity in FMPP is caused by a constitutively activated LH receptor.

Differences in phenotypes seen among patients with FMPP may be correlated with differences in the constitutive activation of various mutant LH receptors. For example, the D578Y mutation was identified in a patient who presented with signs of pubertal development at 1 year of age. When this mutant LH receptor gene was expressed in vitro, transfected cells showed higher basal levels of cAMP than cells transfected with normal and various other mutant LH-r genes (123).

Male Pseudohermaphroditism due to Leydig Cell Hypoplasia.
At the other end of the spectrum, mutations that inactivate the LH receptor have been linked to male pseudohermaphroditism due to Leydig cell hypoplasia (116). This is a rare autosomal recessive condition, first described by Berthezene et al. (17), associated with interference of normal development of male external genitalia in 46,XY individuals. The clinical spectrum ranges from extreme forms, where patients present as 46,XY females, to milder forms, in which males present with hypergonadotropic hypogonadism and a micropenis (213, 214). Most patients have female external genitalia, primary amenorrhea, lack of breast development, a short blind-ending vagina, and no uterus or fallopian tubes. Serum levels of testosterone and testosterone precursors are abnormally low and do not respond to human chorionic gonadotropin (hCG) stimulation. Basal levels of LH are markedly increased, but FSH is within the normal range (141).

Mutations that Inactivate the Luteinizing Hormone (LH) Receptor.
Mutations that inactivate the LH receptor have been identified as homozygous missense mutations in the sixth transmembrane domain (Ala593Pro) and nonsense mutations in exon 11 (A1635C), which introduces a stop codon at residue 545 in the fifth transmembrane helix (116, 124). In vitro studies show that the receptor with an A593P mutation in the sixth transmembrane domain binds hCG with a normal K_D, whereas ligand binding does not result in increased cAMP production. In vitro studies show that surface expression of the truncated receptor, caused by the stop codon at residue 545, is reduced compared to that of the wild-type receptor. In addition, stimulation of cAMP production by hCG was impaired in cells transfected with the mutant receptor.

Adrenocorticotropic Hormone Receptor/Familial Glucocorticoid Deficiency

Mountyjoy et al. (151) reported the sequence of the human adrenocorticotropic hormone (ACTH) receptor cDNA in 1992. The cDNA encodes a 297-amino-acid protein that is most closely related to a small family of melanotropic receptors. Members of this family are among the smallest G protein–coupled receptors so far identified; they have a short amino-terminal extracellular domain, a short C-terminal intracellular domain, unusually short fourth and fifth transmembrane-spanning domains, and a small second extracellular loop. The receptor locus has been mapped to between markers D18S53 and D18S66 on the short arm of chromosome 18 (reviewed in ref. 45).

Familial Glucocorticoid Deficiency.
Familial glucocorticoid deficiency (FGD), also known as unresponsiveness to ACTH, was first described by Shepard et al. (200). Patients have hypocortisolism with preserved mineralocorticoid production. The condition is characterized by hypoglycemic episodes, convulsions, progressive hyperpigmentation, weakness, emaciation, hypotension, gastrointestinal symptoms, failure to thrive, and excessively frequent and severe infections in early childhood.

Among 50 published cases, 18 patients died within the first 2 years of life (228). Biochemical findings in untreated patients include elevated endogenous plasma ACTH levels, low or undetectable basal levels of serum cortisol, which are subnormally responsive to exogenous ACTH, and an abnormal response to corticotrophin-releasing hormone (CRH). Plasma renin and aldosterone levels are normal, in striking contrast to classical Addison's disease, where levels are usually very low or undetectable. While presentation is typically in the first year of life, the disorder may appear in later life. Features of hypoadrenalism are always accompanied by deep pigmentation of the skin as a result of the unopposed action of ACTH on cutaneous melanocyte-stimulating hormone (MSH) receptors. Pathological examination of the adrenal glands removed postmortem from patients with FGD reveals atrophy of the zonae fasciculata and reticularis, with preservation of the zona glomerulosa and a normal medulla. These findings have led to proposals that developmental defects of the adrenals, abnormalities of the ACTH receptor, or intracellular signaling defects downstream of the receptor are responsible (228).

Adrenocorticotropic hormone receptor gene mutations. Familial glucocorticoid deficiency is usually inherited in an autosomal recessive pattern. Several point mutations in the ACTH receptor gene have been linked to FGD. One mutation occurs in the sequence coding for the second transmembrane domain, S74I, in a codon that is not conserved among other GTP-binding protein–linked receptors, although this residue seems to be present in all members of the melanotrophic receptor family. The effect of this mutation on receptor function is to increase the concentration of ACTH required for cAMP response (EC_{50} for the normal receptor is 5.5×10^{-9} vs. 67×10^{-9} for the S74I mutant form) (228, 229). This mutation has been shown to segregate with FGD in several patients, four of whom were homozygous for S741 from two different families and one of whom had a compound heterozygote for S741/R128C. Other FGD patients with ACTH receptor gene mutations that have been characterized were homozygous for Y254C or heterozygous for the I44M/L192 frameshift (229). Parents and family members of patients with FGD who were carriers of one of the mutant alleles did not show subclinical ACTH resistance by CRH testing, suggesting that this is not likely to be of value in identifying carriers (229).

Mutations within the coding regions of the ACTH receptor are not found in all cases of FGD (86, 207, 227, 237). Weber and Clark (227) used a highly polymorphic repeat marker (D18S40) that is closely linked to the ACTH receptor locus to confirm that some cases of FGD result from defects at another locus. This disorder provides an example of a single, relatively homogeneous, clinical syndrome resulting from two different molecular etiologies. The second molecular defect has not been clearly identified.

Arginine Vasopressin/Nephrogenic Diabetes Insipidus

Receptors for antidiuretic hormone (ADH) and the related arginine vasopressin (AVP) are structurally different and located in different organs. Both belong to the seven-transmembrane family of receptors. The antidiuretic effect of AVP is mediated by renal-type (V2) receptors linked to adenylyl cyclase, whereas the V1a receptor for vasopressin is expressed in the liver. The cDNA for the AVP (V2) receptor has been cloned and characterized (19). A 371-amino-acid protein having seven transmembrane segments is predicted to be encoded by the cDNA. The gene for the V2 receptor (AVPR2) has been mapped to Xq28 and contains three exons and two small introns (19, 131, 195).

Diabetes Insipidus. The distinction between diabetes mellitus and diabetes insipidus in patients with polyuria is the glucose content of the urine (138). There are three major defects which cause diabetes insipidus: deficient secretion of AVP (the neurogenic or hypothalamic form), resistance to AVP (insipidus), and excessive water intake, which suppresses AVP (primary polydipsia). (For a review of the clinical spectrum of diabetes insipidus, see ref. 88.) Familial forms account for less than 10% of cases of diabetes insipidus. Diabetes insipidus may be inherited in an autosomal dominant or an autosomal recessive manner in addition to the X-linked mode of inheritance described above. Mutations in the AVP precursor/neurophysin II gene have been linked to the autosomal dominant form (12, 96, 97, 118, 137, 240). Homozygous mutations in the aquaporin-2 gene, which encodes a water channel of the renal collecting duct (218), have been linked to the autosomal recessive form (43, 219).

Nephrogenic Diabetes Insipidus. Loss of function mutations in the vasopressin (V2) receptor gene cause the rare X-linked congenital disorder called nephrogenic diabetes insipidus (NDI). This disease is characterized by the inability of the kidney to concentrate urine. The renal collecting duct is unresponsive to AVP; thus, urine is consistently hypotonic to plasma. Affected individuals suffer from episodes of severe dehydration and hypernatremia. Polyuria is strongly associated with dilation of the urinary tract in NDI patients (217). Symptoms of dehydration occur soon after birth in affected male infants and, if untreated, can cause physical and mental retardation (reviewed in ref. 88).

V2 Receptor Gene Mutations. Over 30 V2 receptor gene mutations have been reported in 37 families, without any significant differences in the phenotypic expression of the disease (18). Most of the mutations identified to date are point mutations and include 13 missense mutations, six nonsense mutations, one in-frame deletion, five deletions, and two insertions causing a frameshift and premature stop codon. In one study, more than half (58%) of the nucleotide substitutions in 26 families seemed to be a consequence of 5-methylcytosine deamination at a CpG dinucleotide, while most of the small deletions and insertions could be attributed to slipped mispairing during DNA replication (18). Three large deletions or gene rearrangements, all different, also have been partially characterized (19). Several of these mutations have been expressed in vitro and the receptor defects analyzed biochemically. A missense mutation in the third extracellular domain (R202C) reduced both binding affinity (15% of normal) and capacity (30% of normal) (215). In biosynthesis and localization studies, it was found that receptors expressing this mutation reach the cell surface (216). A frameshift mutation causing termination at codon 258 (a G insertion at nucleotide 804), removing one-third of the carboxyl terminus of the receptor, also has been characterized. No receptor protein could be detected when this mutant receptor cDNA was expressed in vitro, indicating that it was not effectively translated or that it was rapidly degraded. Receptors with R143P and δV278 mutations were expressed intracellularly but were not localized on the cell surface. Receptors with the R113W change in the first extracellular loop of the V2 receptor next to a frequently conserved cysteine are thought to interact via a disulfide bridge with a cysteine of the second extracellular loop. In vitro studies of receptors expressing the R113W mutation showed that the mutant had a 20-fold reduced affinity for AVP. Two females heterozygous for an AVPR2 mutation had clinical features resembling the phenotype in males. Skewed X-inactivation is the most likely explanation for the disease in female carriers (220).

Rhodopsin/Retinitis Pigmentosa

Mutations in rhodopsin cause an autosomal dominant form of retinitis pigmentosa, a clinically and genetically diverse group of inherited retinopathies characterized by loss of night and peripheral vision followed by progressive degeneration of the retina, sometimes resulting in tunnel vision or complete loss of sight. It is inherited at a frequency of one in 3000 and has been estimated to affect 1.5 million people worldwide (28, 29, 112).

Rhodopsin is the photoreceptor in rod cells which mediates vision in dim light. Rhodopsin is formed when opsin, a 348-amino-acid proenzyme, binds 11-*cis* retinal at lysine 296. Rhodopsin excites the visual system when light induces photoisomerization of the 11-*cis* form of retinal to the all-trans form. Upon photoactivation rhodopsin becomes phosphorylated and undergoes a conformational change which activates transducin, a G protein, which in turn activates a cyclic guanosine monophosphate (cGMP) phosphodiesterase. The resulting decline in free intracellular cGMP closes cGMP-activated channels, leading to membrane hyperpolarization (reviewed in ref. 158). The cDNA sequence was determined and the gene mapped to the long arm of chromosome 3 by Nathans and Hogness (160). Bovine rhodopsin was the first G protein–coupled receptor to be cloned and sequenced (84, 159, 169).

The mechanism by which defects in rhodopsin cause retinitis pigmentosa is unknown. No disease is seen in heterozygote carriers with one null allele. Presumably one normal allele and 50% of the normal amount of rhodopsin is enough to support normal vision and to prevent retinal deterioration. Most of the mutations linked to retinitis pigmentosa and characterized in vitro make mutant receptors in less than the normal amount, and much of the mutant protein is retained in the endoplasmic reticulum, perhaps due to improper folding of the receptor. Mutant receptors also do not regenerate normally with 11-*cis* retinal. Rhodopsin constitutes approximately 80% of the protein in the membrane of photoreceptor disks. Accumulation of rhodopsin in the endoplasmic reticulum or destabilization of the membrane by aberrant receptors may initiate the deterioration of rod cells which make up the photoreceptor disks. The death of rod cells appears to precipitate more extensive tissue damage, causing cone cells to die off, though rhodopsin is not expressed in these cells. As photoreceptor cells die, the retinal epithelium becomes thin and accumulates pigment on its surface. This abnormal pigmentation is the sign for which the disease is named (reviewed in ref. 95).

Rhodopsin Gene Mutations. Over 50 mutations in the rhodopsin gene have been linked to retinitis pigmentosa since the cDNA was cloned and characterized in 1984 (160). The overwhelming number of these are point mutations that alter the receptor but do not lead to null alleles. Mutations that alter residues in the transmembrane domain or in either of two cysteine residues that form a disulfide bond result in severe disease. Milder forms of the disease are associated with mutations that alter amino acids in the C-terminal tail region. In general, mutations in the rhodopsin gene cause two types of disease: a form with diffuse pigmentary changes accompanied by severe loss of rod and cone function and a nonprogressive sectorial type with normal rod and cone function but detectable pigment changes in the inferonasal and inferior retina. (For comprehensive clinical reviews, see refs. 85, 170; for a review of rhodopsin mutations linked to retinitis pigmentosa, see ref. 197.)

Other Mechanisms for Inheritance of Retinitis Pigmentosa. Retinitis pigmentosa can be inherited in an autosomal dominant, an autosomal recessive, or in an X-linked manner. The relative proportions of cases associated with the three different types of transmission have been estimated (85); autosomal recessive or sporadic cases account for more than half, and X-linked and autosomal dominant cases account for 10%–15% each. Two types of X-linked disease have been linked to the short arm of the X chromosome, and three types of autosomal dominant disease have been mapped. One form of autosomal dominant disease maps to the pericentric region of chromosome 8. Disease genes for the other two mapped autosomal dominant loci have been identified as the rhodopsin gene, mapped to the short arm of chromosome 3, and the perpherin gene, mapped to the short arm of chromosome 6 (48, 60, 101). Linkage to these two genes accounts for about 30% of autosomal dominant cases. Autosomal dominant forms of retinitis pigmentosa tend to be less severe than other forms but are highly variable. Humphries (94) reported a three-base-pair deletion in the peripherin-RDS gene in one form of retinitis pigmentosa.

Retinitis pigmentosa is incurable and unpreventable. Characterization of other genes would be helpful in determining the cause of the retinal pathology. Genetic tests to characterize mutations for predicting disease outcome would be invaluable since retinitis pigmentosa is so heterogeneous, ranging from the mildest form, which affects only part of the retina and is nonprogressive, to severe forms that cause debilitating visual handicaps by the second decade.

Parathyroid Hormone/Parathyroid Hormone–Related Peptide Receptor/Jansen-Type Metaphyseal Chondrodysplasia

The parathyroid hormone (PTH)/parathyroid hormone–related peptide (PTHrP) receptor belongs to a family of G protein–coupled receptors. Members of this subfamily include calcitonin, secretin, growth hormone–releasing hormone (GHRH), glucagon, CRH, and the pituitary adenyl cyclase–activating peptide.

These receptors bind peptides that are 27–46 amino acids in length. In addition to the classical seven transmembrane-spanning domains, members of this family share an identical 48-amino-acid region which includes eight extracellular cysteines plus at least two conserved N-linked glycosylation sites (107). The PTH/PTHrP receptor is expressed in a variety of fetal and adult tissues, predominantly bone and kidney, and activates both the adenyl cyclase and phospholipase C second-messenger systems (reviewed in ref. 98). The PTH/PTHrP receptor was cloned and a cDNA expressed by Adams et al. (2) in 1995. The same workers have carried out photoaffinity labeling of the receptor as the first step in directly identifying the amino-acid residues that constitute the binding sites for PTH and PTHrP (2). The gene has been mapped to the short arm of human chromosome 3 in the 3p21.1–p24.2 region (69). The cDNA was cloned and a functional receptor expressed by this group. Mutational analysis of PTH/PTHrP receptors with five different C-terminal truncations revealed that only when the complete tail region (127 amino acids) was deleted was proper targeting to the cell surface and response to cAMP abolished. Ligand binding was unaffected by any of the C-terminal deletions (92).

Gene Mutations. A constitutively active mutant of the PTH/PTHrP receptor was identified in a patient with a rare type of short-limbed dwarfism, called Jansen-type metaphyseal chondrodysplasia (JMC) (190). This disease is associated with asymptomatic but often profound hypercalcemia and hypophosphatemia, despite a lack of parathyroid gland abnormalities and the presence of normal amounts of PTH and PTHrP. The phenotype is similar to that seen in diseases in which PTH and PTHrP are overproduced, such as primary hyperparathyroidism and the syndrome of hypercalcemia of malignancy. A heterozygous mutation (H223R) was identified in a JCM patient which would alter amino acid 223, a residue found at the junction between the first intracellular loop and the second membrane-spanning helix. Both unaffected parents were homozygous for the normal allele. This finding, along with evidence of abnormalities in many tissues, suggests that the patient inherited a germ-line mutation or developed a somatic mutation early in life. Receptors carrying the H223R mutation were tested in vitro and found to have ligand-independent constitutive accumulation of cAMP but failed to accumulate inositol phosphate in the presence or absence of ligand.

Mutations that inactivate the PTH/PTHrP receptor have been sought as the cause of pseudohypoparathyroidism type Ib. However, none was identified in samples from 17 patients with the disease (190). Mutations that completely inactivate the PTH/PTHrP receptor may be lethal in utero, as is the case for transgenic mice that lack the PTH/PTHrP receptor (65).

β3-Adrenergic Receptor/Obesity

A specific mutation in the β3-adrenergic receptor is a candidate for a genetic alteration leading to obesity. This missense mutation in codon 64 (W64R) was associated with early onset of NIDDM in obese Pima Indians. This group also had a tendency for low metabolic rates. In a Finnish population, the mutation also was associated with early onset of NIDDM and clinical features of the insulin resistance syndrome—high serum concentrations of insulin, glucose, and lipids—and hypertension. In French subjects, the mutation was associated with an increased capacity to gain weight in the morbidly obese. Although these studies suggest that the adrenergic system is important for the development of insulin resistance and other metabolic complications of obesity, there is no evidence that the mutation is more frequent among obese than normal subjects. Moreover, differences in receptor expression between mutated and normal genes were small and sometimes of only borderline statistical significance (reviewed in ref. 10).

Growth Hormone–Releasing Hormone Receptor

The GHRH receptor is a member of the G protein–coupled receptor family that is expressed on pituitary somatotroph cells and mediates actions of GHRH in stimulating growth hormone synthesis and secretion. Acromegaly is caused by a pituitary adenoma secreting growth hormone, which arises following a somatic mutation within the somatotroph. Promotion of tumor growth also appears to be regulated by GHRH, which exerts a trophic action on the pituitary cell (reviewed in ref. 143). While a mutation of the GHRH receptor gene is another possible cause of pituitary acromegaly, such a defect has not been associated with growth hormone excess. There are, however, some genetic defects in GHRH receptor function in experimental animals which lead to dwarfism—namely, the little (lit) mouse, in which homozygosity for a missense mutation leads to reduced growth hormone secretion and dwarfism phenotype, and a rat model (dw rat), where the defect is reduced GHRH signal transduction, which is independent of a generalized defect in the stimulatory G protein $G\alpha_s$ (105). In humans, a nonsense mutation in the GHRH receptor which causes growth failure analogous to the little mouse model has been identified (223).

Somatostatin Receptor

The diverse biological effects of somatostatin (SST) are mediated through a family of G protein–coupled receptors, of which five members (SSTR 1–5) have been identified by molecular cloning. The receptors are encoded by a family of five genes, which have been mapped to separate chromosomes and which, with one exception, lack introns. Pituitary and islet tumors express several SST receptor genes, suggesting that multiple SST receptor subtypes are co-expressed in the same cell. (For a review of SST receptors, see ref. 173.) To date, no mutations in the SST receptors have been associated with clinical syndromes.

MUTATIONS OF G PROTEINS

Heterotrimeric G proteins are a subfamily within the large superfamily of GTP-binding proteins that includes ras and ras-like proteins, as well as elongation and initiation factors of ribosomal protein synthesis. Although there is substantial diversity within the G protein subfamily, members have common structural and functional features. The α-, β-, and γ-subunits are encoded by separate genes. The apparent molecular weight ranges are 39–52 kd for the α-subunit, 35–36 kd for the β-subunit, and 5–10 kd for the γ-subunit. Ninety percent of the amino-acid sequences of the α-subunit are conserved but vary for different protein species. The α-subunit has structural and functional properties similar to those of the superfamily of GTP-binding proteins.

G proteins transduce information across cell membranes by coupling receptors with effectors. They act as molecular switches, with the active and inactive states governed by GTP/GDP binding and hydrolysis. In the resting state, the three subunits are bound in complexes with GDP. Ligand-activated receptors bind to the α-subunit, causing GDP to be released and replaced by GTP. Binding of GTP releases the β- and γ-subunits as a dimer. Both the β-γ dimer and the α-subunit bound to GTP modulate key signaling enzymes and channels. The cycle ends when GTP hydrolyzes to GDP. The β-γ dimer then reassociates with the GDP-bound α-subunit, reforming the original complex. G proteins can either stimulate (G_s) or inhibit (G_i) the formation of cAMP through adenyl cyclase. They also activate the phospholipase C second-messenger system.

The primary structure of the human $G\alpha_s$ gene has been deduced from characterization of cDNA and genomic clones (24). The gene is 20 kb in length, has 13 exons, and maps to chromosome 20q13 (68).

$G\alpha_s$ Mutations/Albright Hereditary Osteodystrophy

Albright hereditary osteodystrophy (AHO) is a rare autosomal dominant syndrome comprising short stature, obesity, a round face, brachydactyly, subcutaneous calcifications, and mild mental retardation (108). Most patients with AHO have associated pseudohypoparathyroidism type la (PHPla) characterized by normal to elevated serum concentrations of PTH and primary target cells—bone and kidney—which are unable to respond to either endogenous or exogenously administered hormone. Resistance to a number of other hormones that induce intracellular cAMP as second messenger, such as TSH, gonadotrophins, and glucagon, is observed frequently (reviewed in ref. 108). Interestingly, signaling through other G_s pathways, such as vasopressin in the renal medulla or ACTH in the adrenal cortex, is not clinically affected. Patients with PHPla have renal resistance to PTH, hypocalcemia, hyperphosphatemia, and deficient urinary excretion of cAMP following administration of PTH. The remaining patients, who respond normally to exogenous PTH, have so-called pseudopseudohypoparathyroidism (PPHP).

Mutations in the $G\alpha_s$-gene GNAS1 have been identified in patients with AHO and typically are expressed on only one allele, consistent with the dominant pattern of inheritance (reviewed in ref. 41). Mutations associated with AHO are heterogeneous, comprising point mutations or small deletions that result in reduced expression of the $G\alpha_s$ protein (133, 146, 174, 193, 231). Interestingly, a 50% reduction in $G\alpha_s$ activity can be measured in erythrocyte membranes from patients with PHPla or PPHP. Almost all of the defects in the $G\alpha_s$ gene described to date are due to mutations that result in abnormal RNA processing, production of a nonfunctional mRNA, or synthesis of a truncated protein. An exception is a point mutation (R385H); mutant $G\alpha_s$ proteins in which residue 385 was altered (R385H) could stimulate adenyl cyclase directly but were unable to interact with hormone receptors (193).

Molecular heterogeneity of $G\alpha_s$ mutations is not sufficient to explain the phenotypic differences in hormone responsiveness seen in PHPla and PPHP. Within five separate kindreds, either PHPla or PPHP co-segregated with the same $G\alpha_s$ mutation (235). Parental origin of the mutated allele may influence the phenotype since 66 of 66 offspring with PHPla resulted from maternal transmission and six of six cases with PPHP resulted from paternal transmission (41). Data to support this hypothesis have been reported by Wilson et al. (235), who used an intragenic $G\alpha_s$ FokI polymorphism to determine the parental origin of $G\alpha_s$ gene mutations. Their data show that the phenotypic

"switch" is dependent on the sex of the transmitting parent across two generations. They suggest that genomic imprinting may explain the alternative phenotypes.

Liri et al. (130) characterized a $G\alpha_s$ mutation in two unrelated boys who had the paradoxical combination of PHPla-la and testotoxicosis. Receptors with the A366S alteration, when tested in vitro, were shown to constitutively activate adenyl cyclase in a temperature-dependent manner. The A366S mutation results in synthesis of a temperature-sensitive GTPase which is destabilized at normal body temperature, accounting for the PHP-la phenotype resulting from a loss of $G\alpha_s$ activity. The authors show that the mutant GTPase is stable and constitutively active at lower temperatures and speculate that the G protein remains constitutively active at the lower temperature found in the testis. Hormone-independent cAMP accumulation probably accounts for the testotoxicosis phenotype since cAMP stimulates Leydig cell hyperplasia and overproduction of testosterone.

SINGLE-TRANSMEMBRANE-RECEPTOR–COUPLED DISEASES

Insulin Receptor/Leprechaunism/Rabson-Mendenhall Syndrome/Type A Insulin Resistance

Cloning and characterization of the insulin receptor cDNA has provided insight into its structure and function. The receptor has a 27-amino-acid hydrophobic signal peptide and two repeating domains—one at the N-terminus and one in the middle of the α-subunit—which appear to play an important role in ligand binding. The two sets of four repeating sequences resemble sequences found in the EGF receptor family. Amino acids 155–312 contain a cysteine-rich domain which may play a role in ligand-binding specificity. The C-terminal domain of the α-subunit variably includes the 12 amino acids encoded by exon 11 due to alternative splicing. Four basic amino acids, at positions 732–735, likely provide a proteolytic cleavage site which releases the α-subunit from the proreceptor. The β-subunit contains an extracellular domain which is O-glycosylated, a 23-amino-acid transmembrane domain, and an intracellular tyrosine kinase domain. The insulin receptor gene, which has 22 exons, has been mapped to chromosome 19 (p13.2–13.3). The X-ray crystal structure of the insulin receptor tyrosine kinase domain has been determined (93). The insulin receptor is a heterotetramer with two α- and two β-subunits, both of which are encoded by the same gene. The α- and β-subunits are produced by proteolytic cleavage of a single high molecular weight precursor molecule (190 kd). The α-subunit (135 kd) is entirely extracellular and provides the insulin-binding site. The α-subunit (95 kd) has a single transmembrane domain and anchors the α-subunit to the plasma membrane. The β-subunit also contains a tyrosine kinase domain which is activated by ligand binding, stimulating autophosphorylation of tyrosine residues on the β-subunit. Autophosphorylation activates the receptor to phosphorylate other intracellular proteins, which in turn mediate insulin action.

Mutations in the insulin receptor gene have been linked to several distinct clinical syndromes associated with insulin resistance, including leprechaunism, Rabson-Mendenhall syndrome, type A insulin resistance, and non-insulin-dependent diabetes mellitus (NIDDM) (reviewed in ref. 212). The signs and symptoms seen in these disorders reflect a continuum of insulin resistance from extreme, in leprechaunism, to milder, in NIDDM. Two of the disorders, leprechaunism and Rabson-Mendenhall syndrome, are very similar, being distinguished only by how early symptoms are detected and how long patients survive. Leprechaunism is a rare autosomal recessive disease characterized clinically by intrauterine growth retardation, elf-like facial features, reduced amounts of muscle and adipose tissue, acanthosis nigricans, hyperinsulinemia, and extreme insulin resistance. Patients usually die within the first year of life. In Rabson-Mendenhall syndrome, symptoms are not seen until a few weeks after birth and patients generally survive into childhood. Features of this syndrome include extreme insulin resistance, acanthosis nigricans, abnormalities of the teeth and nails, and pineal hyperplasia.

Over 30 mutations in the insulin receptor gene have been reported, and the effects of these mutations on receptor expression can be grouped into five categories: mutations that impair synthesis of insulin receptor mRNA, mutations that impair transport of receptors to the plasma membrane, mutations that alter insulin binding, mutations that decrease tyrosine kinase activity, and mutations that increase receptor degradation (reviewed in refs. 1, 27, 212). Patients with leprechaunism or Rabson-Mendenhall syndrome generally have two mutant alleles of the insulin receptor gene. In some cases, dominant negative mutations have been characterized. Defective receptors may form dimers with wild-type receptor subunits and cause trans-dominant inhibition of insulin receptor function.

Type A insulin resistance has three characteristic features: insulin resistance, acanthosis nigricans, and hyperandrogenism without obesity or lipoatrophy. Several patients with type A insulin resistance have been reported to have one or two mutant insulin receptor alleles. Patients with two mutant alleles appear to be more insulin-resistant than patients with a single null

allele. However, mutations in the domain encoding the tyrosine kinase may cause insulin resistance in a dominant negative manner (147, 212).

Several studies have suggested that a small number of patients with NIDDM have defects in the insulin receptor gene (reviewed in ref. 212). One of the most common endocrine diseases, NIDDM affects 5%–7% of the population. These patients have both insulin deficiency and insulin resistance. Linkage studies in 51 Japanese NIDDM patients found three patients with insulin receptor gene missense mutations (T831A) that were linked with the disease and one missense mutation (T1334C) that did not co-segregate with the disease (102). Several polymorphisms have been identified in the region of the insulin receptor gene that encodes the intracellular portion of the β-subunit, though these variations are not linked to NIDDM (139). It appears that NIDDM is a syndrome comprising multiple diseases with different causes. Mutations in some genes (for example, those encoding the insulin receptor and insulin receptor substrate-1) appear to cause insulin resistance, while mutations in other genes (for example, insulin, glucokinase) impair β-cell function. However, in the majority of cases, the specific defect has not been identified (reviewed in ref. 211).

Growth Hormone Receptor/Laron Dwarfism

The growth hormone receptor is a 620-amino-acid protein which has a single central hydrophobic membrane-spanning domain. Its primary structure has been deduced from the cDNA clone and was the first member of the cytokine superfamily of receptors to be identified (126). Members of the cytokine superfamily include receptors for prolactin, erythropoietin, granulocyte colony-stimulating factor (CSF), granulocyte/macrophage CSF, TNF-α, leukemia-inhibitory factor, oncostatin M, interleukin (IL)-7, and IL-9. In addition to a single membrane-spanning domain, members of this family share significant homology (about 20% in the extracellular domain) and the absence of a consensus sequence for tyrosine kinase activity. Generation of multiple transcripts of the growth hormone and prolactin genes results from alternative splicing and utilization of multiple promoters. The growth hormone receptor gene, which contains nine exons, has been mapped to chromosome 5p13.1–p12 (reviewed in ref. 184). The receptor is widely expressed in human tissues (144). The X-ray crystallographic structures of growth hormone and its receptor reveal that one growth hormone ligand binds to the extracellular domain of two growth hormone receptor molecules, leading to receptor homodimerization (46).

Primary growth hormone insensitivity, known as

Laron dwarfism or growth hormone receptor deficiency, is linked to mutations in the receptor gene. Laron dwarfism is an autosomal recessive condition characterized by severe growth failure, which was first described by Laron et al. in 1966 (121). In addition to being very short, patients are resistant to growth hormone, have elevated serum levels of growth hormone, low serum levels of IGF-1, and little or no growth hormone–binding protein. Growth hormone receptor deficiency has been reported in different ethnic populations, with major concentrations in Asian Jews and descendants of Spanish settlers in southern Ecuador. Berg et al. (16) found 55 Laron dwarfism patients from Ecuador to be homozygous for the E180 splice mutation. A single A to G mutation which does not change the glutamate codon introduces a new 5' splice site, which is used exclusively and leads to an in-frame 24 base pairs deletion from exon 6. Most of the mutations characterized to date have been found in exons 4, 6, and 7 (reviewed in ref. 16). One nonsense mutation has been identified in each of these exons, producing truncated receptor proteins (R43X, E183X, R217X). Two frameshift mutations which also cause premature terminations have been found at positions 46 and 230. In addition to the E180 splice mutation described above, splice site mutations at positions 71 and 189 have been described. Amino-acid substitutions in codons 422, 560, and 561 of the intracellular region of the receptor in a child with Laron dwarfism were described by Kou et al. (113); in this case, the mutations were localized to exon 10 on the same chromosome and were inherited from the patient's mother. A very interesting missense mutation in the extracellular domain (D152H) has been shown to abolish receptor homodimerization, clearly establishing that monomeric receptors are inactive (50).

Mutations in the growth hormone receptor also have been identified in some children with idiopathic short stature who were not growth hormone–deficient but had reduced serum concentrations of growth hormone–binding protein (72). Growth hormone receptor mutations were found in four of 14 children with idiopathic short stature but in none of 24 normal controls. All four of the affected children were partially resistant to growth hormone therapy. The authors speculate that there may be a continuum of growth hormone binding to various mutant forms of the receptor, the more normal the binding, the less severe the phenotype. One of the affected children was a compound heterozygote, with one mutation that reduced binding 330-fold (E44K) and a second mutation in the other allele which may have prevented proper localization to the plasma membrane (R161C). Another child was heterozygous

for the R211H allele, which reduces receptor expression by 10,000-fold, while another was heterozygous for a null allele (C122 stop). The fourth patient was heterozygous for a missense mutation (E224D).

Insulin-Like Growth Factor-1 Receptor

Insulin-like growth factor-1 is involved in normal erythropoiesis, granulopoiesis, and lymphopoiesis and is mitogenic for cell lines of myeloid and lymphoid leukemia and Burkitt's lymphoma (201). It is an anabolic hormone and causes hypertrophy of skeletal muscle. It acts in synergism with growth hormone and displays considerable mutual interference with thyroid hormones. It has been used to treat cases of primary insulin receptor mutations (type A resistance, leprechaunism, Rabson-Mendehall syndrome) with some success (104). As described in 1 below, IGF-1 and insulin receptors are, to some extent, cross-reactive. Although IGF-1 receptor numbers were shown to be high in glomerular epithelial cells in one study (163), no mutations or other genetic abnormalities of the IGF-1 receptor have been described.

FOUR-TRANSMEMBRANE-SEGMENT RECEPTOR DISEASES

Gamma-Aminobutyric Acid and Serotonin Receptors

Although members of the GABA and serotonin (5-HT) receptor families have been implicated in a number of neuropsychiatric illnesses, no close linkage between these receptor genes and specific genetic disorders has been found. The GABA receptor subtypes $\alpha 1$–6, $\beta 1$ and -3, and $\gamma 2$ were excluded from linkage to manic-depressive illness (37, 56, 177). Mutations in the GABA receptor $\beta 1$ gene were sought as a possible link between receptor defects and schizophrenia. One polymorphism was found in two of three affected sibs in one family but in none of 155 unrelated schizophrenics, and the sequence variant was found in 1.1% of normals (38). The GABA receptor $\beta 3$-subunit gene has been excluded as the Angelman's syndrome gene (178). The $\beta 1$ receptor locus has been excluded from linkage to panic disorders in five Icelandic pedigrees (191). The 5-HT1A receptor was found to be intact in mood disorder patients (236). This same gene was excluded from linkage with Tourette's syndrome, chronic motor tics, and obsessive-compulsive behavior (25). An association between a 5-HT2A receptor gene, silent polymorphism, and clozapine-responsive schizophrenia has been reported (6, 162), but the finding was not replicated in two other studies (11, 30, 81).

Acetylcholine Receptor/Slow-Channel Syndrome

The skeletal muscle Ach receptor is a ligand-gated ion channel that mediates signaling at the neuromuscular junction. It is a pentameric complex of four different subunits, assembled with a stoichiometry of α-2, β, γ, and δ. All four subunits, encoded by different genes, have been cloned and characterized (reviewed in ref. 103). They are related in sequence, displaying pairwise similarities of 35%–50%. The α-subunit has adjacent Cys residues at positions 192 and 193, which are highly conserved among species and thought to be located at or near the Ach-binding site.

Slow-channel syndrome (SCS) is a dominantly inherited myasthenic syndrome linked to mutations in the Ach receptor gene (reviewed in ref. 55). Patients have muscle weakness, progressive muscle atrophy, fatigue, and pathological electrophysiological features such as prolonged end-plate potentials, although the clinical, electrophysiological, and pathological abnormalities differ from family to family. These abnormalities arise from delayed closure of the Ach receptor ion channel due to mutations in one of the four genes that encode Ach receptor subunits. Phenotypic variability is likely due to the heterogeneous nature of the mutations and the altered properties of the mutant receptors encoded by them. Two populations of receptors operate in patients with SCS, normal and those containing a defective subunit. Closing of the ion channel occurs two- to tenfold more slowly when measured in this mixed population of receptors. The progressive weakness and degeneration of the motor end-plate seen in many cases of SCS is attributed to overload of the junctional sarcoplasm by calcium ions and activation of calcium-sensitive degradative enzymes. Antibodies against the Ach receptor are absent, distinguishing this disorder from myasthenia gravis.

Mutations in the genes encoding the Ach receptor subunits have been characterized in several families with SCS. The majority of these mutations cause alterations in the ion channel. Cells expressing the ϵT264P mutation receptors were shown to have prolonged openings of the channel in the presence of agonist and even opened in the absence of agonist (164). This mutation alters a highly conserved residue in the domain lining the channel pore and is likely to disrupt the transmembrane α helix. Linkage of ϵL269F to SCS has been reported (74). The αG153S mutation increases binding affinity for Ach in vitro, causing prolonged activation of the channels due to a decreased rate of Ach release from the receptor (202). A transgenic mouse model of SCS has been developed and characterized for a mutation in the δ-subunit S262T (73).

One of a family of Ach receptor disorders, SCS is the only one in which the precise molecular defect has been characterized. Other congenital myasthenic syndromes result from Ach receptor deficiency and short channel open time, kinetic abnormalities that cause high conductance, fast-channel syndrome, and a syndrome attributed to abnormal interactions of Ach with its receptor (reviewed in ref. 55). In addition, several other human hereditary muscle diseases have been linked to mutations in muscle ion channels: sodium channel/hyperkalemic periodic paralysis, chloride channel/myotonia congenita, and calcium channel/hypokalemic periodic paralysis (reviewed in ref. 90).

Abnormal Recognition, Regulation, and Signaling Pathways

Membrane receptors are normally down-regulated or desensitized in response to a sudden increase in ligand. The number of receptors returns to normal after ligand levels equilibrate. If exposure to ligand becomes chronic due to a pathologic excess of hormone or agonist, the number of receptors on the cell surface may decline, leaving cells resistant to the ligand.

Abnormal down-regulation of the insulin receptor has been well characterized in patients with obesity or NIDDM. Reduced levels of insulin receptors are inversely correlated with elevated serum levels of insulin. If levels of insulin are lowered by diet or drugs that interfere with insulin secretion, the number of receptors returns to normal. The decreased number of insulin receptors seen in obese or NIDDM patients may be due to the down-regulation of receptors induced by chronic overexposure to insulin. Down-regulation of insulin receptors in response to insulin has been well characterized in vitro. Chronic overexposure to insulin decreases the number of insulin receptors on target cell membranes by at least two mechanisms, namely, accelerated degradation and inhibition of receptor biosynthesis (166). Reduction of insulin receptors is believed to play a role in insulin resistance.

NIDDM affects 5%–7% of the population and is characterized by two major defects: insulin resistance, as measured by impaired glucose tolerance, and insulin deficiency due to impaired pancreatic β cells. Susceptibility to insulin resistance has a strong genetic association, as seen in studies of identical twins which show 60%–90% concordance for NIDDM (186). Environmental factors such as body weight and physical activity also play a role in susceptibility to NIDDM (87).

Insulin resistance can lead to chronic hyperglycemia, which may be toxic to pancreatic β cells and impair their ability to secrete insulin, resulting in insulin deficiency. Plasma insulin levels are usually low in patients with chronic disease. It has been proposed that β-cell defects are due to poor fetal and early postnatal nutrition. There is a strong inverse correlation between NIDDM and low weight at birth and at 1 year (82).

RECEPTOR-SPECIFIC CROSS-OVER DISEASE

Members of some hormone receptor families are structurally sufficiently similar that the hormone for one member can bind to a related receptor, though usually with a lower affinity than to its own receptor (reviewed in ref. 62). For example, insulin will bind to and activate the IGF-1 receptor at a 100-fold lower potency than needed for its own receptor. In diseases associated with elevated levels of hormone, cross-over hormone binding can account for the activation of receptors for one hormone through low-affinity binding of a different hormone that is present in excess.

Hyperprolactinemia Syndrome

An example of one such type of cross-over binding occurs in patients with acromegaly, who sometimes also have symptoms of hyperprolactinemia (galactorrhea, amenorrhea, and infertility) but normal levels of serum prolactin. In one study of 500 patients with acromegaly, 43 had galactorrhea, 11 of whom (25.6%) had hyperprolactinemia (57). In a previous study, ten of 28 patients with acromegaly and galactorrhea had normal prolactin levels (44). The authors speculate that excess growth hormone activates prolactin receptors sufficiently to induce galactorrhea in the absence of elevated prolactin. Growth hormone and prolactin bind lactogenic receptors with similar affinities. Human growth hormone is lactogenic and binds to the human prolactin receptor (39). Normally, the cross-reactive effect of growth hormone binding to prolactin receptors is not apparent since physiological levels of growth hormone are much lower than those of prolactin. However, levels of growth hormone in patients with acromegaly may become sufficiently increased to contribute to galactorrhea.

Trophoblastic Tumors/Human Chorionic Gonadotropin

Another example of receptor cross-reactivity occurs in patients with trophoblastic tumors who exhibit altered thyroid function in association with goiter or hyperthyroidism but no other features of Graves' disease, such as exophthalmos and dermopathy, which cannot be explained by circulating levels of TSH, TSH receptor-stimulating antibodies, or thyroid hormones. Symptoms of hyperthyroidism are alleviated in patients after tumor removal. In vitro studies have shown that tumor extracts and patient sera have thyroid-stimulating properties. Trophoblastic neoplasms secrete hCG, which binds to the luteinizing hormone/hCG receptor. Increasing evidence indicates that hCG stimulates thyroid function in patients with trophoblastic tumors. Elevated plasma levels of hCG correlate with increased thyroid hormone production (161). Purified hCG has been shown to bind to the TSH receptor and to activate adenyl cyclase in thyroid cells, though with much lower affinity and at higher concentrations than for TSH (9). However, levels of hCG are sufficiently elevated in some patients with gestational neoplasms to induce a substantial release of thyroid hormone.

Non-Islet Cell Neoplasms/Type II Insulin-Like Growth Factor

A third example of receptor cross-over occurs in some hypoglycemic patients with non-islet cell neoplasms. Fasting hypoglycemia may result from an excess secretion of IGF-2 from large tumors of mesenchymal origin (75, 100). Symptoms in patients with fasting hypoglycemia are the same as those seen in patients with insulinomas, except that insulin levels are suppressed. Other reasons for fasting hypoglycemia were ruled out, and serum levels of IGF-2 were found to be elevated (132). Glucose regulation returns to normal after removal of tumors (59).

Other examples of specificity spillover include the hyperandrogenism sometimes associated with certain forms of severe insulin resistance due to the cross-reactivity of insulin with ovarian IGF-1 receptors and, possibly, macrosomia in infants of diabetic mothers, reflecting cross-reactivity with IGF-1 in somatic tissues (reviewed in ref. 100). The main features of receptor cross-over syndromes are summarized in Table 12.1.

ONCOGENIC RECEPTOR DEFECTS

Thyroid-Stimulating Hormone Receptor/ Thyroid Adenomas

Apparently normal TSH receptor expression in various thyroid tumors correlates with the histological features of thyroid dedifferentiation (23). However, the TSH receptor is not an oncogene for thyroid tumors (142). The DNA for TSH receptor has large insertions or deletions in thyroid adenomas (148). Somatic mutations which result in constitutive activation of the TSH

TABLE 12.1. *Receptor-Specific Cross-Over Syndromes*

Reactive Hormone	Cross-Reacting Receptor	Primary Disorder	"Spillover" Disorder
Growth hormone	Prolactin, other "lacto-genic" receptors	Acromegaly	Galactorrhea, amenorrhea, infertility
Human chorionic gonadotropin	TSH*	Trophoblastic tumors	Hyperthyroidism
Insulin	IGF-1† in ovary	Insulin resistance, diabetes mellitus	Hyperandrogenism
Insulin	IGF-1 in somatic tissues	Mother with diabetes mellitus	Macrosomia in newborns
IGF-2	Insulin	Some large mesenchymal tumors	Hypoglycemia

*TSH, thyroid-stimulating hormone.   †IGF, insulin-like growth factor.

receptor have been found in human hyperfunctioning thyroid adenomas (reviewed in refs. 125, 185). Such mutations were first described by Parma et al. (171). Hyperfunctioning thyroid adenomas are discrete encapsulated neoplasms that are activated independently of TSH, leading to hyperthyroidism and, as a result of the negative feedback exerted by thyroid hormones on TSH release, to suppression of thyroid function in extraadenomatous tissue. Such adenomas are identified in vivo by ^{131} scanning and, after removal, by encapsulation and high-iodide trapping in vitro compared with the quiescent surrounding tissue. When the cAMP cascade is stimulated in human thyroid cells in primary culture, differentiated gene expression is induced; that is, thyroglobulin and thyroid peroxidase are expressed and iodide transport increased. Cells also respond to cAMP by proliferating and hyperfunctioning (that is, they generate H_2O_2, increase protein iodination and iodotyrosine coupling, and secrete increased amounts of thyroid hormone). Mutations are exclusive to the adenoma and are not found in normal surrounding thyroid tissue.

Several of the TSH receptor gene mutations characterized in hyperfunctioning adenomas—namely, D619G, A623I/V, F631C, and T632I—have been shown to confer constitutive activation to TSH receptor receptors expressed in vitro (171, 172, 175, 176). Seven of the mutations identified cluster in the region of the sixth transmembrane domain or in the very nearby third extracellular domain (D619G, A623I/V, F631C, D633Y/E, and T632I) (171, 172, 176). The third intracellular loop is involved in the interaction of the receptor and downstream heterotrimeric G proteins. A similar mutation in the α1-adrenergic receptor (Ala 293 in the third cytoplasmic loop) leads to constitutive activation of the receptor. Ohno et al. (165) have identified five TSH receptor mutations in thyroid adenomas but have not tested the effect of these muta-

tions on receptor function in vitro. Two of these mutations (F197I, D219G) map to the extracellular domain and may alter TSH binding. Two of the mutations (N715, K723M) map to the cytoplasmic tail region and may be involved in receptor internalization. The fifth mutation may be an allelic variant since it has been detected in normal thyroid and encodes a conservative amino-acid change (77).

Constitutive activation of another part of the cAMP cascade, heterotrimeric G proteins, has been identified in some thyroid tumors (205). The effect of mutations of $G\alpha_s$ is to permanently activate adenyl cyclase, causing cells to secrete hormone and proliferate in an autonomous way. The various genetic disorders of the TSH receptor and their effects are summarized in Table 12.2, and the sites of mutations are depicted in Figure 12.1.

$G\alpha_s$ Mutations/McCune-Albright Syndrome

McCune-Albright syndrome (MAS) is a sporadic disease which comprises polyostotic fibrous dysplasia, *cafe-au-lait* spots, precocious puberty, and various hyperfunctional endocrinopathies. Endocrine tissues commonly affected include the gonads, thyroid, adrenal cortex, and pituitary somatotrophs. Acromegaly associated with pituitary adenoma has been reported in several MAS patients (33).

Polyostotic fibrous dysplasia is characterized histologically by the persistence of woven bone where lamellar bone would normally develop. Marrow fibrosis is intense, and the rate of bone turnover is increased. The progressive replacement of normal bone with a mixture of calcified cartilage and woven bone accounts for its poor mechanical strength and the severe deformities that result. Bone lesions expand, causing pathological fractures, pain, and nerve compression (188). Deformities of the chest wall and arteriovenous shunting through dysplastic bone may contribute to cardiopul-

TABLE 12.2. *Thyroid Disorders Caused by Genetic Abnormalities of the TSH * Receptor*

Mode Of Inheritance	Genetic Abnormality	Site Of Abnormality	Effect Of Mutation/Abnormality	Disorder	Clinical Features
Autosomal dominant	Germ-line point mutation (50% of cases), deletions, insertions	Exon 10, 3rd and 7th TM† domains	Activates adenyl cyclase	Toxic thyroid hyperplasia/hereditary hyperthyroidism	Goiter, hyperthyroidism
Autosomal recessive	Point mutations, heterozygous polymorphisms, no abnormalities	Exon 6, extracellular domain	Resistance to TSH, constitutive activation of adenyl cyclase	TSH resistance	Usually euthyroid, normal T_4,‡ increased TSH
Variable	Gene mutations (most), somatic mutations, mutations of Gαs, deletions, insertions	6th and 3rd TM domains	Constitutive activation of the receptor (most), alters TSH binding, receptor internalization	Thyroid adenomas, multinodular goiter	Nodule, goiter, hyperthyroidism
Autosomal recessive	Unknown	Unknown but not due to mutations in receptor gene	Absent in vivo response to TSH, low ^{123}I uptake, no features of thyroid autoimmunity	Congenital hypothyroidism	Hypothyroidism at birth, cretinism, goiter

* TSH, thyroid-stimulating hormone.   † TM, transmembrane.   ‡ T_4, thyroxine.

monary insufficiency in some MAS patients. Increased expression of the c-fos proto-oncogene, likely due to increased adenyl cyclase activity, may be important in the pathogenesis of the bone lesions (31).

The sporadic occurrence, the myriad developmental abnormalities, and the curious pattern of skin pigmentation led to the hypothesis that this disorder is secondary to a dominant somatic mutation occurring early in embryogenesis (83). It also has been suggested that MAS is the result of a lethal gene surviving by mosaicism (83). Molecular studies support this view since an activating missense mutation in the gene for the α-subunit of G_s has been found in affected but not normal tissues of these patients (179, 187). Replacement of the arginine residue at position 201 of the $G\alpha_s$ gene subunit by either histidine or cysteine results in an abnormal $G\alpha_s$ protein that stimulates adenyl cyclase in a constitutive fashion. These missense mutations introduce a novel NIaIII restriction site, which simplifies the detection of such mutations. The R201H/C mutation has been identified in regions of bone with fibrous dysplasia and other affected tissues of patients with MAS (140, 188, 192, 232). The $G\alpha_s$ gene R201C mutation was identified in an infant with ACTH-independent Cushing's syndrome and fibrous dysplasia (22). A subset of patients also may manifest nonendocrine abnormalities associated with sudden or premature death due to hepatobiliary or cardiac disease (187).

Disorders of Ras and Ras-Like Proto-oncogenes

The *ras* genes are a ubiquitous eukaryotic gene family comprising three members that are structurally related to the α-subunit of heterotrimeric G proteins: H-*ras*, K-*ras,* and N-*ras*. Ras proteins are involved in the control of cell growth and differentiation. Somatic mutations in the three *ras* genes have been identified in several types of malignancy, including tumors of the endocrine system. Mutations at three loci convert *ras* genes into oncogenes when codons 12, 13, and 61 are altered. Mutations at these sites inhibit the intrinsic GTPase activity, resulting in constitutive activation of ras proteins. (For reviews, see refs. 14, 36, 180.)

Ras proteins are part of the signal-transduction pathway for several membrane-bound receptors that have intrinsic tyrosine kinase activity. Anti-ras antibodies block the mitogenesis induced by platelet-derived growth factor (PDGF) and insulin. Dominant negative ras mutations inhibit the actions of NGF, fibroblast growth factor (FGF), PDGF, EGF, and insulin. Overexpression of c-*ras* increases the sensitivity to several growth factors and insulin.

Somatic mutations in the α-subunit of the G_s protein (gsp mutations) occur in about 40% of human growth hormone–secreting pituitary adenomas. Such mutations lead to constitutive activation of adenyl cyclase and thus increased intracellular levels of cAMP and disruption of the GHRH receptor–G protein–adenyl cyclase pathway. Activating mutations identified to date are R201C/H and Q227R/L. When expressed in vitro, cells with gsp mutations have up to 24-fold higher levels of cAMP than normal cells (120). Such mutations are thought to be the cause of excessive growth hormone secretion and tumor growth. Surprisingly, since cAMP levels are already elevated, some somatotrophinomas with gsp mutations respond to GHRH, possibly because GHRH exerts its effect through multiple pathways and cells may be re-

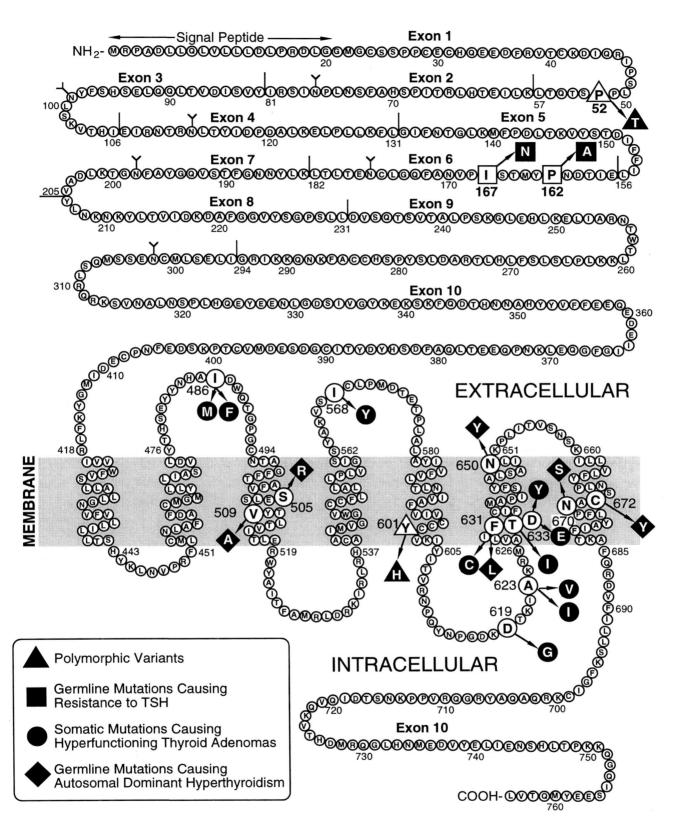

FIG. 12.1. Model of the thyroid-stimulating hormone *(TSH)* receptor molecule showing amino-acid residues, orientation of the receptor in respect to the thyroid cell plasma membrane, its seven-transmembrane loops, and positions of known germ-line and somatic mutations. [Reprinted with permission from ref. 177a.]

sponding via the phosphoinositol system, which activates protein kinase C and raises intracellular calcium. Many pituitary tumors with gsp mutations also respond well to factors and drugs, such as dopamine and somatostatin analogs, that inhibit growth hormone secretion (4). This result suggests that inhibition of growth hormone secretion by somatostatin may be mediated by G_i, a G protein that negatively regulates adenyl cyclase (58). These mutations are found at a low frequency, about 6%, in ACTH-secreting pituitary adenomas (234) and in about 6% of thyroid tumors (32).

Mutations in $G\alpha_{i2}$ (gip), the G protein which negatively regulates adenylyl cyclase, have been described in various endocrine tumors, such as those of the adrenal gland and ovary. $G\alpha_{i2}$ may stimulate cell proliferation via coupling to the IGF-2 receptor or through mitosis-activating kinases (167, 79).

ANTIRECEPTOR ANTIBODIES AND AUTOIMMUNE DISEASE

Antireceptor autoantibodies play a key role in the development of several endocrine and nonendocrine disorders. They are produced in the context of an autoimmune reaction and may be associated with a variety of other tissue-specific and tissue nonspecific autoantibodies. While most autoantibodies associated with autoimmune diseases do not cause tissue damage, those reactive with hormone receptors often have a dramatic effect in vivo. The model for receptor disease caused by autoantibodies is Graves' hyperthyroidism, in which antibodies against TSH receptor stimulate thyroid cell function via the adenylyl cyclase system, leading to increased thyroid cell size, numbers, and function, manifested by increased blood levels of thyroid hormones and a variety of signs and symptoms which comprise the clinical syndrome of "thyrotoxicosis" or hyperthyroidism (3, 203). The other classical antireceptor disorder is myasthenia gravis, in which autoantibodies targeting the nicotinic Ach receptor block neurotransmission, leading to skeletal muscle weakness. Some cases of insulin resistance, so-called type A insulin resistance, also are due to antibodies reactive to the insulin receptor (15). Less common disorders caused by antireceptor antibodies include a type of asthma associated with antibodies reactive with the β-adrenergic receptor and ataxia telangiectasia linked, in an unknown way, with insulin receptor antibodies and associated with immunodeficiency. Finally, many experimental antireceptor antibodies have been produced which have not yet been linked to a human disease. A summary of the best understood disorders associated with receptor antibodies is given in Table 12.3.

Effect of Antireceptor Antibodies

Receptor-reactive autoantibodies may stimulate function of the corresponding target cell; for example, thyroid epithelial cells in Graves' hyperthyroidism, block action of the corresponding trophic hormone, which is the most common effect, or, theoretically, by accelerating receptor turnover, induce receptor or postreceptor desensitization to ligand, with which no disorders have been associated (20).

Thyroid-Stimulating Hormone Receptor Antibodies and Graves' Disease

Antibodies reactive with the TSH receptor may stimulate the thyroid cell (in Graves' hyperthyroidism), block access to TSH and cause hypothyroidism, or induce thyroid cell growth and thus play a role in goiter, adenoma, and possibly thyroid cancer.

The TSH receptor is a single polypeptide chain in which two to six potential glycosylation sites are important in expressing a functional epitope for autoantibodies. Disulfide bonds contribute to the three-dimensional structure of the receptor. For reasons that are not clear, the production of antibodies against the TSH receptor is a common occurrence in humans and the cause of several well-defined disorders, including Graves' disease, a classical autoimmune disorder which affects as many as 1% of the adult population. The molecular nature of the TSH receptor and the relationship between its TSH-binding site and autoantibody-reactive epitopes have been extensively studied (59). The TSH-specific sequences of the TSH receptor are multiple discontinuous regions of the extracellular part of the molecule and highly homologous with the LH receptor (150). Although not proven, it seems likely that TSH- and antibody-binding domains on the receptor are overlapping but different.

While autoantibody binding to the TSH receptor appears to be heterologous, (154, 155) there is a consensus that the main site of high-affinity binding of anti-TSH receptor antibodies is to the extracellular domain of the molecule (156), where several putative epitopes on the receptor molecule have been recognized, especially in the first exon (residues 1–55) (111). Cysteines 494 and 569 of the first and second exoplasmic loops, respectively, of the transmembrane domain of the TSH receptor are involved in binding of both TSH and TSH receptor antibodies and in coupling ligand binding to signal generation; mutation of cysteine to serine leads to the production of a TSH receptor molecule which does not bind to TSH or induce cAMP response to TSH (80) or TSH receptor antibodies (110). Cysteine 301 seems to be important in TSH

TABLE 12.3. *Clinical Disorders Associated with Antibodies Against Receptors*

Disorder	Receptor/Target Cell	Antibody Activity	Clinical Features
Graves' hyperthyroidism	TSH[a]/thyroid cell	Stimulating	Hyperthyroidism
Atrophic thyroiditis/ transient hypothyroidism	TSH/thyroid cell	Blocking	Hypothyroidism
Graves' disease	TSH/thyroid cell	Growth stimulation	Goiter, thyroid nodules
Type B insulin resistance	Insulin/β islet cell	Blocking	Diabetes, acanthosis nigricans
Ataxia telangiectasia	Insulin/β islet cell	Blocking	Diabetes, ataxia telangiectasia, immunodeficiency, neoplasia
Asthma	β-adrenergic receptor/ bronchial muscle cell	Blocking	Bronchospasm
Myasthenia gravis	Nicotinic acetylcholine/neuromuscular junction	Blocking	Muscle weakness, fatigability
Idiopathic diabetes insipidus	Vasopressin/AVP[b] cell	Binding to AVP cells	None identified
Addison's disease	ACTH[c]	Binding	None identified
Idiopathic hypoparathyroidism	PTH[d]/renal tubular cell	Blocking	None identified
Thyroid-associated ophthalmopathy	TSH/orbital fat, fibroblast	Stimulating	Possibly fibroblast proliferation, GAGs,[e] and collagen overproduction, exophthalmos

[a] TSH, thyroid-stimulating hormone. [b] AVP, arginine vasopressin. [c] ACTH, adrenocorticotropic hormone. [d] PTH, parathyroid hormone. [e] GAGs, glycosaminoglycans.

binding and receptor tertiary structure (6). In one study, a point mutation in an extracellular domain of the TSH receptor, which was involved with Graves' immunoglobulin interactions, was reported (21), though this has not been confirmed. While glycosylation sites on the TSH receptor molecule generally are thought to be important in antibody binding, Morgenthaler et al. (149) found that binding of anti-TSH receptor autoantibodies to nascent, in vitro translated receptor was not influenced by the lack of glycosylation of the translated extracellular region of the receptor. While the main site of binding of TSH and anti-TSH receptor autoantibodies is the extracellular domain, there is also some high-affinity binding of both to the transmembrane region of the receptor molecule (156). Despite a good understanding of the general nature of the interaction between the TSH receptor and circulating autoantibodies, the sequences of individual epitopes and their conformations have not been defined clearly.

Receptor antibodies to TSH may stimulate or block receptor activation and thyroid hormone synthesis and secretion. The different activities of TSH receptor antibodies can be measured using a TSH receptor–binding assay modified to demonstrate binding, blocking, or stimulation (79) (Fig. 12.2). In the classical radiorecep-

tor assay, inhibition of ^{131}I-labeled TSH binding to its receptor in thyroid membranes, slices, homogenates, whole cells, or recombinant TSH receptor protein is measured. Antibodies which stimulate the TSH receptor pathways via adenyl cyclase are determined from their effects on cAMP, thyroid cell size or number, colloid droplet formation, or various derived parameters of thyroid cell function, such as serum triiodothyronine (T_3) and Thyroxine (T_4) levels and ^{131}I uptake by thyroid cells, homogenates, or slices as thyroid-stimulating antibody (TSAb) (78). Antibodies which block TSH binding to the receptor are determined by measuring the inhibition of TSH-stimulated cAMP production by human thyroid cells or by the FRTL-5 rat thyroid cell line and expressed as a percentage of inhibition. Activity can shift from stimulating to blocking and back to stimulating (8), possibly reflecting the production of autoantibodies recognizing different domains of the TSH receptor molecule. Because anti-TSH receptor antibodies block each step of TSH action—namely, binding, receptor activation, and thyroid cell stimulation—this must result directly from antibody binding.

Although it is well established that TSH activates a cAMP-dependent pathway in the thyroid follicular cell,

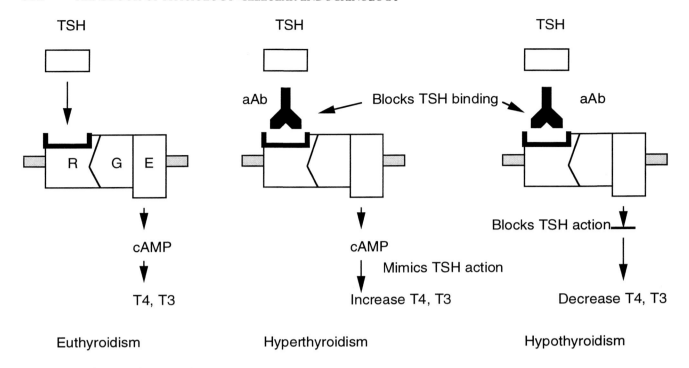

FIG. 12.2. Mechanism of action of thyroid-stimulating hormone *(TSH)* receptor antibodies. Antibodies bind to the TSH receptor, where they block access of TSH, causing hyperthyroidism as a result of stimulation of cAMP or hypothyroidism by blocking TSH action. *T4,* thyroxine; *T3,* triiodothyronine; *aAb,* autoantibody; *R,* receptor; *G,* G protein; *E,* effector.

leading to thyroid hormone synthesis and release, there is evidence that TSH also activates a non-cAMP-dependent signal-transduction system. This involves phosphoinositide turnover and protein kinase C (PKC) activation. Receptor antibodies to TSH may selectively activate cAMP while having no effect on phosphoinositide turnover. However, TSH-blocking antibodies appear to activate PKC, which may be an important mediator of both TSH and TSH receptor autoantibody actions (71).

Graves' disease comprises four different disorders which occur in various combinations in individual patients—namely, hyperthyroidism, ophthalmopathy, pretibial myxedema (dermopathy), and acropachy. Most patients have hyperthyroidism, while about 50% have, or will develop, the eye disorder. The other two features are uncommon and may reflect a generalized connective tissue inflammation; indeed, there is some evidence that Graves' disease may be a multisystem, collagen-like disorder of the skeletal muscle, thyroid, and connective tissue (reviewed in ref. 225), which, for reasons that are unclear, localizes mainly in the orbit, thyroid, and skin. While the pathogenesis of the extrathyroidal manifestations of Graves' disease is undetermined (224), the hyperthyroidism is almost certainly caused by the action of TSH receptor antibodies which stimulate the thyroid cell in a prolonged and uncon-trolled manner, leading to the production of large amounts of thyroid hormone. There is a close temporal relationship between the antibodies and the development of hyperthyroidism in predisposed subjects, such as first-degree relatives, and serum levels usually correlate closely with parameters of hyperthyroidism, such as ^{131}I uptake and serum T_4 and T_3 levels (168). The antibodies are of the IgG isotype and, therefore, can cross the placenta, where they may cause transient neonatal thyrotoxicosis; in this uncommon disorder, symptoms disappear within a few weeks, consistent with the half-life of the molecule (135, 241, 242). There is no experimental model for Graves' disease, and the effects of antibodies reactive with the TSH receptor are known only from clinical syndromes of hyper- and hypothyroidism. Measurement of serum levels of TSAb provides an important aid to the diagnosis and management of Graves' disease—namely, the differential diagnosis of hyperthyroidism, the prediction of possible development of neonatal thyrotoxicosis in children born of mothers with past or present Graves' disease, and the monitoring of treatment of hyperthyroidism with antithyroid drugs, remission typically being associated with disappearance of serum antibodies.

Thyroid-stimulating hormone receptor-blocking antibodies, measured as thyroid-stimulating blocking antibodies (TSBAbs), are implicated in some cases of autoimmune hypothyroidism. These antibodies are found in 0%–20% of patients with idiopathic hypothyroidism and in 0%–40% with atrophic hypothyroidism, in different series, though their role in these disorders is unclear. It is generally thought that TSBAbs play a major role in the development of hypothyroidism and thyroid atrophy in the great majority of patients with nongoitrous autoimmune thyroiditis, both adults (35) and some newborns with transient hypothyroidism (in which case the antibodies cross the placenta from mothers with Graves' disease) (26). While TSAbs are immunoglobulin class-restricted, indicating some oligoclonality, this is not the case for TSBAbs, which are polyclonal (115). The role of dietary iodine may be important in determining the effect of these antibodies (239); in Japan, iodine restriction is associated with recovery in 50% of patients with idiopathic hypothyroidism, presumably due to Hashimoto's thyroiditis (8), whereas in other populations this disorder is usually considered to be irreversible. The serum level of TSBAbs may be critical; when the level exceeds 1500 μ/I, transient hypothyroidism may occur (8). Both TSAbs and TSBAbs appear to react with the same epitope(s) on the TSH receptor molecule.

Thyroid Growth–Stimulating Antibodies

The existence of thyroid growth–stimulating antibodies which are different from TSH receptor antibodies, and postulated by some workers (47) to cause thyroid cell growth and goiter, is a subject of controversy. Serum antibodies with putative growth-promoting activity are quantitated as ^{3}H-thymidine uptake by FRTL-5 thyroid cells or by flow-cytometric measurement of the proportion of thyroid cells in the S and G_2/M phases of the cell cycle. Most workers believe, however, that these activities can be explained by the effects of stimulating TSH receptor antibodies and that a separate family of growth-stimulating antibodies does not exist. The putative role of TSH receptor antibodies in thyroid cell growth and goiter in nonautoimmune thyroid disorders, such as endemic goiter, colloid and multinodular goiter, and thyroid cancer (233), has been challenged in the absence of other autoimmune phenomena or disorders in these patients and the failure to demonstrate serum immunoglobulin with growth-potentiating or TSH receptor–stimulating activities in most studies (40, 222).

Possible Role of Thyroid-Stimulating Hormone Receptor Antibodies in Thyroid-Associated Ophthalmopathy.
Thyroid-associated ophthalmopathy (TAO) is an autoimmune disorder of the extraocular (eye) muscle and orbital connective tissue which is closely associated with Graves' hyperthyroidism and, to a lesser extent, Hashimoto's thyroiditis. Typical histological abnormalities in the periorbital tissues of patients with TAO include lymphocytic infiltration, extraocular muscle damage, and orbital fibroblast stimulation manifested as glycosaminoglycan (GAG) accumulation, fibroblast proliferation, and collagen overproduction (106, 109). While T-lymphocyte reactivity against extraocular muscle and orbital connective tissue antigens is expected to be the primary event in the development of ophthalmopathy, most workers have focused on the role of circulating autoantibodies reactive with various orbital antigens (106). The principal autoantigens are not clearly defined, though there are many candidates. The TSH receptor, or a TSH receptor-like protein, expressed in both thyroid and orbital tissues has been postulated by some (61, 64, 89) to be a target of cross-reactive antibodies and T cells in TAO. However, this notion has been disputed (42). Stimulation of collagen production by monoclonal anti-TSH receptor antibodies was reported in one study (182), though these results have not been confirmed by others (210). In vitro TSH does not stimulate GAG synthesis (93). Moreover, clinical observations of TAO in patients without detectable serum anti-TSH receptor antibodies contradict this hypothesis. While the presence of TSH receptor mRNA in orbital connective tissue has been reported (89), other studies have not confirmed this (61). Indeed, since the TSH receptor is expressed in many tissues (54, 181), it is unlikely that antibody (or T-cell) targeting of shared epitopes would be restricted to the orbital connective tissue, thyroid, and perhaps skin. Finally, there is no close correlation between anti-TSH receptor antibody titers and parameters of TAO (106).

T Lymphocytes Binding to Thyroid-Stimulating Hormone Receptor.
The TSH receptor also is targeted by T lymphocytes in patients with thyroid autoimmunity, though the nature and sites of the T-cell epitopes, which appear to be multiple (7, 157), are even less well understood (209). One group has suggested that the T-cell sites may change during the course of the disease (157).

Insulin Receptor Antibodies

There are many causes of the insulin resistance/diabetes mellitus syndrome, including genetic and acquired factors (67). The characteristics of the various disorders are summarized in Table 12.4. Serum autoantibodies against the insulin receptor have been identified in patients with so-called type B insulin resistance syndrome, which comprises glucose intolerance, high plasma insulin levels, and resistance to exogenous insu-

TABLE 12.4. *Causes of the Insulin Resistance/Diabetes Mellitus Syndrome*

Syndrome	Underlying Abnormality	Blood Insulin Level	Diabetes	Insulin Resistance	Associated Clinical Features	Insulin Receptor	Insulin Receptor Antibodies
IDDM*	Autoimmunity against β islet cells	Low/very low	Yes	No	Other autoimmunity	Normal	<10% of cases
NIDDM† + obesity	Mutation of β 3-adrenergic receptor	Increased	Yes	Yes	Hypertension, hyperlipidemia	Normal	No
NIDDM + insulin resistance	Mutations of insulin receptor	Increased/ normal	Yes	Yes	Disorders of growth, skin, teeth, nails, muscle	Abnormal	No
Common NIDDM in adults	Unknown in most cases, mutations of insulin receptor in 10% of cases	Increased then low	Yes	Yes	Obesity	Abnormal in 10% of cases	No
Type B insulin resistance	Insulin receptor antibodies	Increased	Sometimes	Yes	Acanthosis nigricans, other autoimmune disorders, antibodies, hyper- or hypoglycemia	Normal	Yes
NIDDM + ataxia telangiectasia	Insulin receptor antibodies	Increased	Sometimes	Yes	Ataxia, telangiectasis, immunodeficiency, neoplasia	Normal	Yes
Type I IDDM	Insulin receptor (idiotypic) antibodies	Increased	Sometimes	Yes	Nil usually	Normal	30% of cases

*DDM, insulin-dependent diabetes mellitus.   †NIDDM, non-insulin-dependent diabetes mellitus.

lin and is associated with, in many cases *(1)* acanthosis nigricans (thickening and pigmentation of the skin in selected parts of the body; *(2)* evidence of other autoimmune disorders or phenomena such as alopecia, arthritis, and multisystem autoimmune disease; and *(3)* a variety of organ nonspecific autoantibodies. As is the case for most other autoimmune disorders, the mechanism for loss of tolerance to the insulin receptor protein is unclear, though induction of insulin resistance by autoantibodies to insulin receptors sometimes follows an acute Coxsackie B4 infection (53). The precise epitopes are not well defined, though a region of the insulin receptor (residues 450–601) which is important for ligand binding is recognized by autoantibodies in serum from patients with insulin resistance, NIDDM, and certain inhibitory monoclonal antibodies (243). The antibodies are usually polyclonal and of the IgG isotype, which binds to and blocks the insulin receptor (Fig. 12.3). The effects of the antibodies are complicated and poorly understood but appear to lead to a down-regulated state with chronic unresponsiveness to insulin and clinical and biochemical features of adult-onset-type diabetes. The antibodies appear to

mimic the action of insulin and may, in some cases, lead to excess receptor stimulation and hypoglycemia. The action of antiinsulin receptor autoantibodies has been cited as a model for the action of such receptor antibodies in human disease.

Ataxia Telangiectasia. In patients with ataxia telangiectasia, type B insulin resistance is associated with a characteristic, but heterogeneous, syndrome comprising ataxia, telangiectasis, various immune abnormalities including very low levels of serum IgA and E, and an increased prevalence of neoplasia. The insulin receptor antibodies in this case are of the IgM class and functionally abnormal. Other immunological characteristics of this syndrome include reduced serum and salivary gland secretion levels of IgA, decreased rate of blastic transformation of lymphocytes, and increased serum levels of α-fetoprotein but normal levels of carcinoembryonic antigen. The ataxia telangiectasia locus has been mapped to chromosome 11q22-q23 (134). The immune abnormalities seem to reflect a fairly severe immunodeficiency. The basic genetic defect is a disorder in DNA repair mechanisms. This is autosomal

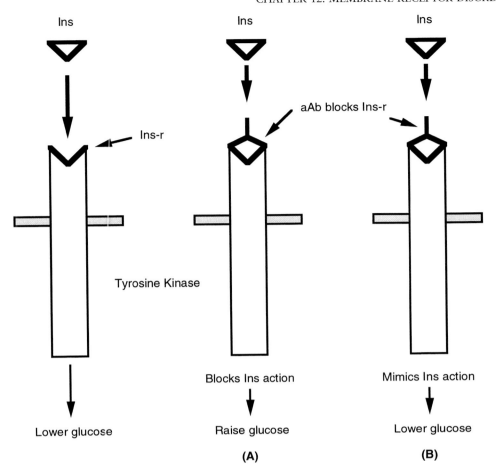

FIG. 12.3. Mechanism of action of insulin receptor antibodies. Antibodies bind to the insulin receptor, where they block access of insulin, causing hyperglycemia with or without insulin resistance and diabetes melitus *(A)* or hypoglycemia by mimicking insulin action *(B)*. *Ins,* insulin; *aAb,* autoantibody; *Ins-r,* insulin receptor.

recessive and linked to some other disorders, including xeroderma pigmentosa, Fanconi syndrome, Bloom's syndrome, and Cockayne's syndrome (136). The disorder can be diagnosed from an abnormal response of ataxia telangiectasia cells to ionizing radiation (34). The mechanism for production of antiinsulin antibodies is unclear but may relate to a general abnormality in immunoglobulin synthesis and immunodeficiency. The ensuing insulin resistance, which is sometimes extreme, is due to a defect in the affinity of insulin receptors, possibly caused by antibodies which inhibit insulin binding (13).

Antiidiotypic Antiinsulin Antibody Syndrome. A third syndrome associated with serum antiinsulin receptor autoantibodies has been described (15, 52). This comprises insulin resistance, type I diabetes mellitus, and circulating antibodies which appear to be an idiotypic

response to antiinsulin receptor antibodies. In one case report of a child with severe hypoglycemia despite low or normal secretion of insulin, serum IgM class antiinsulin receptor antibodies were neutralized by antiinsulin antibodies in another (diabetic) patient's serum, indicating that antiinsulin antibodies with a common idiotype may arise in both diabetes mellitus and hypoglycemia (51). There have been no other reports of disorders associated with such antibodies, and their significance is uncertain.

β-Adrenergic Receptor Antibodies

Classical childhood-onset bronchial asthma is associated with dysfunction of the β-adrenergic receptor adenylyl cyclase signal-transduction pathway. Most cases of so-called intrinsic asthma are due to abnormalities of the β-adrenergic receptor and caused by IgE class antibodies reactive with environmental allergens. One mechanism for β-adrenergic receptor dysfunction is blockade due to autoantibodies with specificity toward the receptor. Autoantibodies to the β-adrenergic receptor in humans are associated with decreased sensitivity to $\beta2$ receptor functions and increased responsiveness of α-adrenergic and muscarinic cholinergic receptors (221). Such antibodies may be the cause of asthma in patients who do not have IgE class antibodies in the context of an atopic etiology (84a), though the mechanism for this is poorly understood and complex. Because of the link between allergies and autoimmunity, both of which are very common, it is possible that such antibodies are a more frequent cause of asthma than is recognized. The effect of binding of the antibodies to the β-adrenergic receptor may be bronchodilation or bronchoconstriction.

Myasthenia Gravis

Myasthenia gravis is an organ-specific autoimmune disorder caused by an antibody-mediated attack on the skeletal muscle nicotinic Ach receptor at the neuromuscular junction. It is the best studied autoimmune disorder caused by autoantibodies against the Ach receptor (129). Antibodies bind to the Ach receptor, leading to loss of functional receptors and impairment of neuromuscular signal transmission, resulting in weakness and fatigability in selected skeletal muscles. Extraocular muscle weakness and double vision are present in about 90% of patients and are the initial complaints in about 20% of cases. Serum antibodies against the Ach receptor are detected in 90% of patients with generalized myasthenia gravis but in only 65% with the ocular variety. Although there are several well-characterized animal models for this disease and while much is known about the mechanism of action of the antibodies, the underlying factors responsible for loss of tolerance to the Ach receptor are, as for most other organ-specific autoimmune disorders, poorly understood (reviewed in ref. 76). Several other autoantibodies against non-Ach receptor skeletal muscle components have been described in myasthenia gravis, including those reactive with the ryanidine receptor (the calcium channel) (151a) and various muscle proteins identified by immunoblotting (119), hemagglutination (91), enzyme-linked immunosorbent assay (119), and immunofluorescence (91, 119); but these are less specific than antibodies against the Ach receptor.

Other Receptor Antibodies

In an unconfirmed study by Weightman et al. (230), IgG from patients with Graves' disease, with or without ophthalmopathy, interacted with IGF-1-binding sites on orbital fibroblasts, whereas IgG from normal subjects did not. A good candidate for another anti-receptor antibody–induced disease is Cushing's disease, due to antibodies which stimulate the ACTH receptor, although, as far as we are aware, such a situation has not been observed nor produced experimentally. The presence of antibodies inhibitory to ACTH-stimulated cortisol secretion was investigated in patients with Addison's disease by Wardle et al. (226). Although IgG preparations from some patients inhibited ACTH-stimulated cortisol secretion, this was not specific and the authors concluded that Addison's disease is not caused by circulating antibodies to the ACTH receptor. Similarly, antibodies reactive with LH and FSH receptors have not been recognized as causes of infertility or other manifestations of gonadal dysfunction, though their existence is also suspected. Scherbaum and Bottazzo (189) described antibodies against AVP cells in some patients with idiopathic diabetes insipidus, while Juppner et al. (99) demonstrated that antibodies against PTH or the PTH receptor could block binding of the hormone to renal tubular membranes and inhibit PTH-mediated cAMP accumulation in the same membranes. These findings have not been confirmed by others, and their significance in diabetes insipidus is unclear.

While polyclonal antibodies in animals and mouse monoclonal antibodies can be produced against many other, perhaps all, receptors, the corresponding clinical syndromes have not been identified.

REFERENCES

1. Accili, D., A. Cama, F. Barbetti, H. Kadowaki, T. Kadowaki, and S. I. Taylor. Insulin resistance due to mutations of the insulin receptor gene: an overview. *J. Endocrinol. Invest.* 15: 857–864, 1992.

2. Adams, A. E., M. Pines, C. Nakamoto, V. Behar, Q. M. Yang, R. Bessalle, M. Chorev, M. Rosenblatt, M. A. Levine, and L. J. Suva. Probing of the bimolecular interactions of parathyroid hormone and the parathyroid hormone-related protein receptor. 2. Cloning, characterization, and photaffinity labeling of the recombinant human receptor. *Biochemistry* 34: 10553–10559, 1995.

3. Adams, D. D. The presence of an abnormal thyroid stimulating hormone in the serum of some thyrotoxic patients. *J. Clin. Endocrinol. Metab.* 18: 699–712, 1958.

4. Adams, E. F., T. R. Lei, M. Buchfelder, B. Petersen, and R. Fahlbusch. Biochemical characteristics of human pituitary somatotropinomas with and without gsp mutations: *in vitro* cell culture studies. *J. Clin. Endocrinol. Metab.* 80: 2077–2081, 1995.

5. Aeschimann, S., P. A. Kopp, E. T. Kimura, J. Zbaeren, A. Tobler, M. F. Fey, and H. Studer. Morphological and functional polymorphism within clonal thyroid nodules. *J. Clin. Endocrinol. Metab.* 77: 846–851, 1993.

6. Akamizu, T., D. Inoue, S. Kosugi, L. D. Kohn, and T. Mori.

Further studies of amino acids (268–304) in thyrotropin (TSH)-lutrotropin/chorionic gonadotropin (LH/CG) receptor chimeras: cysteine-301 is important in TSH binding and receptor tertiary structure. *Thyroid* 4: 43–48, 1994.

7. Akamizu, T., Y. Ueda, J. Okuda, and T. Mori. Establishment and characterization of an antihuman thyrotropin (TSH) receptor-specific CD4+ T cell line from a patient with Graves' disease: evidence for multiple T cell epitopes on the TSH receptor including the transmembrane domain. *Thyroid* 5: 259–264, 1995.

8. Amino, N. Autoimmunity and hypopthyroidism. *Bailliere's Clin. Endocrinol. Metab.* 2: 591–617, 1988.

9. Amir, S., Y. Shimohigashi, P. Carayon, H. C. Chen, and B. Nisula. Role of the carbohydrate moiety of human choriogonadotropin in its thyrotropic activity. *Arch. Biochem. Biophys.* 229: 170–176, 1984.

10. Arner, P. The beta-3-adrenergic receptor—a cause and cure of obesity? *N. Engl. J. Med.* 333: 382–383, 1995.

11. Arranz, M., D. Collier, M. Sodhi, D. Ball, G. Roberts, J. Price, P. Sham, and R. Kerwin. Association between clozapine response and allelic variation in 5-HT2A receptor gene. *Lancet* 346: 281–282, 1995.

12. Bahnsen, U., P. Oosting, D. F. Swaab, P. Nahke, D. Richter, and H. Schmale. A missense mutation in the vasopressin-neurophysin precursor gene cosegregates with human autosomal dominant neurohypophyseal diabetes insipidus. *EMBO J.* 11: 19–23, 1992.

13. Bar, R. S., W. R. Levis, M. M. Rechler, L. C. Harrison, C. Siebert, J. Podskalny, J. Roth, and M. Muggeo. Extreme insulin resistance in ataxia telangiectasia: defect in affinity of insulin receptors. *N. Engl. J. Med.* 289: 1164–1171, 1978.

14. Baracid, M. Ras genes. *Annu. Rev. Biochem.* 56: 779–827, 1987.

15. Batarseh, H., R. A. Thompson, O. Odugbesan, and A. H. Barnett. Insulin receptor antibodies in diabetes mellitus. *Clin. Exp. Immunol.* 71: 85–90, 1988.

16. Berg, M. A., R. Peoples, L. Perez-Jurado, J. Guevara-Aguirre, A. L. Rosenbloom, Z. Laron, R.D.G. Milner, and U. Francke. Receptor mutations and haplotypes in growth hormone receptor deficiency: a global survey and identification of the Ecuadorean E180 splice mutation in an Oriental Jewish patient. *Acta. Paediatr. (Suppl.)* 399: 112–114, 1994.

17. Berthezene, F., M. G. Forrest, J. A. Grimaud, B. Claustrat, and R. Mornex. Leydig cell agenesis: a cause of male pseudohermaphroditism. *N. Engl. J. Med.* 295: 969–972, 1976.

18. Bichet, D. G., M. Birnbaumer, M. Lonergan, M. F. Arthus, W. Rosenthal, P. Goodyer, P. Nivet, H. Benoit, S. Giampietro, and P. Simonetti. Nature and recurrence of AVPR2 mutations in X-linked nephrogenic diabetes insipidus. *Am. J. Hum. Genet.* 55: 278–286, 1994.

19. Bichet, D. G., M. Birnbaumer, M. Lonergan, M. F. Arthus, W. Rosenthal, P. Goodyear, A. Seibold, S. Gilbert, M. Ishido, C. Barberis, A. Antaramian, P. Brabet, and W. Rosenthal. Molecular cloning of the receptor for human antidiuretic hormone. *Nature* 357: 333–335, 1992.

20. Blecher, M. Receptors, antibodies and disease. *Clin. Chem.* 30: 1137–1156, 1984.

21. Bohr, U. R., M. Behr, and U. Loos. A heritable point mutation in an extracellular domain of the TSH receptor involved in the interaction with Graves' immunoglobulins. *Biochim. Biophys. Acta* 1216: 504–508, 1993.

22. Boston B. A., S. Mandel, S. LaFranchi, and M. Bliziotes. Activating mutation in the stimulatory guanine nucleotide-binding protein in an infant with Cushing's syndrome and nodular adrenal hyperplasia. *J. Clin. Endocrinol. Metab.* 79: 890–893, 1994.

23. Brabant G., C. Maenhaut, J. Kohrle, G. Scheumann, H. Dralle, C. Hoang-Vu, R. D. Hesch, A. von zur Muhlen, G. Vassart, and J. E. Dumont. Human thyrotropin receptor gene: expression in thyroid tumors and correlation to markers of thyroid differentiation and dedifferentiation. *Mol. Cell. Endocrinol.* 82: 7–12, 1991.

24. Bray, P., A. Carter, V. Guo, C. Puckett, J. Kamholz, A. Spiegel, and M. Nirenberg. Human cDNA clones for an alpha subunit of G_i signal-transduction protein. *Proc. Natl. Acad. Sci. U.S.A.* 84: 5115–5119, 1987.

25. Brett, P. M., D. Curtis, M. M. Robertson, and H. M. Gurlin. Exclusion of the 5-HT1A serotonin neuroreceptor and tryptophan oxygenase genes in a large British kindred multiply affected with Tourette's syndrome, chronic motor tics, and obsessive-compulsive behavior. *Am. J. Psychol.* 152: 437–440, 1995.

26. Brown, R. S., R. L. Bellisario, E. Mitchell, P. Keating, and D. Botero. Detection of thyrotropin binding inhibitory activity in neonatal blood spots. *J. Clin. Endocrinol. Metab.* 77: 1005–1008, 1993.

27. Brunetti, A., and I. D. Goldfine. Insulin receptor gene expression and insulin resistance. *J. Endocrinol. Invest.* 18: 398–405, 1995.

28. Bundey, S., and S. J. Crews. A study of retinitis pigmentosa in the city of Birmingham. I Prevalence. *J. Med. Genet.* 21: 417–420, 1984.

29. Bunker, C. H., E. L. Berson, W. C. Bromley, R. P. Hayes, and T. H. Roderick. Prevalence of retinitis pigmentosa in Maine. *Am. J. Ophthalmol.* 97: 357–365, 1984.

30. Burnet, P.W.J., and P. J. Harrison. Genetic variation of the 5-HT2A receptor and response to clozapine. *Lancet* 346: 909, 1995.

31. Candeliere, G. A., F. H. Glorieux, J. Prud'homme, and R. St.-Arnaud. Increased expression of the c-fos proto-oncogene in bone from patients with fibrous dysplasia. *N. Engl. J. Med.* 332: 1546–1551, 1995.

32. Challeton, C., A. Bounacer, J. A. Du Villard, B. Caillou, F. De Vathaire, R. Monier, M. Schlumberger, and H. G. Suarez. Pattern of ras and gsp oncogene mutations in radiation-associated human thyroid tumors. *Oncogene* 11: 601–603, 1995.

33. Chanson, P., A. Dib, A. Visot, and P. J. Derome. McCune-Albright syndrome and acromegaly: clinical studies and responses to treatment in five cases. *Eur. J. Endocrinol.* 131: 229–234, 1994.

34. Chessa, L., P. Petrinelli, A. Antonelli, M. Fiorilli, R. Elli, L. Marcucci, A. Federico, and E. Gandini. Heterogeneity in ataxia-telangiectasia: classical phenotype associated with intermediate cellular radiosensitivity. *Am. J. Med. Genet.* 42: 741–746, 1992.

35. Cho, B. Y., W. B. Kim, J. H. Chung, K. H. Yi, Y. K Shong, H. K. Lee, and K. S. Koh. High prevalence and little change in TSH receptor blocking antibody titers with thyroxine and antithyroid drug therapy in patients with non-goitrous autoimmune thyroiditis. *Clin. Endocrinol. (Oxf.)* 43: 465–471, 1995.

36. Conti, C. J. Mutations of genes of the ras family in human and experimental tumors. *Prog. Clin. Biol. Res.* 376: 357–378, 1992.

37. Coon, H., A. A. Hicks, M. E. Bailey, M. Hoff, J. Holik, R. J. Harvey, K. J. Johnson, M. G. Darlison, F. Reimherr, and P. Wender. Analysis of GABAA receptor subunit genes in multiplex pedigrees with manic depression. *Psychiatric Gen.* 4: 185–191, 1994.

38. Coon, H., J. Sobell, L. Heston, S. Sommer, M. Hoff, J. Holik,

F. Umar, M. Robertson, F. Reimherr, and P. Wender. Search for mutations in the beta 1 GABA receptor subunit gene in patients with schizophrenia. *Am. J. Med. Genet.* 54: 12–20, 1994.

39. Cunningham, B. C., S. Bass, G. Fuh, and J. A. Wells, Zinc mediation of the binding of human growth hormone to the human prolactin receptor. *Science* 250: 1709–1712, 1990.

40. Davies, P. R., J. Lawry, V. Bhatia, and A. P. Weetman. Growth stimulating antibodies in endemic goiter: a reappraisal. *Clin. Endocrinol. (Oxf.)* 43: 189–195, 1995.

41. avies, S. J., and H. E. Hughes, Imprinting in Albright's hereditary osteodystrophy. *J. Med. Genet.* 30: 101–103, 1993.

42. Davies, T. D. The thyrotropin receptors spread themselves around [editorial]. *J. Clin. Endocrinol. Metab.* 79: 1232–1233, 1994.

43. Deen, P. M., M. A. Verdijk, N. Y. Knoers, B. Wieringa, L. A. Monnens, C. H. van Os, and B. A. van Oost. Requirement of human renal water channel aquaporin-2 for vasopressin-dependent concentration of urine. *Science* 264: 92–95, 1994.

44. de Pablo, F., R. C. Eastman, J. Roth, and P. Gorden. Plasma prolactin in acromegaly before and after treatment. *J. Clin. Endocrinol. Metab.* 53: 344–352, 1981.

45. Detera-Wadleigh, S. D., S. W. Yoon, W. H. Berrettini, L. R. Goldin, and G. Turner. Adrenocorticotropin receptor/melanocortin receptor-2 maps within a reported susceptibility region for bipolar illness on chromosome 18. *Am. J. Med. Genet.* 60: 317–321, 1995.

46. de Vos, A. M., M. Ultsch, and A. A. Kossiakoff. Human growth hormone and extracellular domain of its receptor: crystal structure of the complex. *Science* 255: 306–312, 1992.

47. Drexhage, H. A., G. F. Botazzo, D. Doniach, L. Bitensky, and J. Chayen. Evidence for thyroid growth stimulating immunoglobulins in some goitrous diseases. *Lancet* 2: 287–292, 1980.

48. Dryja, T. P., T. L. McGee, E. Reichel, L. B. Hahn, G. S. Cowley, D. W. Yandell, M. A. Sandberg, and E. L. Berson. A point mutation of the rhodopsin gene in one form of retinitis pigmentosa. *Nature* 343: 364–366, 1990.

49. Duprez, L., J. Parma, J. Van Sande, A. Allgeier, J. Leclere, C. Schvartz, M. J. Delisle, M. Decoulx, J. Orgiazzi, and J. Dumont. Germline mutations in the thyrotropin receptor gene cause non-autoimmune autosomal dominant hyperthyroidism. *Nat. Genet.* 7: 396–401, 1994.

50. Duquesnoy, P., M. L. Sobrier, B. Duriez, F. Dastot, C. R. Buchanan, M. D. Savage, M. A. Preece, C. T. Craescu, Y. Bloquit, and M. A. Goossens. A single amino acid substitution in the exoplasmic domain of the human growth hormone (GH) receptor confers familial GH resistance (Laron syndrome) with positive GH-binding activity by abolishing receptor homodimerization. *EMBO J.* 13: 1386–1395, 1994.

51. Elias, D., I. R. Cohen, Y. Shechter, Z. Spirer, and A. Golander. Antibodies to insulin receptor followed by anti-idiotype antibodies to insulin in child with hypoglycemia. *Diabetes* 36: 348–354, 1987.

52. Elias, D., M. Rapoport, I. R. Cohen, and Y. Shechter. Desensitization of the insulin receptor by antireceptor antibodies in vivo is blocked by treatment of mice with beta-adrenergic agonists. *J. Clin. Invest.* 81: 1979–1985, 1988.

53. El-Reshaid, K., S. al-Mofti, and N. R. Stepic. Induction of insulin resistance by autoantibodies to insulin receptors following on an acute Coxsackie B4 infection. *Diabetes Res. Clin. Pract.* 25: 207–210, 1994.

54. Endo, T., K. Ohta, K. Haraguchi, and T. Onaya. Cloning and functional expression of a thyrotropin receptor cDNA from fat cells. *J. Biol. Chem.* 270: 10833–10837, 1995.

55. Engel, A. G. Congenital myasthenic syndromes. *Neurol. Clin.* 12: 401–437, 1994.

56. Ewald, H., O. Mors, T. Flint, and T. A. Kruse. Linkage analysis between manic-depressive illness and the region on chromosome 15q involved in Prader-Willi syndrome, including two GABAA receptor subtype genes. *Hum. Hered.* 44: 287–294, 1994.

57. Ezzat, S., M. J. Forester, P. Berchtold, D. A. Redelmeier, V. Boerlin, and A. G. Harris. Acromegaly: clinical and biochemical features in 500 patients. *Medicine (Baltimore)* 73: 233–240, 1994.

58. Faglia, G. Epidemiology and pathogenesis of pituitary adenomas. *Acta Endocrinol.* 129(Suppl. 1): 1–5, 1993.

59. Fairlie, W. D., P. G. Stanton, and M. T. Hearn. Immunochemical characterization of two thyroid-stimulating hormone beta-subunit epitopes. *Biochem. J.* 308: 203–210, 1995.

60. Farrar, G. J., P. Kenna, S. A. Jordan, R. Kumar-Singh, M. M. Humphries, E. M. Sharp, D. M. Sheils, and P. Humphries. A three-base-pair deletion in the peripherin-RDS gene in one form of retinitis pigmentosa. *Nature* 354: 478–480, 1991.

61. Feliciello, A. A. Porcellini, I. Ciullo, G. Bonavolonta, E. V. Avvedimento, and G. Fenzi. Expression of thyrotropin-receptor mRNA in healthy and Graves' disease retro-orbital tissue. *Lancet* 342: 337–338, 1993.

62. Fradkin, J. E., R. C. Eastman, M. A. Lesniak, and J. Roth. Specificity spillover at the hormone receptor—exploring its role in human disease. *New Engl. J. Med.* 320: 640–645, 1989.

63. Francke, U., and M. A. Berg. Genetic heterogeneity in Laron syndrome. *Acta Pediatr. Suppl.* 82: 3–7, 1/993.

64. Franklyn, J. A. Graves' ophthalmopathy and the TSH receptor [editorial]. *Lancet* 342: 318–319, 1993.

65. Fukayama, S., E. Schipani, H. Juppner, B. Lanske, H. M. Kronenberg, A. B. Abou-Samra, and F. R. Bringhurst. Role of protein kinase-A in homologous down-regulation of parathyroid hormone (PTH)/PTH-related peptide receptor messenger ribonucleic acid in human osteoblast-like SaOS-2 cells. *Endocrinology* 134: 1851–1858, 1994.

66. Gammeltoft, S., M. Besser, H. J. Burger, and C. R. Kahn. Principles of hormone action. In: *Endocrinology*, edited by L. J. De Groot *et al.* Philadelphia: Saunders, 1995, p. 17–65.

67. Geffner, M. E., N. Bersch, J. M. Nakamoto, M. Scott, N. B. Johnson, and D. W. Golde. Use of *in vitro* clonogenic assays to differentiate acquired from genetic causes of insulin resistance. *Diabetes* 40: 28–36, 1991.

68. Gejman, P. V., L. S. Weinstein, M. Martinez, A. M. Spiegel, Q. Cao, W. T. Hsieh, M. R. Hoehe, and E. S. Gershon. Genetic mapping of the Gs-alpha subunit gene (GNAS1) to the distal long arm of chromosome 20 using a polymorphism detected by denaturing gradient gel electrophoresis. *Genomics* 9: 782–783, 1991.

69. Gelbert, L., E. Schipani, H. Juppner, A. B. Abou-Samra, G. V. Segre, S. Naylor, H. Drabkin, and H. Heath 3rd. Chromosomal localization of the parathyroid hormone/parathyroid hormone-related protein receptor gene to human chromosome 3p21.1–p24.2. *J. Clin. Endocrinol. Metab.* 79: 1046–1048, 1994.

70. Gerard, C. M., A. Lefort, D. Christophe, F. Libert, J. van Sande, J. E. Dumont, and G. Vassart. Control of thyroperoxidase and thyroglobulin transcription by cAMP: evidence for distinct regulatory mechanisms. *Mol. Endocrinol.* 3: 2110–2118, 1989.

71. Ginsberg, J. Protein kinase C as a mediator of TSH and thyroid autoantibody action. *Autoimmunity* 13: 51–59, 1992.

72. Goddard, A. D., R. Covello, S. M. Luoh, T. Clackson, K. M. Attie, N. Gesundheit, A. C. Rundle, J. A. Wells, and L. M. Carlsson. Mutations of the growth hormone receptor in chil-

dren with idiopathic short stature. *N. Engl. J. Med.* 333: 1093–1098, 1995.

73. Gomez, C. M., B. B. Bhattacharyya, P. Charnet, J. W. Day, C. Labarca, R. L. Wollmann, and E. H. Lambert. A transgenic mouse model of the slow-channel syndrome. *Muscle Nerve* 19: 79–87, 1996.

74. Gomez, C. M., and B. S. Gammack. A leucine-to-phenylalanine substitution in the acetylcholine receptor ion channel in a family with the slow-channel syndrome. *Neurology* 45: 982–985, 1995.

75. Gorden, P.l, C. M. Hendricks, C. P. Kahn, K. Megyesi, and J. Roth. Hypoglycemia associated with non-islet-cell tumor and insulin-like growth factors. *N. Engl. J. Med.* 305: 1452–1455, 1981.

76. Graus, Y. M., and M. H. De Baets. Myasthenia gravis: an autoimmune response against the acetycholine receptor. *Immunol. Res.* 12: 78–100, 1993.

77. Gross, B., M. Misrahi, S. Sar, and E. Milgrom. Composite structure of the human thyrotropin receptor gene. *Biochem. Biophys. Res. Commun.* 177: 679–687, 1991.

78. Gupta, M. K. Thyrotropin receptor antibodies: advances and importance of detection techniques in thyroid diseases. *Clin. Biochem.* 25: 193–9, 1992.

79. Gupta, S. K., C. Gallego, G. L. Johnson, and L. E. Heasley. MAP kinase is constitutively activated in gip2 and src transformed rat 1a fibroblasts. *J. Biol. Chem.* 267: 7987–7990, 1992.

80. Gustavsson, B., B. Westermark, and N. E. Heldin. Point mutations of the thyrotropin receptor determining structural requirements for its ability to bind thyrotropin and to stimulate adenylate cyclase activity. *Biochem. Biophys. Res. Commun.* 199: 612–618, 1994.

81. Gutierrez, B., M. Arranz, L. Fananas, V. Valles, R. Guillamat, J. van Os, and D. Collier. 5HT2A receptor gene and bipolar affective disorder. *Lancet* 346: 969, 1995.

82. Hales, C. N., D. J. Barker, P. M. Clark, L. J. Cox, C. Fall, C. Osmond, and P. D. Winter. Fetal and infant growth and impaired glucose tolerance at age 64. *Br. Med. J.* 303: 1019–1022, 1991.

83. Happle, R. The McCune-Albright syndrome: a lethal gene surviving by mosaicism. *Clin. Genet.* 29: 321–324, 1986.

84. Hargrave, P. A., J. H. McDowell, D. R. Curtis, J. K. Wang, E. Juszczak, S. L. Fong, J. K. Rao, and P. Argos. The structure of bovine rhodopsin. *Biophys. Struct. Mech.* (:235–244, 1983.

84a. Harrison, L. C., J. Callaghan, J. C. Venter, C. M. Fraser, and M. L. Kaliner. Atopy, autonomic function and beta-adrenergic receptor autoantibodies. *Ciba Found. Symp.* 90: 248–262, 1982.

85. Heckenlively, J. R., S. L. Yoser, L. H. Friedman, and J. J. Oversier. Clinical findings and common symptoms in retinitis pigmentosa. *Am. J. Ophthalmol.* 105: 504–511, 1988.

86. Heinrichs, C., C. Tsigos, J. Deschepper, R. Drews, R. Collu, C. Dugardeyn, P. Goyens, G. E. Ghanem, D. Bosson, and G. P. Chrousos. Familial adrenocorticotropin unresponsiveness associated with alacrima and achalasia: biochemical and molecular studies in two siblings with clinical heterogeneity. *Eur. J. Pediatr.* 154: 191–196, 1995.

87. Helmrich, S. P., D. R. Ragland, R. W. Leung, and R. S. Paffenbarger. Physical activity and reduced occurrence of non-insulin-dependent diabetes mellitus. *N. Engl. J. Med.* 325: 147–152, 1991.

88. Hendy, G. N., and D. G. Bichet. Diabetes insipidus. *Baillieres Clin. Endocrinol. Metab.* 9: 509–524, 1995.

89. Heufelder, A. E., C. M. Dutton, G. Sarkar, K. A. Donovan, and R. S. Bahn. Detection of TSH receptor RNA in cultured fibroblasts from patients with Graves' ophthalmopathy and pretibial dermopathy. *Thyroid* 3: 297–300, 1993.

90. Hoffman, E. P., F. Lehmann-Horn, and R. Rudel. Overexcited or inactive: ion channels in muscle disease. *Cell* 80: 681–686, 1995.

91. Hofstad, H., N. E. Gilhus, R. Matre, and J. A. Aarli. Non-receptor muscle antibodies in myasthenia gravis are of Ig1 and Ig4 subclasses. *Autoimmunity* 12: 271–276, 1992.

92. Huang, Z., Y. Chen, S. Pratt, T. H. Chen, T. Bambino, and D. M. Shoback. Nissenson mutational analysis of the cytoplasmic tail of the G protein–coupled receptor for parathyroid hormone (PTH) and PTH-related protein: effects on receptor expression and signaling. *Mol. Endocrinol.* 9: 1240–1249, 1995.

93. Hubbard, S. R., L. Wei, L. Ellis, and W. A. Hendrickson. Crystal structure of the tyrosine kinase domain of the human insulin receptor. *Nature* 372: 746–754, 1994.

94. Humphries, P. A three-base-pair deletion in the peripherin-RDS gene in one form of retinitis pigmentosa. *Nature* 354: 478–480, 1991.

95. Humphries, P., P. Kenna, and G. J. Farrar. On the molecular genetics of retinitis pigmentosa. *Science* 256: 804–808, 1992.

96. Ito, M., Y. Mori, Y. Oiso, and H. Saito. A single base substitution in the coding region for neurophysin II associated with familial central diabetes insipidus. *J. Clin. Invest.* 87: 725–728, 1991.

97. Ito, M., Y. Oiso, T. Murase, K. Kondo, H. Saito, T. Chinzei, M. Racchi, and M. D. Lively. Possible involvement of inefficient cleavage of preprovasopressin by signal peptidase as a cause for familial central diabetes insipidus. *J. Clin. Invest.* 91: 2565–2571, 1993.

98. Juppner, H. Molecular cloning and characterization of a parathyroid hormone/parathyroid hormone-related peptide receptor: a member of an ancient family of G protein–coupled receptors. *Curr. Opin. Nephrol. Hypertension,* 3: 371–378, 1994.

99. Juppner, H., A. A. Bialasiewicz, and R. D. Hesch. Autoantibodies to parathyroid hormone receptor. *Lancet* 2: 122–124, 1978.

100. Kahn, C. R. Insulinoma and non-islet tumors producing hypoglycemia. In: *Current Therapy in Endocrinology*, edited by D. T. Krieger and C. W. Bardin, Philadelphia: Decker, 1983, p. 222–227.

101. Kajiwara, K., L. B. Hahn, S. Mukai, G. H. Travis, E. L. Berson, and T. P. Dryja. Mutations in the human retinal degeneration slow gene in autosomal dominant retinitis pigmentosa. *Nature* 354: 480–483, 1991.

102. Kan, M., F. Kanai, M. Iida, H. Jinnouchi, M. Todaka, T. Imanaka, K. Ito, Y. Nishioka, T. Ohnishi, and S. Kamohara. Frequency of mutations of insulin receptor gene in Japanese patients with NIDDM. *Diabetes* 44: 1081–1086, 1995.

103. Karlin, A. Structure of nicotinic acetylcholine receptors. *Curr. Opin. Neurobiol.* 3: 299–309, 1993.

104. Kasuga, M., and T. Kadowaki. Insulin receptor disorders in Japan. *Diabetes Res. Clin. Pract.* 24: 145–151, 1994.

105. Keitler, P., T. R. Downs, and L. A. Frohman. Impaired growth hormone–releasing signal transduction in the dwarf (dw) rat is independent of a generalized defect in the stimulatory G-protein, Gs alpha. *Endocrinology* 133: 2782–2786, 1993.

106. Kiljanski, J., V. Nebes, and J. R. Wall. The ocular muscle: the target of the immune system in endocrine ophthalmopathy-pro. *Int. Arch. Allergy. Immunol.* 106: 204–212, 1995.

107. Kong, X. F., E. Schipani, B. Lanske, H. Joun, M. Karperien, L. H. Defize, H. Juppner, J. T. Potts, G. V. Segre, and H. M. Kronenberg. The rat, mouse, and human genes encoding the

receptor for parathyroid hormone and parathyroid hormone-related peptide are highly homologous. *Biochem. Biophys. Res. Commun.* 201: 1058, 1994.

108. Koo, B. B., W. F. Schwindinger, and M. A. Levine. Characterization of Albright hereditary osteodystrophy and related disorders. *Acta Paediatr. Sin.* 36: 3–13, 1995.

109. Korducki, J. M., S. J. Loftus, and R. S. Bahn. Stimulation of glycosaminoglycans production in cultured human retroocular fibroblasts. *Invest. Ophthalmol. Vis. Sci.* 33: 2037–2042, 1992.

110. Kosugi S, T. Ban, T. Akamizu, and L. D. Kohn. Role of cysteine residues in the extracellular domain and exoplasmic loops of the TM domain of the TSH receptor: effect of mutation to serine on TSH receptor activity and response to thyroid stimulating autoantibodies. *Biochem. Biophys. Res. Commun.* 189: 1754–1762, 1992.

111. Kosugi, S., T. Ban, and L. D. Kohn. Identification of thyroid-stimulating antibody-specific interaction sites in the N-terminal region of the thyrotropin receptor. *Mol. Endocrinol.* 7: 114–130, 1993.

112. Kosugi, S., C. Van Dop, M. E. Geffner, W. Rabl, J. C. Carel, J. L. Chaussain, T. Mori, J. J. Merendino, and A. Schenker. Characterization of heterogeneous mutations causing constitutive activation of the luteinizing hormone receptor in familial male precocious puberty. *Hum. Mol. Genet.* 4: 183–188, 1995.

113. Kou, K., R. Lajara, and P. Rotwein. Amino acid substitutions in the intracellular part of the growth hormone receptor in a patient with the Laron syndrome. *J. Clin. Endocrinol. Metab.* 76: 54–59, 1993.

114. Kraaij, R., M. Post, H. Kremer, E. Milgrom, W. Epping, H. G. Brunner, J. A. Grootegoed, and A. P. Themmen. A missense mutation in the second transmembrane segment of the luteinizing hormone receptor causes familial male-limited precocious puberty. *J. Clin. Endocrinol. Metab.* 80: 3168–3172, 1995.

115. Kraiem, Z., B. Y. Cho, O. Sadeh, M. H. Shong, P. Pickerill, and A. P. Weetman. The IgG subclass distribution of TSH receptor blocking antibodies in primary hypothyroidism. *Clin. Endocrinol. (Oxf.)* 37: 135–140, 1992.

116. Kremer, H., R. Kraaij, S. P. Toledo, M. Post, J. B. Fridman, C. Y. Hayashida, M. van Reen, E. Milgrom, H. H. Ropers, and E. Mariman. Male pseudohermaphroditism due to a homozygous missense mutation of the luteinizing hormone receptor gene. *Nature Genet.* 9: 160–164, 1995.

117. Kremer, H., E. Mariman, B. J. Otten, G. W. Moll, G. B. Stoelinga, J. M. Wit, M. Jansen, S. L. Drop, B. Faas, and H. H. Ropers. Cosegregation of missense mutations of the luteinizing hormone receptor gene with familial male-limited precocious puberty. *Hum. Mol. Genet.* 2: 1779–1783, 1993.

118. Krishnamani, M. R., J. A. Phillips, and K. C. Copeland. Detection of a novel arginine vasopressin defect by dideoxy fingerprinting. *J. Clin. Endocrinol. Metab.* 77: 596–598, 1993.

119. Kuks, J. B., P. C. Limburg, G. Horst, J. Dijksterhuis, and H. J. Ossterhuis. Antibodies to skeletal muscle in myasthenia gravis. Part I. Diagnostic value for the detection of thymoma. *J. Neurol. Sci.* 119: 183–188, 1993.

120. Landis, C. A., S. B. Masters, A. Spada, A. M. Pace, H. R. Bourne, and L. Valla. GTPase inhibiting mutations activate the alpha chain of Gs and stimulate adenylyl cyclase in human pituitary tumours. *Nature* 340: 692–696, 1991.

121. Laron, Z., A. Pertelan, and S. Mannheimer. Genetic pituitary dwarfism with high serum concentration of growth hormone. *Isr. J. Med. Sci.* 2: 152–155, 1966.

122. Latronico, A. C., J. Anasti, I. J. Arnhold, B. B. Mendonca, S. Domenice, M. C. Albano, K. Zachman, B. L. Wajchenberg, and C. A. Tsigos. A novel mutation of the luteinizing hormone

receptor gene causing male gonadotropin-independent precocious puberty. *J. Clin. Endocrinol. Metab.* 80: 2490–2494, 1995.

123. Laue, L., W. Y. Chan, M. Hsueh, M. Kudo, S. Y. Hsu, S. M. Wu, L. Blomberg, and G. B. Cutler. Genetic heterogeneity of constitutively activating mutations of the human luteinizing hormone receptor in familial male-limited precocious puberty. *Proc. Natl. Acad. Sci. U.S.A.* 92: 1906–1910, 1995.

124. Laue, L., S. M. Wu, M. Kudo, A. J. Hsueh, G. B. Cutler, J. E. Griffin, J. D. Wilson, C. Brain, A. C. Berry, and D. B. Grant. A nonsense mutation of the human luteinizing hormone receptor gene in Leydig cell hypoplasia. *Hum. Mol. Genet.* 4: 1429–1433, 1995.

125. Ledent, C., J. Parma, I. Pirson, M. Taton, P. Roger, C. Maenhaut, J. Van Saude, V. Pohl, F. Lamy, M. Parmentier, G. Vassart, and J. E. Dumont. Positive control of proliferation by the cyclic AMP cascade: an oncogenic mechanism of hyperfunctional adenoma. *J. Endocrinol. Invest.* 18: 120–122, 1995.

126. Leung, D. W., S. A. Spencer, G. Cachianes, R. G. Hammonds, C. Collins, W. J. Henzel, R. Barnard, M. J. Waters, and W. I. Wood. Growth hormone receptor and serum binding protein: purification, cloning and expression. *Nature* 330: 537–543, 1987.

127. Libert, F., A. Lefort, C. Gerard, M. Parmentier, J. Perret, M. Ludgate, J. E. Dumont, and G. Vassart. Cloning, sequencing and expression of the human thyrotropin (TSH) receptor: evidence for binding of autoantibodies. *Biochem. Biophys. Res. Commun.* 165: 1250–1255, 1989.

128. Libert, F., E. Passage, A. Lefort, G. Vassart, and M. G. Mattei. Localization of human thyrotropin receptor gene to chromosome region 14q3 by in situ hybridization. *Cytogenet. Cell. Genet.* 54: 82–83, 1990.

129. Lindstrom, J. Immunobiology of myasthenis gravis, experimental autoimmune myasthenia gravis, and Lambert-Eaton syndrome. *Annu. Rev. Immunol.* 3: 109–131, 1985.

130. Liri, T., P. Herzmark, J. M. Nakamoto, C. van Dop, and H. R. Bourne. Rapid GDP release from Gs alpha in patients with gain and loss of endocrine function. *Nature* 371: 164–168, 1994.

131. Lolait, S. J., A. M. O'Carroll, O. W. McBride, M. Konig, A. Morel, and M. J. Brownstein. Cloning and characterization of a vasopressin V2 receptor and possible link to nephrogenic diabetes insipidus. *Nature* 357: 336–339, 1992.

132. Lowe, W. L., C. T. Roberts, D. LeRoith, M. T. Rojeski, T. J. Merimee, S. T. Fui, H. Keen, D. Arnold, J. Mersey, and S. Gluzman. Insulin-like growth factor-II in nonislet cell tumors associated with hypoglycemia: increased levels of messenger ribonucleic acid. *J. Clin. Endocrinol. Metab.* 69: 1153–1159, 1989.

133. Luttikhuis, M. E., L. C. Wilson, J. V. Leonard, and R. C. Trembath. Characterization of a de novo 43-bp deletion of the Gs alpha gene (GNAS1) in Albright hereditary osteodystrophy. *Genomics* 21: 455–457, 1994.

134. McConville, C. M., P. J. Byrd, H. J. Ambrose, and A. M. Taylor. Genetic and physical mapping of the ataxia-telangiectasia locus on chromosome 11q22-q23. *Int. J. Radiat. Biol.* 66(Suppl. 6): 45–56, 1994.

135. McKenzie, J. M., and M. Zakarija. Fetal and neonatal hyperthyroidism and hypothyroidism due to maternal TSH recepto-recepotor antibodies. *Thyroid* 2: 155–159, 1992.

136. McKinnon, P. J. Ataxia-telangiectasia: an inherited disorder of ionizing-radiation sensitivity in man. Progress in the elucidation of the underlying biochemical defect. *Hum. Genet.* 75: 197–208, 1987.

137. McLeod, J. F., L. Kovacs, M. B. Gaskill, S. Rittig, G. S. Bradley, and G. L. Robertson. Familial neurohypophyseal diabetes insipidus associated with a signal peptide mutation. *J. Clin. Endocrinol. Metab.* 77: 592–595, 1993.

138. Maffly, R. H. Diabetes insipidus. In: *Diabetes Insipidus. Disturbances in Body Fluid Osmolality,* edited by T. E. Andreoli, J. J. Grantham, F. C. Rector, Jr., *et al.,* Bethesda, MD: Am Physiol. Soc., 1977, p. 285–307.

139. Magre, J., A. B. Goldfine, J. H. Warram, A. Krolewski, and C. R. Kahn. Analysis of the insulin receptor gene in noninsulindependent diabetes mellitus by denaturing gradient gel blots: a clinical research center study. *J. Clin. Endocrinol. Metab.* 80: 1882–1887, 1995.

140. Malchoff, C. D., G. Reardon, D. C. MacGillivray, H. Yamase, A. D. Rogol, and D. M. Malchoff. An unusual presentation of McCune-Albright syndrome confirmed by an activating mutation of the Gs alpha-subunit from a bone lesion. *J. Clin. Endocrinol. Metab.* 78: 803–806, 1994.

141. Martinex-Mora, J., J. M. Saez, N. Toran, R. Isnard, M. M. Perez-iribarne, J. Egozcue, and L. Audi. Male pseudohermaphroditism due to Leydig cell agenesis and absence of testicular LH receptors. *Clin. Endocrinol. (Oxf.)* 334: 485–491, 1991.

142. Matsuo, K., E. Friedman, P. V. Gejman, and J. A. Fagin. The thyrotropin receptor (TSH receptor) is not an oncogene for thyroid tumors: structural studies of the TSH receptor and the alpha-subunit of Gs in human thyroid neoplasms. *J. Clin. Endocrinol. Metab.* 76: 1446–1451, 1993.

143. Melmed, S. Etiology of pituitary acromegaly. *Endocrinol. Metab. Clin. North Am.* 21: 539–551, 1992.

144. Mercado, M., N. DaVila, J. F. McLeod, and G. Baumann. Distribution of growth hormone receptor messenger ribonucleic acid containing and lacking exon 3 in human tissues. *J. Clin. Endocrinol. Metab.* 78: 731–735, 1994.

145. Minegishi, T., K. Nakamura, Y. Takakura, K. Miyamoto, Y. Hasegawa, Y. Ibuki, and M. Igarash. Cloning and sequencing of human LH/hCG receptor cDNA. *Biochem. Biophsy. Res. Commun.* 172: 1049–1054, 1990.

146. Miric, A., J. D. Vechio, and M. A. Levine. Heterogeneous mutations in the gene encoding the alpha-subunit of the stimulatory G protein of adenylyl cyclase in Albright hereditary osteodystrophy. *J. Clin. Endocrinol. Metab.* 76: 1560–1568, 1993.

146a. Misrahi, M., H. Loosfelt, M. Atrger, M. T. Vu Hai, B. Gross, G. Meduri, A. Jolivet, and E. Milgrom. LH and TSH receptors. A new family of G-protein-coupled receptors. *Ann. Biol. Clin.* 50: 229–232, 1992 (in French).

147. Moller, D. E., and J. S. Flier. Insulin resistance—mechanisms, syndromes, and implications. *N. Engl. J. Med.* 325:938–948, 1991.

148. Monden, T., M. Yamada, T. Satoh, M. Iizuka, and M. Mori. Analysis of the TSH receptor gene structure in various thyroid disorders: DNA from thyroid adenomas can have large insertions or deletions. *Thyroid* 2: 189–192, 1992.

149. Morgenthaler, N. G., J. Tremble, G. C. Huang, W. S. Scherbaum, A. M. McGregor, and J. P. Banga. Binding of antithyrotropin receptor autoantibodies in Graves' disease serum to nascent, *in vitro* translated thyrotropin receptor; ability to map epitopes recognized by antibodies. *J. Clin. Endocrinol. Metab.* 81: 700–706, 1996.

150. Morris, J. C., E. R. Bergert, and D. J. McCormick. Structure–function studies of the human thyrotropin receptor. Inhibition of binding of labeled thyrotropin (TSH) by synthetic human TSH receptor peptides. *J. Biol. Chem.* 268: 10900–10905, 1993.

151. Mountjoy, K. G., L. S. Robbins, M. T. Mortrud, and R. D. Cone. The cloning of a family of genes that encode the melanocortin receptors. *Science* 257: 1248–1251, 1992.

151a. Mygland, A., O.-B. Tysnes, R. Matre, P. Volpe, J. A. Aarli, and N. E. Gilhus. Ryanodine receptor autoantibodies in myasthenia gravis patients with a thymoma. *Ann. Neurol.* 32: 589–591, 1992.

152. Nagayama, Y., K. D. Kaufman, P. Seto, and B. Rapoport. Molecular cloning, sequence and functional expression of the cDNA for the human thyrotropin receptor. *Biochem. Biophys. Res. Commun.* 165: 1184–1190, 1989.

153. Nagayama, Y., and S. Nagataki. The thyrotropin receptor: its gene expression and structure–function relationships. *Thyroid Today* 17: 1–9, 1994.

154. Nagayama, Y., and B. Rapoport. The thyrotropin receptor 25 years after its discovery: new insight after its molecular cloning. *Mol. Endocrinol.* 6: 145–156, 1992.

155. Nagayama, Y., and B. Rapoport. Thyroid stimulatory autoantibodies in different patients with autoimmune thyroid disease do not all recognize the same component of the human thyrotropin receptor: selective role of the receptor amino acids Ser$_{25}$-Glu$_{30}$. *J. Clin. Endocrinol. Metab.* 75: 1350–1353, 1992.

156. Nagayama, Y., A. Takeshita, W. Luo, K. Ashizawa, N. Yokoyama, and S. Nagataki. High affinity binding of thyrotropin (TSH) and thyroid-stimulating autoantibody for the TSH receptor extracellular domain. *Thyroid* 4: 155–159, 1994.

157. Nagy, E. V., J. C. Morris, H. B. Burch, S. Bhatia, K. Salata, and K. D. Burman. Thyrotropin receptor T cell epitopes in autoimmune thyroid disease. *Clin. Immunol. Immunopathol.* 75: 117–124, 1995.

158. Nathans, J. Rhodopsin: structure, function, and genetics. *Biochemistry* 31: 4923–4931, 1992.

159. Nathans, J., and D. S. Hogness. Isolation, sequence analysis, and intron–exon arrangement of the gene encoding bovine rhodopsin. *Cell* 34: 807–814, 1983.

160. Nathans, J., and D. S. Hogness. Isolation and nucleotide sequence of the gene encoding human rhodopsin. *Proc. Natl. Acad. Sci. U.S.A.* 81: 4851–4855, 1984.

161. Nisula, B. C., G. S. Taliadouros, and P. Carayon. Primary and secondary biologic activities intrinsic to the human chorionic gonadotropin molecule. In: *Chorionic Gonadotropin,* edited by S. J. Segal. New York: Plenum, 1980, p. 17–35.

162. Nothern, M. M., M. Rietschel, J. Erdmann, H. Oberlander, H.-J. Moller, D. Naber, and P. Propping. Genetic variation of the 5-HT2A receptor and response to clozapine. *Lancet* 346: 908–909, 1995.

163. Ohashi, H., K. M. Rosen, F. E. Smith, L. Villa-Komaroff, R. C. Nayak, and G. L. King. Characterization of type 1 IGF receptor and IGF-1 mRNA expression in cultured human and bovine glomerular cells. *Regul. Pep.* 48: 9–20, 1993.

164. Ohno, K., D. O. Hutchinson, M. Milone, J. M. Brengman, C. Bouzat, S. M. Sine, and A. G. Engel. Congenital myasthenic syndrome caused by prolonged acetylcholine receptor channel openings due to a mutation in the M2 domain of the epsilon subunit. *Proc. Natl. Acad. Sci. U.S.A.* 92: 758–762, 1995.

165. Ohno, M., T. Endo, K. Ohta, K. Gunji, and T. Onaya. Point mutations in the thyrotropin receptor in human thyroid tumors. *Thyroid* 5: 97–100, 1995.

166. Kabayashi, Y., B. A. Maddux, A. R. McDonald, C. D. Logsdon, C.J.A. Williams, and I. D. Goldfine. Mechanisms of insulininduced insulin-receptor downregulation. Decrease of receptor biosynthesis and mRNA levels. *Diabetes* 38: 182–187, 1989.

167. Okamoto, T., Y. Ohkuni, E. Ogata, and I. Nishimoto. Distinct mode of G protein activation due to single residue substitution

of active IGF-II receptor peptide Arg2410pLys2423: evidence
for stimulation acceptor region other than C-terminus of G1al-
pha. *Biochem. Biophys. Res. Commun.* 179: 10–16, 1991.

168. Orgiazzi, J., and A. M. Madec. Thyroid-stimulating hormone
receptor and thyroid diseases. *Rev. Prat.* 44: 1184–1191, 1994.

169. Ovchinnikov, I.A., N. G. Abduaev, M. I. Feigina, I. D. Artamo-
nov, and A. S. Bogachuk. Visual rhodopsin. III. Complete
amino acid sequence and topography in a membrane. *Bioorg.
Khim.* 9: 1331–1340, 1983 (in Russian).

170. Pagon, R. A. Retinitis pigmentosa. *Surv. Ophthalmol.* 33: 137–
177, 1988.

171. Parma, J., L. Duprez, J. Van Sande, P. Cochaux, C. Gervy, J.
Mockel, J. Dumont, and G. Vassart. Somatic mutations in
the thyrotropin receptor gene cause hyperfunctioning thyroid
adenomas. *Nature* 365: 649–651, 1993.

172. Paschke, R., M. Tonacchera, J. Van Sande, J. Parma, and G.
Vassart. Identification and functional characterization of two
new somatic mutations causing constitutive activation of the
thyrotropin receptor in hyperfunctioning autonomous adenomas of the thyroid *J. Clin. Endocrinol. Metab.* 79: 1785–1789,
1994.

173. Patel, Y. C., M. T. Greenwood, R. Panetta, L. Demchyshyn,
H. Niznik, and C. B. Srikant. The somatostatin receptor family.
Life Sci. 57: 1249–1265, 1995.

174. Patten, J. L., D. R. Johns, D. Valle, C. Eil, P. A. Gruppuso, G.
Steele, P. M. Smallwood, and M. A. Levine. Mutation in the
gene encoding the stimulatory G protein of adenylate cyclase
in Albright's hereditary osteodystrophy. *N. Engl. J. Med.* 322:
1412–1419, 1990.

175. Porcellini, A., I. Ciullo, L. Laviola, G. Amabile, G. Fenzi, and
E. Avvedimento. Novel mutations of thyrotropin receptor gene
in thyroid hyperfunctioning adenomas. Rapid identification by
fine needle aspiration biopsy. *J. Clin. Endocrinol. Metab.* 79:
657–661, 1994.

176. Porcellini, A., I. Ciullo, S. Pannain, G. Fenzi, and E. Avvedimento. Somatic mutations in the VI transmembrane segment
of the thyrotropin receptor constitutively activate cAMP signalling in thyroid hyperfunctioning adenomas. *Oncogene* 11:
1089–1093, 1995.

177. Puertollano, R., G. Visedo, J. Saiz-Ruiz, C. Llinares, and J.
Fernandez-Piqueras. Lack of association between manic-
depressive illness and a highly polymorphic marker from
GABRA3 gene. *Am. J. Med. Genet.* 60: 434–435, 1995.

178. Reis, A., J. Kunze, L. Ladanyi, H. Enders, U. Klein-Vogler,
and G. Niemann. Exclusion of the GABBA-receptor beta 3
subunit gene as the Angelman's syndrome gene. *Lancet* 341:
122–123, 1993.

179. Rieger, E., R. Kofler, M. Borkenstein, J. Schwingshandl, H. P.
Soyer, and H. Kerl. Melanotic macules following Blaschko's
lines in McCune-Albright syndrome. *Br. J. Dermat.* 130: 215–
220, 1994.

180. Rodenhuis, S. Ras and human tumors. *Semin. Cancer Biol.* 3:
241–247, 1992.

181. Roselli-Rehfuss, L., L. S. Robbins, and R. D. Cone. Thyrotropin receptor messenger ribonucleic acid is expressed in most
brown and white adipose tissues in the guinea pig. *Endocrinology* 130: 1857–1861, 1992.

182. Rotella, C. M., R. Zonefrati, R. Toccafondi, W. A. Valente,
and L. D. Kohn. Ability of monoclonal antibodies to the
thyrotropin receptor to increase collagen synthesis in human
fibroblasts: an assay which appears to measure exophthalmo-
genic immunoglobulins in Graves' sera. *J. Clin. Endocrinol.
Metab.* 62: 357–367, 1986.

183. Rousseau-Merck, M. F., M. Misrahi, H. Loosfelt, M. Atger,

E. Milgrom, and R. Berger. Assignment of the human thyroid
stimulating hormone receptor (TSH-r) gene to chromosome
14q31. *Genomics* 8: 233–236, 1990.

184. Rubtsov, P. M. Structure and gene expression of hormonal
receptors somatotropin and prolactin. *Vest. Ross. Akad. Med.
Nauk.* 12: 19–23, 1994 (in Russian).

185. Russo, D., F. Arturi, R. Wicker, G. D. Chazenbalk, M.
Schlumberger, J. A. DuVillard, B. Caillou, R. Monier, B. Rapoport, and S. Filetti. Genetic alterations in thyroid hyperfunctioning adenomas. *J. Clin. Endocrinol. Metab.* 80: 1347–1351,
1995.

186. Saad, M. F., W. C. Knowler, D. J. Pettitt, R. G. Nelson, M. A.
Charles, and P. H. Bennett. A two-step model for development
of non-insulin-dependent diabetes. *Am. J. Med.* 90: 229–235,
1991.

187. Schenker, A., L. S. Weinstein, A. Moran, O. H. Pescovitz, N.
J. Charest, C. M. Boney, J. J. Van Wyk, M. J. Merino, P. P.
Feuillan, and A. M. Spiegel. Severe endocrine and nonendo-
crine manifestations of the McCune-Albright syndrome associ-
ated with activating mutations of stimulatory G protein Gs. *J.
Pediatr.* 123: 509–518, 1993.

188. Schenker, A., L. S. Weinstein, D. E. Sweet, and A. M. Spiegel.
An activating Gs alpha mutation is present in fibrous dysplasia
of bone in the McCune-Albright syndrome. *J. Clin. Endocrinol.
Metab.* 79: 750–755, 1994.

189. Scherbaum, W. A., and G. F. Botazzo. Autoantibodies to vasopressin cells in idiopathic diabetes insipidus: evidence for an
autoimmune variant. *Lancet* 1: 897–901, 1983.

190. Schipani, E., K. Kruse, and H. Juppner. A constitutively active
mutant PTH-PTHrP receptor in Jansen-type metaphyseal chondrodysplasia. *Science* 268: 98–100, 1995.

191. Schmidt, S. M., T. Zoega, and R. R. Crowe. Excluding linkage
between panic disorder and the gamma-aminobutyric acid beta
1 receptor locus in five Icelandinc pedigrees. *Acta. Psychol.
(Amst.)* 88: 225–228, 1993.

192. Schwindinger, W. F., C. A. Francomano, and M. A. Levine.
Identification of a mutation in the gene encoding the alpha
subunit of the stimulatory G protein of adenylyl cyclase in
McCune-Albright syndrome. *Proc. Natl. Acad. Sci. U.S.A.* 89:
5152–5156, 1992.

193. Schwindinger, W. F., A. Miric, D. Zimmerman, and M. A.
Levine. A novel Gs alpha mutant in patients with Albright
hereditary osteodystrophy uncouples cell surface receptors
from adenylyl cyclase. *J. Biol. Chem.* 269: 25387–25391,
1994.

194. Segaloff, D. L., and M. Ascoli. The lutropin/choriogonadotro-
pin receptor 4 years later. *Endocr. Rev.* 14: 324–347, 1993.

195. Seibold, A., P. Brabet, W. Rosenthal, and M. Birnbaumer.
Structure and chromosomal localization of the human antidiuretic hormone receptor gene. *Am. J. Hum. Genet.* 51: 1078–
1083, 1992.

196. Shankar, R. R., and O. H. Pescovitz. Precocious puberty. *Adv.
Endocrinol. Metab.* 6: 55–89, 1995.

197. Shastry, B. S. Retinitis pigmentosa and related disorders: phenotypes of rhodopsin and peripherin/RDS mutations. *Am. J.
Med. Genet.* 52: 467–474, 1994.

198. Shenker, A. Characterization of heterogeneous mutations causing constitutive activation of the luteinizing hormone receptor
in familial male precocious puberty. *Hum. Mol. Genet.* 4: 183–
188, 1995.

199. Shenker, A., L. Laue, S. Kosugi, J. J. Merendino, T. Minegishi,
and G. B. Cutler. A constitutively activating mutation of the
luteinizing hormone receptor in familial male precocious puberty. *Nature* 365: 652–654, 1993.

200. Shepard, T. H., B. H. Landing, and D. G. Mason. Familial Addison's disease. *Am. J. Dis. Child.* 97: 154–162, 1959.

201. Shimon, I., and O. Shpilberg. The insulin-like growth factor system in regulation of normal and malignant hematopoiesis. *Leukemia Res.* 19: 233–240, 1995.

202. Sine, S. M., K. Ohno, C. Bouzat, A. Auerbach, M. Nmilone, J. N. Pruitt, and A. G. Engel. Mutation of the acetylcholine receptor alpha subunit causes a slow-channel myasthenic syndrome by enhancing agonist binding affinity. *Neuron* 15: 229–239, 1995.

203. Smith, B. R., S. M. McLachlan, and J. Furmaniak. Autoantibodies to the thyrotropin receptor. *Endocr. Rev.* 9: 106–121, 1988.

204. Spiegel, A. M., A. Shenker, W. F. Simonds, and L. S. Weinstein. G protein dysfunction in disease. In: *Molecular Endocrinology: Basic Concepts and Clinical Correlation,* edited by B. D. Weintraub. New York: Raven, 1995, p. 297–317.

205. Suarez, H. G., J. A. du Villard, B. Caillou, M. Schlumberger, C. Parmentier, and R. Monier. gsp mutations in human thyroid tumours. *Oncogene* 6: 677–679, 1991.

206. Sunthornthepvarakui, T., M. E. Gottschalk, Y. Hayashi, and S. Refetoff. Resistance to thyrotropin caused by mutations in the thyrotropin-receptor gene. *N. Engl. J. Med.* 332: 155–160, 1995.

207. Takayanagi, R., Y. Sakai, H. Nawata, S. Nishiyama, T. Ito, M. Kodama, I. Matsuda, and H. Matsuda. Adrenocorticotropin receptor in familial glucocorticoid deficiency. *Nippon Rinsho* 51: 2643-2648, 1993 (In Japanese).

208. Takeshita, A., Y. Nagayama, S. Yamashita, J. Takamatsu, N. Ohsawa, H. Maesaka, K. Tachibana, E. Tokuhiro, K. Ashizawa, and N. Yokoyama. Sequence analysis of the thyrotropin (TSH) receptor gene in congenital primary hypothyroidism associated with TSH unresponsiveness. *Thyroid* 4: 255–259, 1994.

209. Tandon, N., M. A. Freeman, and A. P. Weetman. T cell responses to synthetic TSH receptor peptides in Graves' disease. *Clin. Exp. Immunol.* 89: 468–473, 1989.

210. Tao, T. W., S. L. Leu, and J. P. Kriss. Biological activity of autoantibodies associated with Graves' dermopathy. *J. Clin. Endocrinol. Metab.* 69: 90–99, 1989.

211. Taylor, S. I., D. Accili, and Y. Imai. Insulin resistance or insulin deficiency which is the primary cause of NIDDM? *Diabetes* 43: 735–740, 1994.

212. Taylor, S. I., A. Cama, D. Accili, F. Barbetti, F. Quon, M. J. de la Luz Sierra, M. Suzuki, Y. Koller, E. Levy-Toledano, R. Wertheimer, E. Moncada, V. Y. Kadowaki, and H. Kadowaki. Mutations in the insulin receptor gene. *Endocr. Rev.* 13: 566–595, 1992.

213. Toledo, S. P. Leydig cell hypoplasia leading to two different phenotypes: male pseudohermaphroditism and primary hypogonadism not associated with this [Letter]. *Clin. Endocrinol. (Oxf.)* 36: 521–522, 1992.

214. Toledo, S. P. Spondylar dysplasia (SD)/brachyolmia (BO), type I: search for qualitative anomalies in glycosaminoglycans (GAG) [Letter]. *Clin. Genet.* 42: 213–214, 1992.

215. Tsukaguchi, H., H. Matsubara, and M. Inada. Expression studies of two vasopressin V2 receptor gene mutations, R202C and 804insG, in nephrogenic diabetes insipidus. *Kidney Int.* 48: 554–562, 1995.

216. Tsukaguchi, H., H. Matsubara, S. Taketani, Y. Mori, T. Seido, and M. Inada. Binding-,intracellular transport-, and biosynthesis-defective mutants of vasopressin type 2 receptor in patients with X-linked nephrogenic diabetes insipidus. *J. Clin. Invest.* 96: 2043–2050, 1995.

217. Uribarri, J., and M. Kaskas. Hereditary nephrogenic diabetes insipidus and bilateral nonobstructive hydronephrosis. *Nephron* 65: 346–349, 1993.

218. van Lieburg, A. F., N. Y. Knoers, and P. M. Deen. Discovery of aquaporins: a breakthrough in research on renal water transport. *Pediatr. Nephrol.* 9: 228–234, 1995.

219. van Lieburg, A. F., M. A. Verdijk, V. V. Knoers, A. J. van Essen, W. Proesmans, R. Mallman, L. A. Monnens, B. A. van Oost, C. H. van Os, and P. M. Deen. Patients with autosomal nephrogenic diabetes insipidus homozygous for mutations in the aquaporin 2 water-channel gene. *Am. J. Hum. Genet.* 55: 648–652, 1994.

220. van Lieburg, A. F., M. A. Verdijk, F. Schoute, M. J. Ligtenberg, and B. A. van Oost. Clinical phenotype of nephrogenic diabetes insipidus in females heterozygous for a vasopressin type 2 receptor mutation. *Hum. Genet.* 96: 70–78, 1995.

221. Venter, J. V., and C. M. Fraser. Beta-adrenergic receptor structure, synthesis, antibodies and human disease. *Bull. Eur. Physiol. Respir.* 21: 13–18, 1985.

222. Vitti, P., L. Chiovato, M. Tonacchera, G. Bendinelli, C. Mammoli, A. Capaccioli, M. Giachetti, and A. Pinchera. Use of FRTL-5 for the study of thyroid antibodies involved in goitrogenesis. *Thyroidology* 4: 49–51, 1992.

223. Wajnrajch, M. P., J. M. Gertner, M. D. Harbison, S. C. Chua, and R. L. Leibel. Nonsense mutation in the human growth hormone–releasing hormone receptor causes growth failure analogous to the little (lit) mouse. *Nat. Genet.* 12: 88–90, 1996.

224. Wall, J. R. Extrathyroidal manifestations of Graves' disease [Editorial]. *J. Clin. Endocrinol. Metab.* 80: 3427–3429, 1995.

225. Wall, J. R., J. Kiljanski, V. Nebes, I. Stachura, and J. S. Kennerdell. Should Graves' disease be considered a collagen disorder of the thyroid, skeletal muscle and connective tissue? *Horm. Metab. Res.* 27: 528–532, 1995.

226. Wardle, C. A., A. P. Weetman, R. Mitchell, N. Peers, and W. R. Robertson. Adrenocorticotropic hormone receptor-blocking immunoglobulins in serum from patients with Addison's disease: a reexamination. *J. Clin. Endocrinol. Metab.* 77: 750–753, 1993.

227. Weber, A., and A. J. Clark. Mutations of the ACTH receptor gene are only one cause of familial glucocorticoid deficiency. *Hum. Mol. Genet.* 3: 585–588, 1994.

228. Weber, A., S. Kapas, J. Hinson, D. B. Grant, A. Grossman, and A. J. Clark. Functional characterization of the cloned human ACTH receptor: impaired responsiveness of a mutant receptor in familial glucocorticoid deficiency. *Biochem. Biophys. Res. Commun.* 19: 172–178, 1993.

229. Weber, A., J. Toppari, R. D. Harvey, R. C. Klann, N. J. Shaw, A. T. Ricker, K. Nanto-Salonen, J. S. Bevan, and A. J. Clark. Adrenocorticotropin receptor gene mutations in familial glucocorticoid deficiency: relationship with clinical features in four families. *J. Clin. Endocrinol. Metab.* 80: 65–71, 1995.

230. Weightman, D. R., P. Perros, I. H. Sherif, and P. Kendall-Taylor. Autoantibodies to IGF-1 binding sites in thyroid-associated ophthalmopathy. *Autoimmunity* 16: 251–257, 1993.

231. Weinstein, L. S., P. V. Gejman, E. Friedman, T. Kadowaki, R. M. Collins, E. S. Gershon, and A. M. Spiegel. Mutations of the Gs alpha-subunit gene in Albright hereditary osteodystrophy detected by denaturing gradient gel electrophoresis. *Proc. Natl. Acad. Sci. U.S.A.* 87: 8287–8290, 1990.

232. Weinstein, L. S., A. Schenker, P. V. Gejman, M. J. Merino, E. Friedman, and A. M. Spiegel. Activating mutations of the stimulatory G protein in the McCune-Albright syndrome. *N. Engl. J. Med.* 325: 1688–1695, 1991.

233. Wilders-Truschnig, M. M., H. Warnkross, G. Leb, W. Langsteger, O. Eber, A. Tiran, H. Dobnig, A. Passath, G. Lanzer, and H. A. Drexhage. The effect of treatment with levothyroxine or iodine on thyroid size and thyroid growth stimulating immunoglobulins in endemic goiter patients. *Clin. Endocrinol. (Oxf.)* 39: 281–286, 1993.

234. Williamson, E. A., P. G. Ince, D. Harrison, P. Kendall-Taylor, and P. E. Harris. G-protein mutations in human pituitary adrenocorticotrophic hormone–secreting adenomas. *Eur. J. Clin. Invest.* 25: 128–131, 1995.

235. Wilson, L. C., M.E.M. Luttikhuis, P. T. Clayton, W. D. Fraser, and R. C. Trembath. Parental origin of Gs alpha gene mutations in Albright's hereditary osteodystrophy. *J. Med. Genet.* 31: 835–839, 1994.

236. Xie, D. W., Z. I. Deng, T. Ishigaki, Y. Nakamura, Y. Suzuki, K. Miyasato, and K. Ohara. The gene encoding the 5-HT1A receptor is intact in mood disorders *Neuropsychopharmacology* 12: 263–268, 1995.

237. Yamamoto, Y., Y. Kawada, M. Noda, M. Yamagishi, O. Ishida, T. Fujihira, F. Shirakawa, and I. Morimoto. Siblings with ACTH insensitivity due to lack of ACTH binding to the receptor. *Endocr. J.* 42: 171–177, 1995.

238. Yano, K., A. Hidaka, M. Saji, M. H. Polymeropoulos, A. Okuno, L. D. Kohn, and G. B. Cutler. A sporadic case of male-limited precocious puberty has the same constitutively activating point mutation in luteinizing hormone/choriogonadotropin receptor gene as familial cases. *J. Clin. Endocrinol. Metab.* 79: 1818–1823, 1994.

239. Yokoyama, N., and S. Nagataki. Pathogenesis of Graves' disease. *Nippon Rinsho* 52: 1110–1117, 1994 (in Japanese).

240. Yuasa, H. Y., M. Ito, H. Nagasaki, Y. Oiso, S. Miyamoto, N. Sasaki, and H. Saito. Glu-47, which forms a salt bridge between neurophysin-II and arginine vasopressin, is depleted in patients with familial central diabetes insipidus. *J. Clin. Endocrinol. Metab.* 77: 600–604, 1993.

241. Zakarija, M., and J. M. McKenzie. Pregnancy-associated changes in the thyroid-stimulating antibody of Graves' disease and the relationship to neonatal hyperthyroidism. *J. Clin. Endocrinol. Metab.* 47: 1036–1040, 1983.

242. Zakarija, M., J. M. McKenzie, and W. H. Hoffman. Prediction and therapy on intrauterine and late-onset neonatal hyperthyroidism. *J. Clin. Endocrinol. Metab.* 62: 368–371, 1986.

243. Zhang, B., and R. A. Roth. A region of the insulin receptor important for ligand binding (residues 450–601) is recognized by patients' autoimmune antibodies and inhibitory monoclonal antibodies. *Proc. Natl. Acad. Sci. U.S.A.* 88: 9858–9862, 1991.

13. Cyclic adenosine monophosphate regulation of gene transcription

MARC MONTMINY The Clayton Foundation Laboratories for Peptide Biology, The Salk Institute, La Jolla, California

KEVIN FERRERI VivoRx, Santa Monica, California

ELUCIDATION OF "THE MECHANISM of the hyperglycemic action of epinephrine and glucagon" in the liver began in 1956 (88). In the course of a series of investigations, Sutherland and colleagues found that in response to these hormones glycogen phosphorylase was phosphorylated (75) by a specific kinase (74). This resulted in activation of the phosphorylase, followed by inactivation due to dephosphorylation (92) after hormone withdrawal. These observations were linked to the intracellular production of 3′,5′-cyclic adenosine monophosphate (cAMP) (87) and its activation of phosphorylase kinase by phosphorylase kinase kinase, later known as cAMP-dependent protein kinase A (PKA). These were the first reports clearly linking specific extracellular factors with the cAMP "second-messenger" system, resulting in the activation of specific kinases, all leading to physiological changes within the cell.

This theme of modulating activities by phosphorylation/dephosphorylation cycles is also true for hormonal control of gene expression. In the case of cAMP, several nuclear factors have been implicated as mediators of the transcriptional effects. For example, the cAMP-inducible expression of steroidogenic P450 enzymes is controlled in part by the action of steroidogenic factor 1 (SF-1 or Ad4BP; reviewed in ref. 69). However, the best characterized effectors of cAMP-responsive gene expression are the members of the cAMP-response element–binding protein (CREB) family, which include CREB, activating transcription factor (ATF)-1, and cAMP-response element modulator (CREM). Insight into the mechanism by which these factors mediate hormonal regulation of specific genes has been gained. In this chapter, we discuss some of the advances in our understanding of the structural aspects of control of transcription through phosphorylation and dephosphorylation of these proteins. We also look at modulation of the activity of these factors by other second-messenger systems, as well as by specific protein–protein interactions. Finally, we discuss new evidence for the role of CREB family proteins in two unexpected areas, cell-cycle regulation and memory acquisition.

cAMP-RESPONSE ELEMENT–BINDING/ACTIVATING TRANSCRIPTION FACTOR PROTEINS

Cyclic AMP stimulates the expression of numerous genes via a conserved cAMP-responsive element (CRE). The CREB protein was originally identified as a PKA-regulated factor that bound to the CRE in the somatostatin gene 66, see ref. 63 for an excellent review). Following hormonal stimulation, PKA mediateds transcriptional induction of cAMP-responsive genes via the phosphorylation of CREB at serine 133 (Ser 133) (36). Analysis of the CREB gene revealed the possibility of many splice variants, but only two are commonly found, αCREB and ΔCREB, which differ by a single 14-amino-acid exon (43, 96). The CREB protein is ubiquitous, being found in all cells tested to date, and is therefore the most general mediator of the transcriptional effects of cAMP. Indeed, CREB-like molecules have been described in such diverse species as humans, fruit flies, and hydras.

The ATFs are a group of proteins originally isolated by virtue of their interaction with E1A-response elements within the adenovirus early promoter (40). Only ATF1 has significant homology to CREB, the other ATFs being part of the Jun/Fos family (37). Like CREB, ATF1 appears to be ubiquitously expressed, with no functionally significant splice variants yet described. The major structural distinction of ATF1 from other CREB/ATF family members is the lack of an amino terminal glutamine-rich region (discussed below). Additionally, ATF1 possesses a unique casein kinase II site that regulates DNA binding and, possibly, homodimerization (62).

The CREM proteins are the only members of the family which have functionally distinct isoforms and which show tissue-specific expression. By differential splicing, both repressor proteins (53) (CREM-α and -β) and activator proteins (30) (CREM-τ) are expressed from the same gene. Additionally, use of an alternative intronic promoter generates another repressor form, known as inducible cAMP response element repressor (ICER). Beyond these differences in the activation domains, the CREM gene also codes for two different DNA-binding domains that exhibit slightly different specificities and affinities for promoter elements. The major site of CREM expression appears to be the testes, where it undergoes controlled switching from a repressor to an activator of cAMP-responsive gene expression. The ICER protein is expressed rhythmically in the pineal gland and may function as part of the circadian clock (82).

REGULATION OF PHOSPHORYLATION OF cAMP-RESPONSE ELEMENT–BINDING/ACTIVATING TRANSCRIPTION FACTOR PROTEINS

Since Sutherland's studies on glucagon, many other hormones and growth factors have been shown to stimulate cAMP production. The major steps involved in the cAMP pathway, from an extracellular factor to an intracellular effect, are the subject of numerous reviews so are only summarized here. Briefly, the binding of a hormone such as glucagon to a specific cell-surface receptor results in the dissociation of a heterotrimeric G_s protein coupled to the receptor. The $G\alpha_s$-subunit is then free to interact with and to activate membrane-associated adenylyl cyclase. The cyclase catalyzes the conversion of adenosine triphosphate (ATP) to cAMP, which binds to the regulatory subunit of PKA, bringing about the dissociation of the catalytic subunit from the regulatory subunits. The free catalytic subunits proceed to phosphorylate substrates, which mediate the hormonal effect within the cell.

Cyclic AMP-responsive gene expression results from translocation of the active PKA catalytic subunit to the nucleus. Once in the nucleus, PKA phosphorylates a transcription factor, such as CREB, as well as structural proteins, such as histones (52). About 40% of the CREB molecules are phosphorylated at Ser133 by PKA following maximal stimulation (39). Phosphorylation activated CREB, resulting in increased transcription from genes containing a CRE. Furthermore, the rate and level of transcriptional activation parallel the kinetics and degree of CREB phosphorylation, respectively.

The transcriptional response to cAMP follows "burst-attenuation" kinetics, reaching maximal transcription between 30 and 60 min. The movement of PKA to the nucleus is the rate-limiting step for transcriptional activation, taking 15–30 min to plateau (39). Transcriptional activity steadily declines over the next 4–8 h due to dephosphorylation of CREB at Ser133 by protein phosphatases (PP) 1 and/or 2A (38, 90). This inactivates CREB and down-regulates gene expression.

After about 6–8 h following hormonal treatment, cells become refractory to further cAMP stimulation. This is partially due to down-regulation of the cell-surface receptor, but even postreceptor systems become unresponsive. This refractory period is associated with inactivation of PKA activity by three mechanisms: inhibition of catalytic subunit protein synthesis (6), upregulation of regulatory subunits (76), and up-regulation of the protein kinase inhibitor (PKI) peptide (89). In some cells, cAMP-responsive transcription is further attenuated by the induction of a specific repressor, the CREM ICER isoform (82). Expression of ICER is directed by a cAMP-inducible intronic promoter, which up-regulates its expression with the same time course as other inducible genes (65). The product is a truncated CREM lacking activation domains which competes with other factors for binding to the CRE.

Under certain circumstances, phosphorylation of CREB at Ser133 appears to be sufficient for activated transcription. For example, microinjection of phospho-CREB alone induced expression of a CRE-containing reporter in rat fibroblasts (2). However, stimulation of Jurkat cells through the T-cell receptor (TCR) resulted in phosphorylation of CREB on Ser133 without transactivation (13). Phorbol ester stimulation mimicked the effect of TCR activation, suggesting that CREB was phosphorylated by protein kinase C (PKC). Although PKC alone had no effect, suboptimal doses of the cAMP stimulator forskolin synergized with TCR activation and with phorbol ester to induce transcription from a reporter gene. This indicates that there is a second PKA-dependent event required for transactivation in addition to CREB phosphorylation but with a lower PKA threshold. The observation that CREB phosphorylation is sufficient in some cases suggests that a cell may be primed for cAMP responses by prior completion of the second event. Further studies are needed to clarify these observations.

Other second-messenger systems that activate transcription by phosphorylating CRE-binding proteins at the same site as PKA have been identified. To date, the calcium/calmodulin system is the best characterized of these alternate activation pathways (31). Calcium influx through voltage-gated channels activates calcium/calmodulin-dependent kinases (CaMKs) in neuronal cell lines. Two CaMK isoforms, CaMK-II and CaMK-IV, have been shown to phosphorylate CREB (Ser133) (19, 81) and CREMτ (Ser117) (21) both in vitro and in vivo. Indeed, the calcium-response element (CaRE) in the c-fos gene is equivalent to a CRE and mediates transcriptional induction by both calcium and cAMP. Although both CaMK-II and -IV phosphorylate CREB, only CaMK-IV activates transcription (26).

In another example of pathway convergence, the mitogen-activated protein kinase (MAPK) cascade has been implicated in gene activation through CREB/CREM proteins. In human melanocytes, ribosomal S6 kinase pp90^{RSK}, and to a lesser extent pp70^{S6K}, induces gene expression by phosphorylation of CREB, CREM, and ATF1 in response to endothelin-1, scatter factor, mast cell growth factor, and basic fibroblast growth factor (bFGF) (9). In primary rat cortical cells, CREB is phosphorylated by a ras-dependent protein kinase and induces c-fos expression in response to several growth factors, including nerve growth factor (NGF), epidermal growth factor (EGF), brain-derived neurotrophic factor (BDNF), and bFGF (33). This kinase is estimated to 105 kd and exhibits characteristics of ribosomal S6 kinase pp90^{RSK} but does not co-elute with pp90^{RSK} on an ion exchange column. Similarly, the early growth-response gene 1 (egr-1) is induced by granulocyte-macrophage colony-stimulating factor and by phorbol esters in TF-1 myeloid cells through CREB phosphorylation (54).

MECHANISM AND MODULATION OF cAMP-RESPONSE ELEMENT–BINDING/ACTIVATING TRANSCRIPTION FACTOR ACTIVITY

The activity of transcriptional regulators is a function of two interactions: binding of the factor to a specific site in the gene and interaction with other proteins associated with the gene. Each of these steps can be regulated through second messengers, commonly via phosphorylation/dephosphorylation events (45), to control the expression of various genes. There is increasing evidence that phosphorylation alters the efficiency of transcription by modulating the direct or indirect contact between transcriptional regulatory proteins and the general transcription factors (GTFs) (7) involved in RNA synthesis.

Proteins related to CREB exhibit three distinct activities: constitutive transactivation, phosphorylation-inducible activation, and dimerization with a specific set of partners. Each of these activities is associated with distinct domains and is modulated by phosphorylation events and by protein–protein interactions. It is the interplay between these three domains that determines the specific response mediated by CREB/ATF proteins.

Constitutive Activity: Q-Rich Domains

In addition to mediating a hormonal response, CREB is required for the basal expression of a number of genes (47, 55, 71, 94). This basal transcriptional activity resides in two glutamine (Q)-rich domains, which are similar in composition to the activation domains of the mammalian constitutive activator Sp1 (73). These domains, termed Q1 (amino acids 20–87) and Q2 (amino acids 161–284) in CREB, also are required for the full phosphorylation-dependent activity of these factors. This point is elegantly illustrated by natural splice variants of the CREM gene, which alternate between activators and repressors based on the presence or absence, respectively, of the exons encoding these regions (30, 53, 99).

In CREB, the Q2 domain, which is between the PKA phosphorylation site and the basic leucine zipper domain, accounts for all of the basal activity in the unphosphorylated state. The Q2 domain possesses intrinsic activation potential and can function alone as a constitutive activator when separated from the rest of the CREB molecule (27). Analogous to the Sp1 domains (32), transcriptional activation by Q2 was correlated with binding to dTAF110, a component of the general transcription factor TFIID from Drosophila (44). The importance of this interaction was confirmed subsequently with human TFIID (93) and shown to be independent of phosphorylation. Deletion analysis of Q2 revealed that both the dTAF110-binding and the in vivo transactivation functions are contained within the ten residues between amino acids 204 and 213. This region spans a four-residue motif (leucine–glutamine–threonine–leucine, LQTL), homologous to a region of Sp1 (WQTL), which is required for both binding to dTAF110 and transcriptional activation. By individually changing the amino acids in these motifs to alanine, it was found that it was not the glutamine (Q) but the hydrophobic leucine (L) and tryptophan (W) side chains that were most important for the interaction and resultant activity (32) (K. Ferreri, unpublished data).

The Q-rich regions of CREB, Sp1, and TAF110 appear to define a new class of domain which mediates functional interactions with one another as well as with other transcriptional activators. It was observed that the free activation domains (that is, without DNA-binding domains) of Sp1 could synergize with full-length Sp1 bound at a promoter (17). Later, electron micrographs of DNA looping mediated by Sp1 provided a direct demonstration of the physical association between the activation domains and an explanation for the "superactivation" phenomenon (84). A similar interaction was observed for the Sp1-dependent activity of the BPV-E2 protein (56). We have observed that the Q2 domain is superactivated by the Sp1 activation domain (K. Ferreri, unpublished data), implying that it too is a member of this class of domain. These interactions may be especially important for CREB bound at distal enhancers when there are Sp1 sites located proximal to the transcriptional start site.

The oncogenic tyrosine kinase v-Abl induces transcription from promoters containing a CRE (8). A new type of direct interaction between the Q2 and the SH2 and ATP-binding domains of the v-Abl oncoprotein was demonstrated by glutathione-S-transferase (GST)-pulldown assays and co-immunoprecipitations. However, the interaction did not result in phosphorylation-dependent activation of CREB. This implies either that v-Abl contains a domain that activates the gene when brought into the promoter or that there is another substrate that is phosphorylated, resulting in the increased transcription. In either case, it will be interesting to see if this type of interaction can be generalized to other tyrosine kinases, which may provide another mechanism for CREB regulation.

In contrast to Q2, the Q1 domain exhibits little, if any, independent activity, though it may contribute slightly to the basal activity of Q2 (73). Indeed, the CREM splice isoform containing only the Q1-like domain (CREM-ε), but not Q2, actually represses CRE-mediated activity (12). However, the most notable structural difference between CREB and ATF1 is the lack of a Q1-like region in the latter, and these factors are reported to exhibit markedly different responses to cAMP, depending on the context of the study. Additionally, splice insertion of the Q1 exon into CREM is a regulated phenomenon, implying that it is significant. The exact function of this region is as yet unclear and may depend on a specific cellular context.

Inducible Activity: Kinase-Inducible Domain

Activation of the cAMP cascade results in the phosphorylation of a single serine in CREB/ATF family proteins. This site, Ser133 in CREB, lies within a highly conserved region known variably as the kinase-inducible domain (KID, amino acids 101–160) or phosphorylation box (P-box) because it contains several potential phosphorylation sites for a growing list of kinases, including PKA, PKC, casein kinases-I and -II, and glycogen synthase kinase-3 (21). However, only the PKA site is associated with transcriptional induction, and mutation of this serine to alanine (termed the "M1 mutation") prevents phosphorylation-dependent activation (36).

The reason for this became clearer when another nuclear protein, the CREB-binding protein (CBP) (15), was discovered to bind only to CREB phosphorylated at Ser133. Significantly, it was shown that CBP is required for cAMP-inducible transcription (5) and that overexpression of CBP potentiates the transcriptional effect of PKA mediated through CREB (51). The CBP is a member of a family of transcriptional co-activator proteins that includes the adenovirus E1A-associated p300 protein (24) and an as yet uncharacterized clone from *Caenorhabditis elegans* (4). These proteins are comprised of a bromodomain, which mediates the association with E1A (3); two cysteine/histidine-rich putative Zn fingers; and the KID interaction box (KIX), which binds phosphorylated CREB (59). The KIX domain from each of these proteins binds CREB in a phosphorylation-dependent manner, and p300 also was shown to potentiate CREB activity (51).

However, interaction between phosphorylated KID and KIX is not sufficient for transactivation. The KID is relatively inactive by itself, as exemplified by the CREM repressor isoforms or when attached to a heterologous DNA-binding domain. In both of these cases, the addition of a Q-rich domain restores phosphorylation-dependent activation. Furthermore, other constitutive activation domains can substitute for Q2 in the reconstitution of activity. Importantly, the constitutive activator can be either intermolecular, as with the native CREB/ATF family proteins, or bound to a neighboring site (12). This observation means that CREM proteins which normally act as repressors can be cAMP-responsive activators in the right promoter context.

How does phosphorylation of KID promote the association with CBP and subsequently activate transcription? Initially, we postulated that phosphorylation induced a conformational change in CREB that unmasked its activity. We explored this hypothesis by looking for structural changes by circular dichroism but did not find phosphorylation-dependent changes in the spectra of CREB or the full-length KID peptide. This was supported by nuclear magnetic resonance studies, which indicated that KID was predominantly unstructured, with only a single helical turn on either side of Ser133, and that phosphorylation did not have any detectable effect. Based on the structural analysis, it was likely that the phosphate group directly contacted KIX, reminiscent of the binding of phosphotyrosine by SH2 domains. After thiophosphorylating KID, we were able to specifically cross-link the thiophosphate group to side chains in KIX, thus demonstrating a direct contact (70). This result was confirmed by a phosphatase protection assay in which the phosphoserine 133 on CREB was protected from PP1 or PP2A by binding to KIX. As a control, phosphorylation of the casein kinase-II site (amino acid 151) was not protected. In addition to indicating a specific interaction between the phosphoserine 133 and CBP, this result implies that engagement with CBP may sustain CREB activation by hindering attenuation by phosphatases.

Besides phosphorylation of Ser133, other parts of KID are required for activity. An early study identified a five-amino-acid motif, DLSSD, just C-terminal to the phosphoacceptor, which was also necessary (35), and other regions have been implicated in in vivo activity (73). Binding studies using CREB or KID (amino acids 87–161) and CBP have measured the dissociation constant to be on the order of $10^{-7}M$ (51, 70), but as amino acids are deleted on either side of phosphoserine 133, the affinity progressively drops from 10^{-6} M for the 121–151 peptide to about 10^{-2} M for the tetrapeptide 131–134. A similar drop in transcriptional activity is seen with removal of adjacent sequences but at a more precipitous rate. These data imply that the interaction surfaces between KID and KIX may be extended over more than 30 amino acids. It is not certain which amino-acid side chains are required in addition to those mentioned, but the binding interaction is resistant to high salt concentrations and disrupted by low amounts of detergent. Therefore, hydrophobic interactions are important for stabilizing the complex, once again similar to SH2 domains. Indeed, the single helical turn on either side of the phosphoserine is predicted to bring isoleucine/leucine amino-acid pairs into alignment with the phosphate. Replacement of the distal pair with alanine inhibits binding of phosphoKID to KIX, but the effect of these replacements on activity is yet to be determined.

This region also contains consensus phosphorylation sited for many other kinases which could modulate CREB activity. For example, Sun et al. (85) have demonstrated phosphorylation of CREB by CaMK-II on Ser142 in the $DLS_{142}SD$ motif (85) in addition to Ser133 phosphorylation. Double phosphorylation by CaMK-II inhibits activation by PKA or by CaMK-IV and therefore may modulate CREB activity when the two pathways converge under specific conditions. Both phosphorylation of this site and replacement with aspartic acid inhibit CREB activity but do not prevent association with CBP (86). While the role of CaMK-II in regulating CREB activity is unclear, these observations indicate that the simple binding of CREB to CBP may not be sufficient to transduce the cAMP signal.

There is evidence, for example, that CBP/p300 proteins also may be regulated by phosphorylation. Retinoic acid treatment of the F9 teratocarcinoma cell line induces differentiation and a concomitant acquisition of cAMP-responsive gene expression (61, 78). Interestingly, retinoic acid treatment also results in phosphorylation of both CBP and p300 (49). This parallels the p300-mediated induction of the *c-jun* gene, indicating that phosphorylation of these co-activators may be necessary for transcriptional activation. Phosphorylation of CBP or p300 may be the "second event" required for the transcriptional synergism between forskolin and T-cell activation mentioned above (13).

Dimerization: Basic Leucine Zipper Domain

The CREB/ATF proteins bind to DNA as dimers, so another variable that affects the activity of CREB proteins is dimerization with other factors. A basic leucine zipper (bZIP) domain at the carboxy-terminus provides the specificity of dimerization as well as the binding to specific DNA elements. The CREB-like proteins preferentially dimerize only within their own family, that is, with CREB, ATF1, or the CREMs (42); and despite their similarities, the different dimers appear to have very different activities. For example, it has been reported that ATF1 both mediates (57, 77) and antagonizes (25) cAMP-responsive transcription. This apparent contradiction may be due to the unresponsiveness of ATF-1/CREB heterodimers (46). In fact, F9 teratocarcinoma cells may be refractory to cAMP-induced transcription because a higher concentration of ATF-1 favors ATF-1/CREB heterodimerization (46), and the observed recovery of responsiveness when CREB is overexpressed in these cells supports such a model. However, there also appear to be specific roles for the heterodimer, such as promoting constitutive expression of the Na,K-ATPase α1-subunit (50).

The various CREM isoforms also regulate CREB-dependent transcription by heterodimer formation (29). For the most part, CREM proteins which lack Q-rich domains repress CREB by competition for binding sites or dimerization (53). However, isoforms with KID domains permit partial activation when partnered with

CREB (58) or as a homodimer when bound adjacent to a constitutive activator (12).

Another manner in which the bZIP domain affects CREB/ATF activity is by positioning the factor at specific sites on the DNA. The canonical CRE is the palindromic octamer 5'-TGACGTCA-3'. All members of the CREB/ATF family bind with high affinity (K_d about 5.0×10^{-9}) (91) to consensus CRE sites, which are, therefore, constitutively occupied in vivo; but variation in the site drops the affinity substantially and binding becomes phosphorylation-dependent (67). In terms of gene expression, variations in CRE result in lower basal activity but higher cAMP inducibility.

In addition to CRE, sequences outside of the binding site modulate CREB/ATF activity. Adjacent nucleotides contribute to recognition by specific factors. One instance is the immunoglubulin κ 3' enhancer, which binds ATF-1 and CREM but not CREB (72). Proteins that bind at other sites also can modulate CRE-dependent transcription. Both the glucagon promoter (64) and the lactate dehydrogenase promoter (16) contain CREB-specific silencer elements along with consensus CRE sites. These sites bind as yet unidentified proteins that repress CREB function; but, more commonly, CRE-binding proteins synergize with other factors in the promoter, such as Pax-6 (18), Isl-1 (55), Sp1 (14), and NF-1 (68).

Finally, the bZIP domain is also the target of the viral factors *tax* from HTLV-I (1) and *pX* from hepatitis B virus (60). Tax augments the DNA binding of several transcription factors but shows a marked preference for targeting CREB to the 21-base-pair repeats in the HTLV-I long-terminal repeat region but not to a canonical CRE (100). Tax forms a tenary complex with CREB and the DNA, thus stabilizing the binding of CREB to the 21-base-pair repeat. This stabilization induces expression of the viral genome and may represent the mechanistic switch from viral latency to high-level replication (11). It remains to be determined whether there are cellular factors which aid in defining site specificity in a similar manner.

NEW FUNCTIONS FOR cAMP-RESPONSE ELEMENT–BINDING/ACTIVATING TRANSCRIPTION FACTOR PROTEINS

cAMP-Response Element–Binding Protein/Activating Transcription Factor Factors and the Cell Cycle

The cAMP system has differential effects on proliferation depending on the cell type. In many cells, such as fibroblasts, cAMP inhibits proliferation and induces differentiation. However, in some cell types, such as adrenocortical cells, gonadal cells, hepatocytes, thyrocytes, and others, cAMP induces proliferation, often with a concomitant acquisition of a differentiated phenotype (23). This dichotomy of function has led to the assumption that cAMP plays a modulatory role in the cell cycle. Some studies, however, imply that there may be a more direct role of cAMP and the CREB/ATF proteins in cell-cycle control, at least in some types. It has been shown, for example, that overexpression of a dominant negative form of CREB in pituitary somatotrophs of a transgenic mouse resulted in a specific deficiency of these cells and an ensuing dwarfism (83). Better evidence was provided by the mapping of a CRE in the promoter of the cyclin A gene. Cyclin A associates with cdk2 and cdc2 to control the G1/S and G2/M transitions. Mutation of the CRE substantially decreased cyclin A expression in vascular endothelial cells, and down-regulation of the gene by contact inhibition also was mapped to this site (101). Furthermore, it was shown that ATF1, CREM, and CREB proteins were bound to this site (22) and phosphorylated in Hs 27 cells according to a cell cycle–dependent pattern consistent with regulation of cyclin A. In turn, cdc2 negatively regulates both CREM and CREB by phosphorylation at alternate sites (20). In another study, p300 was shown to be phosphorylated in a cell cycle–dependent pattern (95) in rat kidney cells. T lymphocytes proliferate in response to interleukin-2 (IL-2), which induces a rise in cellular cAMP. It was shown that IL-2 induced phosphorylation of CREB and ATF1 and that rapamycin, which blocked proliferation, also blocked phosphorylation of these factors (28). Overexpression of a dominant negative CREB in thymocytes of a transgenic mouse produced a markedly reduced proliferation of thymocytes and T cells associated with arrest of the cell cycle in G1, similar to the previous observation in somatotrophs. These animals also exhibited reduced mRNA levels of several immediate early genes. These studies indicate a major role of CREB/ATF proteins in the proliferation of certain cells, but other target genes still need to be identified.

cAMP-Response Element–Binding Protein and Memory

The mechanism of memory consolidation involves the strengthening of specific synapses in a process known as "long-term potentiation." This transition from short-term memory to long-term memory requires RNA and protein synthesis (for review, see refs. 34, 80). A role for cAMP in this process has been suspected since the discovery of *Drosophila* mutants with learning deficiency due to changes in either cAMP phosphodiesterase (*dunce* mutant) or adenylyl cyclase (*rutabaga* mutant). This connection has been extended to CREB in three different animal models. In *Aplysia*, 5-hydroxytryptamine, a molecule associated with long-term facilitation, specifically activated expression of a CRE-driven reporter gene (48), showing that this process is at least concomitant with cAMP-responsive gene expression. The transcriptional induction was accompanied by phosphorylation of CREB. In another study, transgenic mice made hypomorphic for CREB experienced a severe loss of long-term memory with no effect on short-term memory (10). This implies that CREB-inducing genes are required for the transition from short-term to long-term memory. A similar conclusion was derived from a study in which a repressor form of dCREB (homologous to the CREM repressors) was overexpressed in *Drosophila*. Transgenic flies experienced a disruption of long-term memory but showed no learning deficit (98). The most exciting result, however, was when the activator dCREB was overexpressed in *Drosophila*. These flies exhibited enhanced long-term memory consolidation, learning in one training session what normal flies failed to learn in ten (97). This is clear evidence for CREB-dependent up-regulation of target genes required for memory acquisition. The next step is to identify these genes.

CONCLUSION

At its heart, regulation of cAMP-responsive transcription is analogous to the regulation of glycogen phosphorylase described by Sutherland and colleagues: activation by phosphorylation, attenuation by dephosphorylation. However, a broad range of responses is available due to activator diversification, generation of splice variants, and interplay between multiple messenger systems.

What is the mechanism underlying cAMP induction of transcription? The answer may lie in the observation that both a constitutive activation domain and an inducible domain are required for the response. The Q2 domain of CREB interacts with TFIID, the general transcription factor that binds to the promoter first and provides a scaffold for the assembly of the RNA polymerase II complex. The Q2 domain may recruit TFIID to the promoter to start the assembly process, thus providing "basal" activity to the promoter. Phosphorylation of KID allows it to interact with the KIX domain in CBP (or p300). Co-activators are associated with RNA polymerase in a large complex known as the "RNA pol II holoenzyme" (41). If CBP is part of the holoPolII complex, phosphoKID would be expected to position the complex at the promoter, increasing the

rate of transcriptional initiation, as observed for cAMP-responsive induction of the *PEPCK* gene (79).

REFERENCES

1. Adya, N., L.-J., Zhao, W. Huang, I. Boros, and C.-Z. Giam. Expansion of CREB's DNA recognition specificity by Tax results from interaction with Ala-Ala-Arg at positions 282–284 near the conserved DNA-binding domain of CREB. *Proc. Natl. Acad. Sci. U.S.A.* 91: 5642–5646, 1994.

2. Alberts, A. S., J. Arias, M. Hagiwara, M. R. Montminy, and J. R. Feramisco. Recombinant cyclic AMP response element binding protein (CREB) phosphorylated on Ser133 is transcriptionally active upon its introduction into fibroblast nuclei. *J. Biol. Chem.* 269: 7623–7630, 1994.

3. Arany, Z., D. Newsome, E. Oldread, D. M. Livingston, and R. Eckner. A family of transcriptional adaptor proteins targeted by the E1a oncoprotein. *Nature* 374: 81–84, 1995.

4. Arany, Z., W. R. Sellers, D. M. Livingston, and R. Eckner. E1A-associated p300 and CREB-associated CBP belong to a conserved family of coactivators. *Cell* 77: 799–800, 1994.

5. Arias, J., A. S. Alberts, P. Brindle, F. X. Claret, T. Smeal, M. Karin, J. Feramisco, and M. Montminy. Activation of cAMP and mitogen responsive genes relies on a common nuclear factor. *Nature* 370: 226–229, 1994.

6. Armstrong, R., W. Wen, J. Meinkoth, S. Taylor, and M. Montminy. A refractory phase in cyclic AMP-responsive transcription requires down regulation of protein kinase A. *Mol. Cell. Biol.* 1826–1832, 1995.

7. Barberis, A., J. Pearlberg, N. Simkovich, S. Farrell, P. Reinagel, C. Bamdad, G. Sigal, and M. Ptashne. Contact with a component of the polymerase II holoenzyme suffices for gene activation. *Cell* 81: 359–368, 1995.

8. Birchenall-Roberts, M. C., F. W. Ruscetti, J. J. Kasper III, Y. D. Yoo, O.-S. Bang, M. S. Roberts, J. M. Turley, D. K. Ferris, and S.-J. Kim. Nuclear localization of v-Abl leads to complex formation with cyclic AMP response element (CRE)–binding protein and transactivation through CRE motifs. *Mol. Cell. Biol.* 15: 6088–6099, 1995.

9. Böhm, M., G. Moellmann, E. Cheng, M. Alvarez-Franco, S. Wagner, P. Sassone-Corsi, and R. Halaban. Identification of p90RSK as the probable CREB-Ser133 kinase in human melanocytes. *Cell Growth Differ* 6: 291–302, 1995.

10. Bourtchuladze, R., B. Frenguelli, J. Blendy, D. Cioffi, G. Schütz, and A. J. Silva. Deficient long-term memory in mice with a targeted mutation of the cAMP-responsive element-binding protein. *Cell* 79: 59–68, 1994.

11. Brauweiler, A., P. Garl, A. A. Franklin, H. A. Giebler, and J. K. Nyborg. A molecular mechanism for the human T-cell leukemia virus latency and Tax transactivation *J. Biol. Chem.* 270: 12814–12822, 1995.

12. Brindle, P., S. Linke, and M. Montminy. Protein-kinase-A-dependent activator in transcription factor CREB reveals a new role for CREM repressors. *Nature* 364: 821–824, 1993.

13. Brindle, P., T. Nakajima, and M. Montminy. Multiple protein kinase A–regulated events are required for transcriptional induction by cAMP. *Proc. Natl. Acad. Sci. U.S.A.* 92: 10521–10525, 1995.

14. Chang, C.-Y., C. Huang, I.-C Guo, H.-M. Tsai, D.-A. Wu, and B.-c. Chung. Transcription of the human ferredoxin gene through a single promoter which contains the 3',5'-cyclic adenosine monophosphate–responsive sequence and Sp1-binding site. *Mol. Endocrinol.* 6: 1362–1370, 1992.

15. Chrivia, J. C., R. P. S. Kwok, N. Lamb, M. Hagiwara, M. R. Montiminy, and R. H. Goodman. Phosphorylated CREB binds specifically to the nuclear factor CBP. *Nature* 365: 855–859, 1993.

16. Chung, K. C., D. Huang, Y. Chen, S. Short, M. L. Short, Z. Zhang, and R. A. Jungmann. Identification of a silencer module which selectively represses cyclic AMP–responsive element–dependent gene expression. *Mol. Cell. Biol.* 15: 6139–6149, 1995.

17. Courey, A. J., D. A. Holtzman, S. P. Jackson, and R. Tjian. Synergistic activation by the glutamine-rich domains of human transcription factor Sp1. *Cell* 59: 827–836, 1989.

18. Cvekl, A., F. Kashanchi, C. M. Sax, J. N. Brady, and J. Piatigorsky. Transcriptional regulation of the mouse αA-crystallin gene: activation dependent on a cyclic AMP–responsive element (DE1/CRE) and a Pax-6 binding site. *Mol. Cell. Biol.* 15: 653–660, 1995.

19. Dash, P. K., K. A. Karl, M. A. Colicos, R. Prywes, and E. R. Kandel. cAMP response element–binding protein is activated by Ca^{2+}/calmodulin- as well as cAMP-dependent protein kinase. *Proc. Natl. Acad. Sci. U.S.A.* 88: 5061–5065, 1991.

20. de Groot, R. P., R. Derua, J. Goris, and P. Sassone-Corsi. Phosphorylation and negative regulation of the transcriptional activator CREM by p34cdc2. *Mol. Endocrinol.* 7: 1495–1501, 1993.

21. de Groot, R. P., J. D. Hertog, J. R. Vandenheede, J. Goris, and P. Sassone-Corsi. Multiple and cooperative phosphorylation events regulate the CREM activator function. *EMBO J.* 12: 3903–3911, 1993.

22. Desdouets, C., G. Matesic, C. A. Molina, N. S. Foulkes, P. Sassone-Corsi, C. Brechot, and J. Sobczak-Thepot. Cell cycle regulation of cyclin A gene expression by the cyclic AMP–responsive transcription factors CREB and CREM. *Mol. Cell. Biol.* 15: 3301–3309, 1995.

23. Dumont, J. E., J.-C. Jauniaux, and P. P. Rogers. The cyclic AMP–mediated stimulation of cell proliferation. *Trends Biochem. Sci.* 14: 67–71, 1989.

24. Eckner, R., M. E. Ewen, D. Newsome, M. Gerdes, J. A. DeCaprio, J. B. Lawrence, and D. M. Livingston. Molecular cloning and functional analysis of the E1A-associated 300-kD protein (p300) reveals a protein with the properties of a transcriptional adaptor. *Genes Dev.* 8: 869–884, 1994.

25. Ellis, M. J. C., A. C. Lindon, K. J. Flint, N. C. Jones, and S. Goobourn. S. Activating transcription factor-1 is a specific antagonist of the cyclic adenosine 3′,5′-monophosphate (cAMP) response element–binding protein-1-mediated response to cAMP. *Mol. Endocrinol.* 9: 255–265, 1995.

26. Enslen, H., P. Sun, D. Brickey, S. H. Soderling, E. Klamo, and T. Soderling. Characterization of Ca^{+2}/calmodulin-dependent kinase IV: role in transcriptional regulation. *J. Biol. Chem.* 269: 15520–15527, 1994.

27. Ferreri, K., G. Gill, and M. Montminy. The cAMP regulated transcription factor CREB interacts with a component of the TFIID complex. *Proc. Natl. Acad. Sci. U.S.A.* 91: 1210–1213, 1994.

28. Feuerstein, N., D. Huang, S. H. Hinrichs, D. J. Orten, N. Aiyar, and M. B. Prystowsky. Regulation of cAMP-responsive enhancer binding proteins during cell cycle progression in T lymphocytes stimulated by IL-2. *J. Immunol.* 154: 68–79, 1995.

29. Foulkes, N. S., E. Borrelli, and P. Sassone-Corsi. CREM gene: use of alternative DNA-binding domains generates multiple antagonists of cAMP-induced transcription. *Cell* 64: 739–749, 1991.

30. Foulkes, N. S., B. Mellström, E. Benusiglio, and P. Sassone-Corsi. Developmental switch of CREM function during sperma-

togenesis: from antagonist to activator. *Nature* 355: 80–84, 1992.

31. Gallin, W. J., and M. E. Greenberg. Calcium regulation of gene expression in neurons: the mode of entry matters. *Curr. Opin. Neurobiol.* 5: 367–374, 1995.

32. Gill, G., E. Pascal, Z. H. Tseng, and R. Tjian. A glutamine-rich hydrophobic patch in transcription factor Sp1 contacts the dTAF110 component of the *Drosophila* TFIID complex and mediates transcriptional activation. *Proc. Natl. Acad. Sci. U.S.A.* 91: 192–196, 1994.

33. Ginty, D. D. A. Bonni, and M. E. Greenberg. Nerve growth factor activates a ras-dependent protein kinase that stimulates c-fos transcription via phosphorylation of CREB. *Cell* 77: 713–725, 1994.

34. Goda, Y. Photographic memory in flies. *Curr. Biol.* 5: 852–853, 1995.

35. Gonzalez, G. A., P. Menzel, J. Leonard, W. H. Fischer, and M. R. Montminy. Characterization of motifs which are critical for activity of the cAMP-responsive transcription factor CREB. *Mol. Cell. Biol.* 11: 1306–1312, 1991.

36. Gonzalez, G. A. and M. R. Montminy. Cyclic AMP stimulates somatostatin gene transcription by phosphorylation of CREB at serine 133. *Cell* 59: 675–680, 1989.

37. Habener, J. F. Cyclic AMP response element binding proteins: a cornucopia of transcription factors. *Mol. Endocrinol.* 4:1087–1094, 1990.

38. Hagiwara, M., A. Alberts, P. Brindle, J. Meinkoth, J. Feramisco, T. Deng, M. Karin, S. Shenolikar, and M. Montminy. Transcriptional attenuation following cAMP induction requires PP-1-mediated dephosphorylation of CREB. *Cell* 70: 105–113, 1992.

39. Hagiwara, M., P. Brindle, A. Harootunian, R. Armstrong, J. Rivier, W. Vale, R. Tsien, and M. R. Montminy. Coupling of hormonal stimulation and transcription via the cyclic AMP-responsive factor CREB is rate limited by the nuclear entry of protein kinase A. *Mol. Cell. Biol.* 13: 4852–4859, 1993.

40. Hai, T., F. Liu, W. J. Coukos, and M. R. Green. Transcription factor ATF cDNA clones: an extensive family of leucine zipper proteins able to selectively form DNA-binding heterodimers. *Genes Dev.* 3: 2083–2090, 1989.

41. Hengartner, C. J., C. M. Thompon, J. Zhang, D. M. Chao, S.-M. Liao, A. J. Koleske, S. Okamura, and R. A. Young. Association of an activator with an RNA polymerase II holoenzyme. *Genes Dev.* 9: 897–910, 1995.

42. Hoeffler, J. P., J. W. Lustbader, and C. Chen. Identification of multiple nuclear factors that interact with cyclic adenosine 3′,5′-monophosphate response element–binding protein and activating transcription factor-2 by protein–protein interactions. *Mol. Endocrinol.* 5: 256–266, 1991.

43. Hoeffler, J. P., T. E. Meyer, G. Waeber, and J. F. Habener. Multiple adenosine 3′,5′-monophosphate response element-binding proteins generated by gene diversification and alternative exon splicing. *Mol. Endocrinol.* 4: 920–930, 1990.

44. Hoey, T., R. O. Weinzierl, G. Gill, J. L. Chen, B. D. Dynlacht, and R. Tjian. Molecular cloning and functional analysis of *Drosophila* TAF110 reveal properties expected of coactivators. *Cell* 72: 247–260, 1993.

45. Hunter, T., and M. Karin. The regulation of transcription by phosphorylation. *Cell* 70: 375–387, 1992.

46. Hurst, H. C., N. F. Totty, and N. C. Jones. Identification and functional characterization of the cellular activating transcription factor 43 (ATF-43) protein. *Nucleic Acids Res.* 19: 4601–4609, 1991.

47. Ishiguro, H., K. T. Kim, T. H. Joh, and K.-S. Kim. Neuron-specific expression of the human dopamine β-hydroxylase gene

requires both the cAMP-response element and a silencer region. *J. Biol. Chem.* 268: 17987–17994, 1993.

48. Kaang, B.-K., E. R. Kandel, and S. G. N. Grant. Activation of cAMP-responsive genes by stimuli that produce long-term facilitation in *Aplysia* sensory neurons. *Neuron* 10: 427–435, 1993.

49. Kitabayashi, I., R. Eckner, Z. Arany, R. Chiu, G. Gachelin, D. M. Livingstone, and K. K. Yokoyama. Phosphorylation of the adenovirus E1A-associated 300 kDa protein in response to retinoic acid and E1A during the differentiation of F9 cells. *EMBO J.* 14: 3496–3509, 1995.

50. Kobayashi, M., and K. Kawakami. ATF-1 CREB heterodimer is involved in constitutive expression of the housekeeping Na,K-ATPase α1 subunit gene. *Nucleic Acids Res.* 23: 2848–2855 1995.

51. Kwok, R. P. S., J. R. Lundblad, J. C. Chrivia, J. P. Richards, H. P. Bächinger, R. G. Brennan, S. G. E. Roberts, and R. H. Goodman. Nuclear protein CBP is a coactivator for the transcription factor CREB. *Nature* 370: 223–226, 1994.

52. Langan, T. A. Phosphorylation of histones *in vivo* under the control of cyclic AMP and hormones. In: *Role of Cyclic AMP in Cell Function,* edited by P. Greengard and E. Costa. New York: Raven, 1970, p. 307–323.

53. Laoide, B. M., N. S. Foulkes, F. Schlotter, and P. Sassone-Corsi. The functional versatility of CREM is determined by its modular structure. *EMBO J.* 12: 1179–1191, 1993.

54. Lee, H. J., R. C. Mignacca, and K. M. Sakamoto. Transcriptional activation of egr-1 by granulocyte-macrophage colony-stimulating factor but not interleukin 3 requires phosphorylation of cAMP response element–binding protein (CREB) on serine 133. *J. Biol. Chem.* 270: 15979–15983, 1995.

55. Leonard, J., P. Serup, G. Gonzales, T. Edlund, and M. Montminy. The LIM family transcription factor Isl-1 requires cAMP response element binding protein to promote somatostatin expression in pancreatic islet cells. *Proc. Natl. Acad. Sci. U.S.A.* 89: 6247–6251, 1992.

56. Li, R., J. D. Knight, S. P. Jackson, R. Tjian, and M. R. Botchan. Direct interaction between Sp1 and the enhancer E2 protein mediates synergistic activation of transcription. *Cell* 65: 493–505, 1991.

57. Liu, F., M. A. Thompson, S. Wagner, M. E. Greenberg, and M. R. Green. Activating transcription factor-1 can mediate Ca²⁺- and cAMP-inducible transcriptional activation. *J. Biol. Chem.* 268: 6714–6720, 1993.

58. Loriaux, M. M., R. G. Brennan, and R. H. Goodman. Modulatory function of CREB-CREMα heterodimers depends upon CREMα phosphorylation. *J. Biol. Chem.* 269: 28839–28843, 1994.

59. Lundblad, J. R., R. P. S. Kwok, M. E. Lawrence, M. L. Harter, and R. H. Goodman. Adenoviral E1A-associated protein p300 as a functional homologue of the transcriptional co-activator CBP. *Nature* 374: 85–88, 1995.

60. Maguire, J. P., J. P. Hoeffler, and A. Siddiqui. HBV X protein alters the DNA-binding specificity of CREB and ATF-2 by protein–protein interactions. *Science* 252: 842–844, 1991.

61. Masson, N., M. Ellis, S. Goodbourn, and K. A. W. Lee, Cyclic AMP response element–binding protein and the catalytic subunit of protein kinase A are present in F9 embryonal carcinoma cells but are unable to activate the somatostatin promoter. *Mol. Cell. Biol.* 12: 1096–1106, 1992.

62. Masson, N., J. John, and K. A. W. Lee. *In vitro* phosphorylation studies of a conserved region of transcription factor ATF1. *Nucleic Acids Res.* 21: 4166–4173, 1993.

63. Meyer, T. E., and J. F. Habener. Cyclic adenosine 3′,5′-mono-

phosphate response element binding protein (CREB) and related transcription-activating deoxyribonucleic acid–binding proteins. *Endocr. Rev.* 14: 269–290, 1993.

64. Miller, C. P., J. C. Lin, and J. F. Habener. Transcription of the glucagon gene by the cAMP-responsive element–binding protein CREB is modulated by adjacent CREB-associated proteins. *Mol. Cell. Biol.* 13: 7080–7090, 1993.

65. Molina, C. A., N. S. Foulkes, E. Lalli, and P. Sassone-Corsi. Inducibility and negative autoregulation of CREM: an alternative promoter directs the expression of ICER, an early response repressor. *Cell* 75: 875–886, 1993.

66. Montminy, M. R., and L. M. Bilezikjian. Binding of a nuclear protein to the cyclic-AMP response element of the somatostatin gene. *Nature* 328: 175–178, 1987.

67. Nichols, M., F. Weih, W. Schmid, C. DeVack, E. Kowenz-Leutz, B. Luckow, M. Boshart, and G. Schütz. Phosphorylation of CREB affects its binding to high and low affinity sites: implications for cAMP induced gene transcription. *EMBO J.* 11: 3337–3346, 1992.

68. Ohlsson, M., G. Leonardsson, X.-C. Jia, P. Feng, and T. Ny. Transcriptional regulation of the rat tissue type plasminogen activatior gene: localization of DNA elements and the nuclear factors mediating constitutive and cyclic AMP-induced expression. *Mol. Cell. Biol.* 13: 266–275, 1993.

69. Omura, T., and K.-i. Morohashi. Gene regulation of steroidogenesis. *J. Steroid Biochem. Mol. Biol.* 53: 19–25, 1995.

70. Parker, D., K. Ferreri, T. Nakajima, V. J. LaMorte, R. Evans, M. Park, W. Fischer, J. Rivier, and M. Montminy. Analysis of a novel phospho-serine recognition motif in the co-activator CBP. *Mol. Cell. Biol.* 16: 694–703, 1996.

71. Pei, L., R. Dodson, W. E. Schoderbek, R. A. Maurer, and K. E. Mayo. Regulation of the α inhibin gene by cyclic adenosine 3′,5′-monophosphate after transfection into rat granulosa cells. *Mol. Endocrinol.* 5: 521–534, 1991.

72. Pongubala, J. M. R., and M. L. Atchinson. Activating transcription factor 1 and cyclic AMP response element modulator can modulate the activity of the immunoglubulin κ 3′ enhancer. *J. Biol. Chem.* 270: 10304–10313, 1995.

73. Quinn, P. G. Distinct activation domains within cAMP response element–binding protein (CREB) mediate basal and cAMP-stimulated transcription. *J. Biol. Chem.* 268: 16999–17009, 1993.

74. Rall, T. W., E. W. Sutherland, and J. Berthet. The relationship of epinephrine and glucagon to liver phosphorylase: IV. Effect of epinephrine and glucagon on the reactivation of phosphorylase in liver homogenate. *J. Biol. Chem.* 224: 463–475, 1957.

75. Rall, T. W., E. W. Sutherland, and W. D. Wosilait. The relationship of epinephrine and glucagon to liver phosphorylase: III. Reactivation of liver phosphorylase in slices and in extracts. *J. Biol. Chem.* 218: 483–495, 1956.

76. Ratoosh, S. L., J. Lifka, L. Hedin, T. Jahnsen, and J. S. Richards. Hormonal regulation of the synthesis and mRNA content of the regulatory subunit of cyclic AMP-dependent protein kinase type II in cultured rat ovarian granulosa cells. *J. Biol. Chem.* 262: 7306–7313, 1987.

77. Rehfuss, R. P., K. M. Walton, M. M. Loriaux, and R. H. Goodman. The cAMP-regulated enhancer-binding ATF-1 activates transcription in response to cAMP-dependent protein kinase A. *J. Biol. Chem.* 266: 18431–18434, 1991.

78. Rickles, R. J., A. L. Darrow, and S. Strickland. Differentiation-responsive elements in the 5′ region of the mouse tissue plasminogen activator gene confer two stage regulation by retinoic acid and cyclic AMP in teratocarcinoma cells. *Mol. Cell. Biol.* 9: 1691–1704, 1989.

79. Sasaki, K., and D. K. Granner. Regulation of phosphoenolpy-

ruvate carboxykinase gene transcription by insulin and cAMP: reciprocal actions on initiation and elongation. *Proc. Natl. Acad. Sci. U.S.A.* 85: 2954–2958, 1988.

80. Schulman, H. Protein phosphorylation in neuronal plasticity and gene expression. *Curr. Opin. Neurobiol.* 5: 375–381, 1995.

81. Sheng, M., G. McFadden, and M. E. Greenberg. Membrane depolarization and calcium induce c-fos transcription via phosphorylation of the transcription factor CREB. *Neuron* 4: 571–582, 1990.

82. Stehle, J. H., N. S. Foulkes, C. A. Molina, V. Simmoneaux, P. Pevét, and P. Sassone-Corsi. Adrenergic signals direct rhythmic expression of transcriptional repressor CREM in the pineal gland. *Nature* 365: 314–320, 1993.

83. Struthers, R. S., W. W. Vale, C. Arias, P. E. Sawchenko, and M. R. Montminy. Somatotroph hypoplasia and dwarfism in transgenic mice expressing a nonphosphorylatable CREB mutant. *Nature* 350: 622–624, 1991.

84. Su, W., S. Jackson, R. Tjian, and H. Echols. DNA looping between sites for transcription activation: self-association of DNA-bound Sp1. *Genes Dev.* 1991.

85. Sun, P., H. Enslen, P. S. Myung, and R. A. Maurer. Differential activation of CREB by Ca^{2+}/calmodulin kinases type II and type IV involves phosphorylation of a site that negatively regulates activity. *Genes Dev.* 8: 2527–2539, 1994.

86. Sun, P., and R. Maurer. An inactivating point mutation demonstrates that interaction of cAMP response element binding protein (CREB) with the CREB binding protein is not sufficient for transcriptional activation. *J. Biol. Chem.* 270: 7041–7044, 1995.

87. Sutherland, E. W., and T. W. Rall. Fractionation and characterization of a cyclic adenine ribonucleotide formed by tissue particles. *J. Biol. Chem.* 232: 1077–1091, 1958.

88. Sutherland, E. W., and T. W. Rall. The relation of adenosine-3′,5′-phosphate and phosphorylase to the actions of catecholamines and other hormones. *Pharmacol. Rev.* 12: 265–299, 1960.

89. Tash, J. S., M. J. Welsh, and A. R. Means. Regulation of protein kinase inhibitor by follicle-stimulating hormone in Sertoli cells *in vitro*. *Endocrinology* 108: 427–433, 1981.

90. Wadzinski, B. E., W. H. Wheat, S. Jaspers, F. Leonard, J. Peruski, R. L. Lickteig, G. L. Johnson, and D. J. Klemm. Nuclear protein phosphatase 2A dephosphorylates protein kinase A, phosphorylates CREB and regulates CREB transcriptional stimulation. *Mol. Cell. Biol.* 13: 2822–2834, 1993.

91. Williams, J. S., J. E. Dixon, and O. M Andrisani. Binding constant determination studies utilizing recombinant ΔCREB protein. *DNA Cell Biol.* 12: 1183–1190, 1993.

92. Wosilait, W. D., and E. W. Sutherland. The relationship of epinephrine and glucagon to liver phosphorylase: II. Enzymatic inactivation of liver phosphorylase. *J. Biol. Chem.* 218: 469–481, 1956.

93. Xing, L., V. K. Gopal, and P. G. Quinn. cAMP response element–binding protein (CREB) interacts with transcription factors IIB and IID. *J. Biol. Chem* 270: 17488–17493, 1995.

94. Xing, L., and P. G. Quinn. Involvement of 3′,5′-cyclic adenosine monophosphate regulatory element binding protein (CREB) in both basal and hormone-medicated expression of the phosphoenolpyruvate carboxykinase (PEPCK) gene. *Mol. Endocrinol.* 7: 1484–1494, 1993.

95. Yaciuk, P., and E. Moran. Analysis with specific polyclonal antiserum indicates that the E1A-associated 300-kDa product is a stable nuclear phosphoprotein that undergoes cell cycle phase–specific modification. *Mol. Cell. Biol.* 11: 5389–5397, 1991.

96. Yamamoto, K. K., G. A. Gonzalez, P. Menzel, J. Rivier, and M. R. Montminy. Characterization of a bipartite activator domain in transcription factor CREB. *Cell* 60: 611–617, 1990.

97. Yin, J. C. P., M. D. Vecchio, H. Zhou, and T. Tully. CREB as a memory modulator: induced expression of a dCREB2 activator isoform enhances long-term memory in *Drosophila*. *Cell* 81: 107–115, 1995.

98. Yin, J. C. P., J. S. Wallach, M. D. Vecchio, E. L. Wilder, H. Zhou, W. G. Quinn, and T. Tully. Induction of a dominant negative CREB transgene specifically blocks long-term memory in *Drosophila*. *Cell* 79: 49–58, 1994.

99. Yin, J. C. P., J. S. Wallach, E. L. Wilder, J. Klingensmith, D. Dang, N. Perriman, H. Zhou, T. Tully, and W. G. Quinn. A *Drosophila* CREB/CREM homolog encodes multiple isoforms, including a cylic AMP–dependent protein kinase–responsive transcriptional activator and antagonist. *Mol. Cell. Biol.* 15: 5123–5130, 1995.

100. Yin, M. J., E. Paulssen, J. Seeler, and R. B. Gaynor. Chimeric proteins composed of jun and CREB define domains required for interaction with the human T-cell leukemia virus type 1 Tax protein. *J. Virol.* 69: 6209–6218, 1995.

101. Yoshizumi, M., C.-M. Hsieh, F. Zhou, J.-C. Tsai, C. Patterson, M. A. Perrella, and M.-E. Lee. The ATF site mediates downregulation of the cyclin A gene during contact inhibition in vascular endothelial cells. *Mol. Cell. Biol.* 15: 3266–3272, 1995.

14. Targeted delivery of hormones to tissues by plasma proteins

WILLIAM M. PARDRIDGE | *Department of Medicine, University of California at Los Angeles, School of Medicine, Los Angeles, California*

CHAPTER CONTENTS

STEROID AND THYROID HORMONES are bound avidly by plasma proteins in a diverse manner among species and these plasma proteins include albumin and specific high-affinity hormone-binding globulins. The functional role of these plasma proteins and the delivery of steroid and thyroid hormones to tissues has been reviewed within the context of in vitro measurements of plasma protein/hormone mass action–binding equilibria. Since the last publication of the *Handbook of Physiology* on this subject, a principal advance has been the recognition that an understanding of the in vivo function of hormone-binding plasma proteins requires a merger of two entirely different disciplines: mass action–binding equilibria and in vivo capillary physiology (Fig. 14.1). Previous *Handbook of Physiology* chapters on capillary physiology did not discuss the role of plasma proteins in the transcapillary passage of steroid or thyroid hormones (40, 123). This chapter reviews steroid- and thyroid hormone–binding plasma proteins within the dual context of capillary physiology and plasma protein hormone binding (Fig. 14.1).

It is important to derive in vivo paradigms for the function of hormone-binding plasma proteins because this component of endocrine physiology is the crucial link between hormonal secretion and action at the end organ nuclear receptor. Indeed, plasma protein binding of steroid or thyroid hormones is the driving force controlling the concentration of cellular free hormone in tissues, and it is the cellular free hormone that determines the occupancy of the nuclear steroid or thyroid hormone receptor, which ultimately controls hormonal action (Fig. 14.2). Hormonal action is a

335

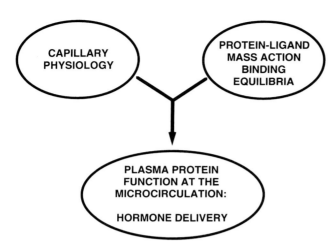

FIG. 14.1. The role of hormone-binding plasma proteins in the targeted delivery of hormones to tissues in vivo emerges from a fusion of two otherwise separate disciplines: capillary physiology and protein–ligand mass action–binding equilibria.

function of nuclear receptor hormone occupancy, and the latter is a function of the concentrations of nuclear receptor and of free (exchangeable) hormone in the nucleus. Since there is no evidence for active transport of steroid or thyroid hormones across the nuclear membrane (see below), the concentration of nuclear free hormone is equal to the concentration of cytosolic free hormone. The cytosolic or cellular free hormone has never been measured directly in vivo since this would require the development of a steroid hormone– or thyroid hormone–specific detection device that could be placed directly into the cell cytosol. However, the concentration of cellular free hormone is a direct function of the capillary bioavailable hormone (Fig. 14.2), and the latter is amenable to direct experimental measurement in vivo (170).

The concentration of capillary exchangeable hormone has been determined, with some exceptions, nearly universally with measurements of free (unbound) hormone in a test tube. An appeal of estimating in vivo bioavailable hormone by in vitro measurements of free hormone is that in vitro methods are easier than in vivo experiments. Moreover, the utility of in vitro measurement is corroborated by frequent clinical correlations between hormonal action in patients and in vitro measurements of free hormone concentrations. The clinical conditions under which free hormone concentration does not predict clinical outcome or the in vivo experiments of transcapillary passage of hormone which show that the hormone flux is far greater than that which can be attributed to free hormone alone traditionally have been dismissed in favor of concepts

embodied by the free hormone hypothesis (53, 213, 217, 233).

There has been much debate in the literature as to how the free hormone hypothesis should be stated. My own view is that the binding or dissociation constant (K_D) governing the hormone/plasma–protein binding reaction in vitro is identical to the K_D that governs the binding between the hormone and the plasma protein in vivo within the capillary lumen perfusing the organ. The free hormone hypothesis posits that, since the K_D controls the concentration of free hormone, the concentration of free hormone measured in vitro is the driving force in controlling the concentration of free cellular hormone in vivo.

The postulates of the free hormone hypothesis are proven invalid when the hypothesis is subjected to direct in vivo empiric testing and when in vivo measurements of the hormone/plasma protein K_D are made. The K_D governing the binding reaction between hormone and plasma protein is a function of the conformational state of the protein around the ligand-binding site. The conformation of the plasma protein is in turn a function of surface interactions between the plasma protein and the capillary endothelium as the plasma protein traverses the organ capillary bed within a single capillary transit. If conformational changes occur

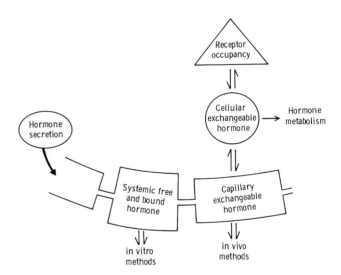

FIG. 14.2. The driving force in nuclear receptor hormone occupancy is the concentration of cellular free (exchangeable) hormone, which is directly proportional to the in vivo capillary bioavailable (exchangeable) hormone. Capillary bioavailable hormone, therefore, is the link between hormonal secretion and hormonal action/receptor occupancy. Although in vitro measurements of free hormone in blood reflect the concentration of free hormone in systemic (arterial or venous) circulation, in vivo methods must be employed to estimate the capillary bioavailable hormone. [From Pardridge (170) with permission.]

around the hormone-binding site on either albumin or the specific globulin, then enhanced dissociation of the hormone from the binding site results, as reflected by an increased K_D in vivo compared to the K_D in vitro. In vivo expansion of the K_D greatly increases the concentration of bioavailable hormone within the capillary lumen in vivo compared to the free hormone in vitro. In vivo bioavailable hormone may be viewed as a free hormone if it is granted that the in vivo free hormone must be measured in vivo. Alternatively, if there is enhanced dissociation of hormone from the albumin- or globulin-binding site in vivo, then the bioavailable hormone may be viewed as being largely determined by the albumin- or globulin-bound fraction of plasma hormone measured in vitro. This terminology, pertaining to the "transport of hormone into tissues from the circulating plasma protein–bound pool," is used within the following context: the transcapillary transfer of steroid or thyroid hormone is much faster in most (but not all) cases than the transcapillary exodus of the plasma protein per se. That is, transport of hormone from the circulating plasma protein–bound pool is a process of enhanced dissociation from the hormone-binding site on the plasma protein. These distinctions are important because it is possible, using in vitro methodologies, to determine the distribution of steroid or thyroid hormones to albumin- or specific globulin-binding sites (Table 14.1).

The distribution of hormone in vitro to the free albumin-, or globulin-bound pools is a function of the binding index of the albumin or specific globulin. The binding index is the ratio of concentration of plasma protein–binding sites divided by the K_D of the plasma protein for the hormone (271). Despite the elaborate distribution of steroid or thyroid hormones to the

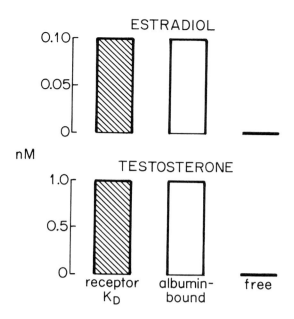

FIG. 14.3. The nuclear receptor dissociation constant (K_D) for estradiol or testosterone approximates the concentration of albumin-bound estradiol or testosterone but is log orders greater than the concentration of free estradiol or testosterone measured in vitro. [From Pardridge (170) with permission.]

albumin- and specific globulin-binding sites, it has been taught for decades that only the free fraction of hormone measured in vitro is available for tissue uptake in vivo (53, 213, 217, 233). The oversimplification by the free hormone hypothesis of hormone physiology is illustrated by comparing the concentration of free steroid or thyroid hormone, the concentration of albumin-bound hormone, and the concentration of hormone required to generate 50% occupancy of the nuclear receptor (Fig. 14.3). A 50% occupancy of the nuclear receptor occurs when the concentration of free cellular hormone is equal to the K_D of the nuclear receptor. The concentration of albumin-bound estradiol or albumin-bound testosterone is, in fact, equal to the K_D of the nuclear receptor for estradiol or testosterone and is manyfold greater than the concentration of free hormone measured in vitro (Fig. 14.3). Similarly, the hepatic nuclear triiodothyronine (T_3) receptor is 50% occupied in vivo, and the K_D of the hepatic nuclear T_3 receptor in rat or human liver is approximately 1 nM (160). Although the concentration of bioavailable T_3 in the hepatic microvasculature is also approximately 1 nM in vivo (181), the concentration of free T_3 measured in vitro is only 3 pM, or 300-fold lower than that required to cause 50% occupancy at the hepatic nuclear T_3 receptor. These considerations illustrate the

TABLE 14.1. *Hormone Distribution to Plasma Proteins*

Hormone	% Globulin-Bound*	% Albumin-Bound	% Free Dialyzable
T_4†	70 (TBG)	10	0.03
T_3	70	30	0.3
Dihydrotestosterone	80	20	2
Testosterone	60 (SHBG)	40	2
Estradiol	40	60	2
Cortisol	75	15	10
Progesterone	10 (CBG)	90‡	2
Aldosterone	10	50	40

*TBG, thyroid hormone–binding globulin; SHBG, sex hormone–binding globulin; CBG, corticosteroid-binding globulin.   †About 20% of plasma thyroxine (T_4) is prealbumin-bound and less than 5% of plasma triiodothyronine (T_3) is prealbumin-bound.   ‡Includes binding to orosomucoid.   [From Pardridge (168) with permission.]

importance of understanding the factors that determine the bioavailable hormone concentration in vivo as the crucial link between hormonal secretion and action.

The different possible mechanisms by which circulating hormone becomes available for uptake by tissues from the capillary compartment may be viewed within the context of three different models of hormonal transport (Fig. 14.4): *(1)* dissociation-limited transport, which embodies the free hormone hypothesis; *(2)* enhanced dissociation transport; and *(3)* receptor-mediated transport of the hormone–plasma protein complex. The latter two mechanisms involve hormonal transport into tissues from the circulating plasma protein–bound pool. This chapter discusses these three models of hormonal transport within the context of in vivo capillary physiology.

ORGAN PHYSIOLOGY OF SOLUTE EXCHANGE THROUGH CAPILLARY WALLS

Quantitation of Capillary Solute Transport: Kety-Renkin-Crone Equation

The Kety-Renkin-Crone (KRC) equation of capillary physiology is as follows (39, 116, 206):

$$E = 1 - e^{-PS/F}$$

where E is the unidirectional extraction of circulating solute by the organ, PS is the microvascular permeability–surface area product, and F is organ blood flow. The units of PS and F are milliliters per minute per gram, and E is a dimensionless fraction. The units of S are centimeters squared per gram of organ, and the units of P are centimeters per minute. The capillary surface area (S) is a function of the average length of the capillary and the extent of capillary recruitment, that is, the fraction of total capillaries perfused under a given physiological state. The permeability coefficient (P) is a function of the intrinsic diffusibility of the solute through the limiting membrane, which is the capillary endothelium in most organs but is the hepatocyte plasma membrane in liver. Organ blood flow (F) is a function of the capillary volume (centimeters cubed per gram) and the capillary transit time (t, min).

Capillary Geometry, Organ Blood Flow, and Capillary Transit Times

The organ-specific microvascular architecture was reviewed in the 1984 *Handbook of Physiology* (274). The angioarchitecture of a given organ has evolved to suit the particular functional needs of that organ. For example, the microvessels in brain are highly anasto-

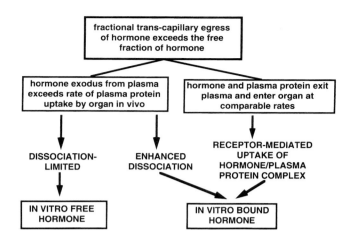

FIG. 14.4. Delivery of hormones to tissues in vivo from the circulating plasma protein–bound pool may be viewed within the context of three distinct models: the dissociation-limited model, the enhanced dissociation model, and the model of receptor-mediated uptake of hormone–plasma protein complex. If the latter two models are operative, then the cellular free hormone is predicted by in vitro measurements of plasma protein–bound hormone. Conversely, when the dissociation-limited model is operative, free cellular hormone is predicted by the free hormone measured in vitro.

mosed and form a complex three-dimensional network, and this architecture allows for immediate equilibration of oxygen throughout the brain. Conversely, the capillaries in skeletal muscle and heart are highly longitudinal in architecture and run parallel to the skeletal muscle fibers. Therefore, capillaries are somewhat longer in cardiac or skeletal muscle and may have average lengths ranging 500–1000 μm (95). The capillary length in brain is shorter, with an average length of 300 μm (104, 105).

Capillary length, plasma velocity, and the solute diffusion coefficient (D, centimeters squared per second) combine to determine the axial dispersion of solute within the microvessel. The KRC equation assumes that axial dispersion effects are negligible and that, under most conditions, the relative values of the solute diffusion coefficient, the plasma velocity, and the capillary length are such as to make axial dispersion equal to approximately zero (125). For example, a typical diffusion coefficient (D) for a small molecule is 3.7×10^{-5} cm^2/s (124). Given a capillary length (l) in brain of 300 μm (0.03 cm) and a plasma velocity (v) of 1,000 μm/s (0.1 cm/s) (124), it can be shown that D$\ll v \times l$. Therefore, convection dominates axial diffusion. The KRC equation has been referred to as the parallel tube (or sinusoidal) model (282), as opposed to a distributed model that accounts for axial dispersion effects (9, 63), or a dispersion model that accounts for convection, axial dispersion, and metabolism (214). When the PS/F ratio is less than or equal to approximately 0.2, the KRC model reduces to $E = PS/(PS + F)$, which is referred to as the well-stirred (or venous equilibrium) model (166, 230).

Erythrocyte velocity in resting dog muscle is approximately 500 μ/s, with a transit time of 3.3 s (Table 14.2). During progressive increases in skeletal muscle exercise, from 0 to 8 twitches/s, red cell velocity increases over 20–fold and transit time decreases to 95 ms (Table 14.2). Since the oxygen release time varies from approximately 50 to 100 ms (94), capillary transit time in a maximally stimulated skeletal muscle decreases to the shortest possible time that allows for oxygenation of the tissue. The data in Table 14.2 illustrate that erythrocyte transit time in skeletal muscle is a function of capillary length and red cell velocity through the capillary (208). In general, plasma transit time in a given organ is slower than erythrocyte transit time, and this accounts for the lower hematocrit in the capillary compartment compared to the arterial compartment (43, 118).

Blood flow is a function of both blood transit time (Table 14.2) and capillary density, as reflected in the capillary surface area. The capillary surface areas in brain, heart, and lung are estimated to be 150, 500, and 3,000 cm^2/g, respectively (207). Capillary surface areas in kidney are estimated to be 1200 cm^2/g for the tubular microvasculature and 50 cm^2/g for the glomerular microvasculature (40). These combined effects of organ-specific capillary surface area, capillary density, and blood flow transit time account for the wide variations in resting organ blood flow (Table 14.3).

tial space (77), the microvascular endothelium of most organs is endowed with a small-pore system that tends to exclude large molecules but permit the rapid passage of small molecules (40, 123). The two pathways of solute transport across the endothelial barrier are the paracellular pathway through leaky junctions between endothelial cells and a transcellular pathway through either micro-pinocytotic vesicles or fenestrations. However, microvascular permeability to large molecules, such as albumin, is essentially the same in fenestrated capillaries (for example, in the small intestine) as in continuous capillaries (for example, in skeletal muscle). Since albumin has a molecular size of 36 Å (195), this observation suggests that if the fenestra do have pores, these are smaller than 36 Å and do not allow for more favorable transport of large proteins through the walls of fenestrated capillaries as compared to continuous capillaries. Unidirectional extractions of raffinose, which has a molecular size of 5.7 Å; inulin, which has a molecular size of 15 Å; and β-lactoglobulin, which has a molecular size of 28 Å, have been measured in feline intestine and are 0.63, 0.41, and 0.07, respectively (196). Therefore, solutes are transported through relatively small pores that exclude molecules such as β-lactoglobulin with a size of 28 Å. The small pores in pulmonary capillaries are permeable to molecules such as cytochrome C, which has a size of 15 Å, but not to horseradish peroxidase, which has a size of 30 Å (195). In brain, the pores for solute exchange are even smaller and resist the free diffusion of molecules as small as urea.

The small effective radius of microvascular endothelial pores allows for selective transport of small molecules relative to plasma proteins. Therefore, it is not

Capillary Membrane Permeability

Differential Capillary Transport of Large and Small Molecules. With the exception of organs such as liver, wherein the sinusoidal microvessels contain large pores that allow for instantaneous equilibration of large molecules (for example, plasma proteins) with the intersti-

TABLE 14.2. *Capillary Flow Parameters in Dog Gracilis Muscle*

Condition	Blood Flow (ml/min/g)	RBC-Velocity (μ/s)	Transit Time (ms)	Perfused Capillaries (number/mm^2)
Rest	0.05	500	3340	510
4 Twitches/s	0.75	4000	330	1050
8 Twitches/s	1.30	11,000	95	615

RBC, red blood cell. [From Honig and Odoroff (94) with permission.]

TABLE 14.3. *Organ Blood Flow in the Rat* *

Organ	Weight (g/wet weight)	Flow (ml/min/g)
Kidney	2.52	6.98
Heart	1.18	3.30
Spleen	0.97	1.41
Liver	13.95	1.40
Intestine	10.38	1.31
Lung	1.77	1.22
Stomach	1.57	0.94
Brain	1.93	0.89
Pancreas	0.62	0.85
Testis	2.95	0.24
Skin	23.3	0.15
Muscle	22.9	0.12

* Conscious male Wistar rats (387 ± 8 g). [From Ishise et al. (103) with permission.]

possible for hormones to escape from the circulation into the organ as a complex with the plasma protein unless there is a specific mechanism for transport of the plasma protein per se. As discussed later in this chapter, such mechanisms do exist for binding proteins such as sex hormone–binding globulin (SHBG) in organs such as the prostate gland or testis.

Extravascular Plasma Protein. The small pores present in microvascular endothelial barriers exclude the transport of plasma proteins, such as albumin or globulin, relative to the rapid rate of transport of small solutes, such as steroid or thyroid hormones. However, plasma proteins do undergo slow exodus from the plasma compartment (44). For example, the *PS* product for albumin in rabbit lung is approximately 2 μl/min/g (114), about 0.1% of the blood flow through that organ. The *PS* product for albumin or globulins in dog hind paw is on the order of 0.1 μl/min/g (10). The protein concentration in the organ interstitium is relatively low compared to plasma because of the dual effects of slow exodus from the plasma compartment into the interstitium and unidirectional movement of plasma proteins into lymph microvessels through one-way valves in the walls of lymph capillaries. Therefore, while a significant amount of body plasma protein is in the extravascular compartment, this protein is largely confined to the space within lymphatic microvessels. While the vascular pool of plasma protein is recycled once per minute, the extravascular pool of plasma protein, that is, the lymphatic pool, is recycled approximately once per day (215). For example, the $t_{1/2}$ of transport of vitamin D–binding protein (DBP), a plasma globulin, into the rat lymphatic system is approximately 15 h (49).

Carrier-Mediated Transport of Thyroid Hormones. Small molecules, such as unbound steroid or thyroid hormones, traverse capillary barriers in most organs via free diffusion through the small-pore system in the endothelial membrane. Owing to the lipid solubility of steroid hormones, these molecules also may undergo a transcellular route of exchange across the capillary barrier via lipid-mediated transport through the endothelial plasma membrane. Thyroid hormones have relatively high lipid/water partition coefficients measured in vitro owing to the lipophilic qualities of the large iodine moieties on thyroxine (T_4) or T_3. However, bulky iodine substituents also retard the free diffusion of iodothyronine through lipid membranes. Therefore, there is minimal free diffusion of T_4 and T_3 through capillary barriers in organs that lack a small-pore pathway for solute exchange. These organs include brain or maternal placenta, wherein the brain capillary endo-

thelium or the syncytiotrophoblast cellular barriers have epithelium-like tight junctions that eliminate the small-pore system (21, 59). In the liver, the hepatocyte plasma membrane acts as the effective capillary barrier, and there is no small-pore system in the hepatocyte plasma membrane for hydrophilic solute exchange (77).

In brain, T_4 and T_3 are transported through the capillary endothelial wall, which makes up the blood–brain barrier (BBB) in vivo, via carrier-mediated transport. Early studies showed that the brain/plasma ratio of T_3 was saturable in the dog (80). Subsequent studies in the rat showed that the BBB transport of T_3 was indeed saturable, with a Michaelis-Menten half-saturation constant (K_m) of 1.1 μM, and that T_4 competed for the BBB T_3 carrier, with an inhibition constant (K_i) of 2.6 μM (167). The maximal velocity (V_{max}) of the BBB T_3 carrier is approximately 0.2 nmol/min/g, which is relatively low compared to the V_{max} of carrier-mediated amino-acid transport through the BBB (169). The BBB T_3 carrier is bi-directional and facilitates the brain-to-blood transport of T_3 (167). The BBB transport of T_3 was not inhibited by high concentrations of large neutral amino acids, such as tyrosine or leucine (167). These results indicate that the BBB T_3 carrier is separate from the lower-affinity/higher-capacity BBB neutral amino-acid transporter (169). The BBB T_3 carrier is also sharply stereospecific as the affinity of the carrier for D-T_3 is ninefold lower than that for L-T_3 (254). Indeed, the stereospecificity of BBB carrier-mediated transport of T_3 may be the principal factor underlying the stereospecificity of L- and D-T_3 as therapeutics in humans. Binding of T_3 either to the nuclear T_3 receptor or to thyroxine-binding globulin (TBG) is not stereospecific (229). Intrathecal administration of T_3 causes a greater restoration of heart rate in hypothyroid rats as compared to intravenously administered hormone (74), which indicates that the central nervous system (CNS) is the principal site of thyroid hormone action with respect to the cardiovascular system. Since T_3 entry into the CNS is a function of the stereospecific BBB T_3 carrier (167), the stereospecificity of this transport process may underlie the stereospecificity of T_3 as a therapeutic in non-brain organs, such as the cardiovascular system.

The evidence for a saturable carrier-mediated transport system for T_3 and T_4 in liver is not as clear as it is in brain. Transport of T_3 into liver is not saturable in vivo (185). Although T_3 uptake in isolated hepatocytes is saturable (52), T_3 readily equilibrates across the hepatocyte plasma membrane and then binds to saturable intracellular binding sites. The failure to experimentally separate transmembrane transport from postmembrane or cytosolic binding may cause a misinterpretation of saturable cytosolic binding as evidence for a saturable cell membrane transport step. Careful measurements of T_3 transport in isolated hepatocytes using an alkaline wash stop technique led to the recording of a saturable, phloretin-sensitive transport system for T_3 entry into hepatocytes (14). The binding constants with respect to the K_m for T_3 transport and the K_i for T_4 or D-T_3 transport in the hepatocyte system are similar to those observed in vivo at the BBB. Thus, T_3 movement across the hepatocyte plasma membrane may be carrier-mediated, similar to that across the BBB. The inability to detect saturability of liver uptake of T_3 in vivo is not incompatible with carrier-mediated transport. For example, glucose undergoes transport across the hepatocyte plasma membrane via carrier-mediated transport on the GLUT2 glucose transporter isoform (258). However, glucose transport into the liver is not saturable in vivo unless extremely high concentrations of glucose are used (36). The very high transport K_m for D-glucose or T_3 at the hepatocyte plasma membrane in vivo may be a function of the kinetic constants that comprise the K_m (34):

$$K_m = \frac{k_{off} + k_{mob}}{k_{on}}$$

where k_{off} and k_{on} are the hormone/carrier dissociation and association rate constants, respectively, and k_{mob} is the rate constant of carrier mobility through the plasma membrane. If $k_{off} \gg k_{mob}$ (as in isolated liver cells in vitro), then $K_m = k_{off}/k_{on}$ and K_m is a true affinity constant. However, if $k_{mob} \gg k_{off}$ (for example, in vivo), then the in vivo K_m may be very high, being dominated by the k_{mob} and giving the appearance of nonsaturability (173).

Lipid-Mediated Transport of Steroid Hormones.

Steroid hormones are lipid-soluble small molecules that traverse biological membranes via lipid mediation in proportion to the lipid solubility of the hormone (184). Steroid hormones are bound actively by cytosolic proteins, and the in vitro measurement of cellular uptake of steroid hormones may be saturable if the experimental design does not separate plasma membrane transport from postmembrane binding. When this separation is done, steroid hormone transport across biological membranes in cells in culture or in vivo is nonsaturable (73, 117, 136, 153). The relative rank order of steroid hormone transport through the BBB in vivo is a function of the number of hydrogen bonds the steroid hormone molecule forms with solvent water (Fig. 14.5). In general, solute transport through biological membranes decreases a log order with each pair of hydrogen bonds formed between the small molecule and solvent water (184). The number of hydrogen bonds formed

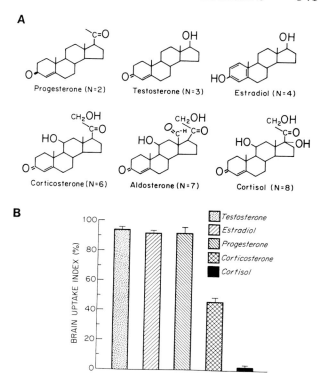

FIG. 14.5. A: Structures of steroid hormones with emphasis on the polar function of groups that form hydrogen bonds with water. The hydrogen bond number (N) is given in parentheses and is equal to the total number of hydrogen bonds formed between solvent water and the individual steroid molecule. B: Brain uptake index of five different [^{3}H]-labeled steroid hormones is shown as means ± SE ($n = 3-5$ rats per point). [From Pardridge (168) and Pardridge and Mietus (184) with permission.]

by steroid hormones with solvent water may be determined from the structure of the molecule using classical rules for hydrogen bonding (239). For example, hydroxyl groups and primary amine groups form two hydrogen bonds with water; secondary amines, carbonyls, and nitriles form one hydrogen bond with water; esters form half-hydrogen bonds; and ethers form zero hydrogen bonds with water. These properties reinforce the idea of Pauling (45): "The significance of the hydrogen bond for physiology is greater than that of any other single structural feature."

CAPILLARY PHYSIOLOGY OF STEROID AND THYROID HORMONE TRANSPORT

Plasma Protein–Binding Kinetics

The K_D values for T_4, T_3, cortisol, testosterone, and estradiol binding to different plasma proteins are given in Table 14.4: $K_D = k_{off}/k_{on}$ (k_{off} units = s^{-1}, k_{on} units

TABLE 14.4. *Rate Constants of Steroid and Thyroid Hormone Dissociation and Association With Plasma Proteins* *

Hormone	Protein	K_D	$t_{1/2}^{diss}$ (s)	k_{off} (s^{-1})	k_{on} ($M^{-1}s^{-1}$)	[C]	$k_{on}[C]$ (s^{-1})
T_4	TBG	0.05 nM	39	0.018	3.6×10^8	250 nM	>80
	Prealbumin	2.3 nM	8	0.087	3.8×10^7	3.4 μM	>100
	HSA	0.6 μM	~0.1	~6.9	1.2×10^7	740 μM	>8000
T_3	TBG	1 nM	4	0.17	1.7×10^8	250 nM	>40
	HSA	4 μM	<1	>0.7	$>2 \times 10^5$	740 μM	>150
Cortisol	CBG	25 nM	0.79	0.88	3.5×10^7	850 nM	>30
Testosterone	SHBG	0.6 nM	22	0.032	5.3×10^7	80 nM	>4
	HSA	28 μM	<0.1	>6.9	$>2.5 \times 10^5$	740 μM	>200
Estradiol	SHBG	2 nM	≤7	>0.1	$>5 \times 10^7$	80 nM	>4

* T_4, thyroxine; T_3, triiodothyronine; TBG, thyroid hormone–binding globulin; HSA, human serum albumin; CBG, corticosteroid–binding globulin; SHBG, sex hormone–binding globulin. $k_{off} = (0.693)/t_{1/2}^{diss}$; $k_{on} = k_{off}/K_D$. K_D values are from references 24, 240, 269. Dissociation half-times ($t_{1/2}^{diss}$) are from references 90, 92, 93, 243.

$= M^{-1} \cdot s^{-1}$); $k_{off} = (0.693)/t_{1/2}^{diss}$, where $0.693 = \ln 2$, and $t_{1/2}^{diss}$ = half-time of hormone dissociation from the binding protein at a given temperature. The k_{on} values in Table 14.4 were calculated from the experimentally determined K_D and k_{off} values. The concentration [C] of binding protein in human plasma is given in Table 14.4, with the product of $k_{on}[C]$ given in the final column. This latter parameter is the rate constant of hormone association with the binding protein and is a dual function of the k_{on} and the binding protein concentration. The data in Table 14.4 show that, in general, the k_{on} value ranges from 10^7 to 10^8 $M^{-1}s^{-1}$. In T_3 or testosterone binding to human serum albumin (HSA), the k_{on} values given in Table 14.4 are minimal estimates since the k_{off} values are too fast to measure experimentally. The finding that the k_{on} values are in the 10^7–10^8 $M^{-1}s^{-1}$ range is in accord with the generally observed observation regarding protein/ligand-binding reactions, that differences in K_D are controlled by differences in k_{off}, not k_{on}. The k_{on} value tends to be diffusion-limited and ranges from 10^6 to 10^8 $M^{-1}s^{-1}$ for a wide variety of protein-binding reactions (227, 236, 279). Since typical k_{on} values range from 10^6 to 10^8 $M^{-1}s^{-1}$ and since a diffusion-limited reaction is on the order of 10^9 $M^{-1}s^{-1}$ (106), approximately 1/10 to 1/1000 collisions leads to an effective complex formation.

Dissociation-Limited Transport

Weisiger (275) advanced the concept that the transport of plasma protein–bound ligands into tissues such as liver is limited by the rate of dissociation of hormone from the albumin- or globulin-binding site. It is hypoth-esized that this situation arises because of enormously high membrane permeability coefficients (that is, *PS* values) in liver and other tissues. It is further posited that the concentration of exchangeable hormone in plasma may greatly exceed the concentration of free (dialyzable) hormone; however, in a dissociation-limited uptake mechanism, the concentration of free cellular hormone still would be driven by the concentration of free hormone measured in vitro by such methods as equilibrium dialysis.

In evaluating the validity of the dissociation-limited hypothesis, there is considerable evidence that refutes its general applicability. First, the term "dissociation-limited" is a misnomer. If the dissociation rate constant (k_{off} in Table 14.4) also is designated k_1 and the membrane permeability coefficient is designated k_3 (units $= s^{-1}$), then dissociation limitation is said to hold forth when $k_1 \ll k_3$. However, what is not emphasized in the dissociation-limited model is that both dissociation and hormone reassociation with the binding protein in the plasma compartment must be slow relative to membrane permeation (172, 179). That is, both $k_1 \ll k_3$ and $k_2 A_F \ll k_3$ must prevail, where A_F is the concentration of unoccupied globulin- or albumin-binding sites in plasma. The $k_2 A_F$ product is identical to the product of $k_{on}[C]$ given in Table 14.4. The data in Table 14.4 show that hormone reassociation rates with the binding protein are enormously fast, even though minimal estimates are given. In the case of T_3 or testosterone reassociation with HSA, the k_{on} values given in Table 14.4 are two to four log orders in magnitude lower than generally ascribed for ligand/protein association rates. Thus, the product $k_{on}[C]$ for these systems is far in excess of 1000 s^{-1}, as is the case for T_4 reassociation with HSA (Table 14.4). These rapid rates of hormone reassociation with HSA nullify the validity of the dissociation-limited model, at least with respect to transport of hormones from albumin-binding sites. Moreover, as discussed later in this section, the dissociation-limited model may be rejected in the case of hormone transport from globulin-binding sites.

Another problem with the dissociation-limited model is that proponents of this hypothesis are forced to propose unphysiologically high values for membrane permeation rate constants (144, 147). Stated differently, the proposed PS values for thyroid or steroid hormones are unphysiologically high, often by several orders of magnitude. For example, in the case of T_4 transport into rat liver, Mendel et al. (144) propose that the PS/F ratio must be 540 to allow for the properties of T_4 transport in vivo to be consistent with the free hormone hypothesis. Yet these workers record an experimentally observed PS/F ratio of only 9.9 in vivo using an unusual perfused liver preparation. When T_4 transport into perfused rat liver was measured under more physiological conditions, the PS/F ratio was 2.2 (91). The PS/F ratio of 9.9 is in itself spuriously high, owing to the unphysiological perfusion conditions used (144). Under these conditions, the rat liver is perfused with a plasma protein-free fluorocarbon solution for 30 min prior to a 4 min perfusion with buffer alone prior to the actual 30 s uptake perfusion. Perfusion of organs with plasma protein-free solution causes a breakdown in microvascular permeability (149). At least 0.1% albumin concentrations are needed to prevent a breakdown of capillary permeability. This increase in capillary PS products caused by perfusion with protein-free buffer was reviewed first by Landis and Pappenheimer (123) in their 1963 chapter in the *Handbook of Physiology*. The organ edema caused by perfusion with plasma protein-free solutions was obseved first by Drinker in 1927 (47). It was hypothesized in the 1940s that plasma proteins absorb to the surface of the capillary endothelium and in this way maintain normal microvascular permeability (30). The phenomenon of increased microvascular permeability caused by perfusion with protein-free solution has been observed in the vascular beds of multiple organs and species, as reviewed by Michel (149).

The dissociation-limited model purports to make in vivo measurements of the capillary physiology of hormone transport compatible with the free hormone hypothesis in the case of T_3 transport in perfused rat liver (147). Under these conditions, rat liver was made edematous with a 30 min perfusion with protein-free fluorocarbon solution and anoxic with a subsequent 4 min preperfusion with buffer containing no protein

and no fluorocarbon, and a PS/F ratio of 6.3 was recorded (147). However, this value was substantially less than the PS/F value of 445 needed to reconcile the transport of T_3 into rat liver with the free hormone hypothesis (147). Therefore, even though the perfusion of edematous, anoxic rat liver gives spuriously high values of PS/F for thyroid hormones, these values are still log orders less than that required to make the experimental observations compatible with the free hormone hypothesis using the dissociation-limited model.

The rapid rates of ligand reassociation with plasma proteins are sometimes ignored. For example, in the case of rat albumin binding of bilirubin, $k_{off} = 0.6$ s^{-1} and $K_D = 6$ nM (288). Therefore, $k_{on} = 10^8$ M^{-1}s^{-1}, and at a physiological albumin concentration of 10^{-4} M, the bilirubin–rat albumin reassociation rate is 10,000 s^{-1}, a value that is log orders greater than the permeation rate constant (k_3) of bilirubin transport into liver. Other studies have concluded that dissociation-limited uptake of plasma protein–bound ligands by organs in vivo is either rare or not possible (72, 219).

Diffusion limitation due to an unstirred water layer has been proposed to explain plasma protein–mediated transport (99). Although diffusion limitation may be important in the transport of substances across the epithelium from the intestinal lumen (99, 138), it has been excluded in organs such as liver and brain (66, 192).

Enhanced Dissociation Mechanism of Plasma Protein–Mediated Transport

In Vivo Measurement of Binding K_D. The K_D governing the plasma protein hormone–binding reaction in vivo within a living capillary may be quantified by adapting the KRC equation of capillary physiology to a solute that is bound by a plasma protein (179):

$$E = 1 - e^{-f(PS/F)}$$

$$f = \frac{K_D^a/n}{A_F + K_D^a/n}$$

where A_F is the unbound plasma protein concentration, for example, the concentration of unoccupied albumin-binding sites; K_D^a is the dissociation constant governing the plasma protein/ligand-binding reaction in vivo within the microcirculation; f is the in vivo bioavailable fraction; and n is the number of ligand-binding sites on the plasma protein. This derivation of the KRC equation assumes that the plasma protein–binding reaction is in steady state in vivo, and this assumption requires only that the rate constant of ligand dissociation from (k_1) and/or association with ($k_2 A_F$) the plasma protein is in excess of the rate constant of ligand permeation (k_3) through the endothelial membrane (179)—that is, either k_1 or $k_2 A_F \gg k_3$. If the capillary transit time is denoted by t (in seconds), then the $k_3 t$ product is identical to the PS/F ratio.

The unidirectional extraction of steroid or thyroid hormones by an organ (E), the microvascular endothelial PS product, the rate of organ blood flow (F), and the in vivo K_D^a may be measured with the tissue-sampling/single-arterial-injection technique called the brain uptake index (BUI) method for brain-transport studies (184). The BUI method has been applied to other organs, including liver (183), uterus (126), kidney (32), salivary gland (28), lymph node (27), testis, and prostate gland (225), by accessing the major artery perfusing the organ. In the case of liver, the tissue-sampling/single-injection technique utilizes portal vein injections following ligation of the hepatic artery. With this method, an approximately 200 μl bolus of buffered Ringer's solution containing radiolabeled hormone and a differentially radiolabeled, highly diffusible internal reference is rapidly injected (<0.5 s) into the artery perfusing the organ. Studies have been performed in anesthetized rats and rabbits or conscious animals following pre-insertion of an external carotid artery catheter for measurement of BBB transport. The single-injection bolus also may contain various concentrations of plasma protein or serum. In this method, the effects of binding proteins in human serum obtained from patients from a wide variety of clinical conditions may be examined in vivo (168). Owing to the rapid common carotid arterial injection, mixing of the bolus with the circulating rat plasma is <5% (182). In brain-transport studies, the bolus passes through the head nearly completely within the first 2 s after injection and the animal is decapitated at 5–15 s after the carotid arterial injection (157). Owing to the large ratio of extravascular to vascular volume in the brain, there is negligible efflux of the radiolabeled substance during the 5–15 s period following injection (187). Therefore, measurement of hormone extraction at 5–15 s after injection represents the unidirectional fractional extraction expressed in the KRC formulation above. This extraction represents actual extravascular distribution in the brain and not simply binding of hormone to the capillary endothelium. Thaw mount autoradiography has been used to demonstrate that distribution of [^{3}H]-estradiol is uniform throughout the organ as compared to the focal distribution of radiolabeled albumin, which is confined to the capillary lumen.

Application of the single-arterial-injection technique to in vivo measurements of K_D is exemplified in the case of brain transport of testosterone (Fig. 14.6).

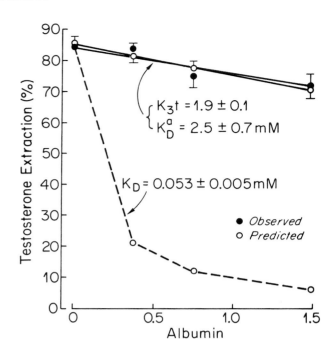

FIG. 14.6. Unidirectional extraction of [^{3}H]-testosterone by rat brain is plotted vs. the concentration of bovine albumin present in carotid arterial injection solution. Experimentally observed extraction values are represented by closed circles (mean ± SE, n = 3–6 animals per point). Extraction values predicted by fitting the experimental data to the KRC equation are shown by open circles, and curve fitting gives the two parameters $k_3 t$ (plasma to tissue influx by time) and K_D^a (in vivo dissociation constant); $t = 1/k_{10}$. Dashed line represents extraction values predicted by substituting into the KRC equation the albumin concentration, the $k_3 t$ product, and the in vitro albumin–testosterone dissociation constant, $K_D = 53 \pm 1 \mu M$. Therefore, the dashed curve gives the expected inhibition of testosterone transport caused by hormone binding to albumin if testosterone was not available for transport into brain from the circulating albumin-bound pool. However, since albumin-bound testosterone is available via an enhanced dissociation mechanism, the upper curve is observed and the K_D^a in vivo (2500 ± 700 μM) is much greater than the K_D in vitro. [From Pardridge and Landaw (179) with permission.]

Unidirectional extraction of [^{3}H]-testosterone by rat brain is plotted against the concentration of bovine serum albumin (BSA) in the carotid arterial-injection solution (179). If only the fraction of testosterone that was free (dialyzable) in vitro was available for transport through the BBB in vivo, then the extraction/albumin concentration curve should conform to the dashed line shown in Figure 14.6. However, the observed testosterone extraction is greatly in excess of that predicted from in vitro measurements of albumin binding of testosterone, and this discrepancy is explicable within the context of the model of enhanced dissociation. That is, owing to conformational changes about the testosterone-binding site on albumin, there is a marked increase in testosterone dissociation from the binding site in vivo within the brain capillary. This enhanced dissociation is reflected by the 50–fold greater K_D value in vivo in the brain circulation as compared to the in vitro K_D value (Fig. 14.6, Table 14.5).

In vivo expansion of the K_D relative to the in vitro value occurs for a variety of plasma protein–bound ligands and different plasma proteins (Table 14.5). However, the K_D of propranolol binding to BSA in vivo within the brain capillary is not significantly different from the in vitro K_D value (Table 14.5). That is, there is no enhanced dissociation of albumin-bound propranolol (189), whereas there is enhanced dissociation of albumin-bound steroid or thyroid hormone (179). Similarly, the in vivo K_D of albumin binding of another lipophilic amine ligand, bupivacaine, is not significantly different from the in vitro K_D value (Table

14.5). These examples illustrate that the single-injection technique may confirm the validity of the free hormone or drug hypothesis in situations where there is no enhanced dissociation of ligand from the protein-binding site in vivo. The difference between the in vivo K_D value and the in vitro K_D value reflects enhanced dissociation from the protein-binding site, and this phenomenon has been termed "plasma protein–mediated transport" (PMT). The PMT phenomenon has been observed by a number of different laboratories (5, 7, 15, 67, 68, 79, 152, 260–262, 280) in addition to those cited in Table 14.5.

The discrepancy between the K_D measured in vivo and the K_D measured in vitro is not a function of using the single-injection technique under non-steady-state conditions. In fact, the single-injection technique approximates the steady-state condition sufficiently to permit steady-state assumptions (232). This is derived from the fact that since $k_2 A_F \gg k_3$ or $\bar{t}$ (Table 14.4), equilibrium of the binding reaction is established all along the capillary (67). Equilibrium binding conditions also exist in tissue culture, and this model system has been used to provide evidence for enhanced dissociation of ligands from albumin-binding sites (61).

Albumin Conformational Analysis. The albumin model of Brown (22), which originally was formulated from the primary amino-acid sequence of the protein, is shown in Figure 14.7. This model has given way to albumin structural models based on X-ray diffraction studies (26), as described in subsequent sections of this chapter. However, the Brown model demonstrates the six binding sites on albumin and allows us to visualize how there might be site-specific conformational changes on the plasma protein. Site-specific conformational changes would explain the enhanced dissociation of steroid or thyroid hormone ligands from the respective albumin-binding sites and the absence of enhanced dissociation of lipophilic amine drugs (propranolol, bupivacaine) from another albumin-binding site (Table 14.5). Albumin is a protein that undergoes reversible conformational states (127). At pH 7.4, albumin exists in two conformations, designated N and B, and equilibrium between these two conformational states is altered by both anions and divalent cations, as well as pH (281). Acid pH favors the N conformation. In the case of binding globulins, such as human corticosteroid-binding globulin (CBG), ligand debinding rates are increased exponentially with small decreases in pH (244). Similarly, acidic pH increases the rate of drug dissociation from the plasma globulin α_1-acid glycoprotein (AAG), also called orosomucoid (264). Apart from pH, simple adsorption of albumin onto surfaces is

TABLE 14.5. *Comparison of Plasma Protein Binding of Hormones and Drugs in Vitro and in Vivo Within the Brain Microvasculature* *

Plasma Protein	Ligand	K_D (μM) (In Vitro)	K_D^a (μM) (In Vivo)
Bovine albumin	Testosterone	53 ± 1	2520 ± 710
	Tryptophan	130 ± 30	1670 ± 110
	Corticosterone	260 ± 10	1330 ± 90
	Dihyrotestosterone	53 ± 6	830 ± 140
	Estradiol	23 ± 1	710 ± 100
	T_3	4.7 ± 0.1	46 ± 4
	Propranolol	290 ± 30	220 ± 40
	Bupivacaine	141 ± 10	211 ± 107
	Imipramine	221 ± 21	1675 ± 600
hAAG	Propranolol	3.1 ± 0.1	19 ± 4
	Bupivacaine	6.5 ± 0.5	17 ± 4
	Isradipine	6.9 ± 0.9	35 ± 2
	Darodipine	2.5 ± 0.5	55 ± 7
	Imipramine	4.9 ± 0.3	90 ± 9
Human albumin	L-663,581	125 ± 16	675 ± 18
	L-364,718	8.2 ± 0.8	266 ± 38
	Diazepam	6.3 ± 0.1	157 ± 36
hVLDL	Cyclosporin	1.9 ± 0.5	$1.8 \pm 0.4 \dagger$
hLDL	Cyclosporin	0.81 ± 0.08	$1.6 \pm 0.4 \dagger$
hHDL	Cyclosporin	0.45 ± 0.10	$0.44 \pm 0.11 \dagger$
HSA	Isradipine	63 ± 8	221 ± 7
	Darodipine	94 ± 5	203 ± 14

*hAAG, human α_1-acid glycoprotein; hVLDL, human very low-density lipoprotein; hLDL, human low-density lipoprotein; hHDL, human high-density lipoprotein; HSA, human serum albumin; T_3, triiodothyronine. †Units are grams per liter. [From refs. 130, 131, 177, 179, 189, 210, 256, 265, 266.]

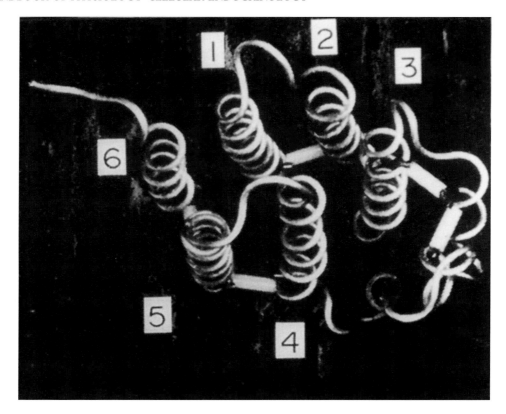

FIG. 14.7. Three-dimensional structure of albumin as deduced from the primary amino-acid sequence by Brown (22, 23). Albumin is composed of three domains and six hemicylinders. Ligand-binding sites are interiors of the six hemicylinders of the albumin molecule. This model illustrates the high flexibility of albumin, and a marked increase in ligand dissociation is expected with a slight uncoiling caused by conformational changes about the binding site. Conformational changes are ligand- and tissue-specific. For example, steroid or thyroid hormone dissociation from albumin is enhanced in brain capillaries, whereas propranolol or lidocaine dissociation is not (Table 14.5). Conversely, the dissociation of propranolol or lidocaine from albumin is markedly enhanced in the liver microcirculation.

known to cause conformational changes about ligand-binding sites, and indeed, conformational changes in plasma albumin have been induced by nonspecific adsorption of albumin on rat hepatocytes (96) and even glass (203) or graphite (60) surfaces.

The phenomenon of surface-mediated conformational changes in albumin is of interest since current concepts of capillary physiology propose that the endothelial glycocalyx lining the microvascular bed normally is adsorbed by a layer of albumin (149). Indeed, specific amino-acid residues on the surface of the albumin molecule are believed to interact with anionic charges on the endothelial glycocalyx (150). Surface modification of crucial arginine, but not lysine, residues alters the ability of albumin to adsorb to the endothelial glycocalyx. The interaction of albumin with membrane phospholipid also may mediate conformational changes in the plasma protein as phospholipid-mediated conformational changes have been demon-

strated for other proteins (56). It is important to emphasize that relatively small changes in conformational state about a ligand-binding site may have profound effects on the rate of ligand dissociation from the binding site and on the K_D of the binding reaction in vivo. X-ray diffraction studies show that removal of a single hydrogen bond from a ligand-binding site may result in an 800-fold increase in the K_D governing the binding reaction (8).

The change in affinity of plasma proteins for different ligands within the microcirculation is analogous to the conformational change that occurs in hemoglobin-binding sites for oxygen at the level of the microcirculation, depending on the relative concentration of 2,3–diphosphoglycerate (DPG). The DPG anion binds to a specific lysine residue on hemoglobin, and this shifts the hemoglobin-binding site between high- and low-affinity states (245). Similarly, oxygen-induced binding of hemoglobin to band 3 of erythrocytes results in an increase in anion exchange at the microcirculation (226). Although it is necessary to hypothesize global conformational changes in band 3, this conformational change has been difficult to prove in vivo (226). The alteration of hemoglobin affinity for oxygen by DPG is of interest to possible biochemical mechanisms of enhanced dissociation of hormones from plasma proteins. Studies in the literature suggest that tissues release dialyzable factors that alter the affinity of plasma proteins for the respective ligands within the organ microcirculation (132, 134). Such dialyzable factors may bind the plasma protein and induce conformational changes about the ligand-binding site that result in enhanced dissociation in vivo.

Stereospecificity of Enhanced Dissociation From Albumin.

The first evidence of stereospecificity of PMT via the enhanced dissociation mechanism was demonstrated in the case of the hepatic uptake of D- and L-T_3 (254). The extravascular hepatic extraction of BSA-bound [^{125}I]-D-T_3, 50 $\pm$ 2%, was nearly half that for BSA-bound [^{125}I]-L-T_3, 93 $\pm$ 12%. There was no significant difference in in vitro binding between [^{125}I]-D-T_3 and [^{125}I]-L-T_3; in the presence of 5 g/dl BSA, free (dialyzable) D-T_3 and L-T_3 were 1.95 $\pm$ 0.16% and 1.79 $\pm$ 0.28% respectively, showing no significant difference. These results indicate a greater degree of enhanced dissociation of L-T_3 from the albumin-binding site relative to D-T_3. The stereospecificity of the enhanced dissociation of T_3 from albumin in vivo within the hepatic microcirculation could take place if there were a different conformational state of the albumin molecule when the plasma protein binds L-T_3 vs. D-T_3. This hypothesis was confirmed by polyacrylamide gel isoelectric focusing of 5 g/dl concentrations of BSA bound by [^{125}I]-D-T_3 or [^{125}I]-L-T_3. The D-T_3–BSA complex had an isoeletric point of 5.0, whereas that of the L-T_3–BSA complex was 5.1 (254). These findings suggest that the surface charge of the albumin molecule is preferentially less acidic in the L-T_3-bound form than in the D-T_3-bound form. Ligand-induced protein conformational changes also have been observed for other plasma proteins (141) and are analogous to classical "induced fit" conformational changes in enzymes caused by substrate binding (119).

Organ Specificity of Plasma Protein–Mediated Transport.

If conformational changes about albumin-binding sites occur owing to interaction of the plasma protein with the endothelial surface, then it would be expected that the extent to which ligands undergo surface-mediated enhanced dissociation may vary from organ to organ. This phenomenon has been observed, as shown in Table 14.6. The K_D governing the binding of testoster-

TABLE 14.6. *In Vivo Dissociation Constant (K_D^a) of Bovine Albumin Binding of Testosterone (T) or Estradiol (E_2) in Three Organs*

Organ	K_D^a (μM)	
	T	E_2
Brain	2500 $\pm$ 700	710 $\pm$ 100
Salivary gland	602 $\pm$ 40	N.D.
Lymph node	300 $\pm$ 90	1500 $\pm$ 500

In vitro K_D values are 53 $\pm$ 1 μM and 23 $\pm$ 1 μM, respectively, for T and E_2. N.D., not determined. [From Pardridge (171) with permission.]

one to BSA may vary over a factor of nearly 10 when comparing different organs such as brain, salivary gland, or lymph node (171). Similarly, the delivery of sex steroid hormones to tissues via SHBG exhibits considerable organ diversity, as shown in Table 14.7 and discussed in subsequent sections of this chapter.

Albumin Receptor Hypothesis.

Prior to proposing the dissociation-limited model of free ligand transport, Weisiger and colleagues (276) proposed an albumin receptor model. This model posited the presence of a specific receptor for albumin on the hepatocyte cell membrane, and evidence for an albumin receptor was obtained from isolated liver or fat cells (19, 276), as well as from in vivo hepatic transport analyses (64, 65). Subsequent studies, however, failed to confirm the presence of a specific albumin receptor on the hepatocyte (242). Extensive PMT of ligands occurs within the brain microcirculation (170), and no albumin receptor exists on the endothelium in this organ (174, 234).

Transcapillary Transport of Protein–Hormone Complex

Plasma protein–mediated transport of ligands into tissues generally occurs through the enhanced dissociation mechanism (Fig. 14.4). However, in some organs

TABLE 14.7. *Sex Hormone–Binding Globulin (SHBG) Delivery of Sex Steroids to Tissues: Organ Diversity in the Rat*

Organ	Estradiol	Testosterone
Brain and uterus	$-$	$-$
Liver, salivary gland, and lymph node	$+$	$-$
Testis	$+$	$+$

($-$), Little, if any, transport of SHBG-bound hormone into tissue under normal conditions; ($+$), SHBG-bound hormone is partially or freely transported into tissue under normal conditions. [From Pardridge (171) with permission.]

and for selective proteins, there are specific mechanisms mediating the transcapillary transport of the plasma protein–hormone complex. Such transport systems exist in the microvasculature of testis or prostate gland for the rapid uptake of SHBG (225). As shown in Figure 14.8, unidirectional extraction of rabbit testosterone-binding globulin (TeBG) is substantially greater than the non-specific exodus of plasma proteins of comparable molecular weight, such as transferrin or albumin. Autoradiographic experiments that follow the fate of the [³H]-testosterone–SHBG complex in prostate gland show that the protein rapidly achieves distribution throughout the stromal compartment in this organ following transcapillary movement of the SHBG–testosterone complex (55), which confirms earlier studies showing high concentrations of SHBG in prostate gland stroma (16, 38) and explains the higher concentrations of testosterone and estradiol in the stromal compartment of the prostate gland than in the epithelium (259).

The presence of a TeBG receptor on the microvessels of certain organs was suggested further by experiments using isolated microvessels obtained from 28-day-old rabbit brain and [³H]-labeled TeBG (176). Radiolabeling of rabbit TeBG with [³H]-sodium borohydride resulted in a physiologically active protein that bound [¹⁴C]testosterone. The [³H]-TeBG was bound avidly by the developing rabbit brain capillaries, and this binding was inhibited by 28-day-old rabbit serum (Fig. 14.9).

The cDNAs to putative SHBG or TeBG receptors have not been isolated to date. However, there is evidence for saturable binding of SHBG to plasma membranes of rat epididymis (122). Saturable binding of [¹²⁵I]-SHBG also has been observed in membranes isolated from human endometruim, liver, prostate gland, and skeletal muscle (69). Other studies provide evidence for saturable binding sites for human CBG in human placental membranes (121).

Physiology-Based Model of Cellular Bioavailable Hormone

Testosterone Availability in Brain. A partly flow–partly compartmental physiology-based mathematical model for testosterone transport into brain from either the free, albumin-bound, or globulin-bound pools is depicted in Figure 14.10. This model of hormone transport into an organ in vivo is comprised of 18 different parameters, each of which represents a discrete physiological event (Table 14.8). The parameters k_1 and k_2 refer to the rates of ligand dissociation from or association with the globulin-binding site in vivo within the brain capillary (180). The parameters k_7 and k_8 refer

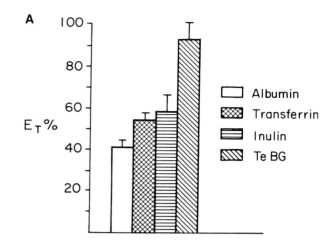

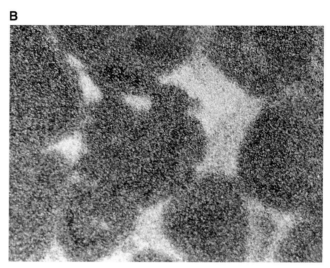

FIG. 14.8. *A:* Percent extraction *(E_T)* of inulin and three plasma proteins across the rat prostate gland microvasculature following a single arterial injection. Data are means ± SE (*n* = 3–7 rats per point). The E_T values of albumin, transferrin, and inulin are comparable, whereas there is a marked increase (*P* < 0.05) of the prostatic extraction of testosterone-binding globulin *(TeBG)*. *B:* Darkfield micrograph of thaw-mount autoradiogram of rat ventral prostate gland obtained 60 s after a descending aortic infusion of [³H]-testosterone bound to the sex hormone–binding globulin (SHBG) in human pregnancy serum. These studies show rapid exodus of the [³H]-testosterone–SHBG complex from prostatic microvessels and rapid distribution into the stromal compartment of the prostate gland. Conversely, when [³H]-testosterone was infused in buffer without SHBG, the steroid molecule uniformly distributed over both the stromal and epithelial compartments. [From Ellison and Pardridge (55) and Sakiyama et al. (225) with permission.]

to the rate of ligand dissociation from and reassociation to albumin within the brain capillary. Since testosterone bound to human SHBG is not available normally for uptake by rat brain, k_1 is set at the in vitro value, 0.03 s⁻¹ (90). The SHBG dissociation constant for testosterone (K_G) is 2 n*M* since $k_2 = k_1/K_G$, $k_2 =$

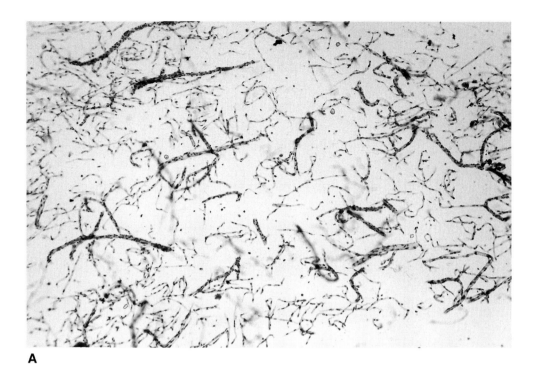

A

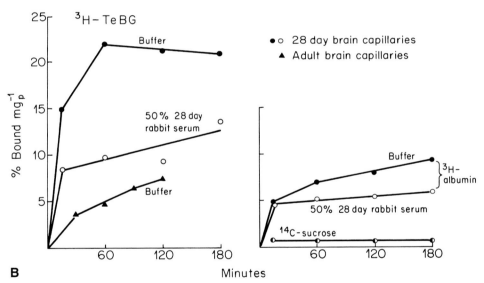

B

Minutes

FIG. 14.9. *A:* Photomicrograph of isolated microvessels obtained from 28-day-old rabbit brain. These capillaries were used in radioreceptor assays to probe for the presence of plasma protein–specific receptors. *B, left:* Binding of [³H]-testosterone-binding globulin *(TeBG)* at 37°C to capillaries isolated from either 28-day-old (open circles) or adult (triangles) rabbits. Inclusion of 50% 28-day-old rabbit serum results in a marked diminution in the uptake of [³H]-TeBG by capillaries isolated from 28-day-old rabbits. *B, right:* Uptake of [³H]-albumin by capillaries isolated from 28-day-old rabbit brain is plotted vs. incubation time in the absence (closed circles) or presence (open circles) of a 50% dilution of 28-day-old rabbit serum. Residual uptake of [¹⁴C]-sucrose, an extracellular fluid marker, is also shown. [From Pardridge et al. (176) with permission.]

TABLE 14.8. *Testosterone Basal Parameters*

Parameter Number	Parameter Symbol (U)	Parameter Name	Parameter Value
1	k_1 (s^{-1})	Capillary globulin–ligand dissociation	0.03
2	k_2 ($M^{-1}\,s^{-1}$)	Capillary globulin–ligand association	1.5×10^7
3	k_3 (s^{-1})	Plasma to tissue influx	1.9
4	k_4 (s^{-1})	Tissue to plasma efflux	0.0271
5	k_5 ($M^{-1}\,s^{-1}$)	Cytosolic protein–ligand association	1.0×10^7
6	k_6 (s^{-1})	Cytosolic protein–ligand dissociation	0.03
7	k_7 (s^{-1})	Capillary albumin–ligand dissociation	2.5×10^3
8	k_8 ($M^{-1} \times 10^6$)	Capillary albumin–ligand association	1.0×10^6
9	k_9 (s^{-1})	Ligand tissue metabolism	0
10	k_{10} (s^{-1})	Plasma transit	1.0
11	K_G (M)	Systemic globulin dissociation constant	2.0×10^{-9}
12	K_A (M)	Systemic albumin dissociation constant	5.3×10^{-5}
13	G_T^O (M)	Total globulin plasma concentration	2.8×10^{-8}
14	A_F (M)	Free (total) albumin plasma concentration	6.4×10^{-4}
15	P_T (M)	Total cytosolic protein concentration	2.5×10^{-9}
16	L_T^O	Total ligand plasma concentration	1.0×10^{-8}
17	V_P (1/kg)	Brain capillary plasma volume	0.01
18	V_T (1/kg)	Brain extravascular water volume	0.70

Assignments of k_7 and k_8 are somewhat arbitrary because only the ratio of k_7/k_8 is known. However, stimulation studies showed that increasing k_7 and k_8 to 2.5×10^5 s^{-1} and 1.0×10^8 $M^{-1}s^{-1}$, respectively, had no effect on the results in Table 14.9. The range in varying k_8 was restricted to 10^6–10^8 $M^{-1}s^{-1}$ because this is the known range of hormone–plasma protein association rate constants (279). However, decreasing k_7 and k_8 to 53 s^{-1} and 21,200 $M^{-1}s^{-1}$, respectively, also had no significant effect on the results in Table 14.9. [From Pardridge and Landaw (180) with permission.]

1.5×10^7 $M^{-1}s^{-1}$. The dissociation constant (K_D^a) of albumin binding of testosterone in the brain capillary is 2500 μM (Fig. 14.6). Assigning a minimal value for k_8 of 1×10^6 $M^{-1}s^{-1}$, $k_7 = K_D^a \times k_8 = 2500$ s^{-1}. The assignments of k_7 and k_8 are arbitrary because only the ratio of k_7/k_8 is known. Simulation studies have shown that increasing k_7 or k_8 by as much as 100–fold has no effect on the results (Table 14.8). The range in varying k_8 was restricted to 10^6–10^8 $M^{-1}s^{-1}$ since this is the known range of hormone–plasma protein association rate constants (236, 279). The concentration of albumin (A_F) or SHBG (G_T^o) is fixed at the normal male serum values of 640 μM and 28 nM, respectively (Table 14.8).

The plasma to organ influx and organ to plasma efflux rate constants are given by k_3 and k_4, respectively. The $k_3 t$ product (which is equivalent to the *PS/F* ratio) for testosterone transport through the rat BBB is 1.9 (Fig. 14.6); given $t = 1$s, $k_3 = 1.9$ s^{-1}. It is assumed that BBB permeability to testosterone is symmetrical and that the ratio of transport rate constants is $k_3/k_4 = V_P/V_T$, where V_P is plasma volume and equals 0.01 ml/g and V_T is extravascular volume in brain and equals 0.70 ml/g. Therefore, given that $k_4 = k_3 (V_P/V_T)$, k_4 is set at 0.027 s^{-1}. The capillary transit time in brain ($\bar{t}$) = $1/k_{10}$, where k_{10} is the rate constant of

plasma transit through the organ and is equal to 1.0 s in brain. Organ blood flow = $V_P \times k_{10}$.

Cytoplasmic hormone binding of testosterone in rat brain has been measured in vivo (187). The rate constant of testosterone dissociation from brain cytosolic proteins in vivo (k_6) is 0.03 s^{-1} (Table 14.8). The P_T/K_P ratio of cytosolic binding of testosterone in brain in vivo is 0.67, where K_P is the dissociation constant of cytoplasmic protein binding of the hormone. Because $K_P = k_6/k_5$ and a typical $k_5 = 10^7$ $M^{-1}s^{-1}$, K_P is set at 3 nM and K_T at 2 nM. Actually, the individual k_5 and k_6 rate constants are not important in the mathematical model as only the k_6/k_5 ratio is used. The cytoplasmic binding system should not be confused with nuclear hormone receptors since the sequestration of hormone by nuclear receptors in brain is trivial compared to the cytoplasmic binding. The cytoplasmic binding proteins that sequester testosterone in the brain may include such proteins as ligandin or Z-protein (115).

The crucial parameter to be determined with this model is L_M, which is the concentration of free cellular hormone, that is, the pool of hormone believed to drive occupancy of the nuclear receptor. For the simplified case of a single plasma protein–binding system, where hormone dissociation and/or reassociation is rapid compared to capillary transit time, the concentrations

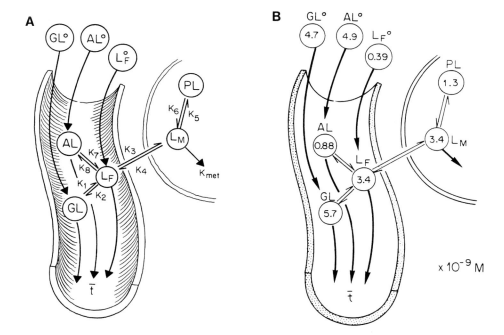

FIG. 14.10. *A:* Steady-state model of testosterone transport through the brain capillary wall and into brain cells. Pools of globulin-bound, albumin-bound, and free ligand in the systemic circulation are denoted as $GL°$, $AL°$, and $L_F°$, respectively; pools of globulin-bound, albumin-bound, and plasma bioavailable hormone in the brain capillary are denoted as GL, AL, and L_F, respectively. Pools of free and cytoplasmic bound steroid hormone in brain cells are denoted as L_M and PL, respectively; t is mean capillary transit time in brain. *B:* Predicted steady-state concentrations of testosterone in the various pools of the brain capillary and in brain cells. Pool sizes represent the basal state, which is simulation 1 in Table 14.9. The concentration of free cytosolic testosterone in brain cells is predicted to approximate the concentration of albumin-bound hormone in the circulation but is more than tenfold greater than the concentration of free hormone measured in vitro by equilibrium dialysis. [From Pardridge and Landaw (180) with permission.]

of free cytoplasmic hormone (L_M) and capillary bioavailable hormone (L_F) are given by the following (171):

$$L_M = \frac{k_3}{k_4 + k_9}\left[\frac{V_p}{V_T}\right]L_F$$

$$L_F = \left[\frac{K_D{}^a}{A_F + K_D{}^a(1 + R)}\right]L_T{}^o$$

$$R = \frac{k_4 k_9}{(k_4 + k_9)k_{10}}$$

These equations are simplified illustrations of important principles. First, when organ metabolism is nil (for example, $k_9 = 0$), $R = 0$ and the plasma bioavailable hormone (L_F) is equal to the free cytosolic hormone (L_M). Second, the concentration of cytoplasmic free hormone is fully independent of cytoplasmic binding proteins and is simply a function of the concentration of capillary bioavailable hormone, rates of membrane transport, and cytoplasmic metabolism. Third, as em-

phasized by Tait and Burstein (250), hormone volume of distribution (V_D) and hormone metabolic clearance rate (MCR) are not linked if cellular enzymes act only on free cytoplasmic hormone, as depicted by the model in Figure 14.10. The hormone V_D is a function of hormone binding to cytoplasmic proteins, but hormone MCR is independent of hormone binding to cytoplasmic proteins if metabolic enzymes act on free cellular hormone (L_M, Fig. 14.10A). However, if enzymes metabolize hormone bound to cytosolic proteins (*PL*, Fig. 14.10A), then hormone MCR and V_D will be linked (163).

Organ MCR is equal to the following (171):

$$MCR = E^{ss} \cdot F$$

$$E^{ss} = \frac{fR}{1 + fR}$$

where E^{ss} is net steady-state hormone extraction by the organ; F is organ blood flow; and f, $K_D{}^a/(A_F +$

$K_D{}^a$) is the fraction of capillary bioavailable hormone. Therefore, the organ MCR, like the free cytoplasmic hormone and nuclear receptor occupancy, is strictly a function of the concentration of capillary bioavailable hormone, membrane transport, and organ metabolism and is fully independent of tissue-binding proteins. If metabolic clearance of steroid hormone by a given organ is essentially nil, then $k_9 = 0$, $R = 0$, and $E^{SS} = 0$. When metabolic clearance by an organ is high, $k_9 \gg k_4$ and R reduces to $k_3/k_{10} = k_3 t$. Under these conditions, hormone transport into the organ from blood is rate-limiting for overall hormone metabolic clearance and the steady-state MCR is equal to the unidirectional transport clearance rate (TCR), as determined by the tissue-sampling/single-injection technique. The correlation between MCR and TCR has been shown for a number of systems and is discussed in subsequent sections of this chapter.

The concentration of testosterone predicted to occupy the various tissue pools is shown in Figure 14.10B under the basal condition, which is simulation 1 in Table 14.9. The free hormone hypothesis is represented by simulations 2 and 11 in Table 14.9. Simulation 1 is the basal state and is described by the parameters listed in Table 14.8. These results show that the concentration of free cellular hormone is equal to the concentration of capillary bioavailable hormone but is nearly tenfold greater than the concentration of free hormone measured in vitro. This discrepancy arises from the fact that albumin-bound testosterone is available for transport through the BBB in vivo (184). In simulation 2, the albumin dissociation constant in vivo within the brain capillary is set at the level measured in vitro and, under these conditions, the concentration of free cellular hormone equals the concentration of free hormone measured in vitro. Simulation 3 shows the effect of a fivefold increase in the velocity of capillary plasma flow, which is equivalent to a fivefold decrease in capillary transit time, and both the capillary bioavailable and cellular free hormones are a function of capillary transit time (168). Simulation 4 is the case of enhanced dissociation of testosterone from the SHBG-binding site within the brain microcirculation. In this situation, testosterone is available for uptake by brain from the circulating SHBG-bound pool, without significant exodus from the capillary compartment of the globulin per se. Simulation 5 represents the case in which the concentration of SHBG is nearly doubled. Simulation 6 shows that a tenfold increase in cellular hormone-binding protein results in a tenfold increase in the concentration of cytoplasm-bound hormone but no change in the concentration of free cellular hormone. This is because the concentration of free cellular hormone is determined solely by the concentration of circulating bioavailable hormone. Simulation 7 represents a case, such as cirrhosis, where the concentration

TABLE 14.9. *Steady-State Model Predictions: Testosterone*

Simulation Number	Parameter* Change	Arterial† G_L^O (nM)	A_L^O (nM)	L_F^O (nM)	Capillary GL (nM)	AL (nM)	L_F (nM)	Cytosolic L_M (nM)	PL (nM)	V_D (l/kg)	E^{SS}
1	Basal	4.7	4.9	0.40	5.7	0.88	3.4	3.4	1.3	0.33	0
2‡	$k_7=53$ s^{-1}	4.7	4.9	0.40	4.7	4.9	0.40	0.40	0.30	0.049	0
3	$k_{10}=5$ s^{-1}	4.7	4.9	0.40	5.0	1.0	4.0	4.0	1.4	0.38	0
4	$k_1=3$ s^{-1}	4.7	4.9	0.40	1.8	1.7	6.5	6.5	1.7	0.58	0
5	$G_T^O=50$ nM	6.3	3.5	0.29	7.4	0.54	2.1	2.1	1.0	0.22	0
6	$P_T=25$ nM	4.7	4.9	0.40	5.7	0.88	3.4	3.4	13.3	1.17	0
7	$G_T^O=50$ nM $A_F=200$ μM	8.1	1.5	0.39	8.7	0.10	1.2	1.2	0.73	0.14	0
8	$k_1=3$ s^{-1} $G_T^O=50$ nM $A_F=200$ μM	8.1	1.5	0.39	3.1	0.51	6.3	6.3	1.7	0.56	0
9	$G_T^O=0$	0	9.2	0.76	0	2.0	8.0	8.0	1.8	0.68	0
10	$k_9=0.1$ s^{-1}	4.7	4.9	0.40	5.2	0.45	1.8	0.38	0.28	0.046	0.26
11‡	$k_7=53$ s^{-1} $k_9=0.1$ s^{-1}	4.7	4.9	0.40	4.7	4.4	0.36	0.078	0.063	0.0098	0.054

* Basal parameters are listed in Table 14.8. Simulations 2–11 include basal parameters plus the respective change in individual parameters for each simulation.   † Because the total ligand concentration is 10 nM (Table 14.8), the percent albumin-bound, globulin-bound, or free hormone in the arterial plasma may be computed by multiplying G_L^O, A_L^O, and L_F^O, respectively, by 10. G_L^O, arterial globulin-bound ligand; A_L^O, albumin-bound fraction; L_F, plasma bioavailable hormone; L_F^O, free hormone in vitro; GL, capillary globulin-bound ligand; AL, capillary albumin-bound ligand; L_M, free cytosolic hormone; PL, cytosolic-bound ligand; V_D, volume of distribution; E^{SS}, net steady-state hormone extraction.   ‡These simulations assume that the hormone-binding protein dissociation constant in the microcirculation is identical to the in vitro constant. [From Pardridge and Landaw (180) with permission.]

of SHBG is increased and that of albumin is decreased (224). In this case, the cytoplasmic free hormone is decreased to 35% of control levels, though there is no change in the concentration of free hormone in vitro. Stimulation 8 is also analogous with cirrhosis, wherein the SHBG concentration is increased, the albumin concentration is decreased, but SHBG-bound hormone is available for uptake by tissues. This has been observed for SHBG-bound estradiol in cirrhosis. Simulation 9 represents the case where SHBG concentrations are essentially 0, as in the adult rat. Simulation 10 gives the hormone pool sizes when metabolism of testosterone by brain is moderate and k_9 is raised from 0 to 0.1. In this simulation, $E^{SS} = 0.26$ and this extraction causes a marked gradient in hormone concentration across the cell membrane as the concentration of free cellular hormone is only 21% of the concentration of plasma bioavailable hormone.

Simulations 2 and 11 reveal two fundamental flaws of the free hormone hypothesis. First, if only free hormone is available for uptake by the organ, then the concentration of free cellular hormone cannot exceed the concen-

tration of free hormone measured in vitro, and this concentration is at least a log order lower than that needed to cause 50% occupancy of the nuclear hormone receptor (Fig. 14.3). This discrepancy would exist even in the presence of dissociation-limited transport. Second, the E^{SS} barely exceeds the dialyzable fraction; thus, the high extraction values for testosterone and other steroid hormones in organs such as liver cannot be generated if only the free hormone is available for uptake by tissues. If dissociation-limited transport of steroid hormones was operative, then high organ extractions could be achieved via the pool of free hormone (4). However, as discussed above, there is no experimental support for the very high membrane permeability coefficients and very low ligand–protein association rate constants required for dissociation-limited transport.

Triiodothyronine Availability in Liver. The model for T$_3$ transport in liver is mathematically identical to that for testosterone transport in brain (181). The T$_3$ model in Figure 14.11 is a partly flow–partly compartmental system, which assumes that events occurring over a

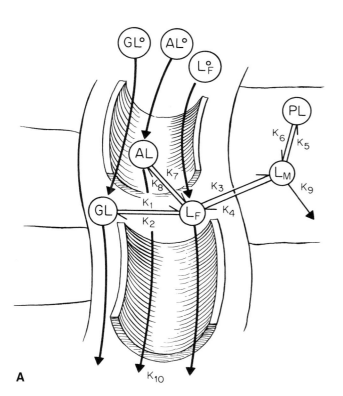
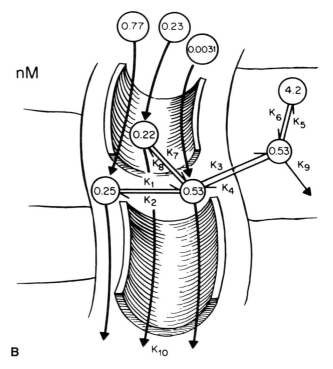

FIG. 14.11. *A:* Steady-state model of triiodothyronine transport in the liver microcirculation in vivo. Rate constants and hormone pools are defined in Table 14.10. *B:* The parameters in Table 14.10 were substituted into the steady-state model equation using a program in BASIC to generate the predicted pool-size concentrations shown in the figure, which correspond to simulation 1 of Table 14.11. *GL°,*

AL°, and *L$_F$°:* pools of globulin-bound, albumin-bound, and free ligand, respectively. *GL, AL,* and *L$_F$:* pools of globulin-bound, albumin-bound, and plasma available hormone, respectively. *L$_M$* and *PL,* pools of free and cytoplasmic bound thyroid hormone, respectively. [From Pardridge (173) and Pardridge and Landaw (181) with permission.]

wide area of the liver microvessel bed can be averaged so that the local plasma compartment behaves as a well-mixed pool. This mixing is facilitated by the large pores in liver sinusoids and the absence of a sinusoidal basement membrane. These anatomical specializations allow for instantaneous equilibration of plasma between the sinusoidal compartment and the interstitial space of the liver. In addition, it is assumed that T_3 transport across the hepatocyte membrane is not active and is symmetrical such that k_3 $(V_P) = k_4$ (V_T). This assumption is supported by previous studies showing that T_3 transport into the liver is nonsaturable up to a concentration of 50 μM (185). It is assumed that there is no significant hepatocyte uptake of circulating albumin or TBG on a single microcirculatory pass. Finally, it is assumed that the K_D values governing T_3 interaction between plasma proteins in vitro are the same in the systemic circulation in vivo but that these K_D values may differ and be much larger in the microvascular compartment.

The parameter values for the basal state for T_3 are given in Table 14.10 and yield the predicted pool sizes shown for simulation 1 in Table 14.11 and Figure 14.11. The rate of T_3 dissociation from albumin within the hepatocyte microvascular pool, 1.83×10^4 s^{-1} (Table 14.10), was estimated numerically from in vivo hepatic extraction data (181). This analysis was compatible with an in vivo K_D of 1.8 mM for albumin binding of T_3 within the hepatocyte microvascular compartment and a hepatic microvascular K_D for TBG binding of T_3 of 530 nM. Based on these parameters, the concentration of free cellular T_3, 0.53 nM, is predicted to be 170-fold greater than the concentration of free T_3 in vitro but to approximate the molar dissociation constant of the hepatic nuclear T_3 receptor, which ranges from 0.6 to 1 nM (160). The hepatic nuclear T_3 receptor is 50% occupied in vivo (160), and the concentration of free cellular T_3 necessary to cause 50% occupancy of the receptor is identical to the receptor K_D, 0.6–1.0 nM. Conversely, if the rates of T_3 dissociation from the albumin- and TBG-binding sites are restricted to the values observed in vitro, then the concentration of free T_3 in the liver cytosol is predicted to be the free (dialyzable) concentration, which is 3 pM (simulation 2, Table 14.11). This concentration of free cellular T_3 is too low by 200-fold to cause 50% occupancy of the hepatic nuclear T_3 receptor. Simulation 3 represents the case where both TBG and total T_3 are increased such that the free T_3 concentration in vitro is unchanged. However, the concentration of plasma bioavailable and cellular free T_3 in the liver is predicted to be increased 49% over basal values for simulation 3 . Simulation 5 models nonthyroidal illness in which there is a fivefold reduction in total T_3 and a

TABLE 14.10. *Triiodothyronine Basal Parameters*

Parameter Number	Parameter Symbol (U)	Parameter Name	Parameter Value
1	k_1 (s^{-1})	Sinusoidal globulin–ligand dissociation	53
2 *	k_2 $(M^{-1}s^{-1})$	Sinusoidal globulin–ligand association	1×10^8
3	k_3 (s^{-1})	Plasma-tissue influx	0.345
4	k_4 (s^{-1})	Plasma-tissue efflux	0.0863
5	k_5 $(M^{-1}s^{-1})$	Cytosolic protein–ligand association	1×10^7
6	k_6 (s^{-1})	Cytosolic protein–ligand dissociation	0.02
7	k_7 (s^{-1})	Sinusoidal albumin–ligand dissociation	1.83×10^4
8 †	k_8 $(M^{-1}s^{-1})$	Sinusoidal albumin–ligand association	1×10^7
9	k_9 (s^{-1})	Ligand tissue metabolism	0
10	k_{10} (s^{-1})	Plasma transit	0.2
11	K_G (M)	Systemic globulin dissociation constant	1×10^{-9}
12	K_A (M)	Systemic albumin dissociation constant	1×10^{-5}
13	G_T^O (M)	Total plasma globulin concentration	2.5×10^{-7}
14	A_F (M)	Free (total) plasma albumin concentration	7.4×10^{-4}
15 †	P_T (M)	Total cytosolic protein concentration	2×10^{-8}
16	L_T^O (M)	Total plasma ligand	1×10^{-9}
17	V_P $(l \cdot kg^{-1})$	Liver sinusoidal plasma volume	0.15
18	V_T $(l \cdot kg^{-1})$	Liver intracellular water volume	0.60

*The k_2 value is set at 10^8 $M^{-1}s^{-1}$ since $K_G = 10^{-9}$ M (181) and $k_1 = 10^{-1}s^{-1}$ in vitro (92) and $k_2 = k_1/K_G$. Simulation studies showed that as long as the k_1/k_2, k_6/k_5, and k_7/k_8 ratios were constant, the individual rate constants may vary over four log orders of magnitude without significantly changing the final results in Figure 14.11 (181).   †The ligand association rate constant was fixed at 10^7 $M^{-1}s^{-1}$ for k_5 and k_8, which is in the range of ligand–protein association rate constants (10^6–10^8 $M^{-1}s^{-1}$) (236, 279).   [From Pardridge and Landaw (181) with permission.]

TABLE 14.11. *Steady-State Model Predictions: Triiodothyronine*

Simulation Number	Parameter Change	Arterial			Sinusoidal			Cytosolic		V_D (l/kg)	E^{SS}
		G_L^O (nM)	A_L^O (nM)	L_F^O (nM)	GL (nM)	AL (nM)	L_F (nM)	L_M (nM)	PL (nM)		
1	Basal	0.77	0.23	0.0031	0.25	0.22	0.53	0.53	4.2	2.8	0
2	$k_1 = 0.1$ s^{-1} $k_7 = 100$ s^{-1}	0.77	0.23	0.0031	0.77	0.23	0.0031	0.0031	0.031	0.020	0
3	$L_T^O = 2$ nM $G_T^O = 600$ nM	1.8	0.22	0.0030	0.89	0.32	0.79	0.79	5.7	1.9	0
4	$L_T^O = 0.8$ nM $A_F = 200$ μM	0.74	0.059	0.0030	0.24	0.055	0.51	0.51	4.0	3.4	0
5	$L_T^O = 0.2$ nM $K_G = 5$ nM $K_A = 50$ μM	0.15	0.045	0.0030	0.051	0.043	0.11	0.11	1.0	3.4	0
6	$G_T^O = 600$ nM $A_F = 200$ μM $L_T^O = 2$ nM	1.9	0.065	0.0032	1.0	0.097	0.89	0.89	6.2	2.1	0
7	$P_T = 1$ nM	0.77	0.23	0.0031	0.25	0.22	0.53	0.53	0.21	0.45	0
8	$L_T^O = 0.5$ nM $G_T^O = 0$	0	0.49	0.0067	0	0.14	0.36	0.36	3.0	4.1	0
9	$k_9 = 0.1$	0.77	0.23	0.0031	0.17	0.14	0.36	0.16	1.5	1.0	0.33
10	$k_9 = 0.1$ $k_{10} = 0.05$ s^{-1}	0.77	0.23	0.0031	0.085	0.072	0.18	0.083	0.80	0.53	0.66

[From Pardridge and Landaw (181) with permission.]

fivefold increase in the dialyzable fraction of T_3 in vitro caused by a fivefold increase in the dissociation constant of T_3 binding to TBG and albumin in vitro. Under these conditions, the concentration of free T_3 in vitro is essentially unchanged from the basal value, but there is an 80% decrease in the concentration of plasma bioavailable and cellular free hormones. Simulation 6 represents the case of acute hepatitis in which there is an approximate doubling of serum TBG, a doubling of total T_3, and a 73% reduction of albumin. Simulation 7 is the case where the concentrations of T_3 cytosolic binding protein is reduced 20–fold. Under these conditions, the concentrations of plasma bioavailable or free cellular T_3 are unchanged but the concentration of cellular bound T_3 is reduced 95%. Simulation 8 is the case of complete TBG deficiency, where the concentration of total serum T_3 is reduced 50%. Simulation 9 is the case where there is rapid hepatic metabolism of T_3 and the k_9 is increased from 0 to 0.1 s^{-1}. Simulation 10 is the case where there is active organ metabolism of T_3 associated with a fourfold increase in transit time. This simulation shows that the concentrations of plasma bioavailable hormone and free cellular T_3 are transit time–dependent as these values are decreased approximately 50% compared to the values shown in simulation 9.

The conclusions of the testostrone/brain (Fig. 14.10, Tables 14.8, 14.9) and the T_3/liver (Fig. 14.11, Tables 14.10, 14.11) models may be summarized as follows.

First, the concentration of cellular free hormone (L_M) is manyfold greater than the concentration of free hormone measured in vitro (L_F^O) but approximates the albumin-bound fraction (A_L^O) measured in vitro. Second, the concentration of free cellular hormone (L_M) is a function of membrane permeability (k_3, k_4), organ metabolism (k_9), and the plasma bioavailable hormone (L_F) but is independent of tissue-binding proteins. Third, the concentrations of plasma bioavailable hormone (L_F) and free cellular hormone (L_M) are transit time–dependent.

Experimental Attempts to Measure Free Cellular Hormone

Dialysis of Tissue Cytosol. To measure free cellular hormone, Oppenheimer and Schwartz (162) dialyzed cytosol of different organ extracts. Free cytosolic T_3 in the liver was measured by multiplying the total hepatic T_3 concentration by the dialyzable fraction of T_3 in hepatic cytosol measured in vitro. However, this approach gives a spuriously false measurement of free cellular T_3 because it is measured under conditions in which the dominant function in vivo, that is, the continuous flow of plasma bioavailable hormone, is absent. In other words, the normal partly flow–partly compartmental model that exists in vivo (Fig. 14.11) is reduced to a simple compartmental model without considering the continuous flow of plasma exchangeable hormone. The concentration of free cellular T_3 in dialyzed liver cytosol is approximately 50-fold greater than the concentration of free T_3 in the nucleus (162). Nuclear free T_3 was measured from the nuclear dissociation constant and the percent occupancy of the nuclear T_3 receptor. For example, the nuclear K_D in liver is 1.0 nM and the receptor is normally 47% occupied (162). Therefore, the nuclear free T_3 concentration was estimated to be 0.9 nM, which approximates the concentration of bioavailable plasma T_3 (Fig. 14.11). However, the low free cellular T_3 recorded with this cytosol dialysis method led these investigators to conclude that there was a 58-fold T_3 concentration gradient between the nucleus and the hepatic cytosol, which led to the postulate that active pumps at the nuclear membrane must exist for T_3. This postulate was made despite the fact that the putative active transport system for T_3 could not be identified in isolated nuclei (151). Moreover, the nuclear membrane is highly permeable and endowed with large pores on the order of 45 Å in size (165). The nuclear membrane is 10^8 times more permeable than the plasma membrane (97). For example, small molecules, such as sucrose (97), readily traverse the nuclear membrane, as do 20 kd proteins (17).

In the intervening years, there has been no experimental corroboration of the idea that there are active transport systems for T_3 at the nuclear membrane. Indeed, there is no precedent in transport biology for active transport pumps at the nuclear membrane for small molecules, such as iodothyronines. In the absence of postulating active pumps for T_3 at the nuclear membrane, it is difficult to reconcile the predictions of the free hormone hypothesis with the experimental observation that the hepatic nuclear T_3 receptor is approximately 50% occupied in vivo (162). This 50% occupancy means that the concentration of free nuclear T_3 is approximately 200-fold greater than the plasma free T_3 measured in vitro. Conversely, owing to enhanced dissociation of T_3 from albumin and TBG-binding sites in the liver microcirculation, the concentration of plasma bioavailable T_3 is approximately 1 nM (Fig. 14.11).

Dialysis Fibers.

Dialysis fibers have been implanted in the brain to measure the in vivo extravascular diazepam concentration (48). The concentration of free diazepam in the intracerebral dialysis fiber effluent was found to be identical to the free diazepam in the microdialysis effluent from a dialysis fiber placed in the inferior vena cava. Subsequent to this study, progress in the dialysis fiber field has shown that it is necessary to *(1)* measure the recovery across the dialysis fiber in vivo (98), not in vitro, as performed by Dubey and co-workers (48), and *(2)* consider the effects of the local injury when

the dialysis fiber is placed into brain tissue. When the drug concentration recovered from the dialysis fiber placed in vitro in a beaker experiment is compared to the recovery measured with the in vivo reference method, in vitro recovery is more than twofold greater with in vivo measurements (251, 252). The discrepancy between the in vivo and in vitro recoveries obtained with dialysis fibers has been attributed to the vasogenic edema and expansion of the extracellular space in brain caused by the injury due to implantation of the dialysis fiber (51). Therefore, the study by Dubey et al. (48) actually confirms the earlier findings of diazepam-enhanced dissociation (107) if in vivo measurements of dialysis fiber recovery are reported. However, a more serious concern with the use of dialysis fibers is the significant tissue injury associated with the implantation of a fiber into brain tissue. Dialysis fibers cause a significant disturbance of brain neurochemistry (11, 159, 285), and implantation of the dialysis fiber is a model of acute brain injury. Studies using a sensitive albumin immunocytochemical approach show exudation of albumin into the parenchyma surrounding the dialysis fiber owing to breakdown of the BBB soon after implantation of the fiber (278). This breakdown persists for at least 24 h and is consistent with persistent brain injury associated with the use of dialysis fibers. Conceivably, this brain injury and breakdown of the normal BBB permeability result in a significant alteration of the normal microcirculatory processes that underlie the enhanced dissociation mechanism.

Salivary Fluid Hormone Concentration Measurements.

Measurement of steroid hormone concentrations in human salivary fluid has been advocated as a method for assessing endocrine function and for providing measurements of free cellular hormone in a given organ, for example, the salivary gland epithelium (209a). Support for using salivary fluid steroid hormone concentrations as indicators of circulating free hormone came from the observation that the concentration of steroid hormone in salivary fluid frequently approximated the concentration of free hormone measured in vitro with techniques such as equilibrium dialysis (209a). In other studies, salivary testosterone exceeded by up to twofold the concentration of free testosterone measured in vitro (235), and salivary progesterone did not correlate with free plasma progesterone (57). Nevertheless, physiological correlates were found in the measurement of salivary testosterone. For example, the saliva/serum ratio of testosterone in normal men was 1.38%, while in hyperthyroid men it was 0.64% (273). The decreases in free and salivary testosterone concentrations in hyperthyroidism were consistent with the increased SHBG in this condition.

Despite the clinical correlations observed with salivary steroid hormone concentrations, the use of this parameter as an index of the circulating bioavailable hormone is flawed because it does not consider the fact that the salivary gland is a depot of active steroid hormone metabolism (28). As revealed by simulation 10 in Table 14.9, the presence of significant organ metabolism (represented by a measurable value for k_9) results in a constriction of the pool size of free cellular hormone (L_M, Fig. 14.10) relative to the concentration of plasma bioavailable hormone (L_F, Fig. 14.10). Moreover, albumin-bound testosterone and estradiol are readily available for transport into the salivary gland in vivo (Table 14.6), and SHBG-bound estradiol also is available for transport into the salivary gland (Table 14.7, Fig. 14.12A). Therefore, in the absence of hormone metabolism in this tissue, the concentration of salivary fluid testosterone should be equal to the free plus albumin-bound testosterone concentrations measured in vitro. The fact that the salivary fluid testosterone concentration approximates the free concentration measured in vitro suggests that there is active organ metabolism of testosterone in salivary gland tissue, which has been confirmed experimentally (Fig. 14.12C). In contrast to salivary gland, there was minimal metabolism of testosterone in brain or lymph node during the short experimental time period of 60 s following a single carotid artery injection of [^{3}H]-testosterone. Two-dimensional thin-layer chromatography showed that the major metabolites formed are androstenedione, at 60 s after injection, and 5α-androstane-3α,17β-diol (3α-diol), at 5 m after injection (28). These studies suggest that enzymes such as 17β-hydroxysteroid dehydrogenase, 5α-reductase, and 3α-hydroxysteroid dehydrogenase are present in salivary gland tissue. The finding that the salivary gland, like the liver or prostate, is an organ of active androgen metabolism contradicts the proposal that only free testosterone is available for transport into the salivary gland because androgen metabolism in this organ is low (209a). Rather, the low concentration of salivary fluid testosterone arises from very active androgen metabolism in this organ.

The salivary testosterone concentration is reduced relative to the albumin-bound concentration owing to active salivary gland metabolism of the hormone. There may be conditions in which salivary gland testosterone metabolism is impaired such that the salivary testosterone concentration increases and approximates the free plus albumin-bound concentrations of testosterone. In fact, the salivary testosterone/blood testosterone ratio in women with hirsutism is 10.3%, as opposed to the free dialyzable testosterone in these women of 1.3% (223). This value approximates the percentage of plasma bioavailable testosterone in salivary gland capillaries in vivo (Fig. 14.12A), which supports the concept that the bioavailable testosterone in the salivary gland includes the free plus albumin-bound testosterone values measured in vitro.

MOLECULAR PHYSIOLOGY OF HORMONE-BINDING PLASMA PROTEINS

Albumin

Structural Features. Bovine serum albumin (BSA) is a 582-amino-acid single polypeptide that is normally not glycosylated (Fig. 14.13). The HSA gene family is comprised of HSA, α-fetoprotein (AFP), DBP (35), and afamin (129). All members of the HSA gene family map to chromosome 4 (198). The albumin gene is comprised of 15 exons and 14 introns and encodes the albumin mRNA, which is a 2.2 kb transcript produced predominantly in liver (198) but also in multiple tissues in the fetus and newborn (154). In a gram of liver, there are 19 μg of poly A+ mRNA for rat serum albumin (RSA). The albumin mRNA is comprised of 2080 nucleotides, with 39 nucleotides in the 5'-untranslated region (UTR) and 210 nucleotides in the 3'-UTR followed by a poly A tail. The translated protein contains a signal peptide of 18 residues, including the methionine initiation amino acid. Proalbumin migrates to the endoplasmic reticulum and contains a hexapeptide leader sequence, which is cleaved prior to secretion of albumin from the cell (198).

There is strong structural amino-acid homology between BSA, HSA, and RSA, which are comprised of 582, 585, and 584 amino acids, respectively (198). The more negatively charged protein of the three is BSA, with a net charge of -18, as opposed to -15 and -12 for HSA and RSA, respectively. It has two tryptophan residues at positions 134 and 212, whereas HSA and RSA have a single tryptophan residue at position 214. This single tryptophan residue participates in the binding of acidic drugs (198). There is 76% amino-acid homology between BSA and HSA. Human serum albumin is comprised of 35 cysteine residues, which form 17 disulfide bridges within the molecule, leaving one free cysteine residue at position 34. Bovine serum albumin has an additional cysteine residue near the amino-terminus and is comprised of 18 disulfide bonds. Analysis of the primary amino-acid sequence of HSA shows that the protein is comprised of six subdomains and three approximately equal repeated domains, each of about 190 amino acids in length (198). The structure is consistent with the evolution of the HSA gene from successive tandem gene duplication. There is a high

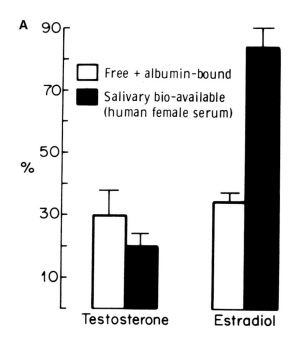

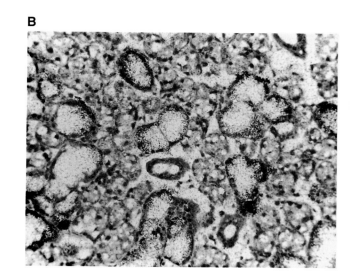

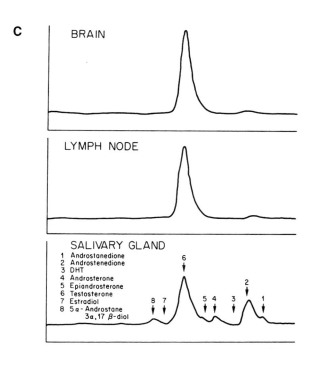

FIG. 14.12. *A*: Fractions of free plus albumin-bound testosterone and estradiol in vitro and bioavailable testosterone and estradiol in rat salivary gland in vivo are compared, showing that sex hormone–binding globulin (SHBG)-bound estradiol, but not SHBG-bound testosterone, is readily available for transport into rat salivary gland. In addition, albumin-bound testosterone or estradiol is bioavailable in salivary gland capillaries. These in vivo measurements were made at 15 s after a single carotid artery injection of [^{3}H]-hormone mixed in human female serum. This short period is sufficient to allow for rapid distribution of hormone into the glandular epithelium, as shown by the autoradiographic studies in *B*. [From Pardridge (170) with permission.] *B*: Thaw-mount autoradiogram of rat salivary gland removed 15 s after single carotid artery injection of [^{3}H]-estradiol dissolved in Ringer-HEPES buffer containing 0.1 g/dl bovine albumin. The [^{3}H]-estradiol is found throughout the gland, with concentration over the salivary gland ductules. The tissue was counterstained after autoradiography with methylgreen-pyronin. [From Cefalu et al. (28) with permission.] *C*: One-dimensional thin-layer chromatographic separation of brain, cervical lymph node, and salivary gland homogenates of tissue obtained 60 s after a single carotid artery injection of [^{3}H]-testosterone (50 μCi/ml) in Ringer-HEPES buffer containing 0.1 g/dl bovine albumin. Migration of testosterone or several other metabolites in the one-dimensional system is shown. The minor peak in the brain and lymph node studies that co-migrated with androstenedione (peak 2) represents an impurity in the isotope, as this was found also in the [^{3}H]-testosterone obtained from the manufacturer. The data show that while testosterone is rapidly metabolized in salivary gland, there is no significant metabolism in the whole brain or lymph node within 60 s after administration in vivo. [From Cefalu et al. (28) with permission.]

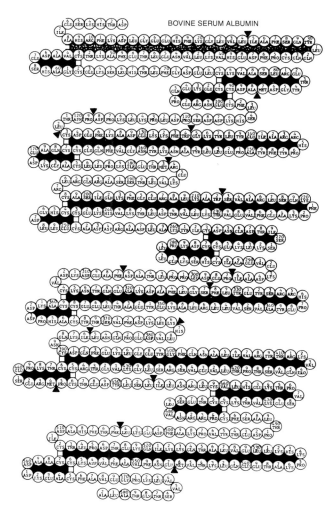

BOVINE SERUM ALBUMIN

FIG. 14.13. Amino-acid sequence of bovine serum albumin, displayed in a model showing the linking of cysteines to form multiple loops as proposed by Brown (22).

helical content of the protein, which ranges from 54% to 68%, and there is a proline residue at the end of each loop. A typical sequence of Arg-His-Pro allows for a 180° turn between two helices (22). Bovine serum albumin can be cleaved with pepsin into two fragments of equal size, which are comprised of residues 1–306 and 307–582 (198).

The three-dimensional structure of HSA has been determined by X-ray diffraction (88), and these data confirm earlier models on the shape of the albumin molecule using circular dichroism (137). The molecule is a V-shaped globular protein with a relatively compact configuration and is comprised of three domains and a total molecular width of approximately 80 Å. The heart-shaped structure of albumin, determined by X-ray diffraction, is shown in Figure 14.14. Domains

I, II, and III are structurally similar and are comprised of two subdomains each, which are designated IA, IB, IIA, IIB, IIIA, and IIIB. Free fatty acids and tryptophan bind to subdomain IIIA, and bilirubin and warfarin bind to subdomain IIA (88). The single free cysteine residue at position 34 is the site of covalent attachment of glutathione or cysteine. The single tryptophan residue conserved in all species at position 212–214 acts as a common interface between domains II and III, and this explains why a ligand bound to domain III affects the conformational state of ligands bound to domain II. The three domains are connected by three α-helical stretches at residues 101–124 (connecting domains IA and IB), 289–316 (connecting domains IIA and IIB), and 487–514 (connecting domains IIIA and IIIB) (Fig. 14.15).

The three-dimensional structure of proteins determined with X-ray diffraction yields a static image of a relatively rigid protein molecule. However, this is not an accurate image as more detailed analyses have shown that proteins should be viewed as "springs" with constant random fluctuations of molecular motion that allow for sudden conformational transitions, sometimes of either a regional or a global nature (112). As reviewed by Peters (198), albumin should not be considered to be in a static state but is a "kicking and screaming stochastic" molecule. Kragh-Hansen (120) has reviewed the flexible nature of the albumin molecule and has classified the conformational changes as being of either large amplitude, similar to a "breathing" molecule, or small amplitude, with conformational changes that have a half-time on the order of nanoseconds. In a series of peptides, albumin conformational changes were found to be the most dynamic (120). The flexibility of the albumin molecule was found to be reduced by either acidic pH or binding by cationic drugs (120). This finding is of interest since the binding of lipophilic amines, such as propranolol or bupivacaine, results in a loss of enhanced dissociation mechanisms of these ligands from the albumin molecule. This loss of enhanced dissociation is shown by the equivalence between the K_D of cationic drug binding to albumin in vivo in the brain capillary vs the K_D found in vitro (Table 14.5).

Familial Dysalbuminemic Hyperthyroxinemia. Familial dysalbuminemic hyperthyroxinemia (FDH) is an autosomal dominant (278) condition that results in approximately one-third of albumin molecules having an unusually high affinity ($K_D = 60$ nM) for (T_4) (6). This K_D is approximately tenfold higher than the affinity of normal albumin for T_4 (6). This is a genetic abnormality that results in a single-amino acid substitution of Arg[218] to His[218] (222). The FDH abnormality provides

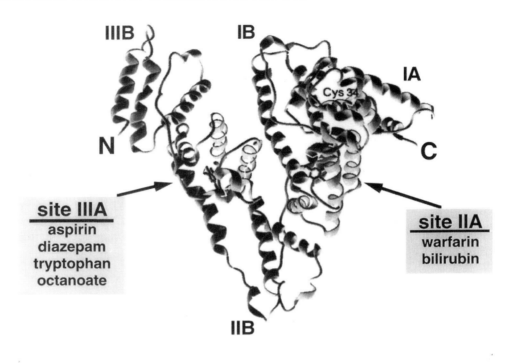

FIG. 14.14. Three-dimensional structure of human serum albumin predicted from X-ray diffraction studies. The amino *(N)* and carboxyl *(C)* termini are shown. The six different putative binding sites on the albumin molecule are shown, designated *IA, IB, IIA, IIB, IIIA,* and *IIIB*. The principal drug-binding sites on albumin are *IIA* and *IIIA*. [From Carter and He (26) with permission.]

an interesting clinical example of the diversity of plasma protein binding of hormones. Thyroxine bound to the normal iodothyronine-binding site on albumin is freely available for transport into the liver in vivo (185), owing to enhanced dissociation of this ligand from the albumin-binding site. However, T_4 bound to the dysalbuminemic binding site in FDH is not available for transport into the liver in vivo via enhanced dissociation (29). That is, the surface interaction between albumin and the hepatocyte in vivo does not cause a conformational change about the dysalbumin T_4-binding site, whereas conformational changes take place around the normal T_4-binding site on albumin.

The differential availability of T_4 bound to either the normal or dysalbuminemic site on HSA may be demonstrated by measuring the unidirectional influx of $[^{125}I]$-T_4 into rat liver in vivo in the presence of either control human or FDH serum using a T_4-loading technique (Fig. 14.16). Loading serum with 25 μM T_4 displaces all radioactive T_4 from the TBG and prealbumin-binding sites to high-capacity albumin sites (29). This results in 100% bioavailability of T_4 in normal serum (Fig. 14.15) but only a marginal increase in bioavailability of T_4 from FDH serum, indicating

that T_4 bound to the dysalbuminemic site on FDH albumin is not readily available for transport into the liver in vivo.

Normally, T_4 is bound at the tryptophan-binding site on albumin (120, 198), which corresponds to domain IIIA (Fig. 14.14). Biochemical studies indicate that the amino-acid residue altered in the FDH albumin corresponds to His^{218} (222), which is located within domain IIA (Fig. 14.15). Domain IIA is normally the binding site for acidic compounds, such as acetylsalicylic acid, bilirubin and warfarin (Fig. 14.14). The decreased hepatic availability of T_4 from the dysalbumin-binding site suggests that the conformational changes about domain IIIA are greater than those about domain IIA in the liver microcirculation when T_4 is bound to that site.

Analbuminemia. The enhanced dissociation model for PMT has been criticized because the genetic condition of analbuminemia (the complete loss of albumin) is not lethal (145). Therefore, it is reasoned that albumin could not play a unique role in hormone or ligand delivery to tissues. However, in this condition, the serum total protein is nearly normal as serum globulins

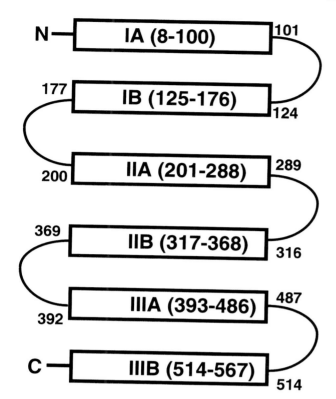

N — IA (8-100) 101

177 IB (125-176)
124

200 IIA (201-288) 289

369 IIB (317-368)
316

IIIA (393-486) 487
392

C — IIIB (514-567)
514

FIG. 14.15. Approximate amino-acid residues comprising the six binding domains in serum albumin. [Drawn from data of Carter and He (26) with permission.]

are increased substantially to offset the diminished plasma albumin concentration (145). Moreover, studies in analbuminemic rats have shown that the serum globulins subserve the function normally carried out by albumin binding of ligands (100). For example, PMT of the dye rose bengal is observed in the liver via the circulating serum γ-globulin pool (263). Similarly, high-density lipoprotein (HDL) transports bilirubin in lieu of albumin in the analbuminemic rat (248). In other studies in these animals, the delivery of acidic drugs, such as furosemide or phenolsulfophthalein (PSP), to kidney was mediated via a complex of albumin and furosemide (101). Thus, urinary secretion of furosemide was significantly reduced in analbuminemic compared to control rats (102). The observation that PMT occurs via the γ-globulins in the analbuminemic rat suggests that these plasma proteins play an important role in ligand delivery to tissues in invertebrates, which lack serum albumin.

α-Fetoprotein. α-Fetoprotein is a 68,000 dalton serum α₁-globulin present in serum (3). This is a sialic acid–containing glycoprotein found in the blood of all mam-

mals. Rat, but not human (249), AFP is a high-affinity binder of estradiol (238). During development, AFP levels in serum may peak at 0.3 g % and represent up to 90% of the plasma globulin fraction (3). Like DBP, AFP is a member of the albumin gene family.

Rat AFP binds estradiol and estrone with high affinity but does not bind other estrogens, 17α-estradiol, progesterone, or testosterone (89, 193). The K_D of estradiol binding to rat AFP at 4°C is 15 nM. Transport of [³H]-estradiol or [³H]-testosterone into adult rat brain has been measured in the presence of newborn rat serum that contains 1–4 μM concentrations of AFP (178). These studies show that brain estradiol uptake is inhibited more than 90% by circulating rat AFP. However, nearly 100% of circulating testosterone is available for uptake by the brain in the presence of newborn rat serum owing to (1) the absence of testosterone binding to AFP and (2) the absence of significant quantities of TeBG in rat serum in the newborn period.

Prealbumin (Transthyretin)

Plasma prealbumin is a high-affinity binder of T₄ (283). The plasma concentration of prealbumin is approximately 1% that of albumin (247). However, the affinity of prealbumin for T₄ (2.9 nM) is approximately 1,000-fold greater than the affinity of albumin for T₄ (247). Therefore, in the rat or rabbit, approximately 86% of T₄ is prealbumin-bound, with approximately 14% albumin-bound and 0.06% free (dialyzable). Unlike humans, the rat or rabbit has low levels of TBG.

Human prealbumin is a homotetramer, comprised of 127 amino-acid subunits and a total molecular weight of approximately 55,000 daltons (13). The protein has two symmetrically related β-sheets containing a pair of helically disposed arms, as described by Blake and Oatley (13) and shown in Figure 14.17. X-ray diffraction studies show that there are two T₄-binding sites on the prealbumin homotetramer and that these sites are deeply buried in the narrow cylindrical channel that runs through the center of the molecule. Prealbumin also has independent high-affinity binding sites for retinol-binding protein (RBP), which is the high-affinity plasma binder of retinol (vitamin A). The dual binding of T₄ and RBP by prealbumin is why this protein is also called transthyretin. There are four RBP-binding sites per prealbumin homotetramer. Although there are two binding sites for T₄, the binding demonstrates negative cooperativity and there is decreased affinity for T₄ at the second site subsequent to binding at the first site (204, 205).

A member of the α₁-acid glycoprotein gene family (197), RBP has a molecular size of 21,000 daltons (75).

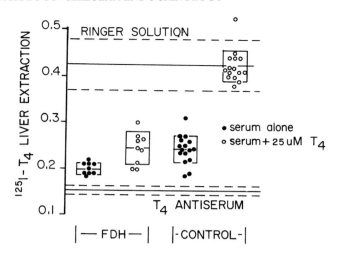

FIG. 14.16. Unidirectional extraction of [^{125}I]-thyroxine *(T$_4$)* into rat liver in vivo is shown for three types of portal vein injection vehicles: Ringer-HEPES buffer plus 0.1 g/100 dl bovine albumin, normal human serum, or serum obtained from patients with familial dysalbuminemic hyperthyroxinemia *(FDH)* in the presence of 0 or 25 μM unlabeled T$_4$, and rabbit anti-T$_4$ antiserum. Extraction of T$_4$ following portal vein injection of Ringer-HEPES buffer represents the situation when approximately 100% of T$_4$ is available for extraction by hepatocytes; extraction of T$_4$ by liver following portal vein injection of the isotope dissolved in the T$_4$ antiserum represents the baseline extraction when the amount of injected T$_4$ available for extraction by hepatocytes is essentially nil. Horizontal bars represent the mean $\pm$ one standard deviation for the extraction of T$_4$ in either Ringer's solution or the T$_4$ antiserum. [From Cefalu et al. (29) with permission.]

Therefore, binding of RBP to prealbumin may retard glomerular filtration of RBP (155). Subsequent to RBP facilitation of retinol transport into tissues, RBP may be modified at the cell membrane such that the protein no longer binds prealbumin, thus releasing it for clearance via glomerular filtration (202).

Rat, rabbit, and human prealbumin have strongly conserved amino-acid sequences (246). There is 85% amino-acid identity between human and rabbit prealbumin, and 83% amino acid identity between human and rat prealbumin. A significant proportion of the substitutions involve charged amino acids. These radical substitutions are listed in Table 14.12. These amino-acid substitutions may account for the major differences in functional delivery of rat and human prealbumin with respect to T$_4$ delivery to the liver. Thyroxine bound to human, but not rat, prealbumin is available for transport into the liver (173, 188). The bioavailable fraction of T$_4$ in rat serum in the hepatic microcirculation is 31% $\pm$ 2%. Rats lack significant plasma concentrations of TBG. Since albumin-bound T$_4$ is freely available for uptake by rat liver (173), the 70% inhibition in bioavailable T$_4$ by rat serum is due to the fact that approximately 70% of T$_4$ is distributed to prealbumin in plasma (247) and that T$_4$ bound to rat prealbumin is not available for uptake by the liver (173). Thus, prealbumin in the rat sequesters T$_4$ in

the plasma of the hepatic microcirculation, a function carried out in human blood by TBG. However, T$_4$ bound to human prealbumin is readily available for transport into the liver in vivo, as shown by the increase in bioavailable T$_4$ in rat liver following portal injection of serum obtained from patients with TBG deficiency (Fig. 14.18). Transport of T$_4$ from the human prealbumin-binding site in rat liver was demonstrated further with portal vein injections of solutions containing purified human prealbumin (Fig. 14.18). The affinities of T$_4$ binding to rat and human prealbumin

TABLE 14.12. *Radical Amino-Acid Substitutions in Rat and Human Prealbumin*

Residue Number	Amino Acid	
	Human	Rat
34	Pro	Lys
39	Asp	Gly
63	Gln	Lys
90	His	Tyr
102	Pro	His
126	Lys	Gln
127	Glu	Asn

[From Dickson et al. (46) and Sundelin et al. (247) with permission.]

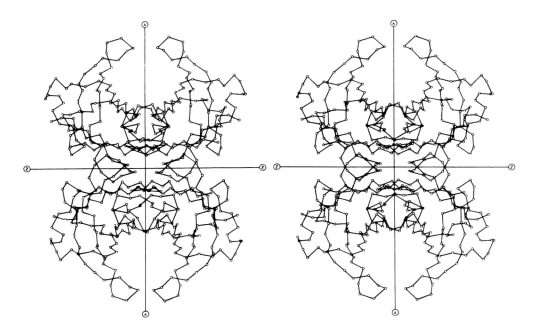

FIG. 14.17. Stereo view of the three-dimensional structure predicted from X-ray diffraction for the prealbumin homotetramer. [From Blake and Oatley (13) with permission.]

are comparable. For example, the K_D of T_4 binding to rat prealbumin is 2.9 nM (247), and that to human prealbumin is 4.4 nM (283). Therefore, the marked differences in T_4 availability in rat liver, depending on whether the molecule is bound to human or rat prealbumin, cannot be ascribed to species differences in binding avidity of T_4 for the protein. An alternate explanation is that there are surface amino-acid residues on human prealbumin that are absent on rat prealbumin. These surface amino acids may trigger adsorption of the protein to the cellular surface of the hepatic microcirculation, causing a conformational change about the T_4-binding site on human prealbumin in vivo. Candidate amino acids are the seven radical substitutions in human prealbumin as compared to rat prealbumin (Table 14.12).

Thyroid Hormone–Binding Globulin

Protein Biochemistry. A product of the X chromosome, TBG is a 54,000 dalton glycoprotein that is a member of the same gene family as CBG and the plasma serine protease inhibitors α_1-antichymotrypsin and α_1-antitrypsin (62). The protein is approximately 20% carbohydrate and there are four consensus N-linked carbohydrate attachment sites at different Asn residues (2, 62). There is a single-copy TBG gene in humans (110).

Differential processing of the primary transcript causes heterogeneity of TBG mRNAs in the liver. Although TBG is increased in patients subjected to estrogen treatment or pregnancy, estradiol may not increase TBG gene transcription (87). Rather, estrogen treatment increases the sialic acid portion of the carbohydrate moiety (1), resulting in inhibition of peripheral degradation of TBG. The increased sialic acid content of TBG causes the protein to be more acidic, as shown by polyacrylamide gel isoelectric focusing (IEF) (Fig. 14.19).

Differential Bioavailability of Thyroid Hormone–Binding Globulin-Bound Triiodothyronine and Thyroxine. The binding of TBG by T_4 is of extremely high affinity, with K_D values ranging from 0.05 to 0.4 nM (237, 284). Although the binding of TBG by T_3 is approximately tenfold less than that by T_4 (237), the overall binding power of circulating TBG by T_3 is substantial. Therefore, in humans, approximately 70% of circulating T_3 is TBG-bound, with 30% albumin-bound and 0.3% free (dialyzable) (284). Approximately 70% of circulating T_4 is TBG-bound, with 20% prealbumin-bound, 10% albumin-bound, and about 0.03% free (dialyzable). The extent to which TBG binds T_3 in vivo was questioned by early studies showing that the $t_{1/2}$ of T_3 removal from the plasma compartment was not altered in patients with either increased TBG (for exam-

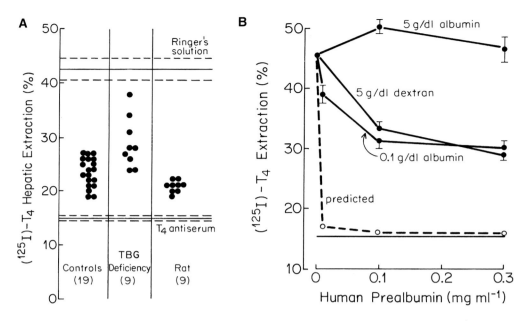

FIG. 14.18. *A:* Extraction of [^{125}I]-thryoxine *(T₄)* into rat liver following portal vein injection of the isotope dissolved in three different solutions: Ringer-HEPES buffer containing 0.1 g/dl bovine albumin *(upper horizontal bar)*, control or thyroid hormone–binding globulin *(TBG)*–deficient human serum or normal rat serum *(closed circles)*, T₄-specific rabbit antiserum *(lower horizontal bar)*. Extractions obtained following injection of Ringer's solution or T₄ antiserum represent the hepatocyte extraction when approximately 100% and 0%, respectively, of labeled hormone is available for transport into liver. Horizontal bars represent mean ± SE (*n* = 3–6 rats per point). The number of subjects in each category is shown in parenthe-

ses. *B:* Extraction of [^{125}I]-T₄ by rat liver in vivo is plotted vs. the concentration of human prealbumin in the portal vein injection solution. Human prealbumin and [^{125}I]-T₄ were mixed with either 5 or 0.1 g/dl bovine albumin or 5 g/dl dextran (65,000 daltons). Dashed line represents the extraction of T₄ predicted on the basis of the bound T₄ fraction as measured in vitro by equilibrium dialysis at each concentration of prealbumin. All concentrations of human prealbumin (0.01–0.3 mg/ml) bound more than 96% of T₄ in vitro. Solid horizontal line represents hepatic extraction of T₄ in the presence of a 10% T₄ antiserum. [From Pardridge et al. (188) with permission.]

ple, by estrogen administration) or congenital TBG deficiency (286, 287). In contrast, the $t_{1/2}$ of T₄ clearance from plasma was increased in patients with elevated TBG and decreased in patients with decreased TBG concentrations in plasma. The TBG independence of hepatic T₃ clearance was confirmed with the portal vein single-injection technique (185), which demonstrated that TBG-bound T₃ is readily available for transport into rat liver in vivo, whereas TBG-bound T₄ is not available (Fig. 14.19). Thus, there is a functional heterogeneity with respect to TBG-mediated delivery of T₄ or T₃ to the liver (173). The presence of TBG in plasma facilitates T₃ delivery but retards T₄ uptake by the liver, making TBG a "T₃ amplifier."

Microheterogeneity of Thyroid Hormone–Binding Globulin Binding of Triiodothyronine and Thyroxine.

The observation, illustrated in Figure 14.19, that TBG selectively delivers T₃, but not T₄, to the liver is difficult to

reconcile with the traditional view that T₃ and T₄ bind to a single competitive binding site on TBG (212). Maberly et al. (139) showed that T₄ and T₃ have different TBG-binding capacities. The functional heterogeneity with respect to T₄ and T₃ delivery to the liver by TBG was correlated with the structural heterogeneity of T₄ and T₃ binding to this plasma protein. The latter was determined with IEF separation of human TBG isoforms carrying either [^{125}I]-T₃ or [^{125}I]-T₄ (Fig. 14.19). These studies show that T₄ is bound selectively to the most acidic isoforms of TBG, whereas T₃ is bound preferentially to the more alkaline isoforms of the protein (255). The IEF results were confirmed with chromatofocusing, showing that T₄ is bound selectively to the more acidic isoforms of TBG. Scatchard analysis showed that the selective binding of T₄ to the acidic isoforms of TBG was due to a reduced affinity of T₃ binding to the most acidic forms of TBG (255). Moreover, T₄ was bound preferentially to the more

STRUCTURE

FUNCTION

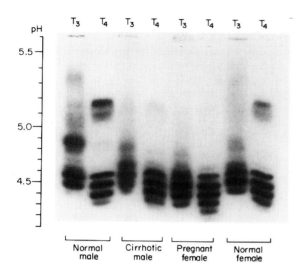

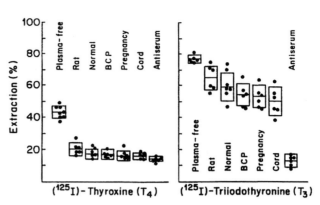

FIG. 14.19. Heterogeneity of thyroid hormone–binding globulin (TBG) structure and function *Right:* Extraction of [^{125}I]-thyroxine (T_4) or [^{125}I]-triiodethyronine (T_3) by rat liver is plotted vs. the type of serum added to the portal vein injection solution. Plasma-free solutions contain 0.1 g/dl bovine albumin; T_4-, or T_4-specific antiserum solutions were diluted to 10%. All other samples were injected at 67% serum solutions. Each point represents a different patient, volunteer, or animal. Boxes represent the mean ± SD.

Normal, human, and cord samples were obtained from both females and males. *BCP,* birth control pills. *Left:* Autoradiogram of [^{125}I]-T_3 or [^{125}I]-T_4 bound to TBG isoforms, albumin isoforms, and prealbumin in serum from normal male subjects, cirrhotic male patients, pregnant subjects, and normal female subjects following separation by isoelectric focusing. The pH values of the gel are shown in the ordinate of the figure. [From Pardridge (173) with permission.]

acidic isoforms of TBG in pregnancy (Fig. 14.19), a condition associated with increased glycosylation of the protein (1). Binding of T_4 advances from more alkaline to more acidic isoforms of TBG in the neonatal rat, which has higher TBG plasma concentrations compared to the adult (218). These combined studies suggest that glycosylation of TBG (71) plays a functional role apart from merely influencing the rate of peripheral catabolism of the binding protein. In fact, glycosylation may allow for microheterogeneity of T_4 and T_3 binding to TBG, and this microheterogeneity may underlie the selective amplification by TBG of T_3 delivery to the liver, relative to T_4 uptake (173).

Nonthyroidal Illness. The free hormone hypothesis predicts that if the concentration of free (dialyzable) hormone is within the normal range, then the endocrine status of the individual is normal (53, 213). Nonthyroidal illness (NTI) provides a clinical test of this hypothesis. In this condition, total T_4 concentration is decreased in parallel with an inhibition of TBG binding

of T_4, which results in a concentration of free (dialyzable) T_4 that is either elevated (12) or normal (33). However, when the bioavailable T_4 in the hepatic microcirculation is measured in vivo with serum obtained from patients with NTI, fractional T_4 delivery to the liver is unchanged (191). Therefore, the flux of T_4 to hepatic tissues is decreased in proportion to the decrease in total T_4 serum concentration. These considerations suggest that patients with NTI are actually hypothyroid in function, and this has been confirmed by studies showing that angiotensin-converting enzyme is decreased in patients with either hypothyroidism or NTI (20). Similarly, measurements of the MCR of T_4 in patients with NTI show that there is no correlation between free T_4 and the MCR in these individuals. In addition, the early disappearance of T_4 is not enhanced in patients with NTI as it is in TBG deficiency (111). Although the free dialyzable fraction of T_4 is increased in both NTI and TBG deficiency, the fractional bioavailable T_4 in the liver is increased only in TBG deficiency (173).

Corticosteroid-Binding Globulin

Protein Biochemistry. The principal corticosteroids of humans and rats are cortisol and corticosterone, respectively. These plasma corticosteroids are approximately 77% CBG-bound, 15% albumin-bound, and 8% free (dialyzable) (216). The dissociation constant of CBG binding of cortisol is 80 nM, and the concentration of CBG in normal serum is 850–1000 nM. A protein of 58,000 daltons, CBG is 23% carbohydrate by weight (83), with six N-linked glycosylation sites (81). The CBG gene is a member of the TBG and α_1-antitrypsin serine protease inhibitor family. The protein is translated from a 1.6 kb mRNA present in liver, kidney, and lung (83). The finding that TBG and CBG are members of the serine protease inhibitor (SERPIN) gene superfamily is somewhat unexpected. Studies have shown that proteolytic cleavage at Val^{344}-Thr^{345} results in the release of a 4000 dalton segment from CBG or TBG (194). This cleavage is mediated by peripheral enzymes, such as elastase (84), and results in conformational changes in the protein (194). These conformational changes are associated with an enhanced dissociation of cortisol from the binding protein. However, it is uncertain that proteolysis is a general mechanism of enhanced hormone dissociation from plasma proteins.

Corticosteroid-Binding Globulin Functions as a Hepatic Cortisol Amplifier.

In peripheral tissues, such as brain, only albumin-bound corticosteroid is available for transport, whereas corticosteroid is not available for transport from the human CBG-bound pool in the rat (190). Conversely, in rat liver, corticosteroid is readily available for transport into this tissue from the human CBG-bound pool of hormone (190). This observation is evidence for enhanced dissociation of corticosteroid from the human CBG-binding site within the hepatic microcirculation. The enhanced dissociation model is invoked because the membrane permeability for cortisol in the hepatic microcirculation is too low to allow for dissociation-limited transport in this tissue. For example, the hepatocyte membrane permeability coefficient (k_3) in the edematous, anoxic perfused rat liver is 2.3 s (146), which is at least 15-fold lower than the rate of cortisol reassociation with CBG (Table 14.4). Selective delivery of cortisol to the liver from the circulating CBG-bound pool in the liver, but not in the brain, allows for CBG to function as a hepatic cortisol amplifier (190). The mechanism underlying the putative enhanced dissociation of cortisol from the CBG-binding site in the hepatic microcirculation is not known. Free fatty acids cause conformational changes in CBG and an increased dissociation of corticosteroids from the CBG-binding site (142). The finding that cortisol is available for uptake from the CBG-bound pool in the liver confirms early studies which suggested that CBG is a hepatic cortisol amplifier (113).

Species Differences in Function. The functional differences in hormone delivery by human and rat prealbumin were discussed previously. Similarly, there are significant species differences between rats and rabbits with respect to CBG function and corticosteroid delivery. Although corticosteroid was not available for uptake by the brain from the human or rat CBG-bound pool in the rat (190), it was readily available for transport into the brain and uterus in the rabbit from the circulating rabbit CBG-bound pool (31, 175). This process represents a mechanism of enhanced dissociation since the transcapillary exodus of the corticosteroid is greatly in excess of the exodus from the capillary of the CBG protein per se. The enhanced dissociation of corticosterone from the CBG-binding site in the rabbit is supported by measurements of the corticosteroid MCR. In the rabbit, CBG has little inhibitory effect on the MCR of corticosterone (42). As discussed elsewhere in this chapter, the steady-state model (Figs. 14.10, 14.11) may be used to show that the free hormone hypothesis, with or without dissociation limitation, predicts that CBG should inhibit the MCR of corticosterone. Failure to observe this inhibition, along with the in vivo transport data (31, 175), indicates there is enhanced dissociation of corticosterone in vivo from the circulating rabbit CBG-binding site.

Sex Hormone–Binding Globulin

Protein Biochemistry. The presence of a high-affinity testosterone-binding protein in human serum, SHBG, was first observed in the 1960s (148). The SHBG in plasma of humans and primates binds both testosterone and estradiol with high affinity, whereas the globulin in the plasma of rabbit, dog, goat, and bull binds only testosterone with high affinity (37, 209). Species such as rat, pig, and horse generally do not have substantial concentrations of an androgen- or estrogen-binding protein in serum, with the exception of neonatal rats, which have high concentrations of the estradiol-binding protein AFP (238). Rat testis secretes an androgen-binding protein (ABP) which is homologous with human SHBG and rabbit TeBG but differs with respect to glycosylation (109). There is 68% amino-acid homology between human SHBG and rabbit ABP. These proteins are members of a gene family that includes laminin and the protein S clotting factor (108).

A cDNA for SHBG was isolated from a λgt11 human liver cDNA library (85). Based on the cDNA sequence, the predicted SHBG polypeptide is comprised of 402 amino acids, with the first 29 residues representing a hydrophobic signal polypeptide (82). The mature protein is comprised of 373 amino acids with two disulfide bridges linking Cys^{164} to Cys^{188} and Cys^{333} to Cys^{361} (82). These structural characteristics are similar for rabbit TeBG, which is 367 amino acids in length, has predicted N-linked carbohydrate sites at Asn^{345} and Asn^{361}, and has disulfide bridges at Cys^{158}–Cys^{182} and Cys^{327}–Cys^{355} (78). There are two consensus sites for N-linked glycosylation and an O-linked site for glycosylation at Thr^7 on human SHBG (82). The protein exists as a homodimer of 90,000–100,000 daltons, wherein the two subunits (52 and 48 kd) apparently differ in glycosylation. Rabbit TeBG (78), like rat ABP (109), has a 79% amino-acid identity with human SHBG. Hammond and Bocchinfuso (82) suggest that SHBG is a modular protein, wherein the amino-terminal domain participates in steroid binding and dimerization, whereas the carboxyl-terminal domain participates in glycosylation and possibly cell surface recognition.

Human SHBG is a high-affinity binder for dihydrotestosterone, testosterone, and estradiol, with K_D values of 0.6, 1, and 2 nM, respectively (268, 269). Testosterone and estradiol also bind to albumin, with K_D values of 28 and 16 μM, respectively (269). The concentration of SHBG in human serum may vary from 20 nM to greater than 200 nM (186, 220). In normal male serum, distributions of estradiol are approximately 61%, 37%, and 2% for the albumin-bound, SHBG-bound, and free (dialyzable) fractions, respectively (50). The corresponding distributions for testosterone in control human female serum are 30%, 66%, and 1.4%. Approximately 2% of testosterone is CBG-bound in control human serum (50).

Sex Hormone–Binding Globulin as an Estradiol Amplifier.

The fact that testosterone and estradiol exist in at least three different states in plasma (free, albumin-bound, SHBG-bound) has been a source of considerable discussion over the years as to which fraction of serum hormone is biologically available for uptake by tissues (272). There also has been debate as to whether SHBG is an important binder of estradiol in vivo. These issues may be addressed by direct in vivo empiric testing of testosterone or estradiol transport into tissues within the context of a quantifiable model of capillary transport physiology. One approach to this end is the use of the single-arterial-injection technique to estimate the bioavailable fraction in an organ capillary bed in vivo (168). When this is done in brain, the K_D of albumin binding of testosterone or estradiol may be measured, and these studies show that there is enhanced dissociation of testosterone or estradiol from the albumin-binding site in vivo (Table 14.5). Therefore, in brain, the bioavailable fraction in plasma includes the free plus albumin-bound testosterone or estradiol. No transport of human SHBG-bound testosterone or estradiol was found in rat brain in vivo. Thus, human SHBG is an important binder of estradiol in vivo, as shown by the studies in Figure 14.20. The BUIs for testosterone and estradiol are plotted in Figure 14.20 for different types of human serum containing various concentrations of SHBG (186). The BUI is essentially identical to the unidirectional extraction of testosterone or estradiol by rat brain in vivo in the presence of varying concentrations of SHBG in different patient groups. The ratio of unidirectional extraction of estradiol relative to that of testosterone is shown in Table 14.13 along with the mean SHBG concentration for the different patient groups. Since (clearance) = (extraction) × (flow) and since the flow cancels in a ratio, the unidirectional clearance ratio is identical to the unidirectional extraction ratio. These data show that as the SHBG concentration increases, the unidirectional clearance of estrogen by the tissue increases relative to testosterone clearance. These studies corroborate the early views of Burke and Anderson (25) that SHBG is an estradiol amplifier, though these authors believed that the bioavailable fraction in vivo was restricted to the free (dialyzable) hormone.

The free and albumin-bound fractions change in parallel when albumin concentrations are constant, and the primary change is in the plasma SHBG concentration. However, the free and albumin-bound fractions may not change in parallel directions in all cases. For example, in cirrhosis, where albumin is decreased and SHBG is increased, these changes have offsetting effects on the free dialyzable fraction, which is relatively unchanged. However, the decreased albumin and increased SHBG both cause the albumin-bound fraction to decrease in cirrhosis (224).

The SHBG amplification of estradiol delivery is even greater in the liver since human SHBG-bound estradiol, but not SHBG-bound testosterone, is available for transport into rat liver in vivo (Fig. 14.21). That is, globulin-bound estradiol, like globulin-bound corticosteroid, is available for transport into the liver in vivo, whereas globulin-bound testosterone is not available for uptake by the liver under normal conditions. The availability of SHBG-bound estradiol to the liver, the principal site of estradiol metabolic clearance, explains the lack of inhibition of estradiol MCR in the rat following infusion of human SHBG (156). Selective transport into the liver of SHBG-bound estradiol, but not SHBG-bound testosterone, is analogous to selective delivery to the liver of TBG-bound T_3 relative to TBG-

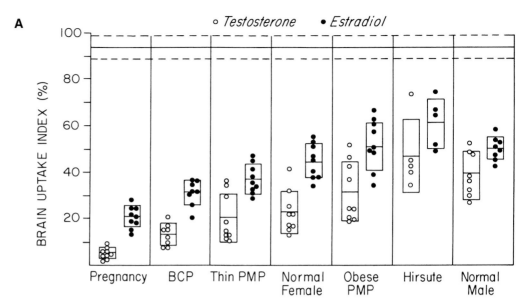

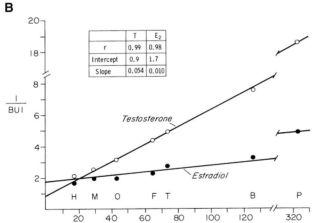

FIG. 14.20. *A:* Brain uptake index (BUI) for [³H]-testosterone and [³H]-estradiol relative to [¹⁴C]-butanol is shown for five to nine patients in seven clinical conditions. Vertical rectangles are means ± SD; horizontal line is mean of testosterone or estradiol BUI in absence of plasma proteins. *BCP,* birth control pill–treated women; *PMP,* postmenopausal women. *B:* Reciprocal of BUI for [³H]-testosterone *(T)* and [³H]-estradiol *(E₂)* is plotted vs. the level of sex hormone–binding globulin *(SHBG)* in human serum. Data for BUI are shown in *A. P,* pregnancy; *B,* birth control pills; *T,* thin postmenopausal female; *F,* normal follicular phase female; *O,* obese postmenopausal female; *M,* normal male; *H,* hirsute female. Data obtained by linear regression are shown in inset for both plots. [From Pardridge et al. (186) with permission.]

bound T_4. Similar to the case with TBG, selective delivery of estradiol to the liver is not compatible with binding of estradiol and testosterone to a single competitive binding site on SHBG. Also similar to TBG, there is evidence for microheterogeneity of estradiol and testosterone binding to human SHBG.

Estradiol bound to human SHBG is also available for transport into peripheral tissues, such as the salivary gland or lymph node in the rat, but not the uterus (171). However, SHBG-bound estradiol was available for transport into both the testis and prostate gland, owing to the uptake of the sex steroid–SHBG-bound complex in these tissues (see earlier sections of this chapter). Thus, the data summarized in Table 14.7 indicate a considerable organ diversity with respect to SHBG delivery of sex steroid to tissues. This remarkable organ diversity in sex steroid uptake allows for organ-specific delivery

of sex steroids to tissues in a way that would not be possible if only the free (dialyzable) hormone was available for uptake by all tissues in vivo.

Correlation of Metabolic Clearance Rate and Transport Clearance Rate.

The unidirectional clearance values for testosterone and estradiol (Table 14.13) are TCRs and reflect the unidirectional transport of the sex steroids into tissues in vivo. The TCR is to be contrasted with the MCR, which is a function of the net extraction of the sex steroid across an organ bed. Net extraction reflects the balance between influx and efflux and the metabolism of the sex steroid and is determined from the arterial/venous difference of sex steroid across the organ bed. If the metabolic clearance of a hormone by a given organ is limited by the transport step (owing to very rapid enzymatic conversion of the sex steroid

TABLE 14.13. *Estradiol (E₂) Amplifier Function of Sex Hormone-Binding Globulin (SHBG)*

Patient Category	SHBG (nM)	E₂/T Unidirectional Clearance Ratio
Pregnancy (9)	323 ± 28	3.9 ± 0.5
Oral contraceptives (8)	126 ± 16	2.6 ± 0.3
Thin postmenopausal (9)	74 ± 9	2.1 ± 0.2
Normal female (9)	65 ± 9	2.1 ± 0.2
Obese postmenopausal (9)	43 ± 4	1.7 ± 0.2
Normal male (8)	28 ± 3	1.3 ± 0.1
Hirsute (5)	17 ± 2	1.3 ± 0.1

Data are mean $\pm$ S.E.M. T, testosterone. Numbers in parentheses are number of patients. [From Pardridge (171) with permission.]

in the organ), then the TCR and MCR are identical. In many cases, metabolic clearance of sex steroid by tissues is limited by transport. In the studies described in Figure 14.20, the TCRs for dihydrotestosterone (DHT) and testosterone were measured in parallel. The TCR ratio for testosterone/DHT in these studies was 2.0–2.2 for human serum, which is identical to the MCR ratio in human subjects (Fig. 14.22).

Role in Feminization of Cirrhosis.

Men with cirrhosis of the liver are feminized and present with gynecomastia and testicular atrophy (128). The basis of this hyperestrogenization is unclear since serum estradiol is generally normal in cirrhosis (267). The feminization picture includes an elevation in SHBG. Since SHBG is an estradiol amplifier, an elevation of SHBG will increase selectively the bioavailability of estradiol to tissues relative to testosterone. However, the MCR for estradiol is not decreased in cirrhosis (158). Conversely, in hyperthyroidism, where there is also an increase in plasma SHBG, there is a parallel decrease in the MCR of estradiol (158, 211). Moreover, there is a decrease in the MCR of testosterone in both cirrhosis (76) and hyperthyroidism (221), which is attributed to the substantial elevation in SHBG in these conditions. Therefore, it remains to be shown why the estradiol MCR is not decreased in cirrhosis.

The failure to observe a decrease in the MCR in estradiol in cirrhosis suggests that SHBG-bound estradiol is available for uptake by tissues in cirrhosis. That is, the SHBG produced by the cirrhotic liver may be modified in such a way that enhanced dissociation of estradiol from the SHBG-binding site occurs within the capillary beds of peripheral tissues. This hypothesis was tested experimentally with the BUI technique, as shown in Figure 14.23. In this study, the SHBG concentration in cirrhotic patients relative to controls more than doubled (224). This increase was associated with

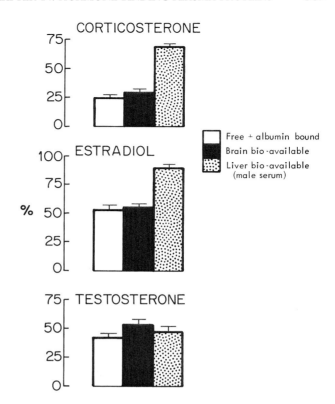

FIG. 14.21. In vitro free plus albumin-bound, in vivo brain bioavailable, and in vivo liver bioavailable fractions for human male serum for three steroid hormones. [From Pardridge (171) with permission.]

a significant decrease in the bioavailable fraction of testosterone in the rat brain capillary in vivo. However, no significant change in the bioavailable fraction of estradiol in the rat brain capillary in vivo was observed, despite the decrease in the non-SHBG-bound fraction of estradiol in sera from these patients (224). This selective delivery of estradiol to tissues from the cirrhotic SHBG-bound pool provides a plausible explanation for the feminization of the peripheral tissues in this condition.

Microheterogeneity of Testosterone and Estradiol Binding.

The findings that SHBG-bound estradiol, but not SHBG-bound testosterone, is available for transport into tissues such as liver, salivary gland, and lymph node, and that SHBG-bound estradiol, but not SHBG-bound testosterone, is available for transport into brain in cirrhosis (171) are difficult to reconcile with the hypothesis of a single competitive binding site for these sex steroid hormones on human SHBG. The possibility of differential binding of testosterone or estradiol to SHBG does exist since SHBG is present in serum in multiple isoforms, owing to differential glycosylation

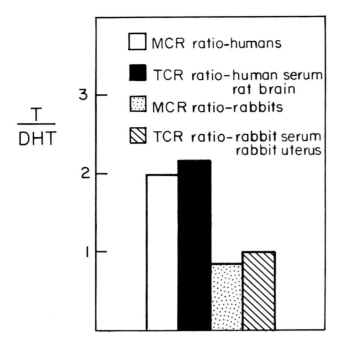

FIG. 14.22. Metabolic clearance rate *(MCR)* and transport clearance rate *(TCR)* ratios for testosterone *(T)*/dihydrotestosterone *(DHT)* are compared for humans and rabbits. Human TCR ratio was measured in rat brain using human male serum. Rabbit TCR ratio was measured in rabbit uterus using rabbit serum (1). Human and rabbit MCR ratios were reported by Vermeulen and Andó (270) and Mahoudeau et al. (140), respectively. The T/DHT MCR ratio in the rhesus monkey (231) is virtually identical to the ratio for humans (270).

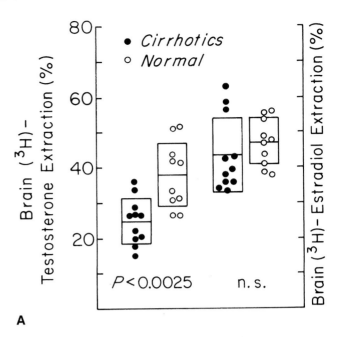

FIG. 14.23. *A:* Rat brain extraction of [³H]-testosterone or [³H]-estradiol after carotid arterial injection of labeled hormone mixed in either male cirrhotic or control human male serum. Rectangles represent means ± SD. The data show that unidirectional testosterone extraction by brain is decreased 33% (*P* < 0.0025) using cirrhotic serum, and this parallels a 2.6-fold increase in sex hormone–binding globulin (SHBG) and a 40% decrease in serum albumin in cirrhosis. However, unidirectional clearance of estradiol by rat brain was not decreased using cirrhotic serum, despite the marked increase in SHBG, the decrease in albumin, and the 41% decrease in the non-SHBG-bound fraction of estradiol in cirrhosis. Brain bioavailable estradiol using cirrhotic serum, 54 ± 4%, exceeds non-SHBG-bound estradiol, 36 ± 6%, in cirrhotic serum, indicating that SHBG-bound estradiol is available for transport into brain from plasma protein–bound pools in cirrhotic serum. Conversely, SHBG-bound estradiol was not available for transport into brain when serum was obtained from other clinical groups (Fig. 14.20). [From Sakiyama et al. (224) with permission.]

of the protein. Similar to previous studies with TBG, it is possible that the differentially glycosylated isoforms of SHBG may have differential binding of testosterone and estradiol. This hypothesis was confirmed with IEF and chromatofocusing studies (253). These results show that testosterone is bound preferentially to the more acidic isoforms of SHBG. This phenomenon was found for normal male serum, normal female serum, and cirrhotic male serum (Fig. 14.23) but not pregnancy serum. When binding of testosterone or estradiol to the different isoforms of SHBG in normal and cirrhotic male sera was compared, there was no difference in the binding pattern for testosterone but there was a shift in estradiol binding to the more acidic isoforms of SHBG (Fig. 14.23). These studies suggest that glycosylation may target estradiol to specific isoforms of SHBG and that these isoforms may more readily release estradiol to peripheral tissues in vivo relative to testosterone. In this way, SHBG may amplify the delivery of estradiol to tissues relative to testosterone, which can cause tissue feminization.

Species Differences. Early studies showed no difference in the MCRs of estradiol and testosterone in rabbits, despite the avid binding of testosterone to rabbit TeBG (18). This observation is inconsistent with the predictions of the free hormone hypothesis since the free (dialyzable) fraction of testosterone is much lower in

FIG. 14.23. *B:* Isoelectric focusing separation of [³H]-testosterone- and [³H]-estradiol-binding isoforms of SHBG in concanavalin-A–glycoprotein fraction of a cirrhotic male serum pool and a normal male serum pool. The pH values of the gel are shown by a diagonal line in the bottom half of the figure. *C:* Profiles of estradiol- or testosterone-binding isoforms of SHBG from *B* are replotted to allow direct comparison of results between normal male and cirrhotic male serum pools. The pH profile is shown by the diagonal line. [From Terasaki et al. (253) with permission.]

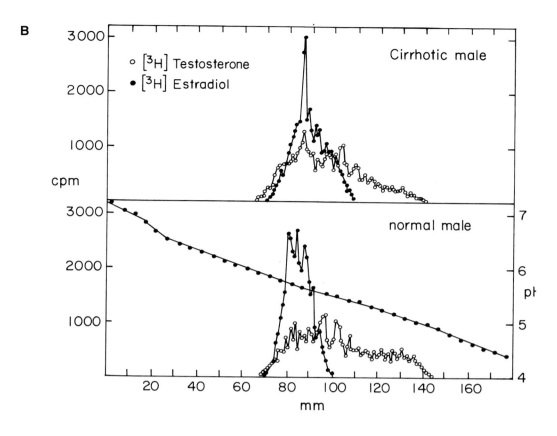

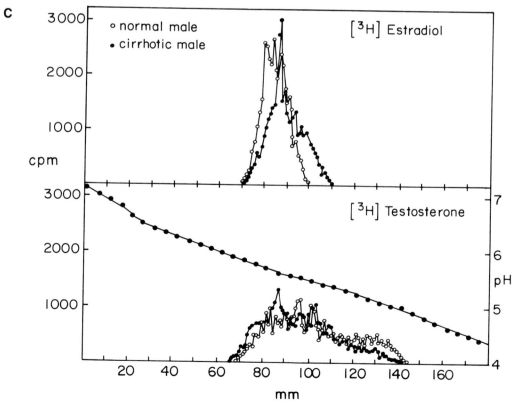

371

rabbit serum than that of estradiol. Similarly, in other studies, no correlation was found between different TeBG concentrations and the MCR of testosterone in rabbits (140). There was no difference in the MCR of DHT or testosterone in rabbits despite the threefold greater affinity of rabbit TeBG for DHT compared to testosterone. Subsequent studies measured the TCR of the sex steroid hormones in rabbits, showing that testosterone and DHT were readily available for uptake by peripheral tissues from the rabbit TeBG-bound pool (31). These results are consistent with enhanced dissociation of androgens from rabbit TeBG within the capillary microcirculation. It is not possible to reconcile these observations with the dissociation-limited model of hormone uptake since the membrane permeability coefficient for androgens is much less than the rates of androgen reassociation with binding globulins or albumin (Table 14.4).

A more compelling reason for excluding the dissociation-limited mechanism is that it can be shown, using the steady-state model (Fig. 14.10), that if the hormone exited from plasma via a dissociation-limited mechanism, the binding globulin should still exert an inhibitory effect on net organ uptake and MCR of the hormone. For example, simulation 2 of Table 14.11 represents the free hormone hypothesis for hepatic uptake, wherein no enhanced dissociation of hormone takes place in vivo. If k_9 is increased from 0 to 10, then the predicted E_{SS} is <1%. That is, in the absence of dissociation limitation, the high net extraction (E_{SS}) of steroid hormones (135, 201) or iodothyronines (58) across organs could not take place. In a dissociation-limited mechanism, for example, one created by increasing membrane permeability by a factor of 1000 and increasing k_3 from 0.345 (Table 14.10) to 345, E_{SS} is predicted to be 26%. That is, dissociation limitation can allow for high net organ extraction. However, the counterargument is twofold. First, there is no evidence for membrane permeability coefficients (that is, k_3) on the order of 345 s^{-1}. Second, even if this high k_3 existed, the MCR should still be related inversely to the globulin fraction. For example, the E_{SS} is predicted to decrease from 26% to 8.7% when $k_3 = 345$, but $G_T°$ is increased threefold, from the value in Table 14.10 to 750 nM, where $G_T° =$ the plasma SHBG or TeBG concentration. In summary, a dissociation-limited mechanism cannot reconcile the avid in vitro binding of testosterone or DHT by rabbit TeBG with the lack of inhibition of the MCRs of these hormones in vivo by TeBG. Conversely, this lack of MCR inhibition by rabbit TeBG is predicted from experimental studies showing enhanced dissociation of androgens from rabbit TeBG in vivo (31).

α_1-Acid Glycoprotein (Orosomucoid)

α_1-Acid glycoprotein (AAG) is a serum glycoprotein with a molecular weight of approximately 40,000 daltons, of which about 45% is carbohydrate (257). This protein is an acute phase reactant produced in the liver that is increased in inflammatory conditions and decreased in estrogen states, such as birth control pill treatment, pregnancy, or cirrhosis (199, 200). It binds a variety of lipophilic amine drugs, progesterone, and the progesterone antagonist RU-486 (241, 243). The normal serum concentration of AAG is high at 75 mg%, or approximately 20 μM (70). Imipramine bound to AAG is readily available for transport through the BBB in vivo through an enhanced dissociation mechanism (210). In these studies, the imipramine PS/F ratio in brain was 2.5, the AAG in vitro K_D value was 4.9 $\pm$ 0.3 μM, and the in vivo K_D of AAG binding to imipramine within the cerebral brain capillary was 90 $\pm$ 9 μM (Table 14.5).

Orosomucoid-bound propranolol or lidocaine are also available for transport into the brain via an enhanced dissociation mechanism (133, 189). Serum was obtained from cord blood, normal subjects, patients with arthritis, and patients with metastatic cancer; and the AAG concentrations in these groups were 0.41 $\pm$ 0.05, 0.78 $\pm$ 0.07, 1.48 $\pm$ 0.10, and 2.93 $\pm$ 0.45 mg/ml, respectively (189). Brain extraction of [^{3}H]-propranolol in the presence of these serum samples was related inversely to the AAG concentration; however, AAG inhibition was much less than predicted by the free drug hypothesis, indicating that AAG-bound drug was less available for transport into the brain in vivo. Brain uptake of [^{3}H]-propranolol from the circulating AAG-bound pool was less when purified human AAG was administered, as opposed to the AAG in human serum (133, 189). This suggests cooperative interactions between HSA and AAG in the microcirculation, similar to interactions detected in vitro (164).

The mechanism for the putative conformational change about the drug-binding site on AAG within the brain capillary is unknown but may involve nonspecific interactions of the protein with the endothelial glycocalyx. Like albumin, AAG is one of the serum proteins that participates in maintaining capillary permeability, owing to absorption of the protein to the endothelial glycocalyx (86, 228).

SUMMARY

Bioavailable steroid or thyroid hormone in plasma is generally much greater than either the free (dialyzable) fraction of hormone measured in vitro or the fraction of plasma protein extracted by an organ (4, 161). These observations are consistent with either a dissociation-limited or an enhanced dissociation mechanism of transcapillary hormone transport. If dissociation-limited transport is operative in vivo, then the fraction of free (dialyzable) hormone measured in vitro is still the driving force of the cellular free hormone. Conversely, if the enhanced dissociation mechanism takes place in vivo, then the cellular free hormone in vivo is driven by the fraction of protein-bound hormone measured in vitro.

The distinction between the dissociation-limited and the enhanced dissociation mechanisms is a classical scientific dialectic (Table 14.14). The dissociation-limited mechanism may be excluded as a general process of hormonal transport on the basis of the following three observations. First, for the dissociation-limited mechanism to be operative in vivo, it is necessary to postulate either unphysiologically high values for membrane permeability (143) or rates of hormonal association with the plasma protein that are orders of magnitude lower than that normally recorded (54). Second, if the dissociation-limited mechanism takes place in vivo, it is necessary to postulate the existence of active transport mechanisms at the nuclear membrane (162); but these putative pumps are not experimentally detectable (151). The postulate of active transport across the nuclear membrane (160) is necessary to account for the vast difference between the concentration of free hormone in the nucleus, which drives occupancy of the hormone nuclear receptor, and the concentration of free (dialyzable) hormone measured in vitro (Fig. 14.3). In fact, there is no experimental precedent for active transport systems for steroid or thyroid hormones at the nuclear membrane. Indeed, there is no experimental precedent for active transport of any small molecular weight solute across this membrane, which has large pores and is freely permeable to small molecules, such as sucrose. Third, the

dissociation-limited mechanism cannot explain many aspects of hormonal metabolic clearance measured in vivo. For example, the metabolic clearance of androgens in rabbits is unrelated to serum concentrations of the high-affinity TeBG in plasma (140). Other examples include the lack of correlation between the metabolic clearance of estradiol in patients with cirrhosis and the elevated serum SHBG concentrations in this condition (158) and the lack of correlation between free T_4 in NTI and the rates of T_4 clearance in these subjects (111).

Conversely, the enhanced dissociation model does not postulate either unphysiologically high values for membrane permeability or extraordinarily low rates of hormonal reassociation with the plasma protein. In addition, this model does not need to postulate active transport systems at the nuclear membrane (Table 14.14). Owing to transport of hormone from the circulating plasma protein–bound pool, the concentration of free cellular hormone is predicted to be approximately equal to the K_D of the steroid or thyroid hormone nuclear receptor, which allows for 50% occupancy of the receptor in vivo. The enhanced dissociation model can explain the independence of hormone metabolic clearance and binding globulin in rabbits or subjects with cirrhosis or NTI.

Enhanced dissociation of hormone from plasma proteins in vivo has been demonstrated repeatedly from a number of different laboratories (5, 7, 15, 68, 79, 152, 260–262, 280) (Table 14.5). These measurements have shown that the dissociation constant governing the hormone ligand-binding reaction in vivo is often many-fold greater than the K_D of the binding reaction measured in vitro (Table 14.5). Since differences in K_D invariably arise from differences in rates of ligand dissociation from the protein, expansion of the K_D in vivo is consistent with enhanced hormonal dissociation from the protein-binding site. Enhanced dissociation arises from conformational changes about the ligand-binding site, which have been verified experimentally during interaction of the plasma protein with cellular surfaces (96). Moreover, the techniques of capillary physiology used to record the increased K_D in vivo, in several circumstances, have recorded values that are not significantly different from the K_D values measured in vitro (Table 14.5). That is, when there is no conformational change about the ligand-binding site and no enhanced dissociation in vivo, the precepts of the free ligand hypothesis are upheld by in vivo empiric testing. However, this is the exception, not the rule.

The challenge to plasma protein–binding research in the future is to identify the modular sites on the plasma protein that are responsible for interactions with the

TABLE 14.14. *Parsimony in Models of Hormonal Transport*

Principal Assumptions	
Enhanced Dissociation Model	Dissociation-Limited Model
Conformational changes in vivo	—
—	Very high membrane permeability coefficients
—	Very low hormone/protein association rates
—	Active pumps at nuclear membrane

cellular surfaces that trigger release of hormones from the plasma protein within the capillary compartment. The cDNAs for virtually all of the hormone-binding plasma proteins have been cloned. Therefore, it is now possible, using the techniques of molecular biology, to perform site-directed mutagenesis of surface residues of hormone-binding proteins, to express these mutated proteins, and to subject the protein to direct in vivo empiric testing with respect to functional changes in hormone delivery to tissues in vivo.

Emily Yu skillfully prepared the manuscript. The author is indebted to numerous collaborators and colleagues over the years who sought to understand the in vivo function of hormone-binding plasma proteins. This work was supported by NIH grant R01–DK25744 from 1980 to 1988.

REFERENCES

1. Ain, K. B., Y. Mori, and S. Refetoff. Reduced clearance rate of thyroxine-binding globulin (TBG) with increased sialylation: a mechanism for estrogen-induced elevation of serum TBG concentration. *J. Clin. Endocrinol. Metab.* 65: 689–696, 1987.
2. Ain, K. B., and S. Refetoff. Relationship of oligosaccharide modification to the cause of serum thyroxine-binding globulin excess. *J. Clin. Endocrinol. Metab.* 66: 1037–1043, 1988.
3. Alpert, E. Human alpha-fetoprotein (AFP) developmental and biological characteristics. In: *Prevention of Neural Tube Defects: The Role of Alpha Feto Protein,* edited by B. F. Crandall and M. A. B. Brazier. New York: Academic, 1978, p. 19–26.
4. Baird, D. T., R. Horton, C. Longcope, and J. F. Tait. Steroid dynamics under steady-state conditions. *Recent Prog. Horm. Res.* 25: 611–664, 1969.
5. Baker, K. J., and S. E. Bradley. Binding of sulfobromophthalein (BSP) sodium by plasma albumin. Its role in hepatic BSP extraction. *J. Clin. Invest.* 45: 281–287, 1966.
6. Barlow, J. W., J. M. Csicsmann, E. L. White, J. W. Funder, and J. R. Stockigt. Familial euthyroid thyroxine excess: characterization of abnormal intermediate affinity thyroxine binding to albumin. *J. Clin. Endocrinol. Metab.* 55: 244–250, 1982.
7. Barnhart, J. L., B. L. Witt, W. G. Hardison, and R. N. Berk. Uptake of iopanoic acid by isolated rat hepatocytes in primary culture. *Am. J. Physiol.* 244 (*Gastrointest. Liver Physiol.* 7): G630–G636, 1983.
8. Bartlett, P. A., and C. K. Marlowe. Evaluation of intrinsic binding energy from a hydrogen bonding group in an enzyme inhibitor. *Science* 235: 569–571, 1987.
9. Bass, L., P. Robinson, and A. J. Braken. Hepatic elimination of flowing substances: the distributed model. *J. Theor. Biol.* 72: 161–184, 1978.
10. Bell, D. R., P. D. Watson, and E. M. Renkin. Exclusion of plasma proteins in interstitium of tissues from the dog hind paw. *Am. J. Physiol.* 239 (*Heart Circ. Physiol.* 10): H532–H538, 1980.
11. Benveniste, H., J. Drejer, A. Schousboe, and N. H. Diemer. Regional cerebral glucose phosphorylation and blood flow after insertion of a microdialysis fiber through the dorsal hippocampus in the rat. *J. Neurochem.* 49: 729–734, 1987.
12. Bernstein, G., and J. H. Oppenheimer. Factors influencing the concentration of free and total thyroxine in patients with nonthyroidal disease. *J. Clin. Endocrinol.* 26: 195–201, 1966.
13. Blake, C. C. F., and S. J. Oatley. Protein–DNA and protein–hormone interactions in prealbumin: A model of the thyroid hormone nuclear receptor? *Nature* 268: 115–120, 1977.
14. Blondeau, J.-P., J. Osty, and J. Francon. Characterization of the thyroid hormone transport system of isolated hepatocytes. *J. Biol. Chem.* 263: 2685–2692, 1988.
15. Bloomer, J. R., P. D. Berk, J. Vergalla, and N. I. Berlin. Influence of albumin on the hepatic uptake of unconjugated bilirubin. *Clin. Sci. Mol. Med.* 45: 505–516, 1973.
16. Bolton, N. J., R. Lahtonen, G. L. Hammond, and R. Vihko. Distribution and concentrations of androgens in epithelial and stromal compartments of the human benign hypertrophic prostate. *J. Endocrinol.* 90: 125–131, 1981.
17. Bonner, W. M. Protein migration into nuclei. 1. Frog oocyte nuclei in vivo accumulate microinjected histones, allow entry to small proteins, and exclude large proteins. *J. Cell Biol.* 64: 421–430, 1975.
18. Bourget, C., C. Flood, and C. Longcope. Steroid dynamics in the rabbit. *Steroids* 43: 225–233, 1984.
19. Brandes, R., R. K. Ockner, R. A. Weisiger, and N. Lysenko. Specific and saturable binding of albumin to rat adipocytes: modulation by epinephrine and possible role in free fatty acid transfer. *Biochem. Biophys. Res. Commun.* 105: 821–827, 1982.
20. Brent, G. A., J. M. Hershman, A. W. Reed, A. Sastre, and J. Lieberman. Serum angiotensin-converting enzyme in severe nonthyroidal illnesses associated with low serum thyroxine concentration. *Ann. Intern. Med.* 100: 680–683, 1984.
21. Brightman, M. W. Morphology of blood–brain interfaces. *Exp. Eye Res.* 25(Suppl.): 1–25, 1977.
22. Brown, J. R. Serum albumin: amino acid sequence. In: *Albumin Structure, Function, and Uses,* edited by V. M. Rosehoer, M. Oratz, and M. A. Rothschild. New York: Pergamon, 1977, p. 27–51.
23. Brown, J. R., and P. Shockley. Serum albumin: structure and characterization of its ligand binding sites. In: *Lipid–Protein Interactions,* edited by P. C. Jost and O. H. Griffith. New York: Wiley, 1982, vol. 1, p. 25–68.
24. Brown-Grant, K., R. D. Brennan, and F. E. Yates. Simulation of the thyroid hormone–binding protein interactions in human plasma. *J. Clin. Endocrinol.* 30: 733–751, 1970.
25. Burke, C. W., and D. C. Anderson. Sex-hormone-binding globulin is an oestrogen amplifier. *Nature* 240: 38–40, 1972.
26. Carter, D. C., and J. X. He. Structure of serum albumin. *Adv. Protein Chem.* 45: 153–203, 1994.
27. Cefalu, W. T., and W. M. Pardridge. Augmented transport and metabolism of sex steroids in lymphoid neoplasia in the rat. *Endocrinology* 120: 1000–1009, 1987.
28. Cefalu, W. T., W. M. Pardridge, G. Chaudhuri, and H. L. Judd. Serum bioavailability and tissue metabolism of testosterone and estradiol in rat salivary gland. *J. Clin. Endocrinol. Metab.* 63: 20–28, 1986.
29. Cefalu, W. T., W. M. Pardridge, and B. N. Premachandra. Hepatic bioavailability of thyroxine and testosterone in familial dysbuminemic hyperthyroxinemia. *J. Clin. Endocrinol. Metab.* 61: 783–786, 1985.
30. Chambers, R., and B. W. Zweifach. Intercellular cement and capillary permeability. *Physiol. Rev.* 27: 436–463, 1947.
31. Chaudhuri, G., K. A. Steingold, W. M. Pardridge, and H. L. Judd. TeBG- and CBG-bound steroid hormones in rabbits are available for influx into uterus in vivo. *Am. J. Physiol.* 254 (*Endocrinol. Metab.* 17): E79–E83, 1988.
32. Chaudhuri, G., C. Verheugen, W. M. Pardridge, and H. L. Judd. Selective availability of protein bound estrogen and estrogen conjugates to the rat kidney. *J. Endocrinol. Invest.* 10: 283–290, 1987.

33. Chopra, I. J., J. M. Hershman, W. M. Pardridge, and J. T. Nicoloff. Thyroid function in nonthyroidal illnesses. *Ann. Intern. Med.* 98: 946–957, 1983.

34. Christensen, H. N. Some special kinetic problems of transport. *Adv. Enzymol.* 32: 1–20, 1969.

35. Cooke, N. E., and E. V. David. Serum vitamin D–binding protein is a third member of the albumin and alpha fetoprotein gene family. *J. Clin. Invest.* 76: 2420–2424, 1985.

36. Cornford, E. M., L. D. Braun, W. M. Pardridge, and W.H. Oldendorf. Determination of blood flow rate and cellular influx of glucose and arginine in mouse liver in vivo. *Am. J. Physiol.* 238 (*Heart Circ. Physiol.* 9): H553–H560, 1980.

37. Corvol, P., and C. W. Bardin. Species distribution of testosterone-binding globulin. *Biol. Reprod.* 8: 277–282, 1973.

38. Cowan, R. A., S. K. Cowan, C. A. Giles, and J. K. Grant. Prostatic distribution of sex hormone–binding globulin and cortisol-binding globulin in benign hyperplasia. *J. Endocrinol.* 71: 121–131, 1976.

39. Crone, C. Permeability of capillaries in various organs as determined by use of the "indicator diffusion" method. *Acta Physiol. Scand.* 58: 292–305, 1973.

40. Crone, C., and D. G. Levitt. Capillary permeability to small solutes. In: *Handbook of Physiology: The Cardiovascular System. Microcirculation,* edited by E. M. Renkin and C. C. Michel. Bethesda, MD: *Am. Physiol. Soc.,* 1984, sect. 2, vol IV, chapt. 10, p. 411–466.

42. Daniel, J.-Y., F. Leboulenger, H. Vaudry, H. H. Floch, and I. Assenmacher. Interrelations between binding affinity and metabolic clearance rate for the main corticosteroids in the rabbit. *J. Steroid Biochem.* 16: 379–384, 1982.

43. Desjardins, C., and B. R. Duling. Microvessel hematocrit: measurement and implications for capillary oxygen transport. *Am. J. Physiol.* 252 (*Heart Circ. Physiol.* 21): H494–H503, 1987.

44. Dewey, W. C. Vascular–extravascular exchange of I^{131} plasma proteins in the rat. *Am. J. Physiol.* 197: 423–431, 1959.

45. Diamond, J. M., and E. M. Wright. Molecular forces governing non-electrolyte permeation through cell membranes. *Proc. R. Soc. Lond. B Biol. Sci.* 172: 276–316, 1969.

46. Dickson, P. W., G. J. Howlett, and G. Schreiber. Rat transthyretin (prealbumin). *J. Biol. Chem.* 260: 8214–8219, 1985.

47. Drinker, C. K. The permeability and diameter of the capillaries in the web of the brown frog (*Rana temporaria*) when perfused with solutions containing pituitary extract and horse serum. *J. Physiol. (Lond.)* 63: 249–269, 1927.

48. Dubey, R. K., C. B. McAllister, M. Inoue, and G. R. Wilkinson. Plasma binding and transport of diazepam across the blood–brain barrier. No evidence for in vivo enhanced dissociation. *J. Clin. Invest.* 84: 1155–1159, 1989.

49. Dueland, S., R. Bouillon, H. van Baelen, J. I. Pederson, P. Helgerud, and C. A. Drevon. Binding protein for vitamin D and its metabolites in rat mesenteric lymph. *Am. J. Physiol.* 249 (*Endocrinol. Metab.* 20): E1–E5, 1985.

50. Dunn, J. F., B. C. Nisula, and D. Rodbard. Transport of steroid hormones: binding of 21 endogenous steroids to both testosterone-binding globulin and corticosteroid-binding globulin in human plasma. *J. Clin. Endocrinol. Metab.* 53: 58–68, 1981.

51. Dykstra, K. H., J. K. Hsiao, P. F. Morrison, P.M. Bungay, I. N. Mefford, M. M. Scully, and R. L. Dedrick. Quantitative examination of tissue concentration profiles associated with microdialysis. *J. Neurochem.* 58: 931–940, 1992.

52. Eckel, J., G. S. Rao, M. L. Rao, and H. Breuer. Uptake of L-triiodothyronine by isolated rat liver cells. *Biochem J.* 182: 473–491, 1979.

53. Ekins, R. P. Methods for the measurement of free thyroid hormones. In: *Free Thyroid Hormones,* edited by R. Ekins, G. Faglia, F. Pennisi, and A. Pinchera. Amsterdam: Excerpta Medica, 1979, p. 72.

54. Ekins, R. P., and P. R. Edwards. Plasma protein–mediated transport of steroid and thyroid hormones: a critique. *Am. J. Physiol.* 255 (*Endocrinol. Metab.* 18): E403–E409, 1988.

55. Ellison, S. A., and W. M. Pardridge. Reduction of testosterone availability to 5α-reductase by human sex hormone-binding globulin in the rat ventral prostate gland in vivo. *Prostate* 17: 281–291, 1990.

56. Endo, T., M. Eilers, and G. Schatz. Binding of a tightly folded artificial mitochondrial precursor protein to the mitochondrial outer membrane involves a lipid-mediated conformational change. *J. Biol. Chem.* 264: 2951–2956, 1989.

57. Evans, J. J. Progesterone in saliva does not parallel unbound progesterone in plasma. *Clin. Chem.* 32: 542–544, 1986.

58. Faber, J., O. Faber, A. Wennlund, and J. Wahren. Splanchnic extraction of 3,3'-diiodothyronine and 3',5'-diiodothyronine in hyperthyroidism. *J. Clin. Endocrinol. Metab.* 59: 147–150, 1984.

59. Farrell, C. L., J. Yang, and W. M. Pardridge. GLUT-1 glucose transporter is present within apical and basolateral membranes of brain epithelial interfaces and in microvascular endothelia with and without tight junctions. *J. Histochem. Cytochem.* 40: 193–199, 1992.

60. Feng, L., C. Z. Hu, and J. D. Andrade. Scanning tunneling microscopic images of adsorbed serum albumin on highly oriented pyrolytic graphite. *J. Colloid Interface Sci.* 126: 650–653, 1988.

61. Fleischer, A. B., W. O. Shurmantine, B. A. Luxon, and E. L. Forker. Palmitate uptake by hepatocyte monolayers. *J. Clin. Invest.* 77: 964–970, 1986.

62. Flink, I. L., T. J. Bailey, T. A. Gustafson, B. E. Markham, and E. Morkin. Complete amino acid sequence of human thyroxine-binding globulin deduced from cloned DNA: close homology to the serine antiproteases. *Proc. Natl. Acad. Sci. U.S.A.* 83: 7708–7712, 1986.

63. Forker, E. L., and B. Luxon. Hepatic transport kinetics and plasma disappearance curves: distributed modeling versus conventional approach. *Am. J. Physiol.* 235 (*Endocrinol. Metab. Gastrointest. Physiol.* 4): E648–E660, 1978.

64. Forker, E. L., and B. A. Luxon. Albumin helps mediate removal of taurocholate by rat liver. *J. Clin. Invest.* 67: 1517–1522, 1981.

65. Forker, E. L., and B. A. Luxon. Albumin-mediated transport of rose bengal by perfused rat liver. *J. Clin. Invest.* 72: 1764–1771, 1983.

66. Forker, E. L., and B. A. Luxon. Effects of unstirred Disse fluid, nonequilibrium binding, and surface-mediated dissociation on hepatic removal of albumin-bound organic anions. *Am. J. Physiol.* 248 (*Gastrointest. Liver Physiol.* 11): G709–G717, 1985.

67. Forker, E. L., B. A. Luxon, and V. S. Sharma. Hepatic transport and binding of rose bengal in the presence of albumin and gamma globulin. *Am. J. Physiol.* 248 (*Gastrointest. Liver Physiol.* 11): G702–G708, 1985.

68. Forker, E. L., B. A. Luxon, M. Snell, and W. O. Shurmantine. Effect of albumin binding on the hepatic transport of rose bengal: surface-mediated dissociation of limited capacity. *J. Pharmacol. Exp. Ther.* 223: 342–347, 1982.

69. Frairia, R., N. Fortunati, F. Fissore, A. Fazzari, P. Zeppegno, L. Varvello, M. Orsello, and L. Berta. The membrane receptor for sex steroid binding protein is not ubiquitous. *J. Endocrinol. Invest.* 15: 617–620, 1992.

70. Ganguly, M., R. H. Carnighan, and U. Westphal. Steroid–protein interactions. XIV. Interaction between human α$_1$-acid glycoprotein and progesterone. *Biochemistry* 6: 2803–2814, 1967.

71. Gärtner, R., R. Henze, K. Horn, C. R. Pickardt, and P. C. Scriba. Thyroxine-binding globulin: investigation of microheterogeneity. *J. Clin. Endocrinol. Metab.* 52: 657–664, 1981.

72. Gillette, J. R. Overview of drug–protein binding. *Ann. N. Y. Acad. Sci.* 226:6–17, 1973.

73. Giorgi, E. P., and W. D. Stein. The transport of steroids into animal cells in culture. *Endocrinology* 108: 688–697, 1981.

74. Goldman, M., M. B. Dratman, F. L. Crutchfield, A. S. Jennings, J. A. Maruniak, and R. Gibbons. Intrathecal triiodothyronine administration causes greater heart rate stimulation in hypothyroid rats than intravenously delivered hormone. *J. Clin. Invest.* 76: 1622–1625, 1985.

75. Goodman, D. S. Vitamin A and retinoids in health and disease. *N. Engl. J. Med.* 310: 1023–1031, 1984.

76. Gordon, G. G., J. Olivo, F. Fafii, and A. L. Southren. Conversion of androgens to estrogens in cirrhosis of the liver. *J. Clin. Endocrinol. Metab.* 40: 1018–1026, 1975.

77. Goresky, C. A., D. S. Daly, S. Mishkin, and I. M. Arias. Uptake of labeled palmitate by the intact liver: role of intracellular binding sites. *Am. J. Physiol.* 234 (*Endocrinol. Metab. Gastrointest. Physiol.* 3): E542–E553, 1978.

78. Griffin, P. R., S. Kumar, J. Shabanowitz, H. Charbonneau, P. C. Namkung, K. A. Walsh, D. F. Hunt, and P. H. Petra. The amino acid sequence of the sex steroid-binding protein of rabbit serum. *J. Biol. Chem.* 264: 19066–19075, 1989.

79. Gumucio, J. J. Functional and anatomic heterogeneity in the liver acinus: impact on transport. *Am. J. Physiol.* 244 (*Gastrointest. Liver Physiol.* 7): G578–G582, 1983.

80. Hagen, G. A., and L. A. Solberg, Jr. Brain and cerebrospinal fluid permeability to intravenous thyroid hormones. *Endocrinology* 95: 1398–1410, 1974.

81. Hammond, G. L. Molecular properties of corticosteroid binding globulin and the sex-steroid binding proteins. *Endocr. Rev.* 11: 65–79, 1990.

82. Hammond, G. L., and W. P. Bocchinfuso. Sex hormone–binding globulin/androgen-binding protein: steroid-binding and dimerization domains. *J. Steroid Biochem. Mol. Biol.* 53: 543–552, 1995.

83. Hammond, G. L., C. L. Smith, I. S. Goping, D. A. Underhill, M. J. Harley, J. Reventos, N. A. Musto, G. L. Gunsalus, and C. W. Bardin. Primary structure of human corticosteroid binding globulin, deduced from hepatic and pulmonary cDNAs, exhibits homology with serine protease inhibitors. *Proc. Natl. Acad. Sci. U.S.A.* 84: 5153–5157, 1987.

84. Hammond, G. L., C. L. Smith, N. A. M. Paterson, and W. J. Sibbald. A role for corticosteroid-binding globulin in delivery of cortisol to activated neutrophils. *J. Clin. Endocrinol. Metab.* 71: 34–39, 1990.

85. Hammond, G. L., D. A. Underhill, C. L. Smith, I. S. Goping, M. J. Harley, N. A. Musto, C. Y. Cheng, and C. W. Bardin. The cDNA-deduced primary structure of human sex hormone–binding globulin and location of its steroid-binding domain. *FEBS Lett.* 215: 100–104, 1987.

86. Haraldsson, B. Physiological studies of macromolecular transport across capillary walls. *Acta Physiol. Scand. Suppl.* 553: 1–40, 1986.

87. Hayashi, Y., Y. Mori, O. E. Janssen, T. Sunthornthepvarakul, R. E. Weiss, K. Takeda, M. Weinberg, H. Seo, G. I. Bell, and S. Refetoff. Human thyroxine-binding globulin gene: complete sequence and transcriptional regulation. *Mol. Endocrinol.* 7: 1049–1060, 1993.

88. He, X. M., and D. C. Carter. Atomic structure and chemistry of human serum albumin. *Nature* 358: 209–215, 1992.

89. Hervé, F., M.-T. Martin, K. Rajkowski, P. Dessen, and N. Cittanova. Participation of the lone tryptophan residue of rat α-foetoprotein in its drug-binding sites. *Biochem. J.* 244: 81–85, 1987.

90. Heyns, W., and P. De Moor. Kinetics of dissociation of 17β-hydroxysteroids from the steroid binding β-globulin of human plasma. *J. Clin. Endocrinol.* 32: 147–154, 1971.

91. Hillier, A. P. The release of thyroxine from serum protein in the vessels of the liver. *J. Physiol. (Lond.)* 203: 419–434, 1969.

92. Hillier, A. P. The rate of triiodothyronine dissociation from binding sites in human plasma. *Acta Endocrinol.* 80: 49–57, 1975.

93. Hillier, A. P., and W. E. Balfour. Human thyroxine-binding globulin and thyroxine-binding pre-albumin: dissociation rates. *J. Physiol. (Lond.)* 217: 625–634, 1971.

94. Honig, C. R., and C. L. Odoroff. Calculated dispersion of capillary transit times: significance for oxygen exchange. *Am. J. Physiol.* 240 (*Heart Circ. Physiol.* 11): H199–H208, 1981.

95. Honig, C. R., C. L. Odoroff, and J. L. Frierson. Capillary recruitment in exercise: rate, extent, uniformity, and relation to blood flow. *Am. J. Physiol.* 238 (*Heart Circ. Physiol.* 9): H31–H42, 1980.

96. Horie, T., T. Mizuma, S. Kasai, and S. Awazu. Conformational change in plasma albumin due to interaction with isolated rat hepatocyte. *Am. J. Physiol.* 254 (*Gastrointest. Liver Physiol.* 17): G465–G470, 1988.

97. Horowitz, S. B. The permeability of the amphibian oocyte nucleus, in situ. *J. Cell Biol.* 54: 609–625, 1972.

98. Hsiao, J. K., B. A. Ball, P. F. Morrison, I. N. Mefford, and P. M. Bungay. Effects of different semipermeable membranes on in vitro and in vivo performance of microdialysis probes. *J. Neurochem.* 54: 1449–1452, 1990.

99. Ichikawa, M., S. C. Tsao, T.-H. Lin, S. Miyauchi, Y. Sawada, T. Iga, M. Hanano, and Y. Sugiyama. "Albumin-mediated transport phenomenon" observed for ligands with high membrane permeability. *J. Hepatol.* 16: 38–49, 1992.

100. Inoue, M. Metabolism and transport of amphipathic molecules in analbuminemic rats and human subjects. *Hepatology* 5: 892–898, 1985.

101. Inoue, M., H. Koyama, S. Nagase, and Y. Morino. Renal secretion of phenolsulfonphthalein: analysis of its vectorial transport in normal and mutant analbuminemic rats. *J. Lab. Clin. Med.* 105: 484–488, 1985.

102. Inoue, M., K. Okajima, K. Itoh, Y. Ando, N. Watanabe, T. Yasaka, S. Nagase, and Y. Morino. Mechanism of furosemide resistance in analbuminemic rats and hypoalbuminemic patients. *Kidney Int.* 32: 198–203, 1987.

103. Ishise, S., B. L. Pegram, J. Yamamoto, Y. Kitamura, and E. D. Frohlich. Reference sample microsphere method: cardiac output and blood flows in conscious rat. *Am. J. Physiol.* 239 (*Heart Circ. Physiol.* 10): H443–H449, 1980.

104. Ivanov, K. P., M. K. Kalinina, and Y. I. Levkovich. Blood flow velocity in capillaries of brain and muscles and its physiological significance. *Microvasc. Res.* 22: 143–155, 1981.

105. Ivanov, K. P., M. K. Kalinina, and Y. I. Levkovich. Microcirculation velocity changes under hypoxia in brain, muscles, liver, and their physiological significance. *Microvasc. Res.* 30: 10–18, 1985.

106. Janin, J., and C. Chothia. The structure of protein–protein recognition sites. *J. Biol. Chem.* 265: 16027–16030, 1990.

107. Jones, D. R., S. D. Hall, E. K. Jackson, R. A. Branch, and G. R. Wilkinson. Brain uptake of benzodiazepines: effects of lipophilicity and plasma protein binding. *J. Pharmacol. Exp. Ther.* 245: 816–822, 1988.

108. Joseph, D. R. Structure, function, and regulation of androgen-

binding protein/sex hormone–binding globulin. *Vitam. Horm.* 49: 197–280, 1994.

109. Joseph, D. R., S. H. Hall, and F. S. French. Rat androgen-binding protein: evidence for identical subunits and amino acid sequence homology with human sex hormone–binding globulin. *Proc. Natl. Acad. Sci. U.S.A.* 84: 339–343, 1987.

110. Kambe, F., H. Seo, Y. Murata, and N. Matsui. Cloning of a complementary deoxyribonucleic acid coding for human thyroxine-binding globulin (TBG): existence of two TBG messenger ribonucleic acid species possessing different 3′-untranslated regions. *Mol. Endocrinol.* 2: 181–185, 1988.

111. Kaptein, E. M., D. A. Grieb, C. A. Spencer, W. S. Wheeler, and J. T. Nicoloff. Thyroxine metabolism in the low thyroxine state of critical nonthyroidal illnesses. *J. Clin. Endocrinol. Metab.* 53: 764–771, 1981.

112. Karplus, M., and J. A. McCammon. The dynamics of proteins. *Sci. Am.* 254: 42–51, 1986.

113. Keller, N., U. I. Richardson, and F. E. Yates. Protein binding and the biological activity of corticosteroids: in vivo induction of hepatic and pancreatic alanine aminotransferases by corticosteroids in normal and estrogen-treated rats. *Endocrinology* 84: 49–62, 1969.

114. Kern, D. F., D. Levitt, and D. Wangensteen. Endothelial albumin permeability measured with a new technique in perfused rabbit lung. *Am. J. Physiol.* 245 (*Heart Circ. Physiol.* 16): H229–H236, 1983.

115. Ketterer, B., T. Carne, and E. Tipping. Ligandin and protein A: intracellular binding proteins. In: *Transport by Proteins,* edited by G. I. Blauer and H. Sund. New York: de Gruyter, 1978, p. 79–92.

116. Kety, S. S. The theory and applications of the exchange of inert gas at the lungs and tissues. *Pharmacol. Rev.* 3: 1–41, 1951.

117. Kilvik, K., K. Furu, E. Haug, and K. M. Gautvik. The mechanism of 17β-estradiol uptake into prolactin-producing rat pituitary cells (GH₃ cells) in culture. *Endocrinology* 117: 967–975, 1985.

118. Klitzman, B., and B. R. Duling. Microvascular hematocrit and red cell flow in resting and contracting striated muscle. *Am. J. Physiol.* 237 (*Heart Circ. Physiol.* 8): H481–H490, 1979.

119. Koshland, D. E., Jr. *The Enzymes,* edited by P. D. Boyer, H. Lardy, and K. Myrbäck. New York: Academic, 1959, vol. 1, p. 305.

120. Kragh-Hansen, U. Molecular aspects of ligand binding to serum albumin. *Pharmacol. Rev.* 33: 17–53, 1981.

121. Krupenko, S. A., O. I. Kolesnik, N.I. Krupenko, and O. A. Strel'chyonok. Organization of the transcortin-binding domain on placental plasma membranes. *Biochim. Biophys. Acta* 1235: 387–394, 1995.

122. Krupenko, S. A., N. I. Krupenko, and B. J. Danzo. Interaction of sex hormone–binding globulin in plasma membranes from the rat epididymis and other tissues. *J. Steroid Biochem. Mol. Biol.* 51: 115–124, 1994.

123. Landis, E. M., and J. R. Pappenheimer. Exchange of substances through the capillary walls. In: *Handbook of Physiology: Circulation.* edited by W. F. Hamilton. Washington D.C.: Am. Physiol. Soc., 1963, sect. 2, vol II, chapt. 29, p. 961–1034.

124. Larson, K. B., J. Markham, and M. E. Raichle. Tracer-kinetic models for measuring cerebral blood flow using externally detected radiotracers. *J. Cereb. Blood Flow Metab.* 7: 443–463, 1987.

125. Lassen, N. A., and W. Perl. *Tracer Kinetic Methods in Medical Physiology.* New York: Raven, 1979, p. 1–189.

126. Laufer, L. R., J. C. Gambone, G. Chaudhuri, W. M. Pardridge, and H. L. Judd. The effect of membrane permeability and binding by human serum proteins on sex steroid influx into the uterus. *J. Clin. Endocrinol. Metab.* 56: 1282–1287, 1983.

127. Lee, J. Y., and M. Hirose. Partially folded state of the disulfide-reduced form of human serum albumin as an intermediate for reversible denaturation. *J. Biol. Chem.* 267: 14753–14758, 1992.

128. Lester, R., P. K. Eagon, and D. H. van Thiel. Feminization of the alcoholic: the estrogen/testosterone ratio (E/T). *Gastroenterology* 76: 415–417, 1979.

129. Lichenstein, H. S., D. E. Lyons, M. M. Wurfel, D. A. Johnson, M. D. McGinley, J. C. Leidli, D. B. Trollinger, J. P. Mayer, S. D. Wright, and M. M. Zukowski. Afamin is a new member of the albumin, α-fetoprotein, and vitamin D–binding protein gene family. *J. Biol. Chem.* 269: 18149–18154, 1994.

130. Lin, T.-H., and J. H. Lin. Effects of protein binding and experimental disease states on brain uptake of benzodiazepines in rats. *J. Pharmacol. Exp. Ther.* 253: 45–50, 1990.

131. Lin, T.-H., Y. Sawada, Y. Sugiyama, T. Iga, and M. Hanano. Effects of albumin and α₁-acid glycoprotein on the transport of imipramine and desipramine through the blood–brain barrier in rats. *Chem. Pharm. Bull.* (*Tokyo*) 35: 294–301, 1987.

132. Lin, T. H., Y. Sugiyama, Y. Sawada, T. Iga, and M. Hanano. Dialyzable serum cofactor(s) required for the protein-mediated transport of DL-propranolol into rat brain. *Biochem. Pharmacol.* 37: 2957–2961, 1988.

133. Lin, T.-H., Y. Sugiyama, Y. Sawada, S. Kawasaki, T. Iga, and M. Hanano. Effect of serum from renal failure and cirrhotic patients on the blood–brain barrier permeability to DL-propranolol in rats. *Drug Metab. Dispos. Biol. Fate Chem.* 16: 290–295, 1988.

134. Listowsky, I., Z. Gatmaitan, and I. M. Arias. Ligandin retains and albumin loses bilirubin binding capacity in liver cytosol. *Proc. Natl. Acad. Sci. U.S.A.* 75: 1213–1216, 1978.

135. Longcope, C., R. B. Billiar, Y. Takaoka, S. P. Reddy, D. Hess, and B. Little. Tissue metabolism of estrogens in the female rhesus monkey. *Endocrinology* 109: 392–396, 1981.

136. Lovell-Smith, C. J., and P. Garcia-Webb. Glucocorticoids and the isolated rat hepatocyte. *Biochem. Biophys. Res. Commun.* 135: 160–165, 1986.

137. Luft, A. J., and F. L. Lorscheider. Structural analysis of human and bovine α-fetoprotein by electron microscopy, image processing, and circular dichroism. *Biochemistry* 22: 5978–5981, 1983.

138. Luxon, B. A., P. D. King, and E. L. Forker. Only free bile acid drives ileal absorption of taurocholate. *Am. J. Physiol.* 250 (*Gastrointest. Liver Physiol.* 13): G648–G652, 1986.

139. Maberly, G. F., K. V. Waite, A. E. Cutten, H. C. Smith, and C. J. Eastman. A reappraisal of the binding characteristics of human thyroxine-binding globulin for 3,5,3′-triiodothyronine and thyroxine. *J. Clin. Endocrinol. Metab.* 60: 42–47, 1985.

140. Mahoudeau, J. A., P. Corvol, and H. Bricaire. Rabbit testosterone-binding globulin. II. Effect on androgen metabolism in vivo. *Endocrinology* 92: 1120–1125, 1973.

141. Mangel, W. F., B. Lin, and V. Ramakrishnan. Characterization of an extremely large, ligand-induced conformational change in plasminogen. *Science* 248: 69–73, 1990.

142. Martin, M. E., C. Benassayag, and E. A. Nunez. Selective changes in binding and immunological properties of human corticosteroid binding globulin by free fatty acids. *Endocrinology* 123: 1178–1186, 1988.

143. Mendel, C. M., R. R. Cavalieri, and R. A. Weisiger. On plasma protein-mediated transport of steroid and thyroid hormones. *Am. J. Physiol.* 255 (*Endocrinol. Metab.* 18): E221–E227, 1988.

144. Mendel, C. M., R. R. Cavalieri, and R. A. Weisiger. Uptake of thyroxine by the perfused rat liver: implications for the free hormone hypothesis. *Am. J. Physiol.* 255 (*Endocrinol. Metab.* 18): E110–E119, 1988.

145. Mendel, C. M., R. R. Cavalieri, L. A. Gavin, T. Pettersson, and M. Inoue. Thyroxine transport and distribution in Nagase analbuminemic rats. *J. Clin. Invest.* 83: 143–148, 1989.

146. Mendel, C. M., R. W. Kuhn, R. A. Weisiger, R. R. Cavalieri, P. K. Siiteri, G. R. Cunha, and J. T. Murai. Uptake of cortisol by the perfused rat liver: validity of the free hormone hypothesis applied to cortisol. *Endocrinology* 124: 468–476, 1989.

147. Mendel, C. M., R. A. Weisiger, and R. R. Cavalieri. Uptake of 3,5,3'-triiodothyronine by the perfused rat liver: return to the free hormone hypothesis. *Endocrinology* 123: 1817–1824, 1988.

148. Mercier, C., A. Alfsel, and E. E. Baulieu. Testosterone binding globulin in human plasma. In: *Proc. 2nd Symp. Steroid Hormones,* Ghent, 1965. New York: Excerpta Med., 1965, p. 212. (Int. Congr. Ser. 101.)

149. Michel, C. C. Capillary permeability and how it may change. *J. Physiol.* 404: 1–29, 1988.

150. Michel, C. C., M. E. Phillips, and M.R. Turner. The effects of native and modified bovine serum albumin on the permeability of frog mesenteric capillaries. *J. Physiol. (Lond.)* 360: 333–346, 1985.

151. Mooradian, A. D., H. L. Schwartz, C. N. Mariash, and J. H. Oppenheimer. Transcellular and transnuclear transport of 3,5,3'-triiodothyronine in isolated hepatocytes. *Endocrinology* 117: 2449–2456, 1985.

152. Moresco, R. M., R. Casati, G. Lucignani, A. Carpinelli, K. Schmidt, S. Todde, F. Colombo, and F. Fazio. Systemic and cerebral kinetics of 16α[^{18}F]fluoro-17β-estradiol: a ligand for the in vivo assessment of estrogen receptor binding parameters. *J. Cereb. Blood Flow Metab.* 15: 301–311, 1995.

153. Müller, R. E., and H. H. Wotiz. Kinetics of estradiol entry into uterine cells. *Endocrinology* 105: 1107–1114, 1979.

154. Nahon, J.-L., I. Tratner, A. Poliard, F. Presse, M. Poiret, A. Gal, and J. M. Sala-Trepat. Albumin and α-fetoprotein gene expression in various nonhepatic rat tissues. *J. Biol. Chem.* 263: 11436–11442, 1988.

155. Navab, M., J. E. Smith, and D. S. Goodman. Rat plasma prealbumin. *J. Biol. Chem.* 252: 5107–5114, 1977.

156. Noé, G., Y. C. Cheng, M. Dabiké, and H. B. Croxatto. Tissue uptake of human sex hormone–binding globulin and its influence on ligand kinetics in the adult female rat. *Biol. Reprod.* 47: 970–976, 1992.

157. Oldendorf, W. H. Measurement of brain uptake of radiolabeled substances using a tritiated water internal standard. *Brain Res.* 24: 372–376, 1970.

158. Olivo, J., G. G. Gordon, F. Rafii, and A. L. Southren. Estrogen metabolism in hyperthyroidism and in cirrhosis of the liver. *Steroids* 26: 47–56, 1975.

159. O'Neill, R. D., J.-L. Gonzalez-Mora, M. G. Boutelle, D. E. Ormonde, J. P. Lowry, A. Duff, B. Fumero, M. Fillenz, and M. Mas. Anomalously high concentrations of brain extracellular uric acid detected with chronically implanted probes: implications for in vivo sampling techniques. *J. Neurochem.* 57: 22–29, 1991.

160. Oppenheimer, J. H. Thyroid hormone action at the nuclear level. *Ann. Intern. Med.* 102: 374–384, 1985.

161. Oppenheimer, J. H., G. Bernstein, and J. Hasen. Estimation of rapidly exchangeable cellular thyroxine from the plasma disappearance curves of simultaneously administered thyroxine-^{131}I and albumin-^{125}I. *J. Clin. Invest.* 46: 762–777, 1967.

162. Oppenheimer, J. H., and H. L. Schwartz. Stereospecific transport of triiodothyronine from plasma to cytosol and from cytosol to nucleus in rat liver, kidney, brain, and heart. *J. Clin. Invest.* 75: 147–154, 1985.

163. Oppenheimer, J. H., M. I. Surks, and H. L. Schwartz. The metabolic significance of exchangeable cellular thyroxine. *Recent. Prog. Horm. Res.* 25: 381–422, 1969.

164. Owens, S. M., M. Mayersohn, and J. R. Woodworth. Phencyclidine blood protein binding: influence of protein, pH, and species. *J. Pharmacol. Exp. Ther.* 226: 656–660, 1983.

165. Paine, P. L. Nucleocytoplasmic movement of fluorescent tracers microinjected into living salivary gland cells. *J. Cell Biol.* 66: 652–657, 1975.

166. Pang, K. S., and M. Rowland. Hepatic clearance of drugs. I. Theoretical considerations of a "well-stirred" model and a "parallel-tube" model. Influence of hepatic blood flow, plasma and blood cell binding, an hepatocellular enzymatic activity on hepatic drug clearance. *J. Pharmacokinet. Biopharm.* 5: 625–653, 1977.

167. Pardridge, W. M. Carrier-mediated transport of thyroid hormones through the rat blood–brain barrier: primary role of albumin-bound hormone. *Endocrinology* 105: 605–612, 1979.

168. Pardridge, W. M. Transport of protein-bound hormones into tissues in vivo. *Endocr. Rev.* 2: 103–123, 1981.

169. Pardridge, W. M. Brain metabolism: a perspective from the blood–brain barrier. *Physiol. Rev.* 63: 1481–1535, 1983.

170. Pardridge, W. M. Plasma protein–mediated transport of steroid and thyroid hormones. *Am. J. Physiol.* 252 (*Endocrinol. Metab.* 15): E157–E164, 1987.

171. Pardridge, W. M. Selective delivery of sex steroid hormones to tissues by albumin and by sex hormone–binding globulin. *Oxf. Rev. Reprod. Biol.* 10: 238–292, 1988.

172. Pardridge, W. M. Hirsutism: free and bound testosterone [Reply]. *Ann. Clin. Biochem.* 27: 93–94, 1990.

173. Pardridge, W. M. Transport of thyroid hormones into tissues in vivo. In: *Thyroid Hormone Metabolism: Regulation and Clinical Implications,* edited by S.-Y. Wu. Boston: Blackwell, 1991, p. 123–143.

174. Pardridge, W. M., J. Eisenberg, and W. T. Cefalu. Absence of albumin receptor on brain capillaries in vivo or in vitro. *Am. J. Physiol.* 249 (*Endocrinol. Metab.* 12): E264–E267, 1985.

175. Pardridge, W. M., J. Eisenberg, G. Fierer, and R. W. Kuhn. CBG does not restrict blood–brain barrier corticosterone transport in rabbits. *Am. J. Physiol.* 251 (*Endocrinol. Metab.* 14): E204–E208, 1986.

176. Pardridge, W. M., J. Eisenberg, G. Fierer, and N. A. Musto. Developmental changes in brain and serum binding of testosterone and in brain capillary uptake of testosterone-binding serum proteins in the rabbit. *Dev. Brain Res.* 38: 245–253, 1988.

177. Pardridge, W. M., and G. Fierer. Transport of tryptophan into brain from the circulating, albumin-bound pool in rats and in rabbits. *J. Neurochem.* 54: 971976, 1990.

178. Pardridge, W. M., R. A. Gorski, B. M. Lippe, and R. Green. Androgens and sexual behavior. *Ann. Intern. Med.* 96: 488–501, 1982.

179. Pardridge, W. M., and E. M. Landaw. Tracer kinetic model of blood–brain barrier transport of plasma protein–bound ligands. *J. Clin. Invest.* 74: 745–752, 1984.

180. Pardridge, W. M., and E. M. Landaw. Testosterone transport in brain: primary role of plasma protein–bound hormone. *Am. J. Physiol.* 249 (*Endocrinol. Metab.* 12): E534–E542, 1985.

181. Pardridge, W. M., and E. M. Landaw. Steady state model of 3,5,3'-triiodothyronine transport in liver predicts high cellular exchangeable hormone concentration relative to in vitro free

hormone concentration. *Endocrinology* 120: 1059–1068, 1987.

182. Pardridge, W. M., E. M. Landaw, L. P. Miller, L. D. Braun, and W. H. Oldendorf. Carotid artery injection technique: bounds for bolus mixing by plasma and by brain. *J. Cereb. Blood Flow Metab.* 5: 576–583, 1985.

183. Pardridge, W. M., and L. J. Mietus. Transport of protein-bound steroid hormones into liver in vivo. *Am. J. Physiol.* 237 (*Endocrinol. Metab. Gastrointest. Physiol.* 6): E367–E372, 1979.

184. Pardridge, W. M., and L. J. Mietus. Transport of steroid hormones through the rat blood–brain barrier. *J. Clin. Invest.* 64: 145–154, 1979.

185. Pardridge, W. M., and L. J. Mietus. Influx of thyroid hormones into rat liver in vivo. *J. Clin. Invest.* 66: 367–374, 1980.

186. Pardridge, W. M., L. J. Mietus, A. M. Frumar, B. J. Davidson, and H. L. Judd. Effects of human serum on transport of testosterone and estradiol in rat brain. *Am. J. Physiol.* 239 (*Endocrinol. Metab.* 2): E103–E108, 1980.

187. Pardridge, W. M., T. L. Moeller, L. J. Mietus, and W. H. Oldendorf. Blood–brain barrier transport and brain sequestration of steroid hormones. *Am. J. Physiol.* 239 (*Endocrinol. Metab.* 2): E96–E102, 1980.

188. Pardridge, W. M., B. N. Premachandra, and G. Fierer. Transport of thyroxine bound to human prealbumin into rat liver. *Am. J. Physiol.* 248 (*Gastrointest. Liver Physiol.* 11): G545–G550, 1985.

189. Pardridge, W. M., R. Sakiyama, and G. Fierer. Transport of propranolol and lidocaine through the rat blood–brain barrier. *J. Clin. Invest.* 71: 900–908, 1983.

190. Pardridge, W. M., R. Sakiyama, and H. L. Judd. Protein-bound corticosteroid in human serum is selectively transported into rat brain and liver in vivo. *J. Clin. Endocrinol. Metab.* 57: 160–165, 1983.

191. Pardridge, W. M., M. F. Slag, J. E. Morley, M. K. Elson, R. B. Shafer, and L. J. Mietus. Hepatic bioavailability of serum thyroid hormones in nonthyroidal illness. *J. Clin. Endocrinol. Metab.* 53: 913–916, 1981.

192. Patlak, C. S., and O. B. Paulson. The role of unstirred layers for water exchange across the blood–brain barrier. *Microvasc. Res.* 21: 117–127, 1981.

193. Payne, D. W., and J. A. Katzenellenbogen. Binding specificity of rat α-fetoprotein for a series of estrogen derivatives: studies using equilibrium and nonequilibrium binding techniques. *Endocrinology* 105: 743–753, 1979.

194. Pemberton, P. A., P. E. Stein, M. B. Pepys, J. M. Potter, and R. W. Carrell. Hormone binding globulins undergo serpin conformational change in inflammation. *Nature* 336: 257–258, 1988.

195. Perry, M. A. Capillary filtration and permeability coefficients calculated from measurements of interendothelial cell junctions in rabbit lung and skeletal muscle. *Microvasc. Res.* 19: 142–157, 1980.

196. Perry, M. A., and D. N. Granger. Permeability of intestinal capillaries to small molecules. *Am. J. Physiol.* 241 (*Gastroint. Liver Physiol.* 4): G24–G30, 1981.

197. Pervaiz, S., and K. Brew. Homology and structure–function correlations between α₁-acid glycoprotein and serum retinol-binding protein and its relatives. *FASEB J.* 1: 209–214, 1987.

198. Peters, T., Jr. Serum albumin. *Adv. Protein Chem.* 37: 161–245, 1985.

199. Piafsky, K. M., and O. Borgå. Plasma protein binding of basic drugs. *Clin. Pharmacol. Ther.* 22: 545–549, 1977.

200. Piafsky, K. M., O. Borgå, I. Odar-Cederlöf, C. Johansson, and F. Sjöqvist. Increased plasma protein binding of propranolol

and chlorpromazine mediated by disease-induced elevations of plasma α₁ acid glycoprotein. *N. Engl. J. Med.* 299: 1435–1439, 1978.

201. Rahman, S. S., R. B. Billiar, R. Miguel, W. Johnson, and B. Little. The metabolic clearance rate, the brain extraction and distribution and the uterine extraction and retention of progesterone and R 5020 in estrogen-treated ovariectomized rabbits. *Endocrinology* 101: 464–468, 1977.

202. Rask, L., and P. A. Peterson. In vitro uptake of vitamin A from the retinol-binding plasma protein to mucosal epithelial cells from the monkey's small intestine. *J. Biol. Chem.* 251: 6360–6366, 1976.

203. Reed, R. G., and C. M. Burrington. The albumin receptor effect may be due to a surface-induced conformational change in albumin. *J. Biol. Chem.* 264: 9867–9872, 1989.

204. Refetoff, S., F. E. Dwulet, and M. D. Benson. Reduced affinity for thyroxine in two of three structural thyroxine-binding prealbumin variants associated with familial amyloidotic polyneuropathy. *J. Clin. Endocrinol. Metab.* 63: 1432–1437, 1986.

205. Reid, D. G., L. K. MacLachlan, M. Voyle, and P. D. Leeson. A proton and fluorine-19 nuclear magnetic resonance and fluorescence study of the binding of some natural and synthetic thyromimetics to prealbumin (transthyretin). *J. Biol. Chem.* 264: 2013–2023, 1989.

206. Renkin, E. M. Transport of potassium-42 from blood to tissue in isolated mammalian skeletal muscles. *Am. J. Physiol.* 197: 1205–1210, 1959.

207. Renkin, E. M. Transport pathways through capillary endothelium. *Microvasc. Res.* 15: 123–135, 1978.

208. Renkin, E. M., S. D. Gray, and L. R. Dodd. Filling of microcirculation in skeletal muscles during timed India ink perfusion. *Am. J. Physiol.* 241 (*Heart Circ. Physiol.* 12): H174–H186, 1981.

209. Renoir, J.-M., C. Mercier-Bodard, and E.-E. Baulieu. Hormonal and immunological aspects of the phylogeny of sex steroid binding plasma protein. *Proc. Natl. Acad. Sci. U.S.A.* 77: 4578–4582, 1980.

209a. Riad-Fahmy, D., G. F. Read R. F. Walker, and K. Griffiths. Steroids in saliva for assessing endocrine function. *Endocr. Rev.* 3: 367–395, 1982.

210. Riant, P., S. Urien, E. Albengres, A. Renouard, and J. P. Tillement. Effects of the binding of imipramine to erythrocytes and plasma proteins on its transport through the rat blood–brain barrier. *J. Neurochem.* 51: 421–425, 1988.

211. Ridgway, E. C., C. Longcope, and F. Maloof. Metabolic clearance and blood production rates of estradiol in hyperthyroidism. *J. Clin. Endocrinol. Metab.* 41: 491–497, 1975.

212. Robbins, J., and J. E. Rall. Effects of triiodothyronine and other thyroxine analogues on thyroxine-binding in human serum. *J. Clin. Invest.* 34: 1331–1338, 1955.

213. Robbins, J., J. E. Rall, and P. Gorden. The thyroid and iodine metabolism. In: *Duncan's Disease of Metabolism,* edited by P. K. Bondy and L. E. Rosenberg. Philadelphia: Saunders, 1974, p. 1009–1023.

214. Roberts, M. S., and M. Rowland. Hepatic elimination-dispersion model. *J. Pharm. Sci.* 74: 585–587, 1985.

215. Rosenoer, V. M., and M. A. Rothschild. The extravascular transport of albumin. In: *Plasma Protein Metabolism,* edited by M. A. Rothschild and T. Waldmann. New York: Academic, 1970, p. 111–127.

216. Rosenthal, H. E., W. R. Slaunwhite, Jr., and A. A. Sandberg. Transcortin: A corticosteroid-binding protein of plasma. X. Cortisol and progesterone interplay and unbound levels of these steroids in pregnancy. *J. Clin. Endocrinol.* 29: 352–367, 1969.

217. Rosner, W. The functions of corticosteroid-binding globulin and sex hormone–binding globulin: recent advances. *Endocr. Rev.* 11: 80–91, 1990.

218. Rouaze-Romet, M., R. Vranckx, L. Savu, and E. A. Nunez. Structural and functional microheterogeneity of rat thyroxine-binding globulin during ontogenesis. *Biochem. J.* 286: 125–130, 1992.

219. Rowland, M., D. Leitch, G. Fleming, and B. Smith. Protein binding and hepatic clearance: discrimination between models of hepatic clearance with diazepam, a drug of high intrinsic clearance, in the isolated perfused rat liver preparation. *J. Pharmacokinet. Biopharmet.* 12: 129–147, 1984.

220. Rudd, B. T., N. M. Duignan, and D. R. London. A rapid method for the measurement of sex hormone binding globulin capacity of sera. *Clin. Chim. Acta* 55: 165–178, 1974.

221. Ruder, H., P. Corvol, J. A. Mahoudeau, G. T. Ross, and M. B. Lipsett. Effects of induced hyperthyroidism on steroid metabolism in man. *J. Clin. Endocrinol.* 33: 382–387, 1971.

222. Rushbrook, J. I., E. Becker, G. C. Schussler, and C. M. Divino. Identification of a human serum albumin species associated with familial dysalbuminemic hyperthyroxinemia. *J. Clin. Endocrinol. Metab.* 80: 461–467, 1995.

223. Ruutiainen, K., E. Sannikka, R. Santti, R. Erkkola, and H. Adlercreutz. Salivary testosterone in hirsutism: correlations with serum testosterone and the degree of hair growth. *J. Clin. Endocrinol. Metab.* 64: 1015–1020, 1987.

224. Sakiyama, R., W. M. Pardridge, and H. L. Judd. Effects of human cirrhotic serum on estradiol and testosterone transport into rat brain. *J. Clin. Endocrinol. Metab.* 54: 1140–1144, 1982.

225. Sakiyama, R., W. M. Pardridge, and N. A. Musto. Influx of testosterone-binding globulin (TeBG) and TeBG-bound sex steroid hormones into rat testis and prostate. *J. Clin. Endocrinol. Metab.* 67: 98–103, 1988.

226. Salhany, J. M., and R. Cassoly. Kinetics of p-mercuribenzoate binding to sulfhydryl groups on the isolated cytoplasmic fragment of band 3 protein. *J. Biol. Chem.* 264: 1399–1404, 1989.

227. Scheider, W. The rate of access to the organic ligand-binding region of serum albumin is entropy controlled. *Proc. Natl. Acad. Sci. U.S.A.* 76: 2283–2287, 1979.

228. Schnitzer, J. E., W. W. Carley, and G. E. Palade. Specific albumin binding to microvascular endothelium in culture. *Am. J. Physiol.* 254 (*Heart Circ. Physiol.* 23): H425–H437, 1988.

229. Schwartz, H. L., D. Trence, J. H. Oppenheimer, N. S. Jiang, and D. B. Jump. Distribution and metabolism of L- and D-triiodothyronine (T_3) in the rat: preferential accumulation of L-T_3 by hepatic and cardiac nuclei as a probable explanation of the differential biological potency of T_3 enantiomers. *Endocrinology* 113: 1236–1243, 1983.

230. Shand, D. G., R. H. Cotham, and G. R. Wilkinson. Perfusion-limited effects of plasma drug binding on hepatic drug extraction. *Life Sci.* 19: 125–130, 1976.

231. Sholl, S. A., P. T. K. Toivola, and J. A. Robinson. The dynamics of testosterone and dihydrotestosterone metabolism in the adult male rhesus monkey. *Endocrinology* 105: 402–405, 1979.

232. Shore, M. L. Biological applications of kinetic analysis of a two-compartment open system. *J. Appl. Physiol.* 16: 771–782, 1961.

233. Siiteri, P. K. Extraglandular oestrogen formation and serum binding of oestradiol: relationship to cancer. *J. Endocrinol.* 89: 119P–129P, 1981.

234. Simionescu, M., N. Ghinea, A. Fixman, M. Lasser, L. Kukes, N. Simionescu, and G. E. Palade. The cerebral microvasculature of the rat: structure and luminal surface properties during early development. *J. Submicrosc. Cytol. Pathol.* 20: 243–261, 1988.

235. Smith, R. G., P. K. Besch, B. Dill, and V. C. Buttram, Jr. Saliva as a matrix for measuring free androgens: comparison with serum androgens in polycystic ovarian disease. *Fertil. Steril.* 31: 513–517, 1979.

236. Smith, T. W., and K. M. Skubitz. Kinetics of interactions between antibodies and haptens. *Biochemistry.* 14: 1496–1502, 1975.

237. Snyder, S. M., R. R. Cavalieri, I. D. Goldfine, S. H. Ingbar, and E. C. Jorgensen. Binding of thyroid hormones and their analogues to thyroxine-binding globulin in human serum. *J. Biol. Chem.* 251: 6489–6494, 1976.

238. Soloff, M. S., M. J. Morrison, and T. L. Swartz. A comparison of the estrone-estradiol-binding proteins in the plasmas of prepubertal and pregnant rats. *Steroids* 20: 597–608, 1972.

239. Stein, W. D. *The Movement of Molecules Across Cell Membranes.* New York: Academic, 1967, p. 65–125.

240. Steiner, R. F., J. Roth, and J. Robbins. The binding of thyroxine by serum albumin as measured by fluorescence quenching. *J. Biol. Chem.* 241: 560–567, 1966.

241. Steingold, K. A., D. W. Matt, L. Dua, T. L. Anderson, and G. D. Hodgen. Orosomucoid in human pregnancy serum diminishes bioavailability of the progesterone antagonist RU 486 in rats. *Am. J. Obstet. Gynecol.* 162: 523–524, 1990.

242. Stollman, Y. R., U. Gärtner, L. Theilmann, and N. Ohmi. Hepatic bilirubin uptake in the isolated perfused rat liver is not facilitated by albumin binding. *J. Clin. Invest.* 72: 718–723, 1983.

243. Stroupe, S. D., S.-L. Cheng, and U. Westphal. Steroid–protein interactions. *Arch. Biochem. Biophys.* 168: 473–482, 1975.

244. Stroupe, S. D., G. B. Harding, M. W. Forsthoefel, and U. Westphal. Kinetic and equilibrium studies on steroid interaction with human corticosteroid-binding globulin. *Biochemistry* 17: 177–182, 1978.

245. Sugihara, J., T. Imamura, S. Nagafuchi, J. Bonaventura, C. Bonaventura, and R. Cashon. Hemoglobin rahere, a human hemoglobin variant with amino acid substitution at the 2,3-diphosphoglycerate binding site. *J. Clin. Invest.* 76: 1169–1173, 1985.

246. Sundelin, J., H. Melhus, S. Das, U. Eriksson, P. Lind, L. Trägårdh, P. A. Peterson, and L. Rask. The primary structure of rabbit and rat prealbumin and a comparison with the tertiary structure of human prealbumin. *J. Biol. Chem.* 260: 6481–6487, 1985.

247. Sutherland, R. L., and M. R. Brandon. The thyroxine-binding properties of rat and rabbit serum proteins. *Endocrinology* 98: 91–98, 1976.

248. Suzuki, N., T. Yamaguchi, and H. Nakajima. Role of high-density lipoprotein in transport of circulating bilirubin in rats. *J. Biol. Chem.* 263: 5037–5043, 1988.

249. Swartz, S. K., and M. S. Soloff. The lack of estrogen binding by human α-fetoprotein. *J. Clin. Endocrinol. Metab.* 39: 589–591, 1974.

250. Tait, J. F., and S. Burstein. In vivo studies of steroid dynamics in man. In: *The Hormones,* edited by G. Pincus, K. V. Thimann, and E. B. Astwood. New York: Academic, 1964, vol. V, p. 441–557.

251. Terasaki, T., Y. Deguchi, Y. Kasama, W. M. Pardridge, and A. Tsuji. Determination of in vivo steady-state unbound drug concentration in the brain interstitial fluid by microdialysis. *Int. J. Pharm.* 81: 143–152, 1992.

252. Terasaki, T., Y. Deguchi, H. Sato, K. Hirai, and A. Tsuji. In vivo transport of a dynorphin-like analgesid peptide, E-2078, through the blood–brain barrier. An application of brain microdialysis. *Pharm. Res.* 8: 815–820, 1991.

253. Terasaki, T., D. M. Nowlin, and W. M. Pardridge. Differential

binding of testosterone and estradiol to isoforms of sex hor-mone–binding globulin: selective alteration of estradiol binding in cirrhosis. *J. Clin. Endocrinol. Metab.* 67: 639–643, 1988.

254. Terasaki, T., and W. M. Pardridge. Stereospecificity of triiodo-thyronine transport into brain, liver, and salivary gland: role of carrier- and plasma protein–mediated transport. *Endocrinol-ogy* 121: 1185–1191, 1987.

255. Terasaki, T., and W. M. Pardridge. Differential binding of thyroxine and triiodothyronine to acidic isoforms of thyroid hormone binding globulin in human serum. *Biochemistry* 27: 3624–3628, 1988.

256. Terasaki, T., W. M. Pardridge, and D. D. Denson. Differential effect of plasma protein binding of bupivacaine on its in vivo transfer into the brain and salivary gland of rats. *J. Pharmacol. Exp. Ther.* 239: 724–729, 1986.

257. Thomas, T., S. Fletcher, G. C. T. Yeoh, and G. Schreiber. The expression of $\alpha(1)$-acid glycoprotein mRNA during rat development. *J. Biol. Chem.* 264: 5784–5790, 1989.

258. Thorens, B., H. F. Lodish, and D. Brown. Differential localiza-tion of two glucose transporter isoforms in rat kidney. *Am. J. Physiol.* 259 (*Cell Physiol.* 28): C296–C302, 1990.

259. Tilley, W. D., D. J. Horsfall, M. A. McGee, D. W. Henderson, and V. R. Marshall. Distribution of oestrogen and androgen receptors between the stroma and epithelium of the guinea-pig prostate. *J. Steroid Biochem.* 22: 713–719, 1985.

260. Tracqui, P., P. Brézillon, J. F. Staub, Y. Morot-Gaudry, M. Hamon, and A. M. Perault-Staub. Model of brain serotonin metabolism. I. Structure determination-parameter estimation. *Am. J. Physiol.* 244 (*Regulatory Integrative Comp. Physiol.* 15): R193–R205, 1983.

261. Tracqui, P., Y. Morot-Gaudry, J. F. Staub, P. Brézillon, A. M. Perault-Staub, S. Bourgoin, and M. Hamon. Model of brain serotonin metabolism. II. Physiological interpretation. *Am. J. Physiol.* 244 (*Regulatory Integrative Comp. Physiol.* 15): R206–R215, 1983.

262. Tsao, S. C., Y. Sugiyama, Y. Sawada, T. Iga, and M. Hanano. Kinetic analysis of albumin-mediated uptake of warfarin by perfused rat liver. *J. Pharmacokinet. Biopharm.* 16: 165–181, 1988.

263. Tsao, S. C., Y. Sugiyama, K. Shinmura, Y. Sawada, S. Nagase, T. Iga, and M. Hanano. Protein-mediated hepatic uptake of rose bengal in analbuminemic mutant rats (NAR). *Drug Metab. Disposit. Biol. Fate Chem.* 16: 482–489, 1988.

264. Urien, S., F. Brée, B. Testa, and J.-P. Tillement. pH-dependency of basic ligand binding to α_1-acid glycoprotein (orosomucoid). *Biochem. J.* 280: 277–280, 1991.

265. Urien, S., J.-L. Pinquier, B. Paquette, P. Chaumet-Riffaud, J.-R. Kiechel, and J. P. Tillement. Effect of the binding of isradipine and darodipine to different plasma proteins on their transfer through the rat blood–brain barrier. Drug binding to lipoproteins does not limit the transfer of drug. *J. Pharmacol. Exp. Ther.* 242: 349–353, 1987.

266. Urien, S., R. Zini, M. Lemaire, and J. P. Tillement. Assessment of cyclosporine A interactions with human plasma lipoproteins in vitro and in vivo in the rat. *J. Pharmacol. Exp. Ther.* 253: 305–309, 1990.

267. van Thiel, D. H. Feminization of chronic alcoholic men: a formulation. *Yale J. Biol. Med.* 52: 219–225, 1979.

268. Vermeulen, A. Influence of anabolic steroids on secretion and metabolism of cortisol. In: *Structure and Metabolism of Corti-costeroids,* edited by J. R. Pasqualini and M. F. Jayle. New York: Academic, 1964, p. 109–116.

269. Vermeulen, A. Transport and distribution of androgens at different ages. In: *Androgens and Antiandrogens,* edited by L. Martini and M. Motta. New York: Raven, 1977, p. 53–65.

270. Vermeulen, A., and S. Andó. Metabolic clearance rate and interconversion of androgens and the influence of the free androgen fraction. *J. Clin. Endocrinol. Metab.* 48: 320–326, 1979.

271. Vermeulen, A., L. Verdonck, M. Van der Straeten, and N. Orie. Capacity of the testosterone-binding globulin in human plasma and influence of specific binding of testosterone on its metabolic clearance rate. *J. Clin. Endocrinol.* 29: 1470–1480, 1969.

272. Vigersky, R. A., S. Kono, M. Sauer, M. B. Lipsett, and D. L. Loriaux. Relative binding of testosterone and estradiol to testosterone–estradiol-binding globulin. *J. Clin. Endocrinol. Metab.* 49: 899–904, 1979.

273. Wang, C., S. Plymate, E. Nieschlag, and C. A. Paulsen. Salivary testosterone in men: further evidence of a direct correlation with free serum testosterone. *J. Clin. Endocrinol. Metab.* 53: 1021–1024, 1981.

274. Weideman, M. P. Architecture. In: *Handbook of Physiology: The Cardiovascular System. Microcirculation,* edited by E. M. Renkin and C. C. Michel. Bethesda, MD: *Am. Physiol. Soc.* 1984, sect. 2, vol. IV., pt. 1, chap. 2, p. 11–40.

275. Weisiger, R. A. Dissociation from albumin: a potentially rate-limiting step in the clearance of substances by the liver. *Proc. Natl. Acad. Sci. U.S.A.* 82: 1563–1567, 1985.

276. Weisiger, R., J. Gollan, and R. Ockner. Receptor for albumin on the liver cell surface may mediate uptake of fatty acids and other albumin-bound substances. *Science* 211: 1048–1051, 1981.

277. Weiss, R. E., T. Sunthornthepvarakul, P. Angkeow, D. Marcus-Bagley, N. Cox, C. A. Alper, and S. Refetoff. Linkage of familial dysalbuminemic hyperthyroxinemia to the albumin gene in a large Amish kindred. *J. Clin. Endocrinol. Metab.* 80: 116–121, 1995.

278. Westergren, I., B. Nyström, A. Hamberger, and B. B. Johans-son. Intracerebral dialysis and the blood–brain barrier. *J. Neu-rochem.* 64: 229–234, 1995.

279. Westphal, U. Steroid-binding serum globulins: recent results. In: *Receptor and Hormone Action,* edited by B. W. O'Malley and L. Birnbaumer. New York: Academic, 1978, vol. 2, p. 443–472.

280. Whittem, T., and D. C. Ferguson. Kinetics of triiodothyronine dissociation from bovine serum albumin: modification of the resin capture method with subsequent computer modeling. *Endocrinology* 127: 2190–2198, 1990.

281. Wilting, J., J. M. H. Kremer, A. P. Ijzerman, and S. G. Schul-man. The kinetics of the binding of warfarin to human serum albumin as studied by stopped-flow spectrophotometry. *Bio-chim. Biophys. Acta* 706: 96–104, 1982.

282. Winkler, K., S. Keiding, and N. Tygstrup. Clearance as a quantitative measure of liver function. In: *The Liver: Quantita-tive Aspects of Structure and Functions,* edited by P. Paumgar-tners and P. Presig. Basel: Karger, 1973, p. 144–155.

283. Woeber, K. A., and S. H. Ingbar. The contribution of thyroxine-binding prealbumin to the binding of thyroxine in human serum, as assessed by immunoadsorption. *J. Clin. In-vest.* 47: 1710–1721, 1968.

284. Yamamoto, T., K. Doi, K. Ichihara, and K. Miyai. Reevaluation of measurement of serum free thyroxine by equilibrium dialysis based on computational analysis of the interaction between thyroxine and its binding proteins. *J. Clin. Endocrinol. Metab.* 50: 882–888, 1980.

285. Yergey, J. A., and M. P. Heyes. Brain eicosanoid formation following acute penetration injury as studied by in vivo micro-dialysis. *J. Cereb. Blood Flow Metab.* 10: 143–146, 1990.

286. Zaninovich, A. A., H. Farach, C. Ezrin, and R. Volpé. Lack of significant binding of L-triiodothyronine by thyroxine-binding globulin in vivo as demonstrated by acute disappearance of ^{131}I-labeled triiodothyronine. *J. Clin. Invest.* 45: 1290–1301, 1966.

287. Zaninovich, A. A., R. Volpé, and C. Ezrin. Effects of variations of thyroxine-binding globulin capacity on the disappearance of triiodothyronine from the plasma. *J. Clin. Endocrinol.* 29: 1601–1607, 1969.

288. Zucker, S. D., W. Goessling, and J. L. Gollan. Kinetics of bilirubin transfer betweenserum albumin and membrane vesicles. *J. Biol. Chem.* 270: 1074–1081, 1995.

15. Steroid hormone receptor families

CLIFF HURD
V. K. MOUDGIL | *Department of Biological Sciences and The Institute for Biochemistry and Biotechnology, Oakland University, Rochester, Michigan*

EARLY WORK ON STEROID HORMONE ACTION utilized mainly the rat uterus as a model system to study the effect of estrogen. A key breakthrough was the development of radiolabeled estrogen, which allowed investigators to trace the tissue-specific retention of this hormone in its target tissues. In the early 1960s Jensen and Jacobson (133) found that when estrogen was injected into female rats, it was concentrated and retained in the uterus. This is regarded as a milestone because they directly demonstrated the selective retention of a hormone by its putative target tissue. They suggested that specific receptors for estrogen were expressed by the uterus.

Another significant observation was made by Edelman et al. (64), who used autoradiography to demonstrate that radiolabeled aldosterone is localized selectively in the nuclei of target bladder epithelial cells. Furthermore, they showed that the physiological effect of this hormone depended on the induction of de novo synthesis of protein. Thus, the intracellular localization of aldosterone within the nucleus coincided with its suspected action—the modulation of gene expression. That the action of a steroid involves the modulation of gene expression was demonstrated by Noteboom and Gorski (193), who found that estrogen administration induced RNA synthesis in the rat uterus.

Although the retention and nuclear uptake of steroid hormones by putative target cells suggested the existence of tissue-specific receptors that might mediate their effects, the direct demonstration and characterization of such a molecule was not accomplished until 1966, when Toft and Gorski (267) labeled uterine tissue extracts with estrogen and separated the radiolabeled receptor from other cellular components by density gradient centrifugation. The molecule that bound estrogen was cleaved by pronase but not by deoxyribonuclease or ribonuclease. This protein moiety sedimented as a 9.5 S species, and the estrogen label was competed for specifically only by estrogens, not glucocorticoids or testosterone. These observations led investigators to speculate that the 9.5 S binder represented a specific estrogen receptor and that it was oligomeric and therefore might be regulated via an allosteric mechanism between receptor subunits. Notides et al. showed this to be the case for the estrogen receptor, which exists as a 4 S species in its monomeric form but readily dimerizes to form a 5 S nuclear bound form in the presence of estrogen (194).

Since the 9.5 S receptor was isolated from the cytosolic fraction of target cells, it was thought to be located in the cytoplasm. The 5 S form was isolated from the nucleus, which suggested that the conversion of the 9.5 S to the 5 S form of the receptor occurred concomitantly with translocation of the estrogen-bound receptor to the nucleus. A two-step model for steroid hormonal action, therefore, was proposed. In this model, steroids bind to receptors in the cytoplasm, forming steroid–receptor complexes which then translocate into the nucleus, where they modify transcription of hormonally regulated genes (134). Subsequently, the search to identify and characterize receptors for other steroid hormones continued. A receptor for progesterone was first isolated from the chicken oviduct by O'Malley and co-workers (197). Using cellular fractionation techniques, a time-dependent gradual retention of the progesterone receptor in the nuclear fraction was observed, with a concomitant decrease in the cytosolic fraction following administration of progesterone. These observations appeared to confirm the two-step model of steroid hormonal action.

However, subsequent studies, which utilized antibodies to localize unbound receptors, indicated that even in the absence of hormone the receptors for estrogen (140) and progesterone (69, 203, 292) are localized predominantly in the nucleus. These observations were in conflict with a generalized hormone-induced cytoplasm-to-nucleus translocation model. It is now generally believed that steroid receptors, with the exception of glucocorticoid receptors (99, 208), are predominantly nuclear whether or not receptors are complexed with hormone. Uncomplexed receptor molecules, although located in the nucleus in vivo, readily leach out of the nucleus during tissue homogenization and are thus isolated in the cytosolic fraction. The widely accepted current model for steroid hormonal action suggests that nascent receptors, independent of their cellular localization, undergo a hormone-induced conformational change (transformation) which results in tight nuclear binding of the receptor. Some of the molecular events which result in a transformed receptor are clear, including subunit dissociation of an oligomeric receptor complex, hetero- or homodimerization, and tight or increased binding to specific DNA sequences called hormone response elements (HREs) located in the hormone-regulated genes (17, 70, 71, 83, 84, 91, 103, 212, 235, 272, 296, 302). What is less clear is the role of phosphorylation/dephosphorylation in modulating the various functions of steroid receptors, how potentially interdependent subdomains of the receptor interact or cooperate to modulate hormone binding, DNA binding and transcriptional activation, and the identity and precise interactions between steroid receptors, basal transcription factors, and/or receptor-specific transcriptional intermediary factors.

Steroid hormones enter target cells by passive processes and bind to receptors in various states of maturation. Functional receptors define the target tissue and mediate the actions of the hormone. In the nascent state, steroid receptors are complexed with a major heat shock protein, HSP-90, which inactivates the innate DNA binding and transacting potential of the receptor. Other protein subunits, including HSP-70 and a 59 kd protein (143, 223, 230, 231, 250, 260), also are associated with nascent steroid receptors; however, the role they play in steroid receptor function is less clear. This 350–400 kd heterooligomeric structure is referred to as the "nontransformed receptor." It sediments in the 8–9 S range, has relatively low affinity for nuclear components (9, 80, 88, 196, 222), and exists as a phosphoprotein (182, 199). Phosphorylation/dephosphorylation of the receptor is thought to modulate the various steroid receptor functions by maintaining or inducing primary, secondary, tertiary, or quaternary structural alterations in the receptor. The phosphorylation state of the receptor is defined by the cell-specific relative activities of terminal kinases or phosphatases, whose activities are regulated by other signal-transduction systems. Ligand binding promotes a conformation in the hormone-binding domain (HBD) that releases and thus relieves the repressor, HSP-90. Dissociation of HSP-90 and homo- or heterodimerization increase the affinity and specificity of the receptor–DNA interaction, resulting in increased complexing of receptors to cis enhancers, the HREs (11, 83, 105, 146, 272–274, 294, 302). These specific DNA-binding sites are located in hormone-regulated genes and show two-fold rotational symmetry, reflecting the subunit structure of a symmetrical homodimer or direct repeats with variable spacing between response element half-sites for heterodimers (104, 254, 272, 302). A stable receptor–DNA interaction and primary structural regions called "activation functions" mediate formation of a transcriptional preinitiation complex (36, 37, 42, 43, 102, 130, 132, 198, 298). Activation functions are thought to interact directly or through transcriptional intermediary factors (TIFs) with basal transcription factors, enhancing the rate of transcriptional initiation of hormonally regulated genes. Theoretically, enhancement or interference with any of these events could be considered receptor agonistic or antagonistic.

The cloning and sequencing of cDNAs of the receptors for steroid hormones, thyroid hormone and its oncogenic derivatives, vitamin D, retinoic acid, and those for which a known ligand has yet to be reported (orphan receptors) have demonstrated a high degree of primary structural homology. Examination of the wild-type primary structures has indicated a number of functionally distinct domains (39, 44, 45, 53, 87, 94, 96, 114, 142, 145, 157, 160, 170, 178, 266, 271, 282). Further analyses of point, deletion, and truncated mutant expression products of the receptor genes (31, 32, 63, 82, 86, 147, 148, 192, 228, 269, 290) along with functional analyses of chimeric receptors (65, 85, 90, 92) have defined a number of autonomous and semiautonomous functional domains. Based on these primary structural homologies, steroid receptors have been classified into a nuclear receptor superfamily of morphogenic gene-regulatory proteins, derived from a single progenitor gene that has replicated and diverged to produce the unique functions of its various members (2, 70, 164).

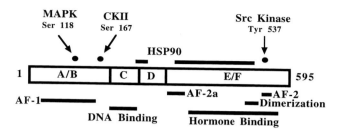

FIG. 15.1. Primary domain structure of human estrogen receptor. Illustrated are regions A–F with subdomains and their functions represented as block lines. Also shown are the kinases that phosphorylate human estrogen receptor and their sites of action. *MAPK,* mitogen-activated protein kinase; *CKII,* casein kinase II; *Src,* tyrosine-specific kinase protooncogene originally isolated as the Rous sarcoma (Src) virus oncogene; *HSP,* heat shock protein; *AF,* activation function.

MOLECULAR COMPOSITION OF RECEPTOR PROTEINS: PRIMARY STRUCTURAL HOMOLOGIES AND FUNCTIONAL DOMAINS

Members of the steroid receptor superfamily have the same modular domain primary structure, divided into regions A–F by their functions. Figure 15.1 illustrates the distinct domains of the human estrogen receptor, their various functions, known phosphorylation sites, and the location of HSP-90 interaction.

The A/B Region of Steroid Receptors Contains a Hormone-Independent Activation Function

At the N-terminus of steroid receptors is a region designated A/B, which is highly variable among members of the superfamily. Analyses of the chromosomal gene structures of the human estrogen receptor (210) and glucocorticoid receptor (68) and the avian progesterone receptor (120) show that the A/B region is encoded in a single divergent exon.

Common among steroid receptors is a hormone-independent activation function (AF-1) in the A/B region which enhances the receptor's ability to activate transcription in a cell- and promoter-dependent manner (112, 169, 237, 268, 270). Under conditions where the receptor is bound to its response element linked to the proper promoters, AF-1 will enhance transcription in the absence of hormone or when receptors are complexed with antagonist ligands. Another activation function located in the HBD (AF-2) must be complexed with agonist ligands to function (24, 26, 262, 285).

The coincidental location of AF-1 and sites of phosphorylation has led to the speculation that covalent

modification of this region by phosphorylation might modify the transacting potential of steroid receptors. This has been demonstrated for the estrogen receptor (1, 5, 135, 139, 151). The exact role of phosphorylation in regulating this function of other receptors is as yet unclear.

The progesterone receptor is expressed as two isoforms, PR-A and PR-B, which are identical except that PR-A lacks the N-terminal 164 amino acids of the A/B region. This segment contains a PR-B-specific activation function (AF-3) and unique basal phosphorylation sites (233, 299). Because of its uniqueness to PR-B and its apparent regulation by phosphorylation, investigations have focused on how it might affect promoter, cellular, and ligand-specific differences in the ability of PR-A and PR-B to transactivate responsive genes and how PR-A, which lacks this region, is able to repress PR-B in a cell- and promoter-specific way (275, 279).

The C Region Encodes a Specific DNA-Binding Function

The region designated C, also called the DNA-binding domain (DBD), is the most highly conserved among the nuclear receptor superfamily, reflecting the fact that DNA binding is the most evolutionarily constrained function of steroid receptors (147, 148). Domain-swapping experiments demonstrate that this region determines the specific DNA-binding activity of steroid receptors (82, 228).

The length of the C domain is approximately 70 amino acids and is divided into subregions C1 and C2, which are separated by a linker region. These subregions, each along with its half of the linker region, are encoded by separate exons (68, 120, 210, 302). Each of these subdomains contains the supersecondary structural motif present in a number of DNA-binding proteins called "zinc fingers" (22, 72, 76). The DBDs of the glucocorticoid and estrogen receptors have been analyzed by nuclear magnetic resonance (106, 241) and the crystal structures determined (161, 240). These studies indicate that the two fingers fold together to form a single structural domain, that they bind DNA as symmetrical homodimers, and that the spacing between half-sites of the palindromic response element is critical for specific interaction between receptors and their response elements.

The relative importance of C1 and C2 in specific DNA binding has been characterized (23, 47, 52, 93, 163, 277, 301, 302). C1 is the N-terminal zinc finger and contains four cysteine residues which tetrahedrally coordinate one zinc atom. Between the third and the fourth cysteine of C1, there are two amino-acid residues which determine the specificity of receptor–DNA interaction by forming hydrogen bonds with two base pairs of the response element. C2 is the C-terminal finger and contains five cysteine residues, the fifth being dispensable for DNA binding. The other four, as with the C1 finger, also tetrahedrally coordinate a zinc atom. This finger does not appear to discriminate particular base pairs of the DNA-binding site through hydrogen bonding but, rather, to affect correct spacing of dimers so that the C1 fingers of a dimer optimally interact with the correct base pairs of the dyadic response element.

The D Region (the Hinge Domain) Contains a Nuclear Localization Signal

The D region shows a low degree of sequence homology and is highly variable with respect to length (147, 148). It is encoded by a single exon, which, of the exons contained in the chromosomal genes of steroid receptors (68, 120, 210), appears to have diverged the most. This suggests that the functional constraints for receptor activity are less for this region. Further evidence for this is the observation that mutational insertions of proline, which disrupt secondary structure, had no effect on estrogen receptor activity (147).

A five-amino-acid-long subregion within the D domain, which is homologous to a nuclear localization signal first identified in the simian virus 40 large T antigen, is conserved absolutely among mammalian progesterone receptors (137). Deletion of this region obliterates constitutive nuclear localization of the receptor but results in a hormone-dependent nuclear translocation (99).

The E/F Region Contains the Hormone-Binding Domain, a Dimerization Motif, Steroid Receptor Repressor Activity, and a Receptor Agonist–Dependent Transcriptional Activation Function

The E/F region is the HBD. It is characteristically 250 amino acids long and is highly conserved among all steroid receptors and even more so for those which bind the same steroid. It contains a high proportion of hydrophobic amino acids, which are thought to form the steroid-binding pocket. Hormone binding is highly vulnerable to even minor mutations in this region (30, 63, 228). In fact, a single point mutation within this region of the estrogen receptor destabilizes estrogen binding (269). This suggests that certain amino acids may be critical either for hormone binding, due to a direct chemical interaction with the steroid, or for maintaining the proper tertiary structure of the binding pocket.

A hormone-dependent activation function (AF-2) in the E/F region is activated by agonist ligands but not by antagonists (36, 37, 102, 169, 198, 285). Another region (AF-2a) in the human estrogen receptor HBD has been distinguished functionally from the original AF-2 (132) (see TRANSACTIVATION BY STEROID RECEPTORS, below). Another function which appears to be determined by the HBD is dimerization. The HBD of the estrogen receptor contains a leucine zipper-like motif and other receptors have a sequence which is highly homologous (73). This region is thought to mediate dimerization and thus to enhance the affinity of the receptor for its response element.

In the unliganded state, the HBD represses other receptor functions, such as DNA binding and transcriptional activation (65, 84, 85, 103). The putative role of hormone binding is to deactivate this repressor function (84, 103). The best evidence for this assertion is that deletion of the HBD renders steroid receptors able to enhance transcription in the absence of hormone, though somewhat less efficiently than an intact receptor does in the presence of hormone (32, 82, 86, 147, 247). In contrast, partial deletions in the HBD of the chicken progesterone receptor or point mutations throughout the region did not yield constitutive activators but, rather, receptors which could not be activated even in the presence of hormone (32, 63). Apparently, point mutations result in a receptor that is unable to respond to hormone but still able to repress the transcriptional activation functions. Thus, the overall general structure, which presumably is not affected by point mutations, is sufficient to repress the receptor.

Exactly how this repressor function works is unclear. One suggestion is that stereospecific contacts made by the unliganded HBD upon the other regions of the receptor repress these domains. However, this seems unlikely since point mutations have no effect on the repressor function (32, 63). Furthermore, chimeric receptors, in which the HBD is fused to entirely different proteins, exhibit repression of the protein's activity (65, 85), which is relieved upon hormone administration. For example, the transcriptional regulatory functions and cellular transformation ability of c-Fos (221, 256), the cellular transformation by c-Abl (131), and the suppression of cellular proliferation by the tumor suppressor *p53* (225) became estradiol-dependent upon fusion of these proteins to the estrogen receptor HBD. The HBD is also capable of repressing steroid receptor activity in a context-independent manner; it can be placed anywhere in the receptor relative to the DBD and still repress receptor activity (207, 297). Again, in all cases, repression of these activities was relieved by adding hormone.

To explain these observations, it has been suggested that this nonspecific repressor activity of the unliganded HBD is mediated by a major heat shock protein, HSP-90 (297). When the receptor is complexed with HSP-90, other protein functions, including DNA binding, dimerization, phosphorylation, and transcriptional activation, are repressed. When hormone-induced dissociation of HSP-90 from the protein occurs, the protein takes on its active structure.

RECEPTOR-ASSOCIATED PROTEINS AND THE OLIGOMERIC STRUCTURE OF STEROID RECEPTORS

Receptor-associated proteins (RAPs) are associated with steroid receptors in their non- or partially activated states. This is in contrast to proteins which interact with steroid receptors after they are activated. Smith and Toft (251) discuss seven known RAPs in descending order of size (HSP-90, HSP-70, p60, p59, p54, p50, and p23) and their functional and structural roles in steroid receptor actions. We highlight below what we believe are the most significant advances in this area.

Major Heat Shock Proteins

The term "heat shock proteins" (HSP) was coined from the observation that their expression was increased dramatically by elevated temperatures in cells and tissues. All organisms express homologs of two of the major HSPs, HSP-70 and HSP-90, which are expressed constitutively under normal cellular conditions but increased dramatically during heat shock or other cellular stresses (155). Some of the suggested roles for these molecular chaperones include prevention of nonspecific

protein aggregation, blockage of proteolytic sites on chaperoned proteins, prevention of misfunctional post-translational modifications, protein misfolding during synthesis (20, 155, 202, 226, 227), and protein transport (144). They also are observed in signal-transduction pathways involving both serine/threonine kinases (46, 257, 281) and tyrosine-specific kinases, including the protooncogene Src (155, 295). A more appropriate term has been applied to HSPs, "molecular chaperones." In their role as regulators of steroid receptors, they are now called RAPs.

HSP-90. There are at least two well-defined functions of HSP-90 in steroid receptor signal transduction: *(1)* to induce and maintain the high-affinity conformation of the receptor for ligand binding and at the same time to repress DNA binding and transcriptional activation and *(2)* to release from the receptor upon hormone binding, a process also referred to as "dissociation of the heterooligomeric steroid receptor complex" or "steroid receptor transformation." A series of reports have demonstrated the necessity of the first of these functions both in vivo and in vitro.

The use of in vitro translation systems, in particular the rabbit reticulocyte lysate system, has helped to clarify the role of HSP-90 in steroid hormone signal transduction. The presence of HSP-90 in the translation system appears to increase the rate of steroid receptor synthesis and to enhance hormone binding by the receptor (48, 51). In contrast, a low number of functional receptors are produced in systems other than reticulocyte lysates, and they have a reduced affinity for ligand. For example, receptors translated in wheat germ extract (48) or *Escherichia (E.) coli* (195) fail to bind HSP-90, and significant specific hormone binding also is not detected. This suggests that receptors which do not associate with HSP-90 during translation are not primed for the hormonal signal. This has been attributed to either low levels of HSP-90 or significant interspecies dishomologies between mammalian and plant or bacterial HSP-90 present in these systems during translation.

For a number of years, the conversion of steroid receptors from their HSP-90-associated, 8–9 S form to the 4 S form was thought to be irreversible due to a lack of success in reassociating HSP-90 with the 4 S form of the receptor in target tissue cytosols. However, a major breakthrough came when the avian progesterone receptor, stripped of HSP-90 by raising the ionic strength of the medium, could be reconstituted with HSP-90 in a rabbit reticulocyte lysate system. This depended on the presence of an intact, unliganded HBD and occurred only in the reticulocyte lysate system; purified or unpurified HSP-90 of target tissue origin did not bind the receptor (252).

Reticulocyte lysates are specialized for efficient protein synthesis and therefore contain high levels of factors involved in this process. Since the association of HSP-90 with steroid receptors appears to be linked to the translational event, it seems plausible that reticulocyte-specific factors which enhance this association during translation are not present in target tissue cytosols (48, 51, 57, 195) or in purified preparations of HSP-90 (51, 252) in sufficiently high amounts to observe the same phenomenon.

The first biological evidence of a role for HSP-90 in steroid hormonal action was obtained from studies in a yeast system which expresses the glucocorticoid receptor and the yeast homolog of HSP-90 (206). The levels of HSP-90 expressed in this particular strain are regulated by the glucose levels in the medium. When expression of HSP-90 was decreased 20-fold, receptors failed to activate transcription in the presence of ligand even though the receptors were in high concentrations and activated. Apparently, receptors which have not associated with HSP-90 are unable to activate transcription.

As stated previously, steroid receptors with the entire HBD deleted are hormone-independent enhancers of transcription. Analyses of these receptors also show that they bind both specific and nonspecific DNA and sediment as 4 S species (33, 38, 214), thus showing characteristics similar to transformed receptors. Under no conditions are these truncated mutants able to associate with HSP-90, either as expression products or by reconstitution (252). However, receptors containing only the HBD apparently are able to interact with HSP-90 (57, 58, 195). A series of studies which functionally dissected the HBD clearly demonstrated that HSP-90 associates with the HBD of steroid receptors (29, 33, 38, 50, 57, 58, 113, 117, 195, 214, 252), though the DBD has been implicated in stabilizing this interaction (38, 214).

Protein modeling of HSP-90 indicates a region that forms mostly α-helices in which the negative charges of the acidic residues mimic the negative charge array of phosphates within the B-DNA backbone (25). This might be the region where the basic residues of the DBD interact electrostatically with HSP-90. This would explain how HSP-90 blocks both specific and nonspecific DNA binding of steroid receptors.

HSP-70 and Assembly of Nascent Steroid Receptors.

Assembly of the heterooligomeric steroid receptor complex is driven by the HSP-70 protein in an adenosine triphosphate (ATP), Mg^{2+}-dependent process (128, 213, 249). Early studies indicated that HSP-70 remained in a stable heterooligomeric complex even after its assembly. However, subsequent reports indicated that, at least for the progesterone receptor from T47D cells, HSP-70 may play only a more transient chaperone role during assembly of the steroid receptor–HSP-90 complex. Cross-linking experiments could not detect the presence of HSP-70 in the heterooligomeric complex of the progesterone receptor (220). The association of HSP-90 with steroid receptors appears to be more stable, and a dynamic equilibrium of associated/dissociated states of the progesterone receptor and HSP-90 has been proposed. Accordingly, hormone binding shifts the disassembly/reassembly process toward the disassembled state by causing conformational changes in the receptor that inhibit the assembly–chaperone function of HSP-70 (249). Thus, HSP-90 has an inherent propensity to dissociate, and it does so unless an energy-requiring chaperone function of HSP-70 occurs.

The Immunophilin p59.

One area of inquiry relates to the RAP p59 (HSP-56). The immunophilin p59, also known as HSP-56 because it is heat-inducible, is associated with nascent steroid receptors and binds the immunosuppressive agents FK506 and rapamycin (258). The immunosuppressive drug FK506 potentiates glucocorticoid receptor–mediated activity in mouse L929 cells (190) and progestin action in T47D cells (175) stably transfected with mouse mammary tumor virus–chloramphenicol acetyltransferase (MMTV-CAT) reporter and mediates transcriptional enhancement of the progesterone/glucocorticoid response element (PRE/GRE) reporter plasmid in a yeast reconstituted system (259). FK506 appears to enhance the hormone-dependent phosphorylation of PR-B (see *Progesterone Receptor Phosphorylation*, below) as measured by the increased quantity of the altered mobility form of PR-B during sodium dodecyl sulfate–polyacrylamide gel electrophoresis (SDS-PAGE). Because this form correlates with its transformed or active state, the transacting capacity of the progesterone receptor may be enhanced by FK506-induced phosphorylation of PR-B (259). The fact that FK506 inactivates the Ca^{2+}-calmodulin-dependent phosphatase calcineurin (154) suggests that the enhanced phosphorylation state of the progesterone receptor may be due to negation of this phosphatase activity. Unactivated mammalian progesterone receptor in an immune complex was dephosphorylated in the presence of Ca^{2+} but not in the presence of Mg^{2+} or Mn^{2+}, suggesting co-purification of a Ca^{2+}-dependent phosphatase in mammalian progesterone receptor immune complexes (127).

CROSS-TALK WITH OTHER SIGNAL-TRANSDUCTION PATHWAYS

Steroid signal transduction exemplifies a convergence of what has come to be called "cross-talk" among previously independent transduction systems. Primary among these are the interactions between members of the steroid receptor superfamily and the activating protein-1 (AP-1) family (for an in-depth review, see ref. 204).

Cyclic Adenosine Monophosphate and Activation of Steroid Receptors

Cascades of kinases that converge on terminal kinases that phosphorylate and thus modulate functions of the receptors for steroid hormones are becoming more clear. For example, casein kinase II (CKII) phosphorylates the estrogen receptor (4, 5), the progesterone receptor (299), and the vitamin D receptor (136), as well as a number of other transcription factors (123). These observations suggest that a common theme in steroid receptor modulation by phosphorylation involves this ubiquitous nuclear kinase.

A number of reports have demonstrated the ability of cyclic adenosine monophosphate (cAMP) to enhance hormonal stimulation of or to independently activate steroid receptors (60, 211). An increase in intracellular cAMP levels activates the cAMP-dependent protein kinase A (PKA). Whether this involves direct phosphorylation of the steroid receptor by PKA is unknown; however, the ability of cAMP-dependent protein kinase to phosphorylate in vitro mammalian (127) and avian (187, 288) progesterone receptors has been demonstrated.

One of the more intriguing findings is that cAMP stimulation of cells converts the progesterone receptor antagonist RU486 and the estrogen receptor antagonist trans-OH tamoxifen to agonists of their respective receptors in a cell- and promoter-specific manner (19, 78, 129, 191, 232, 234). However, it is not clear whether the mechanism involves direct phosphorylation of the steroid receptor or activation of upstream kinases/phosphatases that directly phosphorylate/dephosphorylate steroid receptors. cAMP effects on other enhancing or inhibiting factors of transcription, such as HSP-90, cAMP-inducible transcription factors, basal transcription factors, adapters, or co-activators of transcription, are also possibilities.

Transcriptional Interference

An interesting case of cross-talk between steroid receptors and with other transcription factors is the phenomenon of transcriptional interference, or "squelching." This process was discovered in steroid receptor overexpression systems in which abnormally high levels of expression of one transcription factor interfered with its own ability or the ability of other transcription factors to enhance reporters of transcription. It has been hypothesized that a third limiting factor, perhaps adapters or co-activators (see TRANSACTIVATION BY STEROID RECEPTORS, below) of transcription used in common by various transcription factors, is titrated by direct protein–protein interaction as a result of high levels of a single transcription factor. Whether this occurs under normal physiological conditions, where the levels of transcription factors are lower, is unclear. However, this is one possible explanation for the indirect effects of one class of steroids on another, particularly in cells which express multiple steroid receptors or in cases where one receptor is abnormally high. This argument was strengthened by the discovery of an adapter protein used in common among the various steroid receptors (198).

Pathways That Converge on the Estrogen Receptor

Members of signal-transduction systems involving Src tyrosine kinase, mitogen-activated protein kinase (MAPK), and the erbB2 protooncogene, which is a cell surface tyrosine kinase, appear to converge upon and modulate estrogen receptor activity (see *Estrogen Receptor Phosphorylation*, below). A basal phosphorylation site, tyr[537], of the human estrogen receptor can be phosphorylated by members of the Src family of tyrosine kinases, and ser[118] is phosphorylated by MAPK, which is controlled by cell surface tyrosine kinases such as erbB2 (21). Interestingly, erbB2 can be activated by the estrogen receptor ligand 17β-estradiol (166). An intriguing question is whether activation of erbB2 by estradiol can result in activation of MAPK and phosphorylation of the ser[118] site, which has been shown to up-modulate AF-1 function (see *Estrogen Receptor Phosphorylation*, below). Although the precise mechanism is not understood, estradiol appears to stimulate rapidly but transiently protein tyrosine phosphorylation, which is blocked by antiestrogens (172). Furthermore, antiestrogens decrease the mitogenic activity of epidermal growth factor (EGF) only in estrogen receptor–positive cells, apparently by increasing membrane tyrosine phosphatase activity (77).

ROLE OF PHOSPHORYLATION IN STEROID RECEPTOR STRUCTURE AND FUNCTION

Sites of Phosphorylation, Functional Significance, and Regulatory Kinases

Phosphorylation/dephosphorylation of tyr, ser, or thr residues are perhaps the most common means by which signals are transmitted to modulate the functions of proteins (121–123). Hormones or growth factors acting on cell surface receptors signal cascades of kinases that modulate the functions of transcription factors involved in cellular proliferation or differentiation (56, 109, 123). The multiple target proteins that are substrates for terminal kinases integrate a coordinated response by the cell; each kinase or protein substrate involved in the pathway theoretically can act as an input node, whose activity can be up- or down-modulated by direct phosphorylation/dephosphorylation. Thus, any specific phosphorylation target site on a given protein should be considered cell-specific, depending on the state of activated/inactivated kinases and phosphatases (122). Strategies to decipher the pathways involved in determining the phosphorylation state of proteins involve identification of specific phosphorylation sites and the kinases and phosphatases which modulate the particular site and then working backward to define the upstream kinases/phosphatases that are directly linked spatially and temporally.

The strategy most commonly used to define the function of a given phosphorylation event is to (1) determine the specific serine, threonine, or tyrosine residues modified under various conditions; (2) mutate the site to the amino acid which has the same structure as the phosphoacceptor but lacks the required hydroxyl group; and (3) assess the protein for a loss of phosphorylation at the specific target site and determine how this correlates with the gain or loss of an assayable function of the target protein. In the above analysis, a negatively charged amino-acid residue that mimics phosphorylation is substituted to represent a positive control. In certain cases, the results are clear: for example, a site-directed mutation disrupts a discrete function of the protein, which can be regained upon phosphorylation of that specific site in the wild-type protein. However, loss of function also can occur as a result of an unintended global disruption of protein structure and function as the number of mutated sites increases. Multiple mutations which nonspecifically disrupt protein structure and function may lead to invalid conclusions.

The activities of virtually all of the transcription factors (56, 109, 123), including the steroid receptors (182, 199), are modulated by phosphorylation/dephosphorylation reactions. What sets steroid receptors apart from other transcription factors is that they are also ligand-inducible. Because of this, the effects of ligand as distinct from phosphorylation have been difficult to discern, particularly because steroid receptors undergo hormone-dependent phosphorylation.

An indication that phosphorylation might play a role in steroid receptor function came from studies which showed that lowering the effective concentration of ATP within target cells or treating solubilized receptors with phosphatase in the absence of hormone greatly reduced the specific binding of hormone (189). This suggested that phosphorylation of the receptors for steroids could potentiate the hormonal signal.

A number of in vivo studies have shown that steroid receptors undergo two rounds of phosphorylation (182, 199). The first of these occurs during or subsequent to translation but prior to hormone binding and is referred to as "basal phosphorylation." The second round appears to depend on hormone binding and results in a further increase in the phosphorylation state of the receptor, at least as measured by [^{32}P] incorporation of metabolically labeled cells (59–61, 111, 156, 188, 200, 209, 245, 278). Early studies indicated that the steroid receptor sites for both rounds of phosphorylation were primarily serine residues located in the N-terminus (A/B region) (27, 49, 110, 253, 255); however, it is now clear that phosphorylation is not restricted to this domain and is probably involved in modulating virtually all of the known receptor functions. Progress in this area has been made in spite of the difficulties mentioned above. For background on this topic, the reader is referred to two excellent reviews (182, 199). In this chapter, we highlight some of the progress made since these reviews were published.

Estrogen Receptor Phosphorylation

Early studies utilizing [^{32}P] incorporation of metabolically labeled MCF-7 human adenocarcinoma cells indicated that the estrogen receptor was phosphorylated basally on serine residues. Treatment of cells with estrogen caused increased nuclear retention and [^{32}P] incorporation into the receptor, exclusively on serine residues. When the estrogen receptor was treated with phosphatase, DNA-binding activity was obliterated, suggesting that phosphorylation activated the DNA-binding activity (61). Prior to this demonstration, the estrogen receptor was thought to be phosphorylated predominantly on tyrosine (10, 171, 173, 174). Subsequent findings have provided more insight into this phenomenon.

Published data indicate that the human estrogen receptor is phosphorylated in its AF-1 domain at ser^{118} by MAPK (1, 5, 135, 139), just to the N-terminal side of the DBD at ser^{167} by CKII (4, 5), and in the AF-2 region in the HBD at tyr^{537} by the Src family of tyrosine kinases (3, 6, 7, 35, 171). The ser^{118} site was identified by direct amino-acid and radiolabel sequencing (5), mutational analysis (1, 135, 139, 151), and in vitro phosphorylation (5, 139). In vitro, this site is phosphorylated exclusively by MAPK from a variety of interspecies sources. Conversion of this residue to ala resulted in virtually no incorporation of [^{32}P] into a glutathione-S-transferase (GST) fusion protein used as a substrate for MAPK (139). Loss of a more retarded mobility form of the estrogen receptor in the 118 mutant also indicates that phosphorylation of ser^{118} significantly alters its structure (135).

Phosphorylation in vivo of ser^{118} appears to be stimulated by EGF and insulin-like growth factor (IGF) through a ras-dependent pathway of the MAPK cascade, resulting in up-modulation of estrogen receptor AF-1 activity (139). Because phosphorylation of this site has no effect on the specific DNA-binding function (5, 139), modulation of the AF-1 region by phosphorylation represents the first clear demonstration of a functional module of a steroid receptor that can be regulated independently through extracellular signals.

Ser^{167} was identified by radiolabel and amino-acid sequencing as the major estradiol-induced phosphorylation site on the human estrogen receptor from MCF-7 cells, accounting for 50% of the total [^{32}P] incorporation. Furthermore, the human estrogen receptor from SF9 cells was phosphorylated specifically on this site by CKII in vitro (4). The functional consequence of this event appears to be enhancement of receptor affinity for the estrogen response element (ERE). Addition of increasing quantities of CKII to a DNA-binding reaction resulted in a concentration-dependent increase in the quantity of estrogen receptor–ERE complexes formed in a gel mobility shift assay (5). Confirmatory evidence involving the effects of mutation at this site on DNA binding have not been reported. The potential physiological significance of phosphorylation at this site is so far restricted to human estrogen receptor from MCF-7 cells since this receptor transfected into Cos-1 cells does not appear to be phosphorylated at this site (151).

Phosphorylation of tyr^{537} has been identified by amino-acid and radiolabel sequencing (6) and mutational analysis (7, 35). It is phosphorylated in vitro by two members of the Src family of tyrosine kinases, p60^{c-src} and p56^{lck} (6, 7), and by a Ca^{2+}-calmodulin-dependent tyrosine kinase from calf uterus (35). This is apparently the only site of tyrosine phosphorylation on the estrogen receptor, and it probably represents the site which was previously suggested to be involved in regulating hormone binding (10, 35, 171). Subsequent studies have demonstrated that phosphorylation at tyr^{537} also potentiates dimerization of the estrogen receptor (3, 7). Because the estrogen receptor binds the ERE as a homodimer, the functional consequence of phosphorylation at this site would be to potentiate specific DNA binding. The ability of the human estrogen receptor to bind ERE in a gel mobility shift assay depends on phosphorylation at this site and is reversed

by dephosphorylation (7). Furthermore, a tyr^{537} phosphopeptide containing estrogen receptor sequences flanking tyr^{537} obliterated specific DNA binding in a gel mobility shift assay, whereas unphosphorylated peptide at the same concentration did not have this effect (3). Because of the profound effect of the phosphopeptide on this crucial function, its use as a novel antiestrogen has been suggested (3).

The hormone-binding activity of the estrogen receptor also is regulated by phosphorylation at tyr^{537} by a Ca^{2+}-calmodulin-dependent tyrosine kinase derived form calf uterus (10, 171, 173, 174). Conversion of tyr^{537} to phenylalanine eliminated the ability of the kinase to phosphorylate the human estrogen receptor, resulting in loss of hormone-binding activity (35). This suggests that this function also is regulated by phosphorylation at tyr^{537}. If this is the case, then phosphorylation at this site would determine the capacity of ligand binding, the potentiation of dimerization, and subsequent events, such as DNA binding and transactivation. Since the AF-2 function is hormone-dependent and tyr^{537} phosphorylation controls hormone binding, modification at this site would be required for its activation. Mutation of this site results in the loss of a hyperphosphorylated human estrogen receptor form that migrates more slowly than the dephosphorylated form during electrophoresis (7), indicating the necessity of phosphorylation at this site to observe this phenomenon. Only a subpopulation (60%) of MCF-7 cell estrogen receptors, which may represent basal phosphorylation at this site, undergo a hormone-dependent up-shift (personal observation). The events which alter the receptor structure sufficiently to cause a mobility shift, therefore, may represent a basal phosphorylation of tyr^{537} which potentiates hormone binding, dimerization, and DNA binding in the cell but does not itself cause an up-shift. Subsequently, actions of nuclear kinases, such as CKII and MAPK, which phosphorylate ser^{167} and ser^{118}, respectively, may be directly responsible for the up-shift of estrogen-treated receptors in MCF-7 cells or receptors transfected into Cos cells.

Hormone treatment of MCF-7 cells does not appear to enhance tyrosine phosphorylation of the estrogen receptor (6); therefore, tyr^{537} may represent a basal site of phosphorylation from MCF-7 cells. Furthermore, a requirement of phosphorylation at tyr^{537} for hormone binding would appear to preclude hormone induction of phosphorylation at this site. However, estrogen treatment was shown to induce tyrosine phosphorylation of a number of proteins, including an src-like kinase and possibly the estrogen receptor and HSP-90 in MCF-7 cells (172). All three of these proteins have been implicated in transducing estrogen signals. Although it was suggested that tyrosine phosphorylation of proteins in

MCF-7 cells is estrogen receptor–mediated, it is also possible that estrogen treatment of cells could modulate tyr[537] indirectly and independently of binding to the receptor. For example, the tyrosine kinase erb-B2 protooncogene is activated by estradiol (166) and binds the SRC homology 2 domain of Src kinase (162), the kinase suspected to phosphorylate tyr[537].

Progesterone Receptor Phosphorylation

Results of a number of studies have implicated cAMP-dependent protein kinase in the regulation of progesterone receptor activity. Both avian (187, 288) and mammalian (127) progesterone receptors are good substrates for cAMP-dependent protein kinase. Progesterone treatment of avian oviduct cells was required for phosphorylation of a serine residue located in the D region of the receptor (59). Mutation of ser[530] residing in the hinge region of chicken progesterone receptor to the non-phosphorylatable residue ala resulted in a decrease in hormone responsiveness (13a), indicating that phosphorylation at this site potentiates the hormonal signal. This is particularly relevant to in vivo action where hormone concentrations are below receptor saturation, since differences in the mutated versus wild-type receptors were observed only at less than saturating hormone levels. This region also is phosphorylated by cAMP-dependent protein kinase in vitro and results in a retarded mobility (up-shift) of progesterone receptor in denaturing gels. This upshift is thought to be the result of secondary structural alterations in the receptor protein as a result of phosphorylation (286). However, whether cAMP-dependent protein kinase phosphorylates this site in vivo is not known. Stimulation by forskolin of cAMP levels in avian oviduct mince resulted in increased phosphorylation of both PR-A and PR-B (187), and pharmacological stimulation of cAMP-dependent protein kinase mimics the effect of progesterone on the receptor's transacting capacity (60, 211). Because the catalytic subunit of this enzyme translocates to the nucleus in the presence of sufficiently high concentrations of cAMP, it presumably would have access to the receptor, which is nuclear (167). Although the only known effects of cAMP in vivo are mediated by cAMP-dependent protein kinase, stimulation of this kinase results in the phosphorylation of a broad range of target proteins. The observed effect of cAMP, therefore, may not be due to cAMP-dependent protein kinase directly but, rather, to stimulation of a secondary kinase, which then phosphorylates the progesterone receptor or other factors involved in the process of receptor activation.

In avian oviduct, hormone administration appears to increase the rate at which a number of discrete sites located in the A/B region become phosphorylated. These sites are phosphorylated more slowly in the absence of hormone (255). Thus, progesterone is not a requirement for phosphorylation of the A/B region, but it does accelerate the rate at which phosphorylation occurs.

The progesterone receptors in T47D cells are expressed as a full-length B-receptor and an N-terminally truncated A-receptor. Both forms are phosphorylated in the absence of hormone over a period of 18 h (243, 244, 287). Treatment with the potent progestin R5020 rapidly increases the incorporation of phosphate into both receptor forms five- to tenfold. Treatment with the antiprogestin RU486 increases the phosphorylation state of the receptors 15-fold (245). The B-receptor has a molecular weight of 114 kd in its unphosphorylated state but resolves on denaturing gels as a variently phosphorylated triplet. The two basal sites of phosphorylation unique to the PR-B, ser[81] and ser[162], appear to be responsible for the PR-B-specific basal triplet structure (299). The A-receptor resolves as a single 94 kd species (244). All of the phosphorylation sites mapped in human PR-B are serines residing in the A/B region (299, 300). Four of these, ser[102], ser[162], ser[294], and ser[345], are proline-directed kinase consensus target sites and, thus, potential sites for MAPK or cyclin-dependent kinases (300). The lone exception of ser[81] is a CKII consensus site, and of 11 potential CKII sites in PR-B, it is the only one phosphorylated by this kinase in vitro (299). The homologous PR-B sites of ser[294] and ser[345] also are phosphorylated in PR-A.

Stimulation of T47D cells with progesterone receptor agonist results in a rapid incorporation of [^{32}P] into the receptor and enhanced DNA-binding activity. A subsequent phosphorylation event causes a mobility change (up-shift) in PR-A and PR-B (18). The time course of these events indicates that DNA binding of progesterone receptor in the cell is required and enhances this up-shift.

Two reports have indicated that the up-shift is the result of specific DNA binding by the progesterone receptor to PRE in the cell (13, 261). Progesterone receptor–containing mutations, which inactivate DNA binding or change the capacity to discriminate between EREs and PREs, do not show the mobility shift upon hormone treatment (13, 261). Furthermore, treatment of T47D cells with the type I antagonist ZK98299, which fails to induce DNA-binding activity, does not result in an altered mobility form of the receptor (261). Comparatively, the progestin agonist R5020 and the type II antagonist RU486, both of which appear to enhance specific DNA binding in extracts of T47D cells, induce the altered mobility form of the receptor (13, 261). The drastic changes in the conformation of progesterone receptor detected as a mobility shift during SDS-PAGE, the kinetics of the event, and the requirement of specific DNA binding point to a role for this phosphorylation event in the transmodulation of progestin-regulated genes. However, a direct functional role for phosphorylation has yet to be determined. We have demonstrated that the entire populations of both PR-A and PR-B are up-shifted after treatment of T47D cells with either R5020 or RU486 and that, although progesterone receptor from R5020-treated cells is down-regulated to undetectable levels within 24 h, the receptor population from RU486-treated cells is stable and in the up-shifted form (125, personal observation).

Glucocorticoid Receptor Phosphorylation

A number of studies have shown that the glucocorticoid receptor is phosphorylated primarily within a putative transcriptional activation domain located in the A/B region (27, 49, 110, 111, 200). Like the progesterone receptor, phosphorylation is enhanced three- to fivefold in cells treated with glucocorticoid agonists. However, unlike the progesterone receptor expressed in human breast cancer cells, phosphorylation of the glucocorticoid receptor in NIH 3T3 or mouse thymoma cells treated with the glucocorticoid antagonist RU486 was not increased. Furthermore, RU486 could block the agonist effect (111, 200). Mutant glucocorticoid receptors with their HBD deleted had phosphorylation levels similar to hormone-treated receptors (110). Thus, when conditions prohibit association of the receptor with HSP-90 or favor its dissociation, there is an enhanced phosphorylation of the N-terminal region. Since phosphorylation occurs primarily within a putative transcriptional activation domain (110, 112), it was thought to regulate this function. Subsequent mutational analyses indicate, however, that this may not be the case (165).

Vitamin D Receptor Phosphorylation

The vitamin D receptor (VDR) appears to be phosphorylated by two well-known cellular kinases, protein kinase C (PKC) (118, 119) and CKII (136). Phosphorylation of ser[51] in the DBD linker region of the VDR by PKC has been proposed as a mechanism whereby its DNA-binding activity could be negatively regulated (119). Either substitution of ser[51] by aspartic acid, which would mimic the negative charge of this residue, or phosphorylation by PKC of hVDR from a bacterial expression system abolished the ability of VDR to form a complex with its response element. That gly, but not ala, disrupts its transacting potential may relate to the general disruption of secondary structural properties

in this area of the DBD. This appears to be a basal phosphorylation site since mutation to a nonphosphorylatable residue did not affect the hormone-induced level of VDR phosphorylation. Also intriguing is the observation that this PKC target site is conserved among the subclass of receptors for retinoic acid, thyroid hormone, and estrogen. Whether the DNA-binding activity of any of these receptors can be regulated negatively in a similar manner is not known.

Ser[208] of the hVDR is a consensus site for CKII, is efficiently phosphorylated by this enzyme in vitro, and is a predominant site phosphorylated on VDR transfected into cos cells (136). Conversion of this site to gly dramatically reduces the level of phosphorylation in vitro by CKII. A precise function related to this site has not been determined. Since CKII is a ubiquitous nuclear kinase involved in modulating members of the steroid receptor superfamily and other nuclear transcription factors (3, 123, 299), it may represent an important site of regulatory modulation by phosphorylation of the hVDR.

TRANSACTIVATION BY STEROID RECEPTORS

Members of the steroid receptor superfamily contain at least two defined primary structural motifs called activation functions, one agonist-independent (AF-1) in the A/B region and one hormone agonist–dependent (AF-2) in the E/F (HBD) region. Activated steroid receptors participate in the formation or stabilization of transcriptional preinitiation complexes (43). Activation function primary structural motifs could bind directly the postulated transcriptional intermediary factors (also called adapters or co-activators) and/or interact with general transcription factors. Thus, the DBD may serve only to tether the receptor bound by these factors to the promoter region of the hormonally regulated genes. A direct binding interaction between steroid receptors and intermediary factors was postulated on the basis of early studies suggesting that overexpression of one receptor could squelch the transcriptional activation functions of another. This phenomenon, commonly referred to as "squelching" or transcriptional interference, indicates the necessity of a common, limiting, steroid receptor–titratable factor which mediates steroid-induced transcriptional enhancement.

Direct interactions between steroid receptors and potential intermediary factors have been demonstrated through the use of GST proteins containing the AF-2 regions of the estrogen receptor expressed in *E. coli* (36, 37, 102). Proteins of 160 kd and 140 kd from the estrogen receptor–positive breast cancer cell line MCF-7 and the estrogen receptor–negative cell line MDA-

MB-231 (102) and a 160 kd protein from Cos-1 cells (36) were retained specifically by the HBD. These are referred to as estrogen receptor–associated proteins (ERAPs) or as receptor-interacting proteins (RIPs). Retention of these proteins depends on the HBD being complexed with 17β-estradiol or the potent synthetic estrogen diethylstilbestrol. When the HBD was mutated, uncomplexed or complexed with the antiestrogens 4-OH tamoxifen, ICI 164,384, or ICI 182,780, these proteins were not retained, nor was the AF-2 region active in transient transfection assays. The AF-2 primary structural motif and an estrogen agonist–induced conformation in the HBD thus appear necessary for retention of these suspected transcriptional intermediary factors on the GST protein fusion column. Far Western blotting with radiolabeled HBD-GST (GST-AF2) used as a probe showed a direct estradiol-dependent interaction with these proteins from HeLa, Cos-1, and ZR75-1 cells, as well as from immunoprecipitated estrogen receptor from MCF-7 cells treated with estradiol, but not with tamoxifen (37, 102). The latter evidence indicates an agonist-dependent enhancement of ERAP association with estrogen receptors in vivo. Deletion of amino acids 535–550 of the human estrogen receptor resulted in loss of retention of ERAP[160] (102). Because this region is not required for either hormone binding or dimerization but is apparently required for ERAP binding and AF-2 function, estradiol binding may be necessary, but not sufficient, for the interaction of estrogen receptors with ERAP[160].

In contrast to these transcriptional intermediary factors that require the HBD to be complexed with hormone agonist and appear to interact with estrogen receptor AF-2, another intermediary factor, a TATA-binding protein–associated factor (TAFII30), has been isolated and characterized. It binds in an agonist/antagonist-independent manner to the AF-2a region of the human estrogen receptor (Fig. 15.1) and is required for estrogen receptor–induced transcriptional enhancement. It segregates specifically in a subset of the TFIID complex and may be regulated by posttranslational modification by phosphorylation since it migrates more slowly on SDS gels than it should from its predicted molecular mass (132).

A more general co-activator of steroid receptors has been isolated and characterized (198). Named "steroid receptor co-activator-1" (SRC-1), it specifically enhances agonist-dependent transcriptional activation of all members of the superfamily but does not enhance the activities of other transcriptional factors, such as E2F or cAMP-response element–binding (CREB) protein. Like the interaction of ERAP with estrogen receptor, SRC-1 binds the progesterone receptor HBD only when it is complexed with agonist. Reduced interactions of SRC-1 with the progesterone receptor HBD

were observed when it was complexed with RU486. Increasing the levels of SRC-1 reversed the ability of the estrogen receptor to squelch progesterone receptor activity, indicating that when the estrogen receptor titrates SRC-1 and squelches progesterone receptor activity, reintroduction of high levels of this co-activator restores the transcriptional activation function.

A direct interaction of the estrogen receptor, the progesterone receptor, and the orphan receptor chicken ovalbumin upstream promoter-transcription factor (COUP-TF) with the general transcription factor TFIIB has been demonstrated (130). This factor was retained selectively by a column containing a GST fusion protein containing the progesterone receptor AF-1, AF-2, and DBD or by a construct containing estrogen receptor AF-2; AF-1 alone was not sufficient to observe this binding. Interestingly, TFIIB dissociated from these constructs at a relatively low ionic strength (270 mM). This is well below the strength of buffers used to extract activated nuclear bound steroid receptor and thus explains why factors like TFIIB, which presumably associate only with activated receptors, do not co-precipitate with activated receptors in high-salt (0.4–0.5 M) extracts.

Entry of TFIIB into the preinitiation complex may be a rate-limiting step in its assembly. Transcription factors, particularly those with acidic activation domains, have been proposed to recruit TFIIB to the preinitiation complex by either increasing its association to or decreasing its dissociation from the other proteins in the preinitiation complex (43). Interaction between steroid receptors and TFIIB explains how they might recruit, and thus enhance, formation of the preinitiation complex and in turn initiation of polymerase II transcription. Because this process alone may not be sufficient to initiate transcription, it is likely that direct binding of co-activator by the AF-2 region of steroid receptors is required for stabilization of the TATA binding protein to the promoter. This kind of cooperative effect would not be required on promoters in which antagonists, such as RU486 and 4-OH tamoxifen, activate transcription since they prevent binding of ERAP and SRC-1, both of which are co-activators and apparently interact with the AF-2 function.

Another set of potential co-activators are the human homologs (hSNFa and -b) of the yeast *Saccharomyces cerevisiae* SWI/SNF and brahma genes (42, 298). These genes were discovered to be essential for glucocorticoid receptor function in yeast. Co-transfection of the human homolog along with the estrogen receptor appears to enhance its transacting capacity in transiently transfected HepG2 cells with an estrogen receptor–responsive reporter by approximately a magnitude (42). These genes appear to be members of the helicase family of proteins. It has been speculated that the function of these genes is to enhance transcription by disrupting the closed conformation of the chromatin structure around an enhancer region, thus promoting assembly of the preinitiation complex (42). The helicase protein family also contains a motif which binds the pocket domain of the retinoblastoma protein (pRB). Direct protein–protein interaction between human brahma protein and pRB enhances the transacting activity of the glucocorticoid receptor (248), but how this interaction works is unknown. It is, however, a demonstration of a novel mechanism involving a tumor suppressor's ability to activate a member of the steroid receptor superfamily and that the pRB family of tumor suppressors might influence functions other than cell-cycle regulation.

ANTIHORMONES AND THEIR MODES OF ACTION

A steroid receptor antagonist works at the receptor level to modulate properties attributed to ligand binding (16). Steroid receptor antagonists have been classified into different types. Type-1 antagonists induce DNA-binding activity but disrupt the AF-2 function required for stable preinitiation complex formation on certain promoters (for example, the progesterone receptor antagonist RU486 and the estrogen receptor antagonist 4-OH tamoxifen). Estrogen receptor complexed with 4-OH tamoxifen and progesterone receptor complexed with RU486 bind normally to HREs but are unable to induce the proper conformation in the AF-2 sufficient to activate certain promoters. Aberrant conformations in the HBD when this type of antagonist is bound result in a failure to interact properly with transcriptional intermediary proteins or with the basal transcription factors, but they appear to dimerize normally. Under certain cellular conditions, such as stimulation of cAMP, the partial antagonist RU486, but not ZK98299, shows progesterone receptor–mediated transacting capacity equivalent to that of agonists (19, 191, 232, 234). This effect appears to be mediated by the PR-B isoform, implicating its unique AF-3 function (232). The full antagonist ZK98299 appears to discourage the DNA-binding activity of the progesterone receptor and other subsequent events (141). Estrogen receptor complexed with the partial agonist trans-OH tamoxifen or the full antagonist ICI 164,384 (78, 129) exhibited analogous effects in cAMP-stimulated cells.

RU486, an Agonist/Antagonist of Progesterone Receptor

RU486 was developed by Roussel Uclaf (Romainville, France) to be tested for its clinical effectiveness as an

antiglucocorticoid (205). Preliminary studies showed that it bound to progesterone and glucocorticoid receptors from a number of mammalian species with an affinity as high as or higher than the natural ligand (126, 179, 205, 263, 264). Exceptions were the avian oviduct (67, 186) and hamster uterine (89) progesterone receptors, where it also failed to block progestational effects. RU486 does, however, bind to the avian glucocorticoid receptor (97). The clinical manifestations of this antiprogestin in humans are well documented, and its mode of action at the receptor level is becoming clearer (16).

Early studies which analyzed the effects of RU486 on specific glucocorticoid- or progestin-induced transcription clearly demonstrated its antagonistic properties. It blocked glucocorticoid-dependent gene expression of tyrosine and alanine amino transferase genes in rat hepatoma cells (40), the glutamine synthetase gene in a leukemic cell line (238), and 5'-nucleotidase activity in human lymphoblastoid cells (215). Progesterone-dependent induction of the uteroglobin gene in rabbit uterus also was blocked by RU486 in vivo (216). However, when assayed for its effect in a human breast cancer cell line, it showed partial agonist and antagonist effects (115).

Observations on the misfunction of RU486-bound receptors implicate functions localized in the HBD. These include interactions of the receptor with ligand (183, 184) and with HSP-90, which is stabilized when the receptor is bound to RU486 (62, 75, 98, 150, 176, 185, 224, 229, 242); a variant dimer interface which is not compatible with the dimer interface induced by agonist (169); and failure of RU486 to induce the transcriptional activation function localized within the HBD of the receptor (169, 276, 285).

The effects of RU486 on transcriptional activation have been studied in co-transfection experiments (101, 169, 276, 285). These experiments indicate that RU486-bound receptors are competent to bind response elements but that their ability to enhance transcription of certain promoters is impaired. RU486-bound progesterone and glucocorticoid receptors could enhance transcription only when the hormone-independent transcriptional activation function located in the A/B region of the receptor was sufficient to stimulate promoter activity. Promoter activity, which is dependent on the transcriptional activation function located in the HBD, was not activated by RU486-bound receptors (169, 285).

Apparently, binding of agonist, but not antagonist, induces conformational changes in the HBD necessary for transcriptional activation. However, DNA binding seems to be sufficient to induce the transcriptional activation function located in the A/B domain of the receptor independent of the conformational aspects of the HBD. Similar observations have been made with respect to the activity of the estrogen receptor when it is complexed with the antiestrogen 4-OH tamoxifen (24). In these assays, antagonists induce DNA binding and the transcriptional activation function located in the A/B region but not that in the HBD.

Agonist- or antagonist-bound receptors may interact with DNA in a similar manner (11, 12, 14, 101), but there are indications that interactions at these sites are not identical (28, 66, 81, 169, 236). RU486-bound receptors, upon extraction from DNA, sediment more rapidly than agonist-bound receptors (66, 81). This suggests that when bound to DNA RU486-bound steroid receptor complexes are in a structurally altered form. Progesterone and glucocorticoid receptors show variant association and dissociation kinetics for the interactions with both specific and nonspecific DNA, depending on whether they are liganded with agonist or RU486 (236). Specific and nonspecific associations are accelerated two- to fivefold by agonist and the off-rate is 10–20-fold faster when compared to unliganded receptor. The on-rate for RU486-bound receptor is approximately half that of the agonist and the off-rate is equivalent to that of the unbound receptor, which is significantly slower than that of agonist-bound receptors. This raises the question as to whether occupancy of the response element, which is roughly equivalent for both agonist- and antagonist-bound receptors, is as important as the on-rate.

The studies mentioned above relied on indirect assays and in vitro DNA binding assessments. When the PRE is contained in a more natural context only the agonist induced stable specific DNA binding. In vivo genomic footprinting of stably integrated mouse mammary tumor virus promoter in T47D cells demonstrated protection of PRE when the cells were treated with the progestin, R5020, but not with the antiprogestins, RU486 or ZK98299 (272a). This indicates that although RU486 may exert agonistic actions in vitro, its action in vivo is entirely antagonistic. It is possible that RU486 when complexed with progesterone receptor has agonistic properties that do not require a stable receptor–DNA complex in the cell. Alternatively, other cell-specific factors not present in T47D cells might convert RU486 to an agonist.

ZK98299, a Full Antagonist of Progesterone Receptor

ZK98299 (Schering, Germany) has been shown to block most progesterone receptor–mediated functions and is considered to be a full antagonist. ZK98299 fails to induce DNA-binding activity (95, 141) or DNA-dependent phosphorylation of progesterone receptor (261). Unlike RU486, ZK98299 is not converted to a progesterone receptor agonist upon increase in cellular cAMP (19, 191, 232, 234). By other criteria, ZK98299 appears to act as an agonist (275). When expression vectors for human PR-B were co-transfected with a progesterone receptor–responsive reporter into HeLa cells, RU486 and ZK98299 were capable of inducing reporter activity to levels equivalent to the agonist R5020. This occurred only when B receptors were expressed alone without the A form. Particularly interesting was the demonstration that the antagonists, but not R5020, induced reporter even when the progestin response element was removed (275). Agonistic activity was observed previously for RU486, which induces progesterone receptor DNA-binding activity equivalent to R5020. However, the effects of ZK98299 were surprising because of its reported inability to induce such DNA binding.

Antiestrogens and Estrogen Receptor Function

Among the estrogen receptor antagonists, ICI 164,384 (ICI) originally was thought to block DNA-binding activity in a manner analogous to ZK98299 (74, 95). This seemed to be confirmed by the reported failure of ICI-bound estrogen receptor to activate either AF-1 or AF-2 (95). In contrast, the partial agonistic properties of 4-OH tamoxifen could activate promoters requiring only the activity of AF-1 (24). Early studies of estrogen receptor complexed with ICI in vitro (74) or in cells treated with this compound (218) seemed to confirm this view. Estrogen appeared to induce DNA binding of the originally cloned human estrogen receptor; however, it is now known that this receptor had a point mutation, substituting valine for glycine at position 400 (168). This mutation created an unstable receptor for DNA binding at 37°C but not at 4°C. Furthermore, when estrogen was bound to the receptor, its DNA-binding activity was stabilized but only with this mutant receptor. Subsequent experiments have shown that there is virtually no effect of agonist, partial antagonist, or the full antagonist ICI on the ability of wild-type estrogen receptor to form dimers or the ability of these steroid analogs to disrupt dimer formation (168). This is reflected in the observation that no differences in the quantities of estrogen receptor–ERE complexes are detected in gel mobility assays when receptors are complexed with agonist or antagonist ligands.

The role of ligand binding in vitro is not established. It now appears, at least with respect to the human estrogen receptor, that at the point where in vitro extracts are prepared, ligand has no effect on the dimerization, and thus the DNA-binding potential, of estrogen receptor (168). It appears that ICI induces estrogen receptor DNA-binding activity above the levels of unliganded receptor in vivo (219). However, whether the extent is equivalent to that of estradiol-induced DNA-binding activity is unclear. This leaves open the question of how to explain the full antagonistic properties of estrogen receptor ligands in the class of ICI. Efforts are focusing on the differential conformational changes induced in the HBD of the estrogen receptor by the different classes of antagonist and how this difference might relate to interactions between AF-2 and AF-1 (181). One other explanation for the effects of ICI is that it appears to rapidly down-regulate the receptor in vivo (54, 219). However, some other steroid receptor agonists also down-regulate their receptors. Thus, although ICI actions may include down-regulation of estrogen receptor, this effect may not be sufficient to explain the mechanism of ICI.

There are at least two distinct functions in the HBD of the estrogen receptor. One of these cooperates with the AF-1 function in the N-terminus and is induced by 4-OH tamoxifen and estradiol but not by ICI. Stimulation of cells with cAMP converts partial agonists to agonists (19, 78, 129, 191, 232, 234), indicating the possibility of a functional override of AF-2 activity. Because of the detectable differences in conformations induced by agonist and antagonist ligands, it is possible that cAMP induces a conformation when an antagonist is bound to the receptor in the same way as when the full agonist is bound. Alternatively, cAMP might up-regulate AF-1 sufficiently to overcome the antagonistic effects of known partial antagonists on AF-2 or it may indirectly increase the levels of transcriptional intermediary factors to levels sufficient to induce conformational changes resistant to the partial antagonists.

The partial agonist activity detected in transient transection assays by the estrogen receptor ligands ICI and trans-OH tamoxifen appears to require the F domain. Deletion of this region reduced agonistic activity to zero. In contrast, the F domain is not required for full estrogen receptor agonistic activity when stimulated by estradiol. However, these phenomena are cell type–specific, occurring in the breast cancer cell line MDA-MB-231 and in Chinese hamster ovary cells but not in HeLa or NIH3T3 cells (181). In the latter two cell types, there is no agonistic activity by ICI or trans-OH tamoxifen, and deletion of the E region in this context reduces the transacting potential of the estrogen receptor. Exactly how the factors of cell context and the F domain combine to give this differential response to ER antagonists is unknown. It is possible that the F domain activates the N-terminal AF-1 domain and that other cellular factors are involved which are present in some cells but not in others. The nature of these other cell factors is unknown. The F domain of steroid receptors appears to be the region which mediates this intercooperativity between AF-1 and AF-2 and may explain the cell type and promoter context dependencies of the different classes of antagonist.

STEROID RECEPTORS AND CLINICAL MANAGEMENT OF CANCER

The reported exponential increase in the incidence of breast cancer has led to an all-out effort to determine causation and potential treatments. Since a number of hormones physiologically influence the differentiation, development, and functions of the breast, tumors of the breast generally have been classed into two types: hormone-dependent (receptor-positive) and hormone-independent (receptor-negative). Because of the significant roles estrogen and progesterone play in breast functioning, routine biopsy analyses of tissue involve determining the presence of their receptors. At the time of diagnosis a majority of breast cancers are estrogen receptor–positive (201). However, over a period of time, many become negative, less differentiated, more aggressive, and unresponsive to hormonal therapy (116).

One of the current assumptions in the therapeutic approach to the treatment of hormone-dependent cancers is that the effects of particular hormonal agents are mediated by cognate receptors. It is also believed that the continued growth of receptor-positive breast cancer cells requires stimuli by the cognate hormones. Such breast cancers are considered less malignant and more likely to respond to ablative or antihormonal therapy (201).

Conversely, progesterone- and/or estrogen-resistant tumors generally are correlated with the absence of the cognate receptors. Because of the known proliferative effects of estradiol, the therapeutic approach has been to negate the hormonal effects via endocrine ablative therapy or blockage of estrogen receptor activation by antagonists such as tamoxifen. Because progesterone appears to counter estrogenic stimuli, progestins have been administered therapeutically in the treatment of hormone-sensitive tumors (108). The picture is complicated, however, by the observation that progesterone receptor expression depends on prior estrogenic stimuli; therefore, any therapeutic effect of progestins appears to require estrogenic induction of progesterone receptors. Progression from hormone-dependent to hormone-independent cancers can occur, and the effects of therapeutic treatment of breast cancer involving hormones or antihormones are widely known. Efforts, however, continue to be made in the development of novel antiestrogens and antiprogestins for use in the treatment of receptor-positive cancers.

Cancer: Molecular Aspects

At the level of the base pair sequence, all cancers appear unique. At the cellular level, however, cancer types can be classified. The two levels are linked by the molecules encoded by the genes that are vulnerable to misfunctional mutation. The current dogma for cancer etiology postulates a multiple hit upon the genome, resulting in molecular lesions. These can be inherited or acquired and predispose cells toward a more malignant cancerous state. Carcinogen-induced lesions accelerate this process and account for environmental factors that affect incidence and prevalence. The genes which are vulnerable have been classified into protooncogenes and tumor suppressors. Tumor promoters, in contrast, do not directly cause genetic lesions but, rather, stimulate proliferation of cancer or precancerous cells via extra- or intercellular signals that cause proliferation. Theoretically, any factor involved in the signal-transduction pathways, which control cellular proliferation and genomic stability and whose genes are vulnerable to activating mutations, could be considered a protooncogene; those vulnerable to inactivating mutations could be considered tumor suppressors.

Significant progress toward the identification and characterization of the functions of the factors involving mitogenic stimuli, cell-cycle arrest, and cancer etiology has helped to delineate the precise causes and molecular and cellular mechanisms involved in cancer. For example, the mechanism of the protein product of the retinoblastoma gene is known (291). It is phosphorylated late in the G1 phase of the cell cycle by cyclin-dependent kinases, causing derepression of the mitogenic transcription factor E2F (289). These events are required for transit from G1 to S phase. Misfunctional pRB allows cells to proliferate unchecked (293). In contrast, the protein product of the tumor-suppressor gene *p53* acts as a transcription factor, directly regulating the expression of factors involved in cell-cycle control and programmed cell death (apoptosis) (159, 293). Its ability to act as a transcription factor is determined partially by its sequence-specific DNA-binding activity, which under normal conditions appears to be regulated by an oligomerization inhibitory domain that is relieved by proteolysis or phosphorylation of ser^{392} (124, 177). Its DNA-binding activity is also altered and enhanced when phosphorylated by Cdk2 at a site distinct from the CKII site (283). The function of *p53* under normal conditions is to monitor and correct genetic lesions. If the damage cannot be corrected, *p53* is thought to initiate programmed cell

death and thus greatly reduce the probability of aberrant genomes being passed on to progenitor cells (149).

Steroid hormones have been implicated in the regulation of protooncogenes (239) and programmed cell death (265). What is less clear is the role of steroid hormones in regulating the activities of tumor suppressors and the conditions under which they promote or counter the cancerous state. Only 30% of breast cancers show mutant forms of *p53* (55), compared to 50% when all cancers are considered (107, 153). Screening of inflammatory breast cancer cells for the genetic status and cytoplasmic localization of *p53* has indicated two possible mechanisms which inactivate its tumor-suppressor function. In cells where it was aberrantly retained in the cytoplasmic compartment away from the nucleus, where it exerts its action, *p53* was predominantly wild-type. In contrast, *p53* with missense and nonsense mutations were localized in the nucleus (180). The two distinct mechanisms, nuclear exclusion of wild-type *p53* and nuclear localized mutant *p53*, could account for the lack of functional *p53*. It also appears that a greater number of breast cancers result from misfunctional regulation and not from a genetic lesion per se of the breast cancer gene 1 (BRCA1) protein product (41). In most cases, BRCA1 appears to be a tumor suppressor without a genetic lesion, but it may be regulated aberrantly, causing inappropriate retention in the cytoplasmic fraction of the cell. It is thus crucial to determine not only how mutated genes account for the development of cancer but also how their protein products are regulated functionally. A useful approach to treatment of cancers with wild-type tumor suppressors would be the development of agents or treatments that restore its functional capacity (158).

Inactivation of *p53* protein is thought to be one of the primary events in the evolution of normal tissues to a cancerous state (149). Determining conditions under which *p53* activity is optimal could point to possible therapeutic approaches to both enhancing its activity and combating the proliferative state of cancerous tissues (107, 158). Understanding how steroids and their cognate receptors influence the signal-transduction pathways regulating tumor suppressors should aid this approach (108).

Breast Cancer, Tumor Suppressors, and Estrogen

According to current dogma, antiestrogen therapy is instituted to combat the estrogen receptor–mediated proliferative effects of estrogens. Two human breast cancer cell lines, MCF-7 and T47D, which express relatively high levels of estrogen and progesterone receptors, respectively, have been used extensively to explore estrogen receptor– and progesterone receptor–mediated mechanisms of cell growth. Studies on cells in culture have implicated the tumor suppressors pRB and *p53* in estrogen-dependent breast cancers (Fig. 15.2).

The antiproliferative effects of ICI 182,780 on proliferation appear to involve inhibition in the cell-cycle progression from G1 to S phase in MCF-7 cells (284). Treatment of estrogen receptor–positive MCF-7 cells with this ligand initiates a decreased expression of cyclin D1, a positive stimulator of pRB phosphorylation (289). Decreased levels of cyclin D1 and dephosphorylation of pRB, the state in which it is able to repress the activity of the mitogenic transcription factor E2F (291), occur within a time frame which implicates a direct effect on the G1 to S phase transition of the cell (284). Conversely, estradiol as an agonist induces the G1 to S phase transition and pRB phosphorylation (75a). This is obviously one mode by which estradiol might stimulate proliferation, a phenomenon which is correlated positively with cancer development. In T47D cells this appears to be mediated by the classical estrogen receptor; antiestrogens (ICI 164,384 and 4-OH tamoxifen) competed for estradiol binding and also blocked estradiol-induced hyperphosphorylation of pRB and T47D cell proliferation (125a). Estradiol-dependent cyclin D1 expression appears to be an upstream event leading to pRB phosphorylation and S phase progression. How estradiol initiates cyclin D1 expression is unclear. An estrogen-responsive *cis* element has been mapped within 944 bases upstream of the cyclin D1 gene, although no canonical estrogen-responsive element could be found within this region (17a). This would indicate that transcriptional activation of the cyclin D1 gene occurs either directly via estrogen receptor or indirectly by an estrogen receptor–induced factor. In MCF-7 cells, mitogenic pathways mediated by three classes of receptors—membrane tyrosine kinase activated by epidermal growth factor, estrogen receptor activated by estradiol, and cyclic adenosine monophosphate–dependent signaling from G protein–coupled thyrotropin receptors—converge on the cyclin D1 gene as an upstream integration point controlling the phosphorylation of pRB (161a). Whether other mitogenic signaling pathways potentiate estrogen receptor–mediated pRB phosphorylation is not known. Hypothetically, mitogenic serum factors other than estradiol could potentiate the hormonal signal or directly activate estrogen receptor by phosphorylation at tyr[537] or ser[118] (see *Estrogen Receptor Phosphorylation,* above).

That cyclin D1 and, thus, pRB may be specifically involved in the proliferation of breast cells has been demonstrated utilizing cyclin D1 knock-out mice (246).

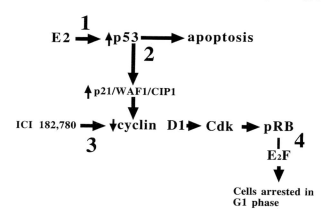

FIG. 15.2. Linkage of estrogen and antiestrogen action to the tumor suppressors, retinoblastoma protein *(pRB),* and *p53. 1,* Increase in the levels/activity of *p53* induced by 17β-estradiol *(E₂); 2,* wild-type *p53* induction of cell-cycle inhibitors and apoptosis; *3,* antiestrogen ICI 182,780 causes down-regulation of cyclin D1, a decrease in the activity of cyclin D1–associated Cdk2 activity, and dephosphorylation of pRB; *4,* dephosphorylated pRB represses E2F, a transcription factor that induces G1 to S phase transition. Cells arrested at G1 phase of the cell cycle. *Cdk,* cylin-dependent kinase; *p53,* protein product of the *p53* gene.

Breast tissue of female mice deficient in cyclin D1 was fully developed, but the mice were unable to nurse because of a defect in pregnancy-associated mammary tissue proliferation. No changes in circulating levels of estrogen and progesterone were detected, nor were differences in the distribution of estrogen receptor, indicating that this defect did not affect directly these known stimulators of breast cell proliferation.

Antiprogestins also affect the phosphorylation state of pRB in T47D cells. This appears to be mechanistically different than effects mediated by estrogen receptor. Antiprogestin increases the expression of the cyclin-dependent kinase inhibitor p21 sufficient to saturate cyclin D1 immunoprecipitates from antiprogestin-treated T47D cells without affecting the expression levels of cyclin D1 (186a). This observation indicates that antiproliferative effects of antiprogestins in T47D cell lines are mediated via increased expression of p21 to modulate the phosphorylation state of pRB.

Much like the effects of antiprogestins on T47D cells, the antineoplastic agent phenylacetate induces accumulation of hypophosphorylated pRB and inhibition of cell growth by increased expression of p21 causing attenuation of cdk2 activity. The demonstration that phenylacetate has no effect on the activity of p42MAPK indicates that the mechanism, like that of the antiprogestins, is primarily by p21 negative regulation of cyclin-dependent kinase activity and not by inactivation of mitogenic stimuli (86a).

The *p53* gene originally was thought to be an oncogene due to a reported correlation between its mutant forms and overexpression of its protein product (55). However, it is now realized that inactivation of *p53* accounts for its lack of tumor-suppressor function (107, 153). Furthermore, overexpression of *p53* mutants can transrepress the function of wild-type *p53* by the formation of misfunctional mixed oligomers (149). It is clear that increased expression of *p53* is not protective in cases where it is inactivated by mutation. Alternatively, increased expression of wild-type *p53* in the absence of other inactivating factors which repress its activity should be protective (158). Such assumptions have prompted investigations on the mechanism of regulation of *p53* levels. Agents or treatments known to enhance the expression of wild-type *p53* appear to be clinically effective, possibly due to *p53*-mediated apoptosis of cancer cells (158). However, a high proportion of breast cancers cannot be attributed to mutant *p53* (55). The cellular environment and growth factors (for example, steroids) may play a critical role in regulating *p53* expression (280).

We have studied estrogen and progesterone regulation of *p53* levels in the estrogen receptor– and progesterone receptor–positive T47D breast cancer cell line (125, 125a). Culturing T47D cells in serum depleted of steroids resulted in approximately a tenfold decrease in levels of *p53* (Fig. 15.3). Furthermore, resupplementation of steroid-depleted media with 0.1 n*M* of estradiol was sufficient to maintain high levels of *p53* (Fig. 15.4). Since physiological levels of estradiol were sufficient to raise *p53* levels, we believe the estrogenic stimulus is estrogen receptor–mediated in T47D cells. Also, there is a correlation between activation of the progesterone receptor as measured by its down-regulation or phosphorylation state and decreased lev-

els of *p53* (125). This occurred only under estrogenized conditions, where progesterone receptor and *p53* levels are high. The precise mechanism for up- and down-regulation of *p53* in these cells is still unclear. However, since T47D cells express high levels of progesterone receptor, estrogenic stimuli could be inhibited by this receptor through transcriptional interference of estrogen receptor–mediated up-regulation of *p53*. In addition, the observation that R5020 and RU486 had similar effects suggests that the AF-1 of progesterone receptor is sufficient to mediate down-regulation of *p53*. Alternatively, the requirement for estrogenized culture conditions could explain how RU486 mimics the effects of R5020. RU486 bound to progesterone receptor could exert agonistic effects due to an estrogen-induced increase in cellular cAMP (8).

Wild-type *p53* appears to inhibit cellular proliferation. For example, transfection of wild-type *p53* into T47D or MDA-MB 468 breast cancer cells, which contain a single copy of an endogenous mutant *p53* gene (15), inhibited cellular proliferation (34). A similar effect was not observed with the MCF-7 breast cancer cell line, which contains endogenous wild-type *p53*. Because we found that estrogen causes proliferation of T47D cells concomitant with a tenfold increase in *p53* protein levels, we suspect that estrogen induction of *p53* serves as a protective mechanism in proliferating breast cells. However, the endogenous mutant *p53* in T47D cells is not sufficient to inhibit cell growth in the presence of estrogen. Whether differences in estrogen-induced *p53* expression levels and the genetic status of *p53* can account for the paradoxical effects of estrogen on proliferation of estrogen receptor–positive cell lines awaits further exploration. That an antiestrogen can convert pRB to the dephosphorylated state in MCF-7 cells (284) and that estrogenic conditions enhance lev-

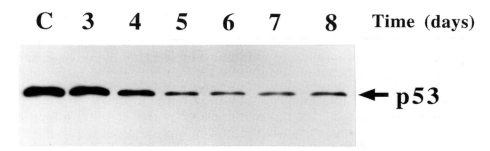

FIG. 15.3. Effect of charcoal treatment on *p53* levels in T47D cells: Western analysis. T47D cells were plated in whole serum for 2 days. Cells were then cultured for various times in medium containing whole *(C)* or charcoal-treated serum (3–8 days). All cells were harvested at the same time after 10 days of culturing. Cells were extracted and analyzed for protein, and a total of 100 μg of protein/lane was applied for SDS-PAGE and Western blot analyses as described (125). [Taken with permission from the American Society for Biochemistry and Molecular Biology for the article *J. Biol. Chem.* 270: 28507–28510, 1995.]

Estradiol (pM)

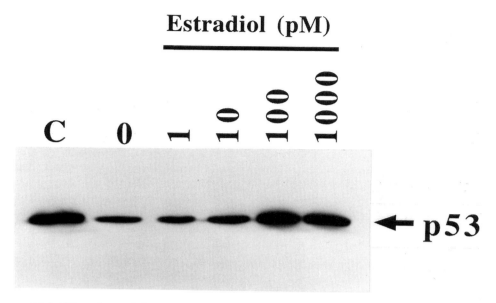

FIG. 15.4. Effect of estradiol concentrations on *p53* levels in T47D cells cultured in charcoal-treated serum: Western blot analysis. T47D cells were plated for 2 days in medium containing whole serum and then for another 6 days in charcoal-treated serum plus estradiol as indicated. Lane *C* represents cells cultured in whole serum for the entire time with no exogenous estradiol treatment. Lane *0* represents a sample with charcoal treatment but no estradiol addition (control). All cells were harvested at the same time after 8 days of culturing. Procedures for SDS-PAGE and Western blot analyses were the same as those used for the experiment described in Figure 15.3 and detailed in reference 125. [Taken with permission from the American Society for Biochemistry and Molecular Biology for the article *J. Biol. Chem.* 270: 28507–28510, 1995.]

els of *p53* in T47D cells suggest an estrogen receptor–mediated release of the G1 to S cell-cycle check point with a concomitant up-regulation of *p53* to insure genomic stability during cell division. The instability of the T47D cell genome also indicates that, in spite of high levels of mutant *p53* in T47D cells, it is incapable of stabilizing the genome during cell division (217).

Paradoxical Effects of Estrogen: Molecular Aspects

It has been suggested that a woman's lifetime exposure to estrogenic stimuli is the best correlative factor in breast cancer development (108). Estrogen receptor agonistic action may be protective under certain conditions. For example, stable transfection of the wild-type receptor into the receptor-negative breast cancer cell line MDA-MB-231 inhibited in vitro cellular proliferation in the presence of estradiol. This effect was reversed by both ICI and 4-OH tamoxifen (79). A number of cell lines exhibit this phenomenon, which indicates that wild-type estrogen receptor may be sufficient to differentiate tumor cells and thus slow their proliferative rate (152). Such experimental results suggest that an approach can be applied in gene therapies

involving introduction of estrogen receptor into receptor-negative breast cancer cells.

Not all estrogenic effects may be estrogen receptor–mediated. The apparent paradoxical effects of agonists and antagonists could involve the erbB2 protooncogene. Estradiol binds directly to the erbB2 protein with a K_D of 2.7 n*M* and enhances erbB2 autophosphorylation on tyrosine and its down-regulation within 15 min (166). Morphological changes also have been reported in NIH 3T3 cells, which contain high levels of erbB2, but not in cells that express little erbB2 (166). Furthermore, these effects could be negated by tamoxifen, raising the possibility that this antagonist has effects on cancer cells that are not directly mediated by estrogen receptors (166). Mechanistically, the intercellular domain of erbB2 as a fusion protein to the EGF receptor extracellular domain activates MAPK upon EGF stimulation (21). In human estrogen receptors, MAPK phosphorylates ser[118] and up-regulates AF-1 (1, 5, 135, 139).

The protooncogene erbB2 is potentially implicated in another pathway that leads to estrogen receptor phosphorylation. The SH2 domain of the protooncogene p60[c-src], implicated in directly modulating estrogen receptor dimerization potential, binds activated erbB2 from human breast carcinoma cell lines (162). Thus, erbB2 activation by estradiol could activate this kinase as well (see *Estrogen Receptor Phosphorylation,* above). Overexpression of erbB2 in breast cancer cells is an indicator of poor prognosis (201). The potential of erbB2 for activating MAPK and p60$^{\text{c-src}}$, suspected to regulate directly the estrogen receptor functions, and the observation that transfection of the v-ras oncogene (an upstream stimulator of the MAPK cascade) could bypass the estrogen-dependent tumorigenicity of the estrogen receptor–positive MCF-7 cells (138) indicate a need to examine how these members of other signal-transduction systems regulate estrogen receptor activation in breast cancer cells.

FUTURE DIRECTIONS

Significant progress has been made in understanding the role of RAPs in modulating the function of nascent steroid receptors. In particular, the role of HSP-90 as a repressor of DNA binding and transcriptional activation but as an activator of steroid binding is widely recognized. Further exploration into the functional roles of the other RAPs is needed and will lead to a better understanding of how steroid receptor functions are potentiated prior to hormone binding. For example, what are the roles of RAPs in defining the basal phosphorylation states of steroid receptors? Are members of RAPs involved in targeting kinases or phosphatases that directly phosphorylate/dephosphorylate steroid receptors, and is this a mechanism by which the hormonal signal is potentiated?

Significant progress also has been made in identifying the steroid receptor regions which interact with the basal transcription factors directly or through intermediary factors. The demonstration of agonist-dependent interaction of estrogen receptors with ERAPs is clearly one explanation of how the cell and promoter context of agonist vs. antagonist transacting capacities may be mediated.

Deciphering the signal-transduction pathways which might be differentially activated or repressed by agonists, agonist/antagonists, and full antagonists of estrogen or progesterone will help in their evaluation as therapeutic agents in hormone-dependent breast cancers. Further work is needed to elucidate distal events, such as the expression and activation of protooncogenes and/or tumor suppressors by steroid hormones. The success of antihormonal therapy for breast cancer may depend on deciphering the differential effects of antihormones on receptor-mediated expression and/or activation of tumor suppressors and protooncogenes. For example,

the use of antihormones that enhance the differentiating capacity of estrogen receptors but not the proliferative estrogen receptor–mediated estrogenic effects could be more effective in the treatment of receptor-positive breast cancers. More importantly, the effects of antihormone treatments on the progression from receptor-dependent to -independent growth needs to be explored. Understanding the pathways that lead into and modulate the activity of steroid receptors, which in turn affects differential transcriptional enhancement of the steroid receptor–regulated genes, will aid in understanding the role of steroid hormones in cancer etiology. The latter can be accomplished by determining the location and significance of phosphorylation sites and defining the terminal or affecter kinases and signal-transduction pathways which activate or inactivate steroid receptors. Further insight into the function as well as the cell specificity of site-specific phosphorylation/dephosphorylation should aid in a better understanding of the cellular context in which steroid receptors function. For example, is the cell specificity of the differential transacting potential due to differential phosphorylation of the receptor? Does maturation by phosphorylation negate nonspecific interactions with other cellular proteins? How do the spatial and temporal aspects of site-specific phosphorylation define the maturation process from the nascent state of the receptor to its transacting potential, down-regulation, and/or recycling? What is the effect of transient vs. sustained activation of signal-transduction pathways leading to phosphorylation on these functions? Could the phosphorylation state and the proteins with which they interact define the specificity of these interactions in a particular cell? What is the role of phosphorylation in such phenomena as transcriptional interference and cross-talk between receptors and other signal-transduction pathways? Answers to these questions will lead to a better understanding of the precise mechanism(s) by which steroid receptors and their cognate hormones determine the pattern of target cell growth and differentiation.

The work in this laboratory is supported by the National Institutes of Health grant DK20893, and in part by the Oakland University Research Excellence Program in Biotechnology. We thank Paul Alban for reading the manuscript and Rita Perris for secretarial assistance.

REFERENCES

1. Ali, S., D. Metzger, J. M. Bornert, and P. Chambon. Modulation of transcriptional activation by ligand-dependent phosphorylation of the human oestrogen receptor A/B region. *EMBO J.* 12: 1153–1160, 1993.
2. Amero, S.A., R. H. Kretsinger, N. D. Moncrief, K. R. Yamamoto, and W. R. Pearson. The origin of nuclear receptor pro-

teins: a single precursor distinct from other transcription factors. *Mol. Endocrinol.* 6: 3–7, 1992.

3. Arnold, S. F., and A. C. Notides. An antiestrogen: a phosphotyrosyl peptide that blocks dimerization of the human estrogen receptor. *Proc. Natl. Acad. Sci., U.S.A.* 92: 7475– 7479, 1995.

4. Arnold, S. F., J. D. Obourn, H. Jaffe, and A. C. Notides. Serine 167 is the major estradiol-induced phosphorylation site on the human estrogen receptor. *Mol. Endocrinol.* 8: 1208–1214, 1994.

5. Arnold, S. F., J. D. Obourn, H. Jaffe, and A. C. Notides. Phosphorylation of the human estrogen receptor by mitogen-activated protein kinase and casein kinase II: consequence on DNA binding. *J. Steroid Biochem. Mol. Biol.* 55: 163–172, 1995.

6. Arnold, S. F., J. D. Obourn, H. Jaffe, and A. C. Notides. Phosphorylation of the human estrogen receptor on tyrosine 537 in vivo and by src family tyrosine kinases in vitro. *Mol. Endocrinol.* 9: 24–33, 1995.

7. Arnold, S. F., D. P. Vorojeikina, and A. C. Notides. Phosphorylation of tyrosine 537 on the human estrogen receptor is required for binding to an estrogen response element. *J. Biol. Chem.* 270: 30205–30212, 1995.

8. Aronica, S. M., W. L. Kraus, and B. S. Katzenellenbogen. Estrogen action via the cAMP signalling pathway: stimulation of adenylate cyclase and cAMP-regulated gene transcription. *Proc. Natl. Acad. Sci., U.S.A.* 91: 8517–8521, 1994

9. Atrache, V., T. Ratajczak, S. Senafi, and R. Hahnel. Purification of the molybdate-stabilized 9–10S estradiol receptor from calf uterus. *J. Biol. Chem.* 260: 5936–5941, 1985.

10. Auricchio, F., A. Migliaccio, M. Di Domenico, and E. Nola. Oestradiol stimulates tyrosine phosphorylation and hormone binding activity of its own receptor in a cell-free system. *EMBO J.* 6: 2923–2929, 1987.

11. Bagchi, M. K., J. F. Elliston, S. Y. Tsai, D. P. Edwards, M. J. Tsai, and B. W. O'Malley. Steroid hormone-dependent interaction of human progesterone receptor with its target enhancer element. *Mol. Endocrinol.* 2: 1221–1229, 1988.

12. Bagchi, M. K., S. Y. Tsai, M. J. Tsai, and B. W. O'Malley. Identification of a functional intermediate in receptor activation in progesterone-dependent cell-free transcription. *Nature* 345: 547–550, 1990.

13. Bagchi, M. K., S. Y Tsai, M. J. Tsai, and B. W. O'Malley. Ligand and DNA-dependent phosphorylation of human progesterone receptor in vitro. *Proc. Natl. Acad. Sci. U.S.A.* 89: 2664–2668, 1992.

13a. Bai, W., S. Tullos, and N. L. Weigel. Phosphorylation of ser[530] facilitates hormone-dependent transcriptional activation of the chicken progesterone receptor. *Mol. Endocrinol.* 8: 1465–1473, 1994.

14. Bailly, A., C. LePage, M. Rauch, and E. Milgrom. Sequence-specific DNA binding of the progesterone receptor to the uteroglobin gene: effects of hormone, antihormone and receptor phosphorylation. *EMBO J.* 5: 3235– 3241, 1986.

15. Bartek, J., R. Iggo, J. Gannon, and D. P. Lane. Genetic and immunochemical analysis of mutant p53 in human breast cancer cell lines. *Oncogene* 5: 893–899, 1990.

16. Baulieu, E. E. Contragestion and other clinical applications of RU486, an antiprogesterone at the receptor. *Science* 245: 1351–1357, 1989.

17. Beato, M. Gene regulation by steroid hormones. *Cell* 56: 335–344, 1989.

17a. Beato, M., V. Sica, F. Bresciani, and A. Weisz. 17-beta estradiol induces cyclin D1 gene transcriptin, p36(D1)–p34(CDK4) complex activation and p105(RB) phosphorylation during mitogenic stimulation of G(1) arrested human breast cancer cells. *Oncogene* 12: 2315–2324, 1996.

18. Beck, C. A., N. L. Weigel, and D. P. Edwards. Effects of hormone and cellular modulators of protein phosphorylation on transcriptional activity, DNA binding, and phosphorylation of human progesterone receptors. *Mol. Endocrinol.* 6: 607–620, 1992.

19. Beck, C. A., N. L. Weigel, M. L. Moyer, S. K. Nordeen, and D. P. Edwards. The progesterone receptor antagonist RU486 acquires agonist activity upon stimulation of cAMP signaling pathways. *Proc. Natl. Acad. Sci., U.S.A.* 90: 4441–4445, 1993.

20. Beckmann, R. P., L. E. Mizzen, and W. J. Welch. Interaction of hsp 70 with newly synthesized proteins: implications for protein folding and assembly. *Science* 248: 850–854, 1990.

21. Ben-Levy, R., H. F. Paterson, C. J. Marshall, and Y. Yarden. A single phosphorylation site confers oncogenicity to the Neu/ErbB-2 receptor and enables coupling to the MAP kinase pathway. *EMBO J.* 13: 3302–3311, 1994.

22. Berg, J. M. Potential metal-binding domains in nucleic acid binding proteins. *Science* 232: 485–487, 1986.

23. Berg, J. M. DNA binding specificity of steroid receptors. *Cell* 57: 1065–1068, 1989.

24. Berry, M., D. Metzger, and P. Chambon. Role of the two activating domains of the oestrogen receptor in the cell-type and promoter-context dependent agonistic activity of the anti-oestrogen 4–hydroxytamoxifen. *EMBO J.* 9: 2811–2818, 1990.

25. Binart, N., B. Chambraud, B. Dumas, D. A. Rowlands, C. Bigogne, J. M. Levin, J. Garnier, E. E. Baulieu, and M. G. Catelli. The cDNA-derived amino acid sequence of chick heat shock protein Mr 90,000 (hsp-90) reveals a "DNA like" structure: potential site of interaction with steroid receptors. *Biochem. Biophys. Res. Commun.* 159: 140–147, 1989.

26. Bocquel, M. T., V. Kumar, C. Stricker, P. Chambon, and H. Gronemeyer. The contribution of the n- and c-terminal regions of steroid receptors to activation of transcription is both receptor and cell specific. *Nucleic Acids Res.* 17: 2581–2595, 1989.

27. Bodwell, J. E., E. Orti, J. M Coull, D. C. J. Pappin, L. I. Smith, and F. Swift. Identification of phosphorylated sites in the mouse glucocorticoid receptor. *J. Biol. Chem.* 266: 7549–7555, 1991.

28. Bourgeois, S., M. Pfahl, and E. E. Baulieu. DNA binding properties of glucocorticosteroid receptors bound to the steroid antagonist RU-486. *EMBO J.* 3: 751–755, 1984.

29. Cadepond, F., G. Schweizer-Groyer, I. Segard-Maurel, N. Jibard, S. M. Hollenberg, V. Giguire, R.M Evans, and E. E. Baulieu. Heat shock protein 90 as a critical factor in maintaining glucocorticosteroid receptor in a nonfunctional state. *J. Biol. Chem.* 266: 5834–5841, 1991.

30. Carlstedt-Duke, J., P. E. Stromstedt, B. Persson, E. Cederlund, J. A. Gustafsson, and H. Jornvall. Identification of hormone-interacting amino acid residues within the steroid-binding domain of the glucocorticoid receptor in relation to other steroid hormone receptors. *J. Biol. Chem.* 263: 6842–6846, 1988.

31. Carlstedt-Duke, J., P. E. Stromstedt, O. Wrange, T. Bergman, J. A. Gustafsson, and H. Jornvall. Domain structure of the glucocorticoid receptor protein. *Proc. Natl. Acad. Sci., U.S.A.* 84: 4437–4440, 1987.

32. Carson, M. A., M. J. Tsai, O. M. Conneely, B. L. Maxwell, J. H. Clark, A. D. W. Dobson, A. Elbrecht, D. O. Toft, W. T. Schrader, and B.W. O'Malley. Structure–function properties of the chicken progesterone receptor A synthesized from complimentary deoxyribonucleic acid. *Mol. Endocrinol.* 1: 791–801, 1987.

33. Carson-Jurica, M. A., A. T. Lee, A. W. Dobson, O. M. Conneely, W. T. Schrader, and B. W. O'Malley. Interaction of the chicken progesterone receptor with heat shock protein (hsp) 90. *J. Steroid Biochem.* 34: 1–9, 1989.

34. Casey, G., M. Lo-Hsueh, M. E. Lopez, B. Vogelstein, and E. J.

Stanbridge. Growth suppression of human breast cancer cells by the introduction of a wild-type p53 gene. *Oncogene* 6: 1791–1797, 1991.

35. Castoria, G., A. Migliaccio, S. Green, M. Di Domenico, P. Chambon, and F. Auricchio. Properties of a purified estradiol-dependent calf uterus tyrosine kinase. *Biochemistry* 32: 1740–1750, 1993.

36. Cavailles, V., S. Dauvois, P. S. Danielian, and M. G. Parker. Interaction of proteins with transcriptionally active estrogen receptors. *Proc. Natl. Acad. Sci., U.S.A.* 91: 10009–10013, 1994.

37. Cavailles, V., S. Dauvois, F. L'Horset, G. Lopez, S. Hoare, J. Kushner, and M. G. Parker. Nuclear factor RIP140 modulates transcriptional activation by the estrogen receptor. *EMBO J.* 14: 3741–3751, 1995.

38. Chambraud, B., M. Berry, G. Redeuilh, P. Chambon, and E. E Baulieu. Several regions of the human estrogen receptor are involved in the formation of receptor–heat shock protein 90 complexes. *J. Biol. Chem.* 265: 20686–20691, 1990.

39. Chang, C., J. Kokontis, and S. Liao. Molecular cloning of human and rat complimentary DNA encoding androgen receptors. *Science* 240: 324–326, 1998.

40. Chasserot-Golaz, S., and G. Beck. An approach to the mechanism of the potent antiglucocorticoid: 17β-hydroxy-11β-4-dimethylaminophenyl-17a-propynyl-estra-4,9-dien-3-one. *J. Steroid Biochem.* 21: 585–591, 1984.

41. Chen, Y., C. F. Chen, D. J. Riley, D. C. Allred, P. L. Chen, D. Von Hoff, C. K. Osborne, and W. H. Lee. Aberrant subcellular localization of BRCA1 in breast cancer. *Science* 270: 789–791, 1995.

42. Chiba, H., M. Muramatsu, A. Nomoto, and H. Kato. Two human homologues of *Saccharomyces cerevisiae* SW12/SNF2 and *Drosophila brahma* are transcriptional coactivators cooperating with the estrogen receptor and the retinoic acid receptor. *Nucleic Acids Res.* 22: 1815–1820, 1994.

43. Choy, B., and M. R. Green. Eukaryotic activators function during multiple steps of preinitiation complex assembly. *Nature* 366: 531–536, 1993.

44. Conneely, O. M., A. D. W. Dobson, M. J. Tsai, W. G. Beattie, D. O. Toft, C. S. Huckaby, T. Zarucki, W. T. Schrader, and B. W. O'Malley. Sequence and expression of a functional chicken progesterone receptor. *Mol. Endocrinol.* 1: 517–525, 1987.

45. Conneely, O. M., W. P. Sullivan, D. O. Toft, M. Birnbaumer, R. G. Cook, B. L. Maxwell, T. Zarucki-Schultz, G. L Green, W. T. Schrader, and B. W. O'Malley. Molecular cloning of the chicken progesterone receptor. *Science* 233: 767–770, 1986.

46. Csermely, P., and R. C. Kahn. The 90–kDa heat shock protein (hsp-90) possesses an ATP binding site and autophosphorylating activity. *J. Biol. Chem.* 266: 4943–4950, 1991.

47. Dahlman-Wright, K., A. Wright, J. A. Gustafsson, and J. Carstedt-Duke. Interaction of the glucocorticoid receptor DNA-binding domain with DNA as a dimer is mediated by a short segment of five amino acids. *J. Biol. Chem.* 266: 3107–3112, 1991.

48. Dalman, F. C., E. H. Bresnick, P. D. Patel, G. H. Perdew, S. J. Watson, and W. B. Pratt. Direct evidence that the glucocorticoid receptor binds to hsp90 at or near the termination of receptor translation in vitro. *J. Biol. Chem.* 64: 9815–9821, 1989.

49. Dalman, F. C., E. R. Sanchez, A. L. Y. Lin, F. Perini, and W.B. Pratt. Localization of phosphorylation sites with respect to the functional domains of the mouse L cell glucocorticoid receptor. *J. Biol. Chem.* 263: 12259–12267, 1988.

50. Dalman, F. C., L. C. Scherrer, L. P. Taylor, H. Akil, and W. B. Pratt. Localization of the 90–kDa heat shock protein–binding

site within the hormone-binding domain of the glucocorticoid receptor by peptide competition. *J. Biol. Chem.* 266: 3482–3490, 1991.

51. Daniel, V., A. B. Maksymowych, E. S. Alnemri, and G. Litwack. Cell-free synthesis of rat glucocorticoid receptor in rabbit reticulocyte lysate. In vitro synthesis of receptor in Mr 90,000 heat shock protein–depleted lysate. *J. Biol. Chem.* 266: 1320–1325, 1991.

52. Danielsen, M., L. Hinck, G. M. Ringold. Two amino acids within the knuckle of the first zinc finger specify DNA response element activation by the glucocorticoid receptor. *Cell* 57: 1131–1138, 1989.

53. Danielsen, M., J. P. Northrop, and G. M. Ringold. The mouse glucocorticoid receptor: mapping of functional domains by cloning, sequencing and expression of wild-type and mutant receptor proteins. *EMBO J.* 5: 2513–2522, 1986.

54. Dauvois, S., P. S. Danielian, R. White, and M. G. Parker. Antiestrogen ICI 164,384 reduces cellular estrogen receptor content by increasing its turnover. *Proc. Natl. Acad. Sci. U.S.A.* 89: 4037–4041, 1992.

55. Davidoff, A. M., P. A. Humphrey, J. D. Iglehart, and J. R. Marks. Genetic basis for p53 overexpression in human breast cancer. *Proc. Natl. Acad. Sci., U.S.A.* 88: 5006–5010, 1991.

56. Davis, R. J. The mitogen-activated protein kinase signal transduction pathway. *J. Biol. Chem.* 268: 14553–14556, 1993.

57. Denis, M., and J. A. Gustafsson. Translation of glucocorticoid receptor mRNA in vitro yields a nonactivated protein. *J. Biol. Chem.* 264: 6005–6008, 1989.

58. Denis, M., J. A. Gustafsson, and A. C. Wikstrom. Interaction of the Mr = 90,000 heat shock protein with the steroid-binding domain of the glucocorticoid receptor. *J. Biol. Chem.* 263: 18520–18523, 1988.

59. Denner, L. A., W. T. Schrader, B. W. O'Malley, and N. L. Weigel. Hormonal regulation and identification of chicken progesterone receptor phosphorylation sites. *J. Biol. Chem.* 265: 16548–16555, 1990.

60. Denner, L. A., N. L. Weigel, B. L. Maxwell, W. T. Schrader, and B. W. O'Malley. Regulation of progesterone receptor–mediated transcription by phosphorylation. *Science* 250: 1740–1743, 1990.

61. Denton, R. R., N. J. Koszewski, and A. C. Notides. Estrogen receptor phosphorylation: hormonal dependence and consequence on specific DNA binding. *J. Biol. Chem.* 267: 7263–7268, 1992.

62. Distelhorst, C. W., and K. J. Howard. Evidence from pulse-chase labeling studies that the antiglucocorticoid hormone RU486 stabilizes the nonactivated form of the glucocorticoid receptor in mouse lymphoma cells. *J. Steroid Biochem.* 36: 25–31, 1990.

63. Dobson, A. D. W., O. M. Conneely, W. Beattie, B. L. Maxwell, P. Mak, M. J. Tsai, W. T. Schrader, and B. W. O'Malley. Mutational analysis of the chicken progesterone receptor. *J. Biol. Chem.* 264: 4207–4211, 1989.

64. Edelman, I. S., R. Bogoroch, and G. A. Porter. On the mechanism of action of aldosterone on sodium transport: the role of protein synthesis. *Proc. Natl. Acad. Sci. U.S.A.* 50: 1169–1177, 1963.

65. Eilers, M., D. Picard, K. R. Yamamoto, and J. M. Bishop. Chimaeras of myc oncoprotein and steroid receptors cause hormone-dependent transformation of cells. *Nature* 340: 66–68, 1989.

66. El-Ashry, D., S. A. Onate, S. K. Nordeen, and D. P. Edwards. Human progesterone receptor complexed with the antagonist RU486 binds to hormone response elements in a structurally altered form. *Mol. Endocrinol.* 3: 1545–1558, 1989.

67. Eliezer, N., C. B. Hurd, and V. K. Moudgil. Immunologically distinct binding molecules for progesterone and RU38486 in the chick oviduct cytosol. *Biochim. Biophys. Acta* 929: 34–39, 1987.

68. Encio, I. J., and S. D. Detera-Wadleigh. The genomic structure of the human glucocorticoid receptor. *J. Biol. Chem.* 266: 7182–7188, 1991.

69. Ennis, B. W., W. E. Stumpf, J. M. Gasc, and E. E. Baulieu. Nuclear localization of progesterone receptor before and after exposure to progestin at low and high temperatures: autoradiographic and immunohistological studies of chick oviduct. *Endocrinology* 119: 2066–2075, 1986.

70. Evans, R. M. The steroid and thyroid hormone receptor superfamily. *Science* 240: 889–895, 1988.

71. Evans, R. M. Molecular characterization of the glucocorticoid receptor. *Recent Prog. Horm. Res.* 45: 1–27, 1989.

72. Evans, R. M., and S. M. Hollenberg. Zinc fingers: gilt by association. *Cell* 52: 1–3, 1988.

73. Fawell, S. E., J. A. Lees, R. White, and M. Parker. Characterization and colocalization of steroid binding and dimerization activities in the mouse estrogen receptor. *Cell* 60: 953–962, 1990.

74. Fawell, S. E., R. White, S. Hoare, M. Sydenham, M. Page, and M. G. Parker. Inhibition of estrogen receptor–DNA binding by the "pure" antiestrogen ICI 164,384 appears to be mediated by impaired receptor dimerization. *Proc. Natl. Acad. Sci. U.S.A.* 87: 6883–6887, 1990.

75. Formstecher, P., P. Lefebvre, and M. Dautrevaux. RU 486 stabilizes the glucocorticoid receptor in a non-transformed high molecular weight form in intact thymus cells under physiological conditions. *J. Steroid Biochem.* 31: 607–612, 1990.

75a. Foster, J. S. and J. Wimalasena. Estrogen regulates activity of cyclin-dependent kinases and retinoblastoma protein phosphorylation in breast cancer cells. *Mol. Endocrinol.* 10: 488–498, 1996.

76. Freedman, L. P., B. F. Luisi, Z. R. Korzun, R. Basavappa, P. B. Sigler, and K. R. Yamamoto. The function and structure of the metal coordination sites within the glucocorticoid receptor DNA binding domain. *Nature* 334: 543–546, 1988.

77. Freiss, G., and F. Vignon. Antiestrogens increase protein tyrosine phosphatase activity in human breast cancer cells. *Mol. Endocrinol.* 8: 1389–1396, 1994.

78. Fujimoto, N., and B. S. Katzenellenbogen. Alteration in the agonist/antagonist balance of antiestrogens by activation of protein kinase A signalling pathways in breast cancer cells: antiestrogen selectivity and promoter dependence. *Mol. Endocrinol.* 8: 296–304, 1994.

79. Garcia, M., D. Derocq, G. Freiss, and H. Rochefort. Activation of estrogen receptor transfected into a receptor-negative breast cancer cell line decreases the metastatic and invasive potential of the cells. *Proc. Natl. Acad. Sci. U.S.A.* 89: 11538–11542, 1992.

80. Gehring, U., and H. Arndt. Heteromeric nature of glucocorticoid receptors. *FEBS Lett.* 179: 138–142, 1985.

81. Geier, A., R. Bella, R. Beery, M. Haimsohn, and B. Lunenfeld. Differences in the association of the progesterone receptor ligated by antiprogestin RU38486 or progestin ORG 2058 to chromatin components. *Biochim. Biophys. Acta* 931: 78–86, 1987.

82. Giguere, V., S. M. Hollenberg, and R. M. Evans. Functional domains of the human glucocorticoid receptor. *Cell* 46: 645–652, 1986.

83. Glass, C. K. Differential recognition of target genes by nuclear receptor monomers, dimers, and heterodimers. *Endocr. Rev.* 15: 391–407, 1994.

84. Godowski, P. J., and D. Picard. Steroid receptors. How to be both a receptor and a transcription factor. *Biochem. Pharmacol.* 38: 3135–3143, 1989.

85. Godowski, P. J., D. Picard, and K. R. Yamamoto. Signal transduction and transcriptional regulation by glucocorticoid receptor-lex A fusion proteins. *Science* 241: 812–816, 1988.

86. Godowski, P. J., S. Rusconi, R. Meisfeld, and K. R. Yamamoto. Glucocorticoid receptor mutants that are constitutive activators of transcriptional enhancement. *Nature* 325: 365–368, 1987.

86a. Gorospe, M., S. Shack, K. Z. Guyton, D. Samid, and N. J. Holbrook. Up regulation and functional role of p21 (WAF1/CIP1) during growth arrest of human breast carcinoma MCF-7 cells by phenylacetate. *Cell growth and differentiation* 7: 1609–1615, 1996.

87. Govindan, M. J., M. Devic, S. Green, H. Gronemeyer, and P. Chambon. Cloning of the human glucocorticoid receptor cDNA. *Nucleic Acids Res.* 13: 8293–8304, 1985.

88. Grandics, P., A. Miller, T. J. Schmidt, D. Mittman, and G. Litwack. Purification of the unactivated glucocorticoid receptor and its subsequent in vitro activation. *J. Biol. Chem.* 259: 3173–3180, 1984.

89. Gray, G. O., and W. W. Leavitt. RU486 is not an antiprogestin in the hamster. *J. Steroid Biochem.* 28: 493–497, 1987.

90. Green, S., and P. Chambon. Oestradiol induction of a glucocorticoid-responsive gene by a chimaeric receptor. *Nature* 325: 75–78, 1987.

91. Green, S., and P. Chambon. Nuclear receptors enhance our understanding of transcription regulation. *Trends Genet.* 4: 309–314, 1988.

92. Green, S., and P. Chambon. Chimeric receptors used to probe the DNA-binding domain of the estrogen and glucocorticoid receptors. *Cancer Res.* 49: 2282s–2285s, 1989.

93. Green, S., V. Kumar, I. Theulaz, W. Wahli, and P. Chambon. The n-terminal DNA-binding "zinc finger" of the oestrogen and glucocorticoid receptors determines target gene specificity. *EMBO J.* 7: 3037–3044, 1988.

94. Greene, G. L., P. Gilna, M. Waterfield, A. Baker, Y. Hort, and J. Shine. Sequence and expression of human estrogen receptor complimentary DNA. *Science* 231: 1150–1154, 1986.

95. Gronemeyer, H., B. Benhamou, M. Berry, M. T. Bocquel, D. Gofflo, T. Garcia, T. Lerouge, D. Metzger, M. E. Meyer, L. Tora, A. Vergezac, and P. Chambon. Mechanisms of antihormone action. *J. Steroid Biochem. Mol. Biol.* 41: 217–221, 1992.

96. Gronemeyer, H., B. Turcotte, C. Quirin-Stricker, M. T. Bocquel, M. E. Meyer, Z. Krozowski, J. M. Jeltsch, T. Lerouge, J. M. Garnier, and P. Chambon. The chicken progesterone receptor: Sequence, expression and functional analysis. *EMBO J.* 6: 3985–3994, 1987.

97. Groyer, A., Y. Le Bouc, I. Joab, C. Radanyi, J. M. Renoir, P. Robel, and E. E. Baulieu. Chick oviduct glucocorticosteroid receptor. Specific binding of the synthetic steroid RU486 and immunological studies with antibodies to chick oviduct progesterone receptor. *Eur. J. Biochem.* 149: 445–451, 1985.

98. Groyer, A., G. Schweizer-Groyer, F. Cadepond, M. Mariller, and E. E. Baulieu. Antiglucocorticosteroid effects suggest why steroid hormone is required for receptors to bind DNA in vivo but not in vitro. *Nature* 328: 624–626, 1987.

99. Guiochon-Mantel, A., H. Loosfelt, P. Lescop, S. Sar, M. Atger, M. Perrot-Applanat, and E. Milgrom. Mechanism of nuclear localization of the progesterone receptor: evidence for interaction between monomers. *Cell* 57: 1147–1154, 1989.

101. Guiochon-Mantel, A., H. Loosfelt, T. Ragot, A. Bailly, M. Atger, M. Misrahi, M. Perricaudet, and E. Milgrom. Receptors

bound to antiprogestin form abortive complexes with hormone responsive elements. *Nature* 336: 695–698, 1988.

102. Halachmi, S., E. Marden, G. Martin, H. MacKay, C. Abbondanza, and M. Brown. Estrogen receptor–associated proteins: possible mediators of hormone-induced transcription. *Science* 264: 1455–1458, 1994.

103. Ham, J., and M. G. Parker. Regulation of gene expression by nuclear hormone receptors. *Curr. Opin. Cell Biol.* 1: 503–511, 1989.

104. Ham, J., A. Thompson, M. Needham, P. Webb, and M. Parker. Characterization of response elements for androgens, glucocorticoids and progestins in mouse mammary tumor virus. *Nucleic Acids Res.* 16: 5263– 5276, 1988.

105. Hard, T., K. Dahlman, J. Carlstedt-Duke, J. A. Gustafsson, and R. Rigler. Cooperativity and specificity in the interactions between DNA and the glucocorticoid receptor DNA-binding domain. *Biochemistry* 29: 5358–5364, 1990.

106. Hard, T., E. Kellenbach, R. Boelens, B. A. Maler, K. Dahlman, L. P. Freedman, J. Carlstedt-Duke, K. R. Yamamoto, J. A. Gustafsson, and R. Kaptein. Solution structure of the glucocorticoid receptor DNA-binding domain. *Science* 249: 157–160, 1990.

107. Harris, C. C. p53: at the crossroads of molecular carcinogenesis and risk assessment. *Science* 262: 1980–1981, 1993.

108. Henderson, B. E., R. K. Ross, and M. C. Pike. Hormonal chemoprevention of cancer in women. *Science* 259: 633–638, 1993.

109. Hill, C. S., and R. Treisman. Transcriptional regulation by extra-cellular signals: mechanisms and specificity. *Cell* 80: 199–211, 1995.

110. Hoeck, W., and B. Groner. Hormone-dependent phosphorylation of the glucocorticoid receptor occurs mainly in the amino-terminal transactivation domain. *J. Biol. Chem.* 265: 5403–5408, 1990.

111. Hoeck, W., S. Rusconi, and B. Groner. Down-regulation and phosphorylation of glucocorticoid receptors in cultured cells. Investigations with a monospecific antiserum against a bacterially expressed receptor fragment. *J. Biol. Chem.* 264: 14396–14402, 1989.

112. Hollenberg, S. M., and R. M. Evans. Multiple and cooperative transactivation domains of the human glucocorticoid receptor. *Cell* 55: 899–906, 1988.

113. Hollenberg, S. M., V. Giguere, and R. M. Evans. Identification of two regions of the human glucocorticoid receptor hormone binding domain that block activation. *Cancer Res.* 49: 2292s–2294s, 1989.

114. Hollenberg, S. M., C. Weinberger, E. S. Ong, G. Cerelli, A. Oro, R. Lebo, E. B. Thompson, M. G. Rosenfeld, and R. M. Evans. Primary structure and expression of a functional human glucocorticoid receptor cDNA. *Nature* 318: 635–641, 1985.

115. Horwitz, K. B. The antiprogestin RU38486: receptor-mediated progestin versus antiprogestin actions screened in estrogen-insensitive T47Dco human breast cancer cells. *Endocrinology* 116: 2236–2245, 1985.

116. Horwitz, K. B. How do breast cancers become hormone resistant. *J. Steroid Biochem. Mol. Biol.* 49: 295–302, 1994.

117. Howard, K. J., S. J. Holley, K. R. Yomamoto, and C. W. Distelhorst. Mapping the hsp90 binding region of the glucocorticoid receptor. *J. Biol. Chem.* 265: 11928–11935, 1990.

118. Hsieh, J. C., P. W. Jurutka, M. A. Galligan, C. M. Terpening, C. A. Haussler, D. S. Samuels, Y. Shimizu, N. Shimizu, and M. R. Haussler. Human vitamin D receptor is selectively phosphorylated by protein kinase C on serine 51, a residue crucial to its trans-activation function. *Proc. Natl. Acad. Sci. U.S.A.* 88: 9315–9319, 1991.

119. Hsieh, J. C., P. W. Jurutka, S. Nakajima, M. A. Galligan, C. A. Haussler, Y. Shimizu, N. Shimizu, G.K. Whitfield, and M.. Haussler. Phosphorylation of the human vitamin D receptor by protein kinase C: biochemical and functional evaluation of the serine 51 recognition site. *J. Biol. Chem.* 268: 15118–15126, 1993.

120. Huckaby, C. S., O. M. Conneely, W. G. Beattie, A. D. W. Dobson, M. J. Tsai, and B. W. O'Malley. Structure of the chromosomal chicken progesterone receptor gene. *Proc. Natl. Acad. Sci. U.S.A.* 84: 8380–8384, 1987.

121. Hunter, T. A thousand and one protein kinases. *Cell* 50: 823–829, 1987.

122. Hunter, T. Protein kinases and phosphatases: the yin and yang of protein phosphorylation and signaling. *Cell* 80: 225–236, 1995.

123. Hunter, T., and M. Karin. The regulation of transcription by phosphorylation. *Cell* 70: 375–387, 1992.

124. Hupp, T. R., D. W. Meek, C. A. Midgley, and D. P. Lane. Regulation of the specific DNA binding function of p53. *Cell* 71: 875–886, 1992.

125. Hurd, C., N. Khattree, P. Alban, K. Nag, S. C. Jhanwar, S. Dinda, and V. K. Moudgil. Hormonal regulation of the p53 tumor suppressor protein in T47D human breast carcinoma cell line. *J. Biol. Chem.* 270: 28507–28510, 1995.

125a. Hurd, C., N. Khattree, S. Dinda, P. Alban and V. K. Moudgil. Regulation of tumor suppressor proteins, p53 and retinoblastoma, by estrogen and antiestrogens in breast cancer cells. *Oncogene,* 15: 991–995, 1997.

126. Hurd, C., and V. K. Moudgil. Characterization of R5020 and RU486 binding to progesterone receptor from the calf uterus. *Biochemistry* 27: 3618–3623, 1988.

127. Hurd, C., M. Nakao, and V. K. Moudgil. Phosphorylation of calf uterine progesterone receptor by cAMP-dependent protein kinase. *Biochem. Biophys. Res. Commun.* 162: 160–167, 1989.

128. Hutchison, K. A., K. D. Dittmar, M. J. Czar, and W. B. Pratt. Proof that hsp70 is required for assembly of the glucocorticoid receptor into heterocomplex with hsp90. *J. Biol. Chem.* 269: 5043–5049, 1994.

129. Ince, B. A., M. M. Montano, and B. S. Katzenellenbogen. Activation of transcriptionally inactive human estrogen receptors by cyclic adenosine 3′,5′-monophosphate and ligands including antiestrogens. *Mol. Endocrinol.* 8: 1397–1406, 1994.

130. Ing, N. H., J. M. Beekman, S. Y. Tsai, M. J. Tsai, and B. W. O'Malley. Members of the steroid hormone receptor superfamily interact with TFIIB (S300–II). *J. Biol. Chem.* 267: 17617–17623, 1992.

131. Jackson, P., D. Baltimore, and D. Picard. Hormone-conditional transformation by fusion proteins of c-Abl and its transforming variants. *EMBO J.* 12: 2809–2819, 1993.

132. Jacq, X., C. Brou, Y. Lutz, I. Davidson, P. Chambon, and L. Tora. Human TAFII30 is present in a distinct TFIID complex and is required for transcriptional activation by the estrogen receptor. *Cell* 79: 107–117, 1994.

133. Jensen, E. V., and H. T. Jacobson. Basic guides to the mechanisms of estrogen actions. *Recent Prog. Horm. Res.* 18: 387–414, 1962.

134. Jensen, E. V., T. Suzuki, T. Kawashima, W. E. Stumpf, P. W. Jungblut, and E. R. Desombre. A two-step mechanism for the interaction of estradiol with rat uterus. *Proc. Natl. Acad. Sci., U.S.A.* 59: 632–638, 1968.

135. Joel, P. B., A. M. Traish, and D. A. Lannigan. Estradiol and phorbol ester cause phosphorylation of serine 118 in human estrogen receptor. *Mol. Endocrinol.* 9: 1041–1052, 1995.

136. Jurutka, P. W., J. C. Hsieh, P. N. MacDonald, C. M. Terpening,

C. A. Haussler, M. R. Haussler, and G. K. Whitfield. Phosphorylation of serine 208 in the human vitamin D receptor: the predominant amino acid phosphorylated by casein kinase II, in vitro, and identification as a significant phosphorylation site in intact cells. *J. Biol. Chem.* 268: 6791– 6799, 1993.

137. Kalderon, D., W. D. Richardson, A. F. Markham, and A. E. Smith. Sequence requirements for nuclear location of simian virus 40 large-T antigen. *Nature* 311: 33–38, 1984.

138. Kasid, A., M. E. Lippman, A. G. Papageorge, D. R. Lowy, and E. P. Gelmann. Transfection of v-ras DNA into MCF-7 human breast cancer cells bypasses dependence on estrogen for tumorigenicity. *Science* 228: 725–728, 1985.

139. Kato, S., H. Endoh, Y. Masuhiro, T. Kitamoto, S. Uchiyama, H. Sasaki, S. Masushige, Y. Gotoh, E. Nishida, H. Kawashima, D. Metzger, and P. Chambon. Activation of the estrogen receptor through phosphorylation by mitogen-activated protein kinase. *Science* 270: 1491–1494, 1995.

140. King, W. J., and G. L. Greene. Monoclonal antibodies localize oestrogen receptor in the nuclei of target cells. *Nature* 307: 745–747, 1984.

141. Klein-Hitpass, L., A. C. B. Cato, D. Henderson, and G. U. Ryffel. Two types of antiprogestins identified by their differential action in transcriptionally active extracts from T47D cells. *Nucleic Acids Res.* 19: 1227–1234, 1991.

142. Koike, S., M. Sakai, and M. Muramatsu. Molecular cloning and characterization of rat estrogen receptor cDNA. *Nucleic Acids Res.* 5: 2499–2513, 1987.

143. Kost, S. L., D. F. Smith, W. P. Sullivan, W. J. Welch, and D. O. Toft. Binding of heat shock proteins to the avian progesterone receptor. *Mol. Cell. Biol.* 9: 3829–3838, 1989.

144. Koyasu, S., E. Nishida, T. Kadowaki, F. Matsuzaki, K. Iida, F. Harada, M. Kasuga, H. Sakai, and I. Yahara. Two mammalian heat shock proteins, hsp90 and hsp100, are actin-binding proteins. *Proc. Natl. Acad. Sci. U.S.A.* 83: 8054–8058, 1986.

145. Krust, A., S. Green, P. Argos, V. Kumar, P. Walter, J. M. Bornert, and P. Chambon. The chicken oestrogen receptor sequence: homology with v-erb-A and the human oestrogen and glucocorticoid receptors. *EMBO J.* 5: 891–897, 1986.

146. Kumar, V., and P. Chambon. The estrogen receptor binds tightly to its responsive element as a ligand-induced homodimer. *Cell* 55: 145–156, 1988.

147. Kumar, V., S. Green, G. Stack, M. Berry, L. R. Jin, and P. Chambon. Functional domains of the human estrogen receptor. *Cell* 51: 941–951, 1987.

148. Kumar, V., S. Green, A. Staub, and P. Chambon. Localisation of the oestradiol-binding and putative DNA-binding domains of the human oestrogen receptor. *EMBO J.* 5: 2231– 2236, 1986.

149. Lane, D.P. p53, guardian of the genome. *Nature* 358: 15–16, 1992.

150. Lefebvre, P., P. M. Danze, B. Sablonniere, C. Richard, P. Formstecher, and M. Dautrevaux. Association of the glucocorticoid receptor binding subunit with the 90K non-steroid binding component is stabilized by both steroidal and nonsteroidal antiglucocorticoids in intact cells. *Biochemistry* 27: 9186– 9194, 1988.

151. Le Goff, P., M. M. Montano, D. J. Schodin, and B. S. Katzenellenbogen. Phosphorylation of the human estrogen receptor: identification of hormone-regulated sites and examination of their influence on transcriptional activity. *J. Biol. Chem.* 269: 4458–4466,1994.

152. Levenson, A. S., and V. C. Jordan. Transfection of human estrogen receptor (ER) cDNA into ER-negative mammalian cell lines. *J. Steroid Biochem. Mol. Biol.* 51: 229–239, 1994.

153. Levine, A. J., J. Momand, and C. A. Finlay. The p53 tumor suppressor gene. *Nature* 351: 453–456, 1991.

154. Li, W., and R. E. Handschumacher. Specific interaction of the cyclophilin–cyclosporin complex with the B subunit of calcineurin. *J. Biol. Chem.* 268: 14040–14044, 1993.

155. Lindquist, S., and E. A. Craig. The heat shock proteins. *Annu. Rev. Genet.* 22: 631–677, 1988.

156. Logeat, F., M. Le Cunff, R. Pamphile, and E. Milgrom. The nuclear-bound form of the progesterone receptor is generated through a hormone-dependent phosphorylation. *Biochem. Biophys. Res. Commun.* 31: 421–427, 1985.

157. Loosfelt, H., M. Atger, M. Misrahi, A. Guiochon-Mantel, C. Meriel, F. Logeat, R. Benarous, and E. Milgrom. Cloning and sequence analysis of rabbit progesterone-receptor complimentary DNA. *Proc. Natl. Acad. Sci. U.S.A.* 83: 9045–9049, 1986.

158. Lowe, S. W., S. Bodis, A. McClatchey, L. Remington, H. E. Ruley, D. E. Fisher, D. E. Housman, and T. Jacks. p53 status and the efficacy of cancer therapy in vivo. *Science* 266: 807–810, 1994.

159. Lowe, S. W., H. E. Ruley, T. Jacks, and D. E. Housman. p53–dependent apoptosis modulates the cytotoxicity of anticancer agents. *Cell* 74: 957–967, 1993.

160. Lubahn, D. B., D. R. Joseph, P. M. Sullivan, H. F. Willard, F. S. French, and E. M. Wilson. Cloning of human androgen receptor complimentary DNA and localization to the X chromosome. *Science* 240: 327–330, 1988.

161. Luisi, B. F., W. X. Xu, Z. Otwinowski, L. P. Freedman, K. R. Yamamoto, and P. B. Sigler. Crystallographic analysis of the interaction of the glucocorticoid receptor with DNA. *Nature* 352: 497–505, 1991.

161a. Lukas, J., J. Bartkova, and J. Bartek. Convergence of mitogenic signalling cascades from diverse classes of receptors at the cyclin D–cyclin-dependent kinase–pRB-controlled G1 checkpoint. *Mol. Cell. Biol.* 16: 6917–6925, 1996.

162. Luttrell, D. K., A. Lee, T. J. Lansing, R. M. Crosby, K. D. Jung, D. Willard, M. Luther, M. Rodriguez, J. Berman, and T. M. Gilmer. Involvement of pp60^c-src^ with two major signalling pathways in human breast cancer. *Proc. Natl. Acad. Sci. U.S.A.* 91: 83–87, 1994.

163. Mader, S., V. Kumar, H. de Verneuil, and P. Chambon. Three amino acids of the oestrogen receptor are essential to its ability to distinguish an oestrogen from a glucocorticoid-responsive element. *Nature* 338: 271–274, 1989.

164. Mangelsdorf, D. J., C. Thummel, M. Beato, P. Herrich, G. Schuts, K. Umesono, B. Blumberg, P. Kastner, M. Mark, P. Chambon, and R. M. Evans. The nuclear receptor superfamily: the second decade. *Cell* 83: 835–839, 1995.

165. Mason, S. A., and P. R. Housley. Site-directed mutagenesis of the phosphorylation sites in the mouse glucocorticoid receptor. *J. Biol. Chem.* 268: 21501–21504, 1993.

166. Matsuda, S., Y. Kadowaki, M. Ichino, T. Akiyama, K. Toyoshima, and T. Yamamoto. 17β-Estradiol mimics ligand activity of the c-erbB2 protooncogene product. *Proc. Natl. Acad. Sci., U.S.A.* 90: 10803–10807, 1993.

167. Meinkoth, J. L., Y. Ji, S. S. Taylor, and J. R. Feramisco. Dynamics of the distribution of cyclic AMP-dependent protein kinase in living cells. *Proc. Natl. Acad. Sci. U.S.A.* 87: 9595–9599, 1990.

168. Metzger, D., M. Berry, S. Ali, and P. Chambon. Effect of antagonists on DNA binding properties of the human estrogen receptor in vitro and in vivo. *Mol. Endocrinol.* 9: 579–591, 1995.

169. Meyer, M. E., A. Pornon, J. Ji, M. T. Bocquel, P. Chambon, and H. Gronemeyer. The agonist and antagonist activities of RU486 on the functions of the human progesterone receptor. *EMBO J.* 9: 3923–3932, 1990.

170. Miesfeld, R., S. Rusconi, P. J. Godowski, B. A. Maler, S. Okret,

A. C. Wikstrom, J. A. Gustafsson, and K. R. Yamamoto. Genetic complimentation of a glucocorticoid receptor deficiency by expression of cloned receptor cDNA. *Cell* 46: 389–399, 1986.

171. Migliaccio, A., M. Di Domenico, S. Green, A. de Falco, E. L. Kajtaniak, F. Blasi, P. Chambon, and F. Auricchio. Phosphorylation on tyrosine of in vitro synthesized human estrogen receptor activates its hormone binding. *Mol. Endocrinol.* 3: 1061–1069, 1989.

172. Migliaccio, A., M. Pagano, and F. Auricchio. Immediate and transient stimulation of protein tyrosine phosphorylation by estradiol in MCF-7 cells. *Oncogene* 8: 2183–2191, 1993.

173. Migliaccio, A., A. Rotondi, and F. Auricchio. Calmodulin-stimulated phosphorylation of 17β-estradiol receptor on tyrosine. *Proc. Natl. Acad. Sci., U.S.A.* 81: 5921–5925, 1984.

174. Migliaccio, A., A. Rotondi, and F. Auricchio. Estradiol receptor: phosphorylation on tyrosine in uterus and interaction with anti-phosphotyrosine antibody. *EMBO J.* 5: 2867–2872, 1986.

175. Milad, M., W. Sullivan, E. Diehl, M. Altmann, S. Nordeen, D. P. Edwards, and D. O. Toft. Interaction of the progesterone receptor with binding proteins for FK506 and cyclosporin A. *Mol. Endocrinol.* 9: 838–847, 1995.

176. Miller, M. M., C. Hurd, and V. K. Moudgil. Transformation of human progesterone receptor in the presence of the progestin (R5020) and the antiprogestin (RU486). *J. Steroid Biochem.* 31: 777–783, 1988.

177. Milne, D. M., R. H. Palmer, and D. W. Meek. Mutation of the casein kinase II phosphorylation site abolishes the antiproliferative activity of p53. *Nucleic Acids Res.* 520: 5565–5570, 1992.

178. Misrahi, M., M. Atger, L. d'Auriol, H. Loosfelt, C. Meriel, F. Fridlansky, A. Guiochon-Mantel, F. Galibert, and E. Milgrom. Complete amino acid sequence of the human progesterone receptor deduced from cloned cDNA. *Biochem. Biophys. Res. Commun.* 143: 740–748, 1987.

179. Moguilewsky, M., and D. Philibert. RU38486: potent antiglucocorticoid activity correlated with strong binding to the cytosolic glucocorticoid receptor followed by an impaired activation. *J. Steroid Biochem.* 1: 271–276, 1984.

180. Moll, U. M., G. Riou, and A. J. Levine. Two distinct mechanisms alter p53 in breast cancer: mutation and nuclear exclusion. *Proc. Natl. Acad. Sci., U.S.A.* 89: 7262–7266, 1992.

181. Montano, M. M., V. Muller, A. Trobaugh, and B. S. Katzenellenbogen. The carboxy-terminal F domain of the human estrogen receptor and the transcriptional activity of the receptor and the effectiveness of antiestrogens as estrogen antagonists. *Mol. Endocrinol.* 9: 814–825, 1995.

182. Moudgil, V.K. Phosphorylation of steroid hormone receptors. *Biochim. Biophys. Acta* 1055: 243–258, 1990.

183. Moudgil, V. K., M. J. Anter, and C. Hurd. Mammalian progesterone receptor shows differential sensitivity to sulfhydryl group modifying agents when bound to agonist and antagonist ligands. *J. Biol. Chem.* 264: 2203–2211, 1989.

184. Moudgil, V. K., and M. Gunda. Hepatic glucocorticoid receptor behaves differently when its hormone binding site is occupied by agonist (triamcinolone acetonide) or antagonist (RU486) steroid ligands. *Biochem. Biophys. Res. Commun.* 174: 1239–1247, 1991.

185. Moudgil, V. K., and C. Hurd. Transformation of calf uterine progesterone receptor: analysis of the process when receptor is bound to progesterone and RU486. *Biochemistry* 26: 4993–5001, 1987.

186. Moudgil, V. K., G. Lombardo, C. Hurd, N. Eliezer, and M. K. Agarwal. Evidence for separate binding sites for progesterone and RU486 in the chick oviduct. *Biochim. Biophys. Acta* 889: 192–199, 1986.

186a. Musgrove, E. A., C. S. L. Lee, A. L. Cornish, A. Swarbrick, and R. L. Sutherland. Antiprogestin inhibition of cell cycle progression in T-47D breast cancer cells is accompanied by induction of the cyclin-dependent kinase inhibitor p21. *Mol. Endocrinol.* 11: 54–66, 1997.

187. Nakao, M., T. Mizutani, A. Bhakta, N. Ribarac-Stepic, and V. K. Moudgil. Phosphorylation of chicken oviduct progesterone receptor by cAMP-dependent protein kinase. *Arch. Biochem. Biophys.* 298: 340–348, 1992.

188. Nakao, M., and V. K. Moudgil. Hormone specific phosphorylation and transformation of chicken oviduct progesterone receptor. *Biochem. Biophys. Res. Commun.* 164: 295–303, 1989.

189. Nielsen, C. J., J. J. Sando, and W. B. Pratt. Evidence that dephosphorylation inactivates glucocorticoid receptors. *Proc. Natl. Acad. Sci. U.S.A.* 74: 1398–1402, 1977.

190. Ning, Y. M., and E. R. Sanchez. Potentiation of glucocorticoid receptor–mediated gene expression by the immunophilin ligands FK506 and rapamycin. *J. Biol. Chem.* 268: 6073–6076, 1993.

191. Nordeen, S. K., B. J. Bona, and M. L. Moyer. Latent agonist activity of the steroid antagonist, RU486, is unmasked in cells treated with activators of protein kinase A. *Mol. Endocrinol.* 7: 731–742, 1993.

192. Northrop, J. P., B. Gametchu, R. W. Harrison, and G. M. Ringold. Characterization of wild type and mutant glucocorticoid receptors from rat hepatoma and mouse lymphoma cells. *J. Biol. Chem.* 260: 6398–6403, 1985.

193. Noteboom, W. D., and J. Gorski. An early effect of estrogen on protein synthesis. *Proc. Natl. Acad. Sci. U.S.A.* 50: 250–255, 1963.

194. Notides, A. C., N. Lerner, and D. E. Hamilton. Positive cooperativity of the estrogen receptor. *Proc. Natl. Acad. Sci. U.S.A.* 78: 4926–4930, 1981.

195. Ohara-Nemoto, Y., P. E. Stromstedt, K. Dahlman-Wright, T. Nemoto, J. A. Gustafsson, and J. Carlstedt-Duke. The steroid-binding properties of recombinant glucocorticoid receptor: a putative role for heat shock protein hsp90. *J. Steroid Biochem. Mol. Biol.* 37: 481–490, 1990.

196. Okret, S., A. C. Wikstrom, and J. A. Gustafsson. Molybdate-stabilized glucocorticoid receptor: evidence for a receptor heteromer. *Biochemistry* 24: 6581–6586, 1985.

197. O'Malley, B. W., M. R. Sherman, and D. O. Toft. Progesterone receptors in the cytoplasm and nucleus of chick oviduct target tissue. *Proc. Natl. Acad. Sci. U.S.A.* 67: 501–509, 1970.

198. Onate, S. A., S. Y. Tsai, M. J. Tsai, and B. W. O'Malley. Sequence and characterization of a coactivator for the steroid hormone receptor superfamily. *Science* 270: 1354–357, 1995.

199. Orti, E., J. E. Bodwell, and A. Munck. Phosphorylation of steroid hormone receptors. *Endocr. Rev.* 13: 105–128, 1992.

200. Orti, E., D. B. Mendel, L. I. Smith, and A. Munck. Agonist-dependent phosphorylation and nuclear dephosphorylation of glucocorticoid receptors in intact cells. *J. Biol. Chem.* 264: 9728–9731, 1989.

201. Pasqualini, J. R. Breast cancer, present and future. *J. Steroid Biochem. Mol. Biol.* 51: V-VI, 1994.

202. Pelham, H. R. B. Speculations on the functions of the major heat shock and glucose-regulated proteins. *Cell* 46: 959–961, 1986.

203. Perrot-Applanat, M., F. Logeat, M.T. Groyer-Picard, and E.

Milgrom. Immunocytochemical study of mammalian progesterone receptor using monoclonal antibodies. *Endocrinology* 116: 1473–1484, 1985.

204. Pfahl, M. Nuclear receptor/AP-1 interaction. *Endocr. Rev.* 14: 651–658, 1993.

205. Philibert, D. RU38486: an original multifaceted antihormone in vivo. In: *Adrenal Steroid Antagonism,* edited by M. K. Agarwal. New York: de Gruyter, 1984, p. 77–101.

206. Picard, D., B. Khursheed, M. J. Garabedian, M. G. Fortin, S. Lindquist, and K. R. Yamamoto. Reduced levels of hsp90 compromise steroid receptor action in vivo. *Nature* 348: 166–168, 1990.

207. Picard, D., S. J. Salser, and K. R. Yamamoto. A movable and regulable inactivation function within the steroid binding domain of the glucocorticoid receptor. *Cell* 54: 1073–1080, 1988.

208. Picard, D., and K. R. Yamamoto. Two signals mediate hormone-dependent nuclear localization of the glucocorticoid receptor. *EMBO J.* 6: 3333–3340, 1987.

209. Pike, J. W., and N. M. Sleator. Hormone-dependent phosphorylation of the 1, 25–di-hydroxyvitamin D3 receptor in mouse fibroblasts. *Biochem. Biophys. Res. Commun.* 131: 378–385, 1985.

210. Ponglikitmongkol, M., S. Green, and P. Chambon. Genomic organization of the human oestrogen receptor gene. *EMBO J.* 7: 3385–3388, 1988.

211. Power, R. F., S. K. Mani, J. Codina, O. M. Conneely, and B. W. O'Malley. Dopaminergic and ligand-independent activation of steroid hormone receptors. *Science* 254: 1636–1639, 1991.

212. Pratt, W. B. Transformation of glucocorticoid and progesterone receptors to the DNA-binding state. *J. Cell. Biochem.* 35: 51–68, 1987.

213. Pratt, W. B. The role of heat shock proteins in regulating the function, folding, and trafficking of the glucocorticoid receptor. *J. Biol. Chem.* 268: 21455–21458, 1993.

214. Pratt, W. B., D. J. Jolly, D. V. Pratt, S. M. Hollenberg, V. Giguere, F. M. Cadepond, G. Schweizer-Groyer, M. G. Catelli, R. M. Evans, and E. E. Baulieu. A region in the steroid binding domain determines formation of the non-DNA-binding, 9S glucocorticoid receptor complex. *J. Biol. Chem.* 263: 267–273, 1988.

215. Rajpert, E. J., F. P. Lemaigre, P. H. Eliard, M. Place, D. A. Lafontaine, I. V. Economidis, A. Belayew, J. A. Martial, and G. G. Rousseau. Glucocorticoid receptors bound to the antagonist RU486 are not downregulated despite their capacity to interact in vitro with defined gene regions. *J. Steroid Biochem.* 26: 513–520, 1987.

216. Rauch, M., H. Loosfelt, D. Philibert, and E. Milgrom. Mechanism of action of an antiprogesterone, RU486, in the rabbit endometrium. Effects of RU486 on the progesterone receptor and on the uteroglobin gene. *Eur. J. Biochem.* 148: 213–218, 1985.

217. Reddel, R. R., I. E. Alexander, M. Koga, J. Shine, and R. L. Sutherland. Genetic instability and the development of steroid hormone insensitivity in cultured T47D human breast cancer cells. *Cancer Res.* 48: 4340–4347, 1988.

218. Reese, J. C., and B. S. Katzenellenbogen. Differential DNA-binding abilities of estrogen receptor occupied with two classes of antiestrogens: studies using human estrogen receptor overexpressed in mammalian cells. *Nucleic Acids Res.* 19: 6595–6602, 1991.

219. Reese, J. C., and B. S. Katzenellenbogen. Examination of the DNA-binding ability of estrogen receptor in whole cells: implications for hormone-independent transactivation and the actions of antiestrogens. *Mol. Cell. Biol.* 12: 4531–4538, 1992.

220. Rehberger, P., M. Rexin, and U. Gehring. Heterotetrameric structure of the human progesterone receptor. *Proc. Natl. Acad. Sci. U.S.A.* 89: 8001–8005, 1992.

221. Reichmann, E., H. Schwarz, E. M. Deiner, I. Leitner, M. Eilers, J. Berger, M. Busslinger, and H. Beug. Activation of an inducible c-fosER fusion protein causes loss of epithelial polarity and triggers epithelial-fibroblastoid cell conversion. *Cell* 71: 1103–1116, 1992.

222. Renoir, J. M., T. Buchou, J. Mester, C. Radanyi, and E. E. Baulieu. Oligomeric structure of molybdate-stabilized, nontransformed 8S progesterone receptor from chicken oviduct cytosol. *Biochemistry* 23: 6016–6023, 1984.

223. Renoir, J. M., C. Radanyi, L. E. Faber, and E. E. Baulieu. The non-DNA binding heterooligomeric form of mammalian steroid hormone receptors contains a hsp90–bound 59–kilodalton protein. *J. Biol. Chem.* 265: 10740–10745, 1990.

224. Renoir, J. M., C. Radanyi, I. Jung-Testas, L. E. Faber, and E. E. Baulieu. The nonactivated progesterone receptor is a nuclear heterooligomer. *J. Biol. Chem.* 265: 14402–4406, 1990.

225. Roemer, K., and T. Friedmann. Modulation of cell proliferation and gene expression by a p53–estrogen receptor hybrid protein. *Proc. Natl. Acad. Sci. U.S.A.* 90: 9252–9256, 1993.

226. Rose, D. W., W. J. Welch, G. Kramer, and B. Hardesty. Possible involvement of the 90–kDa heat shock protein in the regulation of protein synthesis. *J. Biol. Chem.* 264: 6239–6244, 1989.

227. Rothman, J. E. Polypeptide chain binding proteins: catalysts of protein folding and related processes in cells. *Cell* 59: 591–601, 1989.

228. Rusconi, S., and K. R. Yamamoto. Functional dissection of the hormone and DNA binding activities of the glucocorticoid receptor. *EMBO J.* 6: 1309–1315, 1987.

229. Sablonniere, B., P. M. Danze, P. Formstecher, P. Lefebvre, and M. Dautrevaux. Physical characterization of the activated and non-activated forms of the glucocorticoid-receptor complex bound to the steroid antagonist [^{3}H]RU486. *J. Steroid Biochem.* 25: 605–614, 1986.

230. Sanchez, E. R. Hsp 56: a novel heat shock protein associated with untransformed steroid receptor complexes. *J. Biol. Chem.* 265: 22067–22070, 1990.

231. Sanchez, E. R., L. E. Faber, W. J. Henzel. and W. B. Pratt. The 56–59 kilodalton protein identified in untransformed steroid receptor complexes is a unique protein that exists in cytosol in a complex with both the 70– and 90–kilodalton heat shock protein. *Biochemistry* 29: 5145–5152, 1990.

232. Sartorius, C. A., S. D. Groshong, L. A. Miller, R. L. Powell, L. Tung, G. S. Takimoto, and K. B. Horwitz. New T47D breast cancer cell lines for the independent study of progesterone B- and A-receptors: only antiprogestin-occupied B-receptors are switched to transcriptional agonists by cAMP. *Cancer Res.* 54: 3868–3877, 1994.

233. Sartorius, C. A., M. Y. Melville, A. R. Hovland, L. Tung, G. S. Takimoto, and K. B. Horwitz. A third transactivation function (AF3) of human progesterone receptors located in the unique n-terminal segment of the B-isoform. *Mol. Endocrinol.* 8: 1347–1360, 1994.

234. Sartorius, C. A., L. Tung, G. S. Takimoto, and K. B. Horwitz. Antagonist-occupied human progesterone receptors bound to DNA are functionally switched to transcriptional agonists by cAMP. *J. Biol. Chem.* 268: 9262–9266, 1993.

235. Savouret, J. F., M. Misrahi, H. Loosfelt, M. Atger, A. Bailly, M. Perrot-Applanat, M. T. Vu Hai, A. Guiochon-Mantel, A. Jolivet, F. Lorenzo, F. Logeat, M. F. Pichon, P. Bouchard, and E. Milgrom. Molecular and cellular biology of mammalian

progesterone receptors. *Recent Prog. Horm. Res.* 45: 65–120, 1989.

236. Schauer, M., G. Chalepakis, T. Willmann, and M. Beato. Binding of hormone accelerates the kinetics of glucocorticoid and progesterone receptor binding to DNA. *Proc. Natl. Acad. Sci. U.S.A.* 86: 1123–1127, 1989.

237. Schena, M., and K. R. Yamamoto. Mammalian glucocorticoid receptor derivatives enhance transcription in yeast. *Science* 241: 965–967, 1988.

238. Schmidt, T. J. In vitro activation and DNA binding affinity of human lymphoid (CEM-C7) cytoplasmic receptors labeled with the antiglucocorticoid RU38486. *J. Steroid Biochem.* 24: 853–863, 1986.

239. Schuchard, M., J. P. Landers, N. P. Sandhu, and T. C. Spelsberg. Steroid hormone regulation of nuclear proto-oncogenes. *Endocr. Rev.* 14: 659–669, 1993.

240. Schwabe, J. W. R., L. Chapman, J. T. Finch, and D. Rhodes. The crystal structure of the estrogen receptor DNA-binding domain bound to DNA: how receptors discriminate between their response elements. *Cell* 75: 567–578, 1993.

241. Schwabe, J. W. R., D. Neuhaus, and D. Rhodes. Solution structure of the DNA-binding domain of the oestrogen receptor. *Nature* 348: 458–461, 1990.

242. Segniz, B., and U. Gehring. Mechanism of action of a steroidal antiglucocorticoid in lymphoid cells. *J. Biol. Chem.* 265: 2789–2796, 1990.

243. Sheridan, P. L., R. M. Evans, and K. B. Horwitz. Phosphotryptic peptide analysis of human progesterone receptors. New phosphorylated sites formed in nuclei after hormone treatment. *J. Biol. Chem.* 264: 6520–6528, 1989.

244. Sheridan, P. L., M. D. Francis, and K. B. Horwitz. Synthesis of human progesterone receptors in T47D cells. Nascent A- and B-translational maturation step. *J. Biol. Chem.* 264, 7054–7058, 1989.

245. Sheridan, P. L., N. L. Krett, J. A. Gordon, and K. B. Horwitz. Human progesterone receptor transformation and nuclear down-regulation are independent of phosphorylation. *Mol. Endocrinol.* 2: 1329–1342, 1988.

246. Sicinski, P., J. L. Donaher, S. B. Parker, T. Li, A. Fazeli, H. Gardner, S. Z. Haslam, R. T. Bronson, S. J. Elledge, and R. A. Weinberg. Cyclin D1 provides a link between development and oncogenesis in the retina and breast. *Cell* 82: 621–630, 1995.

247. Simental, J. A., M. Sar, M. V. Lane, F. S. French, and E. M. Wilson. Transcriptional activation and nuclear targeting signals of the human androgen receptor. *J. Biol. Chem.* 266: 510–518, 1991.

248. Singh, P., J. Coe, and W. Hong. A role for retinoblastoma protein in potentiating transcriptional activation by the glucocorticoid receptor. *Nature* 374: 562–565, 1995.

249. Smith, D. F. Dynamics of heat shock protein 90–progesterone receptor binding and disactivation loop model for steroid receptor complexes. *Mol. Endocrinol.* 7: 1418–1429, 1993.

250. Smith, D. F., L. E. Faber, and D.O. Toft. Purification of unactivated progesterone receptor and identification of novel receptor-associated proteins. *J. Biol. Chem.* 265: 3996–4003, 1990.

251. Smith, D. F., and D. O. Toft. Steroid receptors and their associated proteins. *Mol. Endocrinol.* 7: 4–11, 1993.

252. Smith, D. F., D. B. Schowalter, S. L Kost, and D. O. Toft. Reconstitution of progesterone receptor with heat shock proteins. *Mol. Endocrinol.* 4: 1704–1711, 1990.

253. Smith, L. I., D. B. Mendel, J. E. Bodwell, and A. Munck. Phosphorylated sites within the functional domains of the 100-kDa steroid-binding subunit of glucocorticoid receptors. *Biochemistry* 8: 4490–4498, 1989.

254. Strahle, U., G. Klock, and G. Schutz. A DNA sequence of 15 base pairs is sufficient to mediate both glucocorticoid and progesterone induction of gene expression. *Proc. Natl. Acad. Sci. U.S.A.* 84: 7871–7875, 1987.

255. Sullivan, W. P., B. J. Madden, D. J. McCormick, and D. O. Toft. Hormone-dependent phosphorylation of the avian progesterone receptor. *J. Biol. Chem.* 263: 14717–14723, 1988.

256. Superti-Furga, G., G. Bergers, D. Picard, and M. Busslinger. Hormone-dependent transcriptional regulation and cellular transformation by fos-steroid receptor fusion proteins. *Proc. Natl. Acad. Sci. U.S.A.* 88: 5114–5118, 1991.

257. Szyszka, R., G. Kramer, and B. Hardesty. The phosphorylation state of the reticulocyte 90-kDa heat shock protein affects its ability to increase phosphorylation of peptide initiation factor 2 alpha subunit by the heme-sensitive kinase. *Biochemistry* 28: 1435–1438, 1989.

258. Tai, P. K. K., M. W. Albers, H. Chang, L. E. Faber, and S. L. Schreiber. Association of a 59–kilodalton immunophilin with the glucocorticoid receptor complex. *Science* 256: 1315–1318, 1992.

259. Tai, P. K. K., M. W. Albers, D. P. McDonnell, H. Chang, S. L. Schreiber, and L. E. Faber. Potentiation of progesterone receptor–mediated transcription by the immunosuppressant FK506. *Biochemistry* 33: 10666–10671, 1994.

260. Tai, P. K. K., Y. Maeda, K. Nakao, N. G. Wakim, J. L. Duhring, and L. E. Faber. A 59-kilo-dalton protein associated with progestin, estrogen, androgen, and glucocorticoid receptors. *Biochemistry* 25: 5269–5275, 1986.

261. Takimoto, G. S., D. M. Tasset, A. C. Eppert, and K. B. Horwitz. Hormone-induced progesterone receptor phosphorylation consists of sequential DNA-independent and DNA-dependent stages: analysis with zinc finger mutants and the progesterone antagonist ZK98299. *Proc. Natl. Acad. Sci. U.S.A.* 89: 3050–3054, 1992.

262. Tasset, D., L. Tora, C. Fromental, E. Scheer, and P. Chambon. Distinct classes of transcriptional activating domains function by different mechanisms. *Cell* 62: 1177–1187, 1990.

263. Teutsch, G. 11 Beta-substituted 19–norsteroids: at the crossroads between hormone agonists and antagonists. In: *Adrenal Steroid Antagonism*, edited by M. K. Agarwal. New York: deGruyter, 1984, p. 43–75.

264. Teutsch, G., T. Ojasoo, and J. P. Raynaud. 11β-Substituted steroids, an original pathway to antihormones. *J. Steroid Biochem.* 31: 549–565, 1988.

265. Thompson, E. B. Apoptosis and steroid hormones. *Mol. Endocrinol.* 8: 665–673, 1994.

266. Tilley, W. D., M. Marcelli, J. D. Wilson, and M. J. McPhaul. Characterization and expression of a cDNA encoding the human androgen receptor. *Proc. Natl Acad. Sci. U.S.A.* 86: 327–331, 1989.

267. Toft, D. O., and J. Gorski. A receptor molecule for estrogens: isolation from the rat uterus and preliminary characterization. *Proc. Natl. Acad. Sci. U.S.A.* 55: 574–1581, 1966.

268. Tora, L., H. Gronemeyer, B. Turcotte, M. P. Gaub, and P. Chambon. The n-terminal region of the chicken progesterone receptor specifies target gene activation. *Nature* 333: 185–188, 1988.

269. Tora, L., A. Mullick, D. Metzger, M. Ponglikitmongkol, I. Park, and P. Chambon. The cloned human oestrogen receptor contains a mutation which alters its hormone binding properties. *EMBO J.* 8: 1981–1986, 1989.

270. Tora, L., J. White, C. Brou, D. Tasset, N. Webster, E. Scheer, and P. Chambon. The human estrogen receptor has two independent nonacidic transcriptional activation functions. *Cell* 59: 477–487, 1989.

271. Trapman, J., P. Klaassen, G. G. J. M. Kuiper, J. A. G. M. van der Korput, P. W. Faber, H. C. J. van Rooij, A. Geurts van Kessel, M. M. Voorhorst, E. Mulder, and A. O. Brinkmann. Cloning, structure and expression of a cDNA encoding the human androgen receptor. *Biochem. Biophys. Res. Commun.* 153: 241–248, 1988.

272. Truss, M., and M. Beato. Steroid hormone receptors: interaction with deoxyribonucleic acid and transcription factors. *Endocr. Rev.* 14: 459–479, 1993.

272a. Truss, M., J. Bartsch, and M. Beato. Antiprogestins prevent progesterone receptor binding to responsive elements *in vivo*. *Proc. Natl. Acad. Sci. U.S.A.* 91: 11333–11337, 1994.

273. Tsai, M. J., S. Y. Tsai, L. Klein-Hitpass, M. Bagchi, J. F. Elliston, J. Carlstedt-Duke, J. K. Gustafsson, and B. W. O'Malley. Cooperative interactions of steroid hormone receptors with their cognate response elements. *Cold Spring Harb. Symp. Quant. Biol.* 53: 829–833, 1988.

274. Tsai, S. Y., J. Carlstedt-Duke, N. L. Weigel, K. Dahlman, J. A. Gustafsson, M. J. Tsai, and B. W. O'Malley. Molecular interactions of steroid hormone receptor with its enhancer element: evidence for receptor dimer formation. *Cell* 55: 361–369, 1988.

275. Tung, L., M. K. Mohamed, J. P. Hoeffler, G. S. Takimoto, and K. B. Horwitz, K. B. Antagonist-occupied human progesterone B-receptors activate transcription without binding to progesterone response elements and are dominantly inhibited by A-receptors. *Mol. Endocrinol.* 7: 1256–1265, 1993.

276. Turcotte, B., M. E. Meyer, M. T. Bocquel, L. Belanger, and P. Chambon. Repression of the alpha-fetoprotein gene promoter by progesterone and chimeric receptors in the presence of hormones and antihormones. *Mol. Cell. Biol.* 10: 5002–5006, 1990.

277. Umesono, K., and R. M. Evans. Determinants of target gene specificity for steroid/thyroid hormone receptors. *Cell* 57: 1139–1146, 1989.

278. Van Laar, J. H., C. A. Berrevoets, J. Trapman, N. D. Zegers, and A. O. Brinkmann. Hormone-dependent androgen receptor phosphorylation is accompanied by receptor transformation in human lymph node carcinoma of the prostate cells. *J. Biol. Chem.* 266: 3734–3738, 1991.

279. Vegeto, E., M. M. Shahbaz, D. X. Wen, M. E. Goldman, B. W. O'Malley, and D. P. McDonnell. Human progesterone receptor A form is a cell- and promoter-specific repressor of human progesterone receptor B function. *Mol. Endocrinol.* 7: 1244–1255, 1993.

280. Vojtesek, B., and D. P. Lane. Regulation of p53 protein expression in human breast cancer cell lines. *J. Cell Sci.* 105: 607–612, 1993.

281. Walker, A. I., T. Hunt, R. J. Jackson, and C. W. Anderson. Double-stranded DNA induces the phosphorylation of several proteins including the 90 000 mol. wt. heat-shock protein in animal cell extracts. *EMBO J.* 4: 139–145, 1985.

282. Walter, P., S. Green, G. Greene, A. Krust, J. M. Bornert, L. M. Jeltsch, A. Staub, E. Jensen, G. Scrace, M. Waterfield, and P. Chambon. Cloning of the human estrogen receptor cDNA. *Proc. Natl. Acad. Sci. U.S.A.* 82: 7889–7893, 1985.

283. Wang, Y., and C. Prives. Increased and altered DNA binding of human p53 by S and G2/M but not G1 cyclin-dependent kinases. *Nature* 376: 88–91, 1995.

284. Watts, C. K. W., A. Brady, B. Sarcevic, A. deFazio, E. A. Musgrove, and R. L. Sutherland. Antiestrogen inhibition of cell cycle progression in breast cancer cells is associated with inhibition of cyclin-dependent kinase activity and decreased retinoblastoma proteinphosphorylation. *Mol. Endocrinol.* 9: 1804–1813, 1995.

285. Webster, N. J. G., S. Green, J. R. Jin, and P. Chambon. The hormone-binding domains of the estrogen and glucocorticoid receptors contain an inducible transcription activation function. *Cell* 54: 199–207, 1988.

286. Wegener, A. D., and L. R. Jones. Phosphorylation-induced mobility shift in phospholamban in sodium dodecyl sulfate-polyacrylamide gels. *J. Biol. Chem.* 259: 1834–1841, 1984.

287. Wei, L. L., P. L. Sheridan, N. L. Krett, M. D. Francis, D. O. Toft, D. P. Edwards, and K. B. Horwitz. Immunological analysis of human breast cancer progesterone receptors. 2. Structure, phosphorylation, and processing. *Biochemistry* 26: 6262–6272, 1987.

288. Weigel, N. L., J. S. Tash, A. R. Means, W. T. Schrader, and B. W. O'Malley. Phosphorylation of hen progesterone receptor by cAMP-dependent protein kinase. *Biochem. Biophys. Res. Commun.* 102: 513–519, 1981.

289. Weinberg, R. A. The retinoblastoma protein and cell cycle control. *Cell* 81: 323–330, 1995.

290. Weinberger, C., S. M. Hollenberg, M. G. Rosenfeld, and R. M. Evans. Domain structure of human glucocorticoid receptor and its relationship to the v-erb-A oncogene product. *Nature* 318: 670–672, 1985.

291. Weintraub, S. J., K. N. B. Chow, R. X. Luo, S. H. Zhang, S. He, and D. C. Dean. Mechanism of active transcriptional repression by the retinoblastoma protein. *Nature* 375: 812–815, 1995.

292. Welshons, W. V., B. M. Krummel, and J. Gorski. Nuclear localization of unoccupied receptors for glucocorticoids, estrogens, and progesterone in GH3 cells. *Endocrinology* 117: 2140–2147, 1985.

293. White, E. p53, guardian of Rb. *Nature* 371: 21–22, 1994.

294. Wrange, O., P. Eriksson, and T. Perlmann. The purified activated glucocorticoid receptor is a homodimer. *J. Biol. Chem.* 264: 5253–5259, 1989.

295. Xu, Y., and S. Lindquist. Heat-shock protein hsp90 governs the activity of pp$^{60V\text{-}src}$ kinase. *Proc. Natl. Acad. Sci. U.S.A.* 90: 7074–7078, 1993.

296. Yamamoto, K. R. Steroid receptor regulated transcription of specific genes and gene networks. *Annu. Rev. Genet.* 19: 209–252, 1985.

297. Yamamoto, K. R., P. J. Godowski, and D. Picard. Ligand-regulated nonspecific inactivation of receptor function: a versatile mechanism for signal transduction. *Cold Spring Harb. Symp. Quant. Biol.* 53: 803–811, 1988.

298. Yoshinaga, S. K., C. L. Peterson, I. Herskowitz, and K. R. Yamamoto. Roles of SWI1, SWI2, and SWI3 proteins for transcriptional enhancement by steroid receptors. *Science* 258: 1598–1603, 1992.

299. Zhang, Y., C. A. Beck, A. Poletti, D. P. Edwards, and N. L. Weigel. Identification of phosphorylation sites unique to the B form of human progesterone receptor: in vitro phosphorylation by casein kinase II. *J. Biol. Chem.* 269: 31034–31040, 1994.

300. Zhang, Y., C.A. Beck, A. Poletti, D. P. Edwards, and N. L. Weigel. Identification of a group of ser-pro motif hormone-inducible phosphorylation sites in the human progesterone receptor. *Mol. Endocrinol.* 9: 1029–1040, 1995.

301. Zilliacus, J., K. Dahlman-Wright, A. Wright, J. A. Gustafsson, and J. Carlstedt-Duke. DNA binding specificity of mutant glucocorticoid receptor DNA-binding domains. *J. Biol. Chem.* 266: 3101–3106, 1991.

302. Zilliacus, J., A. P. H. Wright, J. Carlstedt-Duke, and J. A. Gustafsson. Structural determinants of DNA-binding specificity by steroid receptors. *Mol. Endocrinol.* 9: 389–400, 1995.

16. The roles of cytochromes P-450 in the regulation of steroidogenesis

PETER F. HALL | *Department of Endocrinology and Metabolism, Division of Medicine, Prince of Wales Hospital, Randwick, New South Wales, Australia*

CYTOCHROMES P-450 constitute a superfamily of enzymes that appear to have evolved to serve as agents of detoxification by facilitating removal of lipophilic toxins from the body. At some point in evolution, cytochromes P-450 took on the additional role of steroid hormone synthesis, and six of these enzymes became involved in the synthesis of such hormones. By definition, cytochromes are heme proteins. The archetypal reaction catalyzed by cytochromes P-450 in an atmosphere of $^{18}O_2$ with a substrate RH, can be expressed as follows:

$$R\text{—}H + NADPH + H^+ + {}^{18}O_2 \rightarrow R - {}^{18}OH + H_2{}^{18}O + NADP^+$$

$$(16\text{–}1)$$

A number of important features of P-450 are illustrated in this statement. First, the enzyme uses atmospheric or molecular oxygen and not the oxygen of water. Second, the reaction is called *monooxygenation* (catalyzed by a monooxygenase) since only one of the atoms of oxygen appears in the product while the second is reduced to water, in contrast to *dioxygenases* in which both atoms appear in the product. Third, the product is more polar than the substrate, and this helps to exclude the product from the hydrophobic plasma membrane through which lipophilic toxins enter cells. This effect is greatly magnified when the new hydroxyl group is conjugated to such polar groups as sulfate or glucuronide. This mechanism provides the main defense against lipophilic toxins. Certain lipophilic substances such as steroids and prostaglandins remain in the body after they have served their roles in metabolism. These substances are called *endogenous substrates*, and P-450 helps to remove them from the body in the same way that these enzymes remove xenobiotics or exogenous substrates. The reactions to be discussed in this chapter involve specific cytochromes P-450 that alter steroid substrates in such a way as to provide those features of the steroid hormones that are specifically recognized by receptors and other intra- and extracellular molecules that enable these steroids to act as hormones. The removal of xenobiotics from the body does not require a high degree of specificity so that drug metabolism by P-450 permits a single species of P-450 to act on many substrates and at several atoms in any one substrate molecule. By contrast, the steroidogenic cytochromes P-450 are relatively specific. Fourth, Equation 16–1 shows the characteristic stoichiometry of RH:NADPH: O_2: of 1: 1: 1.

Equation 16–1 does not reveal the need for the reduction of P-450 by NADPH. Microsomal cytochromes P-450 use a single flavoprotein reductase containing flavin mononucleotide (FMN) and flavin adenine dinucleotide (FAD) for this purpose. Mitochondrial cytochromes P-450 use two electron carriers in succession—a flavoprotein reductase and an iron–sulfur protein. The microsomal electron carrier is called *NADPH cytochrome P-450 reductase*. The mitochondrial iron–sulfur proteins are referred to by the suffix *doxin,* for example, *adrenodoxin* for the adrenal protein and *testodoxin* for the testicular protein. The mitochondrial protein that reduces the iron–sulfur protein is referred to as, adrenodoxin *reductase*. Finally, Equation 16–1 should not suggest that the cytochromes P-450 are capable of catalyzing only hydroxylation of substrates. It will be shown later (see INDIVIDUAL CYTOCHROMES P-450) that some of these enzymes are capable of cleaving C—C bonds, although such cleavage requires prior hydroxylation of the substrate. Moreover, in metabolizing toxins hepatic cytochromes P-450 catalyze many other types of reactions.

PROPERTIES OF CYTOCHROMES P-450

Chemical Properties

All cytochromes P-450 contain one molecule of heme per molecule of enzyme. In contrast to other heme proteins, the heme is not covalently bound to the protein but lies in a hydrophobic pocket, which allows the substrate to bind nearby. The manner in which the heme binds the protein moiety gives all cytochromes P-450 certain common properties that are conveniently considered here. The iron of the heme is capable of existing with a valence of 5 or 6 (penta- or hexacoordinate) of which four bonds secure association with the prosthetic group by binding the four pyrrole nitrogens, and one bond is made to a specific cysteine residue in the protein. The sixth (potential) bond is to an unknown group, which may vary from one P-450 to another, and may be water or an amino acid residue in the protein such as histidine. The four Fe—N bonds lie in the plane of the heme ring (planar bonds), whereas the fifth and sixth bonds lie at right angles to the plane of the ring (axial bonds). The fifth bond is made to a thiolate ion associated with the sulfur of the specific cysteine mentioned above. In the pentacoordinate state, the iron is displaced from the plane of the heme ring and the electrons of the *d* orbital in the iron are so arranged as to adopt the so-called high-spin form. In contrast, in the hexacoordinate form, the iron lies in the plane of the ring and assumes the low-spin form as shown below in the diagrams. The fifth thiolate bond is responsible for characteristic spectral properties that distinguish the whole family of cytochromes P-450 from all other heme proteins.

Spectral Properties

Absorption

Native spectra. All cytochromes P-450 show a conspicuous peak at 420 nm in absorption spectroscopy. This is known as the *Soret peak* and results from the conjugated double-bond system of the heme. The molar absorption and the exact location of the peak are influenced by the protein moiety and therefore differ from one P-450 to another. In the absence of substrate, all cytochromes P-450 show low-spin hexacoordinate iron. When any substrate binds any cytochrome P-450 the sixth bond is lost, the iron is displaced from the plane of the ring and assumes the high-spin form. In this form the Soret peak is displaced to approximately 390 nm—the so-called substrate-induced spectral shift, which is illustrated in the graph at the top of the facing page.

This shift can be measured by difference (substrate-induced difference spectrum). The spectrophotometer is set to subtract the absorbance of enzyme plus solvent

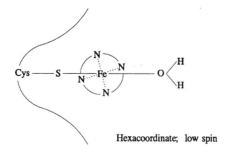

Hexacoordinate; low spin

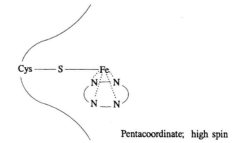

Pentacoordinate; high spin

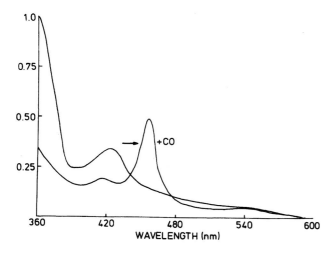

(reference cuvette) from that of enzyme plus substrate (sample cuvette).

The high-spin form (ES) shows a positive peak at 390 nm while the low-spin form (E) shows a negative peak or trough at 420 nm because absorbance of this form is subtracted from that in the sample cuvette. The peak plus trough (A_{390}–A_{420}) is known as a type I difference spectrum and the following diagram illustrates a case in which somewhat less than half of the molecules of P-450 present in the cuvette are bound to substrate. These spectral properties of P-450 can be summarized as follows:

Substrate	Coordination valence	Spin state	Soret peak, nm
Absent	6	Low	420
Present	5	High	390

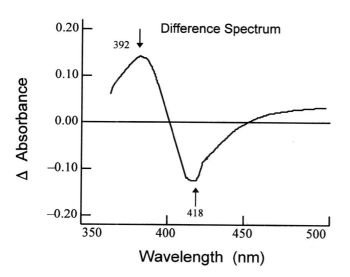

CO spectrum. The most widely used spectral property of all cytochromes P-450 is that which results from the binding of CO. Reduced heme proteins (Fe^{2+}) bind CO as the sixth ligand. This binding is associated with a shift of the Soret peak. Oxidized P-450 does not bind CO. On chemical or biological reduction, all heme proteins bind CO, and in most cases this results in a shift in the Soret peak of a few nanometers to longer wavelength (the so-called red shift). With all cytochromes P-450 this shift with binding of CO is unusually extensive: 420→450 nm. This spectral shift can be measured by difference—reduced P-450–CO complex minus oxidized P-450 plus CO (CO is unbound and does not contribute to the signal at 450 nm). This property is common to all cytochromes P-450 and provides a universal method for identifying any member of the P-450 family. This fundamental property of the spectral shift in the Soret peak gives these enzymes their nickname (pigment-450) and provides an accurate measurement of the concentration of P-450 in a given sample by using a molar extinction coefficient of 91,000 liters · mole^{-1} · cm^{-1} for the absorbance of the P-450–CO complex when the above spectrum is measured by difference.

The P-450 Cycle

To initiate monooxygenation, all cytochromes P-450 must undergo reduction of the heme iron by electrons transported from reduced pyridine nucleotide via the electron carriers described above. P-450, represented here by iron, is oxidized by atmospheric oxygen during monooxygenation. The P-450 is immediately reduced again to permit continued monooxygenase activity. Reduction of P-450 requires the transfer of two electrons to the iron. The cycle of alternating oxidation and reduction constitutes what is conveniently called the P-450 cycle, which can be considered as seven consecutive steps from oxidized P-450 through reduced P-450 and back to the oxidized form to start the cycle again. (See the diagram on page 416.)

Step 1—Binding of substrate. Oxidized P-450 binds substrate with the spectral consequences discussed above. These changes result from displacement of the iron from the plane of the ring with the conversion of the iron to the high-spin state. This step facilitates the delivery of the first electron to the iron, which then becomes reduced.

Step 2—Reduction of enzyme–substrate.

Step 3—Binding of oxygen. The reduced enzyme–substrate complex binds oxygen.

Step 4—Activation of oxygen. A second electron reduces the oxygen bound to the reduced iron as the result of rearrangement of electrons within the complex.

Step 5—Monooxygenation. Monooxygenation begins with reduction of one atom of oxygen to water.

Step 6—Completion of monooxygenation. Monooxygenation is completed with transfer of the remaining atom of oxygen to the substrate, which now becomes the product. The complex Steps 5 and 6 are not fully understood.

Step 7—Completion of the cycle. The hydroxyl group of the product produces repulsive forces within the hydrophobic active site, which facilitates removal of the product. The enzyme is now ready to start the cycle again.

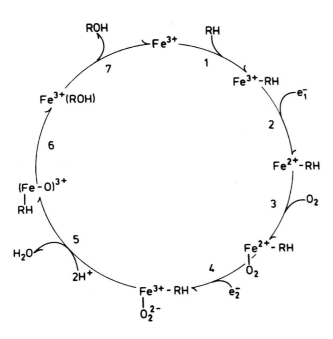

It should be understood that reducing the cycle to seven separate steps, although useful for descriptive purposes, distorts the smooth flow of the overall reaction in which the individual steps do not occur as discrete reactions, as the diagram might suggest.

The Mechanism of P-450 Enzyme Activity

Considerable interest is shown in the mechanisms of the enzymatic activities of cytochromes P-450 because of the possibility of modifying these activities with inhibitors that are based on the steps involved in the monooxygenase reactions (mechanism-based inhibitors). These reactions are thought to begin with hydro-

gen abstraction from a carbon atom of the substrate that is appropriately placed in the active site close to the "active" oxygen bound to the heme iron. Hydrogen abstraction produces two radicals—a carbonyl radical in the substrate and a hydroxyl radical bound to the iron:

$$R—CH_2—CH_2—CH_3 + (Fe—O)^{3+} \rightarrow$$
$$R—CH_2—\dot{C}H—CH_3 + \dot{O}H—Fe^{2+}$$

At this point two alternatives are possible. The first leads to a hydroxylated product, by way of recombination of the two radicals, yielding a hydroxylated substrate—now the product:

$$R—CH_2—\dot{C}H—CH_3 + \dot{O}H—Fe^{2+} \rightarrow$$
$$R—CH_2—\underset{\underset{OH}{|}}{CH}—CH_3 + Fe^{3+}$$

Alternatively, and less frequently, second hydrogen abstraction gives rise to an alkene by way of a two-radical intermediate,

$$R—CH_2—\dot{C}H—CH_3 + \dot{O}H—Fe^{2+} \rightarrow$$
$$R—\dot{C}H—\dot{C}H—CH_3$$

which rearranges to the alkene $R—CH=CH—CH_3$.

It is generally assumed that all reactions catalyzed by cytochromes P-450 represent variations on one or the other of these mechanisms. What directs the reaction one way or the other is not known.

Reduction of Cytochrome P-450

It has been concluded that the rate of reduction of the enzyme by electrons from the electron carriers does not determine the rates of monooxygenase reactions. However, it will be shown that the reduction of particular forms of P-450 can influence the pathways of the reaction(s) catalyzed and hence the nature and number of the products formed (see later under *Pathways to Steroid Hormones*). It should be pointed out here that an additional electron carrier, namely cytochrome b_5, can alter the course of reactions catalyzed by microsomal P-450. Possible mechanisms for these differences will be discussed later with the individual P-450 enzymes.

SYNTHESIS OF STEROID HORMONES

Nomenclature

In general, steroidogenic enzymes are named according to the conventions of classical enzymology. There are three exceptions to these conventions among the steroidogenic P-450 enzymes: *(1)* the conversion of cholesterol to pregnenolone is catalyzed by a single enzyme called "P-450 side-chain cleavage enzyme" or "cytochrome P-450 side-chain cleavage" (P-450$_{scc}$); *(2)* the conversion of progesterone to androstenedione is catalyzed by a single enzyme, 17α-hydroxylase/lyase. To emphasize the important mechanistic similarities between these two enzymes, the terms "C$_{27}$ side-chain cleavage P-450" and "C$_{21}$ side-chain cleavage P-450" (C$_{27scc}$ and C$_{21scc}$) have much to recommend them. Since the lyase activity of C$_{21scc}$ is not always expressed, it is convenient to refer to the two activities as "17α-hydroxylase" and "C$_{17,20}$ lyase." When both activities are expressed the term "hydroxylase/lyase" can be used; *(3)* the conversion of 18-hydroxycorticosterone to aldosterone will be referred to here as "aldehyde synthetase" activity. This reaction constitutes the last step in the synthesis of aldosterone.

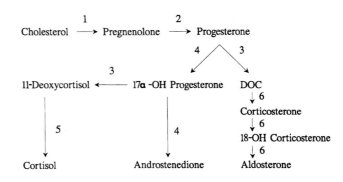

1: Side-chain cleavage P$_{450}$
2: Dehydrogenase/Isomerase
3: 21-Hydroxylase
4: 17α-Hydroxylase/Lyase
5: 11β-Hydroxylase
6: Aldosterone Synthetase

Pathways to Steroid Hormones

The steroid hormones are synthesized from cholesterol by means of the six enzymes shown in the diagram at the top of the next column.

Of these enzymes, numbers 1, 3, 4, 5, and 6 are cytochromes P-450. Number 2, dehydrogenase/isomerase, is not a P-450 and will therefore not be discussed here.

INDIVIDUAL CYTOCHROMES P-450

C$_{27}$ Side-Chain Cleavage P-450

This enzyme catalyzes a reaction that takes place in three steps, of which the first two are typical monooxygenase hydroxylation reactions at C$_{22}$ and C$_{20}$ in that order, and the third step leads to the cleavage of the

intervening C$_{20}$—C$_{22}$ bond resulting in the formation of pregnenolone and isocapraldehyde, as shown below.

Isocapraldehyde was the first cytochrome P-450 to be purified apart from the bacterial (camphor) enzyme. It was isolated from bovine adrenocortical mitochondria by conventional chromatography and was found to be homogeneous by gel electrophoresis and immunological methods. Clearly the three reactions are catalyzed by a single protein. Moreover all of the disappearing cholesterol can be accounted for as pregnenolone. The presence of the two hydroxylated intermediates was first demonstrated by using [^{14}C]cholesterol as substrate so that the very small amounts of these compounds could be detected. This still left open the question of which of the two hydroxylation reactions occurs first. Subsequently, work with mitochondrial extracts on a very large scale was performed to

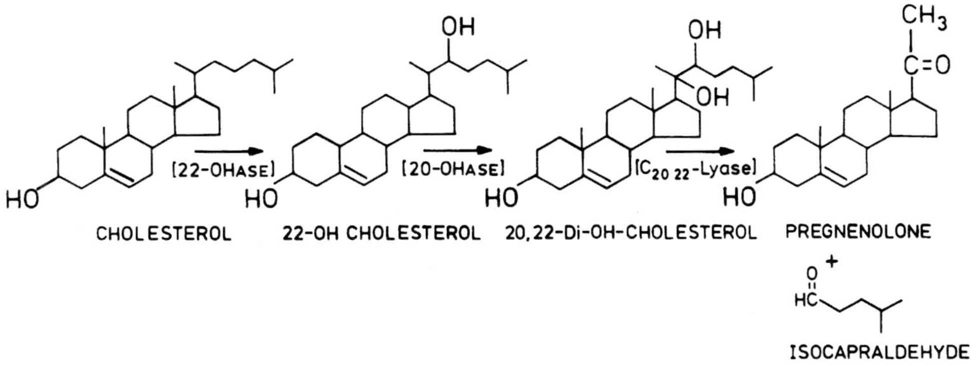

CHOLESTEROL   [22-OHASE]→   22-OH CHOLESTEROL   [20-OHASE]→   20,22-Di-OH-CHOLESTEROL   [C$_{20,22}$-Lyase]→   PREGNENOLONE

ISOCAPRALDEHYDE

determine the order of the two reactions. This work showed that hydroxylation at C_{22} precedes that at C_{20}. In later kinetic and competition studies it was found that isocapraldehyde possesses a single active site. This suggested that the final step involving cleavage of a C—C bond was catalyzed by a cytochrome P-450. Since such a cleavage step was not known to be among the reactions catalyzed by any of the known cytochromes P-450, including those not involved in steroid hormone synthesis, it was important to determine whether the cleavage step uses the heme group in a typical P-450 or monooxygenase reaction. This was demonstrated by showing that each of the three steps gives a typical photochemical action spectrum. The procedure is based upon three properties of P-450–CO: *(1)* this complex is enzymatically inactive, *(2)* it absorbs light with a peak at 450 nm (hence the name P-450), and *(3)* it is light sensitive, that is, light causes breakdown of the P-450–CO complex. For each of the three reactions in side-cleavage it was found that inhibition of enzymatic activity by CO was reversed when the reaction was performed in light of various wavelengths. Of the wavelengths examined, light of 450 nm, being the best absorbed, was most effective in reversing inhibition by CO. Evidently all three steps are typical P-450 reactions, which shows that heme is necessary for the cleavage step.

This is the classical demonstration that P-450 is involved in any enzymatic activity, a conclusion supported by measurement of the stoichiometry of the individual steps and that of the overall reaction. The stoichiometry of each step was that found for P-450 monooxygenation, that is, one mole of substrate plus one mole of NADPH, plus one mole of H^+, plus one mole of O_2, per mole of product. The overall reaction can be written as follows:

$$C_{27}H_{46}O + 3O_2 + 3NADPH + 3H^+ \rightarrow C_{21}H_{32}O_2 + C_6H_{12}O + 4H_2O + 3NADP^+$$

These findings established for the first time the role of typical P-450 monooxygenation in cleavage of a C—C bond. It was known that highly purified P-450$_{scc}$ contains up to 0.8 moles of heme per mole of enzyme. It has sometimes been considered that a heme content of 1.0 moles per mole of enzyme is a criterion of purity in isolated cytochromes P-450. However, the heme is not covalently bound to the protein, so heme is lost during purification, and this criterion therefore is not applicable. It is clear that different cytochromes P-450 lose heme to varying degrees during purification, so it is reasonable to conclude that P-450$_{scc}$ contains one mole of heme per mole of enzyme. This is consistent with a single active site or, at the very least, a region of the molecule capable of binding substrate and inter-

mediates close enough to the heme to permit monooxygenation to proceed three times in succession. This evidence, taken together with that from another P-450 that also cleaves a C—C bond (C_{21scc}), indicates that there is a single active site.

A detailed study of the binding of substrate and the intermediates of C_{27scc} using absorption spectroscopy and electron spin resonance revealed the presence of a single binding site for each of these substances with the dissociation constants (Kd) and dissociation frequency (Df) shown in the accompanying table.

	Kd, nm	Df, S^{-1}
22R-OH cholesterol	4.9	5
20R,22-DiOH cholesterol	81.0	
Pregnenolone	2900.0	

Unfortunately the insolubility of cholesterol has prevented the determination of reliable values for this substrate. Nevertheless it is clear that each of the two intermediates is tightly bound to the active site of the enzyme. This is in marked contrast to the product of the reaction, which dissociates readily from the active site. Because the intermediates are tightly bound and thus have little opportunity to accumulate in the medium, these substances are largely present in stoichiometric amounts—that is, one mole per mole of enzyme—in contrast to the product, which is free to accumulate in the medium. This accounts for the difficulty in isolating the intermediates and is the reason that very large amounts of enzyme are necessary for the isolation of the intermediates of the reaction.

These considerations mean that the P-450 cycle must be modified in such a way that the product of the first step becomes the substrate for the second step without leaving the active site and so on. After the third step, pregnenolone dissociates freely, and the whole process is repeated, beginning with the binding of cholesterol. Evidently, whatever conformational change is precipitated by the binding of the substrate to promote entry of the first electron (step 1), this conformation must be maintained by the retention of the intermediate after the first cycle is complete. Presumably, the enzyme does not change to the conformation of the substrate-free form and back again to the form that starts a new cycle, a pattern that would occur if the intermediates were to dissociate and reassociate.

The product pregnenolone inhibits the side-chain cleavage reaction by binding to a site other than the active site. When this steroid is added to the pure enzyme it induces a spectral shift that is the inverse of the type I or substrate-induced shift—that is, peak at

PROGESTERONE   [17α-OHASE]   17α-OH PROGESTERONE   [C$_{17, 20}$-Lyase]   ANDROSTENEDIONE

420 nm and trough at 390 nm instead of the reverse. This shift is called "inverse type I" and is to be distinguished from a type II shift induced by nitrogenous bases such as aniline and pyridine. The type II shift was put to good effect by Sheets and Vickery, who synthesized steroids with side-chains at C_{17} of various lengths, each with a terminal primary amine. When the amine was sufficiently close to the Fe, a type II shift was recorded. It appears that C_{17} must be within 5.5 Å of the Fe to interact with it. This would mean that C_{22} is close enough to the iron-bound oxygen to interact, which opens the question of possible movement of substrate relative to active site.

C_{20} is an additional 1.54 Å from the Fe. There is some evidence to suggest that a conformational change occurs in the enzyme between the three steps in the reaction. Such a change could bring C_{20} closer to the oxygen molecule and trigger the arrival of the first electron for the next (that is, second) step.

In aqueous buffer, P-450$_{scc}$ aggregates into oligomeric forms—tetramers, octamers, and hexadecamers. The hexadecamers have been studied by electron microscopy. The activities of these forms were investigated by centrifugation through gradients with excess substrate, adrenodoxin, adrenodoxin reductase, and NADPH. It was found that side-chain cleavage activity, that is, production of pregnenolone, is seen only in fractions corresponding to the hexadecamer (16 subunits, MW 850,000). The state of the active form in the inner mitochondrial membrane is unknown.

C_{21} Side-Chain Cleavage P-450 (Hydroxylase/Lyase)

The hydroxylase/lyase reaction represents a second example of C—C bond cleavage catalyzed by a P-450 enzyme. The enzyme converts C_{21} to C_{19} steroids as shown in the reactions above. The same enzyme converts pregnenolone to the corresponding Δ^5 steroid, that is, dehydroepiandrosterone. Since the adrenal synthesizes both C_{19} and 17α-hydroxy-C_{21} steroids, it was originally assumed that the hydroxylase and lyase functions resulted from the activities of two separate

enzymes. Classical enzymology, including purification, immunochemistry, kinetics, and affinity alkylation of the active site, demonstrated conclusively that a single enzyme catalyzes both reactions. How the enzyme permits accumulation of 17α-hydroxy-C_{21} steroids was at first a puzzle: one enzyme should presumably allow both reactions to occur in the absence of specific regulation. It is well known that microsomes from testis produce C_{19} androgens but little or no 17α-hydroxy-C_{21} steroid, whereas adrenal microsomes produce both types of steroids but much more C_{21} steroid than C_{19}. The evidence from protein chemistry indicated that adrenal and testicular microsomes contain one and the same P-450$_{c21scc}$ enzyme. It is also known that there is only a single P-450 reductase. Clearly the difference must lie in the microsomes and not in the proteins. By a process of elimination it was found that testicular microsomes contain much more P-450 reductase and cytochrome b_5 than adrenal microsomes. Cytochrome b_5 can reduce microsomal P-450 with the aid of an additional electron carrier; the role of this cytochrome is considered later.

Reconstitution of the C_{21} side-chain cleavage system from homogeneous proteins revealed that the flavoprotein reductase can support one or both reactions depending on the concentration of the reductase relative to that of P-450. Increasing concentrations of reductase promote increasing production of C_{19} steroids—that is, increasing expression of lyase activity. At low concentrations of reductase, 17α-hydroxy-C_{21} steroid (for example, 17α-hydroxyprogesterone) predominates. Although the K_m of hydroxylase/lyase for the reductase is higher for the lyase activity than for hydroxylase activity, V_{max} is the same for both activities; that is, given enough reductase, the two reactions reach the same velocity. Addition of exogenous reductase to adrenal microsomes causes stimulation of lyase relative to hydroxylase, making these microsomes behave like testicular microsomes, producing high levels of C_{19} androgens. Addition of anti-reductase to testicular microsomes causes them to behave like adrenal microsomes, accumulating high levels of 17α-hydroxy-C_{21} steroid. Clearly the rate of electron transport to this P-450 influences the outcome of the reaction, which is entirely to be expected because lyase activity requires a second turn of the P-450 cycle and hence a second pair of electrons. The greater the concentration of reduced reductase, the greater the electron or reductive drive and hence the greater the production of C_{19} steroids as the result of increased lyase activity. The high K_m for lyase activity sets a limit to the rate of synthesis of the product of lyase activity unless excess reduced reductase is available.

As with C_{27} side-chain cleavage, it is necessary to consider whether the two reactions of hydroxylation and lyase activity are catalyzed by two active sites or one. Studies of competition between substrates for the two reactions by two synthetic inhibitors, inhibition by anti–P-450c_{21scc} together with substrate-induced difference spectra and equilibrium dialysis, all support the existence of a single active site. This conclusion was strongly supported by affinity alkylation of the enzyme by the substrate analogue 17α-bromoacetoxyprogesterone. The active bromine of this substrate analogue causes electrophilic attack on a unique cysteine residue at the active site and causes inactivation of both activities with a first-order rate constant that shows the same value of $t_{1/2}$ for both hydroxylation and lyase activities. Moreover both substrates (progesterone and 17α-hydroxyprogesterone) protect hydroxylation and catalysis against inactivation by the substrate analogue, and the two substrates can be shown to compete for a single active site. This conclusion is in keeping with the fact that both the hydroxylation and the lyase activities of the enzyme require the heme moiety in a typical monooxygenation reaction. Since there is somewhat less than one heme per molecule of enzyme (presumably one heme per molecule in situ), the two reactions must use the same heme in a single active site. This serves to reinforce the similarities between the two side-chain cleavage cytochromes P-450.

It is of interest that in adrenal glands of rat and certain other species, the relevant gene is not expressed, and these species therefore secrete corticosterone instead of cortisol. However, in all species the gene must be expressed in the gonads, both male and female, since both hydroxylase and lyase activities are required for the synthesis of androgens and estrogens by the gonads.

One of the most unusual features of P-450c_{21scc} is seen in the porcine enzyme which, in the presence of cytochrome b_5, forms two entirely unexpected products in the form of Δ^{16} C_{19} steroids, namely 3β-hydroxy-$\Delta^{5,16}$ androstadien-3-one from progesterone. These steroids are formed in the testis of the pig and act as pheromones.

C_{21} HYDROXYLASE

The C_{21} hydroxylase enzyme is essential for the synthesis of corticosteroids—both glucocorticoids and mineralocorticoids. In fact, C_{21} hydroxylase catalyzes a single hydroxylation reaction, in the form of a typical monooxygenation reaction, which results in the conversion of progesterone to 11-deoxycorticosterone (DOC) or that of 17α-hydroxyprogesterone to 11-deoxycortisol. That reaction is shown in the diagram below. There are at least three features of interest concerning this enzyme. First, it was the first cytochrome P-450 in which the monooxygenase mechanism was demonstrated. Second, it is subject to the greatest number of mutations leading to the commonest forms of congenital diseases of the adrenal cortex, namely congenital adrenal hyperplasia. Third, amino acid homology between C_{21scc} and C_{21}-hydroxylase is greater than that between any other pair of steroidogenic cytochromes P-450. It would appear that these two enzymes have evolved from a single microsomal P-450.

It has been proposed that in the synthesis of the 17α-hydroxy-C_{21} steroid cortisol, the 17-hydroxylation must precede 21-hydroxylation. It will be of interest to compare the relative binding affinities of the enzyme for Δ^4-3-ketosteroids—for example, progesterone—as opposed to Δ^5-3β-hydroxysteroids—for example, pregnenolone—since these affinities could determine the specific sequence of reactions in the pathway to cortisol. This sequence would in turn determine the relative importance of the two alternative pathways called Δ^4 and Δ^5, according to which of the two enzymes acts first. The porcine enzyme shows greater affinity for pregnenolone than for progesterone, which is consistent with the known preference for the Δ^5 pathway in this species.

11β-HYDROXYLASE AND ALDEHYDE SYNTHETASE

The last step in the synthesis of cortisol involves the 11β-hydroxylation of 11-deoxycortisol by the 11β-hydroxylase P-450 (P-450$_{11}$) located in the inner mito-

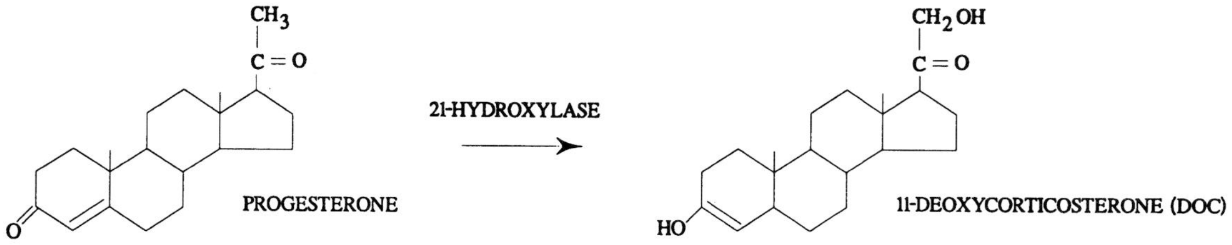

21-HYDROXYLASE

PROGESTERONE

11-DEOXYCORTICOSTERONE (DOC)

Biosynthesis of Aldosterone

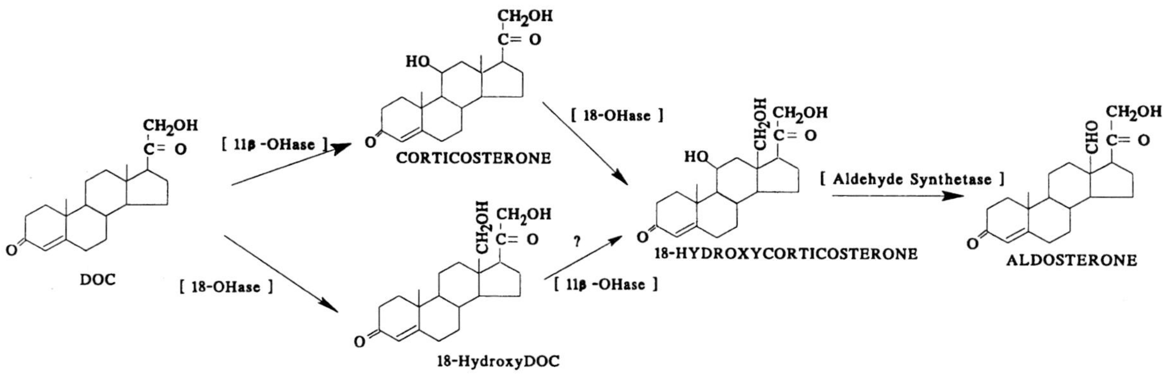

chondrial membrane. This enzyme is essential for synthesis of cortisol and corticosterone in the zona fasciculata, whereas in the zona glomerulosa the synthesis of aldosterone proceeds by way of 11β-hydroxylation and 18-hydroxylation, followed by aldehyde synthetase activity, as shown in the diagram at the top of the page. It is convenient to discuss the synthesis of cortisol, corticosterone, and aldosterone together. When bovine 11β-hydroxylase was first purified from whole adrenal cortex, a single protein was isolated and the pure enzyme was found to catalyze 11β-hydroxylation of DOC and corticosterone, 18-hydroxylation of both steroids, and the synthesis of aldosterone. When the two zones of the cortex were separated by dissection, it was found that mitochondria from glomerulosa produced aldosterone at a considerably greater rate than those from fasciculata, in keeping with the well-known fact that this steroid is synthesized by glomerulosa but not by fasciculata. However, cholate extracts of mitochondria from the two zones produced aldosterone at the same rate. It appears either that mitochondria from fasciculata inhibit an activity (aldehyde synthetase) that is present both in a cholate extract of fasciculata mitochondria and in the pure enzyme, or that mitochondria from glomerulosa contain a factor that specifically stimulates the aldehyde synthetase activity of the enzyme. Both 18-hydroxylation and aldehyde synthetase are inhibited in cholate extracts of mitochondria from fasciculata and granulosa by antibodies raised against the pure enzyme. The same two reactions, catalyzed by extracts of mitochondria from the two zones, were inhibited by two synthetic competitive inhibitors of P-450. The inhibition of the two activities in these experiments showed the same relationship between the degree of inhibition and the concentration of inhibitor (antibodies or synthetic inhibitors). Moreover all three reactions required for the synthesis of aldosterone show classical action spectra of P-450 heme reactions, and the stoichiometry for each of the steps is substrate: $NADPH:O_2:H^+$ of 1:1:1:1. Clearly all the evidence in the bovine adrenal points to the existence of a single enzyme capable of catalyzing the three reactions. Aldehyde synthetase activity in intact mitochondria is confined to the glomerulosa. These findings also apply to the porcine adrenal.

The molecular biology of 11β-hydroxylase is discussed later (see under Cytochrome P-450 11β-Hydroxylase), where it is pointed out that the rat and human systems are quite different from the bovine and the porcine. In rat and human it appears that more than one gene for 11β-hydroxylase is expressed. One gene in glomerulosa expresses a protein capable of synthesizing aldosterone, whereas the corresponding gene expressed in fasciculata gives rise to an enzyme capable of 11β-hydroxylation and 18-hydroxylation but not aldosterone synthetase activity. These findings are in agreement with the known functions of the two zones: the fasciculata produces cortisol and 18-hydroxycorticosterone, whereas glomerulosa produces aldosterone. The function of 18-hydroxycorticosterone, if any, is unknown.

In the meantime an important system for the regulation of the production of aldosterone was revealed in the mitochrondia from glomerulosa. Natarajan and Harding found that ascorbate promotes the synthesis of cortisol by mitochondria from fasciculata over and above maximal levels seen with NADPH. This suggests that additional reductive drive could stimulate the activity of 11β-hydroxylase. The same workers later reported stimulation of the production of aldosterone by ascorbate. The concentrations of the two electron carriers adrenodoxin and adrenodoxin reductase are the same in both inner membranes. Evidently these molecules were not responsible for additional reductive drive. Again, there is a small but significant difference in the concentration of total P-450 and 11β-hydroxylase in the two membranes, both values being higher in membranes from fasciculata. Rotenone shows no effect on any of the three steps involved in the synthesis of aldosterone. It was therefore decided to measure various reductase activities in mitochondria from the two zones when the usual electron-transport system involved in oxidative phosphorylation was inhibited by rotenone. This would determine whether a pathway exists for electron transport capable of reducing P-450_{11}—one that is not inhibited by rotenone.

For this purpose rates of reduction of the chemical electron acceptor DCPIP and the physiological acceptors cytochrome c and cytochrome P-450 were measured. Malate and other Krebs cycle intermediates reduce DCPIP and the two cytochromes in mitochondria from the two zones at the same rates. At the same time, in outer mitochondrial membrane there is a system of electron transport that includes a flavoprotein, a specific outer membrane cytochrome b, and a terminal acceptor in the form of semidehydroascorbate reductase (SDAR). This system shows two important properties, namely that it accepts electrons from ascorbate and that it is not inhibited by rotenone. It was found that NADH causes reduction of SDAR twice as rapidly by the membranes from glomerulosa as by those of fasciculata. Moreover NADH reduces cytochrome c more than three times as rapidly in mitochondria from glomerulosa as in mitochondria from fasciculata. Although the molecular basis for these differences remains to be determined, it is clear that electron or reductive drive from NADH is greater in mitochondria from glomerulosa than in those from fasciculata. It is known that this system of electron transport exists in the outer mitochondrial membranes of other organs, like liver. The question remains, can NADH supply electrons for the synthesis of aldosterone?

It became clear that ascorbate plus NADH but not ascorbate alone, acts synergistically with $NADP^+$ plus malate in supporting aldehyde synthetase. Ascorbate plus NADH alone was without effect, and the complete system (malate, $NADP^+$, ascorbate, and NADH) was without effect on 11β- or 18-hydroxylation in mitochondria from either zone. The complete system increases the low level of production of aldosterone by the organelles from fasciculata incubated with malate and $NADP^+$, whereas with those from glomerulosa there is a doubling of the relatively high levels seen with maximal concentrations of malate plus $NADP^+$.

In considering the role of electron drive in determining the number of turns of the P-450 cycle that can take place, the cycle itself needs to be kept in mind. When a single hydroxylation is performed—for example, 21-hydroxylation—the relatively polar product is readily released from the active site. In contrast, when the initial product of a multistep P-450 reaction, instead of being released, remains to become the substrate for another turn of the cycle, then the fate of the intermediate could be either that of leaving the active site or that of continuing through the P-450 reactions. In the synthesis of aldosterone, if [^{14}C]DOC is used as substrate, addition of unlabeled intermediates (corticosterone, 18-hyroxycorticosterone, or DOC) does not decrease to more than a trivial degree the rate of appearance of [^{14}C] in the product—aldosterone. In other words the [^{14}C] intermediates do not leave the active site to exchange with the exogenous unlabeled intermediates. Each molecule of intermediate must either leave the active site and accumulate in the medium or remain bound in the active site to serve as substrate for another turn of the cycle. Presumably the rate of reduction of P-450 will be one factor in determining the proportion of molecules that stay in the active site; the greater the flow of electrons, the greater the possibility that molecules of intermediate will be swept into the pathway to complete the multistep reaction, and hence the greater the rate of production of aldosterone. It will be recalled that addition of reductase to the C_{21scc} enzyme increased the proportion of molecules that completed both cycles as opposed to those that underwent only the first step and accumulated as 17α-hydroxyprogesterone in the medium. The more rapidly the P-450 is reduced the more molecules it can process through the next step in the pathway.

It would appear that the possibility of a given molecule completing the pathway is the outcome of a balance between the rate of reduction of cytochrome P-450 on the one hand and the rate of dissociation of the enzyme from the active site on the other hand. The synthesis of aldosterone requires three turns of the cycle, so the influx of extra electrons from ascorbate is important to allow sufficient reductive drive to produce significant amounts of aldosterone. It is worthy to note that even fasciculata can produce small amounts of aldosterone with ascorbate and NADH and that mitochondria from this zone produce 18-hydroxycorticosterone as well as the major functional product—cortisol. It is also significant that under all conditions

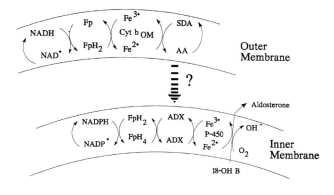

examined, the rate of 11β-hydroxylation is at least one order of magnitude greater than that of either of the last two steps and that aldehyde synthetase is always by far the slowest step, as illustrated above.

It remains to point out that the mechanism of transfer of electrons from outer to inner mitochondrial membrane has not been determined. It has been proposed that transfer of electrons from ascorbate to adrenodoxin allows communication between the auxiliary (ascorbate) pathways to feed into the conventional pathway in the inner mitochondrial membrane electron-transport system (that is, adrenodoxin and reductase). These ideas have recently received strong support from studies showing a direct relationship between the concentration of reduced pyridine nucleotides in glomerulosa cells and the rate of synthesis of aldosterone under the influence of K^+. Once again reductive drive is necessary for completion of multistep P-450 reactions, as in the synthesis of aldosterone.

AROMATASE

The synthesis of estrogens involves the conversion of Δ^4-3-ketosteroids to the corresponding steroids with phenolic A rings. The alternative name "estrogen synthetase" is more appropriate but considerably less popular. The overall pathways involve the conversion of androstenedione to estrone and that of testosterone to estradiol, as shown in the reactions below. Two important changes are involved in these conversions, namely 10-demethylation and conversion of the Δ^4-3-ketone A ring to a phenolic ring. These two reactions indicate that the pathway is another example of a complex multistep reaction catalyzed by a cytochrome P-450. It is now clear that a single P-450 enzyme with a single active site is responsible for catalyzing the conversion of androstenedione to estrone and of testosterone to estradiol. Details of the mechanism of this reaction are not known but are of great importance because of the physiological significance of estrogens and the roles of these steroids in various pathological states, including cancer. The search for a mechanism-based inhibitor to control aromatase activity is at present extremely intense.

It is generally believed that the reaction proceeds by demethylation and aromatization, which is not intended to suggest that the two events occur as two discrete steps, although such separation occurs under certain conditions, as discussed later. The pathway is usually depicted as shown in the illustration at the top of the following page.

The second step is complex and is believed to require hydroxylation to give a gem diol:$C_{19}H—(OH)_2$, which would spontaneously collapse to the aldehyde shown

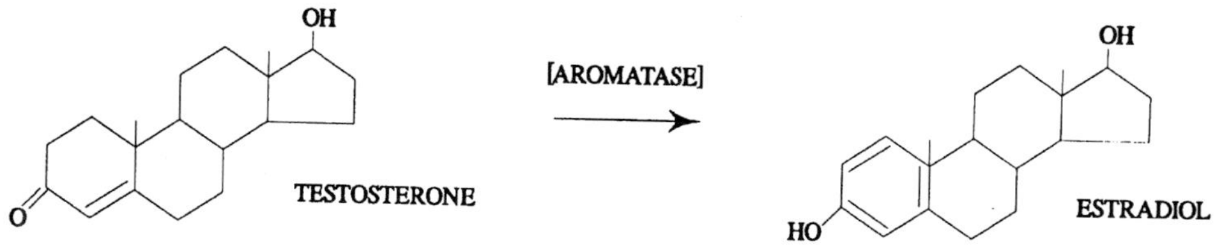

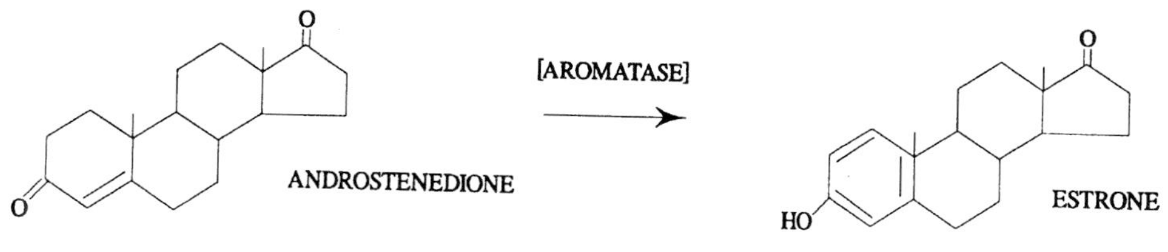

TESTOSTERONE   [AROMATASE] →   ESTRADIOL

ANDROSTENEDIONE   [AROMATASE] →   ESTRONE

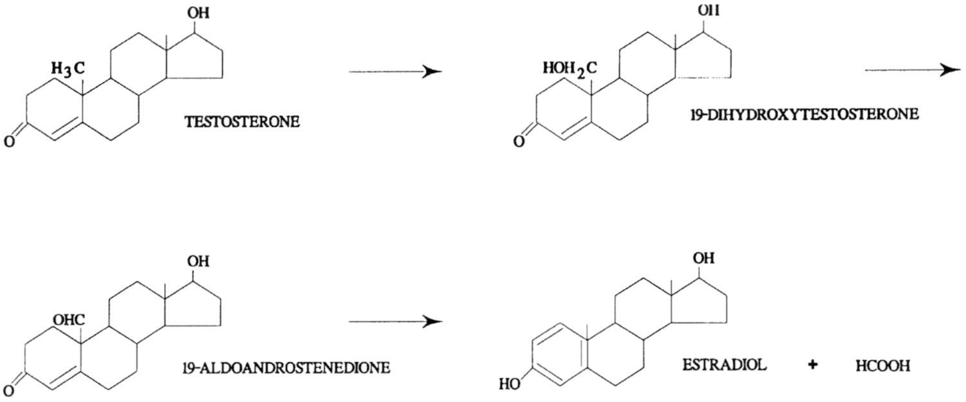

OH

H_3C

TESTOSTERONE

O

→

OH

HOH_2C

19-DIHYDROXYTESTOSTERONE

O

→

OH

OHC

19-ALDOANDROSTENEDIONE

O

→

OH

HO

ESTRADIOL   +   HCOOH

in the diagram above. The process of aromatization involves the loss of formaldehyde from C_{10} and oxidative removal of a hydrogen from both C_1 and C_2. As presented above, there are three successive monooxygenase reactions in keeping with an overall stoichiometry of $NADPH:O_2:H^+$: substrate of 3:3:3:1. Photochemical action spectra to demonstrate involvement of heme in these reactions have not been reported but are hardly necessary at this time.

There are a number of important features of the estrogen synthetase reaction. First, 11β-hydroxylase is capable of limited aromatase activity in that it can convert androstenedione and testosterone to the corresponding estrogens. This is perhaps not surprising since molecular models reveal that C_{18} and C_{19} are equidistant from C_{11}. It is possible to imagine that the C_{19} steroids may enter the active site in such a way that C_{19} is close enough to the heme iron to be subjected to the three monooxygenase steps required for aromatization. It would be predicted that if the substrate entered the active site in the usual manner C_{18} would occupy the site near the iron with the formation of 18-aldoandrostenedione. So far, the production of this steroid does not seem to have been reported.

Second, it has been found that 11β-hydroxylase gives rise to some 19-norandrosterone, a powerful mineralocorticoid. In this case the two steps of the reaction are separated and the conversion stops after removal of the angular methyl group. This process is referred to as non-aromatizing 10-demethylation or more simply as C_{10-19} lyase activity. Similar demethylating reactions are catalyzed by hepatic cytochromes P-450 with cholesterol and other substrates. Evidently a mitochondrial P-450 (11β-hydroxylase) can catalyze the same reaction as a microsomal P-450 (aromatase). Since the fundamental monooxygenase reaction is believed always to proceed by the same mechanism, this observation suggests that if the substrate can fit the active site in such a way as to present a given C atom to the $Fe-O_2$, that C will be subjected to monooxygenation. The C_{10-19} lyase activity provides an interesting contrast to aldehyde synthetase, in which demethylation does not occur because the reaction stops at the aldehyde. The formation of 18-norcorticosterone does not appear to have been reported.

Third, there is an important difference between the aromatase in microsomes from human placenta and that from microsomes of rat ovary. With rat microsomes the conversion of androstenedione to estrone is associated with slow appearance of product, although the two intermediates 19-hydroxy- and 19-aldoandrostenedione accumulate rapidly until the substrate is depleted, at which time rapid formation of estrone is observed. However, when exogenous P-450 reductase (the sole electron carrier in microsomes) is added to ovarian microsomes, this delay is not seen, intermediates do not accumulate in more than small amounts, and the rate of production of estrone is accelerated by a factor of 2.4. This delay in the last steps of the reaction does not occur in the microsomes from human placenta, and in this system exogenous reductase is without effect. The concentration of reductase is higher in microsomes from human placenta than in those from rat ovary. This provides another example of the role of reductive drive in promoting later steps in a multi-step pathway. Whether the difference between the two systems is attributable to a difference between the two organs or between the two species remains to be determined. In any case when reductase is limiting, as in the case of ovarian microsomes, the early steps have first use of available reduced reductase, and the last step becomes rapid only when substrate is exhausted.

Fourth, a major source of aromatase is to be found

in adipose tissue in which the somatic component (cells other than adipocytes) shows high activity. The low activity in adipocytes themselves may be more apparent than real because when lipid droplets are prepared from adipocytes, aromatase activity of the droplets is high. The exogenous steroid substrates added to measure aromatase may not have free access to the enzyme in intact cells. In any event, it is likely that adipose tissue is a major source of estrogens in human subjects. This finding will complicate efforts to treat breast cancer by seeking to remove estrogens from the body by means of oophorectomy.

THE ROLE OF MEMBRANES IN THE ACTIONS OF CYTOCHROMES P-450

Inevitably, early experiments with newly isolated P-450 and homogeneous electron carriers were performed in aqueous buffers. This can clearly offer no more than a hint of the activities of these proteins in vivo where they exist in membranes. The bilayer must greatly influence the rates of interaction of the components of the system by limiting degrees of freedom of the reacting molecules and facilitating interactions between the active sites of the proteins in question. This is especially true in the case of molecules like adrenodoxin, which must accept an electron from one molecule and pass it to another (different) molecule. Conceivably adrenodoxin could rotate during this process to bring a part of the molecule that interacts with reductase to the relevant part of the adjacent P-450 in order to transfer the electron to the P-450. Alternatively, adrenodoxin may be relatively fixed in position, accepting an electron from one side and allowing it to pass through its iron–sulfur structure to the P-450. Furthermore the membrane must shield the electrons from the cytoplasmic water phase in which they would be lost or "shorted out." Such considerations have been studied extensively in the cytochrome chain of oxidative phosphorylation. Although less is known about the steroidogenic system, it is worth considering what is known.

Steroidogenesis takes place within two membranes, namely the inner mitochondrial membrane and the smooth endoplasmic reticulum. Exactly how substrates and intermediates move between these membranes without becoming lost in the cytoplasm remains uncertain.

The Steroidogenic Inner Mitochondrial Membrane

P-450$_{c27scc}$ is found only in the inner mitochondrial membrane of steroid-forming cells, and the enzyme is located on the inner aspect of that membrane. The entire side-chain cleavage system (P-450 plus electron carriers) can be incorporated into membrane vesicles so that it can be studied in an environment that more closely resembles the physiological situation. It appears that cholesterol in one vesicle cannot use P-450 in another vesicle and that the P-450 binding site for cholesterol is on the side of the vesicle that faces the water phase. Moreover it has been proposed that adrenodoxin cycles between the reductase and cytochrome P-450. Oxidized adrenodoxin associates with reduced reductase, and after electron transfer the reduced adrenodoxin dissociates from the now oxidized reductase and binds oxidized P-450, which it reduces. This last step is promoted by the presence of cholesterol bound to the P-450. Adrenodoxin and P-450$_{c27scc}$ are present in the inner membrane in approximately equimolar concentrations while the reductase is present at a lower concentration. This shuttle to and from adrenodoxin may permit the lower concentration of reductase to serve a greater number of molecules of adrenodoxin, which must pass two electrons (e_1 and e_2), to P-450 in two separate steps. An alternative view has been proposed in which a complex is formed between P-450 and the electron carriers. The stable complex is seen as facilitating efficient electron transport, which would enable a small number of molecules of reductase to serve a group of molecules of adrenodoxin in the stable cluster. It is not yet possible to exclude either of these possibilities.

The Steroidogenic Endoplasmic Reticulum

Membrane proteins can be associated with the bilayer by powerful hydrophobic forces within the membrane or more superficially bound to the surface of the membrane by hydrophilic and other forces. To determine the locations of the active sites of membrane proteins and the requirements of these proteins for a boundary of phospholipid, it is possible to use proteolytic and phospholipolytic enzymes, which cannot themselves enter the bilayer, by incubating vesicles isolated from the organelle concerned with these enzymes. If, for example, external trypsin destroys the activity of a particular enzyme it is concluded that the active site of the enzyme faces the external surface of the membrane. To relate this information to the situation in the cell, it is necessary to know whether the vesicles are right side out. If phospholipases A and C destroy activity, it can be concluded that the enzyme requires a phospholipid environment for activity.

Using this approach with testicular microsomes, Samuels and coworkers showed that P-450 reductase faces the cytoplasm. The active site of the dehydrog-

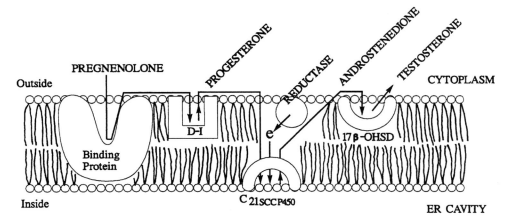

D-I : dehydrogenase/isomerase
OHSD : hydroxysteroid dehydrogenase
e : electrons

enase/isomerase lies at the cytoplasmic surface while P-450 is located within the membrane. Inhibition of activity of hydroxylase/lyase was attributed to destruction of reductase. The binding of pregnenolone to dehydrogenase/isomerase was found to be inhibited by trypsin, suggesting that a binding protein is required for entry of pregnenolone into microsomes in such a way as to bind to the active site of the enzyme. There is independent evidence for the existence of such a protein. Finally, the active site of 17β-hydroxysteroid dehydrogenase is accessible to trypsin. A highly diagrammatic summary of these observations is presented in the illustration at the top of the page. No doubt this scheme will require modification as more evidence comes to light. However, it may assist approaches to exploring the structure of the smooth endoplasmic reticulum of steroidogenic cells.

This membrane was further studied by incubating testicular microsomes with a mixture of [³H]progesterone and 17α-hydroxy-[¹⁴C]progesterone and isolating androstenedione, which showed a higher ratio of [³H]:[¹⁴C] than that of the original substrate mixture. This suggests that hydroxylase/lyase exerts its lyase activity preferentially on the 17α-hydroxyprogesterone generated from progesterone in the active site as opposed to the exogenous intermediate. Yet the two steroids (progesterone and 17α-hydroxyprogesterone) show the same affinity for the active site of the isolated enzyme in an aqueous medium. Moreover, the intermediate generated by the enzyme exchanges freely with exogenous 17α-hydroxy steroid in the water phase. Clearly the hydroxylase/lyase behaves differently in the

membrane than it does in an aqueous buffer, which is not surprising. Presumably progesterone formed in the bilayer from pregnenolone would have access to hydroxylase/lyase without leaving the membrane. Since there is a single active site for the two steps of C_{21scc}, 17α-hydroxyprogesterone would face the alternatives of becoming substrate for lyase in the active site in which it is formed or leaving this site to exchange with the exogenous 17α-hydroxyprogesterone. Possibly the rate of electron transfer would determine what proportion of molecules of intermediate are converted to androstenedione without exchanging (more rapid reduction) and what proportion leave the active site to exchange (slower reduction).

In hepatic microsomes there is a much higher concentration of P-450 than reductase, so that the two views discussed above have been proposed to explain reduction of P-450. The concept of a cluster is based upon Arrhenius plots (that is, enzyme activity versus 1/T) which show a break in an otherwise linear relationship. This is compatible with the cluster hypothesis. It is well known that in plasma membranes protein molecules are extremely mobile in spite of the fact that they are to a large extent restrained by attachment to the cytoskeleton. This would make diffusion of reductase to P-450 a possibility, although it is also true that the microsome is very rich in protein which could limit the freedom of individual protein molecules to diffuse within the membrane. In contrast, spectroscopic and centrifugation studies suggest that a long-lived complex does not occur, so it may be that diffusion accounts for the observed rates of reduction of P-450 by reductase. It is also possible that P-450 may not act as a monomeric species but as an aggregate. Similar studies are needed in steroidogenic microsomes where the molar ratio of P-450 to reductase is much closer to 1.0 than in hepatic microsomes.

MOLECULAR BIOLOGY OF CYTOCHROMES P-450

A major (perhaps the major) focus of interest in the steroidogenic cytochromes P-450 lies in the relevant genes and their transcription. The rates of secretion of the various steroid hormones depend to a considerable extent on the amounts of the various P-450 enzymes present in the steroidogenic cells, which in turn depends on the rates of transcription of the individual genes, which is regulated by the trophic pituitary hormones. This pattern is most clearly seen with the secretion of the ovarian hormones which varies widely during the reproductive cycle. The variations in secretion have been shown to reflect changes in the rates of transcription of the genes concerned. The same can be said of all the cytochromes P-450 in this family. The undoubted importance of transcription in the control of P-450 activities should not be taken to mean that other forms of regulation do not exist and are unimportant.

Much progress has been made in isolating these genes and in measuring the rates of transcription of each gene. Intron/exon maps of the various genes together with DNA sequences are available. In addition much DNA sequence beyond the limits of transcription has been reported, especially that which is upstream or 5' to the start of transcription, which is usually referred to as +1. Much, but not all, regulatory DNA is located upstream of +1. It is possible to attach varying lengths of this upstream DNA to the DNA of a so-called reporter gene and to transfect or inject the relevant cells with such a construct (that is, upstream DNA attached to reporter gene). The reporter gene is usually one that is not normally expressed in the cell in question. The degree of basal or unstimulated expression of the reporter gene is determined by measuring the production of the protein product of the reporter gene. Commonly the reporter gene corresponds to an enzyme that is readily measured—for example, bacterial luciferase. The amount of upstream DNA is progressively shortened in so-called deletion mutants, and the corresponding enzyme activity is determined until too little upstream DNA is present for expression to occur. In this way sequences of 5' DNA necessary for basal transcription can be determined. It is assumed that the reporter gene is expressed under the influence of the 5' upstream DNA of the steroidogenic gene in the same

way as the steroidogenic gene itself is normally expressed with this DNA in the original steroid-forming cell. These studies also enable the investigator to determine accurately the start site of transcription (that is, +1).

Sequences of regulatory DNA are called "elements," and proteins capable of binding specifically to various elements and thereby regulating expression of the gene are called "factors." Sometimes short sequences of DNA with the same base repeated or short runs of repeated bases are called "boxes." Regulation of expression by sequences of DNA without proteins is called *cis* regulation, whereas that resulting from binding of specific proteins is called *trans* regulation.

Upstream base pairs (bp) are designated relative to +1 by a minus sign. This DNA influences transcription in several ways. First, sequences around +1 permit a number of transcription factors to organize the binding site for RNA polymerase; these proteins form what is called the "initiation complex," which secures the correct site for the initiation of transcription. The first 100 or so bases are referred to as "proximal," that is, close to +1. The proximal sequence to which the initiation complex binds is referred to as the "gene promoter," and it is necessary for basal levels of transcription. The number 100 is arbitrary, and examples will be given of promoter sequences that extend beyond −300 (that is, further upstream from +1).

Sequences that are further upstream (>1000 and even >10,000 base pairs) sometimes contain regulatory sequences referred to as "enhancers." *Trans* regulation by promoters and enhancers can be influenced by numerous intracellular and extracellular molecules and physiological conditions—for example, extracellular matrix, cell density, etc.—as well as by such common intracellular signals as cAMP and Ca^{2+}. It is through such mechanisms that the physiological state of the cell is capable of regulating the expression of specific genes. In many cases this form of regulation involves binding of nuclear proteins to promoters and/or enhancers. Altered functional states of the cell that bring about changes in transcription of specific genes may result from the synthesis of new proteins or from posttranslational modification of existing proteins (for example, phosphorylation).

At this point the choice of cells for such expression studies is important. If possible the cell in which the expression of the gene under investigation normally occurs—that is, the steroidogenic cell in the present case—should be used. In mastering the intricacies of molecular biology, it has not always been possible for investigators to learn modern methods of cell biology, with the result that cell lines are frequently used as host cells in the mistaken belief that it is not possible to obtain highly purified samples of the normal cells of interest. The nature and number of mutations in a cell line is never entirely clear, so that important regulatory proteins and other conditions existing in the normal cell may be altered if not entirely missing. In addition to the cells themselves, conditions of growth, including serum-free medium and extracellular matrix, are likely to be important. Attention to these factors has the potential to bring studies of transcription closer to the physiological ideal. For transfection, cells are permeabilized by a variety of methods and the construct is incubated with and taken into the permeabilized cell. The cells seal and repair themselves so that they continue to function in the culture medium. With an appropriate cell and a suitable construct, it is possible to determine the influence of such agents as cAMP on expression of specific genes.

It is generally believed that distal enhancer elements influence transcription as the result of looping around DNA in such a fashion as to bring the distal element to bind at or near the promoter. This looping may be stabilized by protein–protein interactions in which proteins bound to the enhancer also bind to the initiation complex. These protein–protein interactions may be responsible for exerting regulation of gene expression. At present we can only guess at the possible changes taking place in the structural organization of a chromosome during transcription. An interesting start toward resolving this enormous problem has been made by defining sequences of DNA called "insulators." The term refers to specific sequences of DNA that are capable of binding upstream DNA in such a way as to prevent the inappropriate binding of the enhancer to DNA that lies in the linear structure of DNA between enhancer and promoter.

When antibodies to all the steroidogenic P-450 enzymes became available it was only a question of time before the corresponding genes were isolated and sequenced. Since expression studies are for the most part quite straightforward, new information is growing apace. Promoter and enhancer sequences have been defined for each of the genes in various species and expression studies have been reported in cell lines and normal cells. Each month brings new findings concerning the regulation of expression of these genes. To a considerable extent this mass of information is indigestible at this stage and does not provide a clear picture. At present "rules" concerning elements and factors cannot be formulated with confidence. Efforts will be made in this chapter to define promoter and enhancer sequences—sequences necessary for responses to cAMP and the nature of nuclear proteins where these are known. The trophic hormones act by way of cAMP

so that DNA sequences responsible for the action of the cyclic nucleotide are clearly important. Little information is available concerning such stimuli as Ca^{2+}, oxygen tension, and extracellular structures, which are known to be important in the regulation of other genes, and which will no doubt be investigated in future studies in steroidogenic cells. In many cases DNA, to which various proteins are known to bind, has been identified as the result of work performed in systems other than P-450 that have advanced more rapidly. It is proposed to begin by considering the expression of three P-450 genes in a single species, namely mouse, in order to illustrate the information available at present and difficulties in interpreting findings in a single species. The upstream DNA and associated protein factors for the three genes can be summarized as follows:

P-450$_{scc}$:

| | SF-1 | | SF-1 |
| TGAGTTTGGGA—AGGTCA—CAAGGCTA |
| -124 | -14 | -73 | -68 |

P-450$_{21}$:

SF-1 COUP-TF SF-1   SF-1 NGF1-E
AGGTCA——CCAAGGCTG—AGGTCAG
-209 -204 -143   -135 -62   -54

P-450AS:

| SF-1 | | CREBP |
| CCAAGGTCT———————TGACGTGA |
| -307 | -299 | -56 | -49 |

(AS, aldosterone synthetase.)

We can assume that no transcription takes place until an initiation complex is established at +1. It can be seen that all three genes share a promoter element AGGTCA (or something very similar) and that this sequence binds a protein factor called SF-1 (steroidogenic factor 1). This binding is specific and the cDNA for SF-1 has been isolated. It is not yet clear how far a sequence can depart from the above "consensus" sequence and still permit specific binding to SF-1. It will also be seen that the promoter may extend beyond 300 bp (11β-hydroxylase).

It was found that the nucleotide sequence to which SF-1 binds shows high homology to that of three quite different genes, namely embryonal long terminal repeat, a homeobox gene in the fruit fly *Drosophila* called FTZ-F1, which according to current convention corresponds to a protein called ftz, and a sequence to which the superfamily of steroid receptors bind.

The long terminal repeat binds to a protein that

exerts a strong inhibitory effect on the expression of retroviral genes in embryonal carcinoma cells. The significance of this homology with the SF-1 binding sequence is obscure. Homology with FTZ-F1 is intriguing because the synthesis of the steroid hormone ecdysone involves hydroxylation reactions so that the involvement of SF-1 in the regulation of transcription of steroid hydroxylase enzymes may be significant. The significance of homology with homeobox genes is unclear at present. Homology between SF-1 and sequences that bind receptors for steroid hormones includes sequences to which receptors for thyroid hormone, vitamin D, and retinoic acid are known to bind. In addition, this superfamily includes several molecules for which no ligands are known. These molecules resemble other members of this superfamily so closely that it is assumed that such ligands do exist but remain to be identified. These supposed receptors are accordingly referred to as "orphan receptors." Binding of ligands to these receptors at the cell surface causes the receptors (with bound ligand) to move to the nucleus of the target cell, bind to the specific DNA, which shows homology to SF-1, and thereby stimulate transcription. Presumably the homology between these sequences reveals the presence of common sequences that are involved in activation of transcription of various genes the transcription of which is regulated by these receptors.

SF-1 is believed to promote transcription by facilitating cooperative interactions between various transcription factors in such a way as to bring the regulatory domains of these factors together to form a functional initiation complex. The DNA that binds SF-1 varies but usually contains a consensus core CCCGCCC.

It is interesting that SF-1 is expressed in adrenal, Leydig, and ovarian cells. Clearly this protein cannot account for expression of genes that are peculiar to adrenal cells (for example, 21-hydroxylase and 11β-hydroxylase). Additional proteins, not so far isolated, must be involved in securing specificity of transcription of these genes in the various steroidogenic cells.

Two other factors are involved in regulating transcription of the 21-hydroxylase gene, namely COUP-TF (a member of the steroid receptor family so named because it binds to the promoter of the chicken ovalbumin gene) and NGF1-B which is a protein that is induced by nerve growth factor. How these factors work together in regulating transcription of this gene is not clear.

Presumably these and other proteins account for basal or unstimulated expression of these P-450 genes in the mouse. Enhancer elements further upstream capable of stimulating transcription above basal levels

await to be defined. What are we to make of the differences between these three promoter regions in the three mouse genes? The similarities are not great. The number of SF-1 elements varies. One gene requires two additional proteins, and distances of SF-1 elements from +1 vary from −65 to −310. Only time will tell whether such differences are capable of simple interpretation.

The best-studied regulation of these genes is that exerted by ACTH through cAMP. Expression studies have used the potent analogue 8-bromo cAMP or the synthetic agent forskolin, which promotes the synthesis of cAMP. Early studies with these agents in other systems showed that rapid responses to cAMP involve a sequence called cAMP responsive element (CRE) and the cognate factor CRE-binding protein (CREBP). The consensus sequence involved appears with slight modifications in various cells in which cAMP is known to act. These minor variations must be accepted as close enough to the consensus sequence to permit good responses to the cyclic nucleotide. At least in some cases, the response of CREBP to cAMP involves the usual cAMP response via protein kinase A (PKA), resulting in phosphorylation of this CREBP. Presumably phosphorylation of CREBP permits binding to the appropriate element. In other cases a response of transcription to cAMP requires synthesis of new protein.

It has been pointed out that the responses of steroidogenic P-450 genes to cAMP are relatively slow compared to other responses to the cyclic nucleotide in some other cells. It is not surprising to learn that the slower responses do not involve a CRE but different elements instead. Moreover, in some cases, the more slowly responding genes require the synthesis of new protein(s) for a response to cAMP. Whether phosphorylation by PKA is involved in these responses is not known. At least two proteins involved in the regulation of transcription are synthesized at accelerated rates in response to ACTH, namely NGF1-B and c-fos. It appears that NGFI-B is involved in the response of 21-hydroxylase but it is not known whether c-fos is involved in the response of transcription of P-450 genes to ACTH. It should be pointed out that 11β-hydroxylase shows a CRE at −55, which seems to be an exception to the "rule" that CRE is not involved in the slower responses of these genes to cAMP.

So far it appears that differences in the regulation of expression of the individual P-450 genes between different species is often not great. Perhaps regulation of a given gene in various species requires the same or similar conditions whether it is a new protein or a posttranslationally modified protein.

We can now turn to the individual genes to summarize what is known about the requirements for basal transcription, the nature and number of sequences required for a response to cAMP, and where possible, information concerning the roles of nuclear proteins in these responses.

Cytochrome P-450$_{c27scc}$ (CYPII)

The major regulatory hormones for this gene are ACTH and LH, both of which act via cAMP. It was found that these hormones increase the amount of this enzyme using measurements based upon immunoprecipitation. It was surprising to learn that stimulation of transcription of CYPII by cAMP is inhibited by cycloheximide in bovine adrenocortical and JEG-3 choriocarcinoma cells, but not in human granulosa cells or in mouse Leydig cells. Evidently cAMP promotes synthesis of new proteins for this response in the first two species, but not in the last two. This is surprising in view of the similarities between species in the response of steroid synthesis to trophic stimulation. Perhaps the human granulosa and mouse Leydig cells use phosphorylation of existing nuclear proteins to regulate transcription of CYPII.

The cDNA for CYPII shows that translation of the corresponding mRNA yields a preform of the P-450 in which there is a sequence of 39 amino acids at the NH$_2$ terminus that acts as a signal to direct the newly synthesized enzyme to mitochondria. Once inside this organelle the leader sequence is removed by a specific proteolytic enzyme to give the mature form of P-450$_{c27scc}$.

Basal Transcription. Upstream sequences of CYPII were examined for elements necessary for basal levels of transcription with the following results:

Species	Host Cells	Sequences
Human	Adrenal Y-1	−2327 to −605; −152 to −18
Human	Placenta JEG-3	−152 to −142; −79 to +49
Bovine	Adrenal Y-1	−183 to −83
Bovine	Bovine luteal	−186 to −101
Mouse	Adrenal Y-1	−70 to −57; −40 to −27

In most cases the sequences fall within 200 bp of +1. In three cases two sequences are required. Further studies will be necessary to refine these sequences to the shortest possible active elements. It is not possible to account for the role of the far upstream sequence in the human gene for which no equivalent sequence is seen in the other genes. This may be an enhancer but further studies are needed in normal cells. It is, however, reassuring that the distances of at least one element from +1 are similar for the human gene expressed in normal and mutant cells. For the mouse, stimulation of expression above basal level was seen with an additional sequence at −127 which contains an SP1 sequence. An important difference is seen between Y-1 and JEG-3 cells. Presumably the placental cell line uses different proteins and different elements from those involved in the adrenal cell line.

Response to cAMP. Sequences that must be added to the elements required for basal transcription of CYPII in order to permit a response to cAMP have been identified in several species and cells. For the human gene expressed in Y-1 cells two groups have identified the same general region of upstream sequence (−1697 to −1503). A similar region for the response to cAMP was found with the human gene expressed in MA-10 Leydig cells. With JEG-3 cells a rather different region (−108 to −89) is involved.

The response is more complex than appears from these observations. For the human gene three sequences within from −1697 to −1523 are also required for the response to cAMP, and this contains the sequence CGTCA. Another group reported the requirement in JEG placental cells of a distal element (−1621 to −1503) which includes the sequence TCAAGGTCA and an additional proximal element at −117 to −94. In addition an enhancer element was found at −1931 to −1822. It may be significant that when the same (human) gene is expressed in MA-10 cells a sequence for the cAMP response was found in a similar location to that just described for JEG cells (that is, −127 to −110).

The bovine gene when expressed in bovine luteal cells shows a sequence required for response to cAMP at −186 to −101. This sequence contains an AP-1-like sequence and an overlapping GA box. When the same gene is expressed in bovine granulosa cells the sequence involved in the response to cAMP is located in a similar region relative to +1 that is, −118 to −100. This sequence also contains an AP-1 sequence as well as an Sp1 element. When expression studies were performed in Y-1 cells the sequence for the cAMP response is located at −118 to −100 and includes a similar sequence that binds Sp1, although such a sequence is not usually associated with a response to cAMP. However, a DNA-dependent kinase is known to phosphorylate Sp1. Responses exerted through Sp1 may be triggered by phosphorylation. At present, however, responses by

CYPII not inhibited by cycloheximide are not known to involve Sp1.

There appears to be some rationale to these responses but when murine CYPII is expressed in Y-1 cells the sequences required for the cAMP response are -76 to -66 and -40 to -35; the latter includes AGGTC. When the rat enzyme is expressed in rat granulosa cells two elements are necessary for a response to cAMP, namely -79 to -71 and -51 to -43. These sequences have been called scc2 (AGGTCAA) and scc1 (AGCCT), respectively. Neither the locations nor the sequences of these elements resembles the sequences or the locations required for a response of CYPII to cAMP in other species.

Inhibition of Transcription.

An upstream element has been found at -343 to -43 in the human gene that is responsible for inhibition of transcription when that gene is expressed in Y-1 cells treated with phorbol ester and Ca^{2+} ionophore. In the murine gene expressed in Y-1 cells and in bovine adrenal cells, elements have also been found that inhibit responses to forskolin and 8-bromo cAMP.

Cytochrome P-450 C_{21scc} (17α-hydroxylase) (CYP17)

As in the case of P-450 C_{27scc}, hydroxylase/lyase mRNA is increased by LH in rat Leydig cells and by ACTH in adrenocortical cells. The relevant gene is called CYP17.

Basal Transcription.

Considerable interest attaches to basal transcription of this gene. Upstream sequence of the bovine gene as far as -437 nucleotides did not support expression of a reporter gene either in primary cultures of bovine luteal cells or in a subcellular system from Y-1 cells. It appears that in unstimulated cells CYP17 is completely repressed, presumably because of the presence of a negative transcription factor or the absence of a positive factor.

Response to cAMP.

Expression vectors of the bovine gene transfected into Y-1 cells revealed two elements necessary for a cAMP response. These sequences are cAMP responsive sequences I and II (CRSI, II, respectively). Constructs of the bovine gene in bovine granulosa cells revealed a sequence (-118 to -100) that permits a response to forskolin and elements corresponding to AP1 and Sp1 transcription factors, one or both of which are required for the response to forskolin. These findings have been convincingly confirmed by studies of transcription in vitro.

Inhibition of Transcription.

An inhibitory effect of PKC on expression of CYP17 has been reported, and this action has been studied in expression vectors in search of inhibitory upstream sequences. It was found that in the bovine gene the sequence -118 to -110 is responsible for inhibition by PKC as well as stimulation by cAMP in bovine granulosa cells. When inhibition was seen in response to phorbol ester, it was shown that this results from a direct effect on transcription and was not due to such indirect effects as decreased production of cAMP, decreased binding of protein factors to CRSI, or inhibition of PKA. It seems likely that both stimulation by cAMP and inhibition by phorbol ester may result from the actions of one or both of the transcription factors AP1 and Sp1. By contrast, when the upstream DNA from the human gene is attached to a reporter gene and transfected into MA-10 Leydig cells, quite different elements are involved in the inhibitory response.

Nuclear Proteins.

It has been shown that the CRSI sequence described above binds four nuclear proteins in extracts of Y-1 cells. Two of these proteins are homeodomain proteins involved in the development of body segments, PbX1a and PbX1b. Overexpression of these proteins increased the response of Y-1 cells to cAMP. It has been proposed that these proteins, concerned as they are with developmental changes in Drosophila, may be involved in the production of hormones at puberty. On the other hand CRSII binds two nuclear proteins belonging to the steroid receptor superfamily, that is, COUP-TF and SF-I. These proteins are both examples of orphan receptors and they bind part of the CRSII element that includes the two sequences AAGTCA and AGGTCA separated by six nucleotides. Overexpression of these proteins showed that SF-I activates expression of CYP17 in response to CRSII.

The upstream sequence of rat CYP17 contains elements corresponding to CRSI and CRSII described above for the bovine gene. These sequences exert a negative effect in the adrenal and a positive effect in the gonads, which is consistent with the production of corticosterone (17-deoxy-C_{21}-steroid) by mouse adrenal (as opposed to cotisol in most species) and the production of C_{19} and C_{18} steroids in the gonads.

Cytochrome P-450 21-Hydroxylase (CYP21)

Basal Transcription.

For this gene, agreement between species is excellent. An upstream sequence of 40 bp is necessary for basal transcription in human, bovine, and murine genes. This element is located at −210 to −170 in the murine gene and shows the following properties: *(1)* it is required for the response to ACTH, *(2)* it acts specifically in adrenal cells, *(3)* the response of this element to ACTH occurs via PKA, *(4)* it bears no resemblance to the common CRE, and *(5)* it specifically binds nuclear proteins in all three species. This element is part of the CYP21 promoter.

Response to cAMP.

In addition to the proximal promoter sequence there is a far upstream element at −2574 to −2489. This sequence serves as an enhancer acting through the promoter when cAMP is present. Typically enhancers are thought to increase the activities of promoters rather than permitting a direct response of the enhancer to such agents as cAMP. A strict definition of enhancer will not be possible until more is known about the regulation of transcription.

Two cAMP responsive elements have been found in human CYP21 at −126 to −113 and −119 to −110. A sequence in the bovine gene at −129 to −115 is homologous with the more distal of the above two human elements and as expected, is responsive to cAMP. These sequences bind certain nuclear proteins.

Nuclear Proteins.

The two cAMP elements of the human gene mentioned above produce still greater rates of transcription when two nuclear proteins from adrenocortical cells, adrenal specific protein (ASP) and Ad4, in addition to cAMP are also present. Furthermore a maximal response to cAMP requires a combination of elements within the first 300 upstream nucleotides beginning at −170; that is, −170, −65, −140, and −210 in order of descending potency. Although the −170 element is the most potent, it binds numerous proteins and appears to be of general importance rather than specifically involved with the regulation of expression of CYP21. The element at −65 specifically interacts with the orphan receptor NGFI-B. Moreover this sequence confers the ability of the cell to respond to ACTH and cAMP. This element at −65 also binds a second nuclear receptor, SF-1, which occurs only in steroidogenic cells. The interactions of these two proteins with this element may permit complex regulation of the expression of CYP21 so that the enzyme is expressed in the adrenal but not in the gonads. At the same time other regulatory systems determine the rate of expression of this gene.

ASP has been partly purified as a 78 kD protein that promotes synthesis of the mRNA corresponding to CYP21 in the presence of the cAMP responsive sequence at −129 to −96 in the bovine gene in a subcellular system from HeLa cells. However, these cells do not synthesize steroid hormones. Sp1 does not act in this system. It seems that ASP serves as a specific transcription factor for the cAMP-dependent regulation of expression of the CYP21 gene.

A curious observation has been made concerning the regulation of transcription of murine CYP21 gene. An element regulating basal transcription of this gene is located within the DNA sequence of an unrelated (although sex-limited) gene Slp. The evolutionary significance of this conserved linkage remains to be explained.

It is interesting that three steroidogenic genes in the mouse (CYPII, CYP21, and CYP11) share a common promoter element, namely AGGTCA or AGGTCT. It is assumed that the difference between these two sequences is too slight to be of any significance in recognizing the relevant nuclear proteins or other DNA. In any case this element is found in two different places relative to +1 in the CYPII gene—that is, −73 to −68 and −46 to −41; in three places in CYP21—that is, −210 to −205, −143 to −136, and −70 to −65; and one place in CYP11—that is, −316 to −311. These sequences are known to bind several proteins that belong to the superfamily of steroid receptors that are found in the nucleus.

Cytochrome P-450 11β-Hydroxylase (CYP11)

The Genes. Four CYP11 genes have been isolated from the rat genome as follows: CYP11B1 corresponds to 11β-hydroxylase and is involved in the synthesis of corticosterone; B2 corresponds to aldosterone synthetase; B3 of which the corresponding protein shows enzymatic properties that are intermediate between those exhibited by the proteins of B1 and B2 catalyzing both 11β- and 18-hydroxylation without aldehyde synthetase activity; and B4, a pseudogene in which two exons are replaced by unrelated DNA. The genes B1–3 are highly homologous in the amino acid sequences of the corresponding proteins, and the exon structures of the two genes show exact correspondence. In the 5′ upstream DNA, B1 and B3 are almost identical but B2 is significantly different. A putative Ad4 site is found in the promoters of B1 and B2 and indeed in the promoters of most steroidogenic enzymes. This element binds the corresponding factor Ad4BP. Expression of B2 is greater in rats on a diet low in Na⁺ and high in K⁺ in keeping with the known function of the corresponding P-450 in the synthesis of aldosterone.

CYP11B3 is expressed only in neonatal male rats

and expression is decreased by ACTH. The gene is expressed in neonatal fasciculata/reticularis but not in glomerulosa. A possible CRE can be found in the upstream sequence of B3 at −64 (TGACGTA). In B2, the corresponding sequence is altered to TCACATTA. Expression studies of B1 and B2 in COS-7 cells reveal that the steroidogenic activities of the two corresponding proteins are consistent with the activity of the B1 protein as an 11β-/18-hydroxylase and the B2 protein as an aldosterone synthetase. However, only B1 shows 19-hydroxylase activity. Both B1 and B2 proteins are synthesized as preforms with signal peptides for mitochondrial uptake of 24 and 34 amino acids, respectively. It seems that Glu286 and Gly36 are important for aldosterone synthetase activity.

Nuclear Proteins. In analyzing the function of upstream DNA in the CYP11 genes it was found that the promoter of B1 contains six elements that regulate transcription and are called Ad1-6. Ad4 is present in upstream DNA of other steroidogenic genes and binds a protein of MW 51,000 called Ad4BP. This protein is referred to above and is highly homologous to the proteins FTZ-F and ELP that are expressed in *Drosophila* and in embryonal carcinoma cells, respectively. Ad1 (TGACGTGA) closely resembles consensus CRE. Ad3 and Ad4 together with their binding proteins are responsible for the enhanced expression of CYP11B1 by cAMP. The three elements Ad1, 3, and 4 have different functions but all three are necessary for a full response to cAMP. Ad1 together with four copies of Ad4 promotes expression of CYP11B1 in Y-1 cells treated with forskolin. The same response is seen when these cells are transfected with Ad1-(Ad4)4 and the catalytic subunit of PKA. Transfection with Ad1-(Ad4)4 in Leydig cells but not in nonsteroidogenic cells results in expression of CYP11B1, which is not normally expressed in Leydig cells.

Aromatase (CYP19)

CYP19 shows high homology of coding sequences between human, rat, and chicken genes. Studies of experimental mutations reveal that Asp309 is critical for enzyme activity.

The regulation of expression of aromatase is known to involve various hormones. For example, in rat granulosa cells low levels of FSH or cAMP increase production of estradiol by these cells, and this response is enhanced by concomitant administration of estradiol. The same response is seen with forskolin. It is interesting to note that high concentrations of LH or FSH rapidly bring the response to forskolin to a halt.

Changes in the steady state levels of aromatase mRNA have been found both in vivo and in vitro to reflect these changes in the secretion of estradiol. It is also of interest to note that expression of human aromatase is induced in human placental choriocarcinoma cells (JAR) by phorbol esters.

Basal Transcription. In the human, gene −246 to −166 provides *cis* regulation necessary for efficient transcription of the gene. Together with the homologous promoter, this sequence promotes transcription of aromatase in Be Wo choriocarcinoma cells but not in other cell lines including Y-1 adrenal cells and in HeLa cells that do not secrete estrogens.

Response to cAMP. The expression of rat aromatase in the homologous granulosa cell is stimulated by forskolin in keeping with the role of cAMP in the response of the gene to FSH. This hormone is known to increase synthesis of estrogens by these cells. The response to forskolin requires a specific upstream sequence, namely −176 to −31. By contrast, a cell line of Leydig cells (R2C) expresses aromatase constitutively and cAMP is without effect on this expression. In these cells the same element (−176 to −31) is required for constitutive expression of aromatase.

Nuclear Proteins. Binding of various proteins to upstream DNA has been studied with aromatase. For example, nuclear proteins of Be Wo cells bind the sequence −242 to −166 of the human gene. As mentioned earlier this sequence is required for basal expression of the gene in Be Wo cells. Nuclear proteins bind to the cAMP responsive sequence of the rat granulosa cell gene, that is, −176 to −31. This binding is completed by the element −90 to −66 of the same gene, which includes the hexameric sequence AGGTCA (−82 to −77) found in upstream DNA from other steroidogenic genes.

The 5′ upstream DNA of rat aromatase binds the protein SF-1 discussed earlier as a member of the orphan receptor family. SF-1 binds upstream DNA of steroidogenic genes in adrenocortical cells. The SF-1 binding sequence CCAAGGTCA is found at −82 to −74 in the aromatase genes of man and rat. No doubt SF-1, acting through this sequence, is involved in the regulation of expression of aromatase in these two species and possibly others.

Tissue-Specific Expression. The expression of other steroidogenic cytochromes P-450 appears to be confined to those organs known to secrete the relevant hormones, that is, to the various endocrine glands and the placenta. By contrast, it has long been known that a number of tissues are capable of producing estrogens. It is usually assumed that these nonendocrine sources of estrogens use circulating androgens as starting material for the synthesis of estrogens.

The regulation of tissue-specific expression of aromatase is complex and of considerable clinical importance. Tissues that express this gene include ovary, placenta, testis, adipose tissue (both stromal cells and adipocytes), prostate, fetal liver, and fibroblasts. Tissue specificity is determined, at least in part, by means of alternative start sites for transcription together with tissue specific promoters. Regulation results from the use of multiple promoters attached to one of a series of alternative Exons 1. These sequences of DNA are constructed by alternative splicing in the various tissues. A complete account of these specificities is not possible at the present time. However, five species of the aromatase gene have been identified. Of these, four are strongly expressed in the placenta, ovary, and adipose tissue while the fifth is weakly expressed in the placenta. The corresponding mRNAs for the five genes differ one from the other only in the regions corresponding to Exon 1. Specific regulation is secured by the splicing mechanism which puts in place different sequences to act as different Exons 1. Although this form of regulation is unknown in other steroidogenic genes, similar mechanisms of tissue-specific regulation of transcription are known in other genes. The scheme may require further elaboration since a unique aromatase gene has recently been reported in the brain. The nature of two of these specifically spliced sequences is as follows:

1. Expression in the ovary uses Exon 2 with 79 bp of upstream sequence including an initiation site.

2. Adipose tissue employs an 84 bp upstream sequence which is the same as that used in the ovary but with an extension of 5 bp.

The position is complicated by various physiological conditions; for example, some organs (ovary and adipose tissue) are composed of mixtures of various cell types with different aromatase genes expressed. There are changes in the expression of different aromatase genes in some organs during development (for example, liver) and growth conditions in culture can alter the tissue-specific expression of CYP19. The total number of available Exons 1 that could be spliced into Exon 2 appears at present to be 10 or 11. These different Exons 1 are found together with various promoters upstream of Exon 2 to which the required sequence (that is, promoter Exon 1), is spliced to give the mRNA

appropriate for a particular tissue, as shown in the accompanying diagram.

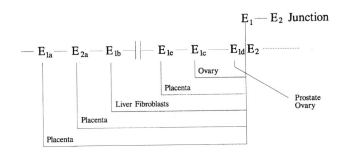

It is not clear why these various forms of the gene have evolved since it would seem likely that different nuclear proteins are available to secure differential expression of aromatase in the various tissues without such a roundabout mechanism of control. Two comments appear relevant to this issue. First, it has been proposed that switching particular Exons 1 may result in the overproduction of estrogens by the adipose tissue of the breast. Such overproduction may be important in the development of cancer of the breast. Second, the rates of expression of these various forms of aromatase are influenced by glucocorticoids and by cAMP.

The author is grateful to Mr. Simon Winter for preparing the figures, to the Department of Medical Illustration at Prince of Wales Hospital, Randwick, NSW, Australia for the photophagraphy and to Mr. Warwick D. G. Hall for typing the manuscript.

READINGS

Dean, W. L., and R. D. Gray. Relationship between state of aggregation and catalytic activity of P450 LM$_2$ and P450 reductase. *J. Biol. Chem.* 257: 14679, 1983.

Griffin, B. W., J. A. Peterson, and R. W. Estabrook. Cytochrome P-450: Biophysical properties and catalytic function. In: *The Porphorins,* edited by D. Dolphin. New York: Academic Press, 1979, p. 333.

Gunsalus, I. C., J. R. Meeks, J. D. Lipscomb, P. De Brunner, and E. Munck. Bacterial monooxygenase—the P450 cytochrome system. In: *Molecular Mechanisms of Oxygen Activation,* edited by O. Hayashi. New York: Academic Press, 1974, p. 559.

Hall, P. F. Cellular organization for steroidogenesis. *Int. Rev. Cytol.* 86: 53, 1984.

Hall, P. F. Trophic stimulation of steroidogenesis: In search of the elusive trigger. *Recent Prog. Horm. Res.* 41: 1, 1985a.

Hall, P. F. The role of cytochromes P450 in the synthesis of steroid hormones. *Vitam. Horm.* 42: 315, 1985b.

Hall, P. F. Cytochromes P450 and the regulation of steroid synthesis. *Steroids* 48: 131, 1986.

Hall, P. F. Testicular steroid synthesis: Organization and regulation. In: *The Physiology of Reproduction,* 2nd ed., edited by E. Knobil and J. D. Neill. New York: Raven Press, 1994, p. 1335.

John, M. E., M. C. Boggaram, V. Simpson, and E. R. Waterman. Transcriptional regulation of steroid hydroxylation genes by corticotropin. *Proc. Natl. Acad. Sci. USA* 83: 4751, 1986.

Johnson, E. F., and S. L. McKnight. Eukaryotic transcriptional regulatory proteins. *Ann. Rev. Biochem.* 58: 799, 1989.

Kimura, T. ACTH stimulation of cholesterol side-chain cleavage. *Mol. Cell. Biochem.* 36: 105, 1981.

Lambeth, J. D., D. W. Seybert, J. R. Lancaster, J. C. Salerno, and H. Kamin. Steroidogenic electron transport in adrenal cortex mitochondria. *Mol. Cell. Biochem.* 45: 13, 1982.

Parker, K. I., and B. P. Schimmer. Transcriptional regulation of the adrenal steroidogenic enzymes. *Trends Endocrinol. Metab.* 4: 46, 1993.

Samuels, L. T., L. Bussman, K. Matsumoto, and R. A. Huseby. Organization of androgen biosynthesis in the testis. *J. Steroid Biochem.* 6: 291, 1975.

Sligar, S. G. Coupling of spin, substrate, and redox equilibria in cytochrome P450. *Biochemistry* 15: 5399, 1976.

White, R. E., and M. J. Coon. Oxygen activation by cytochrome P450. *Annu. Rev. Biochem.* 49: 315, 1980.

17. Cellular localization of receptors mediating the actions of steroid hormones

BARBARA M. JUDY
WADE V. WELSHONS | *Department of Veterinary Biomedical Sciences, University of Missouri-Columbia, Columbia, Missouri*

CHAPTER CONTENTS

THE RECEPTORS FOR STEROID HORMONES are cellular proteins that can act in the cell nucleus as ligand-dependent transcription factors to regulate the expression of specific steroid-responsive genes (Fig. 17.1A). After ligand binding, steroid receptors undergo transformational changes that lead to biologically active complexes. The transformation is accompanied by an increased affinity of the receptor for chromatin and DNA (109) that results from the unmasking of its DNA-binding domain (62, 90). The initial model of steroid hormone action (Fig. 17.1B), based on cell homogenization and fractionation studies, proposed that the unoccupied receptor proteins were cytoplasmic and translocated to the nucleus upon binding of their respective ligands. This model was developed for the estrogen receptor (58, 75, 160) but subsequently was generalized for all steroid receptors (56). The translocation model for all steroid action was widely accepted for a long time and persists in many textbooks.

However, two different techniques, developed in separate laboratories, produced results that led to revision of the translocation model for steroid receptor action (Fig. 17.1A). Evidence obtained by cell enucleation (188, 189) and steroid receptor immunocytochemistry (87, 139) showed almost exclusive nuclear localization of estrogen receptors and progesterone receptors, even in the absence of ligand. Subsequently, many additional studies using receptor-specific antibodies have indicated that in both cases—the absence or the presence of ligand—most steroid receptors are located in the nucleus of the target cells, though the localization of some, particularly the glucocorticoid receptors, remains a subject of controversy. Most studies indicate that the unoccupied glucocorticoid receptors are located in the cytoplasm, while only the occupied receptors are located in the nucleus (59, 133, 190), as in the initial model for all steroid action. However, general agreement has not been reached on the subcellular location of glucocorticoid receptors (17, 46). Both the nuclear receptor model, accepted for most steroid receptors including those for estrogen, progesterone, androgen, and thyroid hormones, and the classic two-step translocation model, still applicable for glucocorticoid receptors, are shown in Figure 17.1.

Despite the importance of steroid receptor nuclear localization, it must be kept in mind that steroid receptors, like all other proteins, are synthesized in the cytoplasm and that, therefore, some of what are described as nuclear steroid receptors must be present also in the cytoplasmic compartment, though perhaps only for a limited time. The majority of nuclear steroid receptors, however, are detected in the nucleus, the site of their action. In general, the genomic response to steroid receptor action is a slow (1 h or more), multistep process. It requires binding of activated steroid receptors to the steroid response element sequences in the DNA, activation of RNA polymerase, transcription, processing and export of the newly synthesized mRNA, translation, and altered cell function by the new protein. In contrast to the relatively slow genomic

steroid actions, rapid biological responses to various steroid hormones have been reported. These rapid steroid responses can be compared to biological responses to the many groups of hydrophilic hormones, the receptors for which are located at the cell surface within the plasma membrane. These transmembrane receptor–mediated responses occur within seconds or minutes, too fast to be mediated through any known genomic pathway. They cannot be blocked by inhibitors of RNA and protein synthesis and may be mediated by nonnuclear steroid receptors associated with plasma membranes. These may represent products of different receptor genes or the classical receptor protein located and acting at a different place in the cell.

In the first part of this chapter we review what is known about the mechanisms of steroid receptor nuclear localization and about steroid receptor trafficking between the nucleus and cytoplasm. The fact that steroid receptors, although predominantly nuclear, also can shuttle between the nuclear and cytoplasmic compartments introduces the possibility of additional receptor functions and interactions with cytoplasmic components. In the second part of this chapter, we describe the nongenomic steroid responses thought to be associated with alternate or nonnuclear steroid receptors localized in the plasma membrane. Although there is limited evidence for connection between genomic and nongenomic responses to steroid hormones, the discovery of steroid receptor trafficking may indicate such a possibility.

A: NUCLEAR RECEPTOR MODEL

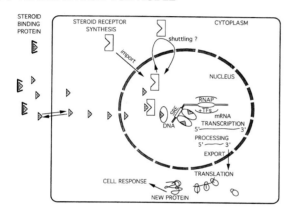

B: TRANSLOCATION MODEL

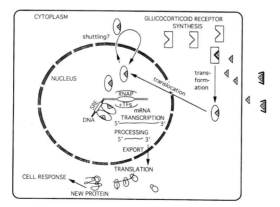

FIG. 17.1. Nuclear receptor model *(A)* and translocation model *(B)* for steroid hormonal action. *RNAP,* RNA polymerase; *TFs,* transcription factors; *SRE,* steroid response element.

NUCLEAR LOCALIZATION OF MOST UNLIGANDED STEROID RECEPTORS

Basis for the Initial Two-Step Translocation Model of Steroid Action and Location

Evidence for the translocation model (Fig. 17.1*B*) was published independently by the labs of Gorski and Jensen beginning in 1968 (58, 75, 160). When immature rat uterus (a model tissue for the study of estrogen action and estrogen receptors) was homogenized, the unoccupied estrogen receptors were found predominantly in the cytosol. If the uterus was exposed to tritiated, high-specific-activity estradiol before homogenization, most of the now occupied estrogen receptors were found in the particulate fraction with the nuclei, from which they could be extracted with buffers containing 0.4–0.6 *M* salt. The apparent translocation of the receptors from the cytosol to the nucleus could be reproduced in cell-free extracts (in vitro), by occupying the cytosolic receptors with estradiol and then incubating them with isolated nuclei. This in vitro translocation process required, first, binding of the hormone to the receptors and, second, incubation at a warmer temperature; 20°–37°C commonly was used. The nuclear location of occupied steroid receptors was not surprising because it had been recognized that a major steroid receptor function was to induce steroid action by modulation of transcription in the nucleus of the cell (120).

The results obtained by subcellular fractionation received apparent confirmation by a morphological technique, autoradiography with techniques for diffusable substances (75, 166). When rat uterus was incubated with tritiated estradiol at 37°C, frozen, and sectioned for autoradiography, the labeled estradiol was observed mostly over the nuclei; when the labeled uterus was homogenized, the radioactive estradiol was recovered mainly in the nuclear pellet. When tissue was incubated with tritiated estradiol at 0°–4°C and processed for autoradiography, radioactivity was distributed generally across the section. This was assumed to represent labeled estradiol bound to cytoplasmic estrogen receptors because if the uterus was homogenized instead, the radioactivity was bound mostly to estrogen receptors in the cytosol.

This evidence for the translocation, or two-step model, of estrogen action and, subsequently, steroid hormonal action obtained from cell fractionation studies was very convincing because it appeared to be confirmed by a morphological technique (autoradiography), it was highly reproducible, and there were no other localization techniques available at the time for steroid receptors that contradicted these observations (reviewed in refs. 182, 183). However, when Sheridan and co-workers reevaluated the autoradiography technique some years later (158, 159), they concluded that the earlier results obtained at 0°–4°C were due to trapped estradiol binding to extracted receptors during homogenization and that for a number of reasons, most estrogen and progesterone receptors were nuclear whether or not they had been occupied by hormone and exposed to "translocation" conditions. These results left the cell fractionation studies as the best evidence for the translocation model, and both of the primary reports noted that this procedure was subject to extraction artifacts (58, 75).

Current Nuclear Localization Model for Most Steroid Receptors

Two additional approaches were applied later. Cell enucleation was used to separate cytoplasm from the nucleus without homogenizing the receptor-containing cells, to avoid the potential extraction artifacts and dilution of the cell contents (188, 189). In addition, after substantial effort over a number of years, reliable antibodies were obtained against the estrogen and progesterone receptor proteins, and these were used to localize the unoccupied steroid receptors by immunocytochemistry with techniques to reduce receptor relocation, loss, or denaturing (47, 87, 98, 139), which had been observed earlier. Both of these very different techniques (cell enucleation and immunocytochemistry) indicated that the unoccupied estrogen and progesterone receptors were located in the nuclei of responsive cells and that few steroid receptors were present in the cytoplasmic compartment.

Glucocorticoid Receptor Localization

Assessing the location of the unoccupied or unliganded glucocorticoid receptors has been more complex (172, 184). The majority of immunocytochemical studies support the translocation model for glucocorticoids (41, 190, and many others), in clear distinction to what is accepted for most of the other steroid receptors. However, Gorski et al. (57) commented on the relatively weak immunostaining of the unoccupied receptors compared to the strong signal of the liganded receptors in glucocorticoid receptor immunocytochemistry and questioned whether the unoccupied receptors were not lost or extracted to some extent in those procedures. When we applied cell enucleation to glucocorticoid receptor localization in earlier studies (188), our results were not consistent with a translocation model. We found instead that few unoccupied, ligand-binding glucocorticoid receptors were present in enucleated GH$_3$ cells (cytoplasts). Immunocytochemical studies that used fixation techniques designed particularly to reduce potential extraction or relocation of unoccupied glucocorticoid receptors [glutaraldehyde fixation (17) and freeze-drying/vapor fixation (138)] also reported that both the unoccupied and occupied glucocorticoid receptors were nuclear.

Many of the studies supporting a translocation model for the glucocorticoid receptors have difficulty demonstrating ligand-dependent translocation of the cytoplasmic immunoreactivity to the nucleus. In principle, this could represent a visible population of extranuclear receptors resident in the cytoplasmic compartment. Most known steroid receptor actions clearly involve activity as ligand-dependent transcription factors acting in the nucleus. However, increased attention has been paid to the possibility of steroid responses through mechanisms which do not directly involve transcription (summarized in ref. 60), and these could involve nonnuclear or membrane-associated steroid receptors working through "nongenomic" action mechanisms. These issues are addressed later in the chapter, but before reviewing nonnuclear and nongenomic steroid receptors, we will review the mechanism of nuclear localization and protein transport and the nuclear localization signals present in the steroid receptor proteins.

NUCLEAR IMPORT AND EXPORT OF STEROID RECEPTORS

Entry of Proteins Into the Nucleus

Nuclear proteins are synthesized in the cytoplasm and transported across the nuclear envelope, which separates the cytoplasm from the nucleoplasm (31). The nuclear envelope consist of two concentric inner and outer membranes, nuclear pore complexes (NPCs), and the nuclear lamina. The inner and outer nuclear membranes, which appear by electron microscopy as conventional lipid bilayers, are separated by a perinuclear space which is continuous with the lumen of the endoplasmic reticulum. The outer nuclear membrane is continuous with, and functionally similar to, the endoplasmic reticulum (48).

Both layers of membrane are perforated by NPCs, which serve as channels for molecular exchanges between the nucleus and cytoplasm. These are organized symmetrically around a central channel and appear to function as rivets that hold the inner and outer layers of membrane together (30). The NPCs have a mass of about 125 megadaltons in higher eukaryotes and are estimated to contain roughly 100 different polypeptides (154). The NPC acts as an aqueous channel, about 9 nm in diameter, allowing free diffusion of small macromolecules at a rate inversely proportional to their mass (14). Small proteins, such as cytochrome c (13kd), can diffuse freely through the pore, whereas diffusion of ovalbumin (43 kd) is delayed and that of bovine serum albumin (BSA; 66 kd) is virtually prevented. Proteins above the size limit for passive diffusion can enter the nucleus based on active processes associated with NPCs (30, 161). Active transport across the NPC can accommodate particles of up to 25 nm in diameter. Transport across the pore occurs in both directions and involves various substrates. For example, all nuclear proteins must be imported from the cytoplasm, where they are synthesized. However, transfer RNAs (tRNAs), ribosomal RNAs (rRNAs), and messenger RNAs (mRNAs) are synthesized in the nucleus and exported to the cytoplasm (rRNAs as assembled ribosomal subunits), where they function in translation.

Nuclear Localization Signals

Active transport of proteins across the nuclear envelope is mediated by a nuclear localization signal (NLS) contained within the transported protein. Some proteins do not possess their own NLS and enter the nucleus via co-transport with another protein (32). In each case, at least one NLS is necessary for import of the protein complex. Experimentally, two criteria are used to establish the presence of NLSs: (1) deletion or mutation causes cytoplasmic accumulation of normally nuclear proteins and (2) when fused to a nonnuclear protein, the NLS directs what are normally cytoplasmic proteins to the nucleus.

The first demonstration that the signal for nuclear import could be restricted to a short, contiguous stretch of amino acids came from studies on nucleoplasmin (molecular weight ~ 33 kd), the major nuclear protein of the Xenopus oocyte (32). A 23 kd fragment of nucleoplasmin missing its C-terminal tail did not enter the nucleus after microinjection into the cytoplasm but remained nuclear when injected directly into the nucleus; however, the C-terminal peptide alone (molecular weight ~ 10kd) was transported efficiently into the nucleus. This experiment demonstrated that the C-terminal portion of nucleoplasmin is necessary for passage of the complete protein into the nucleus, indicating that a subset of amino acids can act as a nuclear determinant. Concurrent with the studies of nucleoplasmin, the NLS was determined for the simian virus 40 (SV40) large T antigen. By deletions, point mutations, and gene fusion, the sequence PKKKRKV (residues 126–132) was defined as the SV40 T antigen minimal NLS (78, 79, 92). A peptide bearing this minimal sequence is sufficient to target a cross-linked carrier protein to the nucleus following microinjection (51). While the SV40 large T antigen-type NLS is composed of a continuous stretch of basic residues (78), further study of nucleoplasmin showed that this protein has a bipartite basic-type NLS, composed of two clusters of basic residues separated by a spacer region (152). Mutation in either region alone has no effect on nuclear localization activity, and the nucleoplasmin NLS is rendered nonfunctional only when both domains are mutated (152). The second cluster of basic residues (AKKKK) in nucleoplasmin shows homology to the minimal NLS of SV40 large T antigen.

It was suggested that bipartite or multiple NLSs increase the efficiency with which proteins interact with the NLS-binding sites at the earliest step of transport into the nucleus (45). The rate of uptake of microinjected protein-coated gold particles into the nucleus increased as a function of the amount of SV40 T antigen NLS per gold particle (37). Also, addition of an extra portion of the T antigen (residues 111–125, which has no homology to minimal NLS) to SV40 T antigen-β-galactosidase hybrid proteins significantly increased the import rate (151). This additional region may function either as a second independent NLS or merely to increase the efficiency of the minimal NLS.

The NLSs for steroid receptors have been identified functionally, but as a group they lack a strict consensus sequence (Table 17.1). However, some general rules can be applied to most NLSs (45): *(1)* they are typically short sequences, usually not more than eight to ten amino acids; *(2)* they are composed of a high proportion of positively charged amino acids (lysine or arginine associated with proline); *(3)* they are not necessarily located at specific sites within the protein; *(4)* they are not removed following nuclear localization; and *(5)* they can be present at more than one site in a given protein. The NLSs of the four steroid receptors have been studied intensively and are described below.

Progesterone Receptors. Studies of NLSs in the progesterone receptor have demonstrated that two major karyophilic mechanisms are involved in nuclear localization of this protein (65, 66). First, a constitutively active karyophilic signal, located around amino acids 638–642 in the hinge region, directs the unoccupied progesterone receptor into the nucleus, and it is similar to the NLS present in SV40 large T antigen. When this signal is deleted, the unoccupied receptors become cytoplasmic. A second localization signal, whose activity is very limited, lies in the steroid-binding domain and requires the binding of hormone to be effective. A receptor mutant containing this signal alone, without karyophilic signals, is cytoplasmic, and treatment with hormone results in only a very small increase in receptor concentration in the nucleus. The putative NLSs in the receptor are shown in Figure 17.2. A second major karyophilic mechanism involved in nuclear localization of

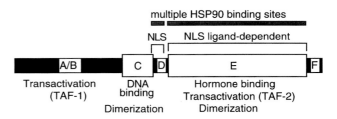

FIG. 17.2. Schematic map of the structural and functional organization of steroid receptors. Conserved regions *C* and *E* are indicated as boxes and a black bar illustrates regions *A/B, D,* and *F.* Domain functions are listed above and below *NLS,* nuclear localization signal; *TAF,* transcription activation function.

the progesterone receptor is activation of the DNA-binding domain through either binding of hormone or deletion of the steroid-binding domain. A mutant in which both the major (amino acids 638–642) and the minor NLSs have been deleted is mainly nuclear because of a constitutively activated DNA-binding domain. Examination of the DNA-binding domain sequence reveals two stretches of basic amino acids which are candidates for NLSs: 614–618 and 624–627. These different signals cooperate. The wild-type progesterone receptor in the presence of hormone (both major karyophilic signals active) is transported more efficiently into the nucleus than proteins containing a single karyophilic signal. The existence of multiple karyophilic signals is observed frequently in nuclear proteins (153) and provides redundant signals to ensure nuclear localization.

Glucocorticoid Receptors. The glucocorticoid receptor also contains two distinct NLSs, NL1 and NL2, that, when fused with heterologous proteins, target them to the nucleus in a hormone-independent and a hormone-dependent manner, respectively (143). The NL1 signal is localized within a 27-amino-acid segment adjacent to the DNA-binding domain, whereas NL2 is located within the C-terminal hormone-binding domain. No additive effect of the two NLSs is seen. Upon hormone addition, the localization rate for the NL1/NL2-fusion protein, which contains both NLSs, displays the same rapid kinetics of localization as the NL2-fusion protein alone. This implies that the NL2 signal is the major kinetic determinant for glucocorticoid receptor localization. In the presence of bound hormone, the glucocorticoid receptor accumulates predominantly in nuclei, but, because the unoccupied glucocorticoid receptor is thought to be cytoplasmic, masking by NL2 of the NL1 function is thought to be responsible for the predominant cytoplasmic localization of unliganded receptors in these studies. An alternative possibility is that in the absence of hormone NLSs within the receptor are not fully functional because they are obscured

TABLE 17.1. *Amino-Acid Sequences or Locations of Potential Nuclear Localization Signals in Steroid Hormone Receptors and SV40 Large T Antigen*

Protein	Species	Sequence and/or Position of Signals*	Reference
SV40 large T antigen	Viral	[126]PKKKRKV	79
Progesterone receptor	Rabbit	[638]RKFKKFNK	66
	Human	[637]RKFKKFNK	66
Glucocorticoid receptor	Rat	497–524	143
	Human	[490]ARKTKKKIK†	68
Estrogen receptor	Human	256–303	143
	Human	[255]IRKDRRGGR†	68
Androgen receptor	Human	[628]RKLKKLGN	66
	Human	[627]ARKLKKLGN†	68

*Position of signal refers to protein region shown to contain a nuclear localization signal (NLS). Large sequences may represent more than one actual signal.   †These NLS sequences were able to target nonnuclear protein (bovine serum albumin) to the nuclear compartment (68).

by the heat shock protein hsp90, bound to the gluco-corticoid receptor in the cytoplasm (142, 155). In this case, dissociation of hsp90 from the glucocorticoid receptor upon hormone binding exposes the NLSs, resulting in receptor translocation into the nucleus. The role of hsp90 in steroid receptor regulation is not clear, but involvement of heat shock protein in protein transport, especially proteins related to the 70 kd heat shock protein, has been proposed (38, 71, 165). However, if unoccupied glucocorticoid receptors are nu-clear, as a number of studies have indicated, then masking of NL1 in cells is not required and the two NLSs may function in glucocorticoid receptors as they do in progesterone receptors.

Estrogen Receptors. The human estrogen receptor con-tains a 48-amino-acid fragment, located in the hinge region between the DNA- and hormone-binding do-mains (amino acids 256–303), which is thought to be responsible for nuclear localization of this protein (141). This portion of the receptor includes three basic stretches of amino acids: 256–260, 266–271, and 299–303. The first two are almost perfectly conserved among the different species. The third stretch is con-served only in charge. In this study, none of these basic stretches alone was sufficient as an NLS and only the whole fragment (amino acids 256–303) mediated nuclear localization of a β-galactosidase-fusion protein. However, in another study, a short synthesized peptide, similar to the first basic stretch of amino acids of the estrogen receptor NLS, was able to direct a different nonnuclear protein (BSA) to the nucleus [Table 17.1; (68)].

Androgen Receptors. Deletion studies on the human androgen receptor have identified that the amino-acid residue 557–653 is important for proper nuclear im-port (76). This part of the androgen receptor contains a signal encoded by two groups of basic residues, separated by a spacer of ten amino-acid residues, which is functionally similar to the bipartite nucleoplasmin NLS. Mutational analysis of the bipartite nucleo-plasmin-like NLS revealed that both basic parts of the signal contribute to nuclear targeting of the androgen receptor. In the presence of hormone, the androgen receptor is located in the nucleus. Interestingly, expres-sion of the wild-type androgen receptor in different cell lines revealed a cell line–specific subcellular distri-bution of the unliganded receptor (76). In the absence of ligand, the androgen receptor was predominantly nuclear when expressed in HeLa cells, more evenly distributed over the cytoplasm and nucleus in CV-1 and Chinese hamster ovary (CHO) cells, and mainly cytoplasmic in COS-1 cells. The dynamic shuttling of

the steroid receptors and their subcellular localization could be influenced by at least three factors: accessibil-ity of the NLS, translocation efficiency, and binding to the nuclear and cytoplasmic components. Transloca-tion efficiency and some components involved in trap-ping the androgen receptor might be cell line–specific, and these factors could explain the contradictory re-ports on the subcellular localization of the unliganded androgen receptor (76, 162, 192).

Mechanism of Nuclear Import

The discovery of multiple, ligand-dependent and -inde-pendent NLSs in the steroid receptor suggested the possibility of their different functions. Two nonhomol-ogous and functionally distinct NLSs have been discov-ered in the nuclear protein MATα2 in yeast (67). Mutation of each signal individually results in different effects and has led to the development of a model in which each signal supports a different step in nuclear import. According to this model, the first signal medi-ates a receptor-dependent association with NPC and the second signal subsequently engages the transport machinery to foster translocation. This model provides a molecular basis for the known two-step model for nuclear import: binding to the NPC, probably to fibrils extending from the cytoplasmic side of the pore, and subsequent energy-dependent translocation through the pore (126, 150).

Nuclear import is a highly specific and saturable process and, therefore, has been postulated to involve specific NLS receptors, either as components of the NPC or as soluble recognition factors (51, 161). Under physiological conditions, the nucleus has a very differ-ent protein composition compared to the cytoplasm, despite the mixing of the cytoplasmic and nuclear contents that takes place during each mitotic cycle in higher eukaryotes. Early experiments in which labeled proteins were injected into frog oocytes showed that the nucleus readily discriminates between nuclear and cytoplasmic proteins (13). The discovery of NLSs in proteins demonstrates the existence of a specific appa-ratus that recognizes these karyophilic signals. Microin-jection of NLS peptide conjugates (cross-linked BSA to the SV40 T antigen NLS) at high concentration led to saturation of the protein-import pathway, providing strong evidence for the existence of a saturable NLS receptor (51). Kinetic competition studies (108) and, later, direct import and binding experiments (54, 181) have shown that the SV40 and nucleoplasmin NLSs use the same receptor, whereas small nuclear ribo-nucleoproteins do not compete with karyophilic pro-teins for import (40, 108) and presumably have distinct receptors.

The development of an in vitro system based on cultured mammalian cells treated with digitonin, which selectively permeabilizes the plasma membrane and depletes cells of their soluble contents (3, 115), led to purification of the four soluble factors essential for active protein import: importin-α (2, 54, 73, 119, 181), importin-β (1, 19, 52, 72, 147), the small guanosine triphosphatase (GTPase) Ran (8, 35, 104, 116), and pp15 (117, 137). The steps of the nuclear protein-import cycle are shown in Figure 17.3 (53). The protein to be imported binds via its NLS to the α-subunit of the importin-α/β heterodimer [originally defined as the NLS receptor (51)] in the cytoplasm (2, 52, 54, 73, 74, 181). This complex then docks with the NPC via importin-β (55, 119) and subsequently is translocated through the pore by an energy-dependent mechanism (126, 150) that also requires Ran and pp15 (116, 117). Translocation involves GTP hydrolysis by Ran and is probably a multistep process. The constituents of the NLS recognition complex become separated as a result of this process. The imported protein and importin-α reach the nucleoplasm, whereas importin-β accumu-

lates at the nuclear envelope (55, 119). Immunoelectron microscopy detects importin-β at both sides of the NPC (55), suggesting that it does not remain at its initial docking site but moves with importin-α and the import substrate through the pore. No importin-β accumulation is seen in the nucleoplasm, presumably because its recycling to the cytoplasm is too rapid. In the nucleus, importin-α has to dissociate from the NLS-containing imported protein. Given the high concentration of NLSs in the nucleus, which would tend to keep the NLS-binding site on importin-α occupied, it is likely that this involves conversion of importin-α to a form with low affinity for the NLS. The different rates of export of the α and β receptor subunits indicate that they return to the cytoplasm separately, possibly by different routes.

Nuclear Export and Nucleocytoplasmic Shuttling

While substantial insight into the molecular basis for nuclear protein import has been obtained, nuclear export remains poorly understood. Nuclear proteins ex-

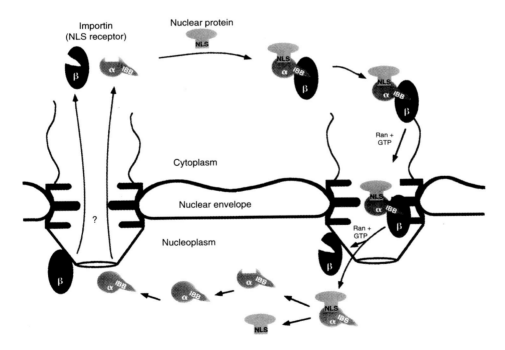

FIG. 17.3. Steps of the nuclear protein-import cycle. Nuclear localization signal *(NLS)*–containing proteins bind to the importin heterodimer (NLS receptor) in the cytosol. The NLS interacts primarily with the α-subunit; the importin-β-binding domain of α mediates heterodimerization. Binding of NLS to α can precede α–β interaction. The β-subunit mediates docking of the complex at the nuclear pore complex. Translocation involves GTP hydrolysis by Ran and is probably a multistep process. The α–β heterodimer dissociates, and α enters the nucleoplasm with the substrate. Dissociation of α from the nuclear protein must then occur. For a further round of import, the subunits of importin are returned to the cytoplasm, possibly separately. [Reprinted with permission from D. Görlich and I. W. Mattaj (53). *Science* 271: 1513–1518. Copyright 1996, American Association for the Advancement of Science.]

change between nuclei in fused cells, and those which are located and act primarily in the nucleus also can be present at some low level in the cytoplasm. The nuclear localization of a number of proteins reflects a dynamic situation, the protein continuously shuttling between the nucleus and the cytoplasm. A number of shuttling proteins have been identified, including members of the 70 kd family of heat shock proteins (96); the heterogeneous nuclear RNA-packaging protein A1 (145); the U1 small nuclear RNA-specific protein U1A (80); and the nucleolar proteins nucleolin, NO38 (15), and Nopp140 (103).

Steroid Receptors. Studies of steroid receptor localization have revealed that the nuclear residency of the receptors reflects a similar situation: although most of the receptor population is nuclear, a portion of the total receptors continuously shuttle between the nucleus and the cytoplasm (18, 65, 95). The fact that steroid receptors are proteins which have NLSs suggests that they should reside in the nucleus, but energy-depletion experiments with progesterone and estrogen receptors have demonstrated that they can exit continuously from the nucleus to the cytoplasm and can be transported constantly and actively back to the nucleus (65). Studies of the migration of the progesterone receptor between nuclei in interspecies heterokaryons have confirmed directly the existence of nucleocytoplasmic trafficking of the receptor. A mouse L-cell line permanently expressing the progesterone receptor was fused with human 293 cells devoid of receptor in the presence of protein-synthesis inhibitors. The progesterone receptor was detected in nuclei of human 293 cells 12 h after fusion. Similar experiments have been performed on ligand-bound glucocorticoid receptors (95) and estrogen receptors (25).

Although earlier studies of progesterone and estrogen receptor exports showed that these processes occur through passive diffusion (65), subsequent research has revealed that the NLSs also may be involved in outward movement of protein through the nuclear membrane (63). The shuttling ability of a construct of bacterial β-galactosidase with progesterone receptor NLS (nlsPR-β-galactosidase) permanently expressed in a mouse L-cell line was compared to complete progesterone receptor or β-galactosidase (63, 65). Both progesterone receptor and nlsPR-β-galactosidase were observed in the nucleus. Administration of sodium azide to reduce intracellular adenosine triphosphate (ATP) provoked an efflux of both proteins from the nucleus to the cytoplasm. When β-galactosidase itself (devoid of any NLS) was microinjected into L-cell nuclei, administration of sodium azide was without effect; in this case, the protein remained inside the nucleus. Similar

results were obtained previously by microinjection of immunoglobulins (65). This property is not specific to progesterone receptor NLS because the same phenomenon was observed with the SV40 large T antigen NLS grafted to β-galactosidase. The amount of protein available for shuttling depends on the interaction of this protein with nuclear or cytoplasmic components. In the SV40 large T antigen, which is a DNA-binding protein, shuttling takes place but at a markedly slower pace (63).

These experiments showed that a large protein devoid of an NLS cannot cross the nuclear membrane in either direction. However, if an NLS is grafted onto this protein, not only does most of it accumulate in the nucleus but the protein also participates in continuous shuttling between the nucleus and the cytoplasm. As mentioned previously, accumulation of protein in the nucleus is signal- and energy-dependent, whereas efflux from the nucleus does not require energy but for some proteins is signal-dependent.

This shuttling phenomenon can explain some contradictory observations in steroid receptor localization; for example, ligand-free progesterone or estrogen receptors which reside in the nucleus after homogenization can be found in the cytosol because in these conditions export of the receptors is not counterbalanced by import, a process which requires energy and is blocked by dilution and low temperature. Furthermore, the ligand-free glucocorticoid receptor found in the cytoplasm in many studies can be explained by less effective or masked constitutive karyophilic signals which lead to an increased time of residency of the receptor in this compartment (64). Although the nuclear import mediated by the putative NLS itself is not regulated by ligand binding, the transport of steroid receptors across the nuclear membrane might be regulated indirectly by ligand. Hormone-induced changes in receptor conformation or dissociation of the receptor complex with heat shock proteins has been proposed to eliminate cytoplasmic retention and expose the receptor NLS, resulting in nuclear translocation (142, 191). Also, phosphorylation in or near the NLS, possibly induced by ligand, might regulate the efficiency of nuclear import (29).

The main conclusion emerging from these studies is that the ability to shuttle between the nucleus and the cytoplasm is not a specific property of a small number of proteins. Instead, most nuclear proteins which contain NLSs are potential shuttling proteins. The steady-state nucleocytoplasmic distribution of a shuttling protein is not governed exclusively by the relative rates of nuclear import and export but also by its relative affinity for nuclear and cytoplasmic binding partners (80).

Other Macromolecules. Shuttling proteins have attracted considerable interest because they might contribute to the coordination of nuclear and cytoplasmic activities (127, 156). Furthermore, it has been speculated widely that shuttling proteins might perform a carrier function in nucleocytoplasmic transport (15, 50, 71, 96, 103). The nucleolar proteins nucleolin, NO38 (15, 157), and Nopp140 (103) have been implicated in the transport of ribosomal proteins to the nucleolus. Moreover, NO38 (49), Nopp140 (102), and the heat shock cognate protein hsc70 (71) have been described as NLS-binding proteins which may function as chaperones during the transport of karyophilic proteins through the nuclear pores. In one plausible model, shuttling proteins contain export signals acting positively to direct export to the cytoplasm. Alternatively, protein export from the nucleus could be a default process, with nonshuttling proteins prevented from leaving the nucleus; nuclear retention might be caused by tight binding to intranuclear structures or by the formation of large complexes.

To distinguish between the above alternatives, a variety of proteins were tested to determine the structural requirements for nuclear export (156). First, HeLa cells were transfected transiently with cDNAs encoding for the wild-type chicken or mutant deletion of nucleolin (a well-characterized nucleolar shuttling protein) and then fused to normal mouse cells in the presence of cycloheximide. Under these conditions, any chicken nucleolin found in the mouse nuclei of the heterokaryon must have been exported from the nuclei of the HeLa cells. Wild-type protein was detectable in the mouse nuclei 24 h after fusion. Analysis of deletion mutants showed that none of the domains of nucleolin was essential for export and shuttling but that individual domains influenced the efficiency of shuttling. Second, rates of nuclear export were measured after wild-type and mutant proteins were injected into Xenopus oocyte nuclei. Export of intact nucleolin was extremely slow, but inactivation of the bipartite NLS resulted in accumulation of 90% of the mutant protein in the cytoplasm within 24 h. This suggested that the lack of observed export of the wild-type protein is due to efflux from the nucleus followed by rapid NLS-dependent reimport. Another protein, a cytoplasmic pyruvate kinase carrying the NLS from SV40 T antigen, introduced experimentally into the nucleus, exhibited shuttling ability. Since it is unlikely that pyruvate kinase has a specific nuclear-export signal, the observed nuclear export is unlikely to be signal-mediated. Addition of the domains of nucleolin required for its retention in the nucleus strongly inhibited the nuclear export of the pyruvate kinase NLS, supporting the view that such retention sequences prevent export and shuttling. Fur-

thermore, a third protein, a nonshuttling lamin B2, which is part of the nuclear lamina, was converted into a shuttling protein by introducing a mutation that impaired its retention within the nucleus.

Taken together, these experiments with three very different proteins establish that shuttling does not necessarily require specific export sequences and that it can be decreased by sequences that promote binding in the nucleus. This model, however, does not explain why some nonnuclear proteins microinjected into the nucleus cannot gain access to the cytoplasm (32, 65, 92, 96).

It is important to emphasize the distinction between the export kinetics of mRNA–protein complexes and the export of nuclear proteins. Before mRNA molecules can be transported to the cytoplasm of eukaryotic cells, they are processed extensively from mRNA precursors in the nucleus (107). Through these maturation events, pre-mRNA and mRNA are associated with a set of over 20 abundant nuclear proteins, collectively termed "heterogeneous nuclear ribonucleoproteins" (hnRNPs) (34). One of the most intriguing aspects of hnRNPs is their intracellular transport. Although primarily nuclear, a subset of hnRNPs (for example, A1, A2, and K) continuously shuttle between the nucleus and cytoplasm, while others (for example, C1, C2, and U) are restricted to the nucleus at all times (145, 146). The observation of Balbiani ring mRNAs by electron microscopy made it clear that the substrate for export is not naked RNA but RNP, implicating RNA-binding proteins as mediators of export (100, 101).

One of the rapid shuttling hnRNPs, A1, is bound to poly(A) + RNA in both the nucleus and cytoplasm, suggesting that it is transported together with the mRNA during export (145). Its nuclear localization domain (38 amino acids long), located near the C-terminus of the protein, has been described (163). This domain, termed M9, also can target heterologous, normally cytoplasmic proteins, such as β-galactosidase and pyruvate kinase. Interestingly, M9 bears no sequence homology to classical NLS sequences, such as the SV40 large T antigen NLS or the nucleoplasmin bipartite basic NLS. As mentioned earlier, the classical NLS sequences, when fused to β-galactosidase, can mediate nuclear egression of these fusion proteins in a non-energy-dependent manner (63). The ability of classical NLSs and of the M9 region of A1 to promote nuclear export has been shown (107). Pyruvate kinase fusion proteins bearing either a classical NLS or M9 are exported to the nucleus at a physiological temperature, but a difference is apparent when export at a low temperature is examined, indicating that separate pathways are utilized. The M9 region of A1 can mediate efficient nuclear export of protein only in a temperature-dependent manner, suggesting an energy-dependent process. Also, a normally nonshuttling protein, the nucleoplasmin core domain, can be exported efficiently when fused to M9 but not when fused to a classical NLS. Therefore, M9 has been identified as a positively acting, transferable nuclear-export signal in a cellular pre-mRNA-binding protein. These data, therefore, suggest that M9 functions as the recognition element that facilitates nuclear export within mRNP particles and support the possibility that shuttling hnRNPs play a role as carriers of mRNA to the cytoplasm.

The ability of M9 to convert pyruvate kinase to the temperature-dependent pathway invokes a comparison between A1 export and classical NLS-mediated nuclear import. Nuclear import of classical NLS-bearing proteins is a multistep process that involves NLS–NLS receptor interaction and docking at the NPC and subsequent translocation through the pore. The translocation, but not the docking step, requires energy and is blocked at low temperature (115, 126, 150). Even small proteins that normally can diffuse freely through the NPC into the nucleus do not efficiently enter the nucleus at low temperature when they include a classical NLS (16). This indicates that a commitment to the classical NLS import pathway overrides diffusion, apparently by interaction of the NLS-containing protein with the relatively large NLS receptor (1, 2, 54, 147, 181). If signal-mediated nuclear export operates by a similar mechanism, it is likely that M9-bearing proteins are blocked in the nucleus at the low temperature because export signal–receptor interactions occur but translocation through the NPC does not. The fact that M9 has NLS activity suggests also that at least some of the factors that mediate nuclear import and export are similar.

Conclusions

Nuclear localization of steroid receptors is brought about by specific sequences in the proteins that are similar to signals of nuclear import and export in other proteins. Nuclear localization is, therefore, a specific, active process, rather than a passive product of steroid receptor interaction with chromatin. The specificity of the process, however, also suggests that either regulation or specific functional deletion of NLSs could, in principle, yield altered forms of the receptor or alternate receptor genes. These protein products might not express NLSs and could function in different places in the cell, for example, in the cytoplasm or associated with plasma membranes, to mediate different hormonal responses. These hypotheses are addressed in the next section.

ALTERNATE STEROID RECEPTORS AND NONGENOMIC STEROID RESPONSES

A great deal of evidence has accumulated on how steroid hormones act through their receptors at the level of nuclear DNA to regulate gene expression. It has become apparent that intracellular steroid receptor proteins, upon activation with their specific cognate ligands, undergo transformational changes to a state in which they are capable of interacting with their hormone response elements on chromatin and regulating the transcription of specific genes. A dual role for steroid hormones has been formulated to explain rapid biological responses. It seems that steroid action may not only control transcription but also trigger rapid cell membrane effects. These rapid changes do not directly involve gene expression and are termed "nongenomic."

In eukaryotes, two major signal-transduction pathways can be distinguished (reviewed in ref. 61). One pathway relies on the receptors for small hydrophobic molecules, such as steroid and thyroid hormones, vitamin D, and retinoids, which are located in or associated with the nucleus and act as ligand-inducible transcription factors. This conventional genomic response is normally slow, requiring 1 h or more to measure effects. The second pathway involves receptors that span the plasma membrane. Ligand binding induces a cascade of rapid events, which, by mechanisms that are still not fully understood, also can modulate activity of certain transcription factors and, thus, genetic programs. Nongenomic steroid responses could fit into the early stage of this pathway. Although the early, rapid, nongenomic and late, much slower, genomic responses are thought of as separate, it is possible that rapid cell membrane effects also indirectly trigger changes in genomic expression.

Nearly all of the major steroid hormone classes have been associated with nongenomic effects. The exact mechanism by which steroids activate such effects is unknown, and there may be multiple mechanisms. Many studies, which have provided evidence of rapid responses to steroids and have localized their action in cell membranes, have not been able to identify the protein responsible for binding these steroids. Factors contributing to the difficulty in identifying these putative membrane-binding sites are their low abundance, the low specific activity of the standard tritiated steroid ligands, and very high nonspecific binding.

Estrogen Receptor-β

The cloning of a novel member of the steroid receptor superfamily, estrogen receptor-β, has been reported (89). The identification of this alternative receptor raises the possibility that potential nongenomic actions of steroids need not rely solely on the properties of the classic receptors and suggests the existence of other, as yet unknown receptors. For example, the estrogen binding reported in plasma membranes might not be due to the classic estrogen receptor, now termed estrogen receptor-α, but could be mediated by estrogen receptor-β or even other as yet undescribed estrogen receptors. Estrogen receptor-β (clone 29) was isolated from a rat prostate cDNA library. The protein, expressed in the reticulolysate system, is 485 amino acids long, with a molecular weight of 54,200 daltons. Estrogen receptor-β displays high homology to the classic estrogen receptor-α, especially in the DNA-binding domain (96%) and in the ligand-binding domain (55%). The main difference from estrogen receptor-α is much shorter A/B- and F-domains at the N- and C-termini, respectively. The hinge region has 29% homology with estrogen receptor-α. By in situ hybridization, estrogen receptor-β mRNA was found in the reproductive tract of both male and female rats, with lower expression in other rat tissues. In male reproductive organs, a high level of expression was seen in epithelial cells of the prostate glands. In female reproductive organs, estrogen receptor-β was expressed only in granulosa cells of primary, secondary, and mature follicles of the ovary (not in the uterus and vagina). It binds estradiol with high affinity [dissociation constant $(K_d) = 0.6$ nM]. Competition curves showed that only estrogens competed efficiently with [^{3}H]-estradiol for binding of estrogen receptor-β. Fifty percent inhibition of specific binding occurred at a 0.6-fold excess of unlabeled estradiol; diethylstilbestrol, estriol, and estrone were 5, 15, and 50 times, respectively, less effective as competitors. Neither testosterone, progesterone, nor corticosterone was an efficient competitor, even at 1000-fold excess. In co-transfection experiments of CHO cells with an estrogen receptor-β expression vector and an estrogen-regulated reporter gene, only estrogen, estrone, and 5α-androstane-3β,17β-diol stimulated reporter gene activity. The biological significance of the existence of two different estrogen receptors has not been determined; however, the discovery of estrogen receptor-β has energized the search for additional binding proteins that could mediate nongenomic actions of estradiol, and this possibility could be extended to other members of the steroid receptor superfamily.

Glucocorticoids

Inhibition of Amphibian Mating Behavior. In some cases, steroid hormones rapidly modulate animal behavior by binding to specific cell-surface receptors on neurons. The evidence comes from research with an amphibian model, *Taricha granulosa* (111–113). In *Taricha*, stress, generally, and corticosterone, specifically, inhibit reproductive behaviors with a rapidity that is inconsistent with traditional models for steroid action (131). The reaction to corticosterone produces multiple neurophysiological effects within 3 min and inhibits mating behavior within 8 min of treatment (Fig. 17.4A). These observations have led to the hypothesis that this rapid effect of corticosterone involves a cell-surface receptor in neuronal membranes.

A series of radioligand-binding assays identified a corticosteroid receptor in neuronal membranes that appears to mediate the rapid behavioral responses in *Taricha* (131). Kinetic and equilibrium saturation binding experiments indicated that corticosterone binding to brain membranes was specific, saturable, and of high affinity ($K_d = 0.16$ and 0.51 nM, respectively). In addition, the ligand specificity for binding to the membrane receptor corresponds to the magnitude of the response (Fig. 17.4A,B). Control experiments showed that exposure of the membrane fraction to high temperature (60°C) or to protease trypsin eliminated corticosterone-specific binding. In a competition study, cortisol was the only other steroid with high affinity (inhibition constant $K_i = 3.75$ nM) for the corticosterone-binding site. The mineralocorticoid aldosterone, the glucocorticoid dexamethasone, and other type I and type II corticoid receptor ligands tested did not display high affinity for this membrane-associated binding site. This indicates that the corticosterone receptor in neuronal membranes is pharmacologically distinct from intracellular corticosteroid receptors (amphibian intracellular corticoid receptors have high affinity for aldosterone, dexamethasone, or both and for corticosterone) (114).

The corticosterone membrane receptor appears to be G protein–coupled (130). This conclusion was based on findings that corticosterone binding in neuronal membranes was modulated negatively by nonhydrolyzable guanine nucleotide analogs, especially GTP-γ-S. Addition of guanyl nucleotide and unlabeled corticosterone induced also a rapid phase. [^{3}H]-corticosterone dissociation from membranes that was not induced by addition of unlabeled ligand alone. Other experiments showed that increasing concentration of Mg^{2+} in the assay buffer enhanced corticosterone binding and the sensitivity of the receptor to modulation by guanyl nucleotides. Therefore, it may be that corticoid-specific G protein–coupled receptors provide a signal-transduction mechanism that mediates rapid behavioral responses in *Taricha*.

Lymphocyte Cytolysis. In mammals, glucocorticoids act on immature or transformed lymphoid tissues through

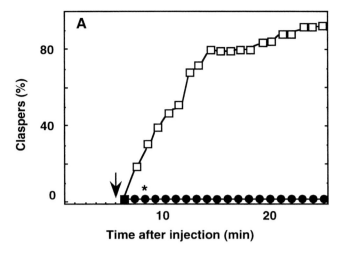

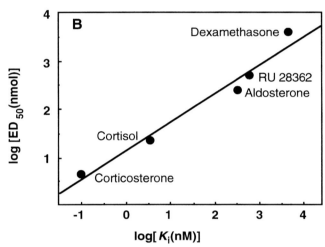

FIG. 17.4. Inhibition of male sexual behavior. *A*: Latency of response to corticosterone. Males were injected with 32 nmol (11 μg) of corticosterone (*filled circles*) or vehicle (*open squares*), *n* = 14. *Arrow* indicates time of addition of females to tanks. Data are reported as cumulative percentage of claspers at 1 min intervals.* Males injected with corticosterone were inhibited significantly within 3 min of testing (Fisher's exact test, $P = 0.025$). *B*: Linear relationship between potency of steroids in inhibition of [^{3}H]corticosterone binding (*ordinate*) and potency in inhibition of sexual behavior (*abscissa*). Males were injected with one of five to seven doses of steroid or vehicle (*n* = 24 for each dose of steroid, except *n* = 14 for RU 28362). Data were recorded as number of claspers in 20 min tests (except cortisol, for which 60 min tests were performed late in the breeding season). [Reprinted with permission from M. Orchinik, T. F. Murray, and F. L. Moore (131). *Science* 252: 1848–1851. Copyright 1991, American Association for the Advancement of Science.]

the glucocorticoid receptor to elicit a series of profound cellular responses which result in cytolysis (164). However, the correlation between the quantity of glucocorticoid receptor and the cytolytic effects of glucocorticoids is imperfect, and resistance to these cytolytic

effects has been described in glucocorticoid receptor–rich rodent lymphomas, normal rodent and human lymphocytes, and cells from a variety of human leukemias (69, 70, 94).

Studies of the mechanisms involved in glucocorticoid-mediated lymphocytolysis in S-49 lymphoma cells have reported a novel glucocorticoid receptor that resides in the plasma membrane (42–44). Plasma membrane localization of this receptor was observed at the ultrastructural level using an immunolabeled colloidal gold-staining technique. In trypsinized cells, however, binding of antibody to the plasma membrane was negligible, suggesting that the immunoreactive membrane antigen is a protein-containing specific proteolytic enzyme cleavage site and that the surface orientation of this antibody-binding domain is extracellular. Further study indicated that removal of the plasma membrane glucocorticoid receptor by trypsin caused cells to be more resistant to the lytic effect of glucocorticoids than untrypsinized cells. Sucrose density gradient analysis using a high salt condition revealed that the cytosolic receptor sedimented as a 4 S protein, while the plasma membrane glucocorticoid receptor sedimented as a multiple protein species with a predominant size of 8–9 S. A molecular size heterogeneity in the sedimentation profile of the competitively radiolabeled membrane receptors shows that the plasma membrane glucocorticoid receptor exists in these cells in various molecular forms. Results from one- and two-dimensional gel analyses corroborated this molecular size heterogeneity and revealed the localization of multiple high-molecular-weight plasma membrane glucocorticoid receptor forms ranging from 97 to 500 kd in S-49 cells. Although the two forms of glucocorticoid receptor described here differ only by size and a slightly altered ability of other steroids to compete for glucocorticoid binding, the results support a role for the plasma membrane glucocorticoid receptor in mediating the lytic effects of glucocorticoids.

Mineralocorticoids

Aldosterone influences the transport of Na$^+$ and K$^+$ in classical (kidney tubules) and nonclassical (hippocampus, arterial smooth muscle cells, mammary gland, and human mononuclear leukocytes) target tissues at the level of the cell membrane. The genomic action of mineralocorticoids involves binding of aldosterone to nuclear type I receptors, which act as transactivating factors to initiate the synthesis of specific aldosterone-induced proteins, including Na–K–ATPase (176). Classical intracellular mineralocorticoid receptors have been cloned (4), and typically these receptors are not specific for aldosterone and bind hydrocortisone and canrenone, the classical mineralocorticoid antagonist, with nearly equal affinity.

Changes in Membrane Electrolyte Transport.

Studies in extrarenal nonepithelial cells, such as rat vascular smooth muscle cells (20, 177) and human lymphocytes (174, 178), have demonstrated that aldosterone produces not only classical genomic effects but also rapid nongenomic effects on transmembrane electrolyte movements. In classical target tissues, aldosterone appears to be involved mainly in stimulating $Na^+–K^+$ exchange (106). In human mononuclear leukocytes, increases of sodium, potassium, and calcium and accompanying shifts of water and volume after aldosterone application appeared to depend on a primary activation of the sodium–proton antiport. Activation of the $Na^+–H^+$ exchanger of the cell membrane occurs at very low physiological concentrations of aldosterone (≈ 0.1 nM), with an acute onset within 1–2 min. Membrane-binding sites highly specific for aldosterone in human lymphocytes were found by radiotracer studies (175), suggesting the presence of novel receptors in membranes. The calculated K_d for aldosterone was 0.04 nM, with maximum binding corresponding to ≈ 150 binding sites per lymphocyte. In contrast to aldosterone, neither canrenone nor cortisol was active at concentrations up to 0.1 μM, whereas deoxycorticosterone acetate had an intermediate activity ($K_d \approx 100$ nM). Association with and dissociation from receptors were rapid, with half-times of about 1 min. These data are consistent with the functional data on aldosterone effects on $Na^+–H^+$ exchange in the same cells. A membrane mineralocorticoid receptor in this affinity range would explain the biological activity of physiological plasma concentrations of free aldosterone in humans (≈ 0.1 nM) rather than a receptor with a K_d greater than 1 nM, such as the classical type I receptor in intact lymphocytes. Mineralocorticoid action on ion flux is thought to be composed of both a primary increase in sodium permeability and an early, secondary stimulation of Na–K–ATPase. Both responses are insensitive to actinomycin D. However, after 1 h, an additional increase in sodium efflux is sensitive to actinomycin D, representing presumably a delayed response of the genome.

Further studies of the rapid intracellular signaling for aldosterone demonstrated that the second messenger inositol-1,4,5-trisphosphate (IP_3) pathway appeared to be involved in intracellular signaling in human mononuclear leukocytes and rat vascular smooth muscle cells (20, 21), as well as free intracellular $[Ca^{2+}]$ (179, 180). Rapid effects of aldosterone were described also on diacylglycerol (DAG), the by-product of phosphoinositide hydrolysis, and protein kinase C (PKC) transloca-tion, presumably mediated through activation of phospholipase C (22).

The effects of aldosterone on electrolyte transport and second messengers and on membrane binding in human mononuclear leukocytes and vascular smooth muscle cells share highly characteristic features: they are rapid and aldosterone-specific, canrenone is inactive, and cortisol is a very weak agonist. These data are summarized in Table 17.2 and compared with the pharmacological data on the classical type I mineralocorticoid receptor, which are quite different. Based on these findings, a two-step model for mineralocorticoid action has been postulated (173):

1. The first step in aldosterone action involves steroid binding to membrane receptors, which triggers changes in membrane electrolyte transport systems. This response is rapid, beginning within 1–2 min. Secondary to this step, the immediate activation of a preexisting electrolyte transport system (Na–K–AT-Pase) is induced in response to changes in electrolyte concentration, which is also rapid and initiated within minutes.

2. A separate response involves a genomic mechanism and provokes ion transport after approximately 1 h, a response which includes production of aldosterone-induced proteins and new Na–K–ATPase molecules.

Similar aldosterone-binding sites have been found in the plasma membrane of porcine kidney and liver microsomes (23, 105). These binding sites are thermolabile and degraded by the protease trypsin, indicating that they are proteins. They have pharmacological properties similar to those described above for aldosterone membrane binding in human lymphocytes and for rapid aldosterone effects on sodium–proton exchange.

Progesterone

Interactions With γ-Aminobutyric Acid A Receptors.

There are several examples of nongenomic actions of progesterone. One well-documented example is the interaction between progesterone or deoxycorticosterone metabolites and the γ-aminobutyric acid A (GABA$_A$) receptor complex. In neuronal tissue, ring A–reduced progesterone and deoxycorticosterone steroids (3α-dihydroxyprogesterone and 5α-tetrahydrodeoxycorticosterone, respectively) have acute cell-surface action mediated via the GABA$_A$ receptor complex, which forms chloride channels in the cell membrane (91, 99). The inhibitory actions of these steroids on neuronal activity by potentiating GABA-induced changes in chloride channel conductance may explain the efficacy of progestational steroids as anesthetic and anticonvulsant agents.

TABLE 17.2. *Comparison of Properties of Cloned Mineralocorticoid Receptor (CMC) and Mineralocorticoid Membrane Receptor (MCM), Rapid Relative Aldosterone Effects on Inositol-1, 4, 5-Trisphosphate (IP₃) Generation in Human Mononuclear Lymphocytes (HML), and Na⁺–H⁺ Exchanger in HML and Rat Vascular Smooth Muscle Cells (VSMC)*

| | CMC | MCM | Na⁺–H⁺ Exchanger | | IP_3 Generation |
			HML	VSMC	
K_d/EC_{50}, nM for aldosterone	1.4	0.05	0.04	0.17	0.1
Aldosterone/cortisol affinity	~1:1	~10,000:1	~10,000:1	>1000:1	~1000:1
Aldosterone/canrenone affinity	~5:1	>1000:1	~10,000:1	>1000:1	≥100:1
Location	Cytosol/ nucleus	Plasma membrane	Plasma membrane	Plasma membrane	Plasma membrane

[From M. Wehling, *Steroids* 60: 153–156, 1995. Reproduced by copyright permission of Elsevier Science Inc.]

Interactions With Oocyte and Sperm Membranes. Some aspects of amphibian oocyte and spermatozoa maturation are regulated by progesterone in a nongenomic manner. In oocytes, progesterone causes a rapid increase in the intracellular free calcium level (171), with onset latencies of 40–60 s and a duration of 5–6 min. Similar to the events occurring in amphibian oocytes, in human spermatozoa during the acrosomal reaction (10), a maturational event involves a progesterone-stimulated influx of extracellular Ca^{2+} (Fig. 17.5). During the acrosomal reaction, a breakdown of the outer acrosomal membrane occurs, allowing secretion of enzymes and revealing internal binding sites that are important in the fertilization process. The acrosomal reaction is initiated when the sperm approach the cumulus oophorus, which secretes progesterone. Progesterone triggers an influx of extracellular calcium into sperm, leading to the acrosomal reaction and preparation of the spermatozoa for fertilization (11, 12, 132).

The cell-surface progesterone-binding site on human sperm (which mediates progesterone-induced changes in Ca^{2+}) is unlike the steroid-binding site on the GABA_A receptor/chloride channel. Stimulation of Ca^{2+} influx by progesterone is not modified by GABA, diazepam, picrotoxin, or pentobarbitol, known regulators of the GABA_A receptor/chloride channel (9, 10). Because picrotoxin, a highly selective inhibitor of GABA_A receptors, inhibits the progesterone-induced acrosomal reaction without preventing the progesterone-stimulated Ca^{2+} influx, it is possible that progesterone interacts with two cell-surface receptors in sperm: one that mediates the rapid Ca^{2+} influx and another which is GABA_A-like and mediates Cl^- flux. Activation of both receptors may be required for the progesterone-induced acrosomal reaction. Alternatively, because this reaction requires a functional GABA_A receptor/chloride channel but not a progesterone-induced Cl^- flux, it is also possible that only the interaction of progesterone with the receptor-mediated Ca^{2+} influx is required.

Desensitization of α_1-Adrenergic Response. Progesterone-induced desensitization of α_1-adrenergic-mediated increases in cyclic adenosine monophosphate (cAMP) in hypothalamic tissue in estrogen-primed rats also lends support to the hypothesis of nongenomic actions of progesterone (140). Two pieces of evidence strongly suggest that progesterone modulates α_1-receptor signaling by acting directly on the plasma membrane. First, the progesterone-dependent decrease in the cAMP re-

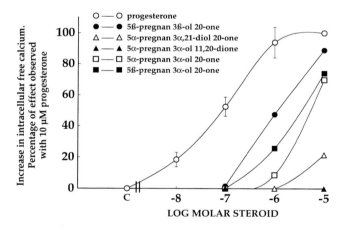

FIG. 17.5. Dose response of progesterone; 5β-pregnan-3β-ol-20-one (epipregnanolone); 5α-pregnane-3α-21-diol-20-one (5α-THDOC); 5α-pregnan-3α-ol-11,20-dione (alfaxalone); 5α-pregnan-3α-ol-20-one (allopregnanolone); and 5β-pregnan-3α-ol-20–one (pregnanolone) to elevate $[Ca^{2+}]_i$ in human sperm. Sperm were loaded with fura-2, and increases in $[Ca^{2+}]_i$ induced by each steroid were determined by measuring the difference between the basal level of $[Ca^{2+}]_i$ (before steroid addition) and the maximum level of $[Ca^{2+}]_i$ attained (usually observed approximately 20 s after steroid addition). Each value shown is the mean of triplicate determinations. Data are expressed as percentage of effect observed with 10 μM progesterone (a maximally effective concentration). [From P. F. Blackmore (10). *Mol. Cell. Endocrinol.* 104: 237–243, 1994. Reproduced by copyright permission of Elsevier Science Ireland Ltd.]

sponse to norepinephrine was rapid in onset, demonstrable within 5 min of progesterone application. Second, incubation of slices from estrogen-primed rats for 5 min in vitro with progesterone conjugated covalently to BSA (rendering this a membrane-impermeable molecule) was sufficient to abolish an α_1-receptor augmentation of β-receptor-stimulated cAMP accumulation. Reduction in norepinephrine-stimulated cAMP formation is a two-step process. First, estradiol inhibits β-adrenoreceptor function, then administration of progesterone eliminates α_{-1}-adrenoreceptor augmentation of cAMP synthesis.

Progesterone Binding in Synaptosomal Membranes.

The conjugation of progesterone to BSA has been used also as a probe to study binding of progesterone to crude synaptosomal membrane preparations derived from hypothalamic tissue of adult female rats (84, 167). These studies showed the specific binding (60%–80%) of the progesterone–BSA conjugate to synaptosomal membrane sites in hypothalamic tissue and identified the 40 to 50 kd protein as a membrane-binding site for progesterone. Expression of the proposed membrane progesterone-binding protein depended on estrogen: specific binding was reduced more the 80% 14 days after ovariectomy and restored again after estrogen treatment. In addition, progesterone rapidly stimulates in vitro release of luteinizing hormone–releasing hormone from hypothalamic tissues and enhances amphetamine-stimulated dopamine release from striatal neurons in rats (33, 83, 148). Both processes are mediated through a progesterone-specific membrane-binding protein, and both require estrogen treatment.

Estrogen

Membrane-Binding Sites.

All of the data described above support the hypothesis that steroids have effects at the membrane level prior to their interaction with the intracellular receptors. Responses to estrogen which are rapid and transient have been characterized in a number of tissues and cell types (36, 93, 136). Steroids immobilized on macromolecules also have been used to identify membrane steroid receptors and membrane steroid action, as well as to isolate receptor-containing cells.

Estrogen immobilized on BSA shows estrogen-specific binding on the surface of MCF-7 (7) and ZR-75-1 (125) breast cancer cells. Osteoblasts show rapid intracellular calcium mobilization with both free estrogen and estrogen conjugated to BSA (93). In another study, estradiol conjugated to derivatized nylon fibers was used to select from heterogeneous liver cell preparations a population of cells responsive to estradiol at the membrane level (144).

Prolactin Secretion and Membrane Estrogen Receptors in GH3/B6 Cells.

In a rat pituitary tumor cell line (GH3/B6), estradiol mediates rapid electrophysiological changes (36) and prolactin release (136). Using an antipeptide antibody to the intracellular estrogen receptor for immunocytochemistry and confocal laser microscopy, the membrane estrogen receptor was identified in 8%–17% of unselected GH3/B6 cells (135, 136). Immunopanning produced populations in which a greater percentage of cells expressed the membrane estrogen receptor antigen with greater intensity than membrane estrogen receptor–depleted cells (Fig. 17.6). The membrane estrogen receptor is antigenically very similar to the intracellular estrogen receptor (cross-reactive at four different epitopes). Co-incubation of cells with anti-estrogen receptor antibody and the fluorescent estrogen–BSA conjugate reveals that these two labels co-localize on cells. Cells immunoenriched for membrane estrogen receptor showed a 100% increase in prolactin secretion with estradiol treatment, while immunodepleted cells lost this response entirely [Fig. 6; (134)]. These data suggest a direct correlation between the presence of membrane estrogen receptor and the rapid estradiol-mediated effect and lend strong support to the hypothesis that the membrane estrogen receptor mediates these effects.

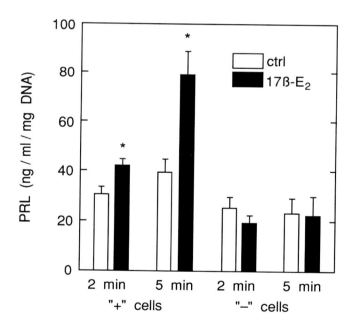

FIG. 17.6. Prolactin release in immunoseparated cell populations. " + " cells are membrane estrogen receptor–enriched; " − " cells are membrane estrogen receptor–depleted. Data are from three independent experiments; error bars are the standard of the mean. *ctrl*, control (ethanol vehicle); *17β-E₂*, 17β-estradiol; *, significantly different from the equivalent time control. [From T. C. Pappas et al. *Endocrine* 3: 743–749, 1995. Reproduced by copyright permission of the Humana Press.]

Intracellular Ca²⁺ Mobilization. Estrogen also generates a rapid signal in granulosa cells, resulting in an increase in free cytosolic calcium (118). The immediate $[Ca^{2+}]_i$ increase is a relatively specific response of granulosa cells to estrogens since progestins and androgens at concentrations as high as 10^{-5} M only minimally affected $[Ca^{2+}]_i$ (Fig. 17.7). This nonclassical response occurs rapidly (less than 5 s) and cannot be blocked by the estrogen receptor antagonist tamoxifen or by the RNA and protein synthesis inhibitors actinomycin D and cycloheximide. The rapid release of Ca^{2+} from intracellular stores is triggered by IP_3 generated by a steroid receptor–induced hydrolysis of membrane phosphatidylinositol-4,5-bisphosphate. This conclusion is based on the observation that the estradiol-17β-triggered $[Ca^{2+}]_i$ surge was not affected by Ca^{2+} channel blockers (lanthanum, cobalt, D600, nifedipine) or Ca^{2+}-free medium containing ethyleneglycoltetracetic acid but was abolished by neomycin, the inhibitor of phospholipase C and phospholipid turnover.

Nonnuclear Estrogen Receptors in MCF-7 Cells. Studies in our lab (184–187) have identified in cytoplasts of MCF-7 human breast cancer cells a subpopulation of estrogen receptors that are nonnuclear and that constitute approximately 15% of the total number of estrogen receptors in intact cells. These nonnuclear estrogen receptors are unable to associate with nuclear components, even in the presence of ligand, and they do not "translocate" to the nucleus in intact cells. Nonnuclear estrogen receptors are not transformed from 4 S to 5 S on high salt/sucrose density gradients, in contrast to nuclear estrogen receptors after binding ligand in intact cells at 37°C. While nuclear and nonnuclear receptors exhibit the same mobilities on sodium dodecyl sulfate-polyacrylamide gel electrophoresis (SDS-PAGE; molecular weight 65,000 daltons for each) and interact with several anti-estrogen receptor antibodies which bind to epitopes in different domains, physical differences between the two forms include different aqueous two-phase partitioning and reduced binding to nonspecific DNA by the nonnuclear receptor. In low salt buffers, the oligomeric form of nonnuclear estrogen receptor migrates 1.2–1.4 S faster than oligomeric estrogen receptor, which suggests a different molecular conformation or that the nonnuclear form is associated in the cytoplasm of the cell with one or more proteins. Considering differences between the two forms, it seems that the nonnuclear receptor is not able to serve as a transcription factor in MCF-7 cells, though it is positioned to mediate potential nongenomic estrogen actions (77). Even if nonnuclear estrogen

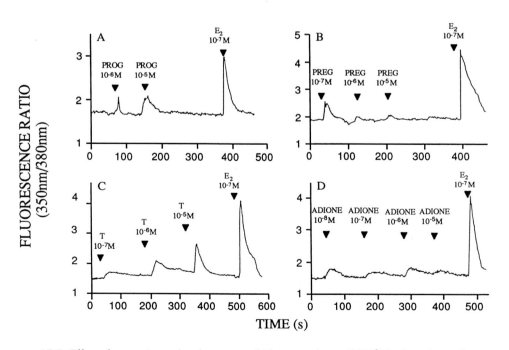

FIG. 17.7. Effect of progestins and androgens on chicken granulosa cell $[Ca^{2+}]_i$. Granulosa cells were treated with progesterone (*PROG*; 10^{-6}–10^{-5}M; *A*), pregnenolone (*PREG*; 10^{-7}–10^{-5}M; *B*), testosterone (*T*; 10^{-7}–10^{-5}M; *C*), or androstenedione (*ADIONE*; 10^{-8}–10^{-5}M; *D*) before stimulation with estradiol-17β (E_2, 10^{-7}M). *Arrowheads* indicate the time of addition of steroids. [From P. Morley et al. (118) *Endocrinology* 131: 1305–1311, 1992. Reproduced by copyright permission of the Endocrine Society.]

receptors are modified intermediates of the classical receptor, the possibility that this molecule may participate in nongenomic pathways is not excluded.

Differences between the cytosolic and nuclear forms of estrogen receptor in the goat uterus also have been observed. Here, deglycosylation of the cytosolic form, using a glycopeptidase, resulted in the conversion of distinct physical features of the cytosolic form to those of the nuclear form (81). The cellular site of localization of the goat uterine nonactivated estrogen receptor may be the plasma membrane (82).

1,25-Dihydroxyvitamin D₃

1,25-Dihydroxyvitamin D_3 [dihydroxycholecalciferol; 1,25-$(OH)_2D_3$] acts as a classical steroid hormone via intracellular receptor binding and subsequent regulation of gene transcription (110, 128). In addition, vitamin D affects a variety of biological responses in various tissues which occur too rapidly to be explained by genomic activation. These include rapid effects of 1,25-$(OH)_2D_3$ on epithelial cell lysosomal enzyme release (123), calmodulin redistribution in muscle cells (26), phospholipid metabolism in intestine and liver (5, 97, 129), $3',5'$-cyclic guanosine monophosphate (cGMP) production by skin fibroblasts (6), and $[Ca^{2+}]$ in osteoblastic cells (24).

Transcaltachia. Experiments investigating *transcaltachia*, the net Ca^{2+} transport from the brush border to the basal lateral membrane of epithelial cells, in chick duodena have demonstrated a rapid response to 1,25-$(OH)_2D_3$ (124). The perfused duodena of normal (vitamin D–replete) chicks responds very rapidly (within 2–4 min) to 1,25-$(OH)_2D_3$ with an increase in net Ca^{2+} transport. This effect occurs only when hormone is directed toward the basal lateral membrane, suggesting the presence of a specific receptor for 1,25-$(OH)_2D_3$. This effect is not inhibited by a wide variety of agents, such as actinomycin D, monesin, cytochalasin B, and pepstatin (121, 122). These data suggest the involvement of 1,25-$(OH)_2D_3$ in the activation of voltage-dependent basal lateral membrane Ca^{2+} channels as an early effect in the transcaltachic response. Nifedipine, a Ca^{2+} channel antagonist, completely abolished the 1,25$(OH)_2D_3$-dependent increase in duodenal Ca^{2+} transport, while the stimulatory response was mimicked by the Ca^{2+} channel agonist BAY K 8644 (27). The acute effects of 1,25-$(OH)_2D_3$ on intestinal Ca^{2+} transport are thought to be mediated indirectly by activation of a second-messenger system. This interpretation is supported by the fact that forskolin (which activates adenylate cyclase to generate cAMP) and the tumor-promoting phorbol esters 12-O-tetradecanoylphorbol-13-acetate and phorbol dibutyrate (shown to be a substi-

tute for DAG in stimulating PKC) were able to reproduce the rapid stimulatory effect of 1,25$(OH)_2D_3$ on intestinal Ca^{2+} transport (Fig. 17.8). It is conceivable that activation of second-messenger systems, such as cAMP-dependent protein kinase and PKC, by 1,25$(OH)_2D_3$ might stimulate Ca^{2+} influx via phosphorylation-dependent activation of voltage-gated Ca^{2+} channels at the basal lateral membrane. The transient increase of intracellular Ca^{2+} in turn may activate exocytosis ofCa^{2+}-containing vesicles as well as Ca^{2+} efflux by the Ca^{2+} pump and the Na^+–Ca^{2+} exchanger, resulting in a net increase of duodenal Ca^{2+} transport (28). Similar results were obtained by 1,25$(OH)_2D_3$ activation of the phosphoinositide signal-transduction cascade in rat colonocytes and the human colon cancer cell line Caco-2. In these studies, 1,25$(OH)_2D_3$ rapidly stimulated membrane phosphoinositide turnover, which generated the second messengers IP_3 and DAG, resulting in a rise in intracellular calcium and translocation of PKC from the cytosol to the membrane (85, 86, 169, 170). This reaction occurred only in the basolateral membrane of colonic cells.

Ca^{2+} Transport in Bone. The study of the role of calcium in bone-resorption processes has shown similar biological responses to 1,25$(OH)_2D_3$. Experiments with a single osteogenic sarcoma ROS 17/2S cell loaded with fura-2 provide evidence that 125$(OH)_2D_3$ rapidly

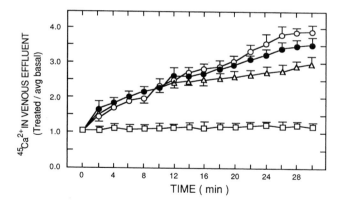

FIG. 17.8. Effect of 1,25$(OH)_2D_3$, the phorbol ester 12-O-tetradecanoyl phorbol=13-acetate (TPA), and forskolin on the appearance of $^{45}Ca^{2+}$ in the venous effluent of perfused duodena from normal chicks. Each duodenum, filled with $^{45}CaCl_2$ (5 μCi/ml) in Grey's balanced saline solution (GBSS), was perfused vascularly (24° C) for the first 20 min with control medium (GBSS containing 0.125% bovine serum albumin and 0.5 μl/ml ethanol) and then with 130 pm 1,25 $(OH)_2D_3$ (*open circles*), 100 nm TPA (*filled circles*), 10 μM forskolin (*open triangles*), or control medium (*open squares*) for up to 30 min. Values are the mean ± SD of four duodena for each treatment. [From A. R. de Boland and A. Norman (28). *Endocrinology* 127: 39–45, 1990. Reproduced by copyright permission of the Endocrine Society.]

affects calcium transport independently from nuclear receptors (24). At high doses (10^{-8}–$10^{-7}M$) of 1,25 $(OH)_2D_3$, the $[Ca^{2+}]$ rise was due to both influx of extracellular Ca^{2+} and release of Ca^{2+} from intracellular stores. At low doses (10^{-9}–10^{-10} M), the effect depended entirely on extracellular Ca^{2+}. The $[Ca^{2+}]$ increase occurred immediately after exposure to the hormone, and the same effect was observed in the ROS 24/1 clone, which does not express an osteoblastic phenotype and is defective in the classical receptor for 1,25$(OH)_2D_3$. Although two metabolites of vitamin D show similar potencies in inducing a $[Ca^{2+}]$ increase in cells, the affinity of 25$(OH)_2D_3$ for 1,25$(OH)_2D_3$ receptors was 100-fold lower than that of 1,25$(OH)_2D_3$ (39). Finally, at doses of 10^{-9} M and higher, 1,25$(OH)_2D_3$ also increased the production of Ins(1,4,5)P_3 and DAG, indicating phospholipase C hydrolysis of phosphatidylinositol bisphosphate (PInsP$_2$), a plasma phospholipid.

Testosterone

Testosterone, as well as all steroid hormones, induces rapid responses in some tissues. In rat pituitary plasma membrane, testosterone, as well as progesterone and estradiol, inhibits gonadotropin-releasing hormone (GnRH) stimulation of G protein GTPase activity within 30 min (149). Gonadal steroids may reduce GTPase activity by inhibiting GnRH binding to its receptor or by disrupting GnRH receptor–G protein coupling. Another study identified and characterized binding sites for testosterone and other gonadal steroids associated with the synaptic plasma membrane from nerve terminals in the rat brain (168). In rat heart cubes and acutely isolated myocytes, nanomolar concentrations of testosterone induce a prompt (5–15 s), short-lived rise in the activity of the enzyme ornithine decarboxylase and in polyamine concentration. This is essential for an acute (30–60 s) stimulation of Ca^{2+} fluxes (Fig. 17.9) and calcium-dependent membrane transport (endocytosis, hexose transport, amino-acid transport) (88). These findings support a model for signal transduction in which newly synthesized polyamines serve as intracellular messengers to regulate transmembrane Ca^{2+} movements, Ca^{2+}-dependent membrane transport functions, and other Ca^{2+}-and polyamine-sensitive processes in cardiac myocytes.

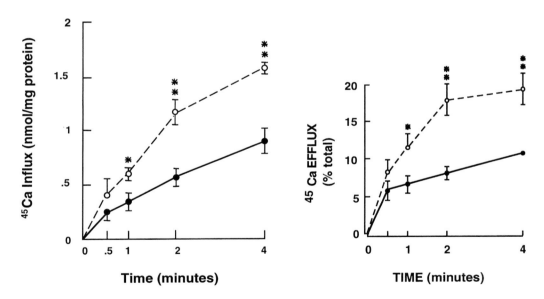

FIG. 17.9. Effect of testosterone on ^{45}Ca influx and efflux in ventricle cubes. *Left panel:* ^{45}Ca influx. Cubes were preincubated in physiological salt solution at 37° C for 10 min. At zero time, ^{45}Ca ($\approx$ 1 μCi/ml) and 10^{-8} M testosterone (*open circles*) or vehicle (*filled circles*) were added, and incubations were terminated at given times. *Right panel:* ^{45}Ca efflux. Cubes were preincubated with ^{45}Ca ($\approx$ 5 μCi/ ml) in physiological salt solution for 20 min, washed, and incubated in fresh medium containing 10^{-8} M testosterone (*open circles*) or vehicle (*filled circles*). ^{45}Ca efflux was determined at given times in supernatant samples and expressed as percentage of total ^{45}Ca in ventricle cubes at the beginning of incubation. Data are mean $\pm$ SEM (n = 3). *P < 0.05; **P < 0.01 (vs. control). [From Koenig et al (88). *Circ. Res.* 64: 417–426, 1989. Reproduced by copyright permission of the American Heart Association.]

CONCLUSIONS

There is increasing evidence for the nongenomic action of steroids. First, many of the responses to steroids are very rapid, within seconds to minutes, too fast to be mediated through the genome. Second, steroids, including progesterone conjugated to BSA, used in several different studies retain hormonal activity. Third, the rapid hormonal responses cannot be blocked by inhibitors of RNA and protein synthesis. Fourth, few potential hormone-specific receptor proteins associated with plasma membranes have been described. While the evidence for the nongenomic action of steroids does not form a complete endocrine link, it suggests that a full understanding of steroid hormonal action may require characterization of the interaction between these two pathways.

We thank Drs. Frederick S. vom Saal, Susan C. Nagel, and Edward M. Curran for critical reading of the manuscript. Supported by NIH Grant R29 CA50354 and by University of Missouri Grant VMFC0018.

REFERENCES

1. Adam, E. H., and S. A. Adam. Identification of cytosolic factors required for nuclear location sequence-mediated binding to the nuclear envelope. *J. Cell Biol.* 125: 547–555, 1994.
2. Adam, S. A., and L. Gerace. Cytosolic proteins that specifically bind nuclear location signals are receptors for nuclear import. *Cell* 66: 837–847, 1991.
3. Adam, S. A., R. Sterne Marr, and L. Gerace. Nuclear import in permeabilized mammalian cells requires soluble cytoplasmic factors. *J. Cell Biol.* 111: 807–816, 1990.
4. Arriza, J. L., C. Weinberger, G. Cerelli, T. M. Glaser, B. L. Handelin, D. Hausman, and R. M. Evans. Cloning of human mineralocorticoid receptor complementary DNA: structural and functional kinship with the glucocorticoid receptor. *Science* 23: 268–275, 1987.
5. Baran, D. T., and A. M. Kelly. Lysophosphatidylinositol: a potential mediator of 1,25–dihydroxyvitamin D-induced increments in hepatocyte cytosolic calcium. *Endocrinology* 122: 930–934, 1988.
6. Barsony, J., and S. L. Marx. Receptor-mediated rapid action of $1\alpha,25$–dihydroxycholecalciferol: increase of intracellular cGMP in human skin fibroblast. *Proc. Natl. Acad. Sci. U.S.A.* 85: 1223–1226, 1988.
7. Berthois, Y., N. Pourreau-Schneider, P. Gandilhon, H. Mittre, N. Tubiana, and P. M. Martin. Estradiol membrane binding sites on human breast cancer cell lines. Use of a fluorescent estradiol conjugate to demonstrate plasma membrane binding system. *J. Steroid Biochem.* 25: 963–972, 1986.
8. Bischoff, F. R., and H. Ponstingl. Mitotic regular protein RCC1 is complexed with a nuclear ras-related polypeptide. *Proc. Natl. Acad. Sci. U.S.A.* 88: 10830–10834, 1991.
9. Blackmore, P. F. Rapid non-genomic actions of progesterone stimulate Ca^{2+} influx and the acrosome reaction in human sperm. *Cell. Signal.* 5: 531–538, 1993.

10. Blackmore, P. F. The cell surface progesterone receptor which stimulates calcium influx in human sperm is unlike the A ring reduced steroid site on the $GABA_A$ receptor /chloride channel. *Mol. Cell. Endocrinol.* 104: 237–243, 1994.
11. Blackmore, P. F., S. J. Beebe, D. R. Danforth, and N. Alexander. Progesterone and 17–alpha hydroxyprogesterone. Novel stimulators of calcium influx in human sperm. *J. Biol. Chem.* 265: 1376–1380, 1990.
12. Blackmore, P. F., and F. A. Lattaanzio. Cell surface localization of a novel non-genomic progesterone receptor on the head of human sperm. *Biochem. Biophys. Res. Commun.* 181: 331–336, 1991.
13. Bonner, W. Protein migration into nuclei. *J. Cell Biol.* 64: 431–437, 1975.
14. Bonner, W. M. Protein migration and accumulation in nuclei. In: *The Cell Nucleus,* edited by H. Busch. New York: Academic, 1978, vol. 6, pt. C, p. 97–148.
15. Borer, R. A., C. F. Lehner, H. M. Eppenberger, and E. A. Nigg. Major nucleolar proteins shuttle between nucleus and cytoplasm. *Cell* 56: 379–390, 1989.
16. Breeuwer, M., and D. Goldfarb. Facilitated nuclear transport of histone H1 and other small nucleophilic proteins. *Cell* 60: 999–1008, 1990.
17. Brink, M., B. M. Humbel, E. R. De Kloet, and R. van Driel. The unliganded glucocorticoid receptor is localized in the nucleus, not in the cytoplasm. *Endocrinology* 130: 3575–3581, 1992.
18. Chandran, U. R., and D. B. DeFranco. Internuclear migration of chicken progesterone receptor, but not simian virus-40 large tumor antigen, in transient heterokaryons. *Mol. Endocrinol.* 6: 837–844, 1992.
19. Chi, N. C., E. J. H. Adam, and S. A. Adam. Sequence and characterization of cytoplasmic nuclear protein import factor p97. *J. Cell Biol.* 130: 265–274, 1995.
20. Christ, M., K. Dauwes, C. Eisen, G. Bechtner, K. Theisen, and M. Wehling. Rapid effects of aldosterone on sodium transport in vascular smooth muscle cells. *Hypertension* 25: 117–123, 1995.
21. Christ, M., C. Eisen, J. Aktas, K. Theisen, and M. Wehling. The inositol-1,4,5–trisphosphate system is involved in rapid effects of aldosterone in human mononuclear leukocytes. *J. Clin. Endocrinol. Metab.* 77: 1452–1457, 1993.
22. Christ, M., C. Meyer, K. Sippel, and M. Wehling. Rapid aldosterone signaling in vascular smooth muscle cells: involvement of phospholipase C, diacylglycerol and protein kinase C α. *Biochem. Biophys. Res. Commun.* 213: 123–129, 1995.
23. Christ, M., K. Sippel, C. Eisen, and M. Wehling. Non-classical receptors for aldosterone in plasma membranes from pig kidneys. *Mol. Cell. Endocrinol.* 99: R31–R34, 1994.
24. Civitelli, R., Y. S. Kim, S. L. Gunsten, A. Fujimori, M. Huskey, L. V. Avioli, and K. A. Hruska. Nongenomic activation of the calcium message system by vitamin D metabolites in osteoblast-like cells. *Endocrinology* 127: 2253–2262, 1990.
25. Dauvois, S., R. White, and M. G. Parker. The antiestrogen ICI182780 disrupts estrogen receptor nucleocytoplasmic shuttling. *J. Cell Sci.* 106: 1377–1388, 193.
26. de Boland, A. R., V. Massheimer, and L. M. Fernandez. 1,25–dihydroxyvitamin D_3 affects calmodulin distribution among subcellular fractions of skeletal muscle. *Calcif. Tissue Int.* 43: 370–375, 1988.
27. de Boland, A. R., I. Nemere, and A. W. Norman. Ca^{2+} agonist Bay K 8644 mimics $1,25(OH)_2$-vitamin D_3 rapid enhancement of Ca^{2+} in chick perfused duodenum. *Biochem. Biophys. Res. Commun.* 166: 217–221, 1990.
28. de Boland, A. R., and A. Norman. Evidence for involvement of

protein kinase C and cyclic adenosine 3′,5′ monophosphate–dependent protein kinase in the 1,25–dihydroxy-vitamin D$_3$-mediated rapid stimulation of intestinal calcium transport (trans-caltachia). *Endocrinology* 127: 39–45, 1990.

29. DeFranco, D. B., M. Qi, M. J. Borror, M. J. Garabedian, and D. L. Brautigan. Protein phosphatase types 1 and/or 2A regulate nucleocytoplasmic shuttling of glucocorticoid receptors. *Mol. Endocrinol.* 5: 1215–1228, 1991.

30. Dingwall, C., and R. Laskey. The nuclear membrane. *Science* 258: 942–947, 1992.

31. Dingwall, C., and R. A. Laskey. Protein import into the cell nucleus. *Annu. Rev. Cell Biol.* 2: 367–390, 1986.

32. Dingwall, C., S. V. Sharnick, and R. A. Laskey. A polypeptide domain that specifies migration of nucleoplasmin into nucleus. *Cell* 30: 449–458, 1982.

33. Dluzen, D. E., and V. D. Ramirez. In-vitro progesterone modulates amphetamine-stimulated dopamine release from the corpus striatum of castrated male rats treated with estrogen. *Neuroendocrinology* 52: 517–520, 1990.

34. Dreyfuss, G., M. J. Matunis, S. Pinol-Roma, and C. G. Burd. hnRNP proteins and the biogenesis of mRNA. *Annu. Rev. Biochem.* 62: 289–321, 1993.

35. Drivas, G. T., A. Shih, E. Coutavas, M. G. Rush, and P. Deustachio. Characterization of four nivel Ras-like genes expressed in a human teratocarcinoma cell line. *Mol. Cell. Biol.* 10: 1793–1798, 1990.

36. Dufy, B., J.-D. Vincent, H. Fleury, P. D. Pasquier, D. Gourdji, and A. T. Vidal. Membrane effects of thyrotropin-releasing hormone and estrogen shown by intracellular recording from pituitary cells. *Science* 204: 509–511, 1979.

37. Dworetzky, S. I., R. E. Lanford, and C. M. Feldherr. The effects of variations in the number and sequence of targeting signals on nuclear uptake. *J. Cell Biol.* 107: 1279–1287, 1988.

38. Ellis, R. J., and S. M. van der Vies. Molecular chaperones. *Annu. Rev. Biochem.* 60: 321–347, 1991.

39. Feldman, D., T. A. McCain, M. A. Hirst, T. L. Chen, and K. W. Colston. Characterization of a cytoplasmic receptor-like binder for 1α,25–dihydroxycholecalciferol in rat intestinal mucosa. *J. Biol. Chem.* 254: 10378–10384, 1979.

40. Fischer, U., E. Darzynkiewicz, S. M. Tahara, N. A. Dathan, R. Luhrmann, and I. W. Mattaj. Diversity in the signals required for nuclear accumulation of U snRNP's and variety in the pathways of nuclear transport. *J. Cell Biol.* 113: 705–714, 1991.

41. Fuxe, K., A.-C. Wikström, S. Okret, L. F. Agnati, A. Härfstrand, Z.-Y. Yu, L. Granholm, M. Zoli, W. Vale, and J.-A. Gustafsson. Mapping of glucocorticoid receptor immunoreactive neurons in the rat tel- and diencephalon using a monoclonal antibody against rat liver glucocorticoid receptor. *Endocrinology* 117: 1803–1812, 1985.

42. Gametchu, B. Glucocorticoid receptor-like antigen in lymphoma cell membranes: correlation to cell lysis. *Science* 236: 456–461, 1987.

43. Gametchu, B., C. S. Watson, and D. Pasko. Size and steroid-binding characterization of membrane-associated glucocorticoid receptor in S-49 lymphoma cells. *Steroids* 56: 402–410, 1991.

44. Gametchu, B., C. S. Watson, C.-Y. Shih, and B. Dashew. Studies on the arrangement of glucocorticoid receptors in the plasma membrane of S-49 lymphoma cells. *Steroids* 56: 411–419, 1991.

45. Garcia-Bustos, J., J. Heitman, and M. N. Hall. Nuclear protein localization. *Biochim. Biophys. Acta* 1071: 83–101, 1991.

46. Gasc, J., F. Delahaye, and E. Baulieu. Compared intracellular localization of the glucocorticoid and progesterone receptors: an immunocytochemical study. *Exp. Cell Res.* 181: 492–504, 1989.

47. Gasc, J.-M., J.-M. Renoir, C. Radanyi, I. Joab, P. Tuohimaa,

and E.-E. Baulieu. Progesterone receptor in the chick oviduct: an immunohistochemical study with antibodies to distinct receptor components. *J. Cell Biol.* 99: 1193–1201, 1984.

48. Gerace, L., and B. Burke. Functional organization of the nuclear envelope. *Annu. Rev. Cell Biol.* 4: 335–374, 1988.

49. Goldfarb, D. S. Karyophilic peptides: applications to the study of nuclear transport. *Cell Biol. Int. Rep.* 12: 809–832, 1988.

50. Goldfarb, D. S. Shuttling proteins go both ways. *Curr. Biol.* 1: 212–214, 1991.

51. Goldfarb, D. S., J. Gariepy, G. Schoolnik, and R. D. Kornberg. Synthetic peptides as nuclear localization signals. *Nature* 322: 641–644, 1986.

52. Görlich, D., S. Kostka, R. Kraft, C. Dingwall, R. A. Laskey, E. Hartman, and S. Prehn. Two different subunits of importin cooperate to recognize nuclear localization signals and bind them to the nuclear envelope. *Cur. Biol.* 5: 383–392, 1995.

53. Görlich, D., and I. W. Mattaj. Nucleocytoplasmic transport. *Science* 271: 1513–1518, 1996.

54. Görlich, D., S. Prehn, R. A. Laskey, and E. Hartmann. Isolation of a protein that is essential for the first step of nuclear protein import. *Cell* 79: 767–778, 1994.

55. Görlich, D., F. Vogel, A. D. Mills, E. Hartmann, and R. A. Laskey. Distinct functions for the two importin subunits in nuclear protein import. *Nature* 377: 246–248, 1995.

56. Gorski, J., and F. Gannon. Current models of steroid hormone action: a critique. *Annu. Rev. Physiol.* 38: 425–450, 1976.

57. Gorski, J., J. R. Malayer, D. W. Gregg, and S. G. Lundeen. Just where are the steroid receptors anyway? *Endocr. J.* 2: 99–100, 1994.

58. Gorski, J., D. Toft, G. Shyamala, D. Smith, and A. Notides. Hormone receptors: studies on the interaction of estrogen with the uterus. *Recent Prog. Horm. Res.* 24: 45–80, 1968.

59. Govindan, M. V. Immunofluorescence microscopy of the intracellular translocation of glucocorticoid-receptor complexes in rat hepatoma (HTC) cells. *Exp. Cell Res.* 127: 293–297, 1980.

60. Griffing, G. T. Dinosaurs and steroids. *J. Clin. Endocrinol. Metab.* 77: 1450–1451, 1993.

61. Gronemeyer, H. Nuclear hormone receptors as transcriptional activators. In: *Steroid Hormone Action,* edited by M. G. Parker. New York: Oxford University Press, 1993, p. 94–117.

62. Groyer, A., G. Schweizer-Groyer, F. Cadepond, M. Mariller, and E.-E. Baulieu. Antiglucocorticoid effects suggest why steroid hormone is required for receptor to bind DNA *in vivo* but not *in vitro*. *Nature* 328: 624–629, 1987.

63. Guiochon-Mantel, A., K. Delabre, P. Lescop, and E. Milgrom. Nuclear localization signals also mediate the outward movement of proteins from the nucleus. *Proc. Natl. Acad. Sci. U.S.A.* 91: 7179–7183, 1994.

64. Guiochon-Mantel, A., K. Delabre, P. Lescop, and E. Milgrom. Intracellular traffic of steroid hormone receptors. *J. Steroid Biochem. Mol. Biol.* 56: 3–9, 1996.

65. Guiochon-Mantel, A., P. Lescop, S. Christin-Maitre, H. Loosfelt, M. Perrot-Applanat, and E. Milgrom. Nucleocytoplasmic shuttling of the progesterone receptor. *EMBO J.* 10: 3851–3859, 1991.

66. Guiochon-Mantel, A., H. Loosfelt, P. Lescop, S. Sar, M. Atger, M. Perrot-Applanat, and E. Milgrom. Mechanisms of nuclear localization of the progesterone receptor: evidence for interaction between monomers. *Cell* 57: 1147–1154, 1989.

67. Hall, M. N., C. Craik, and Y. Hiraoka. Homeodomain of yeast repressor alpha-2 contains a nuclear localization signal. *Proc. Natl. Acad. Sci. U.S.A.* 87: 6954–6958, 1990.

68. Hamy, F., N. Heibecque, and J.-P. Henichart. Comparison between synthetic nuclear localization signal peptides from the steroid/thyroid hormone receptors superfamily. *Biochem. Biophys. Res. Commun.* 182: 289–293, 1992.

69. Homo, F., D. Duval, J. Hatzfeld, and C. Evarard. Glucocorticoid sensitive and resistant cell population in the mouse thymus. *J. Steroid Biochem.* 13: 135–143, 1980.

70. Homo-Delarche, F. Glucocorticoid receptors and steroid sensitivity in normal and neoplastic human lymphoid tissues: a review. *Cancer Res.* 44: 431–437, 1984.

71. Imamoto, N., Y. Matsuoka, T. Kurihara, K. Kohno, M. Miyagi, F. Sakiyama, Y. Okada, S. Tsunasawa, and Y. Yoneda. Antibodies against 70–kD heat shock cognate protein inhibit mediated nuclear import of karyophilic proteins. *J. Cell Biol.* 119: 1047–1061, 1992.

72. Imamoto, N., T. Shimamoto, T. Kose, T. Takao, T. Tachibana, M. Matsubae, T. Sekimoto, Y. Shimonishi, and Y. Yoneda. The nuclear pore-targeting complex binds to nuclear pores after association with a karyophile. *FEBS Lett.* 368: 415–419, 1995.

73. Imamoto, N., T. Shimamoto, T. Takao, T. Tachibana, S. Kose, M. Matsubae, T. Sekimoto, Y. Shimonishi, and Y. Yoneda. In vivo evidence for involvement of a 58 kDa component of nuclear pore-targeting complex in nuclear protein import. *EMBO J.* 14: 3617–3626, 1995.

74. Imamoto, N., T. Tachibana, M. Matsubae, and Y. Yoneda. A karyophilic protein forms a stable complex with cytoplasmic components prior to nuclear pore binding. *J. Biol. Chem.* 270: 8559–8565, 1995.

75. Jensen, E. V., T. Suzuki, T. Kawashima, W. E. Stumpf, P. W. Jungblut, and E. DeSombre. A two-step mechanism for the interaction of estradiol with rat uterus. *Proc. Natl. Acad. Sci. U.S.A.* 59: 632–638, 1968.

76. Jenster, G., J. Trapman, and A. O. Brinkmann. Nuclear import of the human androgen receptor. *Biochem. J.* 293: 761–768, 1993.

77. Judy, B. M., G. L. Greene, and W. V. Welshons. Characterization of non-nuclear estrogen receptors (ER$_{NN}$) in MCF-7 human breast cancer cells by antibody-binding and sedimentation analysis. *Proc. 10th Int. Congr. Endocrinol.*, San Francisco, 1996. Amsterdam: Excerpta Medica, 1996, p. 575.

78. Kalderon, D., W. D. Richardson, A. F. Markham, and A. E. Smith. Sequence requirements for nuclear localization of simian virus 40 large-T antigen. *Nature* 311: 33–38, 1984.

79. Kalderon, D., B. L. Roberts, W. D. Richardson, and A. E. Smith. A short amino acid sequence able to specify nuclear location. *Cell* 39: 499–509, 1984.

80. Kambach, C., and I. W. Mattaj. Intracellular distribution of the U1A protein depends on active transport and nuclear binding to U1 snRNA. *J. Cell Biol.* 118: 11–21, 1992.

81. Karthikeyan, N., and R. V. Thampan. The nuclear estrogen receptor R-II of the goat uterus: distinct possibility that the R-II is the deglycosylated form of the nonactivated estrogen receptor (naER). *Arch. Biochem. Biophys.* 321: 442–452, 1995.

82. Karthikeyan, N., and R. V. Thampan. Plasma membrane is the primary site of localization of the nonactivated estrogen receptor in the goat uterus: hormone binding causes receptor internalization. *Arch. Biochem. Biophys.* 325: 47–57, 1996.

83. Ke, F.-C., and V. D. Ramirez. Membrane mechanism mediates progesterone stimulatory effect on LHRH release from superfused rat hypothalami in vitro. *Neuroendocrinology* 45: 514–517, 1987.

84. Ke, F.-C., and V. D. Ramirez. Binding of progesterone to nerve cell membranes of rat brain using progesterone conjugated to ^{125}I-bovine serum albumin as a ligand. *J. Neurochem.* 54: 467–472, 1990.

85. Khare, S., X.-Y. Tien, D. Wilson, R. K. Wali, B. M. Bissonnette, B. Scaglione-Sewell, M. D. Sitrin, and T. A. Brasitus. The role of protein kinase-C-alpha in the activation of particulate guanylate cyclase by 1-alpha,25–dihydroxy vitamin D-3 in Caco-2 cells. *Endocrinology* 135: 277–283, 1994.

86. Khare, S., D. M. Wilson, X.-Y. Tien, P. K. Dudeja, R. K. Wali, M. D. Sitrin, and T. A. Brasitus. 1,25–Dihydroxycholecalciferol rapidly activates rat colonic particulate guanylate cyclase via a protein kinase C-dependent mechanism. *Endocrinology* 133: 2213–2219, 1993.

87. King, W. J., and G. L. Greene. Monoclonal antibodies localize oestrogen receptor in the nuclei of target cells. *Nature* 307: 745–747, 1984.

88. Koenig, H., C.-C. Fan, A. D. Goldstone, C. Y. Lu, and J. J. Trout. Polyamines mediate androgenic stimulation of calcium fluxes and membrane transport in rat heart myocytes. *Circ. Res.* 64: 415–426, 1989.

89. Kuiper, G. G., E. Enmark, M. Pelto-Huikko, S. Nilsson, and J.-Å. Gustafsson. Cloning of a novel estrogen receptor expressed in rat prostate and ovary. *Proc. Natl. Acad. Sci. U.S.A.* 93: 5925–5930, 1996.

90. Kumar, V., S. Green, G. Stack, M. Berry, J. R. Jin, and P. Chambon. Functional domains of the human estrogen receptor. *Cell* 51: 941–951, 1987.

91. Lan, N. C., M. B. Bolger, and K. W. Gee. Identification and characterization of a pregnane steroid recognition site that is functionally coupled to an expressed GABA$_A$ receptor. *Neurochem. Res.* 18: 347–356, 1991.

92. Landford, R. E., P. Kanda, and R. C. Kennedy. Induction of nuclear transport with a synthetic peptide homologous to the SV40 antigen transport signal. *Cell* 46: 575–582, 1986.

93. Lieberherr, M., B. Grosse, M. Kachkache, and S. Balsan. Cell signalling and estrogen in female rat osteoblasts. *J. Bone Miner. Res.* 8: 1365–1376, 1993.

94. Lippman, M. E., G. K. Yarbro, and B. G. Leventhal. Clinical implications of glucocorticoid receptor in human leukemia. *Cancer Res.* 38: 4251–4256, 1978.

95. Madan, A. P., and D. B. DeFranco. Bidirectional transport of glucocorticoid receptors across the nuclear envelope. *Proc. Natl. Acad. Sci. U.S.A.* 90: 3588–3592, 1993.

96. Mandell, R. B., and C. M. Feldherr. Identification of two HSP70–related *Xenopus* oocyte proteins that are capable of recycling across the nuclear envelope. *J. Cell Biol.* 111: 1775–1783, 1990.

97. Matsumoto, T., O. Fontaine, and H. Rasmussen. Effect of 1,25–dihydroxyvitamin D$_3$ on phospholipid metabolism in chick duodenal mucosal cell. *J. Biol. Chem.* 256: 3354–3360, 1981.

98. McClellan, M. C., N. B. West, D. E. Tacha, G. L. Greene, and R. M. Brenner. Immunocytochemical localization of estrogen receptors in the macaque reproductive tract with monoclonal antiestrophilins. *Endocrinology* 114: 2002–2014, 1984.

99. McEwen, B. S. Non-genomic and genomic effects of steroids on neural activity. *Trends Pharmacol. Sci.* 12: 141–147, 1991.

100. Mehlin, H., B. Daneholt, and U. Skoglund. Translocation of a specific premessenger ribonucleoprotein particle through the nuclear pore studied with electron microscope tomography. *Cell* 69: 605–613, 1992.

101. Mehlin, H., B. Daneholt, and U. Skoglund. Structural interaction between the nuclear pore complex and a specific translocating RNP particle. *J. Cell Biol.* 129: 1205–1215, 1995.

102. Meier, U. T., and G. Blobel. A nuclear localization signal binding protein in the nucleolus. *J. Cell Biol.* 111: 2235–2245, 1990.

103. Meier, U. T., and G. Blobel. Nopp140 shuttles on tracks between nucleolus and cytoplasm. *Cell* 70: 127–138, 1992.

104. Melchior, F., B. Paschal, J. Evans, and L. Gerace. Inhibition of nuclear protein import by nonhydrolyzable analogues of GTP and identification of the small GTPase Ran/TC4 as an essential transport factor. *J. Cell Biol.* 123: 1649–1659, 1993.

105. Meyer, C., M. Christ, and M. Wehling. Characterization and

solubilization of novel aldosterone-binding proteins in porcine liver microsomes. *Eur. J. Biochem.* 229: 736–740, 1995.

106. Meyer, J. W., and D. F. Bohr. Mechanism responsible for the pressure elevation in sodium-dependent mineralocorticoid hypertension. In: *Endocrinology of Hypertension*, edited by F. Mantero, E. G. Biglieri, and C. R. W. Edwards. New York: Raven, 1985, p. 131–148.

107. Michael, W. M., M. Choi, and G. Dreyfuss. A nuclear export signal in hnRNP A1: a signal-mediated, temperature-dependent nuclear protein export pathway. *Cell* 83: 415–422, 1995.

108. Michaud, N., and D. Goldfarb. Multiple pathways in nuclear transport: the import of U2 snRNP occurs by a novel kinetic pathway. *J. Cell Biol.* 112: 215–223, 1991.

109. Milgrom, E. Activation of steroid-receptor complexes. In: *Biochemical action of Hormones*, edited by L. G. Litwack. New York: Academic, 1981, p. 465–492.

110. Minghetti, P. P., and A. W. Norman. Vitamin D_3 receptors: gene regulation and genetic circuitry. *FASEB J.* 2: 3043–3053, 1988.

111. Moore, F. L., C. A. Lowry, and J. D. Rose. Steroid–neuropeptide interactions that control reproductive behaviors in an amphibian. *Psychoneuroendocrinology* 19: 581–592, 1994.

112. Moore, F. L., and L. J. Miller. Stress-induced inhibition of sexual behavior: corticosterone inhibits courtship behaviors of a male amphibian (*Taricha granulosa*). *Horm. Behav.* 18: 400–410, 1984.

113. Moore, F. L., and M. Orchinik. Membrane receptors for corticosterone: a mechanism for rapid behavioral responses in an amphibian. *Horm. Behav.* 28: 512–519, 1994.

114. Moore, F. L., M. Orchinik, and C. Lowry. Functional studies of corticosterone receptors in neuronal membranes. *Receptor* 5: 21–28, 1995.

115. Moore, M. S., and G. Blobel. The two steps of nuclear import, targeting to the nuclear envelope and translocation through the nuclear pore, require different cytosolic factors. *Cell* 69: 939–950, 1992.

116. Moore, M. S., and G. Blobel. The GTP-binding protein Ran-TC4 is required for protein import into the nucleus. *Nature* 365: 661–663, 1993.

117. Moore, M. S., and G. Blobel. Purification of a Ran-interacting protein that is required for protein import into nucleus. *Proc. Natl. Acad. Sci. U.S.A.* 91: 10212–10216, 1994.

118. Morley, P., F. F. Whitfield, B. C. Vanderhyden, B. K. Tsang, and J. L. Schwartz. A new, nongenomic estrogen action: the rapid release of intracellular calcium. *Endocrinology* 131: 1305–1312, 1992.

119. Moroianu, J., M. Hijkata, G. Blobel, and A. Radu. Mammalian karyopherin alpha-1–beta and alpha-2–beta heterodimers: alpha-1 or alpha-2 subunit binds nuclear localization signal and beta subunit interacts with peptide repeat–containing nucleoporins. *Proc. Natl. Acad. Sci. U.S.A.* 92: 6532–6536, 1995.

120. Mueller, G. C., A. M. Herranen, and K. F. Jervell. Studies on the mechanism of action of estrogens. *Recent Progr. Horm. Res.* 14: 95–139, 1958.

121. Nemere, I., and A. W. Norman. Rapid action of 1,25–dihydroxyvitamin D_3 on calcium transport in perfused chick duodenum: effect of inhibitors. *J. Bone Miner. Res.* 2: 99–103, 1987.

122. Nemere, I., and A. W. Norman. The rapid hormonally stimulated transport of calcium (transcaltachia). *J. Bone Miner. Res.* 2: 167–172, 1987.

123. Nemere, I., and C. M. Szego. Early action of parathyroid hormone and 1,25–dihydroxycholecalciferol on isolated epithelial cells from rat intestine. 1. Limited lysosomal enzyme release and calcium uptake. *Endocrinology* 108: 1450–1462, 1981.

124. Nemere, I., Y. Yoshimoto, and A. V. Norman. Calcium trans-

port in perfused duodena from normal chicks: enhancement within fourteen minutes of exposure to 1,25–dihydroxyvitamin D_3. *Endocrinology* 115: 1476–1483, 1984.

125. Nenci, T., G. Fabris, E. Marchetti, and A. Marzola. Cytochemical evidence for steroid binding sites in the plasma membrane of target cells. In: *Perspectives in Steroid Receptor Research,* edited by F. Bresciani. New York: Raven, 1980, p. 61–72.

126. Newmeyer, D. D., and D. J. Forbes. Nuclear import can be separated into distinct steps in vitro: nuclear pore binding and translocation. *Cell* 52: 641–653, 1988.

127. Nigg, E. A. Signal transduction to the cell nucleus. *Adv. Mol. Cell. Biol.* 4: 103–131, 1992.

128. Norman, A. W., J. Roth, and L. Orci. The vitamin D endocrine system: steroid metabolism hormone receptors and biological response. *Endocr. Rev.* 3: 331–336, 1982.

129. O'Doherty, P. J. A. 1,25–Dihydroxyvitamin D_3 increases the activity of the intestinal phosphatidylcholine deacylation–reacylation cycle. *Lipids* 14: 75–80, 1979.

130. Orchinik, M., T. F. Murray, P. H. Franklin, and F. L. Moore. Guanyl nucleotides modulate binding to steroid receptors in neuronal membranes. *Proc. Natl. Acad. Sci. U.S.A.* 89: 3830–3834, 1992.

131. Orchinik, M., T. F. Murray, and F. L. Moore. A corticosteroid receptor in neuronal membranes. *Science* 252: 1848–1851, 1991.

132. Osman, R. A., M. L. Andria, A. D. Jones, and S. Meizel. Steroid induced exocytosis: the human sperm acrosome reaction. *Biochem. Biophys. Res. Commun.* 160: 828–833, 1989.

133. Papamichail, M., C. Ioannidis, N. Tsawdaroglou, and C. E. Sekeris. Translocation of glucocorticoid receptor from the cytoplasm into the nucleus of phytohemmaglutinin-stimulated human lymphocytes in the absence of the hormone. *Exp. Cell Res.* 133: 461–465, 1981.

134. Pappas, T. C., B. Gametchu, and C. S. Watson. Membrane estrogen receptor–enriched GH3/B6 cells have an enhanced nongenomic response to estrogen. *Endocrine* 3: 743–749, 1995.

135. Pappas, T. C., B. Gametchu, and C. S. Watson. Membrane estrogen receptors identified by multiple antibody labeling and impeded-ligand binding. *FASEB J.* 9: 404–410, 1995.

136. Pappas, T. C., B. Gametchu, J. Yannariello-Brown, T. J. Collins, and C. S. Watson. Membrane estrogen receptors in GH3/B6 cells are associated with rapid estrogen-induced release of prolactin. *Endocrine* 2: 813–822, 1994.

137. Paschal, B. M., and L. Gerace. Identification of NTF2, a cytosolic factor for nuclear import that interacts with nuclear pore complex protein p62. *J. Cell Biol.* 129: 925–937, 1995.

138. Pekki, A., J. Koistinaho, P. Vilja, H. Westphal, and P. Tuohimaa. Subcellular location of unoccupied and occupied glucocorticoid receptor by a new immunohistochemical technique. *J. Steroid Biochem. Mol. Biol.* 41: 753–756, 1992.

139. Perrot-Applanat, M., F. Logeat, M. T. Groyer-Picard, and E. Milgrom. Immunocytochemical study of mammalian progesterone receptor using monoclonal antibodies. *Endocrinology* 116: 1473–1484, 1985.

140. Petitti, N., and A. M. Etgen. Progesterone promotes rapid desensitization of α_1 adrenergic receptor augmentation of cAMP formation in rat hypothalamic slices. *Neuroendocrinology* 55: 1–8, 1992.

141. Picard, D., V. Kumart, P. Chambon, and K. R. Yamamoto. Signal transduction by steroid hormones nuclear localization is differentially regulated in estrogen and glucocorticoid receptors. *Cell Regul.* 1: 291–300, 1990.

142. Picard, D., S. J. Salser, and K. R. Yamamoto. A movable and regulable inactivation function within the steroid binding domain of the glucocorticoid receptor. *Cell* 54: 1073–1080, 1988.

143. Picard, D., and K. R. Yamamoto. Two signals mediate hormone-dependent nuclear localization of the glucocorticoid receptor. *EMBO J.* 6: 3333–3340, 1987.

144. Pietras, R. J., and C. M. Szego. Metabolic and proliferative responses to estrogen by hepatocytes selected for plasma membrane binding sites specific for estradiol-17β. *J. Cell Physiol.* 98: 145–160, 1979.

145. Pinol-Roma, S., and G. Dreyfuss. Shuttling of pre-mRNA binding proteins between nucleus and cytoplasm. *Nature* 355: 730–732, 1992.

146. Pinol-Roma, S., and G. Dreyfuss. hnRNP proteins: localization and transport between the nucleus and the cytoplasm. *Trends Cell Biol.* 3: 151–155, 1993.

147. Radu, A., G. Blobel, and M. S. Moore. Identification of a protein complex that is required for nuclear-protein import and mediates docking of import substrate to distinct nucleoporins. *Proc. Natl. Acad. Sci. U.S.A.* 92: 1769–1773, 1995.

148. Ramirez, V. D., K. Kim, and D. E. Dluzen. Progesterone action on the LHRH and the nigrostriatal dopamine neuronal systems: in vitro and in vivo studies. *Recent Prog. Horm. Res.* 41: 421–472, 1985.

149. Ravindra, R., and R. S. Aronstam. Progesterone, testosterone and estradiol-17β inhibit gonadotropin-releasing hormone stimulation of G protein GTPase activity in plasma membranes from rat anterior pituitary lobe. *Acta Endocrinol.* 126: 345–349, 1992.

150. Richardson, W. D., A. D. Mills, S. M. Dilworth, R. A. Laskey, and C. Dingwall. Nuclear protein migration involves two steps: rapid binding at the nuclear envelope followed by slower translocation through nuclear pores. *Cell* 52: 655–664, 1988.

151. Rihs, H. P., and R. Peters. Nuclear transport kinetics depend on phosphorylation-site-containing sequences flanking the karyophilic signal of the simian virus 40 T-antigen. *EMBO J.* 8: 1479–1484, 1989.

152. Robbins, J., S. M. Dilworth, R. A. Laskey, and C. Dingwall. Two interdependent basic domains in nucleoplasmin nuclear targeting sequence: identification of a class of bipartite nuclear targeting sequence. *Cell* 64: 615–623, 1991.

153. Roberts, B. Nuclear localization signal-mediated protein transport. *Biochim. Biophys. Acta* 1008: 263–280, 1989.

154. Rout, M. P., and S. R. Wente. Pores for thought: nuclear pore complex proteins. *Trends Cell Biol.* 4: 357–365, 1994.

155. Sanchez, E. R., D. O. Toft, M. J. Schlesinger, and W. B. Pratt. The 90kD non-steroid binding phosphoprotein that binds to the untransformed gliucocorticoid receptor in molybdate-stabilized L-cell cytosol is the murine 90kD heat shock protein. *J. Biol. Chem.* 260: 12398–12401, 1985.

156. Schmidt-Zachmann, M. S., C. Dargemont, L. C. Kuhn, and E. A. Nigg. Nuclear export of proteins: the role of nuclear retention. *Cell* 74: 493–504, 1993.

157. Schmidt-Zachmann, M. S., B. Hugle-Dorr, and W. W. Franfe. A constitutive nucleolar protein identified as a member of the nucleoplasmin family. *EMBO J.* 6: 1881–1890, 1987.

158. Sheridan, P. J., J. M. Buchanan, V. C. Anselmo, and P. M. Martin. Equilibrium: the intracellular distribution of steroid receptors. *Nature* 282: 579–582, 1979.

159. Sheridan, P. J., J. M. Buchanan, V. C. Anselmo, and P. M. Martin. Unbound progesterone receptors are in equilibrium between the nucleus and cytoplasm in cells of the rat uterus. *Endocrinology* 108: 1533–1537, 1981.

160. Shyamala, G., and J. Gorski. Estrogen receptors in the rat uterus. Studies on the interaction of cytosol and nuclear binding sites. *J. Biol. Chem.* 244: 1097–1103, 1969.

161. Silver, P. A. How proteins enter the nucleus. *Cell* 64: 489–497, 1991.

162. Simental, J. A., M. Sar, M. V. Lane, F. S. French, and E. M. Wilson. Transcriptional activation and nuclear targeting signals of the human androgen receptor. *J. Biol. Chem.* 266: 510–518, 1991.

163. Siomi, H., and G. Dreyfuss. A nuclear localization domain in the hnRNP A1 protein. *J. Cell Biol.* 129: 551–560, 1995.

164. Stevens, J., and Y. W. Stevens. Glucocorticoid receptors in human leukemia and lymphoma: quantitative and clinical significance. In: *Hormonally Responsive Tumors*, edited by V. P. Hollander. San Diego: Academic, 1985, p. 156–182.

165. Stochaj, U., and P. A. Silver. A conserved phosphoprotein that specifically binds nuclear localization sequences is involved in nuclear transport. *J. Cell Biol.* 117: 473–482, 1992.

166. Stumpf, W. E., and L. J. Roth. High resolution autoradiography with dry mounted, freeze-dried frozen sections. Comparative study of six methods using two diffusable compounds ³H-estradiol and ³H-mesobilirubinogen. *J. Histochem. Cytochem.* 14: 274–287, 1966.

167. Tischkau, S. A., and V. D. Ramirez. A specific membrane binding protein for progesterone in rat brain: sex differences and induction by estrogen. *Proc. Natl. Acad. Sci. U.S.A.* 90: 1285–1289, 1993.

168. Towle, A. C., and P. Y. Sze. Steroid binding to synaptic plasma membrane: differential binding of glucocorticoids and gonadal steroids. *J. Steroid Biochem.* 18: 135–143, 1983.

169. Wali, R. K., C. L. Baum, M. D. Sitrin, and T. A. Brasitus. 1,25(OH)$_2$Vitamin D$_3$ stimulates membrane phosphoinositide turnover, activates protein kinase C, and increases cytosolic calcium in rat colonic epithelium. *J. Clin. Invest.* 85: 1296–1303, 1990.

170. Wali, R. K., M. J. G. Bolt, X.-Y. Tien, T. A. Brasitus, and M. D. Sitrin. Differential effect of 1,25–dihydroxycholecalciferol on phosphoinositide turnover in the antipodal plasma membranes of colonic epithelial cells. *Biochem. Biophys. Res. Commun.* 187: 1128–1134, 1992.

171. Wasserman, W. J., L. H. Pinto, C. M. O'Connor, and D. Smith. Progesterone induces an increase in [Ca^{2+}]$_{in}$ of *Xenopus laevis* oocytes. *Proc. Natl. Acad. Sci. U.S.A.* 77: 1534–1536, 1980.

172. Webster, J. C., C. M. Jewell, M. Sar, and J. A. Cidlowski. The glucocorticoid receptor: maybe not all steroid receptors are nuclear. *Endocrine J.* 2: 967–969, 1994.

173. Wehling, M. Nongenomic aldosterone effects: the cell membrane as a specific target of mineralocorticoid action. *Steroids* 60: 153–156, 1995.

174. Wehling, M., D. Armanini, T. Strasser, and P. C. Weber. Effect of aldosterone on sodium and potassium concentration in human mononuclear leukocytes. *Am. J. Physiol.* 252 (*Endocrinol. Metab.* 15): E505–E508, 1987.

175. Wehling, M., M. Christ, and K. Theisen. Membrane receptors for aldosterone: a novel pathway for mineralocorticoid action. *Am. J. Physiol.* 263 (*Endocrinol. Metab.* 26): E974–E979, 1992.

176. Wehling, M., C. Eisen, and M. Christ. Aldosterone-specific membrane receptors and rapid non-genomic actions of mineralocorticoids. *Mol. Cell. Endocrinol.* 90: C5–C9, 1992.

177. Wehling, M., J. Kasmayr, and K. Theisen. Rapid effects of mineralocorticoids on sodium–proton exchanger: genomic or nongenomic pathway? *Am. J. Physiol.* 260 (*Endocrinol. Metab.* 23): E719–E726, 1991.

178. Wehling, M., S. Kuhlas, and D. Armanini. Volume regulation of human lymphocytes by aldosterone in isotonic media. *Am. J. Physiol.* 257 (*Endocrinol. Metab.* 20): E170–E174, 1989.

179. Wehling, M., C. B. Neylon, M. Fullerton, A. Bobik, and J. W. Funder. Nongenomic effects of aldosterone on intracellular Ca^{2+} in vascular smooth muscle cells. *Circ. Res.* 76: 973–979, 1995.

180. Wehling, M., A. Ulsenheimer, M. Schneider, C. Neylon, and M. Christ. Rapid effects of aldosterone on free intracellular calcium in vascular smooth muscle and endothelial cells: subcellular localization of calcium elevations by single cell imaging. *Biochem. Biophys. Res. Commun.* 204: 475–481, 1994.

181. Weis, K., I. W. Mattaj, and A. I. Lamond. Identification of hSRP1a as a functional receptor for nuclear localization signals. *Science* 268: 1049–1053, 1995.

182. Welshons, W. V., E. M. Cormier, V. C. Jordan, and J. Gorski. Biochemical evidence for the exclusive nuclear localization of the estrogen receptor. In: *Gene Regulation by Steroid Hormones,* edited by A. K. Roy and J. H. Clark. New York: Springer-Verlag, 1987, vol. III, p. 1–20.

183. Welshons, W. V., and J. Gorski. Nuclear location of estrogen receptors. In: *The Receptors,* edited by P. M. Conn. Orlando, FL: Academic, 1986, vol. IV, p. 97–147.

184. Welshons, W. V., and B. M. Judy. Nuclear *vs.* translocating steroid receptor models and the excluded middle. *Endocrine* 3: 1–4, 1995.

185. Welshons, W. V., B. M. Judy, R. L. Strnad, and L. H. Grady. Cytoplasmic, non-nucleophilic estrogen receptors in cytoplasts from MCF-7 human breast cancer cells. In: *75th Annual Meeting of the Endocrine Society,* Las Vegas, NV. Bethesda, MD: Endocrine Society Press, p. 517, 1993.

186. Welshons, W. V., L. H. Grady, B. M. Judy, V. C. Jordon, and D. E. Preziosi. Subcellular compartmentalization of MCF-7 estrogen receptor synthesis and degradation. *Mol. Cell. Endocrinol.* 94: 183–194, 1993.

187. Welshons, W. V., B. M. Judy, R. L. Strnad, L. H. Grady, and E. M. Curran. Non-nuclear estrogen receptors (ER_{NN}) in MCF-7 human breast cancer cells. *76th Annual Meeting of the Endocrine Society,* Anaheim, CA. Bethesda, MD: Endocrine Society Press, p. 628, 1994.

188. Welshons, W. V., B. M. Krummel, and J. Gorski. Nuclear localization of unoccupied receptors for glucocorticoids, estrogens and progesterone in GH_3 cells. *Endocrinology* 117: 2140–2147, 1985.

189. Welshons, W. V., M. E. Lieberman, and J. Gorski. Nuclear localization of unoccupied oestrogen receptors. *Nature* 307: 747–749, 1984.

190. Wikström, A.-C., O. Bakke, S. Okret, M. Brönnegård, and J.-A. Gustafsson. Intracellular localization of glucocorticoid receptor: evidence for cytoplasmic and nuclear localization. *Endocrinology* 120: 1232–1242, 1987.

191. Ylikomi, T., M. T. Bocquel, M. Berry, H. Gronemeyer, and P. Chambon. Cooperation of proto-signals for nuclear accumulation of estrogen and progesterone receptors. *EMBO J.* 11: 3681–3694, 1992.

192. Zhou, Z. X., M. Sar, J. A. Simental, M. V. Lane, and E. M. Wilson. A ligand dependent bipartite nuclear targeting signal in human androgen receptor. *J. Biol. Chem.* 269: 13115–13123, 1994.

18. Autocrine/paracrine intermediates in hormonal action and modulation of cellular responses to hormones

CARL DENEF | *Laboratory of Cell Pharmacology, School of Medicine, University of Leuven, Leuven, Belgium*

CHAPTER CONTENTS

THE CONCEPT OF PARACRINE CONTROL was introduced by Feyrter in 1938 (165). He discovered cells dispersed throughout the epithelia of lung and gastrointestinal tract displaying certain morphological characteristics that were homologous to secretory cells in endocrine tissues. Feyrter classified these cell types as belonging to what he called "diffuse endocrine epithelial organs" and suggested that they released substances affecting the function of neighboring epithelial cells in a hormone-like fashion. Feyrter postulated that, in contrast to endocrine cells, which elaborate and secrete specific substances transported to distantly removed target cells by the bloodstream, paracrine substances are released by the producing cell type and travel to the target cell in the neighborhood by diffusion. By 1969 Pearse had incorporated the "Feyrter cells" in a broader family of cells widely distributed throughout the body on the basis of their common ability to take up and decarboxylate amine precursors to biogenic monoamines and to produce biologically active peptides that had been identified also in neurons. He called them APUD (amine precursor uptake and decarboxylation) cells (76, 419, 420). Over the years the APUD cell family expanded to some 40 members, including chromaffin cells in the adrenal medulla and gut, thyroid C cells, cells of the anterior pituitary and the hypothalamus, gut and pancreatic endocrine cells, carotid body chief cells, Merkel cells, melanocytes, endocrine cells of the placenta and thymus, and sympathetic ganglia cells. However, it was later found that the APUD characteristic is absent in certain cells that nevertheless produce bioactive peptides, and since the biological significance of the APUD was poorly understood, the APUD terminology has been replaced by the term "diffuse neuroendocrine system" on the basis of the apparent relationship between these endocrine-like cells and neurons (421). In the 1980s, research on local control reached an explosive phase. In 1980, Sporn and Todaro introduced the concept of *autocrine* control (537). According to its original definition, an autocrine factor is produced and released by a particular cell type, the latter being also the target cell. These factors were discovered as polypeptide growth factors in the spent medium of cultured cells that had been transformed by an oncogene; it was found that, unlike normal cells in culture which need growth factor supplements to grow, transformed cells become independent of these supplements because they start to produce or overproduce the essential growth factors themselves, such as transforming growth factors-α and (TGFs)-β.

This discovery opened an immense field of successful investigations on the role of autocrine growth factors in tumorigenesis and tumor progression. Several of these growth factors appeared to be operative physiologically during embryonic development, when rapid cell growth is required, and pathologically in the adult organism, participating in the pathogenesis of tumors. These growth factors also appeared to influence cellular differentiation and function. During the 1980s a plethora of autocrine and paracrine polypeptides that modulate the differentiation and action of various cells of the immune system were discovered. They are known as interleukins or cytokines. It was found that the same growth factors, originally discovered in cell lines and the immune system, also were essential local regulators of the inflammatory response and tissue repair. Moreover, cytokines and growth factors are produced by specific cells in endocrine glands and the brain as well as in hormone target cells not only during development but also during adult life. In the latter body compartments, they are thought to modulate hormone or neurotransmitter action and to control tissue homeostasis and functional plasticity. Certain autocrine factors in certain conditions do not need to be released by the cell to activate a plasma membrane receptor; they also can exert their biological activity through binding and activating these receptors inside the cell, more precisely within the secretory pathway. The latter mode of local control is called "internal," autocrine or intracrine, action (339, 536). Some growth factors lack a consensus signal peptide sequence at the N-terminal side of the polypeptide chain, impeding their translocation to the secretory pathway. Some of these growth factors appear to be translocated to the nucleolus and possibly affect ribosomal gene transcription, which represents another intracrine action (339). Estrogens and progesterone in the ovary also have been shown to affect the cells in which they are produced by interacting with intracellular receptors.

Still another mode of local control of cells by some of their neighbors is by so-called juxtacrine factors. This mode of control was discovered by Bosenberg and Massagué (60), who observed that pro-TGF-α can be expressed as a plasma membrane–anchored polypeptide on the surface of cells of a mouse bone marrow stromal cell line and binds to an epidermal growth factor (EGF) receptor on adjacent hematopoietic progenitor cells, in this way inducing at the same time cell adhesion and cell division in the progenitor cells. Since then many other examples of juxtacrine communication have been observed. Among them are almost all members of the EGF family, tumor necrosis factor-α, colony-stimulating factor, and platelet-activating factor. Juxtacrine communication provides a mechanism of strict spatial control of activation of one cell type by another which is clearly in contrast with paracrine control, where the paracrine factor acts in the fluid phase within a radius determined by its concentration and diffusion. The active domain of a juxtacrine poly-peptide can be cleaved from the cell surface by regulated proteolytic cleavage, which will abolish spatial specificity.

METHODS TO EXPLORE LOCAL CONTROL

Originally, putative local control of cells by other cells was deduced from morphological data. The putative paracrine cell showed different morphological and, presumably, functional properties from its neighboring cells, as well as features of secretory potential. Local control also has been suggested on the basis of the presence of long cellular extensions reaching or embracing cells in the neighborhood. As shown below, cells producing somatostatin in the mantle area of pancreatic islets extend cellular processes toward A cells, pancreatic polypeptide cells, and the outer layer of the B cells in the core of the islet. In the anterior pituitary, non-hormone-secreting folliculo-stellate cells extend many and long cellular processes between the hormone-secreting cells. Moreover, a topographical affinity between gonadotrophs and cup-shaped lactotrophs has been observed in the rat, the extent of which is regulated negatively by estrogen. In the adrenal cortex, rays and islets of chromaffin cells from the medulla have been observed in close contact with cortical cells at the electron microscopical level.

Experimental evidence that one cell type influences the activity of another can be found by cell separation and recombinations. The cell types in question are separated from each other; established in culture, on the one hand, as separate populations and, on the other, as recombined populations; and then tested for differences in functional responses. In this approach, three-dimensional reaggregate cell cultures have been particularly successful, probably because intimate contacts over the entire cell surface exist, much like the situation in intact tissue (113). As an extension of such studies and to identify paracrine or autocrine factors, purified cell populations are established in culture and the spent culture medium (also called "conditioned medium") is used as a source to extract and purify the secreted putative factor. If the factor can be identified, the following criteria need to be met to establish it as an autocrine or paracrine regulator: the substance should be synthesized in the tissue by a specific cell type, it should be releasable either in a constitutive manner or through the regulated secretory pathway, a receptor for the substance should be present on the producing cell (autocrine mode) or on another cell type (paracrine mode), the amount released should have a typical biological effect on the cells bearing the recep-

tors, and synthesis and release should be under regulatory control. The existence of cell–cell communication also can be assessed by targeted cell ablation in vitro. A known bioactive substance for which the cell type under study is a target is coupled to a cytotoxic agent, and the derivative is incubated with the dispersed tissue cells in vitro. By the mechanism of receptor-mediated endocytosis, the receptor ligand–toxin complex is transported selectively into cells bearing the receptor for the ligand and the toxin selectively kills the targeted cells. For example, the corticotropin-releasing factor (CRF)–gelonin complex has been shown to eliminate CRF responsive corticotrophs from pituitary cell populations in culture (502).

The classical method to determine the local action of bioactive polypeptides in intercellular signaling is to eliminate the action of this polypeptide once secreted in the intercellular spaces by peptide receptor antagonists, monoclonal antibodies blocking the peptide receptor, antibodies immunoneutralizing the putative paracrine or autocrine substance, and recombinant soluble receptors binding the polypeptide and scavenging it from reaching the receptors located on the target cell. Addition to cultures of antisense oligonucleotides which neutralize translation of the polypeptide due to hybridization to the mRNA of the polypeptide also have been used to demonstrate the participation of the polypeptide under study in local control. The latter tool is also capable of inhibiting actions of intracrine factors.

Explorations of local control have been performed mainly in in vitro test systems. For many factors showing local regulatory activity when added to the system, it remains unknown whether they act in a similar way in the intact tissue in vivo. However, in certain cases in vivo assessment of the release and action of locally produced factors has been realized. By microperfusion with microdialysis tubing of the adrenal gland, the ovarian follicular wall, and corpus luteum, it has been possible to measure known substances released under particular conditions and the effect of certain exogenous regulatory factors on this release in the living animal (617). The advent of molecular biology has expanded enormously the possibilities to study the influence of one cell type upon another and local control by known polypeptides in vivo. Toxigenes can be targeted to specific cell types, provided the gene can be fused to a cell-specific promoter, and introduced in the genome of transgenic mice. In this way, selective cell types can be ablated in a particular organ and the consequence of the deletion of that cell type on the development and function of other cell types in that tissue evaluated. For example, ablation of somatotrophs in the pituitary results in a virtual disappearance of lactotrophs without an influence on other cell types

(57). Ablation of gonadotrophs causes hypoplasia of lactotrophs (290). The putative paracrine or autocrine role of known polypeptides can be tested by targeting expression of this polypeptide to a particular cell type or of a dominant negative receptor of this peptide in transgenic mice. A dominant negative receptor is a mutant receptor expressed in high amounts and capable of binding its ligand but devoid of signal-transduction capacity, in this way trapping most of the endogenous paracrine agent and avoiding binding of the agent to normal receptors. Targeting nerve growth factor (NGF) to lactotrophs results in a tremendous hyperplasia of lactotrophs (58). Targeted expression of a dominant negative fibroblast growth factor (FGF) receptor to the epidermis of transgenic mice disrupts the organization of epidermal keratinocytes and causes epidermal hyperthickening (606). Finally, the gene encoding the polypeptide can be deleted in transgenic mice in a tissue-specific manner.

LOCAL CONTROL IN THE ANTERIOR PITUITARY

Endocrine secretion of the anterior pituitary is controlled by the brain through the release in the portal vasculature of peptides and biogenic amines, known as releasing and inhibiting hormones, and through several hormones secreted from the gonads, adrenals, and thyroid into the general circulation. There is a large body of in vitro evidence supporting the hypothesis of paracrine/autocrine regulation in the pituitary. This local regulation operates on various levels. Certain factors modulate or mediate various actions of the hypothalamic and peripheral hormones on pituitary function. Other factors exert a tonic paracrine or autocrine action on basal release of certain hormones. Still other factors transduce activation of one cell type upon another by a releasing hormone, coordinating the release of two pituitary hormones by a single releasing hormone. Finally, locally produced paracrine/autocrine factors seem to affect cellular differentiation and the development of various cell types in the pituitary gland. However, since most data so far have been obtained from in vitro experiments, it is not clear under which physiological conditions the local control systems operate. In this respect, knowledge of the regulatory control of the synthesis and release of the factor may point to the physiological condition in which it operates. Some data obtained from gene and cell targeting in transgenic mice have been collected and probably will be of great importance in testing the significance of the local control factor under various experimental and physiological conditions in vivo. It is important to note that the action of several of these local factors requires the presence of various hormones, such as glucocorticoids, estrogens, and thyroid hormone. Some local interactions are shown in Figure 18.1.

Evidence for Intercellular Communication in the Anterior Pituitary

Gonadotrophs. There are some morphological indications that gonadotrophs interact functionally with lactotrophs. A subpopulation of lactotrophs, the so-called cup-shaped lactotrophs, has the peculiar ability to embrace some gonadotrophs, a topographical affinity which is influenced negatively by estrogen (reviewed in ref. 11). The first in vitro experimental evidence for functional communication in the anterior pituitary was obtained through the introduction of three-dimensional reaggregate cell culture technology. It was shown in such cell cultures of immature rat pituitary that gonadotropin-releasing hormone (GnRH), which is the releasing hormone for luteinizing and follicle-stimulating (FSH) hormones from the gonadotrophs, is capable of provoking a rapid and sustained rise of prolactin (PRL) release from lactotrophs at concentrations similar to those stimulating luteinizing hormone (LH) release (0.01–10 nM) (112). It has been hypothesized that the GnRH action on lactotrophs is not a direct one but that GnRH activates the gonadotrophs, which in turn transmit a signal to the lactotrophs. Support for this hypothesis was found by cell separation and recombination experiments. When GnRH is given to aggregates consisting of a population enriched in lactotrophs but deprived of gonadotrophs, no PRL response is seen. However, when a small percentage of a population consisting of 70% gonadotrophs is co-aggregated with the lactotroph preparation, a clear-cut stimulation of PRL release becomes evident, the magnitude of which depends on the proportional number of gonadotrophs added to the lactotrophs. Thus, the GnRH effect on PRL release appears to be mediated by gonadotrophs, either through a stimulatory paracrine signal or through a signal inducing GnRH receptors in lactotrophs to respond to GnRH. There is some evidence for the former mechanism rather than for the latter since a factor with PRL-releasing activity is secreted by aggregates consisting of 70% gonadotrophs and its amount increases in the presence of GnRH. The PRL response to GnRH is not an artifact of culture as the same response can be elicited in intact pituitary from newborn rats (18). Importantly, the response in the intact pituitary disappears in rats older than 2 weeks, suggesting that signaling from gonadotrophs to lactotrophs may be related to the development of the pituitary.

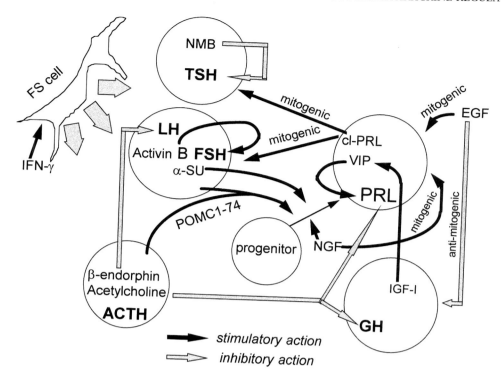

FIG. 18.1 Effect of various paracrine and autocrine factors on anterior pituitary hormone secretion and on cellular proliferation and differentiation. *FS*, folliculo-stellate; *IFN-γ*, interferon-γ; *TSH*, thyroid-stimulating hormone; *LH*, luteinizing hormone; *FSH*, follicle-stimulating hormone; *α-SU*, α-subunit; *POMC*, proopiomela-nocortin; *ACTH*, adrenocorticotrophic hormone; *GH*, growth hormone; *IGF*, insulin-like growth factor; *NGF*, nerve growth factor; *PRL*, prolactin; cleaved product of prolactin; *VIP*, vasoactive intestinal peptide; *cl-PRL*, cleaved product of prolactin; *EGF*, epidermal growth factor; *NMB*, neuromedin B.

Indeed, GnRH may be involved in lactotroph development. In reaggregated cell cultures of 14-day-old rat pituitaries, GnRH at physiological concentrations enhances the number of DNA-replicating lactotrophs and lowers the number of DNA-replicating somatotrophs (565). Cell separation and recombination experiments have shown that this effect occurs only in the presence of gonadotrophs. The participation of a paracrine mechanism in these mitogenic and antimitogenic effects is indicated by observation that medium conditioned by a highly enriched population of gonadotrophs cultured in the presence of GnRH contains different growth factors mimicking the effects of GnRH. At least four substances which display a mitogenic effect on lactotrophs have been partially purified, whereas two other substances inhibit mitosis in somatotrophs (565). None of these growth factors affects the cell cycle of other cell types.

In another study, addition of GnRH to reaggregate cell cultures of 14-day-old rat pituitary resulted in a marked increase in the total number of cells containing PRL mRNA (581). This recruitment of lactotrophs appears to be based on the differentiation of an undefined cell type into PRL-expressing cells, rather than on a mitogenic action on preexisting lactotrophs alone. Furthermore, the total number of cells expressing growth hormone mRNA is reduced significantly by GnRH (582). Interestingly, GnRH also inhibits the mitogenic effect of growth hormone (GH) releasing factor (GRF) on somatotrophs (582).

In further support of paracrine signaling from gonadotrophs in the development of lactotrophs and somatotrophs is the finding that the αT3–1 cell line, a pure cell line of the gonadotroph lineage, can mimic the actions of normal gonadotrophs on the in vitro development of lactotrophs and somatotrophs (22).

Treatment of cultured aggregates from 14-day-old rat pituitaries with medium conditioned with αT3–1 cells increases mitosis in lactotrophs and lowers it in somatotrophs. Different substances that mimic the effect of GnRH on lactotroph and somatotroph development have been partially purified from the αT3–1 cell–conditioned medium (22). The data clearly suggest that gonadotrophs control not only secretion but also development of lactotrophs and somatotrophs through the release of growth factors; inhibition of somatotroph development appears to be mediated by a different set of growth factors from those that stimulate lactotroph development. These findings are most interesting in view of the concepts that lactotrophs may be derived from somatotrophs during fetal and early postnatal development (15) and that somatotrophs may transdifferentiate into lactotrophs even in adult life, such as during pregnancy and lactation (543).

Folliculo-Stellate Cells. Folliculo-stellate cells, which represent 5%–10% of the cells of the anterior pituitary, do not secrete hormones. The origin of these cells remains uncertain; some of these cells express markers of monocytes and dendritic cells of the immune system (10), though there is evidence for an epithelial origin based on the expression of cytokeratins (283, 576). The cells can associate to form small follicles, while others are dispersed throughout the pituitary gland and extend long cytoplasmic processes between other cell types, suggesting a role in intercellular communication (8). There is a body of in vitro experimental evidence supporting this hypothesis. When a cell preparation consisting of up to 65% folliculo-stellate cells is co-aggregated with highly enriched populations of various hormone-secreting anterior pituitary cells, stimulations of growth hormone release by GRF and epinephrine, of PRL release by angiotensin II and thyrotropin-releasing hormone (TRH), and of LH release by GnRH are blunted (32). Folliculo-stellate cells also weaken the secretory response to inhibitory signals, such as dopamine on PRL release and somatostatin on GH release (9). Also, culturing pituitary cells in the presence of interferon-γ (IFN-γ) results in a significant decrease in the secretion of adrenocorticotrophic hormone (ACTH), GH, and PRL in response to various secretagogues (585). This effect is not acute but requires a continuous exposure for 24 h. Evidence was found that folliculo-stellate cells mediate the latter inhibitory actions (584).

Corticotrophs. Observations on individually secreting corticotrophs by means of the reversed hemolytic plaque assay (a method to score the secretion rate of in-

dividual cells dispersed on slides) have suggested the existence of a paracrine factor secreted from corticotrophs rendering a subpopulation of corticotrophs unresponsive to CRF (271). Provided a critical distance between anterior pituitary cells in monolayer culture is not exceeded, the number of corticotrophs secreting ACTH in response to CRF remains relatively constant, but when this critical distance is exceeded, the number of CRF-responsive corticotrophs almost doubles, indicating the existence of a population of corticotrophs, previously repressed by a paracrine factor, which dilutes out and becomes ineffective when the distance between cells becomes too large. The cellular source of the inhibitory factor is the CRF-responsive corticotroph population (271). There is also evidence for the existence of a paracrine system inducing responsiveness to CRF in corticotrophs (502). Exposure to arginine vasopressin (AVP) augments the number of corticotrophs responsive to CRF; it is well known that some of the corticotrophs are target cells of AVP but that these are not the cells that become CRF-responsive; these cells are other corticotrophs, which become CRF targets secondary to a paracrine signal from hitherto unknown AVP target cells (502). As reviewed elsewhere (252), noncorticotroph AVP target cells are thyrotrophs and gonadotrophs. AVP is synthesized in the anterior pituitary, AVP/neurophysin mRNA being located mainly in corticotrophs and AVP immunoreactivity in all hormone-secreting cell types except somatotrophs (563).

Neurointermediate Lobe Cells. Extensive studies have shown that the pituitary neurointermediate lobe (NIL) is involved in the peak phase of the proestrous PRL surge, the suckling-induced rise in PRL release, and the acute estradiol-induced rise in PRL secretion in the rat (43). The mediating mechanism seems to be a humoral factor. The NIL secretes substances capable of releasing PRL and of activating PRL gene expression (43, 545). Co-culturing anterior pituitary and NIL cells results in a marked increase in PRL cell content and release. Co-culturing NIL cells with the PRL- and GH-secreting GH3 cells results in a dramatic stimulation of PRL gene expression, synthesis, and release, whereas cell content of GH is reduced strongly (97). Furthermore, estradiol releases from NIL cells a substance(s) that rapidly augments the relative abundance of lactotrophs in anterior pituitary cell cultures (139). The NIL peptides α-melanocyte-stimulating hormone (MSH) and β-endorphin in their acetylated forms mimic the effect of the substance(s) released by estradiol from NIL cells. Remarkably, the estradiol-induced material from the NIL as well as the NIL peptides recruit PRL-secreting cells exclusively within the central region of the anterior pituitary adjacent to the NIL (441).

Putative Paracrine Factors

Production of some biogenic amines and a very large number of bioactive polypeptides has been detected in the anterior pituitary at both the mRNA and protein levels. Polypeptides belong to almost all known families: the brain–gut peptides vasoactive intestinal peptide (VIP), tachykinins, galanin, neuropeptide Y (NPY), and neurotensin; the bombesin-like peptides gastrin, cholecystokinin, secretin, motilin, and neuromedin U; the proenkephalin-derived, prodynorphin-derived, and proopiomelanocortin (POMC)-derived opioid peptides; peptides related to the cardiovascular system such as atrial natriuretic peptide (ANP), angiotensins, and endothelins; the neurohypophysial peptides oxytocin and vasopressin; the hypothalamic releasing and inhibiting factors GnRH, CRF, GRF, TRH, and somatostatin; and various growth and differentiation factors such as FGFs, insulin-like growth factors (IGFs), members of the EGF family, the TGF-β family, activin, inhibin, members of the neurotrophin family, interleukins, and vascular endothelial growth factor (VEGF). Expression, secretion, regulation, and putative local actions of these peptides have been the subjects of several reviews (252, 276, 398, 422, 423).

Acetylcholine. The synthesis, release, regulation, and paracrine action of acetylcholine by normal and tumoral pituitary corticotrophs have been demonstrated (70–73). Double immunostaining of choline acetyltransferase (CAT), ACTH, GH, PRL, thyroid-stimulating hormone (TSH), S100, LH, and FSH in rat anterior pituitary cells has shown that most of the CAT-immunoreactive cells store ACTH. Incubation of cultured rat pituitary cell aggregates with [^{3}H]-choline yields a derivative identified as [^{3}H]-acetylcholine. Blockers of acetylcholine production, such as hemicholinium and 4-[(1–naphthylvinyl)pyridinium], abolish the formation of [^{3}H]-acetylcholine in pituitary cell aggregates. Both synthesis and release of acetylcholine are increased by the glucocorticoid hormone dexamethasone. The mouse pituitary corticotroph cell line AtT20 also contains CAT immunoreactivity and converts [^{3}H]choline into [^{3}H]-acetylcholine. Perifusion of anterior pituitary cell aggregates with the muscarinic receptor antagonist atropine (Atr) results in dose-dependent (0.1–100 nM) increases in basal PRL and GH secretion; this response requires the presence of dexamethasone in the culture medium. A similar response to Atr is observed in organ-cultured pituitaries. The specificity of the Atr effect has been demonstrated by findings that the highly specific muscarinic receptor blocker dexetimide shows a similar action, whereas its inactive enantiomer levetimide and the nicotinic receptor blocker hexamethonium fail to do so. Also, Atr potentiates stimulation of GH release by the β-adrenergic agonist isoproterenol and of PRL release by VIP. Addition of carbachol, a cholinergic receptor agonist, to pituitary cell aggregates results in an inhibition of PRL and GH release, an effect seen only if a glucocorticoid is present in the culture medium (70, 73). Taken together these data show that acetylcholine meets most of the criteria required to establish this neurotransmitter as a paracrine factor in the anterior pituitary, its paracrine action consisting of a tonic inhibition of basal PRL and growth hormone release.

Vasoactive Intestinal Peptide. Expression of VIP mRNA and peptide has been shown in rat and human anterior pituitary (66, 252, 457). The peptide is released by, receptors for VIP are present in, and expression of the peptide is regulated by thyroid hormone, sex steroids, and adrenal cortex hormones. Moreover, VIP expression is sensitive to changes in osmotic pressure (88), and the number of VIP-immunoreactive cells in the anterior pituitary in cell culture decreases after dopamine treatment (74). Which cell type expresses VIP is unclear. Some authors have located the peptide in lactotrophs (389), whereas others did not find the peptide in lactotrophs but in a cell type with stellate shape still to be identified (216). Expression of VIP may be a matter of plasticity, occurring in more than one cell type depending on hormonal and, perhaps, developmental conditions. For example, after estrogen treatment, VIP is present in a subpopulation of lactotrophs containing galanin-immunoreactive material (541). It is well established that VIP stimulates PRL release from lactotrophs, and the finding that addition of antiserum to VIP in cultured anterior pituitary cells decreases basal PRL release is consistent with an intrapituitary paracrine action of this peptide (316, 389). Furthermore, VIP appears to mediate the action of other bioactive peptides on lactotroph function. In rat anterior pituitary cell cultures, IGF-I increases expression and secretion of VIP together with PRL secretion; the effect of IGF-I on PRL release can be abolished by adding anti-VIP antiserum to the cultures, suggesting that the effect of IGF-I on PRL release is mediated by a paracrine or autocrine action of VIP (318). Still other effects of VIP have been reported when the peptide is added to anterior pituitary in vitro. Both VIP and GRF have no effect on basal ACTH secretion but potentiate CRF-induced ACTH release (332). Also, VIP strongly stimulates GH release in reaggregate pituitary cell cultures provided glucocorticoids are present (114). Whether these effects also are exerted by endogenous VIP in a paracrine manner remains to be studied. Another important finding is that the effect of VIP on

PRL release is not direct but mediated by galanin released from a subpopulation of lactotrophs which does not secrete PRL in response to VIP (618). Thus, VIP, galanin, and IGF-I appear to be related to each other in a complex paracrine network.

Renin–Angiotensin System. Renin, angiotensin II, and angiotensin-converting enzyme have been located in gonadotrophs in the rat and in lactotrophs in the human and the lamb (182, 183, 228, 292, 463, 478, 479). Most of the angiotensinogen in rat anterior pituitary is produced by a separate population of cells. In human and lamb anterior pituitary, angiotensinogen has been found in lactotrophs, co-localized with PRL in the same granules (292, 478). Angiotensin II stimulates PRL and ACTH secretions when added to rat or human pituitary cells in vitro (121, 350, 500, 501) and has a dual effect (stimulatory and inhibitory) on GH secretion (464, 465). It remains, however, uncertain whether endogenous angiotensin II also acts as a PRL or GH release modulator. Indeed, neither angiotensin-converting enzyme inhibitors nor angiotensin II receptor antagonists shows any effect on basal PRL or GH release in perifused pituitary cell aggregates or antagonizes stimulation of PRL or GH release by GnRH used at physiological concentration (462, 463); however, at very high doses of GnRH, PRL release is inhibited or attenuated by the angiotensin II receptor antagonists (275, 313, 463). Thus, so far, there is no evidence that angiotensin II is a paracrine PRL releaser. A putative alternative action of angiotensin II in the anterior pituitary is on growth and differentiation. Angiotensin II increases the percentage of cells that bind CRF and store ACTH (89). The latter may be corticotrophs, cells that store ACTH with gonadotrophins, or cells that store ACTH and TSH (89).

Opioid Peptides. Opioid peptides of all known families are expressed in the anterior pituitary (for review, see ref. 252). In cultured rat pituitary cells morphine exerts a direct inhibitory effect on both basal and GnRH-stimulated LH release whereas treatment with the opiate receptor blocker naltrexone or with β-endorphin antiserum significantly increases basal LH release (49); CRF also decreases basal LH release, an effect that is reversed by naltrexone (49). These data clearly show that intrapituitary opioid peptides released from corticotrophs could exert a paracrine inhibitory action on the gonadotroph. It is well known that stress inhibits gonadotrophin release via an action of CRF at the hypothalamic level. The antigonadotrophic role of CRF may be amplified via an action on corticotrophs which releases β-endorphin thereby inhibiting LH release.

Bombesin-Like Peptides (Gastrin-Releasing Peptide and Neuromedin B). Bombesin immunoreactivity has been detected in the anterior pituitary of rat, guinea pig, cat, dog, pig, cow, monkey, and human, more precisely in somatotrophs (542). Gastrin-releasing peptide (GRP)-immunoreactive material has been found in lactotrophs and corticotrophs in rat pituitary (249). The number of GRP-immunoreactive cells is modulated by estrogen and thyroid hormone (542). By means of RNAse protection hybridization assays, the presence of GRP mRNA, as well as GRP receptor mRNA, in anterior pituitary and cultured anterior pituitary cells has been shown (253). As to its possible local function, GRP was found to stimulate PRL and GH release in vitro (248), an effect strongly potentiated by estradiol (248, 250). Receptors for GRP have been located by autoradiography on lactotrophs and somatotrophs and are up-regulated by estradiol (251). However, a similar stimulatory action of endogenous GRP on PRL or GH release has not been demonstrated since under various experimental conditions addition of a highly potent GRP receptor antagonist to pituitary cell cultures did not affect basal or stimulated release. Thus, the precise conditions leading to release of and/or response to endogenous GRP from lactotrophs or corticotrophs in the pituitary remain to be identified.

Neuromedin B appears to be involved in the local control of TSH release in the rat (453). The peptide is synthesized in the anterior pituitary, where it has been localized in thyrotrophs (274). It directly inhibits TSH release from the anterior pituitary in vitro, whereas incubation of pituitaries with a highly specific antiserum against neuromedin B stimulates TSH release, indicating that it acts in an autocrine fashion to suppress TSH release. In hypothyroid animals, anti-neuromedin B antiserum is ineffective on TSH release, which is consistent with the finding that in hypothyroid rats its expression is drastically reduced (453).

Activin and Follistatin. Expression of activin B has been demonstrated in rat anterior pituitary gonadotrophs (305). Activin stimulates FSH, but not LH gene transcription and FSH production, amplifies the response of FSH to pulses of GnRH (604), stimulates the number of FSH-producing gonadotrophs (287), and inhibits GH gene expression and somatotroph cell proliferation (547). That endogenous activin acts as an autocrine factor on FSH production has been shown clearly in vitro and in vivo: incubation of cultured rat anterior pituitary cells with a monoclonal antibody specific for the activin B homodimer decreases basal secretion of FSH and the level of FSH-β-subunit mRNA without affecting that of LH-β subunit mRNA (98). Administration of a monoclonal antibody against activin B on the evening of proestrus in rats attenuates the rise of serum FSH early in estrus (115). In transgenic mice with deleted activin type II receptors, FSH production is depressed (360).

Some gonadotrophs also express follistatin, an activin-binding protein that inhibits FSH biosynthesis and secretion, suggesting that it has a role in the local regulation of FSH production and release (280). Follistatin suppresses the activin A–stimulated increase in the number of FSH cells (287). However, the finding that follistatin mRNA levels peak before maximal expression of FSH-β-subunit mRNA during the estrous cycle raises the possibility that follistatin is a positive, rather than a negative, regulator of FSH biosynthesis in vivo (217). Follistatin also is expressed in a subpopulation of somatotrophs and lactotrophs early in the rat estrous cycle (323); its role there remains to be established.

Epidermal Growth Factor, Transforming Growth Factor-α, and Heregulins.
Epidermal growth factor and its structural homologue TGF-α are synthesized in the rat, bovine, and human anterior pituitary (147, 153, 383). The anterior pituitary expresses the EGF receptor (82, 153). In situ hybridization coupled with immunocytochemistry experiments in the rat has shown the presence of EGF mRNA in somatotrophs and gonadotrophs; TGF-α mRNA in somatotrophs, gonadotrophs, and lactotrophs; and EGF receptors in all hormone-secreting cells (153). Receptors for EGF have been located in the rat and bovine by autoradiography of labeled ligand, particularly on lactotrophs and somatotrophs (82). Receptors for TGF-α in human pituitary are expressed particularly in somatotrophs (169). Under certain physiological conditions, EGF expression is induced in other cell types: cold stress induces EGF mRNA in corticotrophs and thyrotrophs in the rat (which functionally fits with the activation of these cell types during this type of stress) without affecting the expression of EGF or TGF-α in other cell types and enhances EGF receptor number in thyrotrophs and gonadotrophs (153). In the bovine anterior pituitary, TGF-α has been identified by amino-acid sequencing of purified material (305, 489). Expression of TGF-α also has been shown in human pituitary adenomas (147). According to some investigators (452), TGF-α- and EGF-immunoreactive materials are secreted by nonfunctioning human pituitary adenoma cells, whereas others found only immunoreactive TGF-α in a plasma membrane–bound form, suggesting a juxtacrine mechanism of action in cell growth (147). Expression of TGF-α in its unprocessed, high molecular weight precursor form also has been demonstrated in the MtT/W5, GH1, GH3, and GH4C1 pituitary cell lines (170).

In the normal pituitary, EGF and TGF-α dose-dependently stimulate ^{3}H-thymidine labeling of lactotrophs and decrease ^{3}H-thymidine labeling of somatotrophs (21). Also, EGF is also a mitogen for corticotrophs (90). In rat PRL- and GH–secreting cell lines EGF inhibits mitosis and induces differentiation (447). Treatment of the GH-3 cell line, which lacks functional D2 receptors, with EGF induces expression of this receptor and renders these cells sensitive to inhibition of PRL release by dopamine agonists (188, 370). Also, EGF exerts acute effects on the secretion of anterior pituitary hormones: it stimulates PRL secretion from GH3 cells (1) and TSH release from perfused rat pituitary glands (13). It is a potent inducer of PRL gene transcription (197). Some evidence that TGF-α stimulates lactotroph tumor growth in an autocrine or juxtacrine manner has been given (170).

The anterior pituitary expresses various heregulins, which belong to a family of EGF-like growth factors derived from a single gene by differential splicing of the mRNA of that gene (203). The anterior pituitary expresses the typical members of the EGF receptor family involved in the specific binding of the heregulins: erbB-2 (83) and erbB-4 (438). The action of heregulins in the pituitary remains unknown.

Neurotrophins.
The neurotrophins NGF, brain-derived neurotrophic factor (BDNF), and neurotrophin-3 (NT3) are well known for their trophic action in the central and peripheral nervous systems. These growth factors also are expressed in nonneuronal tissue, including the pituitary gland (307, 368, 416). The finding that targeted overexpression of NGF in lactotrophs of transgenic mice leads to a tremendous hyperplasia (pituitary glands grow up to 50 times their normal volume; 58) inspired investigators to test whether NGF and other neurotrophins are expressed in lactotrophs or other pituitary cell types and whether NGF causes a mitogenic effect on lactotrophs. During pituitary morphogenesis, material cross-reacting with a polyclonal antiserum recognizing NGF, BDNF, and NT3 has been detected in most epithelial cells of the anterior pituitary, NIL, and pars tuberalis of the primate (59); in the adult primate, neurotrophin-immunoreactive cells were fewer in number and found only in the anterior pituitary and pars tuberalis. In the adult rat, NGF immunoreactivity has been found in thyrotrophs by some investigators (96) but in a subpopulation of all pituitary endocrine cell types by others (416). In neonatal rats, NGF and its receptor are found in cultured somato-lactotrophs and lactotrophs (368). In pituitary monolayer cell cultures from neonatal rats, NGF markedly increases the proportional number of lactotrophs, whereas treatment of cultures with antibodies immuno-

neutralizing endogenous NGF prevents the basal recruitment of lactotrophs (368). Also, NGF augments PRL and decreases GH secretion in the PRL- and GH-secreting GH3 cell line and induces expression of the D2 receptor in GH3 cells, which normally lack this receptor; following NGF treatment, GH3 cells become sensitive to inhibition of PRL release by dopamine (371). Also, NGF is capable of converting human prolactinoma cells resistant to dopamine agonist treatment due to an absence of functional D2 receptors in cells expressing the D2 receptor (369); these cells decrease their intrinsic proliferation rate and lose their tumorigenic activity in nude mice. Anterior pituitary cells express different types of neurotrophin receptor (75, 307, 371, 416). Using antiserum specific for NGF, it has been shown that NGF is released from cultured pituitary cells; interleukin-1 increases, whereas GRF and basic FGF (bFGF) inhibit, NGF secretion (417).

The N-Terminal Fragment of Proopiomelanocortin.

Proopiomelanocortin (POMC) was isolated from medium conditioned by gonadotroph-rich aggregates from 14-day-old female rats in a search for the identity of the growth factors mediating the mitogenic action of GnRH on lactotrophs observed in aggregate cell cultures of neonatal rat pituitary (566). From material increasing the number of ^{3}H-thymidine-incorporating lactotrophs in pituitary cell aggregates of 2-week-old rats a substance with a molecular mass of 11 kd was isolated. N-terminal-amino-acid sequence analysis revealed that the substance was a peptide identical to the N-terminal region of rat POMC. Electrospray ionization mass spectrometry suggested that the peptide extends C-terminally at least to amino-acid residue 74, which in the POMC sequence is flanked by an Arg-Arg dibasic residue, a posttranslational cleavage site. The substance increases the number of ^{3}H-thymidine-incorporating lactotrophs in pituitary cell aggregates without affecting ^{3}H-thymidine labeling of other pituitary cell types. Authentic human POMC1–76, in nanomolar concentration, provokes a similar stimulation of the ^{3}H-thymidine-labeled lactotroph number without affecting other cell types. Further evidence for the paracrine action of endogenous POMC1–74 stems from the finding that an antiserum raised against POMC1–74 causes a 50% inhibition of the number of ^{3}H-thymidine-labeled lactotrophs (D. Tilemans and C. Denef, unpublished observation). These data show that POMC1–74 is a growth factor specifically targeting lactotrophs during in vitro development of postnatal rat anterior pituitary and that it may be one of the growth factors mediating the action of GnRH on lactotroph development.

Proopiomelanocortin is the well-known precursor of several hormones and neuropeptides such as ACTH; α-, β-, and γ-MSH; lipotropic hormone; and β-endorphin. Very little is known of the N-terminal POMC fragment. Since POMC is expressed in various other tissues, these data suggest that in these other tissues a hitherto unexplored paracrine function of POMC1–74 may exist.

The Common α-Subunit of the Glycoprotein Hormones.

The pituitary glycoprotein hormones FSH, LH, and TSH consist of a common α-subunit and a hormone-specific β-subunit. Some α-subunit, however, is present in the cell in a free form and is secreted mainly via the constitutive secretory pathway (51). There is evidence that this free α-subunit may be a growth and differentiation factor. It has been reported that the free α-subunit from gonadotrophs participates in the stimulation of lactotroph development in the embryonic rat pituitary (40). Furthermore, when added to pituitary aggregate cell cultures of 14-day-old rats, purified rat α-subunit increases the total number of lactotrophs, as well as ^{3}H-thymidine incorporation in the lactotrophs (580). These effects can be blocked by anti-α-subunit antibodies, showing the specificity of the α-subunit effect. There is growing evidence that the α-subunit is expressed in normal and tumoral pituitary cells other than gonadotrophs and thyrotrophs. Expression of α-subunit mRNA and protein has been demonstrated in the majority of human corticotroph and somatotroph adenomas (116, 224). Another indication for a separate function for free α-subunit in the anterior pituitary is the fact that it is secreted mainly via the constitutive secretory pathway, whereas LH and FSH are secreted primarily via the regulated secretory pathway (51).

Prolactin and a Cleaved Variant of Prolactin.

Using monoclonal antibodies specific to the rat PRL receptor, it has been shown that a subpopulation of all endocrine cell types of the anterior pituitary expresses the PRL receptor, raising the possibility that PRL acts in an autocrine or paracrine manner in regulating anterior pituitary function (380). Evidence for such a role has been presented in the PRL-secreting GH3 and 235-1 cell lines (311). It appears that PRL is an autocrine growth factor in GH3 cells: PRL receptors are present on 40%–50% of GH3 cells, which also contain PRL (as opposed to cells containing only GH in this cell line) (310); addition of anti-rat PRL antiserum, but not control serum, to GH3 cells markedly inhibits proliferation (310). In the 235–1 cell line, PRL receptors are present primarily in the Golgi complex and, only after interleukin-1 treatment, at the cell surface.

In the latter condition, anti-PRL antibodies decrease cellular proliferation. Specific interference with PRL biosynthesis by incubation with PRL mRNA antisense oligonucleotides also inhibits cellular proliferation (311). Also PRL may be an autocrine regulator of its own secretion; PRL secretion from GH3 cells is not normally autoregulated, apparently because a specific charge variant is not produced by these cells, but addition of this isoform to GH3 cells inhibits PRL secretion and induces intracellular storage of PRL (244). Finally, PRL may locally modulate LH and FSH release as it has been shown to stimulate LH and FSH release in rat pituitary cell cultures (315).

A cleaved form of PRL (cl-PRL) has been isolated from conditioned medium of pituitary aggregate cell cultures by means of a monoclonal anti-PRL affinity column (20). By N- and C-terminal amino-acid sequencing, the cleavage site was found between amino acids Tyr_{145} and Leu_{146}. This molecule stimulates ^3H-thymidine incorporation in gonadotrophs and thyrotrophs at nanomolar concentrations without affecting that in other pituitary cell types. The parent PRL, even at a tenfold higher concentration, does not show this effect. The putative paracrine action of cl-PRL was demonstrated by immunoneutralization studies with polyclonal antisera which recognize cl-PRL but not the parent PRL (19). Addition of these antisera to pituitary reaggregate cell cultures significantly decreases ^3H-thymidine incorporation in gonadotrophs and thyrotrophs without affecting that in other cell types, indicating that endogenous cl-PRL has a tonic paracrine mitogenic action on the latter two cell types.

Nitrous Oxide. Gonadotrophs and folliculo-stellate cells express the enzyme nitrous oxide synthase (NOS) (78). This enzyme uses arginine as a substrate to produce the gas nitrous oxide. It has been shown that nitrous oxide can pass from one cell to another and act on the latter through increasing intracellular cyclic guanosine monophosphate (cGMP) levels. Nitrous oxide donor molecules inhibit GH and LH release whereas NOS inhibitors augment such release (78 and references therein). It has been shown that IFN-γ–induced inhibition of pituitary hormone release is mediated, at least in part, by NO (585b).

LOCAL CONTROL IN THE ADRENAL CORTEX AND MEDULLA

Evidence for paracrine control systems in the adrenal cortex has been documented extensively and includes regulation of glucocorticoid and aldosterone secretion as well as growth and differentiation processes (595). Paracrine influences appear to be exerted by adrenal medulla chromaffin cells upon adrenal cortex cells as well as within each of both adrenal gland compartments (242). In the medulla, many of the putative paracrine/autocrine factors are released by acetylcholine of splanchnic nerve terminals, whereas in the adrenal cortex release or expression level is controlled by ACTH and angiotensin II. Their actions may involve effects on basal cellular activities as well as modulation of the influence of ACTH or angiotensin II. Some local interactions are shown on Figure 18.2.

Morphological Correlates of Medulla–Cortex Interactions

Medulla–cortex interactions are clear on microanatomical grounds. Rays and islets of chromaffin cells have been observed in close contact with cortical cells at the electron microscopical level (54, 181). In rat and porcine adrenals, these rays of cells, small chromaffin cell clusters, and single chromaffin cells are detectable in all three zones of the cortex and even spread in the subcapsular area (56). In porcine and bovine adrenals, single cortical cells and small clusters are spread throughout the medulla (56). The close cellular contacts between medullary and cortical cells observed at the ultrastructural level (55, 56) and the finding of an exocytotic process from a chromaffin cell in direct apposition with an adrenocortical cell (54) provide direct evidence in support of a paracrine regulation of the cortex by chromaffin cells. Somatostatin-positive chromaffin cells display short processes similar to those seen in somatostatin-immunoreactive paracrine cells of the gut (594).

Putative Paracrine and Autocrine Factors in the Medulla

Many regulatory peptides have been detected in the adrenal chromaffin cells of several mammalian species, including humans, by means of immunocytochemical techniques and by assessing the presence of the mRNA of the following peptides: the opioid peptides enkephalin (50, 133, 229, 270, 471), dynorphin (320, 331), and β-endorphin (514); the hypothalamic releasing and inhibiting factors CRF (63, 64, 130, 225, 367) and somatostatin-28 (594); NPY (102, 229, 235, 494, 544, 612); neurotensin (343, 426); calcitonin gene–related peptide (CGRP) (306, 426); ANP (379, 612); brain natriuretic peptide (BNP) (325); vasopressin (212, 227); oxytocin (227); parathyroid hormone-like peptide (266); and galanin (362, 471). Also, VIP has been

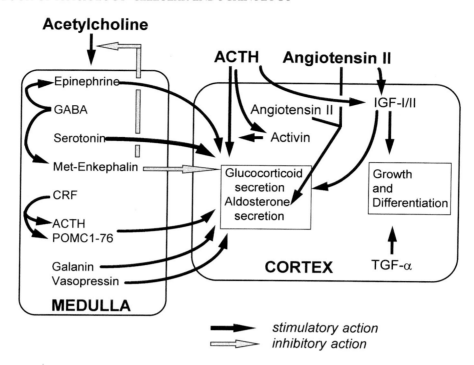

FIG. 18.2 Effect of various paracrine and autocrine factors on hormone secretion from adrenal medulla and cortex and on cellular growth and differentiation. *ACTH,* adrenocorticotrophic hormone; *IGF,* insulin-like growth factor, *TGF-α,* transforming growth factor-α; *GABA,* γ-aminobutyric acid; *CRF,* corticotrophin-releasing factor; *POMC,* proopiomelanocortin.

identified in frog adrenal chromaffin cells (319, 320) but is absent in these cells in mammalian species (361). In the latter, it is found in nerve terminals in the capsule/glomerular zone of the cortex (361). However, when bovine chromaffin cells are dissociated from the adrenal gland and established in culture, they start synthesizing VIP (135, 516). Various POMC-derived peptides, including ACTH1–39, β-lipotropin, and 12 and 14 kd N-terminal POMC fragments have been identified in human adrenal extracts (108, 191, 409) and in adrenal vein effluents upon splanchnic nerve stimulation in functionally hypophysectomized calves (273).

An important question concerns the distribution of expression of these peptides in relation to that of the catecholamines epinephrine and norepinephrine in medullary chromaffin cells. As studied in the pig and bovine, enkephalins co-localize with epinephrine-containing cells (36, 306, 331), some of which in addition contain CGRP (306). Islets of chromaffin cells beneath the capsule co-express enkephalins and CGRP (306). Also, NPY is co-stored with epinephrine in the

rat, mouse, cat, guinea pig, and human (36, 343, 493, 533), though in some species the peptide is co-stored with norepinephrine (36, 349); and it is found in medullary ganglion cells (495) and nerve fibers in the adrenal cortex (343, 349). In the rat, ANP is synthesized primarily in norepinehrine-containing cells, whereas epinephrine-containing cells appear to bind and internalize the peptide (379). In the bovine, dynorphin-derived peptides are located mainly in norepinephrine-synthesizing cells (331). As far as the distribution of galanin is concerned, a striking species difference has been reported (626). Galanin immunoreactivity is found in all medullary cells of guinea pig, duck, and chicken but is missing in these cells in rat and pigeon. In rat, guinea pig, and pigeon, galanin-containing nerve fibers are present instead in subcapsular regions, in cortical layers, and in the medulla. In the chicken, such fibers are seen throughout the gland in close vicinity to both cortical and medullary cells. Species differences have been noted with respect to the distribution of oxytocin and vasopressin over epinephrine- and norepinephrine-containing cells

(227). In the cow, immunostaining is particularly prominent in cortical islands interspersed within the medullary tissue. It should be noted that expression of these peptides may be quite different in submammalian species (320).

In addition to regulatory peptides, several polypeptide growth factors have been identified in the medulla, such as bFGF (207, 243, 540), IGF-1 (221, 243), IGF-2 (221), and TGF-β1 (243). Corticostatin-1 was detected at relatively high levels in the adrenal medulla and increased markedly during acute inflammation (570).

All of these peptides and the classical biogenic amines from the medulla display specific biological effects at physiological doses when added in vitro to adrenal cortex preparations. Evidence that the endogenous peptides exert similar effects to those added to in vitro adrenal preparations and, hence, display paracrine activity has been provided as far as the renin–angiotensin system, the CRF–POMC–glucocorticoid system, and the enkephalins are concerned.

Medullary Biogenic Amines. Locally produced biogenic amines appear to influence adrenocortical function. The cathecholamines epinephrine and norepinephrine stimulate glucocorticoid and aldosterone secretions by a direct action on the cortex (55). The latter effect may be reinforced by NPY from the chromaffin cells, which increases the biosynthesis of catecholamines (246).

An intrinsic γ-aminobutyric acid (GABA)ergic system has been demonstrated in adrenal chromaffin cells (285, 286). Glutamic acid decarboxylase, GABA, and GABA aminotransferase are present in bovine adrenal chromaffin cells; GABA can be taken up and stored by chromaffin cells in culture, and release is stimulated by acetylcholine via nicotinic receptors. Noradrenaline and GABA co-exist within the same chromaffin granules (406), and GABA depolarizes chromaffin cell membranes and augments catecholamine as well as Met-enkephalin releases via GABA-A receptors (177, 285, 300, 301). However, since GABA is also present in autonomic nerve fibers, it is not clear what role it plays within the chromaffin cells.

In the frog, chromaffin cell synthesis of serotonin and a typical neuronal uptake mechanism for this indolamine have been demonstrated (110). In the pig, serotonin histofluorescence is found in norepinephrine-storing chromaffin cells (306). In the human, serotonin is found in adrenal cortex mast cells (326). Addition of serotonin to adrenal cortex in vitro potently enhances corticosterone and aldosterone secretions (12, 326). Dopamine inhibits basal and angiotensin II–induced glucocorticoid secretion in the frog adrenal in vitro

but has no effect on ACTH-induced glucocorticoid secretion (382). The effect of serotonin is potentiated by VIP (319).

A Local Corticotrophin-Releasing Factor–Adrenocorticotrophic Hormone–Glucocorticoid System. Cells containing CRF have a characteristic appearance and are often found at the boundary between the medulla and the cortex (63) and in close association with blood vessels within the adrenal medulla (63, 64). This factor is released from the adrenal medulla upon splanchnic nerve stimulation in the calf (130) and during hemorrhage in the dog (64). The peptide has been reported to stimulate corticosterone secretion from rat adrenal slices, including both the cortex and medulla, but not in adrenal fragments deprived of chromaffin tissue (17). The latter findings suggest that an intermediary compound exists which mediates the effect of CRF. The effect of CRF is completely blocked by corticotrophin-inhibiting peptide, a competitive antagonist of ACTH-stimulated corticosterone secretion, whereas adrenal fragments mainly composed of chromaffin tissue released detectable amounts of ACTH in response to CRF, clearly suggesting that CRF stimulates the adrenal medulla to release ACTH, which in turn stimulates glucocorticoid secretion from the cortex in a paracrine manner. That ACTH is released from the adrenal medulla is in keeping with the findings of others that the POMC gene is expressed in adrenal chromaffin cells (273). Peptides derived from POMC are released upon splanchnic nerve stimulation, resulting in an increased glucocorticoid secretion (273). Thus, the adrenal contains an intrinsic CRF–ACTH–glucocorticoid axis, operating in a paracrine manner. Importantly, a negative feedback may be exerted by ACTH as it decreases CRF secretion induced by splanchnic nerve stimulation (130). In addition, N-terminal fragments of POMC appear to modulate adrenocortical function. Human POMC1–76 and γ3-MSH (POMC51–76) stimulate aldosterone secretion from cultured human aldosteronoma cells (497), stimulate corticosteroid secretion in cultured ovine adrenal cells (128), and potentiate the adrenal steroidogenic effect of ACTH in the rat and human (128). In the rat, POMC1–36 has a mitogenic effect on cortical cells (146). It should be noted, however, that the potentiating effect of N-terminal POMC-derived peptides on the steroidogenic effect of ACTH is not a general phenomenon in mammals (77).

Opioid Peptides. Adrenal medullary opioid peptides may modulate catecholamine secretion from the medulla. Intraadrenal application of Met-enkephalin (via a microdialysis system) reduces acetylcholine-stimulated epinephrine, but not norepinephrine, secretion in the rat, whereas the opioid antagonist naloxone prolongs the epinephrine response to acetylcholine, suggesting that endogenous Met-enkephalin dampens the release of epinephrine in response to splanchnic nerve activation (270). Proenkephalin A mRNA expression is increased by agents enhancing intracellular cyclic adenosine monophosphate (cAMP) levels (135, 442), such as VIP (135, 600), and by acetylcholine, which is released from splanchnic nerve terminals in the medulla (134). There appears to exist a reciprocal regulatory interaction between medullary enkephalins and cortical steroids. On the one hand, the decrease in catecholamine secretion by enkephalins may result in a decrease in glucocorticoid secretion since catecholamines stimulate adrenal corticosteroid secretion. Met-enkephalin also may inhibit steroid production directly as shown by its inhibitory action in aldosterone-producing human adenomas (444). On the other hand, proenkephalin A mRNA expression is increased by exogenous as well as endogenous glucocorticoid (133, 267). Expression of enkephalins is considerably higher during embryonic and early postnatal life in the rat, and the embryonic rise in the proportion of Leu-enkephalin-containing cells correlates with the developmental increase in glucocorticoid production (229).

Galanin. Galanin causes a significant rise in plasma corticosterone levels in hypophysectomized rats and increases both basal and ACTH-stimulated corticosterone production by adrenal quarters and isolated zonae fasciculata/reticularis cells (362). It increases the plasma level of aldosterone in hypophysectomized rats. Remarkably, galanin releases aldosterone from adrenal quarters but not from isolated zona glomerulosa cells, indicating that this action requires the structural integrity of the adrenal or that galanin may affect the release of some medullary peptides, which in turn stimulate aldosterone secretion of the zona glomerulosa in a paracrine manner (362).

Vasopressin. The presence of specific vasopressin-binding sites in zona glomerulosa and zona fasciculata of the human adrenal cortex and the demonstration that the peptide is released from the medulla suggest a local action (212). In glomerulosa cell–enriched primary cultures, vasopressin increases aldosterone secretion as potently as angiotensin-II, whereas in zona fasciculata cell–enriched cultures, it increases cortisol production (212, 418).

Natriuretic Peptides. A paracrine action of ANP is suggested in both the adrenal medulla and cortex as ANP receptor A mRNA is abundantly expressed in the zona glomerulosa, whereas ANP receptor B mRNA is confined to the chromaffin cells (610). Possibly, BNP plays a role in water and electrolyte homeostasis as the peptide is expressed at higher levels in patients with primary hyperaldosteronism (325).

Endothelin. Administration of endothelin causes a decrease in vascular perfusion, whereas the peptide is rapidly released in response to both mechanically increased flow rates through the gland and the increase in flow rate caused by ACTH (67). The finding of binding sites for porcine [^{125}I]endothelin-1 in adrenal zona glomerulosa cells of humans, pigs, and rats suggests a function of the peptide in mineralocorticoid secretion (105).

Trophic Factors. The adrenal medulla is also thought to have a trophic influence on the cortex, particularly on the zona glomerulosa. Some evidence for this stems from the observation that rat adrenals transplanted in the musculus gracilis regenerate cortical tissue but totally lack chromaffin tissue (42). Whereas these regenerated nodules display normal glucocorticoid responses, they show a relative impairment in aldosterone secretion, and this is consistent with the finding of only a few zona glomerulosa-like cells (42). Which of the growth factors present in the medulla are involved in this trophic action remains unknown. Vasopressin stimulates mitotic activity in adrenal zona glomerulosa cells in intact or hypophysectomized rats as well as in glomerulosa cells in culture (418). This peptide, therefore, may exert a trophic action on the cortex.

Putative Paracrine and Autocrine Factors in the Adrenal Cortex

Regulatory peptides and, most notably, polypeptide growth factors or cytokines have been localized in the adrenal cortex. They include the renin–angiotensin system in the zona glomerulosa (152, 620), oxytocin and vasopressin in the zonae glomerulosa and fasciculata (227), bFGF in the three zones (35, 207), IGFs in the zona fasciculata (221, 269, 429, 574), TGF-α (491), activin and inhibin (364, 535, 598), TGF-βs in the three zones (291, 427), and the cytokines interleukin (IL)-1 and IL-6 in the zonae reticularis and glomerulosa (201, 202, 279). Several of these substances also are expressed in the medulla, raising questions about the site of origin of the substances acting upon the adrenal cortex.

Renin–Angiotensin System. The adrenal cortex of various mammalian species, including the human, contains a functional renin–angiotensin system (152, 620). Angiotensin II is released together with renin and aldosterone in perifused adrenal slices; angiotensin-converting enzyme inhibitors decrease the secreted amounts of angiotensin II and aldosterone, which is consistent with a paracrine stimulatory action of angiotensin II on aldosterone secretion from zona glomerulosa cells (152). Stimulation of aldosterone secretion by ACTH and K^+ in rat adrenal cell cultures is associated with an increase in renin activity and secretion (620). The effect of ACTH and K^+ appears to be mediated by angiotensin II as addition of an angiotensin-converting enzyme inhibitor attenuates the effect on aldosterone secretion (620). Angiotensin-stimulated aldosterone secretion is inhibited by somatostatin (320).

Polypeptide Growth Factors. Basic FGF has been localized immunocytochemically in cells of the zonae glomerulosa, fasciculata, and reticularis, and an obvious temporal and spatial distribution among the different cortical zones which closely correlates with developmental changes in the rate of mitosis in these different zones has been observed during postnatal development in the rat (35, 207). These observations strengthen the hypothetical role of bFGF as an autocrine growth factor for adrenocortical cells. Bovine adrenal cortex cells contain, but under normal conditions do not release, bFGF (503), as is the case in other tissues. It has been proposed that bFGF is released upon injury of the adrenal cortex and that it subserves a role in subsequent tissue-repair mechanisms (165). However, some evidence for an intracrine action has been found in other tissues (see above) but remains to be studied in the adrenal. It appears that bFGF is the most potent mitogen for primary cultures of adult adrenocortical cells (162).

In the sheep, bovine, and rat, IGF-1 mRNA and protein have been detected in the zona fasciculata but not in the zona glomerulosa (221, 269, 429, 574). As tested in bovine adrenal fasciculata cells in culture, IGF-1 seems to be required for the maintenance of differentiated functions, such as angiotensin II receptor expression, the cAMP response to ACTH, and the steroidogenic response to ACTH and angiotensin II (428, 429). Further, tissue levels of both IGF-1 and -2 rise during compensatory adrenal growth after unilateral adrenalectomy in the rat (269), supporting a paracrine trophic and growth-regulating role. In the rat, IGF-2 mRNA has been detected in the zonae glomerulosa and fasciculata and in the adrenal capsule (221). The trophic action of ACTH on the adrenal cortex may be mediated at least in part by the IGFs: both ACTH and sodium restriction activate IGF-1 gene expression in the zona glomerulosa; ACTH increases the level of adrenal IGF-2 mRNA (599), and ACTH as well as angiotensin II (429, 430) stimulate basal secretion of IGF-1. Angiotensin II and ACTH also dramatically increase the number of cells immunoreactive to IGF-1 in bovine adrenal cortex cultures (429).

In normal and neoplastic human adrenal cortex, TGF-α, but not EGF, has been detected at both protein and mRNA levels (491). These factors stimulate growth of cultured cortical cells (162) and corticosteroid production (520), in clear contrast to their inhibitory action on testicular, ovarian, and thyroid hormone secretions (171). Since EGF receptors have been observed by autoradiography only on adrenal medulla and capsule (81), it may be that the trophic action of EGF and TGF-α on cortical cells is mediated by medullary cells.

All three activin and inhibin subunit proteins (α, βA, and βB) have been detected in the rat and human fetal and adult adrenal cortex (364, 535, 598). There appears to exist a positive interaction between ACTH and activin on adrenal glucocorticoid secretion in the fetal adrenal. Activin-A enhances ACTH-stimulated cortisol secretion by cultured human fetal zone cells but not by the definitive zone or adult adrenal cortex cells. Inhibin-A, on the contrary, has no such effect (535). However, ACTH stimulates the expression of α- and βA-subunit mRNA in the fetal adrenal and enhances immunoreactive α-subunit secretion by fetal and adult human adrenal cells (535, 598). In human fetal adrenal cells in vitro, activin-A (βA/βA homodimer) inhibits EGF-stimulated fetal zone cell proliferation but not bFGF-stimulated growth (534).

As far as the the *TGF-β* family is concerned, TGF-β2 is expressed specifically in the adrenal cortex of fetal mice (427), whereas TGF-β1-like material is found in the cortex of adult bovine adrenal glands. Immunoreactivity is strong in the zonae fasciculata and reticularis and weaker in the zona glomerulosa (291). Also, TGF-β1 inhibits angiotensin II–stimulated cortisol production (291). In collagenase-dispersed bovine zona glomerulosa cells, TGF-β1 is a potent inhibitor of basal and ACTH-stimulated aldosterone production but enhances the level and release of active renin (213). Also, TGF-β1 has been shown to inhibit ACTH- and angiotensin II–stimulated cortisol production (291, 431). The mechanism of this negative effect of TGF-β1 has been studied in some detail in the bovine adrenal (431). It was found that adrenocortical 17α-hydroxylase activity, a key enzyme in the biosynthetic pathway of corticosteroids, and the cellular content of

17α-hydroxylase mRNA decrease within a few hours after treatment. In addition, TGF-β1 inhibits the induction of the steroidogenic cytochrome P-450(17)α by ACTH but not the induction of P-450scc, another steroidogenic cytochrome.

LOCAL CONTROL IN THE TESTIS

There are three tissue compartments within the testis: the seminiferous tubules, the interstitium, and the vasculature. Interstitial tissue consists of Leydig cells, macrophages, lymphocytes, plasma cells, mast cells, and fibroblasts. Seminiferous tubules consist of peritubular myoid cells, Sertoli cells, and germ cells in various stages of the spermatogenic cycle. Peritubular myoid cells touch each other and are joined by tight junctions, as are Sertoli cells, which creates the blood–testis barrier to the germ cells. Peritubular myoid cells have contractile elements responsible for the contractility of the seminiferous tubules. The site of testosterone production is the Leydig cell. In the immature testis, the main site of estrogen production is the Sertoli cell, but after puberty estrogens are synthesized primarily from androgen in the Leydig cells. The protagonist hormones acting on the testis are FSH and LH. Receptors for the former are expressed on Sertoli cells and for the latter on Leydig cells.

Evidence for Functional Interaction Between Different Testicular Cell Types

There is overwhelming documentation that the three compartments within the testis functionally interact with each other in a complex manner. Interactions have been described between Sertoli cells and Leydig cells, between Sertoli cells and germ cells, between Sertoli cells and peritubular myoid cells, and within the testicular vasculature. However, it is important to realize that local regulation acts in concert with LH and FSH. It is dependent on the presence of these pituitary hormones and results in either an amplification or an inhibition or a transfer of gonadotrophic action on one of the testicular compartments. Furthermore, interactions exist within compartments to control the complex and orderly sequence of events in the spermatogenic cycle (507). Some local interactions are shown in Figure 18.3.

Paracrine Actions of Sertoli Cells on Leydig Cells. It is well known (reviewed in ref. 476) that purified

preparations of FSH not only stimulate seminiferous tubule growth but also cause Leydig cell hyperplasia, augment the number of receptors on Leydig cells, and enhance LH-induced testosterone production. Since FSH receptors are localized exclusively in seminiferous tubules on Sertoli cells and since LH-free recombinant FSH, which unlike purified FSH preparations is not contaminated by traces of LH, elicits similar effects on Leydig cells as purified FSH (321), the effects of FSH on Leydig cells must be mediated by a substance(s) released from the Sertoli cells or other tubular elements. It is well documented that seminiferous tubule elements affect Leydig cell function. This is already evident at the morphological level. The size of peritubular Leydig cells varies with the type of tubules the cells surround. Leydig cells surrounding tubules in stages VII–VIII of the spermatogenic cycle are larger than perivascular Leydig cells (44). This stage-dependent variation in Leydig cell size becomes evident at the onset of puberty (45).

A factor that activates testosterone production in Leydig cells has been demonstrated in spent medium from seminiferous tubules (348). Neither purified nor other substances present in a crude preparation of spent medium of cultured peritubular cells has any effect on basal or gonadotrophin-stimulated testosterone production by Leydig cells (456). In contrast, spent medium from rat Sertoli cell–enriched cultures contains a factor that acutely stimulates the production of testosterone by human interstitial cells and by purified rat and mouse Leydig cells (477, 587, 588). Secretion of the active principle is stimulated by FSH (588). Medium collected from cultures of a Sertoli cell tumor also stimulates testosterone secretion in cultured human testicular cells (460). Homologous or heterologous Sertoli cells when co-cultured with pig Leydig cells enhance luteinizing hormone receptor numbers and responsiveness to LH and cause Leydig cell hypertrophy (477). The identities of the steroidogenic factor and the trophic factors of Sertoli cells remain unknown. Several substances have been partially purified, with molecular weights of 10–80 kd.

Paracrine Actions of Peritubular Cells on Sertoli Cells.
There is compelling evidence for interactions between testicular peritubular cells and Sertoli cells. Peritubular cells appear to secrete a protein, modulating Sertoli cells (P-Mod-S), which modulates the functions of Sertoli cells (526). This protein has an apparent molecular weight of 70 kd. It stimulates certain functional parameters of Sertoli cells such as transferrin and androgen-binding protein production, but not plasminogen activator activity, indicating the specificity of its action.

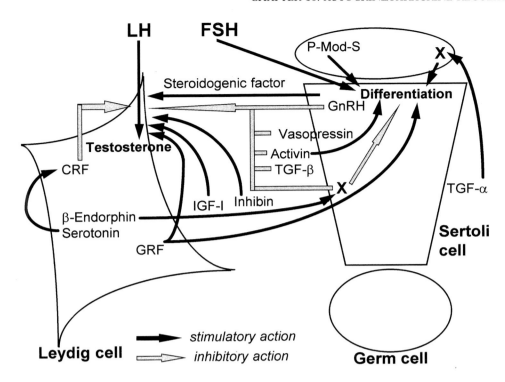

FIG. 18.3 Effect of various paracrine and autocrine factors on hormone secretion and cellular differentiation in various testicular compartments. *LH*, luteinizing hormone; *FSH*, follicle-stimulating hormone; *GnRH*, gonadotrophin-releasing hormone; *TGF-β*, transforming growth factor-β; *CRF*, corticotrophin-releasing factor; *GRF*, growth hormone–releasing factor; *IGF*, insulin-like growth factor.

Most importantly, the magnitude of this action is much larger than that of any other substance known to influence this cell type (FSH, insulin, retinol, and testosterone). Also, P-Mod-S induces the synthesis of several proteins, one of which is an epididymal lactalbumin-like protein (526). It has been purified and appears to consist of two forms, a less hydrophobic 56 kd form (P-Mod-S A) and a more hydrophobic 59 kd form (P-Mod-S B) (525). Developmental studies have shown that FSH facilitates the action of P-Mod-S on Sertoli cells (in terms of induction of transferrin) obtained from 10-day-old rats but not on Sertoli cells from rats older than 35 days (25); however, P-Mod-S remains effective on its own at these later ages, suggesting that it acts together with FSH on Sertoli cell differentiation in the immature testis but that it is sufficient to maintain Sertoli cell function and differentiation in the adult testis. This protein does not use cyclic nucleotides (AMP or GMP), calcium, or inositol phosphates as a signal-transduction pathway (396).

Spent media from peritubular cell cultures also inhibit FSH-inducible aromatase activity in Sertoli cells (550). Similar active principles present in peritubular cell-conditioned media are released by stromal mesenchymal cells from the prostate but not from skin fibroblasts (550). Since peritubular cells are androgen-regulated (26), these findings emphasize the importance of mesenchymal–epithelial cell interactions in endocrine regulation by androgen. Sertoli cells and peritubular myoid cells act in concert in terms of synthesis of the extracellular matrix (448).

Paracrine Interactions Between Sertoli Cells, Peritubular Cells, and Germ Cells.

Sertoli cells exert a trophic action on peritubular myoid cells. Co-culturing peritubular myoid cells with Sertoli cells induces a significant increase in [³H]-thymidine incorporation by peritubular myoid cells, an effect mimicked by secreted factors (449).

Sertoli cells, probably through both a diffusible factor and cell-to-cell contacts, control the multiplication, meiotic reduction, and maturation of germ cells (206). There is evidence that the endocrine regulation of spermatogenesis by FSH and testosterone is mediated through actions on Sertoli cells (206). Indeed, meiotic and postmeiotic germ cells are sequestered in a luminal compartment that is isolated from the serum or lymph by tight junctional complexes between Sertoli cells and, thus, cannot be affected directly by blood-borne FSH. In turn, the activity of Sertoli cells is modulated by the maturational stage of neighboring germ cells. Pachytene spermatocytes and early spermatids secrete a protein stimulating androgen-binding protein and inhibiting estradiol production in the presence of FSH in Sertoli cells (329).

Local Control by Steroids

It is well known that testosterone plays a central role in spermatogenesis. Selective destruction of all Leydig cells in the adult rat testis by ethane dimethane sulfonate causes severe damage to the seminiferous tubule (510). Substitution therapy with testosterone shows that the latter hormone but not the other components of Leydig cells, is the central factor in creating the exact microenvironment for proper spermatogenesis. However, the actions of testosterone are mediated by factors produced by the Sertoli and/or peritubular cells (510). In addition, testosterone is involved in the formation of testicular interstitial fluid, presumably again via the Sertoli and/or peritubular cells.

Local Control by Regulatory Peptides

Different families of regulatory peptides, originally discovered in the brain and other tissues, have been identified in testicular compartments: vasopressin and oxytocin (4, 23, 268, 284, 439, 508, 609); the renin–angiotensin system (403); POMC-derived peptides (87, 294, 333, 351, 353, 514); proenkephalin A–derived peptides (93, 143, 293, 299, 481, 553); prodynorphin-derived peptides (124, 352); the hypothalamic releasing hormones GnRH (46, 259, 480, 508), GRF (92, 148, 432), TRH (163), and CRF (29, 127, 151, 579); GRP (157, 200); ANP (414, 597); NPY (605); endothelin-1 (154, 167); substance P (24, 91); and pituitary adenyl cyclase–activating polypeptide (PACAP) (513). Several of these peptides appear to lack any effect on their own but strongly modulate the action of gonadotrophins on Leydig or Sertoli cells. Depending on the peptide concerned, potentiation or inhibition of gonadotrophin-stimulated testosterone secretion and trophic actions are seen.

Vasopressin and Oxytocin. In testicular extracts, a substance has been identified which behaves in an identical fashion to AVP in radioimmunoassay, radioreceptor assay, and various types of chromatography (284). The peptide is most likely produced by Leydig cells as AVP/neurophysin mRNA has been detected in purified mouse Leydig cells and in rat and mouse Leydig tumor cell lines (268). Neurophysin II and AVP immunoreactivities are also present in Sertoli cells (168). As to its putative intratesticular role, AVP has been reported to stimulate testosterone production but to inhibit human chorionic gonadotrophin (hCG)–stimulated testosterone accumulation (4, 508). These effects are most likely exerted directly on Leydig cells since specific AVP receptors have been identified in purified Leydig cell preparations and on in situ Leydig cells (37, 439). Rat testicular myoid cells also express vasopressin receptors (254). The vasopressin effects are similar to those exerted by GnRH. Another possible role of AVP is regulation of blood flow. Intratesticular injection of AVP causes a decrease in total testicular blood flow (609).

Oxytocin/neurophysin is expressed in Sertoli cells (23) and Leydig cells (392). In cultured rat Leydig cells, oxytocin increases basal testosterone production through a specific oxytocin receptor but, in contrast to AVP, has no effect on LH-stimulated testosterone production (173).

Opioid Peptides. In acid extracts of rat testes, α-, β-, and γ-endorphin immunoreactivities have been detected (353). A POMC mRNA species has been identified in mouse testis, epididymis, and Leydig cell lines. The mRNA, however, is truncated, being approximately 150 bases shorter than in the pituitary or hypothalamus (87). In situ hybridization has shown expression in Leydig cells and interstitial testicular macrophages (333). Leydig cells, but not Sertoli cells or myoid peritubular cells, of many species synthesize and secrete the opioid peptide β-endorphin (149, 352, 514). However, opioid peptide receptors appear to be located on Sertoli cells (149, 352). Secretion of β-endorphin is simulated strongly by hCG (149). Intratesticular injections of β-endorphin significantly decreases the LH-stimulation of testosterone production in various test systems using the rat (84). Both in vivo and in vitro experiments using naloxone to block endogenous opioid peptide action have shown that these peptides inhibit testosterone production (93). The latter effect is not direct and is presumably mediated by the Sertoli cells since β-endorphin does not affect testosterone production by purified Leydig cells, which is consistent with the absence of opioid receptors on these cells but their presence on Sertoli cells (149). Importantly, the effect of β-endorphin on testosterone production occurs only in the presence of LH (93). Also, β-endorphin treatment of Sertoli cells significantly inhibits basal and FSH-stimulated androgen-binding protein production (149). β-Endorphin also inhibits sperm motility via an effect on Sertoli cells (150). Experiments using intratesticular injection of naloxone suggest that endogenous opioids modulate the testicular AVP system by depressing AVP receptor numbers (553).

Opioid peptides derived from POMC exert trophic actions. That β-endorphin may inhibit Sertoli cell proliferation in a paracrine way is indicated by the finding that injection of β-endorphin antiserum directly into the testes of newborn rats dramatically increases the number of Sertoli cells labeled with [^{3}H]-thymidine, whereas in rat fetal testes in organ culture naloxone enhances the FSH-induced rise in Sertoli cell proliferation (408).

Hypothalamic Releasing Factor–Like Peptides.
A GnRH-like substance has been identified in the testis (259), more precisely in Sertoli cells (480). Receptors for GnRH are present on Leydig cells but not on Sertoli cells. Treatment of cultured rat Leydig cells with GnRH as well as intratesticular injection of the peptide in vivo stimulates androgen production under basal conditions but inhibits gonadotrophin-stimulated testosterone production (259, 508), an effect similar to that seen with AVP.

A GRF-like substance has been detected by radioimmunoassay in rat testis, as has a GRF mRNA species which is considerably larger than hypothalamic GRF mRNA (46). Immunoreactivity of GRF, which is indistinguishable from authentic rat GRF by chromatographic analysis, as well as GRF receptors have been located in Leydig cells (92), in the acrosomal region of early and intermediate spermatids at stages III–VI (148, 539), and to a lesser extent in Sertoli cells but not in elongating spermatids or peritubular myoid cells (539). Release of GRF from Leydig cells is stimulated by hCG. It does not affect basal testosterone production but behaves as a potentiator of the acute gonadotrophin stimulation of testosterone production. Thus, LH releases GRF, which in turn amplifies the action of LH on steroidogenesis. Also, GRF stimulates the production of specific Sertoli cell products and potentiates FSH-stimulated cAMP formation in Sertoli cells (148, 538).

Authentic ovine CRF has been identified by direct amino-acid sequencing in extracts of ovine testis and localized in the Leydig cells by immunocytochemistry (29). Cultured rat Leydig cells secrete relatively high amounts of CRF, and secretion is enhanced rapidly by hCG (151). In addition to its well-known antireproductive action at the hypothalamic level (inhibition of sexual behavior and LH secretion), CRF appears to have such a function also by a direct autocrine action in the testis. Rat Leydig cells express high-affinity receptors for CRF. This peptide has no effect on basal testosterone secretion but clearly inhibits hCG-induced androgen production in cultured Leydig cells (579). Incubation of cultured rat Leydig cells with a CRF antagonist results in a rise of basal testosterone production and in an increased response of testosterone production to hCG (151). Another antireproductive action of CRF is the stimulation of β-endorphin release from Leydig cells (127, 145). Enhanced secretion of β-endorphin in turn inhibits FSH actions on Sertoli cells and LH actions on Leydig cells. In the neonatal rat, endogenous CRF seems to act in an autocrine/paracrine manner to stimulate testosterone production, as indicated by the finding that unilateral testicular injection of anti-CRF antiserum results in a significant fall in serum testosterone levels (195).

A prepro-TRH mRNA species considerably larger than that in the hypothalamus as well as TRH immunoreactivity have been detected in rat Leydig cells (163).

Peptides Related to Germ Cell Development and Spermatogenesis.
Several peptides may have some role in the development of germ cells and spermatogenesis in the testis. The proenkephalin-A gene is expressed as a 1700–nucleotide transcript, unique to the testis, in spermatogenic cells of humans, hamsters, rats, mice, and sheep (294), more precisely in pachytene spermatocytes and round spermatids (299). Sertoli cells contain a 1450-nucleotide transcript (293). Proenkephalin-derived peptides have been located in the acrosome and are released during the acrosome reaction, an event required for fertilization (294). High levels of expression of proenkephalin-A in the testis have been achieved in transgenic mice, using a very short promoter region in the transgene construct; these mice display grossly abnormal testicular morphology and a reduced to completely abolished fertility (399).

Leydig cells contain immunoreactive material displaying the features of authentic GRP-like peptides (200). The peptide may have a hitherto undefined function on spermatocyte maturation as a third subtype of bombesin receptor has been discovered which is expressed uniquely in secondary spermatocytes (157).

In mouse and rat testis, ANP mRNA and an ANP peptide corresponding to the 15 kd ANP precursor and a processed 31-residue peptide have been detected (414, 597). Peptide immunoreactivity is localized in the spermatids and elongating spermatozoa (414).

In human testis, NPY-immunoreactive material has

been found in spermatogonia and in primary spermatocytes but not in Sertoli or Leydig cells (605).

In developing germ cells, spermatogonia, and primary spermatocytes, but not in mature spermatids and spermatozoa, PACAP immunoreactivity and mRNA have been detected. They are not found in Sertoli or Leydig cells (513).

Other Peptides. Another POMC-derived peptide found in the testis is α-MSH. This peptide stimulates aromatase activity in rat Sertoli cell–enriched cultures (52). A substance with the characteristics of endothelin-1 has been identified in spent rat Sertoli cell culture medium but not in conditioned medium from rat Leydig cells (154). In immature rats, immunoreactive endothelin-1 is confined to some Sertoli cells, whereas in adult rats it is also found in interstitial cells; binding sites are found on Leydig cells (154) and on myoid cells (167). The tachykinin substance P has been detected by immunocytochemistry in hamster, mouse, and human Leydig cells (24). Preprotachykinin-A (substance P) mRNA has been found in extracts of human, mouse, and bovine testis (91). A putative intratesticular role is plausible based on the finding of specific receptor mRNA (91). Renin and angiotensin II, as well as angiotensin II receptors, have been identified in Leydig cells (117, 298, 403). Angiotensin II inhibits basal and LH-stimulated testosterone production (298).

Local Control by Biogenic Amines and Nitrous Oxide

Leydig cells produce biogenic amines. Adult Leydig cells secrete considerable amounts of serotonin, which is stimulated acutely by hCG (567). Serotonin stimulates the secretion of CRF (through 5HT2 receptors), which in turn inhibits gonadotrophin-induced androgen production (567).

In the rat testis (458), GABA reaches its highest levels just before the onset of puberty (459). It stimulates or inhibits basal and hCG-stimulated testosterone secretion in vitro, depending on the developmental stage of the testis (459).

Human Leydig cells, as well as MA-10 and TM3 mouse Leydig cells, display immunoreactivity for the brain isoform of NOS synthase (106), implying the putative role of nitrous oxide in the regulation of Leydig cells or in the interaction of the latter with other testicular cells.

Local Control by Polypeptide Growth Factors

Insulin-Like Growth Factors. The cellular distribution of IGF-1-like immunoreactivity in rat testis depends on the age of the animal. During the first 2 weeks after birth, it is found in Sertoli cells, Leydig cells, and spermatogenic cells, whereas in adult rats, it is found only in spermatogenic cells (223), suggesting participation in the differentiation, but not the initiation, of cellular proliferation during spermatogenesis. In a test system consisting of 2 mm segments of seminiferous tubules of adult rat testis in culture, addition of IGF-1 stimulates [^{3}H]-thymidine incorporation in DNA of types A4 and B spermatogonia (531). However, most of the IGF-1 mRNA has been localized in Leydig cells in the rat testis (335). Expression of IGF-1, but not IGF-2, mRNA is stimulated by LH, FSH, and GH and inhibited by PRL treatment (95). As demonstrated by co-culture experiments, Leydig and Sertoli cells cooperate in IGF-1 production in response to luteinizing hormone and FSH, respectively (390). Addition of IGF-1 or IGF-2 to cultured rat interstitial cells increases hCG-stimulated testosterone production (111). This effect requires an additional cell–cell communication mechanism as it is seen only at relatively high cell density. Conversely, addition of an anti-IGF-1 antiserum to cultured Leydig cells from immature rats decreases testosterone production capacity (589). Taken together, these data firmly support a trophic paracrine or autocrine role of IGF-1 on Leydig cells.

Basic Fibroblast Growth Factor. Basic FGF protein and mRNA have been demonstrated in Leydig cells, Sertoli cells, and peritubular cells in amounts decreasing with sexual maturity (384). FSH increases expression in Sertoli cells (384). Basic FGF alone does not affect androgen biosynthesis in cultured testicular cells from neonatal rats but significantly decreases LH-stimulated testosterone production in a time-dependent manner (158). Also, bFGF inhibits forskolin and dibutyryl-cAMP-stimulated testosterone production, indicating an effect distal to the LH receptor. Furthermore, bFGF inhibits the conversion of exogenously added progesterone to testosterone in LH-stimulated cultures, indicating that it acts through inhibition of 17α-hydroxylase (158). However, conflicting results have been reported as to the long-term effects of bFGF on testosterone production (476). Better insight into the exact role of bFGF requires further study.

Members of the Epidermal Growth Factor Family. Spent medium of cultures of Sertoli and peritubular myoid cells of developing rat testis contains material competing with labeled EGF in an EGF radioreceptor assay; this material has been identified as TGF-α both immunologically and on the basis of the presence of a TGF-α mRNA transcript in both peritubular and Sertoli cells (528). Immunoreactivity of EGF has been shown in Sertoli cells, pachytene spermatocytes, and round spermatids (445). The target cells of TGF-α are the peritubular cells as high-affinity EGF receptors have been detected on peritubular cells and not or at very low levels on Sertoli and germ cells (385, 528). Transferrin production in Sertoli cells is stimulated by TGF-α, not by a direct action but through the peritubular cells (528). Also, TGF-α stimulates peritubular cellular proliferation and migration (385, 528). The developmental role of TGF-α is further indicated by the fact that the genes for TGF-α and its receptor are expressed predominantly during early testis development and decrease during puberty (385). The level of expression is correlated with certain stages of spermatogenesis (34). In interstitial cells not expressing LH receptors, EGF increases testosterone production (377). In transgenic mice overexpressing TGF-α in the testis, testicular morphology and spermatogenesis are normal (385).

Inhibin and Activin.

Inhibin/activin subunits have been located in Sertoli and Leydig cells in both human and non-human primates (586, 596). High levels of βA-subunit mRNA and some inhibin α-subunit mRNA and βB-subunit mRNA are expressed in cultured rat peritubular myoid cells (118). A polyclonal antiserum against recombinant activin-A has demonstrated the presence of 25 kd activin-A in the medium of cultured rat peritubular myoid cells (108). LH and FSH stimulate biosynthesis of inhibin in Sertoli cells (257, 509). The effect of luteinizing hormone appears to be mediated by testosterone and other Leydig cell factors (509). In primary testicular cell cultures, inhibin enhances androgen biosynthesis stimulated by LH in Leydig cells, whereas activin suppresses androgen production (257). No effect is seen on basal testosterone biosynthesis. As shown in immature testis of rats and primates, Sertoli cells secrete inhibin predominantly from the apical surface of the cell toward the lumen of the seminiferous tubule, suggesting that inhibin has an important paracrine role in spermatogenesis (222). This is supported by the finding that expression of inhibin subunits decreases during sexual maturation (364) but that it is critically up- and down-regulated in relation to spermatogenesis. The highest levels of both α- and βB-subunit mRNAs are seen in stages XIII–I and the lowest in stages VII–VIII of spermatogenesis (48). Inhibin α-subunit mRNA expression is relatively high at stages V and XIII of the spermatogenic cycle, whereas βB-subunit mRNA expression is high at stage XIII but not at stage V, resulting in a high βB/α-subunit mRNA ratio at stage XIII (303). However, as studied in the rat, receptors for [^{125}I]-inhibin co-localize with androgen-producing interstitial cells, whereas [^{125}I]-activin binding is seen on cells in the basal compartment of the

seminiferous tubules and, in 45- and 60-day-old animals, on spermatids in stage VII–VIII tubules (312). Since expression of the activin receptor is high at stages XIII–I, locally formed activin might play a role in the regulation of meiosis (303). In co-cultures of Sertoli and germ cells isolated from immature rats, activins A and B, but not inhibin-A, stimulate proliferation of spermatogonia. Proliferating germ cells, visualized by [^{3}H]Thymidine labeling, localize in clusters adhering to the Sertoli cell monolayer and activin causes reaggregation of the cultures into tubule-like structures (358). Activin-A, secreted by peritubular cells, stimulates both basal and FSH-stimulated inhibin and transferrin production by Sertoli cells in culture. These effects resemble the effects of P-Mod-S on Sertoli cells (118).

Transforming Growth Factor-β.

Germ cells, peritubular cells, and Sertoli cells in the rat express a TGF-β1, -β2, and -β3 mRNA species and protein (386, 527, 559). These factors function primarily during testicular development and spermatogenesis. Strongly staining immunoreactive material is found in Sertoli cells at mid-gestation, becoming weak in late fetal age (192). Intense staining is found in late fetal Leydig cells, whereas adult-type Leydig cells display weak or no staining (559). Expression TGF-β1 and -β3 in Sertoli cells increases during pubertal development; TGF-β2 mRNA is seen only in immature Sertoli cells (386). The fall of TGF-β expression from puberty onward is most probably induced by the pubertal rise in FSH; indeed, FSH treatment causes a dramatic decrease in Sertoli cell TGF-β2 (386). The β1 form inhibits TGF-α-induced [^{3}H]thymidine incorporation into peritubular cell DNA but has no effect on Sertoli cell proliferation (386). Also, TGF-β1 induces changes in shape and increases contractility of peritubular cells in culture (7) and has been reported to enhance proteoglycan production in Sertoli cells of immature rat testis (415). The predominance of TGF-β1 expression and action during early development is consistent with the finding that TGF-β1 mRNA and mRNA for type I and type II TGF-β receptors is essentially limited to the immature testis (330). Expression of TGF-β1 is high in spermatocytes and early round spermatids but decreases as the spermatids elongate (stages VIII–IX); TGF-β2 comes to expression around stages V–VI, and expression is maintained as the spermatids elongate (559).

Neurotrophins.

Nerve growth factor and its corresponding receptors have been implicated in the regulation of spermatogenesis (123). Both the p75 and the *trk* receptors are present, with maximal expression in 10- and 20-day-old rats. The p75 receptor is detected in membranes of Sertoli cells and peritubular myoid cells (123). In rat Sertoli cells, NGF stimulates expression of androgen-binding protein (340).

Local Control by Substances From Testicular Macrophages

Macrophages are an important constituent of the testicular interstitial cell compartment. Their number increases gradually during prepubertal development to reach 15%–20% of the interstitial compartment in the adult rat. These macrophages are in close morphological association with Leydig cells, suggesting a paracrine interaction (295). Leydig cell testosterone production in the presence of LH (but not in its absence) is inhibited by co-culturing these cells with testicular macrophages or with conditioned medium collected from these macrophages through a factor acting distal to the LH receptor (548). This factor may be TNF-α since TNF-α, but not IL-1, has been found to inhibit testosterone production and since in the macrophage-conditioned medium a substance with specific TNF-α bioactivity which can be neutralized by anti-murine TNF-α antiserum is present (265, 548). Lipopolysaccharide (LPS) stimulates expression of TNF-α mRNA and secretion of TNF-α protein from interstitial macrophages in vitro (378, 619). The two major macrophage products, IL-1 and TNF, exert still other effects on Leydig cell function. In cultured Leydig cells from 10- and 20-day-old rats, IL-1 stimulates [^{3}H]thymidine incorporation into DNA but has no effect in cells from adult rats (295), suggesting that this cytokine plays an important role in the proliferation of Leydig cells during prepubertal development.

Also, TNF-α is expressed in mouse spermatogenic cells, more precisely in pachytene spermatocytes and round spermatids (107). Since the TNF-α receptor is expressed in Sertoli cells in the mouse (107), TNF-α may be the paracrine mediator of an as yet unidentified process in germ cell–Sertoli cell interaction. Sertoli cells also produce the cytokine IL-6 (455).

LOCAL CONTROL IN THE OVARY

The preovulatory ovary is composed of two primary tissue components, stroma, and follicles. Stroma contains mesenchymal-like interstitial and thecal cells as well as macrophages. Thecal cells surround the ovarian follicle. Granulosa cells are epithelial-like cells that form the follicle and support the developing oocyte. Thecal/interstitial cells are the specific site of androgen production in response to LH (238). Expression of the cytochrome P450c17α gene (17-hydroxylase/C17-20-

lyase) is specific to thecal/interstitial cells (530). Androgens traverse the basal lamina, enter granulosa cells, and accumulate in antral fluid. Granulosa cells use androgens derived from thecal cells as a substrate for the production of estrogen by the enzyme aromatase. Luteinizing hormone and FSH are the primary stimuli for follicular development. Luteinizing hormone initially acts on thecal/interstitial cells, and FSH acts on granulosa cells to activate their function and proliferation. At the onset of the ovulatory LH surge, proliferation of granulosa cells is inhibited, their aromatase activity (estrogen production) declines, while progesterone production increases and the cells further differentiate to form luteal granulosa cells of the corpus luteum. The latter differentiation is induced by LH, the receptor of which is expressed on granulosa cells from the large antral stage of follicular development. Whereas FSH and LH are the protagonists in ovarian function, there is a body of evidence showing that the different compartments in the ovary functionally interact and that locally produced steroids and polypeptides profoundly modulate the action of the gonadotrophins on folliculogenesis, ovulation, and corpus luteum formation, as well as on follicular atresia and corpus luteum regression. Many of these local factors are released by gonadotrophins and require the presence of the gonadotrophins to be effective. Various local interactions are shown in Figure 18.4.

Evidence for Functional Interaction Between Thecal Cells and Granulosa Cells

Direct evidence for functional interaction between thecal cells and granulosa cells has been shown in culture systems in which the two types of cell are allowed to attach to opposite sides of a collagen membrane (308). Co-culture results in marked changes in the morphology, structure, and growth of both cell types. Androstenedione production of thecal cells in the co-cultured condition increases severalfold, while progesterone formation in granulosa cells is reduced. When granulosa cells are cultured with thecal cells, FSH promotes, whereas LH suppresses, growth of granulosa cells; LH treatment augments their progesterone, but not estradiol, production (actions consistent with the in vivo action of LH on granulosa cell differentiation to corpus luteum cells). LH treatment increases androstenedione production of thecal cells when co-cultured with granulosa cells. The existence of paracrine interaction between granulosa and thecal cells is supported further by the finding that treatment of thecal/interstitial cell cultures from 21-day-old hypophysectomized female rats with conditioned medium from recombi-

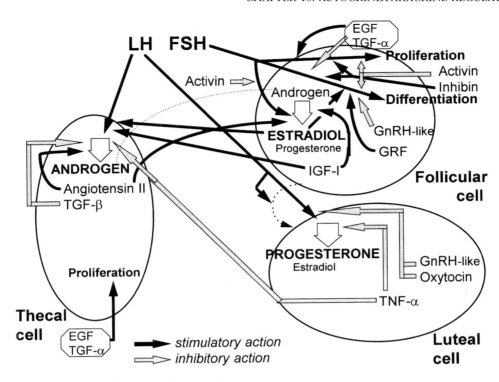

FIG. 18.4 Effect of various paracrine and autocrine factors on hormone secretion and on cellular proliferation and differentiation in various compartments of the ovary. *LH,* luteinizing hormone; *FSH,* follicle-stimulating hormone; *TGF-β,* transforming growth factor-*β;* *EGF,* epidermal growth factor; *IGF,* insulin-like growth factor; *GRF,* growth hormone–releasing factor; *GnRH,* gonadotrophin-releasing hormone; *TNF-α,* tumor necrosis factor-*α.*

nant human FSH (rhFSH)–treated granulosa cell cultures enhances LH-stimulated, but not basal androgen, production in thecal cells (530). Similar co-culture experiments have shown the existence of inhibitory factors in stromal cell–follicular cell interactions on steroidogenesis (532).

Local Control by Steroids

Ovarian steroids have important paracrine actions. Thecal cell steroidogenesis plays a major role in folliculogenesis (236, 571). During early antral stages of follicular development, granulosa cells are exposed to a high local concentration of androgens derived from thecal cells (236). Androgens augment FSH stimulation of estrogen and progesterone biosynthesis in granulosa cells. In the absence of FSH, however, they cause atresia and granulosa cell death (256). Estrogens produced in granulosa cells enhance the stimulation of aromatase activ-

ity by the gonadotrophins in these cells, resulting in a further increase in estrogen production. Moreover, high levels of estrogens are found in follicular fluid which enhance the FSH induction of LH receptors. The paracrine role of estrogens is clearly demonstrated by experiments in which rats primed with pregnant mare serum gonadotrophin (PMSG) are treated with the aromatase inhibitor CGS 16949A (fadrozole). This treatment causes a decrease in the number of healthy antral follicles and a drastic reduction in the ovulatory response to hCG (506). Furthermore, there appears to exist a local positive feedback system between granulosa and thecal cells in as far as estrogen produced by granulosa cells dramatically stimulate androgen production by thecal cells (467, 615). In contrast, estradiol inhibits both basal and LH-stimulated secretions of progesterone in cultured bovine thecal cells (615). Estradiol inhibits 3β-hydroxysteroid dehydrogenase, a key enzyme of progesterone synthesis, in porcine thecal cells (571).

Autocrine effects of progesterone in the ovary also have been described. The activity of 3β-hydroxysteroid dehydrogenase is stimulated by progesterone itself (556): the increase in activity of this enzyme at ovulation (induced by treatment of immature rats with hCG after priming with PMSG) was blocked when the progesterone antagonist RU486 was administered 2 h before hCG. As studied by histochemical staining, RU486 inhibits 3β-hydroxysteroid dehydrogenase in granulosa, but not in thecal, cells (556). In contrast, 3β-hydroxysteroid dehydrogenase in thecal cells is inhibited by progesterone (571).

Local Control by Regulatory Peptides

A variety of regulatory peptides have been identified in ovarian compartments. They belong to a broad range of different families: vasopressin and oxytocin (136, 137, 174, 296, 297, 437, 492); the renin–angiotensin system (65, 100, 328); pituitary hormones such as PRL (137) and POMC-derived peptides (341, 490); the hypothalamic releasing hormones GnRH (28, 41, 94, 144, 400, 472), GRF (33, 381); and CRF (356, 357); GRP (199); proenkephalin A–derived peptides (474); prodynorphin-derived peptides (124); ANP (214); parathyroid hormone–related protein (215); endothelin-1 (314); and galanin (172).

Evidence of local synthesis of these peptides is based on their high tissue concentration and levels in ovarian vein compared to their concentration in the general circulation, immunodetection of material eluting from high-performance liquid chromatographic (HPLC) columns with the same retention time as the authentic peptide, and the identification of the mRNA encoding the propeptide amino-acid sequence. Most of these paracrine actions have been inferred from effects observed after treatment with these peptides in various test systems.

Oxytocin and Vasopressin.

The oxytocin–neurophysin gene is expressed in granulosa cells and granulosa-derived luteal cells but not in thecal cells of all species so far studied, including humans (174). However, immunoreactive oxytocin also was demonstrated in thecal cells (136). Gene expression in granulosa/luteal cells initiates at ovulation, peaks in the early luteal phase, and falls to low levels in the late luteal phase (174). In porcine luteal cell cultures, but not in granulosa cell cultures, oxytocin inhibits basal as well as LH-stimulated progesterone secretion (137, 437). Vasopressin has the same effect but is more potent. Each of these peptides was shown to act through its own receptor (437). Oxytocin and vasopressin also inhibit androstenedione secretion, but no effect is seen on estrogen

secretion (437). When added to intact corpus luteum, however, oxytocin stimulates progesterone and estradiol secretions (617). These data point to a participation of oxytocin and vasopressin in the differentiation and regression of the corpus luteum.

Renin–Angiotensin System.

Renin and angiotensin II have been identified in human follicular fluid (100). In humans, synthesis of prorenin, renin, and angiotensin II is confined to the thecal cells of preovulatory follicles (328). Synthesis is controlled by LH. In the rat ovary, angiotensin II receptors of the AT2 type are found only in a discrete subpopulation of follicles, where the receptor is located primarily in the theca interna and granulosa cells (65, 328). Receptors are down-regulated by FSH and up-regulated by LH (328). The peptide stimulates both androgen and estrogen secretions from rat ovarian slices (65). The ratio of androgen to estrogen is increased, suggesting a role in follicular atresia (328).

Opioid Peptides

Proenkephalin A mRNA has been detected primarily in thecal cells of preovulatory follicles and, to a lesser extent, in granulosa cells (474), and POMC mRNA has been detected in cells of the antral follicles and corpus luteum (490). The percentage of follicles containing these cells increases after treatment with PMSG, suggesting a role of POMC-derived peptides in follicular development and corpus luteum formation (490). One of these peptides may be β-endorphin (341).

Hypothalamic Releasing Factor–Like Peptides.

A peptide with GnRH-like activity, but not GnRH (distinguished by differences in HPLC retention times), has been found in extracts of bovine granulosa cells and corpus luteum but not follicular fluid (28). A GnRH-like protein has been detected in ovarian extracts of the rat, human, cow, and ewe in amounts much higher than GnRH (41). The highest levels of this protein are found in granulosa cells, but a significant amount is present in luteal, thecal, and stromal tissues but not in follicular fluid (28, 41). The GnRH-like protein inhibits LH-stimulated cAMP accumulation in rat luteal cells (28) as well as the action of LH in cultures of rat luteal cells and of FSH in granulosa cells, suggesting an antigonadotrophic function (41). A similar effect is displayed by GnRH but to a much smaller extent than GnRH-like protein. The antigonadotrophic action of GnRH is evident from the finding that treatment of immature hypophysectomized, estrogen-primed rats with a GnRH agonist in vivo causes a dramatic decrease in the mitotic index of the granulosa cells of all preantral follicles and increases pyknosis (144). By means of in situ hybridization with an oligonucleotide probe complementary to the GnRH coding sequence, it has become clear that the GnRH gene is expressed in rat granulosa and thecal cells at all stages of follicular development as well as in the corpus luteum (94). Also, GnRH receptor mRNA has been located in granulosa cells of the rat at different stages of follicular development and in the corpus luteum (607). Treatment of immature hypophysectomized female rats with a GnRH agonist inhibits basal and PMSG-induced inhibin secretions, while a GnRH antagonist augmented the stimulatory effect of PMSG on inhibin release, clearly suggesting that a GnRH-like peptide of ovarian origin plays a physiological paracrine role in regulating inhibin secretion in the rat (461).

In contrast, no effects of GnRH agonists on granulosa cells are found in human tissue (472). In the normal human ovary, neither GnRH nor GnRH mRNA is detectable, but they have been demonstrated in human ovarian adenocarcinoma and the ovarian adenocarcinoma cell line SK-OV3 (400). Thus, whereas in nonhuman species a GnRH-like poplypeptide and GnRH may have a paracrine role, in the human this appears to be the case only in tumoral development.

A GRF-like peptide has been detected by immunostaining in the human ovary and by radioimmunoassay in follicular fluid (33). Immunoreactivity of GRF co-eluting on gel filtration chromatography with authentic rat GRF has been detected in rat ovarian extracts. In rat ovarian RNA extract, Northern blot hybridization reveals the presence of two GRF mRNA species, the major one being much larger than that present in the hypothalamus but similar to that in the testis (33). In addition to an effect mediated by GH, GRF appears to have a direct effect on the ovary. A common receptor for GRF and VIP has been detected in granulosa cells from immature estrogen-treated rats, while in cultured granulosa cells, GRF stimulates cAMP formation and potentiates FSH-induced cAMP formation, progesterone biosynthesis, aromatase activity, and LH receptor formation (381), suggesting a paracrine maturational role for GRF in follicular development.

Immunoreactive CRF, not distinguishable from authentic CRF, has been demonstrated in rat thecal and stromal cells and in a subpopulation of cells in the corpus luteum, and CRF receptors have been found in thecal cells and stroma (357). A similar distribution is found in the human ovary (356). In polycystic ovary syndrome, CRF levels are decreased (356). The local function of CRF is at present not clear.

Other Peptides. Specific staining for GRP has been found in porcine granulosa cells (199). In rats, ANP

mRNA has been detected in interstitial cells surrounding the follicles (164). Endothelin-1 mRNA and peptide have been demonstrated in cultured porcine granulosa cells in human follicular fluid (314); the peptide significantly increases DNA synthesis in the cells and shows a dual effect on progesterone secretion: at short incubation time it stimulates basal and FSH-stimulated secretions of progesterone, whereas at longer times it is inhibitory. In the rat, hCG administration increases galanin mRNA levels in the ovary (172); little is known about its putative local action. In granulosa cell cultures, the peptide slightly increases levels of estradiol, with no effect on progesterone (172).

Local Control by Polypeptide Growth Factors

A large number of polypeptide growth factors are expressed in the ovary: IGFs (2, 69, 140, 193, 218, 219, 233, 234, 255, 376, 404, 486, 623, 629); bFGF (204, 262, 317, 624); members of the EGF family, such as EGF (220, 354, 504) and TGF-α (86, 272, 338, 355, 504, 524, 560); members of the TGF-β family, such as inhibin (240, 257, 336, 364, 461, 614), activins (239, 336, 364, 443, 614, 625), Mullerian inhibiting substance (608), and TGF-β (3, 232, 347, 504); platelet-derived growth factor (PDGF) (230); follistatin (336); the cytokines TNF-α (16, 469, 616) and IL-1 (263, 264, 519); plasminogen activator inhibitor-1 and -2 (436); and the neurotrophin NGF (401). A body of evidence suggests a putative paracrine/autocrine action of these growth factors in a dose- and time-dependent manner on both steroid synthesis and follicular development and/or atresia and corpus luteum formation and/or regression. Most of these data, however, concern effects obtained after in vitro or in vivo treatment with the growth factors.

Insulin-Like Growth Factors. Granulosa cells appear to be the site of production of IGF-1 (256), the mRNA of which has been located in granulosa cells of developing preantral and antral follicles but not in atretic follicles or corpus luteum (404). In preovulatory follicles, there are high levels of IGF-1 mRNA in the antral cell layers and the cells of the cumulus oophorus (404). Secretion of IGF-I in cultured immature porcine granulosa cells is stimulated by FSH and LH, the effect being enhanced by estradiol (255). The site of action of IGF-1 appears to be the granulosa cells as well as the thecal/interstitial cells (2, 233). Its primary action is to amplify the actions of gonadotrophins. In rat and porcine granulosa cells, IGF-1 synergizes with FSH in the induction of aromatase activity (2, 218). Through interaction with the adjacent thecal/interstitial cells, the growth factor also enhances androgen biosynthesis and potentiates the hCG-stimulated accumulation of androgen in that compartment (233). Thus, IGF-1 may function in both an autocrine and a paracrine fashion. More evidence for this was found by using immunoneutralizing anti-IGF-1 antibodies. Porcine follicular fluid collected from large follicles (and charcoal-treated to remove steroids) stimulates progesterone production in cultured granulosa cells from immature porcine follicles, and this can be inhibited specifically by an anti-IGF monoclonal antibody (376). Furthermore, the anti-IGF antibody inhibits the effects of FSH, estradiol, and GH on progesterone production. Also, IGF-1 is involved in follicular growth. The cellular distribution of IGF-1 mRNA is the same as that of granulosa cells showing mitotic figures (404). Stimulation of granulosa cell growth by FSH and estradiol is blocked by an anti-IGF monoclonal antibody (376). The expression level of IGF-1 mRNA correlates in time with the presumptive function of this growth factor, to amplify the effects of gonadotrophins on follicular development and ovulation. During the rat estrous cycle, levels of IGF-1 and IGF-1 mRNA are lowest at proestrus and highest at estrus (69). In the human, IGF-1 mRNA and IGF-1 are found in thecal cells of small antral follicles (140) but not in either thecal or granulosa cells of dominant follicles (140). The receptor mRNA for IGF-1 is expressed in granulosa cells (140), particularly of antral and atretic follicles (629), and at low levels in thecal and interstitial cells (629). In the infant ovary, IGF-1 and its receptors are expressed in growing oocytes (629).

In the rat, expression of IGF-2 is not confined to granulosa cells but to the thecal/interstitial cells (234). The action of the growth factor, however, appears to involve both ovarian compartments, as indicated by the finding of type 1 and type 2 IGF receptor gene mRNA in both granulosa and thecal/interstitial cells (140, 234). Regulation of expression also seems to be opposite to that of IGF-1. Estrogens down-regulate IGF-2 and, as already mentioned, up-regulate IGF-1 expression (234). The situation is quite different in humans: IGF-2 mRNA is present in granulosa cells collected immediately before ovulation (140, 193), whereas it is restricted to thecal cells in small antral follicles (140). Levels of IGF-2 mRNA are high in the granulosa cells of atretic follicles (629); it is also present in follicular blood vessels (629).

Ovarian cells secrete a heterogeneous family of IGF-binding proteins which evoke effects generally opposite to those of the IGFs themselves (219).

Basic Fibroblast Growth Factor. Basic FGF is expressed in germinal epithelial cells and stimulates cellular proliferation (204); therefore, it may be involved in the development of early follicles. However, at later stages of development, bFGF displays clear-cut antigonadotrophic activity. When added to cultured rat ovary cells, it strongly attenuates androgen biosynthesis stimulated by hCG and IGF-1 through an inhibitory effect on the steroidogenic enzyme 17α-hydroxylase/17-20-lyase in thecal/interstitial cells (262). The latter action together with an inhibitory effect on aromatase activity in granulosa cells decrease estrogen production and, hence, follicular maturation.

Members of the Epidermal Growth Factor Family. As studied by immunological techniques, there is an impressive change in the expression of EGF and EGF receptor in oocytes, granulosa cells, thecal cells, and stromal cells during follicular growth and regression in the human ovary (354). In primordial follicles, immunostaining for EGF and EGF receptor is negative. In preantral follicles, EGF and EGF receptor immunoreactivities become detectable in the oocyte, with increased intensity at the preovulatory stage. In the antral follicle, immunostaining becomes apparent in the granulosa and theca interna cell layers and persists in preovulatory follicles and the corpus luteum. In atretic follicles, the theca interna cells show intense staining for EGF and EGF receptor. However, immunostaining for EGF and its receptor reveals the presence of EGF in thecal cells but not in granulosa cells, while the receptor is found in both cell types (504). In the porcine ovary, EGF-binding sites are found in granulosa and luteal cells but not in thecal cells (179). In the bovine, no EGF expression has been found at the mRNA level (524); however, serum-free conditioned medium from bovine thecal cells, but not from granulosa cells, contains a substance that specifically binds to the EGF receptor (524); this substance is most probably TGF-α as thecal cells express the TGF-α gene (524). Expression of the TGF-α gene in thecal cells has been confirmed at the protein level by immunostaining in the bovine, rat, and human (338, 504, 560). Expression of TGF-α has been observed in oocytes of the primary follicles, in granulosa cells, and in luteal cells (86). As to its putative paracrine/autocrine function, TGF-α stimulates the growth of cultured granulosa and thecal cells (524). Morphological correlates for this observation are the findings that TGF-α staining is most intense in the theca of small follicles at a developmental stage corresponding with rapid granulosa cell growth and weak in large preovulatory follicles, in which granulosa cell mitosis declines (338). However, EGF and TGF-α have negative effects on differentiation parameters in granulosa cells. It has been shown that EGF reduces hCG-induced secretion of estradiol and progesterone in the perfused rabbit ovary (141) and in in vivo-treated sheep (387). Also, EGF strongly reduces ovulation efficiency in the latter experimental setup (141). As to the mechanism involved, EGF decreases expression of aromatase in granulosa cells and attenuates the stimulatory effect of rhFSH on the expression of 17β-hydroxysteroid dehydrogenase type 1, another key enzyme in estrogen biosynthesis (196). That TGF-α has similar negative actions on follicular development has been shown in transgenic mice overexpressing the TGF-α gene (344).

Inhibin and Activin. In the human ovary, activin-A has been located in the granulosa and cumulus cells of follicles and in granulosa luteal cells of the corpus luteum (443). Inhibin α- and βA-subunit mRNA expression is confined to granulosa cells; it is not found in other follicular or stromal cells (62). Secretion of inhibin is stimulated by FSH (625) and by estrogens probably of local origin (524). Binding of [^{125}I]-inhibin-A is restricted to the antral granulosa cells in rats and sheep (142, 613), but receptors also may be present on thecal cells since inhibin exerts effects on isolated thecal cells. Activin receptors are expressed in rat oocytes and in corpus luteum and granulosa cells, activin type II receptor being the predominant form (68). [^{125}I]-Activin-A-binding sites locate to the granulosa cells of all stages of follicles, whereas binding to thecal cells is found in developing follicles of the rat (613). The available evidence is consistent with the idea that ovarian inhibin and activin act in a paracrine manner to regulate follicular development, ovulation, and corpus luteum formation. Immunization of ewes against the N-terminal peptide of the inhibin α-subunit disturbs corpus luteum formation and decreases follicular gelatinase activity, indicating that inhibin may have a role in tissue-remodeling during ovulation and corpus luteum formation (475). There is a sequential appearance and disappearance of inhibin α and βA mRNAs during follicular development and atresia, respectively (62, 568). Inhibin unilaterally injected into the ovarian intrabursal space of immature rats allows a greater accumulation of follicles than in the contralateral control ovary, and the size of the follicles is similar to that seen after treatment with PMSG (614). Activin, on the contrary, causes follicular atresia and blocks the follicular development induced by PMSG (614). In addition, inhibin stimulates and activin decreases granulosa cell proliferation in the rat (614). In contrast, in cultured human luteal follicular cells, inhibin-A has no effect on mitogenesis, while activin stimulates mitogenic activity (443).

Inhibin and activin also modulate steroid hormone production (239, 240, 257, 615). Treatment of human thecal cells in monolayer culture with inhibin provokes a modest increase of androgen production, comparable in magnitude to the maximal stimulation by LH but much lower in magnitude than that by IGF-1. Combined treatment with LH + inhibin elicits additive effects; LH + IGF-1 are synergistic, whereas the additional presence of inhibin dramatically augments the response to this combination without effects on progesterone and estrogen production (240, 443). In cultured bovine thecal cells, inhibin enhances basal as well as LH- and estradiol-stimulated androgen production (615). In contrast, activin inhibits androgen synthesis induced by LH + IGF-1 in human cultured thecal cells (239, 240) but this inhibition is completely overcome by inhibin (240). In bovine thecal cells, activin inhibits both LH- and estradiol-stimulated androgen secretions (615). Activin also reverses the positive effect of inhibin on basal and LH- and estradiol-stimulated androgen production (615). As far as granulosa cell steroidogenesis is concerned, little effect is provoked by inhibin, whereas activin has pronounced modulatory effects that alter with the stage of follicular development. In cultured human follicular cells, activin causes a dose- and time-dependent inhibition of basal and gonadotrophin-stimulated progesterone secretion and aromatase activity (334, 443). In contrast, activin enhances gonadotrophin-stimulated aromatase activity and simultaneously suppresses progesterone production by mature granulosa cells, an event mimicking what occurs physiologically in the preovulatory follicle (237). The action of activin on the ovary has been documented in vivo: treatment of monkeys with activin stimulated ovarian estrogen secretion during the early follicular phase but disrupted subsequent events in the menstrual cycle (546).

Müllerian Inhibiting Substance and Transforming Growth Factor-β. The mRNA of Müllerian inhibiting substance has been detected in the granulosa cells of primordial, primary, and antral human follicles, as well as within the cytoplasm of oocytes and stroma (608).

In the rat and human, TGF-β is produced by thecal/interstitial cells (232, 504). In immature rats, TGF-β does not change basal androgen production but causes a marked inhibition of LH-stimulated androgen secretion (232, 347). Inhibition is probably caused at the level of the steroidogenic enzyme 17α-hydroxylase/17-20-lyase. Also, the synergistic stimulation of LH action on androgen accumulation by IGF-1 is blocked by TGF-β (232, 347). Treatment of mouse thecal/interstitial cells with TGF-β fails to affect either basal or hCG-stimulated androgen production. In contrast, added to granulosa cells, TGF-β augments FSH-induced aromatase activity (3).

Cytokines. Resident ovarian macrophages have long been recognized as potential local regulators of ovarian function, presumably through paracrine regulatory molecules (263). At the end of the luteal phase, macrophages producing TNF-α invade the corpus luteum, which is indicative of their role in corpus luteum regression (luteolysis) (reviewed in ref. 617). This has initiated studies on the production and effects of inflammatory cytokines. Immunoreactive TNF-α has been detected in the ovary and is confined to granulosa cells of human antral and atretic follicles and to large granulosa-lutein cells but not preantral follicles (469). It appears to be secreted since it is present in follicular fluid. In highly purified thecal/interstitial cells from immature rats, TNF-α does not affect basal accumulation of androgens but strongly inhibits hCG-stimulated androgen biosynthesis, most likely through inhibition of cAMP accumulation, the second messenger of gonadotrophin action, and through an effect on key enzymes of androgen biosynthesis (16). Furthermore, TNF-α inhibits estradiol and progesterone production in luteal cells, in this way counteracting the luteotrophic action of various polypeptides. Another cytokine explored in the ovary is IL-1. In the rat, it is expressed exclusively in thecal/interstitial cells, the level being markedly up-regulated after hCG treatment (264). It mimics the effect of TNF-α described above (263). A more detailed study in the mouse has revealed that IL-1-immunoreactive material is present in thecal/interstitial cells but that immediately after follicle rupture intense staining also occurs in granulosa cells and in granulosa/luteal cells of the corpus luteum (519). These data point to a role for these cytokines in follicular atresia and luteolysis.

PARACRINE FACTORS MEDIATING ACTIONS OF THYROID AND STEROID HORMONES

Thyroid hormones stimulate the rate of cell division in various organs. Thyroid hormone is an absolute requirement for proliferation of GH4C1 rat pituitary tumor cells plated at low density. In one study, conditioned medium from triiodothyronine (T_3)-treated cells (from which T_3 previously had been removed) was as active as T_3 itself in inducing GH4C1 cell division, suggesting that the mitogenic action of T_3 is brought about by stimulating the secretion of an autocrine growth factor(s) (241). At least one of the T_3-induced growth factors appears to be apotransferrin (521). The estrogen-induced increase in basal PRL release in rat anterior pituitary cell cultures appears to be mediated by a paracrine action of galanin (618): galanin is secreted by a minority of lactotrophs, but estrogen treatment increases the number of galanin-secreting cells and stimulates the galanin mRNA level in the anterior

pituitary more than 1000-fold, while the estrogen-induced increase in PRL secretion is completely abolished by immunoneutralization with an antigalanin antiserum. The mitogenic effect of estrogen in PRL-secreting cell lines also is abolished completely by galanin antiserum (618). Another putative growth factor involved in estradiol-induced lactotroph growth is TGF-α. Estradiol treatment induces TGF-α mRNA in the anterior pituitary preceding macroscopic growth (53).

Various growth factors also seem to mediate at least part of the trophic actions of estradiol in other tissues. Both IGF-1 and EGF are involved in the induction of uterine growth by estradiol (120): EGF is expressed in the uterus, and estradiol treatment in vivo augments the expression of EGF and the EGF receptor in the uterus (120, 391). Administration of an anti-EGF antiserum in vivo markedly inhibits the induction of uterine and vaginal growth induced by estrogen treatment in the mouse (391). Moreover, EGF administered in slow-release pellets stimulates uterine and vaginal growth and induces estrogen-dependent uterine lactoferrin in the absence of estradiol (391). Estrogen is also known to stimulate growth of normal mammary epithelial and breast cancer cells. Again, this growth depends on the induction of various growth factors, acting in an autocrine or juxtacrine fashion, including IGF-1 and the EGF-like growth factors TGF-α, amphiregulin, and the heregulins (122, 395, 485).

LOCAL CONTROL IN PANCREATIC ENDOCRINE CELLS

The endocrine pancreas consists of islets of aggregated cells, the so-called islets of Langerhans, which are dispersed throughout the exocrine tissue. Classically, four main endocrine cell types have been distinguished: the A cells, producing glucagon; the B cells, producing insulin; the D cells, synthesizing somatostatin; and the pancreatic polypeptide cells. About 9% of all endocrine cells are found as single cells or in small groups outside the islets distributed among the epithelial lining of exocrine acini or excretory ducts and the connective tissue (450). Some of the endocrine pancreatic cells are located close to the excretory ducts as islets or small clusters, while others are associated with the ducts as single cells scattered through the ductal epithelium (47). Buds of mainly B cells protruding from the ducts have been found in the rat pancreas, which may be a manifestation of "neohistogenesis" because the embryological origin of islets is the ductal epithelium (47). There is an obvious heterogeneity in cell type composition among different islets. In the rabbit, some islets are composed of all established endocrine cells, others contain only B and A cells or B and D cells, whereas still others are monocellular, that is, exclusively made up of B cells (277).

Are Insulin, Glucagon, Somatostatin, and Pancreatic Polypeptide Paracrine and Autocrine Factors in the Pancreatic Islets?

The microanatomy of islets has intrigued scientists for decades. In regular islets, most of the cells are B cells and are located in the center (core) of the islet, whereas A cells, D cells, and pancreatic polypeptide cells are located in the mantle area, where they appear to be distributed randomly. The latter microanatomical organization has tempted many to speculate about the existence of functional communication between the different endocrine cell types. In fact, D cells extend cellular processes toward A and pancreatic polypeptide cells and toward the outer part of the core B cells. Pancreatic polypeptide cells also have long cytoplasmic extensions. Although the anatomical distribution of cell types and the morphology of D cells are compatible with a putative paracrine interaction within the mantle and with at least certain cells in the periphery of the B cells in the core, the intraislet blood flow and, presumably, the flow of fluids through canaliculi and intercellular spaces are in the opposite direction from that expected to enable paracrine interaction from mantle cells to core cells. Indeed, there exists a portal microcirculation within the islets, the direction of flow being from core to mantle, more precisely from B cells to A cells and then to D cells (488). It remains unclear, therefore, whether communication between these cell types is via humoral factors diffusing from the releasing cell to neighboring cells or via humoral factors secreted from certain cells and reaching other islet cells via the intrainsular circulation or along the perivascular spaces.

Nevertheless, at least some cells may communicate locally. Although the majority of D cells are located in close apposition to the capillaries and intracellular immunoreactive somatostatin is concentrated in the compartment of the cell facing the capillaries or perivascular spaces, about 15% of D cells are not in close contact with capillaries and display much lower somatostatin immunostainability (208). These cells thus may interact with neighboring A cells.

The existence of interaction at a local (paracrine) level between A and B cells has some experimental support. It has been reported that under conditions of maintaining plasma glucose levels constant by the glucose clamp technique, infusion of insulin to humans provokes B-cell suppression (as shown by a fall in the plasma C-peptide level), and this is associated with an enhanced release of glucagon in response to arginine (27); in C-peptide-negative diabetics, the acute glucagon response to arginine also is inhibited by insulin infusion. These data suggest an inhibitory autocrine effect of insulin on insulin secretion and an inhibitory effect of insulin on glucagon secretion.

On the basis of close cellular contacts and many observations in various in vitro and in vivo pancreatic preparations that somatostatin treatment provokes a clear-cut inhibition of insulin and glucagon release, somatostatin secreted from D cells has been considered to function as a paracrine factor tonically inhibiting the secretion of glucagon and insulin from the neighboring A and B cells. An endocrine route of somatostatin to the B and A cells via the general bloodstream seems unlikely as the contribution of islet somatostatin is minimal compared to the contribution of somatostatin from the gastrointestinal tract. Long-term immunization of rabbits against somatostatin increases the proportion of D cells and lowers the content of insulin in B cells and the ultrastructural features of increased metabolic activity in A and B cells (209, 278). When the somatostatin analog D-Ala5-D-Trp8-somatostatin (which is not recognized by somatostatin antiserum and which, in contrast to somatostatin itself, at the doses used does not inhibit glucagon or insulin release) is infused intravenously into anesthetized dogs in vivo, secretion of somatostatin is inhibited by the analog but secretions of glucagon and insulin increase (552), supporting the hypothesis that endogenous islet somatostatin inhibits insulin and glucagon release. Since intrainsular blood flow is from B cells in the core to A and D cells in the mantle, somatostatin cannot reach the B cells through the microvasculature; therefore, a paracrine route of communication has been postulated. Using the same somatostatin analog, evidence was found that pancreatic somatostatin also mediates the well-known inhibition of glucagon secretion by hyperglycemia (302): hyperglycemia causes suppression of glucagon secretion and stimulates insulin and somatostatin release, whereas the somatostatin analog reverses the stimulation of somatostatin and suppression of glucagon secretion without affecting plasma glucose level and insulin secretion.

However, inhibition of glucagon release by insulin and stimulation of somatostatin secretion by glucagon appear to be exerted by an endocrine mode of action of these hormones via the intraislet vascular route (that is, from B cells to A cells to D cells). This was shown elegantly by perfusion experiments in which various immunoneutralizing antibodies were delivered by perfusing the islets in the anterograde (normal) direction and the retrograde direction (487). Infusion of insulin antibody in the anterograde direction increases glucagon and somatostatin secretions, whereas retrograde infusion is without effect. Anterograde infusion of glucagon antibody decreases somatostatin secretion without influencing insulin, whereas retrograde infusion decreases insulin without changing somatostatin secretion. Similar infusion experiments failed to support a paracrine mode of action of somatostatin in inhibiting insulin and glucagon release; indeed, anterograde infusion of somatostatin antibody has no effect on insulin or glucagon secretion, though (as expected) retrograde infusion increases both (487).

Another concept supported by experimental evidence is that each islet hormone may affect its own function in an autocrine way (209). It has been reported that long-term immunization against glucagon results in hyperplasia of A cells and a decrease in the cellular content of glucagon, while immunization against somatostatin causes an increase in the proportion of D cells.

A possible additional determinant in targeting the islet hormones to the endocrine or the paracrine route is the existence of polarity of secretion (99). Morphological studies have suggested that pancreatic islet cells display different domains for signal reception and secretion (99). That at least insulin is secreted vectorially has been demonstrated by functional studies (99).

The putative paracrine role of pancreatic polypeptide cells was first suggested on the basis of the finding in normal and tumoral human endocrine pancreas that these cells extend long cytoplasmic processes in close contact with other endocrine cells as well as with acinar cells (446). In vivo treatment of rats with pancreatic polypeptide slightly augments basal insulin and glucagon release (551). Infusion of pancreatic polypeptide in rat pancreas, however, lowers basal and glucose- or arginine-stimulated insulin release without affecting glucagon output. The inhibitory effect of pancreatic polypeptide on arginine-induced insulin release is accompanied by an increase in somatostatin release (109).

Others have proposed that the D cell is not a paracrine regulator of islet hormone secretion but may be so in the regulation of pancreatic exocrine function (488).

Local Control by Other Regulatory Peptides

In addition to the classical hormonal peptides present in the typical cell types, different families of regulatory peptides have been identified in the endocrine pancreas: glucagon-like peptide-1 (289, 512); vasopressin and oxytocin (14, 186, 413); the renin–angiotensin system (85); POMC-derived peptides (101, 261, 304, 393); proenkephalin A–derived peptides (80, 591); dynorphin-derived peptides (79); protachykinin A–derived peptides (363); the hypothalamic releasing hormones TRH (322), GRF (61, 337), and CRF (468); NPY (388, 601); CGRP (178, 435); and gastric inhibitory polypeptide (529). A striking characteristic in the action of these peptides when added to in vitro pancreatic islets or perfused pancreas is that they modulate glucose-dependent insulin or glucagon release and often are inactive on insulin release at low glucose. Whether the endogenous peptides act in a similar fashion to the peptides added to the in vitro system has been documented only for some peptides.

Glucagon-like peptide-1 is a cleavage product of proglucagon precursor peptide (372). It is stored in A cells and released together with glucagon (289, 512). The truncated peptide-7–37 also is released and strongly and potently stimulates insulin secretion and inhibits glucagon secretion in rats and humans (159, 359, 372, 407). It is approximately 100 times more potent than glucagon in the stimulation of insulin secretion, and its action is highly dependent on glucose concentration (104, 603). Glucagon-like peptide-2 and the intervening peptide-2, two other peptides encoded by the glucagon gene, have no effect on insulin secretion (603). Glucagon-like peptide-1 stimulates somatostatin and pancreatic polypeptide release at low glucose levels, at which the peptide is ineffective on insulin secretion (159).

Neuropeptide Y has been localized in B, A, and D cells (388) and is releasable from isolated rat pancreatic islets (601). In perifused rat islets and in perifused rat pancreas in situ, the peptide decreases basal and glucose-stimulated insulin releases (375, 601), whereas immunoneutralization of endogenous NPY with NPY antiserum increases insulin secretion (601). These observations suggest that NPY can control B cells in an autocrine manner, though it remains uncertain whether it is released from all cell types in which it is expressed.

Oxytocin and AVP augment secretions of insulin, glucagon, and somatostatin from mouse islets (184, 185, 187). Importantly, whereas the effect of oxytocin on glucagon and somatostatin release is seen at low and high glucose levels, the effect on insulin release is present only at high glucose levels. In isolated mouse islets, AVP is ineffective at low glucose levels and amplifies the insulin-releasing effect of higher glucose levels (185). At both low and high glucose levels, AVP increases somatostatin and glucagon releases even in the absence of glucose (186).

The *5' truncated 800-base POMC mRNA* as well as the *full-length POMC mRNA* have been demonstrated in pancreatic islets (261). β-Endorphin immunoreactivity has been localized in pancreatic islets (393), more precisely in the D cell of the rat, guinea pig, and human (602). Binding sites have been found on A, B, and D cells (628). The peptide transiently potentiates glucose-stimulated insulin secretion by the isolated perfused rat pancreas (101). However, in isolated rabbit pancreatic islets, β-endorphin inhibits glucose-stimulated insulin secretion (498). In vivo in the mouse, the responses are complicated: at low doses the peptide inhibits and at high doses it augments stimulated insulin secretion (5). In the rat pancreas, all A cells immunostain for both β-neoendorphin and dynorphin A (79). As far as proenkephalin A–derived peptides are concerned, Met-enkephalin is confined exclusively to B cells (80). Glucose-stimulated, but not basal, insulin secretion and synthesis are increased by low concentrations of enkephalin (484, 591), but in vivo treatment evokes an opposite effect (5). In the isolated perfused dog pancreas, Met-enkephalin inhibits somatostatin release and stimulates insulin secretion at 8.3 mM glucose (231); however, the opioid antagonist naloxone does not affect somatostatin or insulin secretion, indicating that endogenous opioid peptides have no tonic activity on islet cell function.

The preprotachykinin A–derived peptides *substance P and neurokinin A* are expressed in both insulin-containing and non-insulin-containing endocrine cells of the fetal and neonatal rat pancreas but are undetectable in the adult (363), suggesting a role as growth factors during islet development.

In A cells of many species, including humans, CRF-immunoreactive material has been observed (433, 434). The in vitro effects of CRF on pancreatic islets are unclear. In rat pancreas perfused in situ, CRF causes a rapid inhibition of insulin release but has no significant effect on glucagon release (373). In isolated rat pancreatic islets, CRF increases glucagon release, though only over a narrow range of concentration, and has no effect on insulin release (374).

Prepro-TRH immunoreactivity has been located exclusively within B cells of the rat (322). The target cell of TRH has not been found but is not the B cell itself (30). Also, GRF has been located in pancreatic polypeptide cells (61). Overexpression of GRF in pancreatic islets in transgenic mice results in increased numbers of B cells (337).

Pancreastatin is a peptide probably derived by proteolytic processing from chromogranin A, an acidic protein present in secretory granules in endocrine and neuronal cells (499), and is found in A, B, and D cells (499). It has been shown in several species to inhibit basal and glucose-induced insulin release in the perfused pancreas as well as insulin secretion induced by glucagon, VIP, gastric inhibitory peptide, and 8-cholecystokinin (CCK-8) without any effect on glucagon or somatostatin output (6, 410, 424, 425, 499, 518, 522).

Amylin, a peptide showing 46% identity in amino-acid sequence with CGRP, is expressed abundantly in pancreatic islets but is not present in many other tissues (327, 342). It is secreted by B cells (160, 342), augments glucose- and arginine-stimulated insulin releases, and inhibits glucagon and somatostatin releases from the isolated perfused rat pancreas (161).

In the mouse, CGRP is found in B cells, whereas in the rat, the peptide is located in D cells (178, 435). It inhibits GRP- and CCK-8–stimulated insulin release from isolated rat islets in vitro (178) and carbachol-stimulated insulin secretion in vivo (435). After infusion in calves, CGRP produces a significant rise in plasma pancreatic polypeptide levels without having an effect on plasma levels of insulin (129).

Immunocytochemical localization of *gastric inhibitory polypeptide (GIP)* is within A cells (529). In isolated rat pancreatic islets, GIP significantly augments glucose-stimulated insulin secretion, an effect also seen after in vivo treatment, and counteracts glucose inhibition of glucagon release (496, 555).

An important question is whether the effects of the above-mentioned peptides on the cell type releasing the hormone are direct or indirect. For example, are inhibitory actions on insulin release mediated by somatostatin? This problem has been explored only in a few cases. For example, the inhibitory action of CGRP on insulin release does not seem to be mediated by somatostatin as no stimulation of somatostatin release from isolated rat islets in vitro is seen after CGRP administration (178).

Local Control by Biogenic Amines

Although pancreatic islets are innervated by adrenergic, cholinergic, and peptidergic nerves, certain biogenic amines are also synthesized in particular endocrine cells and may have a local regulatory function. For example, GABA as well as the GABA-synthesizing enzyme glutamate decarboxylase and the GABA-metabolizing enzyme GABA-transaminase are present in B cells of several species, including humans (189, 402, 483, 557, 593). Also, GABA is present in synapse-like microvesicles, and glutamic acid decarboxylase is localized around the synapse-like microvesicles much like in neurons (451). In culture some B cells extend neurite-like processes, and the synapse-like microvesicles are concentrated in the distal portions of these processes (451). These microvesicles also express a GABA transporter driven by a proton pump (451). In peripheral islet cells (mantle cells), GABA is not present; these cells appear to be the target of GABA (451, 592). Perfusion with muscimol, a specific GABA agonist, inhibits glucose-stimulated somatostatin release, whereas glucose-stimulated insulin release is not affected (466). When glucose is present, GABA inhibits arginine-induced insulin secretion from the isolated perfused rat pancreas but does not affect arginine-induced insulin secretion in the absence of glucose (211). Muscimol slightly inhibits basal glucagon release from the isolated perfused rat pancreas (198). There is evidence that GABA may mediate part of the well-known inhibitory action of glucose on glucagon secretion (473), though some controversy exists over this matter (198).

Pancreatic islet cells also express tyrosine hydroxylase, the rate-limiting enzyme of cathecholamine biosynthesis (226, 562). During embryogenesis, islet precursor cells co-express insulin, glucagon (226, 561, 562), and the neuronal proteins tyrosine hydroxylase and NPY (562).

Another biogenic amine, serotonin, is produced in A and pancreatic polypeptide cells in the cat pancreatic islets (180).

Local Control by Polypeptide Growth Factors

Relatively little information is available concerning the role of local growth factors in pancreatic islets. In the pancreas of humans, dogs, and rats, IGF-1 is localized in A cells, whereas IGF-2 is found in B cells (345). Treatment of cultured islets with IGF-1 inhibits insulin secretion in rats but not in humans (138). However, others have found stimulatory effects of IGF-1 on insulin biosynthesis and secretion in isolated pancreatic rat islets, as well as on [^{3}H]-thymidine incorporation and DNA content (517).

Nerve growth factor has been identified in and is secreted by nonendocrine cells surrounding the islets, suggesting a paracrine action on the adjacent islet cells. Receptors for NGF have been identified on A and B cells (282). Islet morphogenesis is retarded in the presence of K252a, an inhibitor of the tyrosine kinase activity of the NGF receptor (282).

In a small number of human B cells, TGF-β1, TGF-β2, and TGF-β3 and their mRNAs are found (621). Both TGF-β1 and TGF-β2 increase basal and, even more so, glucose-stimulated insulin releases in isolated rat pancreatic islets (572); TGF-β counteracts the mitogenic action of glucose in fetal rat pancreatic islets in tissue culture without affecting glucose-induced insulin secretion (523). Expressing TGF-β1 in B cells directed by human insulin promoter in transgenic mice results in fibroblast proliferation, abnormal deposition of extracellular matrix in exocrine pancreas from birth onward, inhibition of proliferation of acinar cells, and development of only small islet cell clusters (324).

The mRNAs of the α-, βA-, and βB-subunits of inhibin and activin have been detected in rat pancreatic islets (397). Activin-A-immunoreactive material has been identified in A and D cells (622). Activin-A, but not inhibin-A, augments glucose-stimulated insulin secretion in perifused rat pancreatic islets (511, 573, 622). It also affects glucagon secretion, but the direction of the effect depends on the concentration of glucose: it decreases glucagon secretion at 3.0 mM, has no effect at 8.3mM, and increases secretion at 16.7 mM glucose (590).

LOCAL CONTROL IN THE THYROID GLAND

In the thyroid gland, several cell types exist which functionally interact: thyroid follicular cells (TFCs), calcitonin-producing cells, parafollicular cells, mast cells, and stromal fibroblasts. There exists spatial integration of follicular and parafollicular cells (281): parafollicular cells are located in the central regions of the thyroid gland lobes, where follicular cell activity seems to be greater than in the periphery of the lobes. Local control in the thyroid primarily consists of clear-cut modulation of TSH action on thyroid hormone production and thyroid growth.

Local Control by Regulatory Peptides

One of the better studied peptides with putative paracrine function in the thyroid is somatostatin. Somatostatin-immunoreactive cells display characteristic morphological features, particularly cytoplasmic elongations, which supports the postulated paracrine role for this peptide (440). In thyroid organ cultures, somatostatin significantly depresses the mitotic rates of TFCs, both basal and that stimulated by TSH (627). Somatostatin inhibits T$_3$ and thyroxine (T$_4$) production and secretion (119). In the majority of Hashimoto thyroiditis patients, an elevated number of somatostatin-immunoreactive cells is found (119) among cells also positive for neuron-specific enolase but not among calcitonin-producing cells, suggesting that somatostatin is responsible, at least in part, for the hypothyroid state in that disease. In thyroid organ cultures, somatostatin significantly depresses the mitotic rate of TFCs stimulated by TSH (627). Somatostatin inhibits DNA synthesis and cellular proliferation induced by both TSH and IGF-1 in the cell line FRTL5, a line of differentiated and nontransformed rat TFCs (578). Somatostatin mRNA and somatostatin receptors are detected in medullary thyroid carcinomas, as is the case for a large proportion of neuroendocrine tumors, suggesting an autocrine negative feedback on growth rate (454). This hypothesis is supported by the finding that calcitonin cells in rat and human thyroid also contain somatostatin (166). In spontaneous medullary thyroid carcinomas occurring in old rats, high levels of both somatostatin-immunoreactive material and its mRNA have been detected in a subpopulation of tumoral calcitonin cells, located preferentially at the periphery of the tumor (411). These cells also express high levels of calcitonin and its mRNA. The proliferative activity of the somatostatin-containing areas is low compared to the areas lacking somatostatin production, again suggesting a negative role in cellular proliferation.

Another neuropeptide with wide tissue distribution found in the thyroid is *GRP* (549). This gene is expressed in human thyroidal calcitonin-containing cells and at high levels in calcitonin cell hyperplasias and neoplasias (medullary carcinomas of the thyroid). Levels of GRP and calcitonin are linearly correlated during development, GRP content being up to 20 times higher in infants during the first months of life than in adults (549). The mRNA and peptide of GRP co-localize to the majority of calcitonin cells in fetuses and neonates but to only a few calcitonin cells in normal adults. Moreover, developing, but not adult, calcitonin cells have a dendritic morphology, consistent with a paracrine role during postnatal growth. Calcitonin cells positive for GRP occur in normal thyroid areas adjacent to follicular adenomas and papillary carcinomas, which themselves are GRP-negative (549). These data support the hypothesis that GRP may function as a paracrine growth factor of TFC in normal and tumoral development.

Human and porcine TFCs produce endothelin and express endothelin receptors, both being up-regulated by TSH (575, 577). As studied in porcine tissue, endothelin receptors are of type A (577). There is good evidence for a paracrine or autocrine role of endothelin in the thyroid (577). In porcine thyroid cells, endothelin-1 and endothelin-2 increase c-fos mRNA expression, the significance remaining unclear since no effect on DNA synthesis stimulated by either EGF or IGF-1 is seen. However, endothelin-1 inhibits TSH-induced iodide uptake. Antibody to endothelin-1, however, increases TSH-induced iodide uptake. Endothelin appears to be secreted as immunoreactive endothelin-1 has been detected in medium conditioned by porcine thyroid cells.

As in several other endocrine organs, immunoreactive ANP, probably identical to circulating ANP, as well as ANP mRNA have been identified in intact human thyroid tissue and in cultured thyroid cells, strongly suggesting that immunoreactivity is locally produced (194, 260). Since high-affinity ANP receptors also are found, an autocrine action of ANP is plausible. Secretion of immunoreactive ANP from rat FRTL-5 cells also has been shown, accumulation of the peptide in granules being dependent upon the presence of TSH in the medium (505).

Local Control by Polypeptide Growth Factors

A major growth and differentiation factor, TSH, is blood-borne from the pituitary gland. However, there is a body of evidence that locally produced growth factors participate in these processes either by synergizing with the action of TSH or by inhibiting it. Moreover, TSH enhances the synthesis and release of several of these growth factors. The putative local role of several polypeptide growth factors in the thyroid has been the subject of intensive investigation, the best documented being studies on IGFs, FGFs, and members of the EGF and TGF-β families.

Thyroid tissue produces and secretes IGF-1 and IGF-2, and their synthesis is stimulated by TSH (31, 131). In addition, intrinsic thyroid factors seem to augment IGF secretion. There is evidence that conditioned medium from isolated porcine thyroid follicles stimulates IGF-1 production in fibroblasts, resulting in fibroblast and thyrocyte growth (190). By in situ hybridization, it was found that IGF-1 mRNA is predominantly present in mouse follicular cells and C cells (564). In porcine thyroid follicles established in culture, no IGF-1 mRNA was found by Northern hybridization (perhaps because low levels may have escaped detection), but in follicles stimulated with TSH, IGF-1 mRNA was detected after 24 h (245). Human thyroid follicular cells not contaminated by fibroblasts in primary culture secrete IGF-1, and, again, secretion is stimulated by TSH (also by GH) (569). Abundant IGF-2, but not IGF-1, is found in spent media of rat FRTL5 cell cultures (346). Expression of IGF-1 and -2 genes has been demonstrated in rat medullary thyroid carcinoma (247) and in human thyroid carcinoma (405) cell lines. Specific IGF receptors have been identified on sheep thyroid cell membranes (31). In normal thyroid cells and in the rat FRTL5 cell line, IGFs stimulate DNA synthesis (31, 131). Also, IGFs synergize with the mitogenic effect of TSH and other agents that increase intracellular cAMP concentration (346). This effect is mediated by a secreted factor which is not IGF-1 itself (554). That endogenous IGFs are autocrine mitogens in the rat thyroid is shown by the finding that a monoclonal antibody recognizing IGF-1 and IGF-2 but not insulin, inhibits basal DNA synthesis in FRTL5 cells and blocks the synergizing action of TSH (346). In humans, normal thyroid follicles do not seem to produce sufficient amounts of IGF-1 and culturing these cells requires addition of IGF-1 to the medium (611). However, follicular adenoma cells can be cultured without the growth factor supplement. Conditioned medium from follicular adenoma cells can confer IGF-1 independence on normal thyroid cells, and this activity is abolished by immunoadsorption with an anti-IGF-1 antibody (611).

There have been many more data reported in favor of an autocrine activity of IGFs. Addition of a monoclonal antibody to IGF-1 receptors in cultures of a human thyroid carcinoma cell line significantly reduces the growth of cancer cells (405). The modest increase in thymidine incorporation stimulated by TSH in wild-type FRTL5 cells is markedly increased in the presence of exogenous IGF-1 (103). By transfecting FRTL5 cells with the IGF-1 gene under the control of the mouse metallothionein-1 or IGF-2 5' genomic promoter region, stable IGF-1 secreting cell lines have been generated in which the mitogenic response to TSH was indistinguishable from that stimulated by combined TSH and IGF-1 in wild-type cells (103). Moreover, TSH-stimulated DNA synthesis is blocked by a monoclonal antibody to IGF (103). The autocrine mitogenic effect of IGFs has raised the question of whether the polypeptide could play a pathogenic role in thyroid tumorigenesis. This problem was tested in transgenic mice in which high plasma levels of IGF-2 (20- or 30-fold increase above normal) were obtained by IGF-2 overexpression (470). Mice developed diverse tumors at a higher frequency than controls after 18 months of age, including thyroid carcinomas. The growth-promoting role of thyroid IGFs is further demonstrated by the finding that IGF-1 mRNA and peptide expressions in follicular cells in normal mice are significantly higher during postnatal thyroid growth and during the growth response to goitrogen than in adults (564).

Also, IGFs appear to be involved in thyroid hormone synthesis. As is the case in thyroid growth, IGFs strongly amplify the action of TSH on thyroid hormone synthesis, and their action depends on the presence of TSH. In cultured ovine thyroid follicles, TSH alone displayed a modest stimulatory effect on iodine uptake and organification but this was potentiated by physiological concentrations of IGF-1 or IGF-2, which on their own have no effect (38). Expression of IGF-1 mRNA is under the negative control of iodide (245), which is in keeping with the inhibitory action of iodide on thyroid hormone secretion.

In normal thyroid, EGF, prepro-EGF mRNA, TGF-α, and the EGF receptors are widely expressed (412, 583). The level of EGF expression is increased by T_4 (412). In human thyroid follicles cultured in suspension in which the follicular three-dimensional structure is retained, EGF attenuates TSH-stimulated iodide uptake and organification and T_3 secretion but enhances TSH-stimulated cAMP formation (309). In the latter culture system, EGF enhances cellular proliferation on its own,

but this effect is inhibited by TSH (309). In filter-cultured monolayers of porcine thyrocytes, EGF stimulates cellular proliferation (394).

As shown by the presence of its mRNA and protein in TFCs, TGF-β is produced in the human thyroid gland (210). It behaves as a negative regulator of thyroid growth stimulated by TSH, IGF-1, EGF, and TGF-α (210). It may be involved in the pathogenesis of iodine-deficient nontoxic goiter (210). Treatment of porcine thyroid follicular cells in monolayer culture with TGF-β over a 7-day period has been reported to reduce IGF-1 release as well as [^{3}H]thymidine incorporation (39). Preincubation of cells with iodide also reduced [^{3}H]thymidine incorporation. This effect is reversed partially when the iodide-containing preincubation medium is immunoadsorbed with a neutralizing TGF-β antiserum and subsequently re-added to the cells (39), indicating that iodide inhibition of thyroid growth is mediated by endogenous TGF-β.

An endothelial cell growth factor which is regulated by TSH, EGF, and iodide in parallel with the effect of these substances on thyroid cell growth is released from cultured porcine thyroid follicles, suggesting that thyroid angiogenesis during thyroid enlargement may be due to paracrine mitogenic factors released by the thyroid epithelial cells when exposed to TSH and iodine (205).

LOCAL CONTROL IN THE PARATHYROID GLAND

It is well known that both parathyroid hormone (PTH) secretion and cell growth are regulated negatively by extracellular calcium (Ca^{2+}) (482). Local regulation in the parathyroid gland is related primarily to the efficacy of this extracellular signal.

Chromogranin-A (CgA) is a ubiquitous 50 kd protein which co-localizes in secretory granules of endocrine tissues and is co-secreted with peptide hormones. There is ample evidence that CgA is co-stored and co-secreted with PTH (126, 156). A 26 kd N-terminal fragment of CgA has been identified as a natural breakdown product in bovine parathyroid cells, and this fragment also is secreted (126). Since this fragment inhibits the low Ca^{2+}-stimulated secretion of PTH, it is thought to function as an autocrine regulator (126). CgA contains a sequence identical to pancreastatin, suggesting that it is the precursor of pancreastatin. The latter peptide is a potent inhibitor of PTH secretion when added to the incubation medium of an in vitro preparation of parathyroid tissue at 0.5 mM Ca^{2+} (155). Since antiserum directed against CgA or pancreastatin potentiates the secretion of PTH at 0.5 mM, but not 3.0 mM, Ca^{2+}, it is believed that fragments of

CgA act in an autocrine fashion on PTH release in response to decreasing extracellular Ca^{2+} (155).

Endothelin-1 is synthesized and released by bovine and rat parathyroid epithelium (175, 558) and bovine chief cells (175). Expression of preproendothelin-1 mRNA and peptide production are up-regulated by extracellular Ca^{2+} (changes from high to low or vice versa) (175). The peptide stimulates PTH secretion through specific endothelin-A receptors (175, 176). Taking these data together, it is likely that endothelin-1 may mediate, at least in part, the effects of extracellular Ca^{2+} on the parathyroid system. In human parathyroid adenoma, expression of both endothelin-A and endothelin-B receptor mRNA has been demonstrated, as well as expression of prepro-PTH (132); in the latter cells, endothelin-1 inhibits basal PTH secretion. Cell growth is not affected by endothelin-1 (176).

Evidence exists that an autocrine acidic FGF (aFGF) system is the main mechanism by which Ca^{2+} regulates parathyroid cell growth (482); aFGF mRNA and peptide and aFGF receptors have been demonstrated in the cells. Expression of both aFGF mRNA and peptide is suppressed by Ca^{2+}, and the number of aFGF receptors is reduced. Decreasing extracellular Ca^{2+} as well as administration of aFGF result in an increase in [^{3}H]thymidine incorporation. Treatment with anti-aFGF antibody, however, inhibits thymidine incorporation in cells exposed to 0.05 mM Ca^{2+} but is without effect at 0.7 mM Ca^{2+}.

REFERENCES

1. Aanesad, M., J. S. Rotnes, P. A. Torjesen, E. Haug, O. Sand, and T. Bjoro. Epidermal growth factor stimulates the prolactin synthesis and secretion in rat pituitary cells in culture (GH4C1 cells) by increasing the intracellular concentration of free calcium. *Acta Endocrinol. (Copenh.)* 128: 361–366, 1993.
2. Adashi, E. Y., C. E. Resnick, A. J. D'Ercole, M. E. Svoboda, and J. J. Van Wyk. Insulin-like growth factors as intraovarian regulators of granulosa cell growth and function. *Endocr. Rev.* 6: 400–420, 1985.
3. Adashi, E. Y., C. E. Resnick, E. R. Hernandez, J. V. May, A. F. Purchio, and D. R. Twardzik. Ovarian transforming growth factor-beta (TGF beta): cellular site(s), and mechanism(s) of action. *Mol. Cell. Endocrinol.* 61: 247–256, 1989.
4. Adashi, E. Y., E. M. Tucker, and A. J. Hsueh. Direct regulation of rat testicular steroidogenesis by neurohypophysial hormones. Divergent effects on androgen and progestin biosynthesis. *J. Biol. Chem.* 259: 5440–5446, 1984.
5. Ahren, B. Effects of beta-endorphin, met-enkephalin, and dynorphin A on basal and stimulated insulin secretion in the mouse. *Int. J. Pancreatol.* 5: 165–178, 1989.
6. Ahren, B., S. Lindskog, K. Tatemoto, and S. Efendic. Pancreastatin inhibits insulin secretion and stimulates glucagon secretion in mice. *Diabetes* 37: 281–285, 1988.
7. Ailenberg, M., P. S. Tung, and I. B. Fritz. Transforming growth factor-beta elicits shape changes and increases contractility of testicular peritubular cells. *Biol. Reprod.* 42: 499–509, 1990.
8. Allaerts, W., P. Carmeliet, and C. Denef. New perspectives in the function of pituitary folliculo-stellate cells. *Mol. Cell. Endocrinol.* 71: 73–81, 1990.
9. Allaerts, W., and C. Denef. Regulatory activity and topological distribution of folliculo-stellate cells in rat anterior pituitary cell aggregates. *Neuroendocrinology* 49: 409–418, 1989.
10. Allaerts, W., P. H. Jeucken, F. T. Bosman, and H. A. Drexhage. Relationship between dendritic cells and folliculo-stellate cells in the pituitary: immunohistochemical comparison between mouse, rat and human pituitaries. *Adv. Exp. Med. Biol.* 329: 637–642, 1993.
11. Allaerts, W., A. Mignon, and C. Denef. Selectivity of juxtaposition between cup-shaped lactotrophs and gonadotrophs from rat anterior pituitary in culture. *Cell Tissue Res.* 263: 217–225, 1991.
12. Alper, R. H. Evidence for central and peripheral serotonergic control of corticosterone secretion in the conscious rat. *Neuroendocrinology* 51: 255–260, 1990.
13. Altschuler, L. R., M. N. Parisi, L. F. Cageao, S. R. Chiocchio, J. A. Fernandez-Pol, and A. A. Zaninovich. Epidermal growth factor stimulates thyrotropin secretion in the rat. *Neuroendocrinology* 57: 23–27, 1993.
14. Amico, J. A., F. M. Finn, and J. Haldar. Oxytocin and vasopressin are present in human and rat pancreas. *Am. J. Med. Sci.* 296: 303–307, 1988.
15. Andersen, B., and M. G. Rosenfeld. Pit-1 determines cell types during development of the anterior pituitary gland. A model for transcriptional regulation of cell phenotypes in mammalian organogenesis. *J. Biol. Chem.* 269: 29335–29338, 1994.
16. Andreani, C. L., D. W. Payne, J. N. Packman, C. E. Resnick, A. Hurwitz, and E. Y. Adashi. Cytokine-mediated regulation of ovarian function. Tumor necrosis factor alpha inhibits gonadotropin-supported ovarian androgen biosynthesis. *J. Biol. Chem.* 266: 6761–6766, 1991.
17. Andreis, P. G., G. Neri, A. Mazzocchi, F. Musajo, and G. G. Nussdorfer. Direct secretagogue effect of corticotropin-releasing factor on the rat adrenal cortex: the involvement of the zona medullaris. *Endocrinology* 131: 69–72, 1992.
18. Andries, M., and C. Denef. Gonadotropin-releasing hormone influences the release of prolactin and growth hormone from intact rat pituitary in vitro during a limited period in neonatal life. *Peptides* 16: 527–532, 1995.
19. Andries, M., G. F. Jacobs, D. Tilemans, and C. Denef. In vitro immunoneutralization of a cleaved prolactin variant: evidence for a local paracrine action of cleaved prolactin in the development of gonadotrophs and thyrotrophs in rat pituitary. *J. Neuroendocrinol.* 8: 423–427, 1996.
20. Andries, M., D. Tilemans, and C. Denef. Isolation of cleaved prolactin variants that stimulate DNA synthesis in specific cell types in rat pituitary cell aggregates in culture. *Biochem. J.* 281: 393–400, 1992.
21. Andries, M., D. Tilemans, and C. Denef. Modulation of epidermal growth factor receptor binding and action by N-acetyl-TGF alpha (34–43) methyl ester. *Peptides* 15: 619–625, 1994.
22. Andries, M., V. Vande Vijver, D. Tilemans, C. Bert, and C. Denef. Interaction of alpha T3–1 cells with lactotropes and somatotropes of normal pituitary in vitro. *Neuroendocrinology* 61: 326–336, 1995.
23. Ang, H. L., R. Ivell, N. Walther, H. Nicholson, H. Ungefroren, M. Millar, D. Carter, and D. Murphy. Over-expression of oxytocin in the testes of a transgenic mouse model. *J. Endocrinol.* 140: 53–62, 1994.
24. Angelova, P., and M. Davidoff. Immunocytochemical demonstration of substance P in hamster Leydig cells during ontogenesis. *Z. Mikrosk. Anat. Forsch.* 103: 560–566, 1989.

25. Anthony, C. T., M. Rosselli, and M. K. Skinner. Actions of the testicular paracrine factor (P-Mod-S) on Sertoli cell transferrin secretion throughout pubertal development. *Endocrinology* 129: 353–360, 1991.

26. Anthony, C. T., and M. K. Skinner. Cytochemical and biochemical characterization of testicular peritubular myoid cells. *Biol. Reprod.* 40: 811–823, 1989.

27. Asplin, C. M., T. L. Paquette, and J. P. Palmer. In vivo inhibition of glucagon secretion by paracrine beta cell activity in man. *J. Clin. Invest.* 68: 314–318, 1981.

28. Aten, R. F., J. J. Ireland, C. W. Weems, and H. R. Behrman. Presence of gonadotropin-releasing hormone-like proteins in bovine and ovine ovaries. *Endocrinology* 120: 1727–1733, 1987.

29. Audhya, T., C. S. Hollander, D. H. Schlesinger, and B. Hutchinson. Structural characterization and localization of corticotropin-releasing factor in testis. *Biochim. Biophys. Acta* 995: 10–16, 1989.

30. Awouters, P., H. P. Meissner, and J. C. Henquin. Thyrotropin-releasing hormone and insulin release: in vitro studies with islets of normal and dysthyroid mice. *Diabetes Res.* 2: 105–110, 1985.

31. Bachrach, L. K., M. C. Eggo, R. L. Hintz, and G. N. Burrow. Insulin-like growth factors in sheep thyroid cells: action, receptors and production. *Biochem. Biophys. Res. Commun.* 154: 861–867, 1988.

32. Baes, M., W. Allaerts, and C. Denef. Evidence for functional communication between folliculo-stellate cells and hormone-secreting cells in perifused anterior pituitary cell aggregates. *Endocrinology* 120: 685–691, 1987.

33. Bagnato, A., C. Moretti, J. Ohnishi, G. Frajese, and K. J. Catt. Expression of the growth hormone-releasing hormone gene and its peptide product in the rat ovary. *Endocrinology* 130: 1097–1102, 1992.

34. Bartlett, J. M., J. Spiteri-Grech, and E. Nieschlag. Regulation of insulin-like growth factor I and stage-specific levels of epidermal growth factor in stage synchronized rat testes. *Endocrinology* 127: 747–758, 1990.

35. Basile, D. P., and M. A. Holzwarth. Basic fibroblast growth factor may mediate proliferation in the compensatory adrenal growth response. *Am. J. Physiol.* 265 (*Regulatory Integrative Comp. Physiol.* 36): R1253–R1261, 1993.

36. Bastiaensen, E., J. De Block, and W. P. De Potter. Neuropeptide Y is localized together with enkephalins in adrenergic granules of bovine adrenal medulla. *Neuroscience* 25: 679–686, 1988.

37. Bathgate, R. A., and C. Sernia. Characterization and localization of oxytocin receptors in the rat testis. *J. Endocrinol.* 141: 343–352, 1994.

38. Becks, G. P., D. K. Buckingham, J. F. Wang, I. D. Phillips, and D. J. Hill. Regulation of thyroid hormone synthesis in cultured ovine thyroid follicles. *Endocrinology* 130: 2789–2794, 1992.

39. Beere, H. M., J. Soden, S. Tomlinson, and S. P. Bidey. Insulin-like growth factor-I production and action in porcine thyroid follicular cells in monolayer: regulation by transforming growth factor-beta. *J. Endocrinol.* 130: 3–9, 1991.

40. Begeot, M., F. J. Hemming, M. L. Aubert, and P. M. Dubois. Differentiation of pituitary cells in culture. *Ann. Endocrinol. (Paris)* 48: 367–377, 1987.

41. Behrman, H. R., R. F. Aten, J. J. Ireland, and R. A. Milvae. Characteristics of an antigonadotrophic GnRH-like protein in the ovaries of diverse mammals. *J. Reprod. Fertil. Suppl.* 37: 189–194, 1989.

42. Belloni, A. S., G. Neri, F. G. Musajo, et al. Investigations on the morphology and function of adrenocortical tissue regenerated from gland capsular fragments autotransplanted in the musculus gracilis of the rat. *Endocrinology* 126: 3251–3262, 1990.

43. Ben-Jonathan, N., and J. W. Liu. Pituitary lactotrophs. Endocrine, paracrine, juxtacrine and autocrine interactions. *Trends Endocrinol. Metab.* 3: 254–258, 1992.

44. Bergh, A. Paracrine regulation of Leydig cells by the seminiferous tubules. *Int. J. Androl.* 6: 57–65, 1983.

45. Bergh, A. Development of stage-specific paracrine regulation of Leydig cells by the seminiferous tubules. *Int. J. Androl.* 8: 80–85, 1985.

46. Berry, S. A., and O. H. Pescovitz. Identification of a rat GHRH-like substance and its messenger RNA in rat testis. *Endocrinology* 123: 661–663, 1988.

47. Bertelli, E., M. Regoli, and A. Bastianini. Endocrine tissue associated with the pancreatic ductal system: a light and electron microscopic study of the adult rat pancreas with special reference to a new endocrine arrangement. *Anat. Rec.* 239: 371–378, 1994.

48. Bhasin, S., L. A. Krummen, R. S. Swerdloff, B. S. Morelos, W. H. Kim, G. S. di Zerega, N. Ling, F. Esch, S. Shimasaki, and J. Toppari. Stage dependent expression of inhibin alpha and beta-B subunits during the cycle of the rat seminiferous epithelium. *Endocrinology* 124: 987–991, 1989.

49. Blank, M. S., A. Fabbri, K. J. Catt, and M. L. Dufau. Inhibition of luteinizing hormone release by morphine and endogenous opiates in cultured pituitary cells. *Endocrinology* 118: 2097–2101, 1986.

50. Bloch, B., D. Le Guellec, and Y. de Keyzer. Detection of the messenger RNAs coding for the opioid peptide precursors in pituitary and adrenal by "in situ" hybridization: study in several mammal species. *Neurosci. Lett.* 53: 141–148, 1985.

51. Blomquist, J. F., and J. U. Baenziger. Differential sorting of lutropin and the free alpha-subunit in cultured bovine pituitary cells. *J. Biol. Chem.* 267: 20798–20803, 1992.

52. Boitani, C., D. Farini, R. Canipari, and C. W. Bardin. Estradiol and plasminogen activator secretion by cultured rat Sertoli cells in response to melanocyte-stimulating hormones. *J. Androl.* 10: 202–209, 1989.

53. Borgundvaag, B., J. E. Kudlow, S. G. Mueller, and S. R. George. Dopamine receptor activation inhibits estrogen-stimulated transforming growth factor-alpha gene expression and growth in anterior pituitary, but not in uterus. *Endocrinology* 130: 3453–3458, 1992.

54. Bornstein, S. R., and M. Ehrhart-Bornstein. Ultrastructural evidence for a paracrine regulation of the rat adrenal cortex mediated by the local release of catecholamines from chromaffin cells. *Endocrinology* 131: 3126–3128, 1992.

55. Bornstein, S. R., M. Ehrhart-Bornstein, W. A. Scherbaum, E. F. Pfeiffer, and J. J. Holst. Effects of splanchnic nerve stimulation on the adrenal cortex may be mediated by chromaffin cells in a paracrine manner. *Endocrinology* 127: 900–906, 1990.

56. Bornstein, S. R., M. Ehrhart-Bornstein, H. Usadel, M. Bockmann, and W. A. Scherbaum. Morphological evidence for a close interaction of chromaffin cells with cortical cells within the adrenal gland. *Cell Tissue Res.* 265: 1–9, 1991.

57. Borrelli, E., R. A. Heyman, C. Arias, P. E. Sawchenko, and R. M. Evans. Transgenic mice with inducible dwarfism. *Nature* 339: 538–541, 1989.

58. Borrelli, E., P. E. Sawchenko, and R. M. Evans. Pituitary hyperplasia induced by ectopic expression of nerve growth factor. *Proc. Natl. Acad. Sci. U.S.A.* 89: 2764–2768, 1992.

59. Borson, S., G. Schatteman, P. Claude, and M. Bothwell. Neurotrophins in the developing and adult primate adenohypophysis: a new pituitary hormone system? *Neuroendocrinology* 59: 466–476, 1994.

60. Bosenberg, M. W., and J. Massagué. Juxtacrine cell signaling molecules. *Curr. Opin. Cell Biol.* 5: 832–838, 1993.

61. Bosman, F. T., C. Van Assche, A. C. Nieuwenhuyzen Kruseman, S. Jackson, and P. J. Lowry. Growth hormone releasing factor (GRF) immunoreactivity in human and rat gastrointestinal tract and pancreas. *J. Histochem. Cytochem.* 32: 1139–1144, 1984.

62. Braw-Tal, R. Expression of mRNA for follistatin and inhibin/activin subunits during follicular growth and atresia. *J. Mol. Endocrinol.* 13: 253–264, 1994.

63. Bruhn, T. O., W. C. Engeland, E. L. Anthony, D. S. Gann, and I. M. Jackson. Corticotropin-releasing factor in the adrenal medulla. *Ann. N.Y. Acad. Sci.* 512: 115–128, 1987.

64. Bruhn, T. O., W. C. Engeland, E. L. Anthony, D. S. Gann, and I. M. Jackson. Corticotropin-releasing factor in the dog adrenal medulla is secreted in response to hemorrhage. *Endocrinology* 120: 25–33, 1987.

65. Bumpus, F. M., A. G. Pucell, A. I. Daud, and A. Husain. Angiotensin II: an intraovarian regulatory peptide. *Am. J. Med. Sci.* 295: 406–408, 1988.

66. Byrne, J. M., P. M. Jones, S. F. Hill, W. M. Bennet, M. A. Ghatei, and S. R. Bloom. Expression of messenger ribonucleic acids encoding neuropeptide-Y, substance-P, and vasoactive intestinal polypeptide in human pituitary. *J. Clin. Endocrinol. Metab.* 75: 983–987, 1992.

67. Cameron, L., S. Kapas, and J. P. Hinson. Endothelin-1 release from the isolated perfused rat adrenal gland is elevated acutely in response to increasing flow rates and ACTH(1–24). *Biochem. Biophys. Res. Commun.* 202: 873–879, 1994.

68. Cameron, V. A., E. Nishimura, L. S. Mathews, K. A. Lewis, P. E. Sawchenko, and W. W. Vale. Hybridization histochemical localization of activin receptor subtypes in rat brain, pituitary, ovary, and testis. *Endocrinology* 134: 799–808, 1994.

69. Carlsson, B., L. Carlsson, and H. Billig. Estrus cycle–dependent co-variation of insulin-like growth factor-I (IGF-I) messenger ribonucleic acid and protein in the rat ovary. *Mol. Cell. Endocrinol.* 64: 271–275, 1989.

70. Carmeliet, P., M. Baes, and C. Denef. The glucocorticoid hormone dexamethasone reverses the growth hormone-releasing properties of the cholinomimetic carbachol. *Endocrinology* 124: 2625–2634, 1989.

71. Carmeliet, P., and C. Denef. Immunocytochemical and pharmacological evidence for an intrinsic cholinomimetic system modulating prolactin and growth hormone release in rat pituitary. *Endocrinology* 123: 1128–1139, 1988.

72. Carmeliet, P., and C. Denef. Synthesis and release of acetylcholine by normal and tumoral pituitary corticotrophs. *Endocrinology* 124: 2218–2227, 1989.

73. Carmeliet, P., P. Maertens, and C. Denef. Stimulation and inhibition of prolactin release from rat pituitary lactotrophs by the cholinomimetic carbachol in vitro. Influence of hormonal environment and intercellular contacts. *Mol. Cell. Endocrinol.* 63: 121–131, 1989.

74. Carretero, J., F. Sanchez, M. Rubio, C. M. Francos, J. Blanco, and R. Vazquez. In vitro and in vivo evidence for direct dopaminergic inhibition of VIP-immunoreactive pituitary cells. *Neuropeptides* 27: 1–6, 1994.

75. Carroll, S. L., J. B. Schweitzer, D. M. Holtzman, M. L. Miller, G. M. Sclar, and J. Milbrandt. Elements in the 5′ flanking sequences of the mouse low-affinity NGF receptor gene direct appropriate CNS, but not PNS, expression in transgenic mice. *J. Neurosci.* 15: 3342–3356, 1995.

76. Carvalheira, A. F., U. Welsch, and A. G. Pearse. Cytochemical and ultrastructural observations on the argentaffin and argyrophil cells of the gastro-intestinal tract in mammals, and their place in the APUD series of polypeptide-secreting cells. *Histochemie* 14: 33–46, 1968.

77. Cathiard, A. M., P. Durand, M. G. Seidah, M. Chretien, and J. M. Saez. Effects of several pro-opiomelanocortin derived peptides on steroidogenesis in ovine and bovine adrenal cells. *J. Steroid Biochem.* 23: 185–190, 1985.

78. Ceccatelli, S., A. L. Hulting, X. Zhang, L. Gustafsson, M. Villar, and T. Hokfelt. Nitric oxide synthase in the rat anterior pituitary gland and the role of nitric oxide in regulation of luteinizing hormone secretion. *Proc. Natl. Acad. Sci. U.S.A.* 90: 11292–11296, 1993.

79. Cetin, Y. Immunohistochemistry of beta-neoendorphin and dynorphin in the endocrine pancreas of rat and man. *Histochemistry* 83: 369–373, 1985.

80. Cetin, Y. Immunohistochemistry of opioid peptides in the guinea pig endocrine pancreas. *Cell Tissue Res.* 259: 313–319, 1990.

81. Chabot, J. G., P. Walker, and G. Pelletier. Distribution of epidermal growth factor binding sites in the adult rat adrenal gland by light microscope autoradiography. *Acta Endocrinol. Copenh.)* 113: 391–395, 1986.

82. Chabot, J. G., P. Walker, and G. Pelletier. Distribution of epidermal growth factor binding sites in the adult rat anterior pituitary gland. *Peptides* 7: 4 5–50, 1986.

83. Chaidarun, S. S., M. C. Eggo, M. C. Sheppard, and P. M. Stewart. Expression of epidermal growth factor (EGF), its receptor, and related oncoprotein (erbB-2) in human pituitary tumors and response to EGF in vitro. *Endocrinology* 135: 2012–2021, 1994.

84. Chandrashekar, V., and A. Bartke. The influence of beta-endorphin on testicular endocrine function in adult rats. *Biol. Reprod.* 47: 1–5, 1992.

85. Chappell, M. C., A. Millsted, D. I. Diz, K. B. Brosnihan, and C. M. Ferrario. Evidence for an intrinsic angiotensin system in the canine pancreas. *J. Hypertens.* 9: 751–759, 1991.

86. Chegini, N., and R. S. Williams. Immunocytochemical localization of transforming growth factors (TGFs) TGF-alpha and TGF-beta in human ovarian tissues. *J. Clin. Endocrinol. Metab.* 74: 973–980, 1992.

87. Chen, C. L., J. P. Mather, P. L. Morris, and C. W. Bardin. Expression of pro-opiomelanocortin-like gene in the testis and epididymis. *Proc. Natl. Acad. Sci. U.S.A.* 81: 5672–5675, 1984.

88. Chew, L. J., K. Pardy, D. Murphy, and D. A. Carter. Osmotic stimuli attenuate vasoactive intestinal peptide gene expression in the rat anterior pituitary gland. *Mol. Cell. Endocrinol.* 92: 9–14, 1993.

89. Childs, G. V. Structure–function correlates in the corticotropes of the anterior pituitary. *Front. Neuroendocrinol.* 13: 271–317, 1992.

90. Childs, G. V., D. Rougeau, and G. Unabia. Corticotropin-releasing hormone and epidermal growth factor: mitogens for anterior pituitary corticotropes. *Endocrinology* 136: 1595, 1995.

91. Chiwakata, C., B. Brackmann, N. Hunt, M. Davidoff, W. Schulze, and R. Ivell. Tachykinin (substance-P) gene expression in Leydig cells of the human and mouse testis. *Endocrinology* 128: 2441–2448, 1991.

92. Ciampani, T., A. Fabbri, A. Isidori, and M. L. Dufau. Growth hormone-releasing hormone is produced by rat Leydig cell in culture and acts as a positive regulator of Leydig cell function. *Endocrinology* 131: 2785–2792, 1992.

93. Cicero, T. J., M. L. Adams, L. H. O'Connor, and B. Nock. In vivo evidence for a direct effect of naloxone on testicular steroidogenesis in the male rat. *Endocrinology* 125: 957–963, 1989.

94. Clayton, R. N., L. Eccleston, F. Gossard, J. C. Thalbard, and G. Morel. Rat granulosa cells express the gonadotrophin-releasing hormone gene: evidence from in-situ hybridization histochemistry. *J. Mol. Endocrinol.* 9: 189–195, 1992.

95. Closset, J., A. Gothot, B. Sente, M. L. Scippo, A. Igout, M. Vandenbroeck, D. Dombrowicz, and G. Hennen. Pituitary hormones dependent expression of insulin-like growth factors I and II in the immature hypophysectomized rat testis. *Mol. Endocrinol.* 3: 1125–1131, 1989.

96. Conner, J. M., and S. Varon. Nerve growth factor immunoreactivity in the anterior pituitary of the rat. *Neuroreport* 4: 395–398, 1993.

97. Corcia, A., R. Steinmetz, J. W. Liu, and N. Ben-Jonathan. Coculturing posterior pituitary and GH3 cells: dramatic stimulation of prolactin gene expression. *Endocrinology* 132: 80–85, 1993.

98. Corrigan, A. Z., L. M. Bilezikjian, R. S. Carroll, L. N. Bald, C. H. Schmelzer, B. M. Fendly, A. J. Mason, W. W. Chin, R. H. Schwall, and W. Vale. Evidence for an autocrine role of activin B within rat anterior pituitary cultures. *Endocrinology* 128: 1682–1684, 1991.

99. Cortizo, A., J. Espinal, and P. Hammonds. Vectorial insulin secretion by pancreatic beta-cells. *FEBS Lett.* 272: 137–140, 1990.

100. Culler, M. D., B. C. Tarlatzis, A. Lightman, L. A. Fernandez, A. H. Decherney, A. Negro-Vilar, and F. Naftolin. Angiotensin II-like immunoreactivity in human ovarian follicular fluid. *J. Clin. Endocrinol. Metab.* 62: 613–615, 1986.

101. Curry, D. L., L. L. Bennett, and C. H. Li. Stimulation of insulin secretion by beta-endorphins (1-27 & 1-31). *Life Sci.* 40: 2053–2058, 1987.

102. Dagerlind A., and M. Schalling. Localization of dopamine beta-hydroxylase (DBH) and neuropeptide tyrosine (NPY) mRNA in the grey monkey locus coeruleus and adrenal medulla. *Acta Physiol. Scand.* 134: 563–564, 1988.

103. Dai, Z., S. I. Takahashi, J. J. Van Wyk, and A. J. D'Ercole. Creation of an autocrine model of insulin-like growth factor-I action in transfected FRTL-5 cells. *Endocrinology* 130: 3175–3183, 1992.

104. D'Alessio, D. A., W. Y. Fujimoto, and J. W. Ensinck. Effects of glucagonlike peptide I-(7-36) on release of insulin, glucagon, and somatostatin by rat pancreatic islet cel monolayer cultures. *Diabetes* 38:1534–1538, 1989.

105. Davenport, A. P., D. J. Nunez, J. A. Hall, A. J. Kaumann, and M. J. Brown. Autoradiographical localization of binding sites for porcine [^{125}I]endothelin-1 in humans, pigs, and rats: functional relevance in humans. *J. Cardiovasc. Pharmacol.* 13 (Suppl. 5): S166–S170, 1989.

106. Davidoff, M. S., R. Middendorff, B. Mayer, and A. F. Holstein. Nitric oxide synthase (NOS-I) in Leydig cells of the human testis. *Arch. Histol. Cytol.* 58: 17–30, 1995.

107. De, S. K., H. L. Chen, J. L. Pace, J. S. Hunt, P. F. Terranova, and G. C. Enders. Expression of tumor necrosis factor-alpha in mouse spermatogenic cells. *Endocrinology* 133: 389–396, 1993.

108. DeBold, C. R., J. K. Menefee, W. E. Nicholson, and D. N. Orth. Proopiomelanocortin gene is expressed in many normal human tissues and in tumors not associated with ectopic adrenocorticotropin syndrome. *Mol. Endocrinol.* 2: 862–870, 1988.

109. Degano, P., E. Peiro, P. Miralles, R. A. Silvestre, and J. Marco. Effects of rat pancreatic polypeptide on islet-cell secretion in the perfused rat pancreas. *Metabolism* 41: 306–309, 1992.

110. Delarue, C., D. Becquet, S. Idres, F. Hery, and H. Vaudry. Serotonin synthesis in adrenochromaffin cells. *Neuroscience* 46: 495–500, 1992.

111. De Mellow, J. S., D. J. Handelsman, and R. C. Baxter. Short-term exposure to insulin-like growth factors stimulates testos-terone production by testicular interstitial cells. *Acta Endocrinol. (Copenh.)* 115: 483–489, 1987.

112. Denef, C., and M. Andries. Evidence for paracrine interaction between gonadotrophs and lactotrophs in pituitary cell aggregates. *Endocrinology* 112: 813–822, 1983.

113. Denef, C., P. Maertens, W. Allaerts, A. Mignon, W. Robberecht, L. Swennen, and P. Carmeliet. Cell-to-cell communication in peptide target cells of anterior pituitary. *Methods Enzymol.* 168: 47–71, 1989.

114. Denef, C., C. Schramme, and M. Baes. Stimulation of growth hormone release by vasoactive intestinal peptide and peptide PHI in rat anterior pituitary reaggregates. Permissive action of a glucocorticoid and inhibition by thyrotropin-releasing hormone. *Neuroendocrinology* 40: 88–91, 1985.

115. DePaolo, L. V., L. N. Bald, and B. M. Fendly. Passive immunoneutralization with a monoclonal antibody reveals a role for endogenous activin-B in mediating FSH hypersecretion during estrus and following ovariectomy of hypophysectomized, pituitary-grafted rats. *Endocrinology* 130: 1741–1743, 1992.

116. Desai, B., J. M. Burrin, C. A. Nott, J. F. Geddes, E. J. Lamb, S. J. Aylwin, D. F. Wood, C. Thakkar, and J. P. Monson. Glycoprotein hormone alpha-subunit production and plurihormonality in human corticotroph tumours; an in vitro and immunohistochemical study. *Eur. J. Endocrinol.* 133: 25–32, 1995.

117. Deschepper, C. F., S. H. Mellon, F. Cumin, J. D. Baxter, and W. F. Ganong. Analysis by immunohistochemistry and in situ hybridization of renin and its mRNA in kidney, testis, adrenal and pituitary in the rat. *Endocrinology* 119: 36–43, 1986.

118. de Winter, J. P., H. M. Vanderstichele, G. Verhoeven, M. A. Timmerman, J. G. Wesseling, and F. H. de Jong. Peritubular myoid cells from immature rat testes secrete activin-A and express activin receptor type II in vitro. *Endocrinology* 135: 759–767, 1994.

119. Dhillon, A. P., J. Rode, A. Leathem, and L. Papadaki. Somatostatin: a paracrine contribution to hypothyroidism in Hashimoto's thyroiditis. *J. Clin. Pathol.* 35: 764–770, 1982.

120. Di Augustine, R. P., P. Petrusz, G. I. Bell, C. F. Brown, K. S. Korach, J. A. McLachlan, and C. T. Teng. Influence of estrogen on mouse uterine epidermal growth factor precursor protein and messenger robonucleic acid. *Endocrinology* 122: 2355–2363, 1988.

121. Diaz-Torga, G. S., D. Becu-Villalobos, and C. Libertun. Ontogeny of angiotensin-II-induced prolactin release in vivo and in vitro in female and male rats. *Neuroendocrinology* 59: 57–62, 1994.

122. Dickson, R. B., and M. E. Lippman. Estrogenic regulation of growth and polypeptide growth factor secretion in human breast carcinoma. *Endocr. Rev.* 8: 29–43, 1987.

123. Djakiew, D., B. Pflug, C. Dionne, and M. Onoda. Postnatal expression of nerve growth factor receptors in the rat testis. *Biol. Reprod.* 51: 214–221, 1994.

124. Douglass, J., B. Cox, B. Quinn, O. Civelli, and E. Herbert. Expression of the prodynorphin gene in male and female mammalian reproductive tissues. *Endocrinology* 120: 707–713, 1987.

126. Drees, B. M., J. Rouse, J. Johnson, and J. W. Hamilton. Bovine parathyroid glands secrete a 26–kDa N-terminal fragment of chromogranin-A which inhibits parathyroid cell secretion. *Endocrinology* 129: 3381–3387, 1991.

127. Dufau, M. L., J. C. Tinajero, and A. Fabbri. Corticotropin-releasing factor: an antireproductive hormone of the testis. *FASEB J.* 7: 299–307, 1993.

128. Durand, P., A. M. Cathiard, N. G. Seidah, M. Chretien, and

J. M. Saez. Effects of proopiomelanocortin-derived peptides, methionine-enkephalin and forskolin on the maturation of ovine fetal adrenal cells in culture. *Biol. Reprod.* 31: 694–704, 1984.

129. Edwards, A. V., and S. R. Bloom. Pancreatic endocrine responses to substance P and calcitonin gene-related peptide in conscious calves. *Am. J. Physiol.* 267 (*Endocrinol. Metab.* 30): E847–E852, 1994.

130. Edwards, A. V., and C. T. Jones. Secretion of corticotrophin releasing factor from the adrenal during splanchnic nerve stimulation in conscious calves. *J. Physiol. (Lond.)* 400: 89–100, 1988.

131. Eggo, M. C., L. K. Bachrach, and G. N. Burrow. Role of non-TSH factors in thyroid cell growth. *Acta Endocrinol. Suppl. (Copenh.)* 281: 231–237, 1987.

132. Eguchi, S., Y. Hirata, T. Imai, K. Kanno, T. Akiba, A. Sakamoto, M. Yanagisawa, T. Masaki, and F. Marumo. Endothelin receptors in human parathyroid gland. *Biochem. Biophys. Res. Commun.* 184: 1448–1455, 1992.

133. Eiden, L. E. The enkephalin-containing cell: strategies for polypeptide synthesis and secretion throughout the neuroendocrine system. *Cell. Mol. Neurobiol.* 7: 339–352, 1987.

134. Eiden, L. E., P. Giraud, J. R. Dave, A. J. Hotchkiss, and H. U. Affolter. Nicotinic receptor stimulation activates enkephalin release and biosynthesis in adrenal chromaffin cells. *Nature* 312: 661–663, 1984.

135. Eiden, L. E., and A. J. Hotchkiss. Cyclic adenosine monophosphate regulates vasoactive intestinal polypeptide and enkephalin biosynthesis in cultured bovine chromaffin cells. *Neuropeptides* 4: 1–9, 1983.

136. Einspanier, A., R. Ivell, G. Rune, and J. K. Hodges. Oxytocin gene expression and oxytocin immunoactivity in the ovary of the common marmoset monkey (*Callithrix jacchus*). *Biol. Reprod.* 50: 1216–1222, 1994.

137. Einspanier, R., L. Pitzel, W. Wuttke, G. Hagendorff, K. D. Preuss, E. Kardalinou, and K. H. Scheit. Demonstration of mRNAs for oxytocin and prolactin in porcine granulosa and luteal cells. Effects of these hormones on progesterone secretion in vitro [published erratum appears in *FEBS Lett.* 207: 307, 1986]. *FEBS Lett.* 204: 37–40, 1986.

138. Eizirik, D. L., A. Skottner, and C. Hellerstrom. Insulin-like growth factor I does not inhibit insulin secretion in adult human pancreatic islets in tissue culture. *Eur. J. Endocrinol.* 133: 248–250, 1995.

139. Ellerkmann, E., G. Nagy, and L. S. Frawley. Alpha-melanocyte-stimulating hormone is a mammotrophic factor released by neurointermediate lobe cells after estrogen treatment. *Endocrinology* 130: 133–138, 1992.

140. el-Roeiy, A., X. Chen, V. J. Roberts, D. Le Roith, C. T. Roberts, Jr., and S. S. Yen. Expression of insulin-like growth factor-I (IGF-I) and IGF-II and the IGF-I, IGF-II, and insulin receptor genes and localization of the gene products in the human ovary. *J. Clin. Endocrinol. Metab.* 77: 1411–1418, 1993.

141. Endo, K., S. J. Atlas, J. D. Rone, V. L. Zanagnolo, T. C. Kuo, A. M. Dharmarajan, and E. E. Wallach. Epidermal growth factor inhibits follicular response to human chorionic gonadotropin: possible role of cell to cell communication in the response to gonadotropin. *Endocrinology* 130: 186–192, 1992.

142. Engelhardt, H., K. B. Smith, A. S. McNeilly, and D. T. Baird. Expression of messenger ribonucleic acid for inhibin subunits and ovarian secretion of inhibin and estradiol at various stages of the sheep estrous cycle. *Biol. Reprod.* 49: 281–294, 1993.

143. Engelhardt, R. P., P. Saint-Pol, G. Tramu, and J. Leonardelli. Immunohistochemical localization of enkephalinlike peptides during testicular development in rats. *Arch. Androl.* 17: 49–56, 1986.

144. Erickson, G. F., D. Li, R. Sadrkhanloo, X. J. Liu, S. Shimasaki, and N. Ling. Extrapituitary actions of gonadotropin-releasing hormone: stimulation of insulin-like growth factor-binding protein-4 and atresia. *Endocrinology* 134: 1365–1372, 1994.

145. Eskeland, N. L., C. J. Molineaux, and B. S. Schachter. Regulation of beta-endorphin secretion by corticotropin-releasing factor in the intact rat testis. *Endocrinology* 130: 1173–1179, 1992.

146. Estivariz, F. E., M. Carino, P. J. Lowry, and S. Jackson. Further evidence that N-terminal pro-opiomelanocortin peptides are involved in adrenal mitogenesis. *J. Endocrinol.* 116: 201–206, 1988.

147. Ezzat, S., I. A. Walpola, L. Ramyar, H. S. Smyth, and S. L. Asa. Membrane-anchored expression of transforming growth factor-alpha in human pituitary adenoma cells. *J. Clin. Endocrinol. Metab.* 80: 534–539, 1995.

148. Fabbri, A., D. R. Ciocca, T. Ciampani, J. Wang, and M. L. Dufau. Growth hormone-releasing hormone in testicular interstitial and germ cells: potential paracrine modulation of follicle-stimulating hormone action on Sertoli cell function. *Endocrinology* 136: 2303–2308, 1995.

149. Fabbri, A., and M. L. Dufau. Hormonal regulation of beta-endorphin in the testis. *J. Steroid Biochem.* 30: 347–352, 1988.

150. Fabbri, A., E. A. Jannini, L. Gnessi, S. Ulisse, C. Moretti, and A. Isidori. Neuroendocrine control of male reproductive function. The opioid system as a model of control at multiple sites. *J. Steroid Biochem.* 32: 145–150, 1989.

151. Fabbri, A., J. C. Tinajero, and M. L. Dufau. Corticotropin-releasing factor is produced by rat Leydig cells and has a major local antireproductive role in the testis. *Endocrinology* 127: 1541–1543, 1990.

152. Fallo, F., M. Pistorello, F. Pedini, D. D'Agostino, F. Mantero, and M. Boscaro. In vitro evidence for local generation of renin and angiotensin II/III immunoreactivity by the human adrenal gland [published erratum appears in *Acta Endocrinol. (Copenh.)* 126: 191–192, 1992]. *Acta Endocrinol. (Copenh.)* 125: 319–330, 1991.

153. Fan, X., and G. V. Childs. Epidermal growth factor and transforming growth factor-alpha messenger ribonucleic acids and their receptors in the rat anterior pituitary: localization and regulation. *Endocrinology* 136: 2284–2293, 1995.

154. Fantoni, G., P. L. Morris, G. Forti, G. B. Vannelli, C. Orlando, T. Barni, R. Sestini, G. Danza, and M. Maggi. Endothelin-1: a new autocrine/paracrine factor in rat testis. *Am. J. Physiol.* 265 (*Endocrinol. Metab.* 28): E267–274, 1993.

155. Fasciotto, B. H., S. U. Gorr, A. M. Bourdeau, and D. V. Cohn. Autocrine regulation of parathyroid secretion: inhibition of secretion by chromogranin-A (secretory protein-I) and potentiation of secretion by chromogranin-A and pancreastatin antibodies. *Endocrinology* 127: 1329–1335, 1990.

156. Fasciotto, B. H., S. U. Gorr, and D. V. Cohn. Autocrine inhibition of parathyroid cell secretion requires proteolytic processing of chromogranin A. *Bone Miner.* 17: 323–333, 1992.

157. Fathi, Z., M. H. Corjay, H. Shapira, E. Wada, R. Benya, R. Jensen, J. Viallet, E. A. Sausville, and J. F. Battey. BRS-3: a novel bombesin receptor subtype selectively expressed in testis and lung carcinoma cells. *J. Biol. Chem.* 268: 5979–5984, 1993.

158. Fauser, B. C., A. Baird, and A. J. Hsueh. Fibroblast growth factor inhibits luteinizing hormone–stimulated androgen production by cultured rat testicular cells. *Endocrinology* 123: 2935–2941, 1988.

159. Fehmann, H. C., B. J. Hering, M. J. Wolf, H. Brandhorst, D. Brandhorst, R. G. Bretzel, K. Federlin, and B. Goke. The effects of glucagon-like peptide-I (GLP-I) on hormone secretion from isolated human pancreatic islets. *Pancreas* 11: 196–200, 1995.

160. Fehmann, H. C., V. Weber, R. Goke, B. Goke, and R. Arnold. Cosecretion of amylin and insulin from isolated rat pancreas. *FEBS Lett.* 262: 279–281, 1990.

161. Fehmann, H. C., V. Weber, R. Goke, B. Goke, R. Eissele, and R. Arnold. Islet amyloid polypeptide (IAPP; amylin) influences the endocrine but not the exocrine rat pancreas. *Biochem. Biophys. Res. Commun.* 167: 1102–1108, 1990.

162. Feige, J. J., and A. Baird. Growth factor regulation of adrenal cortex growth and function. *Prog. Growth Factor. Res.* 3: 103–113, 1991.

163. Feng, P., J. Gu, U. J. Kim, N. E. Carnell, and J. F. Wilber. Identification, localization and developmental studies of rat prepro thyrotropin-releasing hormone mRNA in the testis. *Neuropeptides* 24: 63–69, 1993.

164. Ferrara, N., J. Winer, T. Burton, A. Rowland, M. Siegel, H. S. Phillips, T. Terrell, G. A. Keller, and A. D. Levinson. Expression of vascular endothelial growth factor does not promote transformation but confers a growth advantage in vivo to Chinese hamster ovary cells. *J. Clin. Invest.* 91: 160–170, 1993.

165. Feyrter, F. *Uber diffuse endocrine epitheliale Organe.* Leipzig: Ambrosius Barth, 1938.

166. Fierabracci, A., M. Castagna, and L. Baschieri. Calcitonin and somatostatin containing C cells in rat and human thyroid. Immunohistochemical study by a double-staining method. *Pathologica* 85: 467–474, 1993.

167. Filippini, A., A. Tripiciano, F. Palombi, A. Teti, R. Paniccia, M. Stefanini, and E. Ziparo. Rat testicular myoid cells respond to endothelin: characterization of binding and signal transduction pathway. *Endocrinology* 133: 1789–1796, 1993.

168. Fillion, C., A. Malassine, A. Tahri-Joutei, A. M. Allevard, M. Bedin, C. Gharib, J. N. Hugues, and G. Pointis. Immunoreactive arginine vasopressin in the testis: immunocytochemical localization and testicular content in normal and in experimental cryptorchid mouse. *Biol. Reprod.* 48: 786–792, 1993.

169. Finley, E. L., J. S. King, and J. S. Ramsdell. Human pituitary somatotropes express transforming growth factor-alpha and its receptor. *J. Endocrinol.* 141: 547–554, 1994.

170. Finley, E. L., and J. S. Ramsdell. A transforming growth factor-alpha pathway is expressed in GH4C1 rat pituitary tumors and appears necessary for tumor formation. *Endocrinology* 135: 416–422, 1994.

171. Fisher, D. A., and J. Lakshmanan. Metabolism and effects of epidermal growth factor and related growth factors in mammals. *Endocr. Rev.* 11: 418–442, 1990.

172. Fox, M. D., J. F. Hyde, K. N. Muse, S. C. Keeble, G. Howard, S. N. London, and T. E. Curry, Jr. Galanin: a novel intraovarian regulatory peptide. *Endocrinology* 135: 636–641, 1994.

173. Frayne, J., and H. D. Nicholson. Effect of oxytocin on testosterone production by isolated rat Leydig cells is mediated via a specific oxytocin receptor. *Biol. Reprod.* 52: 1268–1273, 1995.

174. Fuchs, A. R. Oxytocin and ovarian function. *J. Reprod. Fertil. Suppl.* 36: 39–47, 1988.

175. Fujii, Y., J. E. Moreira, C. Orlando, M. Maggi, G. D. Aurbach, M. L. Brandi, and K. Sakaguchi. Endothelin as an autocrine factor in the regulation of parathyroid cells. *Proc. Natl. Acad. Sci. U.S.A.* 88: 4235–4239, 1991.

176. Fujii, Y., M. Tomic, S. S. Stojilkovic, T. Iida, M. L. Brandi, Y. Ogino, and K. Sakaguchi. Effects of endothelin-1 on Ca^{2+} signaling and secretion in parathyroid cells. *J. Bone Miner. Res.* 10: 716–725, 1995.

177. Fujimoto, M., Y. Kataoka, A. Guidotti, and I. Hanbauer. Effect of gamma-aminobutyric acid A receptor agonists and antagonists on the release of enkephalin-containing peptides from dog adrenal gland. *J. Pharmacol. Exp. Ther.* 243: 195–199, 1987.

178. Fujimura, M., G. H. Greeley, Jr., M. B. Hancock, A. Alwmark, A. Santos, C. W. Cooper, K. J. Reumont, J. Ishizuka, and J. C. Thompson. Colocalization of calcitonin gene-related peptide and somatostatin in pancreatic islet cells and inhibition of insulin secretion by calcitonin gene-related peptide in the rat. *Pancreas* 3: 49–52, 1988.

179. Fujinaga, H., M. Yamoto, R. Nakano, and K. Shima. Epidermal growth factor binding sites in porcine granulosa cells and their regulation by follicle-stimulating hormone. *Biol. Reprod.* 46: 705–709, 1992.

180. Furuzawa, Y., Y. Ohmori, and T. Watanabe. Immunohistochemical colocalization of serotonin, aromatic L-amino acid decarboxylase and polypeptide hormones in islet A- and PP-cells of the cat pancreas. *J. Vet. Med. Sci.* 56: 911–916, 1994.

181. Gallo-Payet, N., P. Pothier, and H. Isler. On the presence of chromaffin cells in the adrenal cortex: their possible role in adrenocortical function. *Biochem. Cell Biol.* 65: 588–592, 1987.

182. Ganong, W. F. Blood, pituitary, and brain renin–angiotensin systems and regulation of secretion of anterior pituitary gland. *Front. Neuroendocrinol.* 14: 233–249, 1993.

183. Ganong, W. F., C. F. Deschepper, M. K. Steele, and A. Intebi. Renin–angiotensin system in the anterior pituitary of the rat. *Am. J. Hypertens.* 2: 320–322, 1989.

184. Gao, Z. Y., G. Drews, and J. C. Henquin. Mechanisms of the stimulation of insulin release by oxytocin in normal mouse islets. *Biochem. J.* 276: 169–174, 1991.

185. Gao, Z. Y., G. Drews, M. Nenquin, T. D. Plant, and J. C. Henquin. Mechanisms of the stimulation of insulin release by arginine-vasopressin in normal mouse islets. *J. Biol. Chem.* 265: 15724–15730, 1990.

186. Gao, Z. Y., M. Gerard, and J. C. Henquin. Glucose- and concentration-dependence of vasopressin-induced hormone release by mouse pancreatic islets. *Regul. Pept.* 38: 89–98, 1992.

187. Gao, Z. Y., and J. C. Henquin. Arginine vasopressin and oxytocin effects in mouse pancreatic beta-cells. Receptors involved in stimulation of insulin release. *Endocrinology* 87: 439–444, 1993.

188. Gardette, R., R. Rasolonjanahary, C. Kordon, and A. Enjalbert. Epidermal growth factor treatment induces D2 dopamine receptors functionally coupled to delayed outward potassium current (IK) in GH4C1 clonal anterior pituitary cells. *Neuroendocrinology* 59: 10–19, 1994.

189. Garry, D. J., R. L. Sorenson, R. P. Elde, B. E. Maley, and A. Madsen. Immunohistochemical colocalization of GABA and insulin in beta-cells of rat islet. *Diabetes* 35: 1090–1095, 1986.

190. Gartner, R., G. Bechtner, D. Stubner, and W. Greil. Paracrine interaction between thyrocytes and fibroblasts. *Acta Endocrinol. Suppl. (Copenh.)* 281: 225–230, 1987.

191. Gaspar, L., J. S. Chan, N. G. Seidah, and M. Chretien. Peptides related to the N-terminus of pro-opiomelanocortin in the human adrenal medulla. *Clin. Invest. Med.* 12: 90–98, 1989.

192. Gautier, C., C. Levacher, O. Avallet, M. Vigier, V. Rouiller-Fabre, L. Lecerf, J. Saez, and R. Habert. Immunohistochemical localization of transforming growth factor-beta 1 in the fetal and neonatal rat testis. *Mol. Cell. Endocrinol.* 99: 55–61, 1994.

193. Geisthovel, F., I. Moretti-Rojas, R. H. Asch, and F. J. Rojas. Expression of insulin-like growth factor-II (IGF-II) messenger ribonucleic acid (mRNA), but not IGF-I mRNA, in human

preovulatory granulosa cells. *Hum. Reprod.* 4: 899–902, 1989.

194. Gerbes, A. L., L. Dagnino, T. Nguyen, and M. Nemer. Transcription of brain natriuretic peptide and atrial natriuretic peptide genes in human tissues. *J. Clin. Endocrinol. Metab.* 78: 1307–1311, 1994.

195. Gerendai, I., A. Nemeskeri, and V. Csernus. Effect of intratesticular administration of anti-corticotropin-releasing factor antiserum (a-CRF) on testicular function in neonatal rats. *Andrologia* 25: 211–215, 1993.

196. Ghersevich, S., M. Poutanen, J. Tapanainen, and R. Vihko. Hormonal regulation of rat 17 beta-hydroxysteroid dehydrogenase type 1 in cultured rat granulosa cells: effects of recombinant follicle-stimulating hormone, estrogens, androgens, and epidermal growth factor. *Endocrinology* 135: 1963–1971, 1994.

197. Gilchrist, C. A., and J. D. Shull. Epidermal growth factor induces prolactin mRNA in GH4C1 cells via a protein synthesis–dependent pathway. *Mol. Cell. Endocrinol.* 92: 201–206, 1993.

198. Gilon, P., G. Bertrand, M. M. Loubatieres-Mariani, C. Remacle, and J.C. Henquin. The influence of gamma-aminobutyric acid on hormone release by the mouse and rat endocrine pancreas. *Endocrinology* 129: 2521–2529, 1991.

199. Gnessi, L., S. Altamura, M. Arizzi, C. Tei, C. La Torre, V. Bonifacio, F. Facchinetti, and G. Spera. Gastrin-releasing peptide-like immunoreactivity in porcine follicular fluid and ovary. *Mol. Cell. Endocrinol.* 66: 115–118, 1989.

200. Gnessi, L., A. Isidori, M. Bolotti, S. Altamura, S. Ulisse, E. A. Jannini, A. Fabbri, and G. Spera. Identification of immunoreactive gastrin-releasing peptide related substances in adult rat Leydig cells. *Endocrinology* 124: 558–560, 1989.

201. Gonzalez-Hernandez, J. A., S. R. Bornstein, M. Ehrhart-Bornstein, J. E. Gschwend, A. Gwosdow, G. Jirikowski, and W. A. Scherbaum. IL-1 is expressed in human adrenal gland in vivo. Possible role in a local immune–adrenal axis. *Clin. Exp. Immunol.* 99: 137–141, 1995.

202. Gonzalez-Hernandez, J. A., S. R. Bornstein, M. Ehrhart-Bornstein, E. Spath-Schwalbe, G. Jirikowski, and W. A. Scherbaum. Interleukin-6 messenger ribonucleic acid expression in human adrenal gland in vivo: new clue to a paracrine or autocrine regulation of adrenal function. *J. Clin. Endocrinol. Metab.* 79: 1492–1497, 1994.

203. Goodearl, A. D., J. B. Davis, K. Mistry, L. Minghetti, M. Otsu, M. D. Waterfield, and P. Stroobant. Purification of multiple forms of glial growth factor. *J. Biol. Chem.* 268: 18095–18102, 1993.

204. Gospodarowicz, D., J. Plouet, and D. K. Fujii. Ovarian germinal epithelial cells respond to basic fibroblast growth factor and express its gene: implications for early folliculogenesis. *Endocrinology* 125: 1266–1276, 1989.

205. Greil, W., M. Rafferzeder, G. Bechtner, and R. Gartner. Release of an endothelial cell growth factor from cultured porcine thyroid follicles. *Mol. Endocrinol.* 3: 858–867, 1989.

206. Griswold, M. D. Interactions between germ cells and Sertoli cells in the testis. *Biol. Reprod.* 52: 211–216, 1995.

207. Grothe, C., and K. Unsicker. Immunocytochemical mapping of basic fibroblast growth factor in the developing and adult rat adrenal gland. *Histochemistry* 94: 141–147, 1990.

208. Grube, D., and R. Bohn. The microanatomy of human islets of Langerhans, with special reference to somatostatin (D-) cells. *Arch. Histol. Jpn.* 46: 327–353, 1983.

209. Grube, D., and A. Jorns. The endocrine pancreas of glucagon- and somatostatin-immunized rabbits. I. Light microscopy and immunohistochemistry. *Cell Tissue Res.* 265: 251–260, 1991.

210. Grubeck-Loebenstein, B., G. Buchan, R. Sadeghi, et al. Transforming growth factor beta regulates thyroid growth. Role in the pathogenesis of nontoxic goiter. *J. Clin. Invest.* 83: 764–770, 1989.

211. Gu, X. H., T. Kurose, S. Kato, K. Masuda, K. Tsuda, H. Ishida, and Y. Seino. Suppressive effect of GABA on insulin secretion from the pancreatic beta-cells in the rat. *Life Sci.* 52: 687–694, 1993.

212. Guillon, G., M. Trueba, D. Joubert, et al. Vasopressin stimulates steroid secretion in human adrenal glands: comparison with angiotensin-II effect. *Endocrinology* 136: 1285–1295, 1995.

213. Gupta, P., R. Franco-Saenz, L. E. Gentry, and P. J. Mulrow. Transforming growth factor-beta 1 inhibits aldosterone and stimulates adrenal renin in cultured bovine zona glomerulosa cells [published erratum appears in *Endocrinology* 132: 326, 1993]. *Endocrinology* 131: 631–636, 1992.

214. Gutkowska, J., J. Tremblay, T. Antakly, R. Meyer, S. Mukaddam-Daher, and M. Nemer. The atrial natriuretic peptide system in rat ovaries. *Endocrinology* 132: 693–700, 1993.

215. Gutmann, J. N., W. J. Burtis, B. E. Dreyer, P. Andrade-Gordon, A. S. Penzias, M. L. Polan, and K. L. Insogna. Human granulosa-luteal cells secrete parathyroid hormone-related protein in vivo and in vitro. *J. Clin. Endocrinol. Metab.* 76: 1314–1318, 1993.

216. Hagen, T. C., M. A. Arnaout, and W. J. Schertzer. Antisera to vasoactive intestinal peptide inhibit basal prolactin release from dispersed anterior pituitary cells. *Neuroendocrinology* 43: 641–645, 1986.

217. Halvorson, L. M., J. Weiss, A. C. Bauer-Dantoin, and J. L. Jameson. Dynamic regulation of pituitary follistatin messenger ribonucleic acids during the rat estrous cycle. *Endocrinology* 134: 1247–1253, 1994.

218. Hammond, J. M., C. J. Hsu, J. Klindt, B. K. Tsang, and B. R. Downey. Gonadotropins increase concentrations of immunoreactive insulin-like growth factor-I in porcine follicular fluid in vivo. *Biol. Reprod.* 38: 304–308, 1988.

219. Hammond, J. M., J. S. Mondschein, S. E. Samaras, and S. F. Canning. The ovarian insulin-like growth factors, a local amplification mechanism for steroidogenesis and hormone action. *J. Steroid Biochem. Mol. Biol.* 40: 411–416, 1991.

220. Hammond, J. M., S. E. Samaras, R. Grimes, J. Leighton, J. Barber, S. F. Canning, and H. D. Guthrie. The role of insulin-like growth factors and epidermal growth factor-related peptides in intraovarian regulation in the pig ovary. *J. Reprod. Fertil. Suppl.* 48: 117–125, 1993.

221. Han, V. K., F. Lu, N. Bassett, K. P. Yang, P. J. Delhanty, and J. R. Challis. Insulin-like growth factor-II (IGF-II) messenger ribonucleic acid is expressed in steroidogenic cells of the developing ovine adrenal gland: evidence of an autocrine/paracrine role for IGF-II. *Endocrinology* 131: 3100–3109, 1992.

222. Handelsman, D. J., J. A. Spaliviero, and A. F. Phippard. Highly vectorial secretion of inhibin by primate Sertoli cells in vitro. *J. Clin. Endocrinol. Metab.* 71: 1235–1238, 1990.

223. Hansson, H. A., H. Billig, and J. Isgaard. Insulin-like growth factor I in the developing and mature rat testis: immunohistochemical aspects. *Biol. Reprod.* 40: 1321–1328, 1989.

224. Harris, P. E., J. M. Alexander, H. A. Bikkal, D. W. Hsu, E. T. Hedley-Whyte, A. Klibanski, and J. L. Jameson. Glycoprotein hormone alpha-subunit production in somatotroph adenomas with and without Gs alpha mutations. *J. Clin. Endocrinol. Metab.* 75: 918–923, 1992.

225. Hashimoto, K., K. Murakami, T. Hattori, M. Niimi, K. Fujino, and Z. Ota. Corticotropin-releasing factor (CRF)-like immunoreactivity in the adrenal medulla. *Peptides* 5: 707–711, 1984.

226. Hashimoto, T., H. Kawano, S. Daikoku, K. Shima, H. Tani-

guchi, and S. Baba. Transient coappearance of glucagon and insulin in the progenitor cells of the rat pancreatic islets. *Anat. Embryol. (Berl.)* 178: 489–497, 1988.

227. Hawthorn, J., S. S. Nussey, J. R. Henderson, and J. S. Jenkins. Immunohistochemical localization of oxytocin and vasopressin in the adrenal glands of rat, cow, hamster and guinea pig. *Cell Tissue Res.* 250: 1–6, 1987.

228. Healy, D. P., M. Q. Ye, L. X. Yuan, and B. S. Schachter. Stimulation of angiotensinogen mRNA levels in rat pituitary by estradiol. *Am. J. Physiol.* 263 (*Endocrinol. Metab.* 26): E355–E361, 1992.

229. Henion, P. D., and S. C. Landis. Asynchronous appearance and topographic segregation of neuropeptide-containing cells in the developing rat adrenal medulla. *J. Neurosci.* 10: 2886–2896, 1990.

230. Henriksen, R., K. Funa, E. Wilander, T. Backstrom, M. Ridderheim, and K. Oberg. Expression and prognostic significance of platelet-derived growth factor and its receptors in epithelial ovarian neoplasms. *Cancer Res.* 53: 4550–4554, 1993.

231. Hermansen, K. Enkephalins and the secretion of pancreatic somatostatin and insulin in the dog: studies in vitro. *Endocrinology* 113: 1149–1154, 1983.

232. Hernandez, E. R., A. Hurwitz, D. W. Payne, A. M. Dharmarajan, A. F. Purchio, and E. Y. Adashi. Transforming growth factor-beta 1 inhibits ovarian androgen production: gene expression, cellular localization, mechanisms(s), and site(s) of action. *Endocrinology* 127: 2804–2811, 1990.

233. Hernandez, E. R., C. E. Resnick, M. E. Svoboda, J. J. Van Wyk, D. W. Payne, and E. Y. Adashi. Somatomedin-C/insulin-like growth factor I as an enhancer of androgen biosynthesis by cultured rat ovarian cells. *Endocrinology* 122: 1603–1612, 1988.

234. Hernandez, E. R., C. T. Roberts, Jr., A. Hurwitz, D. LeRoith, and E. Y. Adashi. Rat ovarian insulin-like growth factor II gene expression is theca-interstitial cell-exclusive: hormonal regulation and receptor distribution. *Endocrinology* 127: 3249–3251, 1990.

235. Higuchi, H., K. Yokokawa, A. Iwasa, H. Yoshida, and N. Miki. Age-dependent increase in neuropeptide Y gene expression in rat adrenal gland and specific brain areas. *J. Neurochem.* 57: 1840–1847, 1991.

236. Hillier, S. G. Intrafollicular paracrine function of ovarian androgen. *J. Steroid Biochem.* 27: 351–357, 1987.

237. Hillier, S. G., and F. Miro. Inhibin, activin, and follistatin. Potential roles in ovarian physiology. *Ann. N.Y. Acad. Sci.* 687: 29–38, 1993.

238. Hillier, S. G., C. D. Smyth, P. F. Whitelaw, F. Miro, and C. M. Howles. Gonadotrophin control of follicular function. *Horm. Res.* 43: 216–223, 1995.

239. Hillier, S. G., E. L. Yong, P. J. Illingworth, D. T. Baird, R. H. Schwall, and A. J. Mason. Effect of recombinant activin on androgen synthesis in cultured human thecal cells. *J. Clin. Endocrinol. Metab.* 72: 1206–1211, 1991.

240. Hillier, S. G., E. L. Yong, P. J. Illingworth, D. T. Baird, R. H. Schwall, and A. J. Mason. Effect of recombinant inhibin on androgen synthesis in cultured human thecal cells [published erratum appears in *Mol. Cell. Endocrinol.* 79: 177, 1991]. *Mol. Cell. Endocrinol.* 75: R1–R6, 1991.

241. Hinkle, P. M., and P. A. Kinsella. Thyroid hormone induction of an autocrine growth factor secreted by pituitary tumor cells. *Science* 234: 1549–1552, 1986.

242. Hinson, J. P. Paracrine control of adrenocortical function: a new role for the medulla? *J. Endocrinol.* 124: 7–9, 1990.

243. Ho, M. M., and G. P. Vinson. Endocrine control of the distribution of basic fibroblast growth factor, insulin-like growth

factor-I and transforming growth factor-beta 1 mRNAs in adult rat adrenals using non-radioactive in situ hybridization. *J. Endocrinol.* 144: 379–387, 1995.

244. Ho, T. W., J. R. Greenan, and A. M. Walker. Mammotroph autoregulation: the differential roles of the 24K isoforms of prolactin. *Endocrinology* 124: 1507–1514, 1989.

245. Hofbauer, L. C., M. Rafferzeder, O. E. Janssen, and R. Gartner. Insulin-like growth factor I messenger ribonucleic acid expression in porcine thyroid follicles is regulated by thyrotropin and iodine [see comments]. *Eur. J. Endocrinol.* 132: 605–610, 1995.

246. Hong, M., S. Li, A. Fournier, S. St.-Pierre, and G. Pelletier. Role of neuropeptide Y in the regulation of tyrosine hydroxylase gene expression in rat adrenal glands. *Neuroendocrinology* 61: 85–88, 1995.

247. Hoppener, J. W., P. H. Steenbergh, R. J. Slebos, P. de Pagter-Holthuizen, B. A. Roos, M. Jansen, J. L. Van den Brande, J. S. Sussenbach, H. S. Jansz, and C. J. Lips. Expression of insulin-like growth factor-I and -II genes in rat medullary thyroid carcinoma. *FEBS Lett.* 215: 122–126, 1987.

248. Houben, H., and C. Denef. Stimulation of growth hormone and prolactin release from rat pituitary cell aggregates by bombesin- and ranatensin-like peptides is potentiated by estradiol, 5 alpha-dihydrotestosterone, and dexamethasone. *Endocrinology* 126: 2257–2266, 1990.

249. Houben, H., and C. Denef. Evidence for the presence of gastrin-releasing peptide immunoreactivity in rat anterior pituitary corticotrophs and lactotrophs, AtT20 cells, and GH3 cells: failure to demonstrate participation in local control of hormone release. *Endocrinology* 128: 3208–3218, 1991.

250. Houben, H., and C. Denef. Negative regulation by dexamethasone of the potentiation of neuromedin C-induced growth hormone and prolactin release by estradiol in anterior pituitary cell aggregates. *Life Sci.* 50: 775–780, 1992.

251. Houben, H., and C. Denef. Autoradiographic localization of bombesin receptors in anterior pituitary. *Peptides* 15: 1–5, 1994a.

252. Houben, H., and C. Denef. Bioactive peptides in anterior pituitary cells. *Peptides* 15: 547–582, 1994b.

253. Houben, H., A. T. Vandenbroucke, A. M. Verheyden, and C. Denef. Expression of the genes encoding bombesin-related peptides and their receptors in anterior pituitary tissue. *Mol. Cell. Endocrinol.* 97: 159–164, 1993.

254. Howl, J., S. A. Rudge, R. A. Lavis, A. R. Davies, R. A. Parslow, P. J. Hughes, C. J. Kirk, R. H. Michell, and M. Wheatley. Rat testicular myoid cells express vasopressin receptors: receptor structure, signal transduction, and developmental regulation. *Endocrinology* 136: 2206–2213, 1995.

255. Hsu, C. J., and J. M. Hammond. Gonadotropins and estradiol stimulate immunoreactive insulin-like growth factor-I production by porcine granulosa cells in vitro. *Endocrinology* 120: 198–207, 1987.

256. Hsueh, A. J. Paracrine mechanisms involved in granulosa cell differentiation. *Clin. Endocrinol. Metab.* 15: 117–134, 1986.

257. Hsueh, A. J., K. D. Dahl, J. Vaughan, E. Tucker, J. Rivier, C. W. Bardin, and W. Vale. Heterodimers and homodimers of inhibin subunits have different paracrine action in the modulation of luteinizing hormone-stimulated androgen biosynthesis. *Proc. Natl. Acad. Sci. U.S.A.* 84: 5082–5086, 1987.

259. Hsueh, A. J., and J. M. Schaeffer. Gonadotropin-releasing hormone as a paracrine hormone and neurotransmitter in extra-pituitary sites. *J. Steroid Biochem.* 23: 757–764, 1985.

260. Hughes, C. E., and D. F. Sellitti. Thyroidal ANF: a possible mediator of autocrine regulation in the porcine thyroid gland. *Peptides* 12: 705–714, 1991.

261. Hummel, A., and H. Zuhlke. Expression of two proopiomelanocortin mRNAs in the islets of Langerhans of neonatal rats. *Biol. Chem. Hoppe Seyler* 375: 811–815, 1994.

262. Hurwitz, A., E. R. Hernandez, C. E. Resnick, J. N. Packman, D. W. Payne, and E. Y. Adashi. Basic fibroblast growth factor inhibits gonadotropin-supported ovarian androgen biosynthesis: mechanism(s) and site(s) of action. *Endocrinology* 126: 3089–3095, 1990.

263. Hurwitz, A., D. W. Payne, J. N. Packman, C. L. Andreani, C. E. Resnick, E. R. Hernandez, and E. Y. Adashi. Cytokine-mediated regulation of ovarian function: interleukin-1 inhibits gonadotropin-induced androgen biosynthesis. *Endocrinology* 129: 1250–1256, 1991.

264. Hurwitz, A., E. Ricciarelli, L. Botero, R. M. Rohan, E. R. Hernandez, and E. Y. Adashi. Endocrine- and autocrine-mediated regulation of rat ovarian (theca-interstitial) interleukin-1 beta gene expression: gonadotropin-dependent preovulatory acquisition. *Endocrinology* 129: 3427–3429, 1991.

265. Hutson, J. C. Secretion of tumor necrosis factor alpha by testicular macrophages. *J.Reprod. Immunol.* 23: 63–72, 1993.

266. Ikeda, K., E. C. Weir, M. Mangin, P. S. Dannies, B. Kinder, L. J. Deftos, E. M. Brown, and A. E. Broadus. Expression of messenger ribonucleic acids encoding a parathyroid hormone-like peptide in normal human and animal tissues with abnormal expression in human parathyroid adenomas. *Mol. Endocrinol.* 2: 1230–1236, 1988.

267. Inturrisi, C. E., A. D. Branch, H. D. Robertson, R. D. Howells, S. O. Franklin, J. R. Shapiro, S. E. Calvano, and B. C. Yoburn. Glucocorticoid regulation of enkephalins in cultured rat adrenal medulla. *Mol. Endocrinol.* 2: 633–640, 1988.

268. Ivell, R., N. Hunt, M. Hardy, H. Nicholson, and B. Pickering. Vasopressin biosynthesis in rodent Leydig cells. *Mol. Cell. Endocrinol.* 89: 59–66, 1992.

269. Jackson, S., S. Hodgkinson, F. E. Estivariz, and P. J. Lowry. IGF1 and 2 in two models of adrenal growth. *J. Steroid Biochem. Mol. Biol.* 40: 399–404, 1991.

270. Jarry, H., M. Dietrich, A. Barthel, A. Giesler, and W. Wuttke. In vivo demonstration of a paracrine, inhibitory action of met-enkephalin on adrenomedullary catecholamine release in the rat. *Endocrinology* 125: 624–629, 1989.

271. Jia, L. G., B. J. Canny, and D.A. Leong. Paracrine communication regulates adrenocorticotropin secretion. *Endocrinology* 130: 534–539, 1992.

272. Jindal, S. K., D. M. Snoey, D. K. Lobb, and J. H. Dorrington. Transforming growth factor alpha localization and role in surface epithelium of normal human ovaries and in ovarian carcinoma cells. *Gynecol. Oncol.* 53: 17–23, 1994.

273. Jones, C. T., and A. V. Edwards. Release of adrenocorticotrophin from the adrenal gland in the conscious calf. *J. Physiol. (Lond.)* 426: 397–407, 1990.

274. Jones, P. M., D. J. Withers, M. A. Ghatei, and S. R. Bloom. Evidence for neuromedin-B synthesis in the rat anterior pituitary gland. *Endocrinology* 130: 1829–1836, 1992.

275. Jones, T. H., B. L. Brown, and P. R. Dobson. Evidence that angiotensin II is a paracrine agent mediating gonadotrophin-releasing hormone-stimulated inositol phosphate production and prolactin secretion in the rat. *J. Endocrinol.* 116: 367–371, 1988.

276. Jones, T. H., B. L. Brown, and P. R. Dobson. Paracrine control of anterior pituitary hormone secretion. *J. Endocrinol.* 127: 5–13, 1990.

277. Jorns, A., E. Barklage, and D. Grube. Heterogeneities of the islets in the rabbit pancreas and the problem of "paracrine" regulation of islet cells. *Anat. Embryol. (Berl.)* 178: 297–307, 1988.

278. Jorns, A., and D. Grube. The endocrine pancreas of glucagon- and somatostatin-immunized rabbits. II. Electron microscopy. *Cell Tissue Res.* 265: 261–273, 1991.

279. Judd, A.M., and R. M. MacLeod. Adrenocorticotropin increases interleukin-6 release from rat adrenal zona glomerulosa cells. *Endocrinology* 130: 1245–1254, 1992.

280. Kaiser, U. B., B. L. Lee, R. S. Carroll, G. Unabia, W.W. Chin, and G.V. Childs. Follistatin gene expression in the pituitary: localization in gonadotropes and folliculostellate cells in diestrous rats. *Endocrinology* 130: 3048–3056, 1992.

281. Kalisnik, M., O. Vraspir-Porenta, T. Kham-Lindtner, M. Logonder-Mlinsek, Z. Pajer, D. Stiblar-Martincic, R. Zorc-Pleskovic, and M. Trobina. The interdependence of the follicular, parafollicular, and mast cells in the mammalian thyroid gland: a review and a synthesis [published erratum appears in *Am. J. Anat.* 185: 101, 1989]. *Am. J. Anat.* 183: 148–157, 1988.

282. Kanaka-Gantenbein, C., E. Dicou, P. Czernichow, and R. Scharfmann. Presence of nerve growth factor and its receptors in an in vitro model of islet cell development: implication in normal islet morphogenesis. *Endocrinology* 136: 3154–3162, 1995.

283. Kasper, M. Cytokeratins in intracranial and intraspinal tissues. *Adv. Anat. Embryol. Cell Biol.* 126: 1–82, 1992.

284. Kasson, B. G., R. Meidan, and A. J. Hsueh. Identification and characterization of arginine vasopressin-like substances in the rat testis. *J. Biol. Chem.* 260: 5302–5307, 1985.

285. Kataoka, Y., M. Fujimoto, H. Alho, A. Guidotti, M. Geffard, G. D. Kelly, and I. Hanbauer. Intrinsic gamma aminobutyric acid receptors modulate the release of catecholamine from canine adrenal gland in situ. *J. Pharmacol. Exp. Ther.* 239: 584–590, 1986.

286. Kataoka, Y., Y. Gutman, A. Guidotti, P. Panula, J. Wroblewski, D. Cosenza-Murphy, J. Y. Wu, and E. Costa. Intrinsic GABAergic system of adrenal chromaffin cells. *Proc. Natl. Acad. Sci. U.S.A.* 81: 3218–3222, 1984.

287. Katayama, T., K. Shiota, H. Sugino, and M. Takahashi. Paracrine effect of follicculo-stellate cells on the growth factor-like action of activin A in anterior pituitary cultures. *Endocrinol. Jpn.* 39: 289–297, 1992.

289. Kauth, T., and J. Metz. Immunohistochemical localization of glucagon-like peptide 1. Use of poly-and monoclonal antibodies. *Histochemistry* 86: 509–515, 1987.

290. Kendall, S. K., T. L. Saunders, L. Jin, R. V. Lloyd, L. M. Glode, T. M. Nett, R. A. Keri, J. H. Nilson, and S. A. Camper. Targeted ablation of pituitary gonadotropes in transgenic mice. *Mol. Endocrinol.* 5: 2025–2036, 1991.

291. Keramidas, M., J. J. Bourgarit, E. Tabone, P. Corticelli, E. M. Chambaz, and J. J. Feige. Immunolocalization of transforming growth factor-beta 1 in the bovine adrenal cortex using anti-peptide antibodies. *Endocrinology* 129: 517–526, 1991.

292. Kettani, S., V. Beldent, M. C. Rousselet, P. Ronco, P. Verroust, and J. P. Saint-Andre. Presence of renin, angiotensinogen, angiotensin II in the lamb anterior pituitary gland: immunocytochemical study after cryoultramicrotomy. *Histochemistry* 95: 561–566, 1991.

293. Kew, D., and D. L. Kilpatrick. Expression and regulation of the proenkephalin gene in rat Sertoli cells. *Mol. Endocrinol.* 3: 179–184, 1989.

294. Kew, D., K. E. Muffly, and D. L. Kilpatrick. Proenkephalin products are stored in the sperm acrosome and may function in fertilization. *Proc. Natl. Acad. Sci. U.S.A.* 87: 9143–9147, 1990.

295. Khan, S. A., S. J. Khan, and J. H. Dorrington. Interleukin-1 stimulates deoxyribonucleic acid synthesis in immature rat Leydig cells in vitro. *Endocrinology* 131: 1853–1857, 1992.

296. Khan-Dawood, F. S., and M. Y. Dawood. Paracrine regulation of luteal function. *Clin. Endocrinol. Metab.* 15: 171–184, 1986.

297. Khan-Dawood, F. S., L. T. Goldsmith, G. Weiss, and M. Y. Dawood. Human corpus luteum secretion of relaxin, oxytocin, and progesterone. *J. Clin. Endocrinol. Metab.* 68: 627–631, 1989.

298. Khanum, A., and M. L. Dufau. Angiotensin II receptors and inhibitory actions in the Leydig cells. *J. Biol. Chem.* 263: 5070–5074, 1988.

299. Kilpatrick, D. L., and C. F. Millette. Expression of proenkephalin messenger RNA by mouse spermatogenic cells. *Proc. Natl. Acad. Sci. U.S.A.* 83: 5015–5018, 1986.

300. Kitayama, S., Y. Koyama, K. Morita, T. Dohi, and A. Tsujimoto. Increase in catecholamine release and $^{45}Ca^{2+}$ uptake induced by GABA in cultured bovine adrenal chromaffin cells. *Eur. J. Pharmacol.* 131: 145–147, 1986.

301. Kitayama, S., K. Morita, T. Dohi, and A. Tsujimoto. Enhancement by GABA of the stimulation-evoked catecholamine release from cultured bovine adrenal chromaffin cells. *Naunyn Schmiedebergs Arch. Pharmacol.* 341: 414–418, 1990.

302. Klaff, L. J., and G. J. Taborsky, Jr. Pancreatic somatostatin is a mediator of glucagon inhibition by hyperglycemia. *Diabetes* 36: 592–596, 1987.

303. Klaij, I. A., A. M. van Pelt, M. A. Timmerman, L. J. Blok, D. G. de Rooij, and F. H. de Jong. Expression of inhibin subunit mRNAs and inhibin levels in the testes of rats with stage-synchronized spermatogenesis. *J. Endocrinol.* 141: 131–141, 1994.

304. Knudtzon, J. Effects of pro-opiomelanocortin-derived peptides on plasma levels of glucagon, insulin and glucose. *Horm. Metab. Res.* 18: 579–583, 1986.

305. Kobrin, M. S., S. L. Asa, J. Samsoondar, and J. E. Kudlow. Alpha-transforming growth factor in the bovine anterior pituitary gland: secretion by dispersed cells and immunohistochemical localization. *Endocrinology* 121: 1412–1416, 1987.

306. Kong, J. Y., A. Thureson-Klein, and R. L. Klein. Differential distribution of neuropeptides and serotonin in pig adrenal glands. *Neuroscience* 28: 765–775, 1989.

307. Kononen, J., S. Soinila, H. Persson, J. Honkaniemi, T. Hokfelt, and M. Pelto-Huikko. Neurotrophins and their receptors in the rat pituitary gland: regulation of BDNF and trkB mRNA levels by adrenal hormones. *Brain Res. Mol. Brain Res.* 27: 347–354, 1994.

308. Kotsuji, F., and T. Tominaga. The role of granulosa and theca cell interactions in ovarian structure and function. *Microsc. Res. Tech.* 27: 97–107, 1994.

309. Kraiem, Z., O. Sadeh, M. Yosef, and A. Aharon. Mutual antagonistic interactions between the thyrotropin (adenosine 3',5'-monophosphate) and protein kinase C/epidermal growth factor (tyrosine kinase) pathways in cell proliferation and differentiation of cultured human thyroid follicles. *Endocrinology* 136: 585–590, 1995.

310. Krown, K. A., Y. F. Wang, T. W. Ho, P. A. Kelly, and A. M. Walker. Prolactin isoform 2 as an autocrine growth factor for GH3 cells. *Endocrinology* 131: 595–602, 1992.

311. Krown, K. A., Y. F. Wang, and A. M. Walker. Autocrine interaction between prolactin and its receptor occurs intracellularly in the 235–1 mammotroph cell line. *Endocrinology* 134: 1546–1552, 1994.

312. Krummen, L. A., A. Moore, T. K. Woodruff, R. Covello, R. Taylor, P. Working, and J. P. Mather. Localization of inhibin and activin binding sites in the testis during development by in situ ligand binding. *Biol. Reprod.* 50: 734–744, 1994.

313. Kubota, T., A. M. Judd, and R. M. MacLeod. The paracrine role of angiotensin in gonadotrophin-releasing hormone-stimulated prolactin release in rats. *J. Endocrinol.* 125: 225–232, 1990.

314. Kubota, T., S. Kamada, and T. Aso. Endothelin-1 as a local ovarian regulator in porcine granulosa cells. *Horm. Res.* 41 (Suppl. 1): 29–35, 1994.

315. Kugu, K., Y. Taketani, and M. Mizuno. Stimulatory action of prolactin on gonadotropin secretion in vitro. *Endocrinol. Jpn.* 36: 509–514, 1989.

316. Lam, K. S., F. M. Lechan, N. Minamitani, and S. Reichlin. Vasoactive intestinal peptide in the anterior pituitary is increased in hypothyroidism. *Endocrinology* 124: 1077–1084, 1989.

317. LaPolt, P. S., M. Yamoto, M. Veljkovic, C. Sincich, T. Ny, A. Tsafriri, and A. J. Hsueh. Basic fibroblast growth factor induction of granulosa cell tissue-type plasminogen activator expression and oocyte maturation: potential role as a paracrine ovarian hormone. *Endocrinology* 127: 2357–2363, 1990.

318. Lara, J. I., M. J. Lorenzo, L. Cacicedo, R. M. Tolon, J. A. Balsa, J. Lopez-Fernandez, and F. Sanchez-Franco. Induction of vasoactive intestinal peptide gene expression and prolactin secretion by insulin-like growth factor I in rat pituitary cells: evidence for an autoparacrine regulatory system. *Endocrinology* 135: 2526–2532, 1994.

319. Leboulenger, F., M. Benyamina, C. Delarue, S. Netchitailo, S. Saint-Pierre, and H. Vaudry. Neuronal and paracrine regulation of adrenal steroidogenesis: interactions between acetylcholine, serotonin and vasoactive intestinal peptide (VIP) on corticosteroid production by frog interrenal tissue. *Brain Res.* 453: 103–109, 1988.

320. Leboulenger, F., Y. Charnay, P. M. Dubois, J. Rossier, D. H. Coy, G. Pelletier, and H. Vaudry. The coexistence of neuropeptides and catecholamines in the adrenal gland. Research on paracrine effects on adrenal cortex cells. *Ann. Endocrinol. (Paris)* 45: 217–227, 1984.

321. Lecerf, L., V. Rouiller-Fabre, C. Levacher, C. Gautier, J. M. Saez, and R. Habert. Stimulatory effect of follicle-stimulating hormone on basal and luteinizing hormone-stimulated testosterone secretions by the fetal rat testis in vitro. *Endocrinology* 133: 2313–2318, 1993.

322. Leduque, P., M. Bulant, P. M. Dubois, P. Nicolas, and H. Vaudry. Processing of thyrotropin-releasing hormone prohormone (pro-TRH) in the adult rat pancreas: identification and localization of pro-TRH-related peptides in beta-cells of pancreatic islets. *Endocrinology* 125: 1492–1497, 1989.

323. Lee, B. L., G. Unabia, and G. Childs. Expression of follistatin mRNA by somatotropes and mammotropes early in the rat estrous cycle. *J. Histochem. Cytochem.* 41: 955–960, 1993.

324. Lee, M. S., D. Gu, L. Feng, et al. Accumulation of extracellular matrix and developmental dysregulation in the pancreas by transgenic production of transforming growth factor-beta 1. *Am. J. Pathol.* 147: 42–52, 1995.

325. Lee, Y. J., S. R. Lin, S. J. Shin, Y. H. Lai, Y. T. Lin, and J. H. Tsai. Brain natriuretic peptide is synthesized in the human adrenal medulla and its messenger ribonucleic acid expression along with that of atrial natriuretic peptide are enhanced in patients with primary aldosteronism. *J. Clin. Endocrinol. Metab.* 79: 1476–1482, 1994.

326. Lefebvre, H., V. Contesse, C. Delarue, M. Feuilloley, F. Hery, P. Grise, G. Raynaud, A. A. Verhofstad, L. M. Wolf, and H. Vaudry. Serotonin-induced stimulation of cortisol secretion from human adrenocortical tissue is mediated through activation of a serotonin4 receptor subtype. *Neuroscience* 47: 999–1007, 1992.

327. Leffert, J. D., C. B. Newgard, H. Okamoto, J. L. Milburn, and K. L. Luskey. Rat amylin: cloning and tissue-specific expression

in pancreatic islets. *Proc. Natl. Acad. Sci. U.S.A.* 86:3127–3130,1989.

328. Le Gall, S., C. Feral, and P. Leymarie. Renin–angiotensin system of the uterus and ovary in mammalian females. *Reprod. Nutr. Dev.* 33: 185–198, 1993.

329. Le Magueresse, B., and B. Jegou. Paracrine control of immature Sertoli cells by adult germ cells, in the rat (an in vitro study). Cell–cell interactions within the testis. *Mol. Cell. Endocrinol.* 58: 65–72, 1988.

330. Le Magueresse-Battistoni, B., A. M. Morera, I. Goddard, and M. Benahmed. Expression of mRNAs for transforming growth factor-beta receptors in the rat testis. *Endocrinology* 136: 2788–2791, 1995.

331. Lemaire, S., R. Day, M. Dumont, L. Chouinard, and R. Calvert. Dynorphin and enkephalins in adrenal paraneurones. Opiates in the adrenal medulla. *Can. J. Physiol. Pharmacol.* 62: 484–492, 1984.

332. Leonard, J. F., M. T. Bluet-Pajot, C. Oliver, and C. Kordon. Interaction of vasoactive intestinal peptide (VIP) and growth hormone releasing factor (GRF) with corticotropin releasing factor (CRF) on corticotropin secretion in vitro. *Neuropeptides* 12: 131–133, 1988.

333. Li, H., G. P. Risbridger, and J. A. Clements. Pro-opiomelanocortin (POMC) gene expression, as identified by in situ hybridization, in purified populations of interstitial macrophages and Leydig cells of the adult rat testis. *Reprod. Fertil. Dev.* 5: 545–554, 1993.

334. Li, W., B. H. Yuen, and P. C. Leung. Inhibition of progestin accumulation by activin-A in human granulosa cells. *J. Clin. Endocrinol. Metab.* 75: 285–289, 1992.

335. Lin, T., D. L. Wang, J. H. Calkins, H. Guo, R. Chi, and P. R. Housley. Regulation of insulin-like growth factor-I messenger ribonucleic acid expression in Leydig cells. *Mol. Cell. Endocrinol.* 73: 147–152, 1990.

336. Ling, N., L. V. DePaolo, T. A. Bicsak, and S. Shimasaki. Novel ovarian regulatory peptides: inhibin, activin, and follistatin. *Clin. Obstet. Gynecol.* 33: 690–702, 1990.

337. Lloyd, R. V., L. Jin, A. Chang, E. Kulig, S. A. Camper, B. D. Ross, T. R. Downs, and L. A. Frohman. Morphologic effects of hGRH gene expression on the pituitary, liver, and pancreas of MT-hGRH transgenic mice. An in situ hybridization analysis. *Am. J. Pathol.* 141: 895–906, 1992.

338. Lobb, D. K., M. S. Kobrin, J. E. Kudlow, and J. H. Dorrington. Transforming growth factor-alpha in the adult bovine ovary: identification in growing ovarian follicles. *Biol. Reprod.* 40: 1087–1093, 1989.

339. Logan, A. Intracrine regulation at the nucleus—a further mechanism of growth factor activity? *J. Endocrinol.* 125: 339–343, 1990.

340. Lonnerberg, P., O. Soder, M. Parvinen, E. M. Ritzen, and H. Persson. Beta-nerve growth factor influences the expression of androgen-binding protein messenger ribonucleic acid in the rat testis. *Biol. Reprod.* 47: 381–388, 1992.

341. Lovegren, E. S., S. J. Zimniski, and D. Puett. Ovarian contents of immunoreactive beta-endorphin and alpha-N-acetylated opioid peptides in rats. *J. Reprod. Fertil.* 91: 91–100, 1991.

342. Lukinius, A., E. Wilander, G. T. Westermark, U. Engstrom, and P. Westermark. Co-localization of islet amyloid polypeptide and insulin in the B cell secretory granules of the human pancreatic islets. *Diabetologia* 32: 240–244, 1989.

343. Lundberg, J. M., T. Hokfelt, A. Hemsen, E. Theodorsson-Norheim, J. Pernow, B. Hamberger, and M. Goldstein. Neuropeptide Y-like immunoreactivity in adrenalin cells of adrenal medulla and in tumors and plasma of pheochromocytoma patients. *Regul. Pept.* 13: 169–182, 1986.

344. Ma, Y. J., G. A. Dissen, G. Merlino, A. Coquelin, and S. R. Ojeda. Overexpression of a human transforming growth factor-alpha (TGF alpha) transgene reveals a dual antagonistic role of TGF alpha in female sexual development. *Endocrinology* 135: 1392–1400, 1994.

345. Maake, C., and M. Reinecke. Immunohistochemical localization of insulin-like growth factor 1 and 2 in the endocrine pancreas of rat, dog, and man, and their coexistence with classical islet hormones. *Cell Tissue Res.* 273: 249–259, 1993.

346. Maciel, R. M., A. C. Moses, G. Villone, D. Tramontano, and S. H. Ingbar. Demonstration of the production and physiological role of insulin-like growth factor II in rat thyroid follicular cells in culture. *J. Clin. Invest.* 82: 1546–1553, 1988.

347. Magoffin, D. A., B. Gancedo, and G. F. Erickson. Transforming growth factor-beta promotes differentiation of ovarian thecal-interstitial cells but inhibits androgen production. *Endocrinology* 125: 1951–1958, 1989.

348. Maillard, N., S. Wolczynski, A. Argyriou, M. A. Drosdowsky, P. Foucault, and S. Carreau. Steroidogenesis in the two enriched-Leydig cell populations of human testis: evidence for a positive control by seminiferous tubules secreted factor(s). *Arch. Androl.* 33: 187–199, 1994.

349. Majane, E. A., H. Alho, Y. Kataoka, C. H. Lee, and H. Y. Yang. Neuropeptide Y in bovine adrenal glands: distribution and characterization. *Endocrinology* 117: 1162–1168, 1985.

350. Malarkey, W. B., B. J. Zvara, and V. L. DeGroff. Angiotensin II promotes prolactin release from normal human anterior pituitary cell cultures in a calcium-dependent manner. *J. Clin. Endocrinol. Metab.* 64: 713–717, 1987.

351. Mann, D. R., and T. E. Orr. Effect of restraint stress on gonadal proopiomelanocortin peptides and the pituitary–testicular axis in rats. *Life Sci.* 46: 1601–1609, 1990.

352. Margioris, A. N., G. Koukoulis, M. Grino, and G. P. Chrousos. In vitro-perfused rat testes secrete beta-endorphin and dynorphin: their effect on testosterone secretion. *Biol. Reprod.* 40: 776–784, 1989.

353. Margioris, A. N., A. S. Liotta, H. Vaudry, C. W. Bardin, and D. T. Krieger. Characterization of immunoreactive proopiomelanocortin-related peptides in rat testes. *Endocrinology* 113: 663–671, 1983.

354. Maruo, T., C. A. Ladines-Llave, T. Samoto, H. Matsuo, A. S. Manalo, H. Ito, and M. Mochizuki. Expression of epidermal growth factor and its receptor in the human ovary during follicular growth and regression. *Endocrinology* 132: 924–931, 1993.

355. Mason, H. D., L. Carr, R. Leake, and S. Franks. Production of transforming growth factor-alpha by normal and polycystic ovaries. *J. Clin. Endocrinol. Metab.* 80: 2053–2056, 1995.

356. Mastorakos, G., C. D. Scopa, A. Vryonidou, T. C. Friedman, D. Kattis, C. Phenekos, M. J. Merino, and G. P. Chrousos. Presence of immunoreactive corticotropin-releasing hormone in normal and polycystic human ovaries. *J. Clin. Endocrinol. Metab.* 79: 1191–1197, 1994.

357. Mastorakos, G., E. L. Webster, T. C. Friedman, and G. P. Chrousos. Immunoreactive corticotropin-releasing hormone and its binding sites in the rat ovary. *J. Clin. Invest.* 92: 961–968, 1993.

358. Mather, J. P., K. M. Attie, T. K. Woodruff, G. C. Rice, and D. M. Phillips. Activin stimulates spermatogonial proliferation in germ–Sertoli cell cocultures from immature rat testis. *Endocrinology* 127: 3206–3214, 1990.

359. Matsumura, T., H. Itoh, N. Watanabe, Y. Oda, M. Tanaka, M. Namba, N. Kono, T. Matsuyama, R. Komatsu, and Y. Matsuzawa. Glucagonlike peptide-1(7–36)amide suppresses glucagon secretion and decreases cyclic AMP concentration in

cultured In-R1–G9 cells. *Biochem. Biophys. Res. Commun.* 186: 503–508, 1992.

360. Matzuk, M. M., T. R. Kumar, and A. Bradley. Different phenotypes for mice deficient in either activins or activin receptor type II [see comments]. *Nature* 374: 356–360, 1995.

361. Maubert, E., G. Tramu, D. Croix, J. C. Beauvillain, and J. P. Dupouy. Co-localization of vasoactive intestinal polypeptide and neuropeptide Y immunoreactivities in the nerve fibers of the rat adrenal gland. *Neurosci. Lett.* 113: 121–126, 1990.

362. Mazzocchi, G., L. K. Malendowicz, P. Rebuffat, and G. G. Nussdorfer. Effects of galanin on the secretory activity of the rat adrenal cortex: in vivo and in vitro studies. *Res. Exp. Med. (Berl.)* 192: 373–381, 1992.

363. McGregor, G. P., R. Hartel, R. Haberberger, W. Kummer, and K. Voigt. Preprotachykinin-A gene expression occurs transiently in the developing rat endocrine pancreas and can be regulated in RINm5F cells. *Endocrinology* 136: 2538–2546, 1995.

364. Meunier, H., C. Rivier, R. M. Evans, and W. Vale. Gonadal and extragonadal expression of inhibin alpha, beta A, and beta B subunits in various tissues predicts diverse functions. *Proc. Natl. Acad. Sci. U.S.A.* 85: 247–251, 1988.

367. Minamino, N., A. Uehara, and A. Arimura. Biological and immunological characterization of corticotropin-releasing activity in the bovine adrenal medulla. *Peptides* 9: 37–45, 1988.

368. Missale, C., F. Boroni, M. Frassine, A. Caruso, and P. Spano. Nerve growth factor promotes the differentiation of pituitary mammotroph cells in vitro. *Endocrinology* 136: 1205–1213, 1995.

369. Missale, C., F. Boroni, M. Losa, M. Giovanelli, A. Zanellato, R. Dal Toso, A. Balsari, and P. Spano. Nerve growth factor suppresses the transforming phenotype of human prolactinomas. *Proc. Natl. Acad. Sci. U.S.A.* 90: 7961–7965, 1993.

370. Missale, C., F. Boroni, S. Sigala, L. Castelletti, P. Falardeau, R. Dal Toso, M. G. Caron, and P. Spano. Epidermal growth factor promotes uncoupling from adenylyl cyclase of the rat D2S receptor expressed in GH4C1 cells. *J. Neurochem.* 62: 907–915, 1994.

371. Missale, C., F. Boroni, S. Sigala, A. Zanellato, R. Dal Toso, A. Balsari, and P. Spano. Nerve growth factor directs differentiation of the bipotential cell line GH-3 into the mammotroph phenotype. *Endocrinology* 135: 290–298, 1994.

372. Mojsov, S., G. C. Weir, and J. F. Habener. Insulinotropin: glucagon-like peptide I (7–37) co-encoded in the glucagon gene is a potent stimulator of insulin release in the perfused rat pancreas. *J. Clin. Invest.* 79: 616–619, 1987.

373. Moltz, J. H., and C. P. Fawcett. Corticotropin-releasing factor inhibits insulin release from perfused rat pancreas. *Am. J. Physiol.* 248 (*Endocrinol. Metab.* 11): E741–E743, 1985.

374. Moltz, J. H., and C. P. Fawcett. Corticotropin-releasing factor: its action on the islets of Langerhans. *Endocr. Res.* 11: 87–93, 1985.

375. Moltz, J. H., and J. K. McDonald. Neuropeptide Y: direct and indirect action on insulin secretion in the rat. *Peptides* 6: 1155–1159, 1985.

376. Mondschein, J. S., S. F. Canning, D. Q. Miller, and J. M. Hammond. Insulin-like growth factors (IGFs) as autocrine/paracrine regulators of granulosa cell differentiation and growth: studies with a neutralizing monoclonal antibody to IGF-I. *Biol. Reprod.* 41: 79–85, 1989.

377. Moore, A., and I. D. Morris. Paracrine effects via the epidermal growth factor receptor in the rodent testis may be mediated by non-Leydig interstitial cells. *J. Endocrinol.* 136: 439–446, 1993.

378. Moore, C., and J. C. Hutson. Physiological relevance of tumor

necrosis factor in mediating macrophage–Leydig cell interactions. *Endocrinology* 134: 63–69, 1994.

379. Morel, G., J. G. Chabot, T. Garcia-Caballero, F. Gossard, F. Dihl, M. Belles-Isles, and S. Heisler. Synthesis, internalization, and localization of atrial natriuretic peptide in rat adrenal medulla. *Endocrinology* 123: 149–158, 1988.

380. Morel, G., A. Ouhtit, and P. A. Kelly. Prolactin receptor immunoreactivity in rat anterior pituitary. *Neuroendocrinology* 59: 78–84, 1994.

381. Moretti, C., A. Bagnato, N. Solan, G. Frajese, and K. J. Catt. Receptor-mediated actions of growth hormone releasing factor on granulosa cell differentiation. *Endocrinology* 127: 2117–2126, 1990.

382. Morra, M., F. Leboulenger, and H. Vaudry. Dopamine inhibits corticosteroid secretion from frog adrenal gland, in vitro. *Endocrinology* 127: 218–226, 1990.

383. Mueller, S. G., M. S. Kobrin, A. J. Paterson, and J. E. Kudlow. Transforming growth factor-alpha expression in the anterior pituitary gland: regulation by epidermal growth factor and phorbol ester in dispersed cells. *Mol. Endocrinol.* 3: 976–983, 1989.

384. Mullaney, B. P., and M. K. Skinner. Basic fibroblast growth factor gene expression and protein production during pubertal development of the seminiferous tubule: follicle stimulating hormone induced Sertoli cell bFGF expression. *Endocrinology* 131: 2928–2934, 1992.

385. Mullaney, B. P., and M. K. Skinner. Transforming growth factor-alpha and epidermal growth factor receptor gene expression and action during pubertal development of the seminiferous tubule. *Mol. Endocrinol.* 6: 2103–2113, 1992.

386. Mullaney, B. P., and M. K. Skinner. Transforming growth factor-beta (beta 1, beta 2, and beta 3) gene expression and action during pubertal development of the seminiferous tubule: potential role at the onset of spermatogenesis. *Mol. Endocrinol.* 7: 67–76, 1993.

387. Murray, J. F., J. A. Downing, G. Evans, J. K. Findlay, and R. J. Scaramuzzi. Epidermal growth factor acts directly on the sheep ovary in vivo to inhibit oestradiol-17 beta and inhibin secretion and enhance progesterone secretion. *J. Endocrinol.* 137: 253–264, 1993.

388. Myrsen, U., and F. Sundler. Neuropeptide Y is expressed in islet somatostatin cells of the hamster pancreas: a combined immunocytochemical and in situ hybridization study. *Regul. Pept.* 57: 65–76, 1995.

389. Nagy, G., J. J. Mulchahey, and J. D. Neill. Autocrine control of prolactin secretion by vasoactive intestinal peptide. *Endocrinology* 122: 364–366, 1988.

390. Naville, D., P. G. Chatelain, O. Avallet, and J. Saez. Control of production of insulin-like growth factor-I by pig Leydig and Sertoli cells cultured alone and together. Cell–cell interactions. *Mol. Cell. Endocrinol.* 70: 217–224, 1990.

391. Nelson, K. G., T. Takahashi, N. L. Bossert, D. K. Walmer, and J. A. McLachlan. Epidermal growth factor replaces estrogen in the stimulation of female genital tract growth and differentiation. *Proc. Natl. Acad. Sci. U.S.A.* 88: 21–25, 1991.

392. Nicholson, H. D., and M. P. Hardy. Luteinizing hormone differentially regulates the secretion of testicular oxytocin and testosterone by purified adult rat Leydig cells in vitro. *Endocrinology* 130: 671–677, 1992.

393. Niendorf, W. R., and H. Zuhlke. Biosynthesis of beta-endorphin in pancreatic islets of neonatal Wistar rats. *Biomed. Biochim. Acta* 44: K51–K54, 1985.

394. Nilsson, M., and L. E. Ericson. Effects of epidermal growth factor and phorbol ester on thyroid epithelial integrity. *Exp. Cell Res.* 219: 626–639, 1995.

395. Normanno, N., F. Ciardiello, R. Brandt, and D. S. Salomon. Epidermal growth factor-related peptides in the pathogenesis of human breast cancer. *Breast Cancer Res. Treat.* 29: 11–27, 1994.

396. Norton, J. N., J. L. Vigne, and M. K. Skinner. Regulation of Sertoli cell differentiation by the testicular paracrine factor PModS: analysis of common signal transduction pathways. *Endocrinology* 134: 149–157, 1994.

397. Ogawa, K., K. Abe, N. Kurosawa, M. Kurohmaru, H. Sugino, M. Takahashi, and Y. Hayashi. Expression of alpha, beta A and beta B subunits of inhibin or activin and follistatin in rat pancreatic islets. *FEBS Lett.* 319: 217–220, 1993.

398. O'Halloran, D. J., P. M. Jones, and S. R. Bloom. Neuropeptides synthesised in the anterior pituitary: possible paracrine role. *Mol. Cell. Endocrinol.* 75: C7–C12, 1991.

399. O'Hara, B. F., D. M. Donovan, I. Lindberg, et al. Proenkephalin transgenic mice: a short promoter confers high testis expression and reduced fertility. *Mol. Reprod. Dev.* 38:275–284, 1994.

400. Ohno, T., A. Imai, T. Furui, K. Takahashi, and T. Tamaya. Presence of gonadotropin-releasing hormone and its messenger ribonucleic acid in human ovarian epithelial carcinoma. *Am. J. Obstet. Gynecol.* 169: 605–610, 1993.

401. Ojeda, S. R., G. A. Dissen, and M. P. Junier. Neurotrophic factors and female sexual development. *Front. Neuroendocrinol.* 13: 120–162, 1992.

402. Okada, Y., H. Taniguchi, and C. Schimada. High concentration of GABA and high glutamate decarboxylase activity in rat pancreatic islets and human insulinoma. *Science* 194: 620–622, 1976.

403. Okuyama, A., N. Nonomura, M. Nakamura, M. Namiki, and T. Sonoda. Renin–angiotensin system. *Arch. Androl.* 21: 169–180, 1988.

404. Oliver, J. E., T. J. Aitman, J. F. Powell, C. A. Wilson, and R. N. Clayton. Insulin-like growth factor I gene expression in the rat ovary is confined to the granulosa cells of developing follicles. *Endocrinology* 124: 2671–2679, 1989.

405. Onoda, N., E. Ohmura, T. Tsushima, Y. Ohba, N. Emoto, O. Isozaki, Y. Sato, K. Shizume, and H. Demura. Autocrine role of insulin-like growth factor (IGF)-I in a human thyroid cancer cell line. *Eur. J. Cancer* 28A: 1904–1909, 1992.

406. Oomori, Y., H. Iuchi, K. Nakaya, H. Tanaka, K. Ishikawa, Y. Satoh, and K. Ono. Gamma-aminobutyric acid (GABA) immunoreactivity in the mouse adrenal gland. *Histochemistry* 100: 203–213, 1993.

407. Orskov, C. Glucagon-like peptide-1, a new hormone of the entero–insular axis. *Diabetologia* 35: 701–711, 1992.

408. Orth, J. M. FSH-induced Sertoli cell proliferation in the developing rat is modified by beta-endorphin produced in the testis. *Endocrinology* 119: 1876–1878, 1986.

409. Osamura, R. Y., Y. Tsutsumi, N. Yanaihara, H. Imura, and K. Watanabe. Immunohistochemical studies for multiple peptide-immunoreactivities and co-localization of met-enkephalin-Arg6-Gly7-Leu8, neuropeptide Y and somatostatin in human adrenal medulla and pheochromocytomas. *Peptides* 8: 77–87, 1987.

410. Ostenson, C. G., S. Sandler, and S. Efendic. Effects of porcine pancreastatin on secretion and biosynthesis of insulin and glucose oxidation of isolated rat pancreatic islets. *Pancreas* 4: 441–446, 1989.

411. Ouazzani, L., J. C. Reubi, G. E. Volle, S. Lausson, E. Pidoux, M. S. Moukhtar, and F. Treilhou-Lahille. Evaluation of somatostatin biosynthesis, somatostatin receptors and tumor growth in murine medullary thyroid carcinoma. *Eur. J. Endocrinol.* 131: 522–530, 1994.

412. Ozawa, S., L. G. Sheflin, and S. W. Spaulding. Thyroxine increases epidermal growth factor levels in the mouse thyroid in vivo. *Endocrinology* 128: 1396–1403, 1991.

413. Page, S. R., V. T. Ang, R. Jackson, and S. S. Nussey. The effect of oxytocin on the plasma glucagon response to insulin-induced hypoglycaemia in man. *Diabete. Metab.* 16: 248–251, 1990.

414. Pandey, K. N., and M. C. Orgebin-Crist. Atrial natriuretic factor in mammalian testis: immunological detection in spermatozoa. *Biochem. Biophys. Res. Commun.* 180: 437–444, 1991.

415. Panthou, P., P. Barbey, B. Thiebot, and J. Bocquet. Effects of transforming growth factor-beta 1, interleukin-1 alpha and interleukin-6 on rat Sertoli cell proteoglycan synthesis. *Biochem. Mol. Biol. Int.* 34: 603–612, 1994.

416. Patterson, J. C., and G. V. Childs. Nerve growth factor and its receptor in the anterior pituitary. *Endocrinology* 135: 1689–1696, 1994.

417. Patterson, J. C., and G. V. Childs. Nerve growth factor in the anterior pituitary: regulation of secretion. *Endocrinology* 135: 1697–1704, 1994.

418. Payet, N., Y. Deziel, and J. G. Lehoux. Vasopressin: a potent growth factor in adrenal glomerulosa cells in culture. *J. Steroid Biochem.* 20: 449–454, 1984.

419. Pearse, A. G. Common cytochemical and ultrastructural characteristics of cells producing polypeptide hormones (the APUD series) and their relevance to thyroid and ultimobranchial C cells and calcitonin. *Proc. R. Soc. Lond. B Biol. Sci.* 170: 71–80, 1968.

420. Pearse, A. G. The cytochemistry and ultrastructure of polypeptide hormone-producing cells of the APUD series and the embryologic, physiological and pathologic implications of the concept. *J. Histochem. Cytochem.* 17: 303–313, 1969.

421. Pearse, A. G. The diffuse neuroendocrine system and the apud concept: related "endocrine" peptides in brain, intestine, pituitary, placenta, and anuran cutaneous glands. *Med. Biol.* 55: 115–125, 1977.

422. Peillon, F., M. Le Dafniet, P. Pagesy, J. Y. Li, C. Benlot, A. M. Brandi, and D. Joubert. Neuropeptides of anterior pituitary origin. Autocrine or paracrine functions? *Pathol. Res. Pract.* 187: 577–580, 1991.

423. Peillon, F., M. Le Dafniet, P. Pagesy, J. Y. Li, C. Benlot, A. Lagoguey, A. M. Brandi, and D. Joubert. Neuropeptides of anterior pituitary origin. *Ann. Endocrinol. (Paris)* 51: 133–136, 1990.

424. Peiro, E., P. Degano, P. Miralles, R.A. Silvestre, and J. Marco. Homologous pancreastatin inhibits insulin secretion without affecting glucagon and somatostatin release in the perfused rat pancreas. *Regul. Pept.* 34: 159–167, 1991.

425. Peiro, E., P. Miralles, R. A. Silvestre, M. L. Villanueva, and J. Marco. Pancreastatin inhibits insulin secretion as induced by glucagon, vasoactive intestinal peptide, gastric inhibitory peptide, and 8–cholecystokinin in the perfused rat pancreas. *Metabolism* 38: 679–682, 1989.

426. Pelto-Huikko, M. Immunocytochemical localization of neuropeptides in the adrenal medulla. *J. Electron Microsc. Tech.* 12: 364–379, 1989.

427. Pelton, R. W., B. Saxena, M. Jones, H. L. Moses, and L. I. Gold. Immunohistochemical localization of TGF beta 1, TGF beta 2, and TGF beta 3 in the mouse embryo: expression patterns suggest multiple roles during embryonic development. *J. Cell Biol.* 115: 1091–1105, 1991.

428. Penhoat, A., P. G. Chatelain, C. Jaillard, and J. M. Saez. Characterization of insulin-like growth factor I and insulin receptors on cultured bovine adrenal fasciculata cells. Role of

these peptides on adrenal cell function. *Endocrinology* 122: 2518–2526, 1988.

429. Penhoat, A., P. Leduque, C. Jaillard, P. G. Chatelain, P. M. Dubois, and J.M. Saez. ACTH and angiotensin II regulation of insulin-like growth factor-I and its binding proteins in cultured bovine adrenal cells. *J. Mol. Endocrinol.* 7: 223–232, 1991.

430. Penhoat, A., D. Naville, C. Jaillard, P. G. Chatelain, and J. M. Saez. Hormonal regulation of insulin-like growth factor I secretion by bovine adrenal cells. *J. Biol. Chem.* 264: 6858–6862, 1989.

431. Perrin, A., O. Pascal, G. Defaye, J. J. Feige, and E. M. Chambaz. Transforming growth factor beta 1 is a negative regulator of steroid 17 alpha-hydroxylase expression in bovine adrenocortical cells. *Endocrinology* 128: 357–362, 1991.

432. Pescovitz, O. H., S. A. Berry, M. Laudon, N. Ben-Jonathan, A. Martin-Myers, S. M. Hsu, T. J. Lambros, and A. M. Felix. Localization and growth hormone (GH)-releasing activity of rat testicular GH-releasing hormone-like peptide. *Endocrinology* 127: 2336–2342, 1990.

433. Petrusz, P., I. Merchenthaler, J. L. Maderdrut, S. Vigh, and A. V. Schally. Corticotropin-releasing factor (CRF)-like immunoreactivity in the vertebrate endocrine pancreas. *Proc. Natl. Acad. Sci. U.S.A.* 80: 1721–1725, 1983.

434. Petrusz, P., I. Merchenthaler, P. Ordronneau, J. L. Maderdrut, S. Vigh, and A. V. Schally. Corticotropin-releasing factor (CRF)-like immunoreactivity in the gastro-entero-pancreatic endocrine system. *Peptides 5* (Suppl. 1): 71–78, 1984.

435. Pettersson, M., B. Ahren, G. Bottcher, and F. Sundler. Calcitonin gene-related peptide: occurrence in pancreatic islets in the mouse and the rat and inhibition of insulin secretion in the mouse. *Endocrinology* 119: 865–869, 1986.

436. Piquette, G. N., M. E. Crabtree, I. el-Danasouri, A. Milki, and M. L. Polan. Regulation of plasminogen activator inhibitor-1 and -2 messenger ribonucleic acid levels in human cumulus and granulosa-luteal cells. *J. Clin. Endocrinol. Metab.* 76: 518–523, 1993.

437. Pitzel, L., I. Probst, H. Jarry, and W. Wuttke. Inhibitory effect of oxytocin and vasopressin on steroid release by cultured porcine luteal cells. *Endocrinology* 122: 1780–1785, 1988.

438. Plowman, G. D., J. M. Culouscou, G. S. Whitney, J. M. Green, G. W. Carlton, L. Foy, M. G. Neubauer, and M. Shoyab. Ligand-specific activation of HER4/p180erbB4, a fourth member of the epidermal growth factor receptor family. *Proc. Natl. Acad. Sci. U.S.A.* 90: 1746–1750, 1993.

439. Pointis, G., and A. Tahri-Joutei. Intragonadal control of testicular function by neurohypophyseal-like peptides. *Ann. Endocrinol. (Paris)* 51: 209–217, 1990.

440. Polak, J. M., and S. R. Bloom. Somatostatin localization in tissues. *Scand. J. Gastroenterol. Suppl.* 119: 11–21, 1986.

441. Porter, T. E., and L. S. Frawley. Neurointermediate lobe peptides recruit prolactin-secreting cells exclusively within the central region of the adenohypophysis. *Endocrinology* 131: 2649–2652, 1992.

442. Quach, T. T., F. Tang, H. Kageyama, I. Mocchetti, A. Guidotti, J. L. Meek, E. Costa, and J. P. Schwartz. Enkephalin biosynthesis in adrenal medulla. Modulation of proenkephalin mRNA content of cultured chromaffin cells by 8–bromo-adenosine 3′,5′-monophosphate. *Mol. Pharmacol.* 26: 255–260, 1984.

443. Rabinovici, J., S. J. Spencer, N. Doldi, P. C. Goldsmith, R. Schwall, and R. B. Jaffe. Activin-A as an intraovarian modulator: actions, localization, and regulation of the intact dimer in human ovarian cells. *J. Clin. Invest.* 89: 1528–1536, 1992.

444. Racz, K., I. Varga, E. Glaz, R. Kiss, S. Vida, G. Lada, K. di Gleria, K. Medzihradszky, K. Lichtwald, and P. Vecsei. Met-enkephalin inhibits mineralocorticoid production in isolated

human aldosteronoma cells. *J. Clin. Endocrinol. Metab.* 54: 656–660, 1982.

445. Radhakrishnan, B., B. O. Oke, V. Papadopoulos, R. P. DiAugustine, and C.A. Suarez-Quian. Characterization of epidermal growth factor in mouse testis. *Endocrinology* 131: 3091–3099, 1992.

446. Rahier, J., and J. Wallon. Long cytoplasmic processes in pancreatic polypeptide cells. *Cell Tissue Res.* 209: 365–370, 1980.

447. Ramsdell, J. S. Transforming growth factor-alpha and -beta are potent and effective inhibitors of GH4 pituitary tumor cell proliferation. *Endocrinology* 128: 1981–1990, 1991.

448. Raychoudhury, S. S., A. W. Blackshaw, and M. G. Irving. Hormonal modulation of the interactions of cultured rat testicular Sertoli and peritubular myoid cells. Effects on glycosaminoglycan synthesis. *J. Androl.* 14: 9–16, 1993.

449. Raychoudhury, S. S., E. W. Thompson, A. W. Blackshaw, and M. G. Irving. Sertoli cells as paracrine modulators of DNA synthesis in rat peritubular myoid cells in culture. *J. Reprod. Fertil.* 99: 513–518, 1993.

450. Redecker, P., A. Seipelt, A. Jorns, G. Bargsten, and D. Grube. The microanatomy of canine islets of Langerhans: implications for intra-islet regulation. *Anat. Embryol. (Berl.)* 185: 131–141, 1992.

451. Reetz, A., M. Solimena, M. Matteoli, F. Folli, K. Takei, and P. De Camilli. GABA and pancreatic beta-cells: colocalization of glutamic acid decarboxylase (GAD) and GABA with synaptic-like microvesicles suggests their role in GABA storage and secretion. *EMBO J.* 10: 1275–1284, 1991.

452. Renner, U., J. Mojto, E. Arzt, M. Lange, J. Stalla, O. A. Muller, and G. K. Stalla. Secretion of polypeptide growth factors by human nonfunctioning pituitary adenoma cells in culture. *Neuroendocrinology* 57: 825–834, 1993.

453. Rettori, V., C. C. Pazos-Moura, E. G. Moura, J. Polak, and S. M. McCann. Role of neuromedin B in control of the release of thyrotropin in hypothyroid and hyperthyroid rats. *Proc. Natl. Acad. Sci. U.S.A.* 89: 3035–3039, 1992.

454. Reubi, J. C., B. Waser, S. W. Lamberts, and G. Mengod. Somatostatin (SRIH) messenger ribonucleic acid expression in human neuroendocrine and brain tumors using in situ hybridization histochemistry: comparison with SRIH receptor content. *J. Clin. Endocrinol. Metab.* 76: 642–647, 1993.

455. Riccioli, A., A. Filippini, P. De Cesaris, E. Barbacci, M. Stefanini, G. Starace, and E. Ziparo. Inflammatory mediators increase surface expression of integrin ligands, adhesion to lymphocytes, and secretion of interleukin 6 in mouse Sertoli cells. *Proc. Natl. Acad. Sci. U.S.A.* 92: 5808–5812, 1995.

456. Risbridger, G. P., and M. K. Skinner. Evaluation of the effect of peritubular cell secretions and the testicular paracrine factor P-Mod-S on Leydig cell steroidogenesis and immunoactive inhibin production. *Int. J. Androl.* 15: 73–83, 1992.

457. Riskind, P. N., J. M. Allen, S. M. Gabriel, J. I. Koenig, and J. Audet-Arnold. Sex differences in vasoactive intestinal peptide (VIP) concentrations in the anterior pituitary and hypothalamus of rats. *Neurosci. Lett.* 105: 215–220, 1989.

458. Ritta, M. N., and R. S. Calandra. Occurrence of GABA in rat testis and its effect on androgen production. *Adv. Biochem. Psychopharmacol.* 42: 291–297, 1986.

459. Ritta, M. N., M. B. Campos, and R. S. Calandra. Effect of GABA and benzodiazepines on testicular androgen production. *Life Sci.* 40: 791–798, 1987.

460. Rivarola, M. A., A. Belgorosky, E. Berensztein, and M. T. de Davila. Human prepubertal testicular cells in culture: steroidogenic capacity, paracrine and hormone control. *J. Steroid Biochem. Mol. Biol.* 53: 119–125, 1995.

461. Rivier, C., and W. Vale. Immunoreactive inhibin secretion

by the hypophysectomized female rat: demonstration of the modulating effect of gonadotropin-releasing hormone and estrogen through a direct ovarian site of action. *Endocrinology* 124: 195–198, 1989.

462. Robberecht, W., M. Andries, and C. Denef. Stimulation of prolactin secretion from rat pituitary by luteinizing hormone-releasing hormone: evidence against mediation by angiotensin II acting through a (Sar1–Ala8)-angiotensin II-sensitive receptor. *Neuroendocrinology* 56: 185–194, 1992.

463. Robberecht, W., M. Andries, and C. Denef. Angiotensin II is retained in gonadotrophs of pituitary cell aggregates cultured in serum-free medium but does not mimic the effects of exogenous angiotensins and luteinizing hormone–releasing hormone on growth hormone release. *Neuroendocrinology* 56: 550–560, 1992.

464. Robberecht, W., and C. Denef. Stimulation and inhibition of pituitary growth hormone release by angiotensin II in vitro. *Endocrinology* 122: 1496–1504, 1988.

465. Robberecht, W., and C. Denef. Evidence for a pertussis toxin-sensitive signalling pathway in the dual action of angiotensin II on growth hormone release in pituitary cell aggregates. *Cell Biol. Int. Rep.* 14: 1001–1011, 1990.

466. Robbins, M. S., L. H. Grouse, R. L. Sorenson, and R. P. Elde. Effect of muscimol on glucose-stimulated somatostatin and insulin release from the isolated, perfused rat pancreas. *Diabetes* 30: 168–171, 1981.

467. Roberts, A. J., and M. K. Skinner. Mesenchymal–epithelial cell interactions in the ovary: estrogen-induced theca cell steroidogenesis. *Mol. Cell Endocrinol.* 72: R1–R5, 1990.

468. Robichon, A., and P. Nicolas. Evidence for the synthesis of pro-CRF (corticotropin-releasing factor) in cultured fetal pancreatic islets of rats. *Exp. Cell Res.* 185: 283–291, 1989.

469. Roby, K. F., J. Weed, R. Lyles, and P. F. Terranova. Immunological evidence for a human ovarian tumor necrosis factor-alpha. *J. Clin. Endocrinol. Metab.* 71: 1096–1102, 1990.

470. Rogler, C. E., D. Yang, L. Rossetti, J. Donohoe, E. Alt, C. J. Chang, R. Rosenfeld, K. Neely, and R. Hintz. Altered body composition and increased frequency of diverse malignancies in insulin-like growth factor-II transgenic mice. *J. Biol. Chem.* 269: 13779–13784, 1994.

471. Rokaeus, A., R. M. Pruss, and L. E. Eiden. Galanin gene expression in chromaffin cells is controlled by calcium and protein kinase signaling pathways. *Endocrinology* 127: 3096–3102, 1990.

472. Rommerts, F. F., and A. P. Themmen. LHRH, the role of LHRH (agonists) in the regulation of gonadal function. *Acta Endocrinol. Suppl. (Copenh.)* 276: 76–84, 1986.

473. Rorsman, P., P. O. Berggren, K. Bokvist, H. Ericson, H. Mohler, C. G. Ostenson, and P. A. Smith. Glucose-inhibition of glucagon secretion involves activation of GABAA-receptor chloride channels. *Nature* 341: 233–236, 1989.

474. Rosen, H., A. Itin, R. Schiff, and E. Keshet. Local regulation within the female reproductive system and upon embryonic implantation: identification of cells expressing proenkephalin A. *Mol. Endocrinol.* 4: 146–154, 1990.

475. Russell, D. L., L. A. Salamonsen, and J. K. Findlay. Immunization against the N-terminal peptide of the inhibin alpha 43–subunit (alpha N) disrupts tissue remodeling and the increase in matrix metalloproteinase-2 during ovulation. *Endocrinology* 136: 3657–3664, 1995.

476. Saez, J. Leydig cells: endocrine, paracrine and autocrine regulation. *Endocr. Rev.* 15: 574–626, 1994.

477. Saez, J. M., M. H. Perrard-Sapori, P.G. Chatelain, E. Tabone, and M. A. Rivarola. Paracrine regulation of testicular function. *J. Steroid Biochem.* 27: 317–329, 1987.

478. Saint-Andre, J. P., V. Rohmer, F. Alhenc-Gelas, J. Menard, J. C. Bigorgne, and P. Corvol. Presence of renin, angiotensinogen, and converting enzyme in human pituitary lactotroph cells and prolactin adenomas. *J. Clin. Endocrinol. Metab.* 63: 231–237, 1986.

479. Saint-Andre, J. P., V. Rohmer, F. Pinet, M. C. Rousselet, J. C. Bigorgne, and P. Corvol. Renin and cathepsin B in human pituitary lactotroph cells. An ultrastructural study. *Histochemistry* 91: 291–297, 1989.

480. Saint Pol, P., E. Hermand, and G. Tramu. Paracrine factors in adult rat testis gonadotrophin control of opioids and LHRH like peptide. *Andrologia* 20: 173–181, 1988.

481. Saint-Pol, P., J. P. Peyrat, R. P. Engelhardt, and B. Leroy-Martin. Immunohistochemical localization of enkephalins in adult rat testis: evidence for a gonadotrophin control. *Andrologia* 18: 485–488, 1986.

482. Sakaguchi, K. Acidic fibroblast growth factor autocrine system as a mediator of calcium-regulated parathyroid cell growth. *J. Biol. Chem.* 267: 24554–24562, 1992.

483. Sakaue, M., N. Saito, and C. Tanaka. Immunohistochemical localization of gamma-aminobutyric acid (GABA) in the rat pancreas. *Histochemistry* 86: 365–369, 1987.

484. Salazar, R., and H. Zuhlke. Expression of the insulin gene is regulated by opioid peptides. *Biomed. Biochim. Acta* 49: 1165–1170, 1990.

485. Salomon, D. S., N. Normanno, F. Ciardiello, R. Brandt, M. Shoyab, and G. J. Todaro. The role of amphiregulin in breast cancer. *Breast Cancer Res. Treat.* 33: 103–114, 1995.

486. Samaras, S. E., H. D. Guthrie, J. A. Barber, and J. M. Hammond. Expression of the mRNAs for the insulin-like growth factors and their binding proteins during development of porcine ovarian follicles. *Endocrinology* 133: 2395–2398, 1993.

487. Samols, E., and J. I. Stagner. Intra-islet regulation. *Am. J. Med.* 85: 31–35, 1988.

488. Samols, E., and J. I. Stagner. Islet somatostatin—microvascular, paracrine, and pulsatile regulation. *Metabolism* 39: 55–60, 1990.

489. Samsoondar, J., M. S. Kobrin, and J. E. Kudlow. Alpha-transforming growth factor secreted by untransformed bovine anterior pituitary cells in culture. I. Purification from conditioned medium. *J. Biol. Chem.* 261: 14408–14413, 1986.

490. Sanders, S. L., M. H. Melner, and T. E. Curry, Jr. Cellular localization of ovarian proopiomelanocortin messenger RNA during follicular and luteal development in the rat. *Mol. Endocrinol.* 4: 1311–1319, 1990.

491. Sasano, H., T. Suzuki, S. Shizawa, K. Kato, and H. Nagura. Transforming growth factor alpha, epidermal growth factor, and epidermal growth factor receptor expression in normal and diseased human adrenal cortex by immunohistochemistry and in situ hybridization. *Mod. Pathol.* 7: 741–746, 1994.

492. Schaeffer, J. M., J. Liu, A. J. Hsueh, and S. S. Yen. Presence of oxytocin and arginine vasopressin in human ovary, oviduct, and follicular fluid. *J. Clin. Endocrinol. Metab.* 59: 970–973, 1984.

493. Schalling, M., A. Dagerlind, S. Brene, H. Hallman, M. Djurfeldt, H. Persson, L. Terenius, M. Goldstein, D. Schlesinger, and T. Hokfelt. Coexistence and gene expression of phenylethanolamine N-methyltransferase, tyrosine hydroxylase, and neuropeptide tyrosine in the rat and bovine adrenal gland: effects of reserpine. *Proc. Natl. Acad. Sci. U.S.A.* 85: 8306–8310, 1988.

494. Schalling, M., A. Franco-Cereceda, A. Hemsen, A. Dagerlind, K. Seroogy, H. Persson, T. Hokfelt, and J. M. Lundberg. Neuropeptide Y and catecholamine synthesizing enzymes and their mRNAs in rat sympathetic neurons and adrenal glands:

studies on expression, synthesis and axonal transport after pharmacological and experimental manipulations using hybridization techniques and radioimmunoassay. *Neuroscience* 41: 753–766, 1991.

495. Schalling, M., K. Seroogy, T. Hokfelt, et al. Neuropeptide tyrosine in the rat adrenal gland—immunohistochemical and in situ hybridization studies. *Neuroscience* 24: 337–349, 1988.

496. Schauder, P., J. C. Brown, H. Frerichs, and W. Creutzfeldt. Gastric inhibitory polypeptide: effect on glucose-induced insulin release from isolated rat pancreatic islets in vitro. *Diabetologia* 11: 483–484, 1975.

497. Schiffrin, E. L., M. Chretien, N. G. Seidah, M. Lis, J. Gutkowska, M. Cantin, and J. Genest. Response of human aldosteronoma cells in culture to the N-terminal glycopeptide of pro-opiomelanocortin and gamma 3-MSH. *Horm. Metab. Res.* 15: 181–184, 1983.

498. Schleicher, R. L. Beta-endorphin inhibits insulin secretion from isolated pancreatic islets. *Endocrinology* 124: 1254–1258, 1989.

499. Schmidt, W. E., and W. Creutzfeldt. Pancreastatin—a novel regulatory peptide? *Acta Oncol.* 30: 441–449, 1991.

500. Schramme, C., and C. Denef. Stimulation of prolactin release by angiotensin II in superfused rat anterior pituitary cell aggregates. *Neuroendocrinology* 36: 483–485, 1983.

501. Schramme, C., and C. Denef. Stimulation of spontaneous and dopamine-inhibited prolactin release from anterior pituitary reaggregate cell cultures by angiotensin peptides. *Life Sci.* 34: 1651–1658, 1984.

502. Schwartz, J., T. Pham, A. Rao, and J. W. Funder. Effect of AVP on susceptibility of ovine pituitary cells to a cytotoxic analogue of CRF. *Am. J. Physiol.* 260 (*Endocrinol. Metab.* 23): E905–E909, 1991.

503. Schweigerer, L., G. Neufeld, J. Friedman, J. A. Abraham, J. C. Fiddes, and D. Gospodarowicz. Basic fibroblast growth factor: production and growth stimulation in cultured adrenal cortex cells. *Endocrinology* 120: 796–800, 1987.

504. Scurry, J. P., K. A. Hamand, S. B. Astley, R. E. Leake, and M. Wells. Immunoreactivity of antibodies to epidermal growth factor, transforming growth factors alpha and beta, and epidermal growth factor receptor in the premenopausal ovary. *Pathology* 26: 130–133, 1994.

505. Sellitti, D. F., C. E. Hughes, S. A. Hensen, and M. M. Vincent. Secretion of immunoreactive ANF from FRTL-5 rat thyroid cells: regulation by calcium ionophore A23187. *Regul. Pept.* 41: 257–273, 1992.

506. Selvaraj, N., G. Shetty, K. Vijayalakshmi, A. S. Bhatnagar, and N. R. Moudgal. Effect of blocking oestrogen synthesis with a new generation aromatase inhibitor CGS 16949A on follicular maturation induced by pregnant mare serum gonadotrophin in the immature rat. *J. Endocrinol.* 142: 563–570, 1994.

507. Sharpe, R. M. Paracrine control of the testis. *Clin. Endocrinol. Metab.* 15: 185–207, 1986.

508. Sharpe, R.M., and I. Cooper. Comparison of the effects on purified Leydig cells of four hormones (oxytocin, vasopressin, opiates and LHRH) with suggested paracrine roles in the testis. *J. Endocrinol.* 113: 89–96, 1987.

509. Sharpe, R. M., J. B. Kerr, and S. Maddocks. Evidence for a role of the Leydig cells in control of the intratesticular secretion of inhibin. *Mol. Cell. Endocrinol.* 60: 243–247, 1988.

510. Sharpe, R. M., S. Maddocks, and J. B. Kerr. Cell–cell interactions in the control of spermatogenesis as studied using Leydig cell destruction and testosterone replacement. *Am. J. Anat.* 188: 3–20, 1990.

511. Shibata, H., H. Yasuda, N. Sekine, T. Mine, Y. Totsuka, and I. Kojima. Activin A increases intracellular free calcium concen-

trations in rat pancreatic islets. *FEBS Lett.* 329: 194–198, 1993.

512. Shima, K., M. Hirota, C. Ohboshi, M. Sato, and T. Nishino. Release of glucagon-like peptide 1 immunoreactivity from the perfused rat pancreas. *Acta Endocrinol. (Copenh.)* 114: 531–536, 1987.

513. Shioda, S., G. Legradi, W.C. Leung, S. Nakajo, K. Nakaya, and A. Arimura. Localization of pituitary adenylate cyclase-activating polypeptide and its messenger ribonucleic acid in the rat testis by light and electron microscopic immunocytochemistry and in situ hybridization. *Endocrinology* 135: 818–825, 1994.

514. Shu-Dong, T., D. M. Phillips, N. Halmi, D. Krieger, and C. W. Bardin. Beta-endorphin is present in the male reproductive tract of five species. *Biol. Reprod.* 27: 755–764, 1982.

516. Siegel, R. E., L. E. Eiden, and R. M. Pruss. Multiple populations of neuropeptide-containing cells in cultures of the bovine adrenal medulla. *Brain Res.* 349: 267–270, 1985.

517. Sieradzki, J., H. Fleck, A. K. Chatterjee, and H. Schatz. Stimulatory effect of insulin-like growth factor-I on [³H]thymidine incorporation, DNA content and insulin biosynthesis and secretion of isolated pancreatic rat islets. *J. Endocrinol.* 117: 59–62, 1988.

518. Silvestre, R. A., E. Peiro, P. Miralles, M. L. Villanueva, and J. Marco. Effects of pancreastatin on insulin, glucagon and somatostatin secretion by the perfused rat pancreas. *Life Sci.* 42: 1361–1367, 1988.

519. Simon, C., A. Frances, G. Piquette, and M. L. Polan. Immunohistochemical localization of the interleukin-1 system in the mouse ovary during follicular growth, ovulation, and luteinization. *Biol. Reprod.* 50: 449–457, 1994.

520. Singh-Asa, P., and M. J. Waters. Stimulation of adrenal cortisol biosynthesis by epidermal growth factor. *Mol. Cell. Endocrinol.* 30: 189–199, 1983.

521. Sirbasku, D. A., R. Pakala, H. Sato, and J. E. Eby. Thyroid hormone regulation of rat pituitary tumor cell growth: a new role for apotransferrin as an autocrine thyromedin. *Mol. Cell. Endocrinol.* 77: C47–C55, 1991.

522. Sjoholm, A., A. Funakoshi, S. Efendic, C. G. Ostenson, and C. Hellerstrom. Long term inhibitory effects of pancreastatin and diazepam binding inhibitor on pancreatic beta-cell deoxyribonucleic acid replication, polyamine content, and insulin secretion. *Endocrinology* 128: 3277–3282, 1991.

523. Sjoholm, A., and C. Hellerstrom. TGF-beta stimulates insulin secretion and blocks mitogenic response of pancreatic beta-cells to glucose. *Am. J. Physiol.* 260 (*Cell Physiol.* 29): C1046–C1051, 1991.

524. Skinner, M. K., and R. J. Coffey, Jr. Regulation of ovarian cell growth through the local production of transforming growth factor-alpha by theca cells. *Endocrinology* 123: 2632–2638, 1988.

525. Skinner, M. K., P. M. Fetterolf, and C. T. Anthony. Purification of a paracrine factor, P-Mod-S, produced by testicular peritubular cells that modulates Sertoli cell function. *J. Biol. Chem.* 263: 2884–2890, 1988.

526. Skinner, M. K., and I. B. Fritz. Identification of a non-mitogenic paracrine factor involved in mesenchymal–epithelial cell interactions between testicular peritubular cells and Sertoli cells. *Mol. Cell. Endocrinol.* 44: 85–97, 1986.

527. Skinner, M. K., and H. L. Moses. Transforming growth factor beta gene expression and action in the seminiferous tubule: peritubular cell–Sertoli cell interactions. *Mol. Endocrinol.* 3: 625–634, 1989.

528. Skinner, M. K., K. Takacs, and R. J. Coffey. Transforming growth factor-alpha gene expression and action in the seminif-

erous tubule: peritubular cell–Sertoli cell interactions. *Endocrinology* 124: 845–854, 1989.

529. Smith, P. H., F. W. Merchant, D. G. Johnson, W. Y. Fujimoto, and R. H. Williams. Immunocytochemical localization of a gastric inhibitory polypeptide-like material within A-cells of the endocrine pancreas. *Am. J. Anat.* 149: 585–590, 1977.

530. Smyth, C. D., F. Miro, P. F. Whitelaw, C. M. Howles, and S. G. Hillier. Ovarian thecal/interstitial androgen synthesis is enhanced by a follicle-stimulating hormone-stimulated paracrine mechanism. *Endocrinology* 133: 1532–1538, 1993.

531. Soder, O., P. Bang, A. Wahab, and M. Parvinen. Insulin-like growth factors selectively stimulate spermatogonial, but not meiotic, deoxyribonucleic acid synthesis during rat spermatogenesis. *Endocrinology* 131: 2344–2350, 1992.

532. Soendoro, T., M. P. Diamond, J. R. Pepperell, and F. Naftolin. The in vitro perifused rat ovary: III. Interrelationship of the follicular and stromal compartments on steroid release. *Gynecol. Endocrinol.* 7: 1–6, 1993.

533. Solcia, E., L. Usellini, R. Buffa, G. Rindi, L. Villani, A. Aguzzi, and E. Silini. Endocrine cells producing regulatory peptides. *Experientia* 56 *(Suppl.)* 220–246, 1989.

534. Spencer, S. J., J. Rabinovici, and R. B. Jaffe. Human recombinant activin-A inhibits proliferation of human fetal adrenal cells in vitro. *J. Clin. Endocrinol. Metab.* 71: 1678–1680, 1990.

535. Spencer, S. J., J. Rabinovici, S. Mesiano, P. C. Goldsmith, and R. B. Jaffe. Activin and inhibin in the human adrenal gland. Regulation and differential effects in fetal and adult cells. *J. Clin. Invest.* 90: 142–149, 1992.

536. Sporn, M. B., and A. B. Roberts. Autocrine secretion—10 years later. *Ann. Intern. Med.* 117: 408–413, 1992.

537. Sporn, M. B., and G. J. Todaro. Autocrine secretion and malignant transformation of cells. *N. Engl. J. Med.* 303: 878–880, 1980.

538. Srivastava, C. H., P. R. Breyer, J. K. Rothrock, M. J. Peredo, and O. H. Pescovitz. A new target for growth hormone releasing-hormone action in rat: the Sertoli cell. *Endocrinology* 133: 1478–1481, 1993.

539. Srivastava, C. H., M. W. Collard, J. K. Rothrock, M. J. Peredo, S. A. Berry, and O. H. Pescovitz. Germ cell localization of a testicular growth hormone-releasing hormone-like factor. *Endocrinology* 133: 83–89, 1993.

540. Statuto, M., M. G. Ennas, G. Zamboni, F. Bonetti, M. Pea, F. Bernardello, A. Pozzi, M. Rusnati, A. Gualandris, and M. Presta. Basic fibroblast growth factor in human pheochromocytoma: a biochemical and immunohistochemical study. *Int. J. Cancer* 53: 5–10, 1993.

541. Steel, J. H., G. Gon, D. J. O'Halloran, P. M. Jones, N. Yanaihara, H. Ishikawa, S. R. Bloom, and J. M. Polak. Galanin and vasoactive intestinal polypeptide are colocalised with classical pituitary hormones and show plasticity of expression. *Histochemistry* 93: 183–189, 1989.

542. Steel, J. H., D. J. O'Halloran, M. A. Emson, S. Van Noorden, S. R. Bloom, and J. M. Polak. Identification of bombesin-immunoreactive cells in rat, human, and other mammalian pituitaries, their ontogeny and the effect of endocrine manipulations in the rat. *Endocrinology* 130: 2587–2596, 1992.

543. Stefaneanu, L., K. Kovacs, R. V. Lloyd, B. W. Scheithauer, W. F. Young, Jr., T. Sano, and L. Jin. Pituitary lactotrophs and somatotrophs in pregnancy: a correlative in situ hybridization and immunocytochemical study. *Virchows Arch. B Cell Pathol. Incl. Mol. Pathol.* 62: 291–296, 1992.

544. Steiner, H. J., K. W. Schmid, R. Fischer-Colbrie, G. Sperk, and H. Winkler. Co-localization of chromogranin A and B, secretogranin II and neuropeptide Y in chromaffin granules of rat adrenal medulla studied by electron microscopic immunocytochemistry. *Histochemistry* 91: 473–477, 1989.

545. Steinmetz, R., A. Gutierrez-Hartmann, R. M. Bigsby, and N. Ben-Jonathan. Activation of the prolactin promoter in transfected GH3 cells by posterior pituitary cells. *Endocrinology* 135: 2737–2741, 1994.

546. Stouffer, R. L., T. K. Woodruff, K. D. Dahl, D. L. Hess, J. P. Mather, and T. A. Molskness. Human recombinant activin-A alters pituitary luteinizing hormone and follicle-stimulating hormone secretion, follicular development, and steroidogenesis, during the menstrual cycle in rhesus monkeys. *J. Clin. Endocrinol. Metab.* 77: 241–248, 1993.

547. Struthers, R. S., D. Gaddy-Kurten, and W. W. Vale. Activin inhibits binding of transcription factor Pit-1 to the growth hormone promoter. *Proc. Natl. Acad. Sci. U.S.A.* 89: 11451–11455, 1992.

548. Sun, X. R., M. P. Hedger, and G. P. Risbridger. The effect of testicular macrophages and interleukin-1 on testosterone production by purified adult rat Leydig cells cultured under in vitro maintenance conditions. *Endocrinology* 132: 186–192, 1993.

549. Sunday, M. E., H. J. Wolfe, B. A. Roos, W. W. Chin, and E. R. Spindel. Gastrin-releasing peptide gene expression in developing, hyperplastic, and neoplastic human thyroid C-cells. *Endocrinology* 122: 1551–1558, 1988.

550. Swinnen, K., J. Cailleau, W. Heyns, and G. Verhoeven. Stromal cells from the rat prostate secrete androgen-regulated factors which modulate Sertoli cell function. *Mol. Cell. Endocrinol.* 62: 147–152, 1989.

551. Szecowka, J., K. Tatemoto, G. Rajamaki, and S. Efendic. Effects of PYY and PP on endocrine pancreas. *Acta Physiol. Scand.* 119: 123–126, 1983.

552. Taborsky, G. J., Jr. Evidence of a paracrine role for pancreatic somatostatin in vivo. *Am. J. Physiol.* 245 *(Endocrinol. Metab.* 8): E598–E603, 1983.

553. Tahri-Joutei, A., C. Fillion, M. Bedin, J. N. Hugues, and G. Pointis. Local control of Leydig cell arginine vasopressin receptor by naloxone. *Mol. Cell. Endocrinol.* 79: R21–R24, 1991.

554. Takahashi, S., M. Conti, and J. J. Van Wyk. Thyrotropin potentiation of insulin-like growth factor-I dependent deoxyribonucleic acid synthesis in FRTL-5 cells: mediation by an autocrine amplification factor(s). *Endocrinology* 126: 736–745, 1990.

555. Taminato, T., Y. Seino, Y. Goto, Y. Inoue, and S. Kadowaki. Synthetic gastric inhibitory polypeptide. Stimulatory effect on insulin and glucagon secretion in the rat. *Diabetes* 26: 480–484, 1977.

556. Tanaka, N., J. Iwamasa, K. Matsuura, and H. Okamura. Effects of progesterone and anti-progesterone RU486 on ovarian 3 beta-hydroxysteroid dehydrogenase activity during ovulation in the gonadotrophin-primed immature rat. *J. Reprod. Fertil.* 97: 167–172, 1993.

557. Taniguchi, H., Y. Okada, H. Seguchi, C. Shimada, M. Seki, A. Tsutou, and S. Baba. High concentration of gamma-aminobutyric acid in pancreatic beta cells. *Diabetes* 28: 629–633, 1979.

558. Tanini, A., P. Failli, M. Maggi, F. Franceschelli, U. Frediani, L. Becherini, A. Giotti, C. Ruocco, and M. L. Brandi. Effects of endothelin-1 on bovine parathyroid cells. *Biochem. Biophys. Res. Commun.* 193: 59–66, 1993.

559. Teerds, K. J., and J. H. Dorrington. Localization of transforming growth factor beta 1 and beta 2 during testicular development in the rat. *Biol. Reprod.* 48: 40–45, 1993.

560. Teerds, K. J., and J. H. Dorrington. Immunolocalization of transforming growth factor alpha and luteinizing hormone

receptor in healthy and atretic follicles of the adult rat ovary. *Biol. Reprod.* 52: 500–508, 1995.

561. Teitelman, G. On the origin of pancreatic endocrine cells, proliferation and neoplastic transformation. *Tumour Biol.* 14: 167–173, 1993.

562. Teitelman, G., S. Alpert, J. M. Polak, A. Martinez, and D. Hanahan. Precursor cells of mouse endocrine pancreas coexpress insulin, glucagon and the neuronal proteins tyrosine hydroxylase and neuropeptide Y, but not pancreatic polypeptide. *Development* 118: 1031–1039, 1993.

563. Terrier, C., J. G. Chabot, G. Pautrat, L. Jeandel, D. Gray, B. Lutz-Bucher, H.H. Zingg, and G. Morel. Arginine-vasopressin in anterior pituitary cells: in situ hybridization of mRNA and ultrastructural localization of immunoreactivity. *Neuroendocrinology* 54: 303–311, 1991.

564. Thomas, G. A., H. G. Davies, and E. D. Williams. Site of production of IGF1 in the normal and stimulated mouse thyroid. *J. Pathol.* 173: 355–360, 1994.

565. Tilemans, D., M. Andries, and C. Denef. Luteinizing hormone–releasing hormone and neuropeptide Y influence deoxyribonucleic acid replication in three anterior pituitary cell types. Evidence for mediation by growth factors released from gonadotrophs. *Endocrinology* 130: 882–894, 1992.

566. Tilemans, D., M. Andries, P. Proost, B. Devreese, J. Van Beumen, and C. Denef. In vitro evidence that an 11-kilodalton N-terminal fragment of proopiomelanocortin is a growth factor specifically stimulating the development of lactotrophs in rat pituitary during postnatal life. *Endocrinology* 135: 168–174, 1994.

567. Tinajero, J. C., A. Fabbri, D. R. Ciocca, and M. L. Dufau. Serotonin secretion from rat Leydig cells. *Endocrinology* 133: 3026–3029, 1993.

568. Tisdall, D. J., N. Hudson, P. Smith, and K. P. McNatty. Localization of ovine follistatin and alpha and beta A inhibin mRNA in the sheep ovary during the oestrous cycle. *J. Mol. Endocrinol.* 12: 181–193, 1994.

569. Tode, B., M. Serio, C. M. Rotella, G. Galli, F. Franceschelli, A. Tanini, and R. Toccafondi. Insulin-like growth factor-I: autocrine secretion by human thyroid follicular cells in primary culture. *J. Clin. Endocrinol. Metab.* 69: 639–647, 1989.

570. Tominaga, T., J. Fukata, Y. Hayashi, Y. Satoh, N. Fuse, H. Segawa, O. Ebisui, Y. Nakai, Y. Osamura, and H. Imura. Distribution and characterization of immunoreactive corticostatin in the hypothalamic–pituitary–adrenal axis. *Endocrinology* 130: 1593–1598, 1992.

571. Tonetta, S. A., R. S. De Vinna, and G. S. diZerega. Thecal cell 3–beta hydroxysteroid dehydrogenase activity: modulation by human chorionic gonadotropin, progesterone, estradiol-17 beta and dihydrotestosterone. *J. Steroid Biochem.* 28: 77–82, 1987.

572. Totsuka, Y., M. Tabuchi, I. Kojima, Y. Eto, H. Shibai, and E. Ogata. Stimulation of insulin secretion by transforming growth factor-beta. *Biochem. Biophys. Res. Commun.* 158: 1060–1065, 1989.

573. Totsuka, Y., M. Tabuchi, I. Kojima, H. Shibai, and E. Ogata. A novel action of activin A: stimulation of insulin secretion in rat pancreatic islets. *Biochem. Biophys. Res. Commun.* 156: 335–339, 1988.

574. Townsend, S. F., M. F. Dallman, and W. L. Miller. Rat insulin-like growth factor-I and -II mRNAs are unchanged during compensatory adrenal growth but decrease during ACTH-induced adrenal growth. *J. Biol. Chem.* 265: 22117–22122, 1990.

575. Tseng, Y. C., S. Lahiri, S. Jackson, K. D. Burman, and L. Wartofsky. Endothelin binding to receptors and endothelin production by human thyroid follicular cells: effects of transforming growth factor-beta and thyrotropin. *J. Clin. Endocrinol. Metab.* 76: 156–161, 1993.

576. Tsuchida, T., R. H. Hruban, B. S. Carson, and P. C. Phillips. Folliculo-stellate cells in the human anterior pituitary express cytokeratin. *Pathol. Res. Pract.* 189: 184–188,1993.

577. Tsushima, T., M. Arai, O. Isozaki, Y. Nozoe, K. Shizume, H. Murakami, N. Emoto, M. Miyakawa, and H. Demura. Interaction of endothelin-1 with porcine thyroid cells in culture: a possible autocrine factor regulating iodine metabolism. *J. Endocrinol.* 142: 463–470, 1994.

578. Tsuzaki, S., and A. C. Moses. Somatostatin inhibits deoxyribonucleic acid synthesis induced by both thyrotropin and insulin-like growth factor-I in FRTL5 cells. *Endocrinology* 126: 3131–3138, 1990.

579. Ulisse, S., A. Fabbri, and M. L. Dufau. Corticotropin-releasing factor receptors and actions in rat Leydig cells. *J. Biol. Chem.* 264: 2156–2163, 1989.

580. Van Bael, A., and C. Denef. Evidence for a trophic action for the glycoprotein homone alpha-subunit in rat pituitary. *J. Neuroendocrinol.* 8: 99–102, 1996.

581. Van Bael, A., R. Huygen, B. Himpens, and C. Denef. In vitro evidence that LHRH stimulates the recruitment of prolactin mRNA-expressing cells during the postnatal period in the rat. *J. Mol. Endocrinol.* 12: 107–118, 1994.

582. Van Bael, A., M. Proesmans, D. Tilemans, and C. Denef. Interaction of LHRH with growth hormone-releasing factor-dependent and -independent postnatal development of somatotrophs in rat pituitary cell aggregates. *J. Mol. Endocrinol.* 14: 91, 1995.

583. van der Laan, B. F., J. L. Freeman, and S. L. Asa. Expression of growth factors and growth factor receptors in normal and tumorous human thyroid tissues. *Thyroid* 5: 67–73, 1995.

584. Vankelecom, H., M. Andries, A. Billiau, and C. Denef. Evidence that folliculo-stellate cells mediate the inhibitory effect of interferon-gamma on hormone secretion in rat anterior pituitary cell cultures. *Endocrinology* 130: 3537–3546, 1992.

585. Vankelecom, H., P. Carmeliet, H. Heremans, J. Van Damme, R. Dijkmans, A. Billiau, and C. Denef. Interferon-gamma inhibits stimulated adrenocorticotropin, prolactin, and growth hormone secretion in normal rat anterior pituitary cell cultures. *Endocrinology* 126: 2919–2926, 1990.

585b. Vankelecom, H., P. Matthÿs, and C. Denef. Involvement of nitric oxide in the interferon-γ induced growth hormone and prolactin secretion in anterior pituitary cell cultures. *Mol. Cel. Endocrinol.* 129: 157–167, 1997.

586. Vannelli, G. B., T. Barni, G. Forti, A. Negro-Vilar, W. Vale, M. Serio, and G. C. Balboni. Immunolocalization of inhibin alpha-subunit in the human testis. A light- and electron-microscopy study. *Cell Tissue Res.* 269: 221–227, 1992.

587. Verhoeven, G., and J. Cailleau. A factor in spent media from Sertoli-cell-enriched cultures that stimulates steroidogenesis in Leydig cells. *Mol. Cell. Endocrinol.* 40: 57–68, 1985.

588. Verhoeven, G., and J. Cailleau. A Leydig cell stimulatory factor produced by human testicular tubules. *Mol. Cell. Endocrinol.* 49: 137–147, 1987.

589. Verhoeven, G., and J. Cailleau. Influence of coculture with Sertoli cells on steroidogenesis in immature rat Leydig cells. *Mol. Cell. Endocrinol.* 71: 239–251, 1990.

590. Verspohl, E. J., H. P. Ammon, and M. A. Wahl. Activin A: its effects on rat pancreatic islets and the mechanism of action involved. *Life Sci.* 53: 1069–1078, 1993.

591. Verspohl, E. J., U. Berger, and H. P. Ammon. The significance

of mu- and delta-receptors in rat pancreatic islets for the opioid-mediated insulin release. *Biochim. Biophys. Acta* 888: 217–224, 1986.

592. Vincent, S. R., and J. C. Brown. Autoradiographic studies of the gamma-aminobutyric acid (GABA) system in the rat pancreas. *Histochemistry* 88: 171–173, 1988.

593. Vincent, S. R., T. Hokfelt, J. Y. Wu, R. P. Elde, L. M. Morgan, and J. R. Kimmel. Immunohistochemical studies of the GABA system in the pancreas. *Neuroendocrinology* 36: 197–204, 1983.

594. Vincent, S.R., C.H. McIntosh, P.B. Reiner, and J.C. Brown. Somatostatin immunoreactivity in the cat adrenal medulla. Localization and characterization. *Histochemistry* 87:483–486,1987.

595. Vinson, G. P., R. Teja, M. M. Ho, and J. R. Puddefoot. Zonation, paracrine function, and aldosterone secretion in the rat adrenal cortex. *Endocr. Res.* 21: 1, 1995.

596. Vliegen, M. K., S. Schlatt, G. F. Weinbauer, M. Bergmann, N. P. Groome, and E. Nieschlag. Localization of inhibin/activin subunits in the testis of adult nonhuman primates and men. *Cell Tissue Res.* 273: 261–268, 1993.

597. Vollmar, A. M., A. Friedrich, and R. Schulz. Atrial natriuretic peptide precursor material in rat testis. *J. Androl.* 11: 471–475, 1990.

598. Voutilainen, R., M. Eramaa, and O. Ritvos. Hormonally regulated inhibin gene expression in human fetal and adult adrenals. *J. Clin. Endocrinol. Metab.* 73: 1026–1030, 1991.

599. Voutilainen, R., and W. L. Miller. Coordinate tropic hormone regulation of mRNAs for insulin-like growth factor II and the cholesterol side-chain-cleavage enzyme, P450scc, in human steroidogenic tissues [published erratum appears in *Proc. Natl. Acad. Sci. U.S.A.* 84: 6194, 1987]. *Proc. Natl. Acad. Sci. U.S.A.* 84: 1590–1594, 1987.

600. Wan, D. C., and B. G. Livett. Vasoactive intestinal peptide stimulates proenkephalin A mRNA expression in bovine adrenal chromaffin cells. *Neurosci. Lett.* 101: 218–222, 1989.

601. Wang, Z. L., W. M. Bennet, R. M. Wang, M. A. Ghatei, and S. R. Bloom. Evidence of a paracrine role of neuropeptide-Y in the regulation of insulin release from pancreatic islets of normal and dexamethasone-treated rats. *Endocrinology* 135: 200–206, 1994.

602. Watkins, W. B., J. F. Bruni, and S. S. Yen. Beta-endorphin and somatostatin in the pancreatic D-cell colocalization by immunocytochemistry. *J. Histochem. Cytochem.* 28: 1170–1174, 1980.

603. Weir, G. C., S. Mojsov, G. K. Hendrick, and J. F. Habener. Glucagonlike peptide I (7–37) actions on endocrine pancreas. *Diabetes* 38: 338–342, 1989.

604. Weiss, J., W. F. Crowley, Jr., L. M. Halvorson, and J. L. Jameson. Perifusion of rat pituitary cells with gonadotropin-releasing hormone, activin, and inhibin reveals distinct effects on gonadotropin gene expression and secretion. *Endocrinology* 132: 2307–2311, 1993.

605. Wenger, T., M. Bouhdiba, P. Saint Pol, P. Ciofi, G. Tramu, and J. Leonardelli. Presence of neuropeptide—Y and its C-terminal flanking peptide immuno-reactivity in the seminiferous tubules of human testis. *Andrologia* 22: 299–303, 1990.

606. Werner, S., W. Weinberg, X. Liao, K. Peters, M. Blessing, S. A. Yuspa, R. L. Weiner, and L. T. Williams. Targeted expression of a dominant-negative FGF receptor mutant in the epidermis of transgenic mice reveals a role of FGF in keratinocyte organization and differentiation. *EMBO J.* 12: 2635–2643, 1993.

607. Whitelaw, P. F., K. A. Eidne, R. Sellar, C. D. Smyth, and S. G. Hillier. Gonadotropin-releasing hormone receptor messenger ribonucleic acid expression in rat ovary. *Endocrinology* 136: 172–179, 1995.

608. Whitman, G. F., and C. G. Pantazis. Cellular localization of Mullerian inhibiting substance messenger ribonucleic acid during human ovarian follicular development. *Am. J. Obstet. Gynecol.* 165: 1881–1886, 1991.

609. Widmark, A., J. E. Damber, and A. Bergh. Arginine-vasopressin induced changes in testicular blood flow. *Int. J. Androl.* 14: 58–65, 1991.

610. Wilcox, J. N., A. Augustine, D. V. Goeddel, and D. G. Lowe. Differential regional expression of three natriuretic peptide receptor genes within primate tissues. *Mol. Cell. Biol.* 11: 3454–3462, 1991.

611. Williams, D. W., E. D. Williams, and D. Wynford-Thomas. Evidence for autocrine production of IGF-1 in human thyroid adenomas. *Mol. Cell. Endocrinol.* 61: 139–143, 1989.

612. Wolfensberger, M., W. G. Forssmann, and M. Reinecke. Localization and coexistence of atrial natriuretic peptide (ANP) and neuropeptide Y (NPY) in vertebrate adrenal chromaffin cells immunoreactive to TH, DBH and PNMT. *Cell Tissue Res.* 280: 267–276, 1995.

613. Woodruff, T. K., L. Krummen, G. McCray, and J. P. Mather. In situ ligand binding of recombinant human [^{125}I] activin-A and recombinant human [^{125}I]inhibin-A to the adult rat ovary. *Endocrinology* 133: 2998–3006, 1993.

614. Woodruff, T. K., R. J. Lyon, S. E. Hansen, G. C. Rice, and J. P. Mather. Inhibin and activin locally regulate rat ovarian folliculogenesis. *Endocrinology* 127: 3196–3205, 1990.

615. Wrathall, J. H., and P. G. Knight. Effects of inhibin-related peptides and oestradiol on androstenedione and progesterone secretion by bovine theca cells in vitro. *J. Endocrinol.* 145: 491–500, 1995.

616. Wu, S., C. M. Boyer, R. S. Whitaker, A. Berchuck, J. R. Wiener, J. B. Weinberg, and R. C. Bast, Jr. Tumor necrosis factor alpha as an autocrine and paracrine growth factor for ovarian cancer: monokine induction of tumor cell proliferation and tumor necrosis factor alpha expression. *Cancer Res.* 53: 1939–1944, 1993.

617. Wuttke, W., H. Jarry, I. Pitzel, I. Knoke, and S. Spiess. Luteotrophic and luteolytic actions of ovarian peptides. *Hum. Reprod.* 8 (Suppl. 2): 141–146, 1993.

618. Wynick, D., P. J. Hammond, K. O. Akinsanya, and S. R. Bloom. Galanin regulates basal and oestrogen-stimulated lactotroph function. *Nature* 364: 529–532, 1993.

619. Xiong, Y., and D. B. Hales. Expression, regulation, and production of tumor necrosis factor-alpha in mouse testicular interstitial macrophages in vitro [published erratum appears in *Endocrinology* 134: 1597, 1994]. *Endocrinology* 133: 2568–2573, 1993.

620. Yamaguchi, T., Z. Naito, G. D. Stoner, R. Franco-Saenz, and P. J. Mulrow. Role of the adrenal renin–angiotensin system on adrenocorticotropic hormone- and potassium-stimulated aldosterone production by rat adrenal glomerulosa cells in monolayer culture. *Hypertension* 16: 635–641, 1990.

621. Yamanaka, Y., H. Friess, M. Buchler, H. G. Beger, L. I. Gold, and M. Korc. Synthesis and expression of transforming growth factor beta-1, beta-2, and beta-3 in the endocrine and exocrine pancreas. *Diabetes* 42: 746–756, 1993.

622. Yasuda, H., K. Inoue, H. Shibata, et al. Existence of activin-A in A- and D-cells of rat pancreatic islet. *Endocrinology* 133: 624–630, 1993.

623. Yeh, J., F. T. Danehy, R. Osathanondh, and L. Villa-Komaroff.

mRNAs for insulin-like growth factor-II (IGF-II) and variant IGF-II are co-expressed in human fetal ovary and uterus. *Mol. Cell. Endocrinol.* 80: 75–82, 1991.

624. Yeh, J., and R. Osathanondh. Expression of messenger ribonucleic acids encoding for basic fibroblast growth factor (FGF) and alternatively spliced FGF receptor in human fetal ovary and uterus. *J. Clin. Endocrinol. Metab.* 77: 1367–1371, 1993.

625. Ying, S. Y. Inhibins, activins and follistatins. *J. Steroid Biochem.* 33: 705–713, 1989.

626. Zentel, H. J., D. Nohr, S. Muller, N. Yanaihara, and E. Weihe. Differential occurrence and distribution of galanin in adrenal nerve fibres and medullary cells in rodent and avian species. *Neurosci.Lett.* 120: 167–170, 1990.

627. Zerek-Melen, G., A. Lewinski, M. Pawlikowski, E. Sewerynek, and J. Kunert-Radek. Influence of somatostatin and epidermal growth factor (EGF) on the proliferation of follicular cells in the organ-cultured rat thyroid. *Res. Exp. Med. (Berl.)* 187: 415–421, 1987.

628. Zhang, M., M. Zheng, and R. L. Schleicher. Autoradiographic localization of beta-endorphin binding in the pancreas. *Mol. Cell. Neurosci.* 5: 684–690, 1994.

629. Zhou, J., and C. Bondy. Anatomy of the human ovarian insulin-like growth factor system. *Biol. Reprod.* 48: 467–482, 1993.

19. Role of pulsatility in hormonal action

ROSALIND P. MURRAY-McINTOSH | *Institute of Molecular Biosciences, Massey University*
Palmerston North, New Zealand

THE DYNAMICS OF CELLULAR STIMULATION and response is now recognized as an essential feature of endocrinology and pharmacology. Information on timing is required for understanding mechanisms of stimulant action, inhibitor action, and their dysfunction. Knowledge of dynamics is essential also for appropriate intervention. On a broader scale, understanding the mechanisms underlying the dynamics of interacting systems provides a basis for approaching functional organization in biology.

In the last edition of this series, the concept of rhythms, particularly in the reproductive and endocrine systems, was well established; but these rhythms related to clearly visible annual, monthly, and lifetime cycles. Within these rhythms, those hormonal, biochemical, and physiological causes of events giving rise to periodicity which could be observed and measured were researched and described thoroughly and elegantly (for example, ref. 61). However, the pulsatile appearance of many hormones in general circulation as an essential part of the endocrine signaling mechanism between organs was not yet understood to be the pervasive norm that many subsequent studies have shown, nor had the neural contribution to the function of endocrine systems been fully investigated.

One example will suffice. Dynamics received no comment in descriptions of the mechanisms of stimulus coupling with secretion in the neurohypophysis (39) or in neurohypophysis structure related to function (94). The electrical excitability of neurons and neurosecretory fibers, that is, the capacity to generate and propagate impulses, was known to provide impulses stimulating release of neurotransmitters and causing exocytosis of granules containing hormones, but how the dynamics of this release was translated into control of the activity of more distant organs had yet to be explored.

Investigating time series of hormone concentrations requires replicated measurement of many samples from the same individual. Earlier measures of bioactivity, for example, assaying responses of cultured cells stimulated with the unknown hormone sample, posed considerable experimental difficulty. In studies of responses of target organs and tissues in vivo and in vitro, this problem was eased greatly by the development of the radioimmunoassay—for example, the first assay for luteinizing hormone (125). Refinements and developments in techniques for measuring hormones with greater accuracy, convenience, and sensitivity and in smaller volumes continue to improve access to the large amounts of data necessary for exploring pulsatile patterns of hormone concentration. Development of a direct and continuous readout of hormone levels using biosensors remains an exciting possibility for the future.

Along with investigations of hormone clearance rates from the blood, time series measurements have revealed varying and apparently unstable concentrations of luteinizing hormone circulating in castrated animals. By sampling repeatedly at closer intervals (about 20 min) in the same individual, the existence of oscillations in hormone level, termed "circhoral pulses," was discovered in plasma of castrated rats and monkeys (37, 55). There appeared to be a burst of hormone release, causing rapid elevation of concentration over 10 min, followed by cessation of release and clearance according to the expected half-life of metabolism of the hormone. After an interval of 1–2 h, the process repeated in a fairly regular fashion. As surmised by McCann (108) in the last edition of this *Handbook*, these pulses represented a pituitary release of luteinizing hormone into the general circulation in response to periodic pulsatile discharges of gonadotropin-releasing factors from the hypothalamic neurons into the portal vessels bathing the pituitary, "but further work is needed to confirm this view."

Later, it was demonstrated that continuous infusion into animals of either the gonadotropin-releasing hormone (GnRH) decapeptide or an agonist, far from stimulating luteinizing hormone output and reproductive function, paradoxically prevented them (20); however, both could be restored by reinstating pulsatile delivery of releasing hormone (12). This evidence made it clear that pulsatile stimulation was not just a physiologically convenient mode of delivery but actually an essential requirement for normal function.

Over the intervening years, the measurement of pulsatile rhythms in endocrine systems and the determination of their effects on target cells has become a fundamental part of the study of both the classical hormones and the many new biologically active substances, including pulsatility associated with secretion of releasing hormones from the hypothalamus (52, 90, 91, 133) and factors influencing this (40, 63, 130, 197), effects of hypothalamic pulses and modulators on release of pituitary hormones [for example, in animals (30) and in tissues and cells (113)], and the influence of pulses of pituitary hormones on the cells they stimulate at target organs (9, 120). In addition, pulsatility in tissues not directly related to the pituitary has been studied, including, for example, release of insulin from the pancreas (173).

Some of the basic principles underlying a very large published literature on these subjects are described here, using necessarily just a few illustrative examples taken predominantly from reproductive endocrinology.

RHYTHMICITY, CYCLICITY, AND ORGANIZATION OF FUNCTION

Context of Pulsatile Events

Hormonal pulses are part of a dynamic web of fluctuating interactions between the individual organism and both its internal and external environments. The outcome produces function adapted to circumstances. For example, pulses of hormone released by the hypothalamus into the portal blood system bathing the pituitary contain signals from the brain which integrate neural and chemical messages from a host of developmental, environmental, sensual, body, and organ feedback states. The natural world and the biological entities responding and adapting to it abound in pulsatility. Indeed, pulsatility may be considered our experiential norm. Rather than acting to produce differences within constant surroundings, biological systems have needed to develop highly sophisticated mechanisms to smooth or hold near constant responsive elements (for example, acidity or blood glucose levels) in the face of bombardment by natural physical and biological pulsatility. Yet within this fluctuation, we observe structure and function developing and declining in a stable, almost predictable way.

Figure 19.1 shows some of the cycles, rhythms, and pulses of widely different frequencies involved in mammalian ovulation, a remarkably rich range of events, each of which must exist and have accurate timing in relation to all of the others for ovulation to occur repeatedly. The simultaneous energy and subtlety of the factors driving and shaping the organization of such events is illustrated not only from the necessity of the mutual placing and timing of components and the support systems providing them but also from the frequency and reliability with which it has occurred in order to populate the earth with the great variety and numbers of sexually produced beings now here.

Exciting concepts and perceptions of rhythms and their relationship to biological organization have developed; a selection of formative views by several leading protagonists can be found in references 51, 75, 107, 140, 144, 146, 149, 151, 188, 204, 205, 210 and are summarized briefly in rerference 109.

Mathematical Models With the Properties of Biological Rhythms

Such pulsatile events as ovulation, as shown by the frequency of their success, clearly represent a form of "(thermodynamic) energy minimum." Are there models which describe an energy minimum with properties of stable repetition? In classical thermodynamics, rhythmicity in an isolated system, that is, one which does not

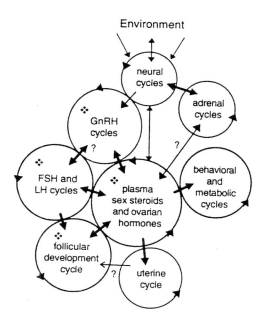

Ovulatory time cascade

Brain
neural pulses (milliseconds)

Intracellular Ca⁺⁺
pulses and waves (seconds)

❖ Circhoral rhythms
*GnRH, LH, FSH, ovarian steroid pulses
hormone synthesis and release dynamics
(several min - several hours)*

❖ Daily cycles
*pulse frequency alters with darkness or sleep,
controls rat LH surge*

❖ Ovulation cycles
Human - monthly

❖ Yearly cycles
anestrous in animals

❖ Life cycles
*development, puberty, fertility, menopause, etc.
(decades)*

FIG. 19.1. Coordinated cycles/pulses of major components in cyclic ovulation, and some of their interactions. Some of the different frequencies of action and response in cycles/pulses are indicated. [Adapted from McIntosh and McIntosh (109) with permission from Springer-Verlag.]

exchange matter or energy with its environment, decays to a stable minimum energy and maximum entropy (Fig. 19.2). This stable state has neither organization nor structure. Such a view is manifestly in contrast to our experience of open, highly organized biological systems which continually arise and develop while showing repeated oscillatory behaviors for long periods in a stable fashion. Mathematical models describing limit cycles, however, do exhibit properties which are remarkably similar to pulsatile biological systems (as described in ref. 109): namely, they exhibit a stable rhythmic oscillation which, when disturbed by outside events, will return to its rhythmic behavior. Important also, limit cycles can entrain to external rhythms with a different period by taking up the new frequency.

To illustrate that we do not require very complex systems and equations to generate these characteristics, a relatively simple set of equations describing one system is developed here in more detail. The example in Figures 19.3 and 19.4 illustrates the simplest known interactions forming a limit cycle, the Zhabotinski-Zaikin chemical reaction, with the following equations:

$$dy/dt = A - (B+1)y + y^2z$$
$$dz/dt = By - y^2z$$

This system has two variables (y and z) and two constants (A and B), with a nonlinear term (y^2) arising

from autocatalysis. The equations describe behavior which can vary in both space and time (t), one example being oscillations and waves in the colors of interacting chemicals disturbed from homogeneous solution. The exact form of the outcome depends on the values of A and B (144, 201). Starting from apparently simple equations and interactions, we find self-organizing behavior with emergent dynamic properties, which, to say the least, are not intuitively obvious.

Figures 19.3 and 19.4 illustrate some of the properties of solutions to these equations. Figure 19.3 shows stable pulses in y and a stable oscillation in z with time when $A = 1$ and $B = 3$. In this example, the values of y and z are plotted against time with a regular cycle established. In Figure 19.4, the same equation is plotted with y and z as the axes and time is shown as equal intervals along the trajectories. Five different starting points outside or inside the limit cycle are shown; the variables cycle toward the stable periodicity. However, when A and B take different values (dashed line) the variables may show damped oscillations toward an invariant state.

Another aspect of this model's behavior of interest for endocrinology is the change in variation of the parameters with time resulting from imposing a sinusoidal oscillation at a different frequency, illustrated in Figure 19.5. The period of 7.1 arbitrary time units (from Fig. 19.3) rapidly approaches that of the imposed

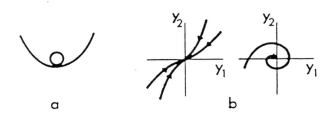

FIG. 19.2. Stability in a closed dynamic system. *a:* Topological metaphor. *b:* Trajectories of a stable system in phase space showing monotonic or oscillatory movement to a steady state. This metaphor does not describe most biological behavior.

rhythm, 6.7 time units. There are many examples in endocrine systems where similar periodicity and frequency entrainment may be operating. Synchronization of biological rhythms with the 24 h clock is an obvious one; a free-running rhythm with a period longer than 24 h is entrained to 24 h by the daily light/dark cycle. Organization of the interactions to produce functional ovulatory cycles (Fig. 19.1) could be based on such principles, involving also harmonics because of the disparate frequencies involved.

These three figures illustrate how one set of relatively simple model equations can describe several cyclic phenomena, including a homogeneous approach to stability (Fig. 19.4), stable space-independent oscillations of

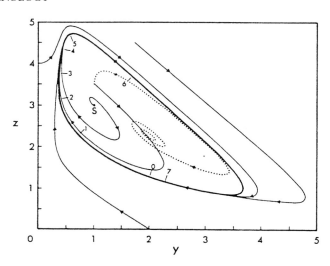

FIG. 19.4. Further limit cycle behaviors. The limit cycle of Figure 19.3 has been plotted with axes y and z in phase space. Equal time intervals are marked on the cycle *(0–7)*. Also shown *(light lines)* are changes in y and z with time when started from values either inside or outside the stable cycle values; the limit cycle is approached. When begun at precisely $y = 1$ and $z = 3$, their values remain constant at this point (S, an unstable steady state). However, on displacing the values slightly to $y = 1.001$ and $z = 3.003$, y and z spiral out to the limit cycle. The *dotted line* represents changes in values of y and z when $A = 2$ and $B = 4.5$. With these different parameters, damped oscillations move the variables toward a stable, constant steady state. [Adapted from McIntosh and McIntosh (109) with permission from Springer-Verlag.]

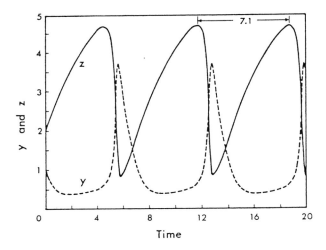

FIG. 19.3. Limit cycle stability in an open system. Values of two variable components y and z showing limit cycle behavior with time, as defined by the Zhabotinski-Zaikin equations with diffusion terms omitted. In the equations, A and B equal *1* and *3*, respectively. The period of the cycle/pulses is approximately *7.1* time units. Such stable cyclicity is typical of many biological behaviors. [Adapted from McIntosh and McIntosh (109) with permission from Springer-Verlag.]

components (Fig. 19.3, 19.4), and entrainment (Fig. 19.5). In addition, spatial variation of component values with time (standing waves) and many different kinds of change dependent on space and time (propagated waves) are possible. Such mathematical descriptions with nonlinear interactions may result in any of these dynamic outcomes. As well, more complex interactions of frequencies are possible, including chaotic variation of variables defined by equations with totally deterministic relationships (171). Clearly, identifying kinds and types of interaction which may produce stable cyclical and pulsatile behavior in endocrine systems is essential to understanding functional organization in biology.

Several known biological interactions have properties that are able to contribute to limit cycle-type outcomes. These include diffusion combined with biochemical reactions obeying mass action laws, diffusion combined with substrate inhibition, and nonlinear feedback loops with several steps containing time delays. With endocrine systems the situation may be complex; the parameters and variables of such equations may not easily be identified directly with specific biochemical or physiological structural components,

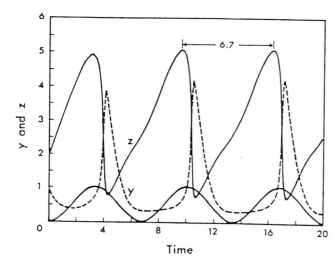

FIG. 19.5. Entrainment of a limit cycle. A continuous forcing function, $dz/dt = E\sin(2\pi / P)$ with amplitude $(E) = 0.5$ and period $(P) = 6.7$ (*lowest curve*), is added to the cycle shown in Figure 19.1. Initial values of $y = 1$ and $z = 2$ were on the original cycle. A new cycle was rapidly approached (*upper curves*), having the same period as the forcing function (6.7 *time units*). [Adapted from McIntosh and McInosh (109) with permission from Springer Verlag].

and it is possible that they may be composites of these components. Overall combined internal rhythms of cells (of hormone synthesis, receptor sensitivity, receptor initiation of response to stimulation, and other biochemical and morphological outcomes) along with transport of signals (hormone-release characteristics, transport delays, and clearance) and feedback exchange between endocrine cells and their target tissue, are the possible contributors to parameters and variables responsible for limit cycle type outcomes, but the details of crucial elements of the steps involved and their dynamics are still being elucidated. We know the general behavior of endocrine systems but not usually the precise biochemical, cellular, and physiological steps crucial in shaping stable cyclic behavior.

In general, however, the mathematical concept of rhythm as a form of stability acts as a metaphor of our experience, confirming acceptance of the potential of rhythms and pulses for playing a major role in biological organization and development.

Modeling of Endocrine Systems to Show Rhythmic Behavior

Based on the available information about particular endocrine systems, so-called whole-system modeling has been carried out to illustrate known relationships. The hope is that equations describing the significant

parts will reflect self-organizing behavior with emergent dynamic properties caused by the nature of the mathematical description, as in the example of the limit cycle above.

A summary and critique of early attempts to model the ovulatory cycle in women is given in reference 109, the most informative description being that of Bogumil et al. (19). This model included pulsed hormones and was also developed further to simulate introduction of random variations to produce differences in cycle outcome resembling physiological situations, such as occasional anovulatory cycles (17, 18, 44). Sometimes mathematical models have been designed merely to describe the end behavior of a system so that little new information or tests of mechanism can emerge. Nevertheless, such modeling has been effective in defining known relationships in endocrine systems by articulating their description and in showing where deficiencies in this information need to be remedied by further experiments. However, the critical test of a model is whether it predicts new features beyond the initial description. These new aspects then require experimental confirmation, in turn refining and then expanding the depth of our understanding.

One example of systems-level analysis concerns the factors influencing growth hormone levels in blood (27). Figure 19.6 illustrates the interactions and feedback relationships considered relevant to this outcome, gleaned from decades of intensive research in many laboratories. Equations describing parts of the system were combined, and the resulting output simulated physiological responses in growth hormone pulses in rats after several types of disturbance. Direct physiological outcomes were associated with particular mathematical properties of the model used.

A mathematical model that included the major mechanisms involved in glucose regulation investigated whether oscillations in the variables insulin and glucose could result from feedback loops between them (172). Two negative-feedback loops were included to describe the effects of insulin on glucose utilization and production, and both loops included the stimulatory effect of glucose on insulin secretion, using parameter values from clinical determinations. Sustained insulin and glucose oscillations depended on (1) a time delay of 30–45 min for the effect of insulin on glucose production and (2) a sluggish effect of insulin on glucose utilization. Numerical simulations mimicked experimental findings, including constant glucose infusion at various rates producing self-sustained ultradian oscillations (with periods in the range of fractions of hours to several hours).

The neuroendocrine pulse generator has been modeled based on a simple dynamical network and knowl-

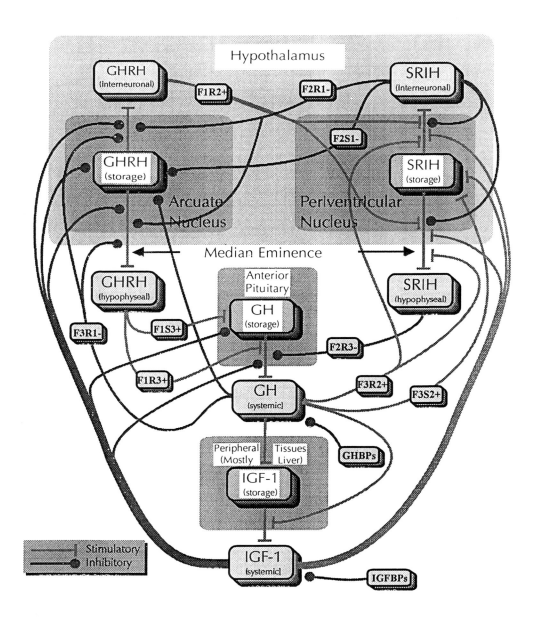

FIG. 19.6. Model showing network of known interactions, neuroendocrine, pituitary, and systemic, which determine secretion of growth hormone *(GH)*. This was used to design equations producing stable pulsatile behavior of growth hormone release in rats. Up-regulatory interactions are indicated by *lines with T endings* (—⊢); down-regulatory interactions are indicated by *lines with ball endings* (—●). *GHRH*, growth hormone–releasing hormone; *SRIH*, somatostatin; *IGF*, insulin-like growth factor; *BP*, binding proteins; *F+* and *F−*, modifier functions, up-regulatory and down-regulatory, respectively; *R*, release; *S*, synthesis. [Adapted from Chen et al. (27) with permission from Academic Press Inc.]

edge of neural behavior (23). Experimental investigations are difficult because the neurons regulating reproductive functioning are scattered sparsely within the hypothalamus. The minimal component required to simulate pulsatile luteinizing hormone secretion was a combination of GnRH-releasing neurons with recip-

rocally connected inhibitory interneurons and an external stimulatory input. Local gamma-aminobutyric acid (GABA) neurons (79) and ascending noradrenergic and/or adrenergic inputs were used as the biological bases for these components. The network displayed a repertoire of behaviors comparable with experimental observations, including some which were apparently paradoxical (23).

We can anticipate that further efforts to combine mathematical approaches with known physiological interactions within endocrine systems will lead to new insights into the role of dynamics in adapted, functional organization. This undoubtedly will lead to innovative experimental tests of new hypotheses.

Pulses as Signals

Although early workers did not anticipate that hormones would be detected as pulses, it is easy in retrospect to see the advantages of pulsatility for cellular communication. Hormones are signals for cell activation or inhibition (Fig. 19.7). The binding of a molecule of hormone to an appropriate receptor either on the plasma membrane of a cell or intracellularly is a signal for the cell to act. Responses may be immediate in the short term and can accumulate over time. Such responses may take every form of cell activity, including electrical changes; release of secreted granules; transport of cell particles, receptors, ions or metabolites; transcription; protein synthesis; cell differentiation; contraction; replication; apoptosis; etc. The outcome depends on the state of preparedness of the cell and the function served both by its state of differentiation and by the hormone. Clearly, interpretation of the hormonal signal must depend on the receptive condition of the target tissue rather than on properties of the channel conveying the signal. The signal must be able to transcend variability in the means of its dispersion.

If an abrupt but temporary change in hormone level is effective in altering cell behavior, then it would be expected that *(1)* the amount of hormone secreted by the stimulating organ into the channel in which it is transferred (for example, the general circulation) could be minimal, *(2)* to maintain precise high concentrations would not be crucial, and *(3)* feedback from the target organ could be monitored with fine tuning of subsequent pulse characteristics. Also, the timing of the response may be entrained to the rhythm of the stimulating signal (compare Figs. 19.5 and 19.3). The maximum rate at which pulses can be discerned, however, depends on how rapidly the hormone is cleared from the circulation, to allow the next pulse to be distinguished from baseline (112).

In contrast, if the signal were an incremental and sustained increase in concentration, rather than pulsatile, a larger amount of secreted hormone would be required and there would seem to be limited possibility for rapid feedback modulation. Further, blood flow is used for many purposes and provides a noisy, variable channel for detecting signals based on detection of

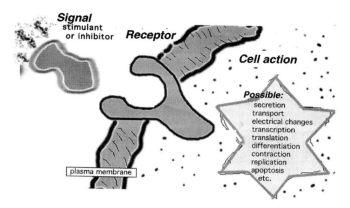

FIG. 19.7. A hormone (or any stimulant or inhibitor) interacts with a cell receptor. The biochemistry of this event and its many possible consequences depend on the state of the cell. Also, there are dynamic aspects. The signal for action is encoded in how the hormone is presented over time to the cellular response mechanisms, which have their own inherent timing. Dynamic aspects of this interaction are the focus of this chapter.

sustained hormone concentration; hormone level would have to be continuously higher than minimally effective to be sure of overriding hindrances to delivery.

Which aspects of the delivery of the hormonal signal are effective in inducing the response? A train of pulses contains several attributes that may influence cell activation (Fig. 19.8), namely, amplitude and interval of pulses, the rate at which each pulse rises from baseline, the time that each pulse continues, and possibly a baseline continuous stimulation signal. ("Interval" is also called "period" and is equal to 1/frequency.) Studies are described below which investigated each of these possibilities in cells perifused with a constant flow of medium in a controlled environment to which selected stimulatory hormonal signals could be added.

There may be an enormous differential between the energy of a response and the stimulation signal. The latter could be as slight as momentary activation of the optic nerve or a pulse of hormone. Information from external and internal stimulation signals is coupled to endogenous power sources through highly evolved functional structures and activities so that actions appropriate to survival are performed.

The pituitary appears to act as such an amplification system. The integrated response to internal and external stimulations of the brain is expressed in tiny amounts of peptide hormones secreted in pulses into the pituitary portal system. The pituitary interprets these signals in amplified form so that transport of its secreted hormones in the general circulation throughout the body can reach and activate distant target tissues. From the perspective of the target organ, how-

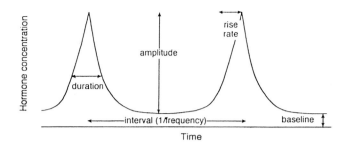

FIG. 19.8. Characteristics of a hormone pulse which may be significant to the form of cell responses. [Adapted from McIntosh and McIntosh (113) with permission from the *Journal of Endocrinology* Ltd.]

ever, the ways in which the pulsatility of the pituitary hormones are significant are still being clarified, apart from pulses being an efficient mechanism for transport of the hypothalamic signal.

EXPERIMENTAL STUDIES IN ENDOCRINE PULSATILITY

Three categories of physiological preparation have been developed for studying pulsatility in endocrine action: live animals, organs, and isolated cells. These approaches are complementary, each being appropriate for investigating specific questions where interpretation is least affected by inherent methodological difficulties.

In vivo studies have involved blood sampling from the general circulation of humans, or live animals, or, in animals, from specific vessels draining the organ of investigation. In addition, electrical measurements, manipulation of electrical impulses, and microdialysis techniques have been used in animals to investigate the involvement of brain and neural tissue. Limitations related to the use of these methods in whole animals include greater difficulty in defining direct causal effects which exclude the possibility of intermediates and possible contributions to the outcome arising from stress, anesthesia, or other manipulations.

At the tissue level, responses from perfused (media circulated through blood vessels in the organ) or perifused intact organs or slices of tissue allow more control of selected components but require skill in maintaining the tissue in a near natural, viable state. Other results have been obtained from perifusing separated cells (or even cells in static culture), where contributing factors can be defined more directly and replication of identical samples for controls and measurement is easier. However, there is a lack of natural support from surrounding tissues and of possible biochemical and physiological influences from neighboring cells. Both

of these tissue preparations require the methodology to be investigated particularly thoroughly, to avoid contributions from interference of the mechanical or chemical attributes of the system or from slow or selective cell death processes (126, 128, 164).

Hypothalamic Studies

The characteristics of the different endocrine pulse systems and their neurological generators have been studied intensively in live animals for several decades. In an extensive literature, the factors influencing these pulses, their effects on target tissue, and their responses feeding back to the brain and pituitary are described also. The following descriptions illustrating particular concepts represent just a few examples and have a bias toward the female ovulatory cycle.

A highly simplified picture of endocrine processes in the adult reproductive system would include the following. Integrated neurological signals within the brain activate release of GnRH from the hypothalmus. This hormone is secreted into the portal blood system bathing the pituitary to cause release into the general circulation of luteinizing hormone and follicle-stimulating hormone (FSH) from specialized gonadotrope cells. The latter hormones stimulate the gonads to produce and release ova in the female or mature sperm in the male. Hormones produced by the gonads feed back to modify both the release of GnRH from the hypothalamus and the responses of the pituitary gonadotropes (61). Most other endocrine systems have equivalent anatomical features and feedback systems.

By the mid-1970s, the expectation was that central control of initiation of all hormonal pulses released from the pituitary resided in the hypothalamus. For luteinizing hormone in the monkey, in particular, the controller was localized to the arcuate nucleus in the mediobasal region of the hypothalamus, as shown from classical neuroendocrine techniques of radiofrequency lesions and surgical disconnection (summarized in ref. 89). Determination of the dynamic characteristics of this generator linked to luteinizing hormone release has been attempted by several means:

1. through exploration of the hypothalamus with both lesions and electrodes to find correlates with and controls of GnRH and luteinizing hormone release (131),

2. by measurements of the dynamics of GnRH appearance in samples of the extracellular fluid bathing the hypothalamus by "push–pull" or micro-perfusion (96),

3. by similar determination of GnRH concentrations in the cerebrospinal fluid of the third ventricle (180),

4. through time series measurement of GnRH in pituitary portal blood (30), and

5. through frequent assessment of luteinizing hormone concentration in peripheral blood, the only method possible with humans (35, 114).

The first, fourth, and fifth of these methods are described briefly below.

Hypothalamic Electrical Activity Correlating With Pulses of Circulating Pituitary Hormones.

In the laboratory of Knobil, GnRH pulse generator activity was studied in the brains of rhesus monkeys using electrophysiological techniques. Sharp increases were detected in the frequency of hypothalamic multiunit electrical activity (MUA) (133). Animals were fitted with arrays of recording electrodes consisting of multiple nichrome wires precisely implanted by stereotaxic means into the mediobasal region of the hypothalamus. After testing each electrode for synchrony of its emitted volleys with the appearance of pulses of luteinizing hormone in peripheral blood, an appropriate one was selected for radiotelemetric monitoring. The battery-powered FM transmitter used could operate continuously for over a month, allowing long-term (chronic) studies. The MUA volley frequency was recorded in caged monkeys tethered to a swivel joint but otherwise able to behave freely. Measurement of luteinizing hormone concentration in peripheral blood used a bioassay of Leydig cells from gerbil testes.

It was discovered that precipitous increases in the MUA were invariably synchronous with the initiation of pulses of luteinizing hormone. Activity varied during the menstrual cycle: there was a slower frequency of MUA and luteinizing hormone pulses in the luteal phase after ovulation than in the phase of follicular development prior to ovulation. However, during the luteinizing hormone surge immediately prior to and essential for ovulation, volleys and distinct hormone peaks unexpectedly ceased. This appeared to be caused by the preovulatory rise in plasma estrogen concentration (133). In contrast, studies in women have claimed to show both frequent luteinizing hormone pulses at this time of the cycle (38) and ones at the same constant pulse frequency as observed in the follicular development phase of the cycle (2). Despite this effect in monkeys, pulsatile administration of GnRH at constant frequency and amplitude can reestablish menstrual cycles when hypothalamic GnRH has been disabled (91). A similar constant pulsatile administration of GnRH to women deficient in activity of this hormone can restore fertility (see later under *Pulses and Pathology*).

Figure 19.9 shows experimental measurements of MUA volleys and accompanying luteinizing hormone in peripheral blood of monkeys during the ovulatory cycle. While variation over the menstrual cycle is well illustrated, these particular results show only a correlation of GnRH and luteinizing hormone pulsatility; additional evidence was needed to establish the direction and mechanisms of causation.

Factors Interacting With Hypothalamic Electrical Activity Related to Pulsatile Releasing Hormones.

The following descriptions give examples of factors shown to interact with GnRH release from the hypothalamus in this monkey model and thereby expected to modulate reproductive development and function. Similar investigations are being carried out with other endocrine systems.

The duration of MUA volleys was 1–3 min in intact monkeys, but following castration and the resultant removal of ovarian sex steroids, duration increased slowly over the next 6 weeks to 20 min. Similar changes are likely to occur during reduction of ovarian steroid production in menopausal women.

A significant reduction in GnRH pulse generator frequency was observed at night during the follicular phase, but not the luteal phase, of the menstrual cycle (133). This is similar to observations of circadian luteinizing hormone pulse frequency in women. In rhesus monkeys, this reduction in frequency was influenced both directly by light and indirectly by an inherent diurnal rhythm independent of light (132).

To initiate puberty, it appears that maturation of the neuroendocrine control system, which directs the pulsatile secretion of GnRH from the hypothalamus, is required. Normal ovulatory cycles could be produced in prepubertal female rhesus monkeys by infusion of GnRH for 6 min once every hour. However, when this regimen was discontinued, the animals promptly reverted to an immature state, demonstrating that pituitary and ovarian competences were insufficient for puberty (196).

Neurotransmitter elements acting on GnRH characteristics included α-adrenergic, α 1–adrenoceptor, and dopaminergic blockers (86), while morphine was found to inhibit MUA with a differential effect on frequency and duration (198).

High concentrations of peripheral luteinizing hormone did not influence MUA, providing evidence against a short feedback loop from pituitary luteinizing hormone secretions inhibiting levels of its own stimulant from the hypothalamus (87).

In the same experimental system, interactions have been studied between MUA controlling GnRH pulses and the endocrine hormones mediating responses to stress. The effects of the hypothalamic stress-related hormone corticotropin-releasing factor (CRF) on the

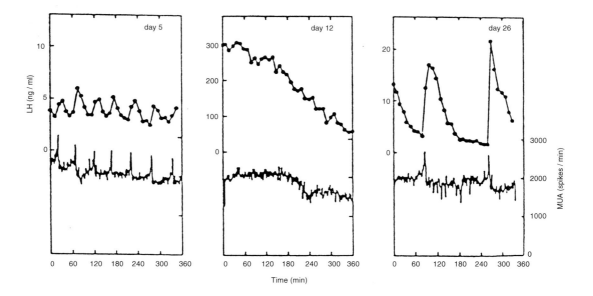

FIG. 19.9. Synchrony between hypothalamic and pituitary activities. Volleys of hypothalamic multiunit electrical activity (*MUA*) and luteinizing hormone *(LH)* pulses in the peripheral circulation were measured during the follicular phase (day 5), mid-cycle luteinizing hormone surge (day 12), and luteal phase (day 26) of the menstrual cycle of a rhesus monkey. On day 12 there was an absence of both luteinizing hormone peaks (using "cluster methods" of analysis) and volleys during the sampling period. [Adapted from O'Byrne et al. (133) with permission from *Endocrinology.*]

hypothalamic GnRH pulse generator in monkeys were to decrease the frequency of pulse generator activity, to decrease duration of MUA volleys, and to raise circulating cortisol levels. An inhibitor of adrenal steroidogenesis preventing rise in serum cortisol levels did not reverse the inhibitory effects of CRF. Effects of the opiate antagonist naloxone suggested that endogenous opioids may mediate the action of CRF on pulse generator frequency but not on duration (197). Hypoglycemic "stress" inhibited the GnRH pulse generator by a nonopioidergic mechanism, while ovarian products, probably estradiol, exacerbated the effect (28). Insulin-induced hypoglycemia also profoundly inhibited the activity of the hypothalamic GnRH pulse generator. Arginine vasopressin (AVP) is another neurosecretion that stimulates release of pituitary stress-related hormones. When this hormone was infused intravenously by cannula it failed to decrease pulse generator activity but did decrease mean serum luteinizing hormone concentrations and increase serum cortisol. However, a CRF antagonist infused intravenously delayed inhibition of the pulse generator frequency in response to insulin. These results suggest that AVP does not mediate the hypoglycemia-induced inhibition of GnRH pulse generator frequency in the rhesus monkey but that CRF may be involved in this response (29).

With regard to signal characteristics, it was concluded that initiation of MUA caused release of GnRH,

with further duration not influencing GnRH output (199). This is similar to the observation of the relatively greater effectiveness of the rising side of a GnRH pulse on stimulation of luteinizing hormone release from pituitary cells (115). Both results coincide with the hypothesis that a sharply rising pulse allows for effective signal transmission. From spike analysis it was determined that the MUA volleys arose from synchronous increases in firing rates of single units coordinating within the hypothalamus (131). Dynamical network modeling of the kinds of interaction necessary to produce some of these responses has been carried out (23) and shows complex behaviors similar to those described here.

Similar electrical stimulation experiments on the brains of rats also have been carried out (60). Measurement of plasma growth hormone concentrations in anesthetized rats during electrical stimulation of the arcuate nucleus showed large pulses of secretion. Stimulation of the median eminence was ineffective. It appears that growth hormone release is not linearly related to the activation of growth hormone–releasing hormone (GRH) neurons but is strongly facilitated with increased burst duration (26). In rats intravenous injection of endotoxin lipopolysaccharide has been shown to suppress GnRH pulse generator activity (MUA) through a mechanism involving TNF-α (208a).

The above examples give an idea of the kinds of

investigation of electrical activity in the hypothalamus of intact animals used to define influences on endocrine function which stimulate pulsatile release of the hypothalamic releasing hormones. To understand more about causal mechanisms, other experimental approaches have been made.

Hormone Pulse Release From Hypothalamic Cells.

Studies on isolated cells allow investigation of cycles inherent to individual cells. It is of interest that GnRH secretory neurons are likely to have an inherent pulsatile secretion that is synchronized. Cultures of a cell line of immortalized GT1 GnRH-secreting cells placed on two coverslips were found in perifusion to have synchronized spontaneous release of hormone at a frequency of 25.8 ± 1.6 min, an average peak width of 18.8 min, and an average height of $150.5 \pm 6.0\%$ above the preceding low point (nadir) (106). This was maintained in two different cell culture media and when cells were cultured on Cytodex beads. Few of the cells had formed gap junctions so that a paracrine effect was proposed to be transmitted through the medium. The shape of the pulse was defined by the perifusion system, but the frequency of GnRH release was close to that observed in castrated rats and mice. This system has provided a means for investigating modulators and intracellular mechanisms in GnRH secretion. In vivo GnRH cells are dispersed and few in number; for example, in the rat only ~1300 cells are distributed in the forebrain.

Spontaneous high-frequency/low-amplitude pulses of luteinizing hormone released from pieces of human pituitary in vitro also have been observed (54). The mechanisms causing these releases need further investigation.

Studies have been carried out also on hypothalamic slice explant tissue in roller-tube cultures which reduce to one to three cells thick. This allows electrophysiological, immunohistochemical, and in situ hybridization methodologies to be applied (93).

Measurement of Releasing Hormones in Pituitary Portal Blood.

An example of this approach is the work of Clarke and Cummins, who aimed to demonstrate directly that the pulsatile nature of luteinizing hormone from the pituitary gland is the direct result of pulsatile GnRH release from the hypothalamus into the hypothalamo–hypophyseal portal vessels (30). Their method involved collection of hypophyseal portal blood from conscious sheep and simultaneous measurement of secretions of GnRH and luteinizing hormone. An artificial sinus was built with dental acrylic on the anterior face of the pituitary. A stab incision made in the portal vessels thus exposed drained into the sinus and was collected at the same time as sampling from the jugular vein draining the pituitary. Lesions of the portal vessels were sufficiently discrete to allow the remainder of the pituitary to continue functioning. They demonstrated an exact temporal relationship between GnRH and luteinizing hormone, which always occurred together.

Similar measurements were made of portal GHRH and somatostatin in unanesthetized sheep and compared to growth hormone in the jugular vessels. While GHRH secretion was pulsatile, with a mean pulse interval of 71 min, the mean interval between pulses of somatostatin secretion was 54 min. The resultant growth hormone pulse interval was 62 min, and GHRH and growth hormone secretory peaks were associated. However, those for GHRH were not correlated with somatostatin pulses, nor was somatostatin release correlated with initiation of growth hormone pulse output from the pituitary. Insulin hypoglycemia resulted in a brief stimulation of somatostatin secretion followed by a decline in growth hormone levels and, after 90 min, a slight increase in GHRH. The results suggested the presence of an independent neural rhythmicity of GHRH and somatostatin secretion. It appears that GHRH has a primary role in determining pulsatile growth hormone secretion, while somatostatin has more of a modulatory role (52).

In the hypophyseal-portal circulation of the conscious sheep, CRF and AVP were investigated in another example of this technique. In the basal state, pulsatile secretion of stress-related hormones—CRF and AVP from the hypothalamus, proopiomelanocortin peptides from the pituitary, and cortisol from the adrenal target organ—were measured. A 3 min audiovisual stress (barking dog) rapidly increased the plasma levels of all of the measured substances. Insulin-induced hypoglycemia increased AVP and CRF concentrations in portal plasma, while a strict 1:1 concordance between CRF/AVP pulse secretion and that of adrenocorticotropin hormone (ACTH) was not seen (40). Prolactin release from the pituitary was shown to be independent of portal thyrotropin-releasing hormone (TRH) (174) in this same experimental system, despite the response of lactotropes to TRH in culture.

Many more investigations have been carried using the experimental systems described above and others like them to study the endocrine systems controlled and modulated from the hypothalamus. These approaches have large potential for clarifying influences of neurological interactions, external environmental factors, internal feedback systems, developmental aspects, and interaction between systems in endocrine function, as well as the intermediate processes, mechanisms and dynamics involved. A review of all of these matters is beyond the scope of this chapter, so only selected results are presented to show some interesting possibilities and conclusions related to pulsatility.

Pulses of Pituitary Hormones in Peripheral Blood

Specialized cells in the pituitary synthesize hormones, package them in secretory granules, and then release them into the circulation. Signals influencing these processes include pulsatile neurohypophyseal hormones delivered through the portal blood vessels and feedback from responses of target organs delivered in blood. Hypothalamic activity, as shown by pulses of releasing hormones in the portal vessels, has been well studied particularly in the rat, sheep, horse, and monkey. Obviously, it is not possible to investigate hypothalamic control of secretion in humans using the same interactive approach. In humans, the study of pituitary hormone pulses in the peripheral blood is the closest way to view the neuroendocrine activity influencing their output. In general, while pulse frequency appears to be modulated by the hypothalamic releasing hormones, pulse amplitude is strongly influenced by other factors, including stage of development and response hormones feeding back from the target tissue. In the female reproductive cycle, sex steroids, estrogens, and progesterone have a marked effect on pituitary responses.

General Characteristics of Pulses in Blood. Figure 19.10 illustrates important aspects of hormonal pulses in the peripheral blood. The shape of the pulse is determined by both the secretory activity of the pituitary in response to stimulation from the hypothalamus and the rate of clearance of the hormone from the circulation as it is metabolized. Where pulse interval is long compared to clearance [as usually occurs with lutenizing hormone in the luteal phase of the menstrual cycle after ovulation ($M-3$ and $M-6$ in Fig. 19.10)], the pulses often can be distinguished easily from each other and directly characterized. Where the pulses are more rapid, as occurs in the preovulatory follicular phase of the cycle ($M+2$, $M+6$), the pulses become less distinct and hormonal levels do not fall below the sensitivity of the assay. In this situation, there is a question of whether there is a basal mode of continuous secretion of hormone from the pituitary in addition to pulses stimulated by the hypothalamic releasing hormone (114, 122). Figure 19.10 illustrates differences in luteinizing hormone secretion patterns during progression from the luteal to the follicular phases of the menstrual cycle. Also demonstrated is the variation found when sampling the same normally ovulating woman several times at the same phases of the cycle; this is presented quantitatively in Figure 19.11 after

deconvolution analysis (see later under *Methods of Analyzing Pulses*). There is a considerable range of pulse amplitude and pulse frequency found in this individual with repeated sampling on the same days of the cycle measured in relation to the start of menstruation (114).

In assaying these blood samples for variation in the concentration of FSH, the precision of the method was found to be too low when combined with the slow clearance rate of this hormone, to allow reliable measurement of peaks.

Figures 19.12 and 19.13 compare the characteristics of luteinizing hormone and growth hormone peaks in the same plasma samples (116). Peaks occurred one-half to one-third less frequently for growth hormone than for luteinizing hormone. There is no correlation in timing of the peaks. While luteinizing hormone peaks rose sharply (median time to maximum was 13 min) and cleared relatively slowly (median clearance -0.012/min), growth hormone peaks rose slowly (median time to maximum 38 min) and cleared more rapidly (median clearance -0.038/min). Circulating pituitary hormones increased at rates which were indistinguishable when GHRH and GnRH were injected simultaneously into a vein of the same woman (though the rise rate was slower because of less efficient delivery of hormones to the pituitary through the general circulation than through portal vessels). Therefore, different mechanisms of stimulation appear to cause the natural luteinizing and growth hormone pulse releases by the pituitary. Probable explanations for differences in pulses of these two hormones are that hypothalamic pulses of a single or dominant releasing hormone cause secretion of luteinizing hormone, whereas for growth hormone, the hypothalamic inhibitor of release (somatostatin) and the releasing hormone have different dynamics of secretion from the hypothalmus which mutually interact on pituitary release. Release of the binding protein for growth hormone (which is the cleaved extracellular part of the receptor) occurs after the peak, and this would be expected to speed clearance of circulating hormone. (Current knowledge of these interactions is illustrated in Figure 19.6; growth hormone control in sheep is discussed earlier under *Measurement of Releasing Hormones in Pituitary Portal Blood*.)

Variation of Pulses in Different Physiological States. There have been many measurements made of the pulsatile patterns of pituitary and other hormones in blood of different mammals in different physiological states. For luteinizing hormone and FSH, results of just a few of these studies are included in references 35, 46–48, 105, 114, 139, 155, and 208. Some examples are given of the

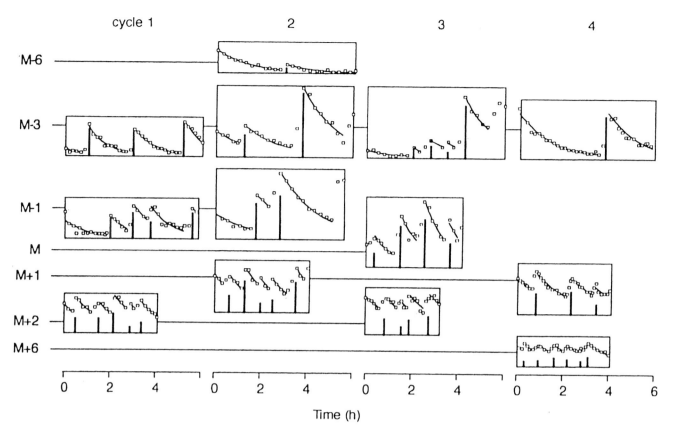

FIG. 19.10. Pituitary hormone pulses in the peripheral circulation. Variation of luteinizing hormone concentration in serial plasma samples *(squares)* from four cycles of one woman measured around onset of menstruation *(M)* on selected days during the transition from the luteal to the follicular phases and the results of fitting a secretory episode model to the data using deconvolution. *Solid lines,* results of fitting the model; *vertical solid lines,* timing and amplitude of secretory episodes seen in plasma. [Adapted from McIntosh and McIntosh (114) with permission from the *Journal of Endocrinology* Ltd.]

many investigations of effects on pulse characteristics of sex steroids (129) and added synthetic GnRH pulses (16, 118, 161, 186), the roles of GnRH pulses in development of the fetal hypothalamo–pituitary–gonadal axis (22), puberty (206), lactation (121, 141), and seasonal anestrus of animals (83). In general, these studies confirm and extend, or are confirmed by, the conclusions reached from the methodologies used in investigating brain and portal blood systems described above.

To illustrate information obtained from investigations of time series measurements of hormones in blood, some studies on the reproductive system are summarized (104). A single GnRH molecular structure differentially regulates luteinizing hormone and FSH production and pulsatile release from the pituitary. The frequency of GnRH stimulation of the gonadotrope is a selective regulator of gonadotropin synthesis, with slow frequency stimuli favoring FSH and faster frequency stimuli favoring luteinizing hormone secretion. In utero and for the first months after birth, GnRH is secreted at approximately 1 pulse/h, but during the first year, both amplitude and frequency of pulses are reduced. Activation of GnRH secretion occurs during sleep at puberty. Some studies show increasing GnRH pulsatile secretion during pubertal maturation, causing the predominant FSH release from gonadotropes to evolve to a predominant luteinizing hormone secretion. Other evidence concludes that a persistent pattern of GnRH release is maintained but with increased amplitude (202). The patterns of GnRH secretion appear reasonably consistent in adult life in men, occurring approximately every 90–110 min. However, in women, cyclic changes which may be important in maintaining cyclic ovulation are clear. Once pubertal maturation

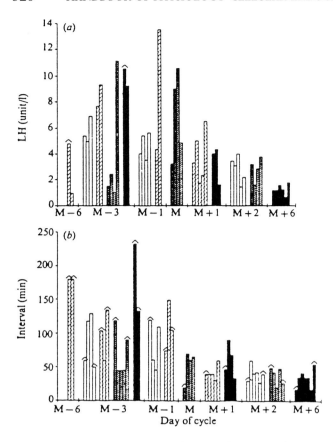

FIG. 19.11. Quantitative variation of pituitary hormone pulses in an individual with peripheral blood sampling repeated in the same healthy physiological conditions. *a:* Amplitudes of episodic luteinizing hormone *(LH)* release. *b:* Intervals between releases on different days of the menstrual cycle around onset of menstruation *(M)*. Raw data are shown in Figure 19.10. Four menstrual cycles sampled are shown: *open bars,* cycle 1; *lightly hatched bars,* cycle 2; *heavily hatched bars,* cycle 3; *solid bars,* cycle 4. *Arrowheads* indicate incomplete peaks at the beginning or end of the sampling period; the size shown is less than actual and has been inferred from trends in the data. [Adapted from McIntosh and McIntosh (114) with permission from the *Journal of Endocrinology* Ltd.]

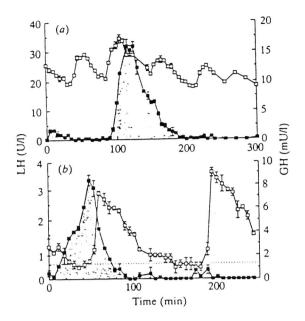

FIG. 19.12. Differences in pulse characteristics of two hormones secreted by the pituitary. Luteinizing hormone *(LH, empty squares)* and growth hormone *(GH, filled squares)* were measured in the same blood samples at two phases of the menstrual cycle: *a,* 10 days after and, *b,* 3 days before menstruation began. Luteinizing hormone peaks rose more rapidly and were cleared more slowly than growth hormone peaks. Timing of pulse onset of the different hormones is not correlated. *Error bars* represent S.E.M. of triplicate assays of each sample. The *dotted line* in *b* is the minimum detectable level of luteinizing hormone in the assay. [Adapted from McIntosh et al. (116) with permission from the *Journal of Endocrinology* Ltd.]

has been established in women, GnRH is secreted at a relatively faster frequency (about 1 pulse/h) with, in repeated ovulatory cycles, a slowing of this GnRH stimulus during the luteal phase to allow subsequent preferential FSH release. This slowing of GnRH secretion appears to be effected by estradiol and progesterone enhancement of hypothalamic opioid activity. There are also direct effects from ovarian estradiol and inhibin to reduce FSH secretion at the pituitary.

Thus, time series measurements in blood provide good descriptions and information on interrelationships. However, aspects of mechanism also need exploration.

Pulses and Pathology.

Various types of reproductive problem in men and women have been associated with the intervals between GnRH pulses being longer or shorter than those observed in the fertile condition. Analogs of the decapeptide GnRH developed since 1971 (177, 207) have allowed therapeutic modification of the hypothalamic–pituitary–gonadal axis (reviewed in refs. 31, 49). For example, portable infusion pumps intravenously delivering regular pulses of GnRH to mimic physiological hypothalamic secretion have been used to restore reproductive potential in both sexes where disorders of endogenous GnRH secretion occur. As mentioned above, it is of interest that delivery of GnRH into the peripheral circulation, using a pump giving pulses at a persistent and constant amplitude and frequency of one per hour, is capable of restoring ovulation and fertility in some anovulatory women, thus permitting pregnancy. This suggests that changes in pituitary output of FSH and luteinizing hormone are controlled predominantly at the pituitary by gonadal feedback and that variation in GnRH pulse rates

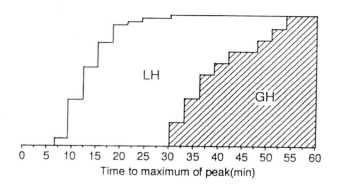

FIG. 19.13. Illustration of the more rapid rise of luteinizing hormone *(LH)* pulses secreted by the pituitary into the peripheral circulation compared to growth hormone *(GH)* pulses. Data are expressed as cumulative frequency distributions of the observed times for the concentrations of the hormones to increase from minimum levels in blood to the maxima of peaks. [Adapted from McIntosh et al. (116) with permission from the *Journal of Endocrinology* Ltd.]

throughout the ovulatory cycle is not crucial, at least in this somewhat artificial situation (91).

In other applications, long-acting agonists of the GnRH receptor have been administered by depot delivery or nasal sprays to maintain high levels of stimulant without pulses, to induce the paradoxical desensitization of pituitary gonadotropin secretion discussed earlier. This results in therapeutic elimination of reproductive function where activity or overactivity of hormones is detrimental to uterine and prostate problems and in precocious puberty. Antagonism of the GnRH receptor has similar potential (24).

Another example of altered pulsatility in pathology concerns menstrual dysfunction related to insulin-dependent diabetes mellitus (IDDM), which occurs in nearly one-third of women suffering from diabetes. The cause of this dysfunction appears to be predominantly changes at the hypothalamus, with intermittent failure of the GnRH pulse generator, similar to the situation observed in some women in endurance training or who suffer from anorexia nervosa. Explanations have focused on increased central opioidergic activity, increased central dopaminergic activity, and central glucose deprivation causing alteration in pulsatile stimulation of the pituitary (62).

An interesting approach toward quantifying endocrine disturbances has been suggested using a different kind of analysis of hormone pulses in blood (140). In this method, the data are analyzed and compared for regularity or noisiness; full characterization of pulses is not essential. The method quantifies the general disturbances in rhythmic secretions often seen intu-itively in pathology when viewing time series of hormones in blood. An example of disturbances in pulsatility of derived insulin secretion rates is seen in patients with diabetes mellitus and impaired glucose tolerance (Fig. 19.14), with the added feature that not only is the secretion rate more noisy with pathology but the system's ability to accommodate a regular disturbance by returning rapidly to stable limit cycle-like behavior appears to be impaired (134). The method of analysis of irregularity (140) discerns abnormal pulsatility in clinical hormonal secretion data given data sets as small as 72 points. The example of analysis of growth hormone pulses in acromegaly has been used to illustrate the method's potential (68). Other analyses and methodologies used for comparison and description of hormone pulses in blood are described below.

There are many examples of tolerance developing with long use of pharmaceutical drugs. It is possible that closer attention to timing of delivery of these drugs, using pulses at intervals specifically designed to suit the response dynamics of the target tissue, may ease this problem (112).

Further Functions of Pulsatile Hormone Secretion. Pulsatile hormones act in a variety of ways in endocrine systems other than the reproductive system. The following gives some experimentally supported examples showing further possibilities of functional organization based on the pulse characteristics of hormonal signals and their interactions.

Growth regulation. Growth regulation illustrates several interesting modes of action and interaction of pulsed secretions. In humans and rats, circulating growth hormone shows strong differences between males and females both in patterns of concentration variation and in levels (reviewed in ref. 181). These differences play a role in regulation of sex-dependent peripubescent growth rates and liver function. In males, circulating pulses of growth hormone are clearly differentiated, with hormone declining to low levels between pulses; in females, while frequency of peaks is similar, there is a much higher baseline (137). The cause of these differences appears to involve the sex steroids combined with variation in inhibition of growth hormone release by the hypothalamic hormone somatostatin. Variation in negative feedback effects also may be involved. A contributing factor could be a lower metabolic clearance rate of growth hormone in women; however, without measurements of volume distribution, growth hormone–binding protein (GHBP) concentration, and other potential influences on clearance, the high baseline of growth hormone cannot be attributed to a longer half-life in women (181).

Sexual differentiation of liver function controlled by

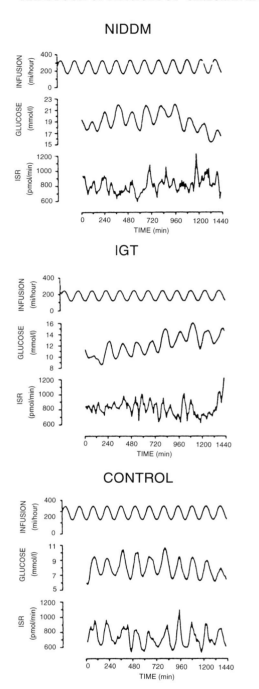

FIG. 19.14. Regularity and entrainment of pulsatile secretion in health compared to disease. Profiles of glucose infusion rates, plasma glucose levels, and insulin secretion rates *(ISR)* from patients with non-insulin-dependent diabetes mellitus *(NIDDM),* or impaired glucose tolerance *(IGT)* and a weight-matched control subject. Glucose was infused in an oscillatory fashion with a period of 144 min. ISRs entrained to the glucose periodicity in control subject but not patients. [Adapted from *The Journal of Clinical Investigation,* 1993, 92: 262–271 (134) by copyright permission from The American Society for Clinical Investigation.]

these different patterns of growth hormone pulses in blood includes expression of the protein steroid hydroxylase cytochrome P-450. A critical element for the rat liver to produce male patterns of cytochrome P-450 is an interval between growth hormone pulses where there is no detectable hormone for at least 2.5 h. It is suggested that hepatocytes undergo an obligatory recovery period which is necessary for resetting a growth hormone–activated intracellular signaling pathway, or which is related to the short-term absence of growth hormone receptors at the hepatocyte surface after a cycle of hormone binding and receptor internalization (190). The intermittent plasma growth hormone pulses occurring in male, but not female, rats activate in liver a latent cytoplasmic transcription factor, Stat 5, by a mechanism that involves tyrosine phosphorylation and nuclear translocation. Physiological levels of growth hormone also can activate other transcription factors, Stat 1 and Stat 3 in liver, but with a dependence on the dose of GH and its temporal plasma profile that is distinct from activation of Stat 5; there is a striking desensitization following a single hormone pulse for Stat 5 only. Growth hormone activation of the two groups of Stats leads to their selective binding either to DNA response elements upstream of the *c-fos* gene (*c-sis*-inducible enhancer element binds Stat 1 and Stat 3), or to the β-casein gene (mammary gland factor element binds Stat 5) (145). The role of a form of Stat 5 in sexual dimorphism of liver gene expression has been substantiated using a mouse gene knockout model (175a).

Further differential responses in growth to peak and trough components of the growth hormone secretion pattern have been shown. Dose-response curves of growth in response to growth hormone given by pulsatile compared to continuous infusion into rats were significantly nonparallel, growth being stimulated primarily by the pulsatile component of a mixed growth hormone infusion pattern. Adding a continuous infusion to a series of pulses did not change weight gain, whereas doubling the dose by adding a pulsatile component significantly enhanced growth. Conversely, a different dynamic of regulation was shown by the hepatic growth hormone receptor and plasma GHBP levels, which were highly sensitive to the continuous element of the infusion pattern and were unaffected by varying the pulsatile component over a wide range of doses (57). During puberty in humans, however, secreted growth hormone pulse characteristics were not found to influence growth (see later under *Pulsatility in Stimulation of End Organ Responses*).

Different mechanisms control the different pulse characteristics of growth hormone release. In rats, the neuroendocrine stimulator of pituitary release of growth hormone, GHRH, appears to regulate both peak and trough components of secretion because administration of antiserum causes a profound suppression of both within 15 min (136). Opioid receptor activation has been shown to reset the hypothalamic mechanism generating pulsatile secretion by shortening both the period and duration of the pulse rhythm (200).

Amplitude rather than frequency of growth hormone pulses is modulated in some conditions. For example, amplitude is reduced by glucocorticoid in Cushing's disease in humans (1), in growth retardation attributed to psychosocial deprivation (4), and with age (71). Strong attenuation of growth hormone pulse amplitude occurs with the negative feedback of insulin-like growth factor (IGF)-1 infused into men, while frequency is reduced to nearly half; these combined effects are compatible with stimulation of secretion of the hypothalamic inhibitor somatostatin (13). Thyroid-stimulating hormone responses to TRH also were greatly reduced, probably from the same cause. The drugs clonidine and L-dopa act on growth hormone release through modulation of GHRH, while hypoglycemia, arginine, and propranolol augment growth hormone release in humans by modulating hypothalamic somatostatin secretion (101). The interaction of GHRH and somatostatin on release of growth hormone pulses from pituitary cells, however, is complex; for example, in perfused rat pituitary cells, somatostatin pulses inhibit growth hormone release but produce a delayed rebound if pulsed during stimulation by GHRH, while somatostatin prior to a GHRH pulse did not affect it (135).

The activity of growth hormone is greatly affected by a circulating binding protein formed from processing of its receptor (152). Each burst of growth hormone pulse release from the pituitary is followed by a wave of receptor turnover and a rapid increase in serum GHBP, which occurs 30 min after the peak. This must influence the rate of disappearance of the pulse and needs to be considered in analyses of growth hormone secretory episodes (72).

Taken together, these examples illustrate the diversity of aspects of pulses important in the control of both secretion and action of growth hormone.

Pulses of hormone responding to stress. Pulses of hormones in the hypothalamo–pituitary–adrenal axis illustrate further interactions and variations in pulse function. The pituitary stress-response hormone ACTH and adrenal cortisol levels in peripheral blood display irregular pulsatile ultradian patterns (pulses at intervals of one-half to several hours). In humans, a variety of numbers of pulses of ACTH per 24 h have been de-

scribed, for example, about 17 (92), about 34 (179), and 3.3 (156) peaks/h. These differences may relate to individual variation or, measurement techniques or be the products of different methods or criteria used in analysis, as described above. Release of cortisol from the adrenals is correlated with the pattern of ACTH pulses but is delayed by up to 10 min. These pulsatile patterns are superimposed on a well-characterized circadian rhythm, leading to a daily rise in blood cortisol in the early morning in humans. It is generally accepted that CRF is released from the hypothalamus in a similar manner to the observed ultradian ACTH and cortisol pulses, which it is expected to stimulate. In rats, the diurnal increase in plasma ACTH has been explained by increased amplitude and duration of CRF pulses secreted from the hypothalamus, while frequency remains constant at 3 pulses/h (103). In this system, there is a particularly clear connection between the circadian pacemaker and episodic release of CRF, though all hypothalamic hormones appear to be similarly modified in some physiological conditions and to some extent.

Perifused pieces of hypothalami of macaque maintain pulsatility of CRF and may contain an inherent pulse generator which controls its release, as discussed previously for GnRH release. A regular pulse interval of 90 ± 11 min was measured in perfusate samples collected at 10 min intervals for 20 h. This interval is described as very similar to the average pulse interval of ACTH and cortisol in the human, but the regular pattern in vitro has not been demonstrated in the intact adrenal axis in vivo. Therefore, to account for the irregularity observed, nonrhythmic factors outside the hypothalamus have been suggested to play a major role in modifying either CRF or its stimulation of adrenal hormone output (123).

These examples illustrate contributions to observed pulses from factors with a range of frequencies, including nonrhythmic ones.

Thyroid metabolism–related stimulation. In humans, secretion of thyroid-stimulating hormone (TSH) from the pituitary has a pronounced circadian rhythm, with an increase in pulse frequency and amplitude clustering around midnight. Clearance from the circulation appears slow relative to pulse frequency at this time so that the baseline is elevated. A tonic secretion as well as a pulsatile release for this hormone and for prolactin (PRL) have been proposed, unlike other pituitary hormones where only pulsatile release appears appropriate (183). In humans, pulses of TSH are significantly concordant with pulses of luteinizing hormone and FSH (153) and PRL (154), indicating common controls in dynamics of stimulation of these pituitary hormones. For example, with 15 min sampling, 36%–45% of TSH pulses occur within 15 min of PRL pulses, while 37%–67% of PRL pulses occur within 15 min of TSH pulses. Releases of PRL and TSH are stimulated by both TRH and dopamine. Because the pulsatility of TSH and PRL remained during constant TRH infusion, factors other than pulsatility of hypothalamic TRH stimulation of the pituitary appear to be involved in the pulse dynamics of the circulating hormones.

Different influences on pulse patterns of baseline secretion, concordance of pituitary release, and non-releasing hormone control of pulsatility are suggested by these results.

Pulsatile secretion in fetus and placenta. Classical studies of fetal development used the chronic fetal sheep model in which continuous in utero studies can be carried out for several weeks, often in unanesthetized ewes and with normal term delivery. This sophisticated surgical approach allowed study of the ontogeny of neuroendocrine pulsatility in this species. A functional pulse generator secreting a luteinizing hormone–releasing factor in the ovine fetus was strongly supported by detection of pulsatile ovine luteinizing hormone secretion in the fetal circulation by 81 days' gestation (term 147 days). Gonadotropin secretion is suppressed by chronic administration of either a luteinizing homrone–releasing factor agonist or an antagonist, while administration of N-methyl-D-aspartate (a neuroexcitatory amino-acid analog) evokes a fetal luteinizing hormone pulse. Sex differences in fetal gonadal function as well as gonadotropin secretion are observed before day 114 (124).

By the last third of gestation, neuroendocrine and pituitary hormones are secreted in a pulsatile fashion (59) with a circadian rhythm for PRL and growth hormone. Also observed was a circadian pattern for the pineal hormone melatonin, which presumably provides information on environmental photoperiod, influencing later development. There is co-pulsatile secretion of luteinizing hormone, FSH, PRL, and, unlike in adults, growth hormone (5). Growth hormone and thyrotropin pulses have exaggerated amplitudes compared to the postnatal pattern. It has been suggested that this enhanced pulsatility is caused by immature feedback loops (58).

Glucocorticoids play a pivotal role in maturation of the fetal organs, which is necessary for survival after birth and during the birth process, particularly functional activity of the lung. Plasma cortisol and ACTH concentrations are pulsatile in the fetus but not interdependent in the same way as in the adult, nor do they change in relation to maternal hormones. During late

gestation, within 72 h of birth, they surge. At this time, there appears to be an absence of regulation of pulsatile ACTH secretion by negative feedback from cortisol. Rather, cortisol appears to exert a positive feedforward influence to create the essential cortisol surge (8). Thus, pulsatile cortisol appears to be driven by a means independent of neuroendocrine secretion.

Classical hypophysiotropic neurohormones are produced and secreted by the human placenta. Indeed, during pregnancy, GnRH and CRF in maternal plasma attain levels high enough to permit measurement, in contrast to levels in nonpregnant subjects. Both releasing factors are secreted in a pulsatile fashion, with GnRH pulses following about 30 min after CRF pulses (158). Human chorionic gonadotropin (hCG), which combines luteinizing hormone– and FSH–like activity, also is secreted in a pulsatile fashion by the placenta stimulated by GnRH (10). The mechanisms of pulsatility and synchrony in this organ require exploration.

Parathyroid hormone. Pulsatile secretion into the general circulation has been reported for parathyroid hormone, which influences bone metabolism. In early postmenopausal women, the pulse count per hour was 5.1 ± 2.2. After 6 months of hormone replacement therapy, a 30% reduction in secretion of both baseline and amplitude, but not frequency, was observed, which could relate to the beneficial effects of replacement therapy in reducing osteoporosis (102). Mechanisms of secretion and action allowing more direct support of the significance of the pulsatility of this hormone, however, remain to be explored.

Secretion from the pancreas. Secretion from the pancreas is controlled by neither pituitary nor hypothalamic hormones. Nevertheless, pulsatile release of insulin and glycogen occurs in vivo and from isolated islets and cells in vitro. Several explanations have been proposed. A pacemaker may be present in the gland itself. Modeling, as discussed above, indicates feedback mechanisms causing this pulsatility to arise. At the level of the individual mouse pancreatic cell, however, cytoplasmic Ca^{2+} concentrations respond to constant 3 mM glucose, with slow oscillations with a period of 2.5–10 min (15). Pulsatile insulin release could be generated from these cells also in the absence of stimulated entry of Ca^{2+}. A tentative explanation given for this phenomenon was inherent fluctuations in the adenosine triphosphate (ATP) production of the beta cells (195).

One analysis of individual 24 h insulin secretory profiles in humans (143) showed about 11 pulses in each 24 h period, with up to eight occurring after meals and about four during the period of overnight sampling. In obese subjects, the amplitude of the pulses was greater. Profound alterations in the temporal organization and the amount of stimulated insulin secretion were suggested to be important in the pathophysiology of beta-cell dysfunction in diabetes mellitus (142) (from illustrations such as Figure 19.14). Here, the entrainment of pulsatile insulin secretion by a sinusoidal infusion of glucose is shown in normal humans; the ability of insulin secretion to respond to this stimulus in diabetes is markedly impaired. Ultradian oscillations may represent optimal functioning of this pancreatic regulatory network (134).

Other studies have shown an approximately 13 min period between natural insulin pulses. This is the interval found to be most effective when injecting pulses of insulin into both healthy and diabetic men for inducing inhibition of endogenous glucose production. Pulsatile delivery of insulin at this frequency is also more effective than continuous infusion or when using longer intervals between peaks (138).

A link between insulin pulsatility and the reproductive system is indicated from pulse frequency, which appears to be an important determinant in the synthesis of sex hormone–binding globulin (SHBG) in normal men (76). This circulating protein binds testosterone and may be important in delivery of the sex steroid to target cells (33).

Interleukin pulsatility. Another pulsatile output which apparently is not controlled by hypothalamic pulsatile secretion is that of interleukin-1 alpha (IL-1α). This cytokine acts as an intermediary between neuroendocrinological and immune systems, exerting numerous actions on both. It is a powerful endogenous pyrogen released, for example, as a response to bacterial endotoxin by monocytes and macrophages. By acting at the hypothalamus, it stimulates ACTH, PRL, and growth hormone release, as well as inhibiting thyrotropin release. In the ovariectomized monkey, it inhibits pulsatile leutinizing hormone and FSH secretions. This inhibitory effect of IL-1α on the gonadotropins is mediated by hypothalamic CRF and AVP through inhibition of prostaglandin E$_2$-mediated release of GnRH and is modulated by estradiol levels (45, 150). Interruption of the menstrual cycle by "stress" also through CRF action on GnRH release, is discussed earlier under *Factors Interacting With Hypothalamic Electrical Activity Related to Pulsatile Releasing Hormones.*

Interleukin-1 alpha acts locally where it is secreted but, interestingly, is also secreted into the circulation in pulses. In healthy women, there are 12.8 ± 0.8 pulses in 24 h, with a mean pulse width of 80.4 ± 2.3 min and an interpulse interval of 105.3 ± 2.8 min. Furthermore IL-1α levels and pulse parameters significantly correlate with those for IL-2 in the same blood samples. Based on these data, it has been speculated that a pulsatile cytokine cascade may exist in the systemic circulation (99). The significance and mechanism of this pulsed interleukin release remains to be elucidated.

Peripheral leptin communicates nutritional status to regulatory centers in the brain. It has been reported to exhibit pulsatile behavior which fluctuates independently of but inversely with ACTH and cortisol (99a).

The illustrations above are just some of many described in the literature showing the capacity for differential control, modulation, and adaptation of function in both tissues and organisms by modifying specific characteristics of pulsatile stimulation. Just a few examples of effects of frequency, multiple frequencies, amplitude, baseline secretion, clearance, positive and negative feedback, and interaction with other pulsatile and nonpulsatile systems were described. An inherent pulsatility of systems, organs, and cells has been proposed, while there remain to be explored many mechanisms of pulsatility and how it relates to function. Much more waits to be revealed about the role of pulsed signals in biological organization. This applies both to systems currently known to be pulsatile and to many others which may yet be shown to be. It is clear that the description of dynamic influences of biologically active factors and the mechanisms controlling them is an essential part of the study of all receptor-modulated biological systems.

Pulsatility in Stimulation of End Organ Responses

Correlation of secretory episodes of end organs with pituitary pulsatile stimulation is often seen. Of more interest is the question of whether pulsatile stimulation is a requirement for optimal function of the target tissue or whether continuous stimulation may serve as well.

With regard to the functioning of the pituitary, pulsatile stimulation by hypothalamic signals usually appears essential to biological function because desensitization of secretion occurs with continuous input. Some examples of different or improved outcomes from pulsatile stimulation in other tissues have been described above. These include effects of growth hormone pulsatility on growth, liver function, and gene transcription in rats and effects of insulin periodicity on inhibiting glucose production and on SHBG production, which modifies the effects of steroid hormones.

Correlations of pulsatile stimulus and ovarian response have been measured in the ovulatory cycle. From measuring sex steroids and luteinizing hormone in the blood of normal women, one study showed that pulsatile release of the ovarian steroids from the corpus luteum in response to luteinizing hormone pulses developed during the second half of the luteal phase after ovulation. However, correlation was detectable only in cases where there were accompanying PRL peaks but not where luteinizing hormone peaks occurred on their own. Prior to menstruation, at the decline of the corpus luteum, luteinizing hormone episodes no longer produced progesterone secretion. The effect was not consistent between individuals; in some women, both gonadal steroids fluctuated greatly, with no discernible correlation to luteinizing hormone fluctuations (70). In another study (56), cross-correlation analysis was used to show concordance between luteinizing hormone and progesterone ($P < 0.05$), with a delay of 0–40 min in normal women, while they were maximally correlated with a 10 min lag.

The necessity of luteinizing hormone pulsatility in stimulation of the ovary (as opposed to correlation with ovarian secretion) is less clear. During the luteal phase of the sheep ovulatory cycle, pulsatile progesterone secretion was shown to be independent of luteinizing hormone because it was not affected by 3 days' treatment with GnRH antagonist, which abolished luteinizing hormone pulses (119). Basal amounts of luteinizing hormone, but not pulses, were thought to be essential for FSH-induced follicular growth in sheep in the preovulatory phase of the cycle. Rather, it was suggested that the function of luteinizing hormone pulses was to cause atresia (breakdown) of those ovarian follicles not selected for ovulation (120).

In correlative studies of gonadal secretion of inhibin and testosterone in men, these hormones were shown to follow a clear diurnal rhythm, with four to seven pulses of inhibin per day correlating with median testosterone levels. A physiological role for the pulsatile nature of inhibin secretion has not been clarified, nor was any relationship to pulsatility of pituitary hormones tested in this study (21). A testosterone frequency of 12.3 ± 0.8 pulses/day and an FSH frequency of 16 ± 1.9 pulses/day were determined, as well as circadian periodicities (185). Cross-correlation analyses showed correlations between luteinizing hormone and testosterone to be maximal at a testosterone lag of 60 min (range 50–70 min). To eliminate high intrinsic autocorrelations within the testosterone and luteinizing hormone time series, stepwise autoregressive fitting was employed. The resulting partial cross-correlation matrices indicated that luteinizing hormone concentrations were correlated significantly to testosterone concentrations at a lag of 10–20 min.

Correlation of the ultradian release of ACTH and cortisol was investigated in male rhesus monkeys (156). There was a 32% concordance of ACTH with cortisol peaks, and 56% percent of ACTH peaks were followed by a cortisol peak within 10 min ($P < 0.02$). A significant correlation between the ACTH and coincident cortisol pulse amplitudes ($P < 0.0001$) was found. The amplitudes of ACTH peaks coincident with cortisol peaks at a 0 min time lag were significantly higher than ACTH peaks not temporally coupled with cortisol peaks. Concordance between secretion of these two hormones appears incomplete.

To study the relation of growth hormone peaks to growth, short children were submitted to tests of nocturnal spontaneous growth hormone secretion and to provocative insulin–arginine tests (191). Growth velocity correlated with growth hormone mean concentration in blood ($r = 0.36$; $P < 0.001$) but not with plasma IGF-1 levels nor with any of the pulsatility indices: number of peaks, main period, and pulse height. The relevance of growth hormone pulsatility to growth is less clear in humans than in rats. In adult men, however, peak concentrations of growth hormone have been suggested to influence the IGF axis, whereas trough values influence body composition and metabolic parameters of growth hormone action (69a).

Thus, in most cases, the roles of the pulsatile nature of pituitary and other signals in facilitating functional responses in end organs and target tissues remain poorly defined.

Cellular Studies

Studies on preparations of cells or individual cells offer the advantage of allowing controlled environments for investigating the specifics of pulsatile stimulation and release, as well as for testing intracellular responses. The methodologies operate on a more detailed time scale than is usually possible in whole animals. Conditions of experimentation can be reproduced readily, and multiple samples from the same cell preparation allow replication of measurements with resultant statistical precision in conclusions. A disadvantage is that essential environmental components and structures may be disrupted during cell preparation. Also, measurements may relate to slow deterioration of the cells rather than to their responses to the experimental test conditions. Artifacts of the methodology may give misleading but reproducible changes. Nevertheless, with care, much useful information on the processes of pulsatility can be obtained from this methodology. The following sections describe principles of perifusion of multiple cells and tissues; the study of single cells requires the use of similar principles on a microscale along with specific aspects peculiar to the microprecision required. The latter are described in the chapter by Dannies in this *Handbook*.

Perifusion Methodology. Using moving fluid, perifusion systems replace nutrients and gases and remove cellular waste products, during investigations of single cells, multiple cells, and tissue pieces of organs. Two articles describe useful methodological aspects of multiple cell and tissue perifusion in detail (126, 128). Figure 19.15 shows a perifusion system which, although used in earlier studies of sheep pituitary cells, illustrates the essential features (111). Reservoirs of medium with and without dissolved stimulants or cell affecters supply a multichannel pump able to deliver the liquid through, in this case, up to 15 columns at constant temperature inside a water jacket. Solenoids controlled by a programmable computer determine the mixing of solutions that shapes the pattern of cell affecters delivered to the columns with time. The computer also runs the fraction collector sampling the perifusate. Cells or tissue pieces can be either layered on a porous medium or filter within the columns or precultured on beads before loading.

Preparation of the cells requires prior experimentation to determine spurious factors influencing the results. Just some of these issues include preculture procedures, the presence of a support matrix, the composition of medium and gaseous phase, the change from in vivo hormonal environment to experimental milieu, the effects of cell dispersion methods, sterilization treatments, methods of loading equal cell numbers, and assessing cell viability at the end of procedures.

Matters relating to the apparatus that affects the outcome include ensuring adequate and constant rates of medium flow, sterility, determining how the shape of the signal is distorted by the diffusion, laminar flow (164), bubbles, binding and other hindrances in the tubes and how the shape of the response is altered in similar ways (128). Of course, all aspects of measurement of the cell responses require normal validation.

An illustration of potential influences of experimental conditions concerns cell culture conditions for a neuronal cell line (GT1). In cells in suspension, stimulation produced a broad intracellular Ca^{2+} increase to about 30 nM. In isolated cells attached to a coverslip the same stimulation produced a sharp peak to about 800 nM, lasting 12 s; and in an interconnected cellular monolayer on a coverslip cultured at higher density, a broad increase occurred to 300 nM, slowly declining over more than 100 s. In isolated pituitary cells on a coverslip, depending on the stimulus, cells exhibited either repeating sharp spikes of intracellular Ca^{2+} or a single broader peak lasting more than five times longer (170).

On-line sensors, such as electrodes, are useful for some types of investigation (126). Sensitive, fast-responding on-line sensors of hormones would be a most welcome innovation for perifusion studies and would lead to rapid advances in knowledge. The cleaner the shape of the signal that can be delivered, and the more continuous, fast, and accurate the mea-

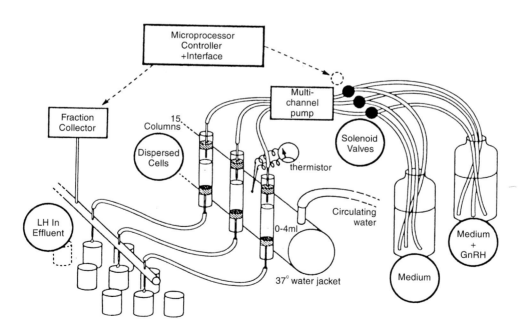

FIG. 19.15. Basic components of apparatus perifusing single cells or tissue pieces. [Adapted from McIntosh et al. (111, 128) with permission from Academic Press, Inc.]

surement of the response, the more detailed can be the characterization of elements involved in the dynamics of stimulation and response and in the consequent intracellular processes.

Influence of Signal Characteristics on Responses.

Detection of repeating pulses in time series measurements gives information (and raises questions) on how the sender of the signal is organized. Even if the pulses appear large by our measurement procedures, their appearance in itself does not tell us about their significance to the functioning of the cells receiving these signals.

The following experiments were designed to test directly the significance of the various aspects of the shape of a hormonal pulse signal (Fig. 19.8) to responses of cells binding the stimulant to expressed receptors. The period, amplitude, and rise rate of the leading edge of a pulse are characteristics which distinguish it from a "continuous or incrementally changing" signal known to desensitize some cells. Tests were made on one kind of tissue; exploration of many other tissues is required to assess other ways in which pulses affect cell outcomes and how generally the conclusions may be applied. In addition, interactions in the dynamics of different stimulants of the same response and between multiple responses to the same stimulant are illustrated.

Pituitary tissue was used because it contains several kinds of secretory cell known to require pulsatility of stimulation by hypothalamic hormones for secretory responses to be maintained. Dispersed cells were perifused because small time scales and differences in measurement needed to be detected reproducibly in one experiment, and to be replicated in several experiments. Sheep pituitaries discarded by a meat-processing plant were readily available from animals of known ages and reproductive state, and these supplied large numbers of cells from a few glands.

When square-wave stimulatory pulses of GnRH were delivered at intervals longer than about 15 min apart to the perifusion column containing the cells, each rising edge of stimulant concentration initiated a sharp increase in luteinizing hormone output. This response, however, started to decline rapidly even while the GnRH continued at the same level and before the stimulation was removed (Fig. 19.16); that is, luteinizing hormone release was desensitized. This occurred even when the concentration of GnRH was well below that causing maximal luteinizing hormone output. With collection of column output fractions at 1 min intervals or less, two maxima of luteinizing hormone release were resolved in this response (for example, Fig. 19.17 and ref. 126). These have been related to different intracellular processes causing elevated cytosolic Ca^{2+} concentrations (6).

The effects of varying duration and interval between input pulses of GnRH on the release of luteinizing hormone from dispersed pituitary cells are illustrated in Figure 19.18 and analyzed in Figures 19.19 and 19.20. The pulse frequency of the stimulant was critical, a recovery time of about 15 min being necessary to avoid disappearance of the release response to GnRH within a few hours. When the interval between pulses was extended (to a maximum of 2 h), the amount of luteinizing hormone release was increased per pulse. Maximum release over 10 h occurred with pulse periods between 15 and 60 min, the specific period being dependent on pulse duration (113).

Above a threshold (5–10 nM GnRH), pulse amplitude had little influence on luteinizing hormone output or the rate of cellular desensitization; this is in marked contrast to the strong effect of the period of the pulses. Desensitization, therefore, is not related to binding of

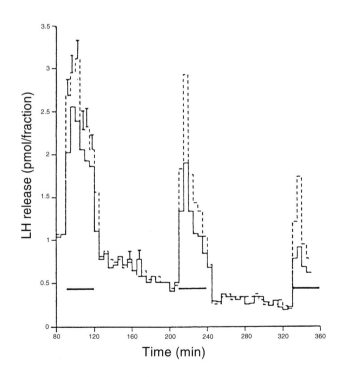

FIG. 19.16. Desensitization of response from pituitary cells within a few minutes of application of a square wave of releasing hormone even at very low stimulant concentration. Sheep pituitary cells were stimulated in perifusion with gonadotropin-releasing hormone at 5 pM *(solid line)* and 10 pM *(dashed line)* for 30 min every 2 h *(heavy bars)*. *Luteinizing hormone (LH)* was measured by radioimmunoassay in fractions collected at 5 min intervals. Representative error bars only are shown (S.E.M.). Maximal luteinizing hormone release was produced by 5–10 nM *GnRH* in similar preparations. [Adapted from McIntosh and McIntosh (115) with permission from *Endocrinology.*]

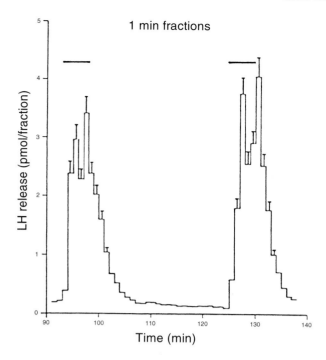

1 min fractions

FIG. 19.17. Biphasic stimulated release of pituitary hormone shown by higher time resolution of output (1 min fractions). Sheep pituitary cells were stimulated in perifusion by two 5 min square-wave pulses of 1 n*M* gonadotropin-releasing hormone *(heavy bars)*. Luteinizing hormone *(LH)* release was measured by radioimmunoassay in each fraction. Error bars are S.E.M. [Adapted from McIntosh and McIntosh (115) with permission from *Endocrinology*.]

more of the available receptors but, rather, depends on the dynamic factor of too frequent stimulation (113).

The rate at which the leading edge of the pulse rises is also important, as shown in Figure 19.21. Increases in concentration of stimulant slower than 17 pg GnRH/ml·min^{-1} altered the shape of the response, allowing increasing release beyond the initial output. This illustrates the sensitivity of the mechanism to the changing aspect of the stimulation. A constant level of stimulant resulted in reduction of luteinizing hormone output past the first few minutes, even with low concentrations of GnRH producing small releases (115). However, the amount of hormone released per unit mass of GnRH stimulation was less with the slowly rising ramped GnRH signal (Fig. 19.21) than with the rapid rise. Interestingly, the shape of the GnRH pulse in pituitary portal vessels in ewes has a contour approximating a square wave, the rising edge increasing as much as 50-fold within 1 min (127). The GnRH signal in portal blood was sustained for a mean of 5.5 min and thereafter fell to prepulse levels within 3 min.

In another tissue (immature rat ovaries stimulated with luteinizing hormone and FSH pulses), the rate of increasing hormone concentration was shown to be important also. Here, it differentially regulated steroid (estradiol and progesterone) output. In contrast, using matured ovaries, the concentrations of these steroids continued to rise following the pulses and did not depend on rise rates (165).

Tests on pituitary cells also combined continuous and pulsatile stimulations with GnRH. Low continuous baselines of stimulatory GnRH (within the physiological range measured in sheep portal blood supplying the pituitary) decreased luteinizing hormone responses to repeated GnRH pulses superimposed on them. Step changes in continuous stimulation also were studied. It was of interest that cells desensitized to continuous GnRH concentrations high enough to produce maximal luteinizing hormone release could, after a time lag, produce a further response to an even higher concentration of GnRH. Initial and additional levels would have produced the same response if applied to previously unstimulated cells (115). A possible explanation links the first response to cytosolic Ca^{2+}, which desensitizes and has a recovery time lag. The later response was proposed to involve activation of protein kinase C at the subsequent step change in stimulation (189). This further illustrates a dominant aspect of the dynamic processes which respond rapidly to changes in signal and decline under constant conditions. Similar responses are illustrated in Figure 19.22*e,f*.

In summary, the cells did not give responses typically expected with simple enzyme/substrate interactions, which exhibit a fixed dose-response curve. Rather, in receptor dynamics, cells exhibited high sensitivity to increases in the level of stimulant, after which an inherent time delay hindered their capacity to respond to further rapid pulses or prolonged stimulation. There are sensitive phases within the rhythm of their response mechanisms during which delivery of stimulant is most effective. The molecular mechanisms determining these receptor-mediated responses of cells must have the same qualitative and dynamic characteristics.

Release of both luteinizing hormone and FSH is stimulated from pituitary cells by the one hypothalamic releasing factor GnRH. Nevertheless, it is essential for reproductive function that their relative concentrations in the circulation change during different reproductive states. When experiments similar to the above were carried out testing the correlation of luteinizing hormone and FSH release in response to GnRH signals, the two hormones responded in the same way to variations in stimulant pulse characteristics (summarized in Fig. 19.19, 19.20). Gonadal feedback and a differential effect of pulse rate on the transcription rates of their

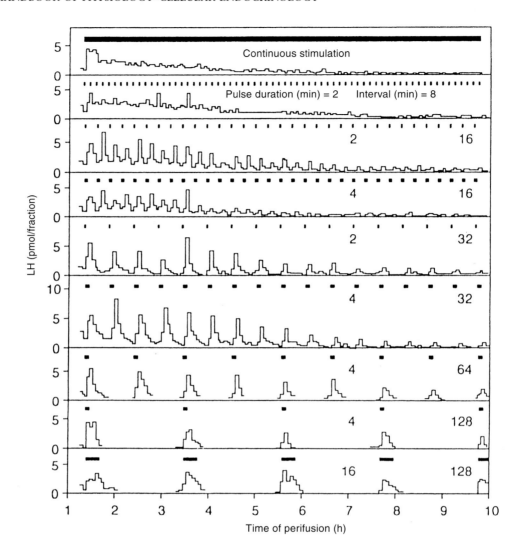

FIG. 19.18. Effects of varying period and duration of stimulatory pulses of releasing hormone on output of hormone from perifused dispersed pituitary sheep cells. Timing and duration of stimulation with 850 pM gonadotropin-releasing hormone are shown *(solid bars)*. Effluent fractions of 0.4 ml were collected for 4 min, and luteinizing hormone *(LH)* was measured by radioimmunoassay. Nine columns were run simultaneously and contained equal aliquots of the same cell preparation. [Adapted from McIntosh and McIntosh (113) with permission from the *Journal of Endocrinology* Ltd.]

subunits (see later under *Dependence of Transcription on Pulsatile Stimulation*) appear to be involved in allowing hormonal levels to be modified independently in whole animals.

Pulses of CRF applied to pituitary cells gave strongly correlated pulsatile releases of the stress-response hormones ACTH, β-endorphin, and β-lipotrophin (42), which is not unexpected for these hormones expressed from one gene in the same type of cell. The effects of the

pulse dynamics of CRF as stimulant were qualitatively similar to the effects of GnRH on luteinizing hormone and FSH, as well as to stimulation of ACTH release by AVP, or by CRF and AVP combined (41). It is generally accepted that the receptors for the hypothalamic hormones CRF and AVP activate the corticotropes of the pituitary by different intracellular transduction mechanisms: CRF stimulates activation of adenylate cyclase, whereas AVP (and GnRH) activates phospho-

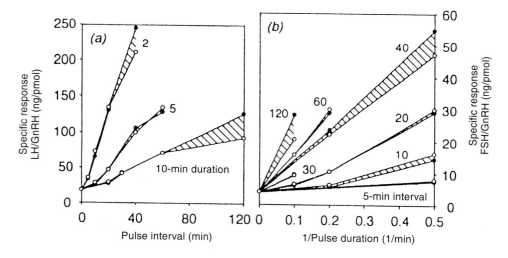

FIG. 19.19. Output of pituitary hormone per unit of applied releasing hormone increases with longer intervals between pulses and decreases with longer duration of pulses, using perifused dispersed pituitary sheep cells. In an experiment similar to that in Figure 19.18, square-wave pulses of 423 p*M* gonadotropin-releasing hormone *(GnRH)*, with a range of durations and intervals between them, were applied for 8 h, using one pulse type for each of 13 columns containing equal aliquots of cells. Luteinizing hormone *(LH, open circles)* and follicle-stimulating hormone *(FSH, filled circles)* were measured by radioimmunoassay in each 4 min output fraction. *a:* Variation of output with *intervals* between pulses. *Numbers* on the graph refer to the *duration* of the GnRH pulse at each interval. *b:* Variation of output with *duration* of pulses. *Numbers* on the graph show *intervals* between pulses. *Hatching* links results for luteinizing hormone and *FSH* measured in the same samples. [Adapted from McIntosh and McIntosh (110) with permission from the *Journal of Endocrinology* Ltd.]

inositidase. Indeed, separate receptors for the two stimulants, CRF and AVP, and different intracellular mechanisms could be inferred because pulse series of submaximal stimulation of each alone desensitized ACTH release, but enhanced release then occurred with a fresh stimulus of the other hormone (Fig. 19.22c,d). Despite these differences, the general dynamic characteristics of stimulus/release processes were shown to be the same.

Quantitative differences in dynamics, however did occur. On withdrawal of GnRH or AVP from the perifusion medium, luteinizing hormone/FSH and ACTH, respectively, took 5 min to fall to baseline levels. After removal of CRF, however, ACTH took 20 min to decay away (Fig. 19.22). Combined stimulation with CRF and AVP produced greater release of ACTH than the sum of amounts from the two stimulants separately; further, this potentiation was caused by an increase in the initial response because the duration of the pulse had the characteristics of AVP stimulation and was less than that observed from application of CRF alone (41). Studies on the secretory responses of individual corticotropes to these two stimulants have

indicated further mechanistic differences, which are undoubtedly related to the dynamic differences (25). While increasing concentrations of AVP stimulated more corticotropes to secrete, and the amount of ACTH secreted by each cell remained relatively fixed, increasing concentrations of CRF stimulated more ACTH secretion per cell, and the number of secretory cells remained relatively constant. Overall, however, the dynamics of the sensitivity of the responses display very similar qualitative characteristics.

Additional experiments using the same perifused pituitary cell experimental system showed that delaying metabolism of inositol phosphates delayed only the desensitization response for GnRH stimulation of luteinizing hormone release and that neither the amounts of releasable hormone nor the presence of intact cytoskeletal function (for example, required for transport of secretory granules) was rate-limiting in the dynamics of any of the processes determining the release characteristics (117, 169).

These similar and additional experimental approaches (particularly single-cell explorations of secretion, intracellular ionic calcium, and other chemicals de-

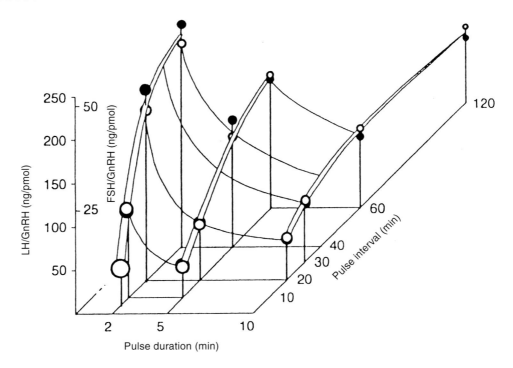

FIG. 19.20. Specific response of luteinizing hormone *(LH, open circles)* and follicle-stimulating hormone *(FSH, filled circles)* release from perifused sheep pituitary cells stimulated with three pulses of gonadotropin-releasing hormone *(GnRH)*, having a range of pulse durations and intervals. Output is plotted as functions of both pulse *interval* and *duration. Smooth curves* emphasize trends. Experimental procedure was similar to that described in Figure 19.19. [Adapted from McIntosh and McIntosh (110) with permission from the *Journal of Endocrinology* Ltd.]

scribed below) are rapidly providing the essentials of mechanisms and will allow construction of mathematical models explaining the above dynamic observations.

Dependence of transcription on pulsatile stimulation. A dramatic advance in understanding endocrine dynamics of pulsatility has been the finding of effects on protein synthesis.

The effects of pulsatile stimulation of rat pituitary cells by GnRH on gene transcription of mRNA coding for luteinizing hormone and FSH have been measured in vivo and in vitro (67). mRNA synthesis for the α-subunit of luteinizing hormone and FSH and for luteinizing hormone β were found to be stimulated three- to five-fold after three pulses of GnRH for 10 min duration once an hour in vitro (162); FSHβ showed less consistent results. While continuous GnRH for 4 h stimulated the α-subunit, pulsatile delivery of stimulant was essential for any increase in luteinizing hormone β mRNA to be detected. Similar results were obtained by others (194) except that increases in FSHβ, rather than luteinizing hormone β, were observed.

In vivo studies provide an important check and com-

plementary information to conclusions from cellular studies. They were used to demonstrate that frequency of GnRH stimulation may be a mechanism that enables a single GnRH peptide to regulate selectively subunit gene expression and secretion of the gonadotropins luteinizing hormone and FSH (36). Pulses of GnRH were administered to male rats at intervals of 8–480 min to cover the range of physiological pulsatile GnRH secretions. Fast-frequency GnRH pulses increased α-subunit mRNA concentrations threefold above those in saline-pulsed controls and luteinizing hormone β mRNA by 50%, but FSHβ mRNA was unchanged. Pulses of GnRH given every 30 min increased all three subunit mRNAs, and acute luteinizing hormone release and serum FSH concentrations were maximal at this frequency. Slower frequency GnRH stimuli did not change α-subunit and luteinizing hormone β mRNA levels but increased FSHβ mRNA 2-to 2.5-fold, while FSH secretion was maintained. Using equal total doses of GnRH given at different intervals over 24 h confirmed the frequency dependence of subunit mRNA expression.

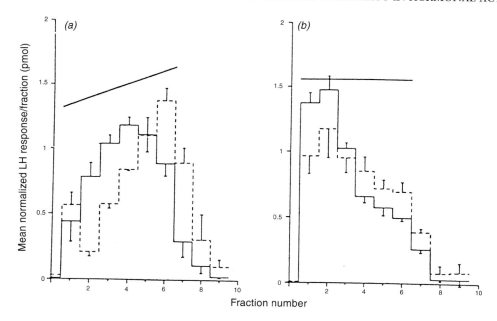

FIG. 19.21. Shapes of responses of pituitary cells to ramped and square-wave stimulations with releasing hormone. Gonadotropin-releasing hormone concentration rose from 0 to 17 pM *(dashed line)* or from 0 to 423 pM *(solid line)* over 30 min *(a)* or within seconds *(b)* in columns containing equal aliquots of dispersed sheep pituitary cells perifused simultaneously. Luteinizing hormone *(LH)* responses from three pulses of stimulation from each column were normalized and combined; results are shown as means and, for illustrative purposes, S.E.M. [Adapted from McIntosh and McIntosh (115) with permission from *Endocrinology.*]

A further influence of hourly pulses of GnRH on the synthesis of gonadotropins used perifusion of rat pituitary cells to determine modifications of polyadenylation. Changes in the lengths of luteinizing hormone β- and α-subunit mRNAs were shown to be due to increased polyadenylation, but there was no observable change in polyadenylation of FSHβ mRNA. Thus, in addition to transcriptional stimulation of the gonadotropin gene, GnRH pulses appear to modify gonadotropin mRNAs at a posttranscriptional level (192).

Follistatin is produced in the gonadotrope and folliculo-stellate cells of the pituitary gland and is thought to indirectly regulate FSH biosynthesis and secretion through its ability to bind, and hence inactivate, activin, a stimulant of FSH activity. The effects of GnRH on follistatin gene expression were examined using an in vitro perifusion model of rat pituitaries. Continuous GnRH treatment resulted in a significant elevation in follistatin mRNA levels, whereas pulsatile GnRH had no effect at either cycle stage. These results suggest that the proestrous GnRH surge is responsible at least in part for the elevation in pituitary follistatin mRNA levels associated with the primary FSH surge (11). Similar results were obtained in whole male ani-

mals, an important check that the results were not an artifact of tissue preparation. Fast-frequency GnRH pulses (8 min), which did not increase FSHβ mRNA, were associated with an increase in follistatin mRNA (2.5-fold). Slower-pulse frequencies ($\geq$120 min), which selectively stimulated a rise in FSHβ mRNA, did not increase follistatin mRNA. Therefore, GnRH frequency modulation of pituitary follistatin provides another mechanism whereby a single hypothalamic hormone can differentially regulate luteinizing hormone and FSH (88).

Following is an illustration of the use of perifusion compared to static cell cultures. With continuous infusion of 50 ng/ml activin in perifusion, a 50-fold increase in FSHβ mRNA was observed in rat pituitary cells. This magnitude of response was unexpected because only a 2.7-fold increase in FSHβ mRNA was measured when activin was administered to cells cultured in dishes. Perifusion columns, unlike culture dishes, are exposed to a continuous supply of fresh medium, and further experiments indicated that endogenous factors produced by cells cultured in dishes inhibited FSHβ mRNA production in a paracrine fashion (193).

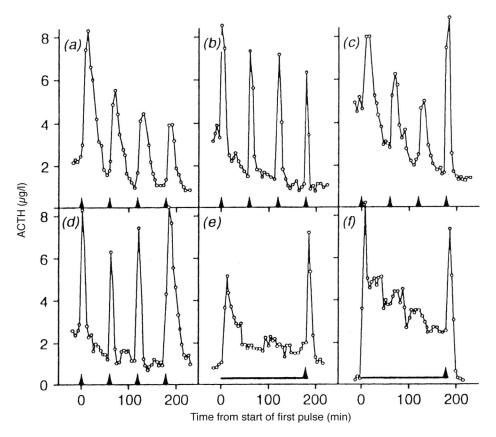

FIG. 19.22. Differences and similarities in dynamics of release of a pituitary hormone from stimulation of the same cells with two releasing hormones activating distinct transduction pathways. *a–d*: Ten minute pulses of stimulant at hourly intervals to perifused aliquots of sheep pituitary cells. Stimulants: *a*, 100 nM corticotropin-releasing factor *(CRF)*; *b*, 200 nM arginine vasopressin *(AVP)*; *c*, three pulses of 100 nM CRF, then one of 200 nM AVP; *d*, three pulses of 200 nM AVP, then one of 100 nM CRF; *e*, continuous infusion of 20 nM CRF followed by 2 μM CRF; *f*, continuous infusion of 100 nM AVP, followed by 2 μM AVP. Five minute fractions were collected and analyzed for adrenocorticotropic hormone *(ACTH)* by radioimmunoassay. Different rates of decline are seen on removal of each releasing hormone, desensitization to one stimulant does not inhibit response to the other, and cells desensitized to one level of stimulant develop responsiveness to a higher concentration of the same stimulant. [Adapted from Evans et al. (41) with permission from the *Journal of Endocrinology* Ltd.]

Using perifusion, pulsatile TRH stimulation has been shown to be more effective than continuous stimulation in producing PRL, TSHβ, and α mRNAs in rat pituitary cells. Different stimulation signals with TRH over 48 h showed differential transcription of these genes, dependent on the amplitude and frequency of the signal (65).

An interesting question concerns the kind of mechanism leading to transcription which requires pulsatile rather than continuous stimulation. Intermittent changes in intracellular second messengers may be a necessary part of the pathway involved in the transduction of signals from the plasma membrane to the nucleus (66). Using perifusion of rat pituitary cells, PRL and α-subunit gene expressions were shown to require intermittent, rather than continuous, changes in cyclic adenosine monophosphate (cAMP) stimulation, whereas TSH-, luteinizing hormone–, and FSHβ were unaltered with this particular stimulant. In similar experiments (67), the Ca^{2+} channel blocker verapamil prevented the stimulatory action of pulsatile TRH on pituitary PRL, α, and TSHβ mRNAs and of GnRH on α and FSHβ mRNAs. This suggests that Ca^{2+} influx is critical to the stimulatory action of TRH and GnRH. As further evidence, pulsatile increases in Ca^{2+} influx by channel openers stimulated elevations in all mRNAs studied except TSHβ, with the magnitudes of changes similar to that observed after TRH and GnRH pulses. These experiments imply that a pulsatile signal is required not just to accommodate receptor dynamics but also for appropriate functioning of intracellular mechanisms stimulated by the receptor.

Further, on the question of intracellular mechanisms, pulses, but not continuous stimulation, are effective in increasing transcription of receptors for GnRH by the action of GnRH on rat pituitaries (85, 203). In other studies, the rat pituitary GH3 cell line was co-transfected with rat GnRH receptor cDNA and with regulatory regions of the common α-, luteinizing hormoneβ–, or FSHβ-subunit genes fused to a luciferase reporter gene. When stimulated with GnRH, an increase in luciferase activity was observed (82). This system was used to show that different cell surface densities of the GnRH receptor resulting from different frequencies of stimulation caused differential regulation of luteinizing hormone– and FSH-subunit gene expression by GnRH, thus providing an additional mechanism by which a single ligand can act through a single receptor to regulate differentially the production of two hormones in the same cell.

Taken together, these studies show that the effects from pulsatility of hormone stimulation at the level of protein synthesis are quite widespread. How are these effects mediated by transduction processes after receptor binding?

Other uses of perifusion. Further examples of the use of perifusion have been described elsewhere in this chapter—for example, to show intrinsic and synchronized pulsatility of secretion in cultured cell lines and hypothalamic tissue.

Interaction of different hormones and feedback from target organ responses have been investigated extensively in tissue in perifusion. For example, much has been published on the effects of steroids on pituitary responsiveness. In one such study, progesterone was shown to inhibit luteinizing hormone release in response to pulsatile administration of GnRH and to change desensitization rates in perifused rat pituitary cells (78).

Sexual dimorphism and the role of sex steroids in growth hormone secretion at the pituitary level were investigated using rat hemipituitaries given two 3-min pulses of GHRH at 3-h intervals and separated by a continuous flow of somatostatin. A neonatal imprint effect of testosterone in the male appeared to induce primarily an increase in pulse amplitude in response to GHRH compared to females. Therefore, sexual differences in growth hormone secretion appear to be induced partially at the pituitary level by modification of the response to hypothalamic hormones (74). The complex effects of pituitary cell stimulation with combinations of somatostatin and GHRH have been examined (135).

Ovarian tissue has been used in perifusion; for example, insulin was shown to have an effect on steroid secretion in rat ovaries exposed to luteinizing hormone/FSH pulsatile stimulation. Decreases in estradiol and testosterone releases and stimulation of progesterone secretion were associated with its presence (166).

The pervasive influence of pulses in organizing biological function by use of dynamic as well as biochemical controls has been clearly demonstrated using perifusion.

Intracellular Effects of Pulsatile Stimulation. The molecular and cellular basis of GnRH action in the pituitary and central nervous system has been reviewed (32), and other chapters in this volume describe advances in the understanding of general hormone receptor function, secretion, calcium transients, action potentials, and other intracellular events, as well as the methodologies developed to study these. Here, briefly, the focus is on the effects of pulsatile signaling on cell function. Above, the importance to transcription of pulses of hormones, cAMP, and Ca^{2+} has been illustrated (see earlier under *Dependence of Transcription on Pulsatile Stimulation*).

Of central importance to the requirement for pulsatile stimulation of cells for continuing responsiveness (for example, gonadotropes by GnRH) are the intracellular mechanisms involved in the desensitization of secretion, synthesis, etc. during continuous stimulation. The causes of desensitization presumably determine also the time lag required before full responsiveness is recovered after cessation of a signal. A large literature on desensitization investigates most of the known components of stimulation and response as limiting factors and will not be analyzed here. Some studies of possible factors involved in the desensitization of GnRH receptor action in cell preparations have focused on cAMP action on Ca^{2+} transients (163, 168), guanyl nucleotide–binding protein (77), inositol phosphate production (69, 169), and GnRH receptor number (69).

Attention is drawn here to the dynamics of intracellular oscillations in Ca^{2+} concentration, which have been observed in single cells in both time and space and are currently under intense investigation. One kind of electrical response of a gonadotrope to continuous GnRH shows oscillatory behavior of the Ca^{2+}-activated K^+ current (163). This has a period of about 6 s, which continues as long as guanosine triphosphate (GTP) and ATP are supplied to the cytoplasm of the recorded cell and for at least 30 min (175). Measurements of intracellular Ca^{2+} responses in a gonadotrope cell line showed an initial transient complete in seconds, with a smaller plateau lasting several minutes (6). Both kinds of pattern are shown in the Ca^{2+} response of gonadotropes to GnRH (95), the particular form depending on individual cell sensitivity to GnRH concentration. Localization of sites at which Ca^{2+} transients begin within single gonadotrope cells also has been reported (147). At the same time as electrophysiological measurements are made, secretion can be assessed in single cells using the changes in membrane capacitance which occur on joining of the membrane of the secretory granule with the external plasma membrane. This method has a sensitivity approaching insertion of one vesicle and a time scale of milliseconds. For example, application of GnRH to a gonadotrope for 1 min may show changes in capacitance equivalent to the release of 400 secretory vesicles (175).

To comprehend the time course of cytosolic Ca^{2+} signaling stimulated by hormones, the kinetics of cooperative and inhibitory steps in the second-messenger cascade need to be known. In cases where the transduction product inositol trisphosphate evokes Ca^{2+} release, single-cell studies can be made by patch-clamp techniques on whole cells combined with microspectrofluorimetry and flash photolytic release of inositol trisphosphate to give quantitative, time-resolved release of Ca^{2+} from intracellular stores. Such studies have shown that the inositol trisphosphate receptor is regulated first by positive and then by negative feedback from the free cytosolic Ca^{2+} concentration, producing a pulse of Ca^{2+} release with characteristics that may be important in the spatial propagation of Ca^{2+} signals within and between cells in communication through gap junctions. A small increment of cytoplasmic Ca^{2+} concentration triggers a large Ca^{2+} pulse or oscillations. This nonlinear regenerative behavior has been attributed to inositol 1,4,5–trisphosphate channels and Ca^{2+}-ATPase transporters on the endoplasmic reticulum membrane. In pituitary cells, Ca^{2+} excitability qualitatively resembles the plasma membrane electrical excitability of neurons and other cells (97) but with differences between tissue types. For example, Purkinje neurons of the cerebellum, when compared to liver cells, require 20–50 times higher inositol trisphosphate concentrations to change the free cytosolic Ca^{2+} con-

centration; this occurs 30 times faster and reaches higher peak concentrations than in the liver (53).

Hormone agonist stimulation of pituitary cells causes electrical activity on the plasma membrane involving such intracellular Ca^{2+} release. Action potentials and Ca^{2+} changes can occur also in unstimulated cells (98). A general model has been elaborated by Berridge and collaborators (50) for Ca^{2+} changes in cells. It has been applied to Ca^{2+} transients in the mouse oocyte upon fertilization or stimulation by hormones. Two pools of Ca^{2+} are included which are regulated differentially by intracellular transduction components and show intracellular calcium buffering. A fourth-order dependence of calcium-induced calcium release on cytosolic Ca^{2+} concentration results in stable limit cycle oscillations of the type described earlier (*Mathematical Models With the Properties of Biological Rhythms*). By changing the parameters of the model in physiologically realistic ways, the single mechanism proposed can generate both sinusoidal and spike-like calcium transients in cells, as observed in mouse oocytes. By contrast, other studies indicate that the slow oscillatory behavior of glucose-stimulated individual beta cells of the pancreas may not depend on inositol 1,4,5-trisphosphate-mediated release of intracellular Ca^{2+} (100).

A few other selected examples of the roles of pulsatile Ca^{2+} transients in the regulation of endocrine function include the following. Because it contains stress responses, inhibitory feedback of ACTH-stimulated adrenal glucocorticoids on pituitary corticotropes has been proposed to act through reducing stimulus-induced Ca^{2+} transients and, hence, release of ACTH (7). The variety of Ca^{2+} transients induced in different kinds of pituitary cell response from lactotropes and somatotropes are illustrated in references 3, 84, and 148 and for the action of FSH and endothelin-1 on Sertoli cells in references 159 and 160.

Entrainment (phase resetting) and desensitization (refractoriness) of intracellular Ca^{2+} transients have been studied. These operate on a smaller time scale (seconds) than responses to pulsatile hormone stimulation in gonadotropes (tens of minutes). A single depolarizing pulse causing Ca^{2+} entry during response of a single cell to GnRH shifted the phase of subsequent endogenous intracellular Ca2 + oscillations, which thereafter continued to occur at their previous frequency before the depolarization. Application of further depolarizing pulses indicated that each endogenous or evoked Ca^{2+} rise cycle left the Ca^{2+} release mechanism of the gonadotrope in a refractory state, requiring a recovery time. A mechanism for this refractoriness was proposed to involve, again, the inositol 1,4,5-trisphosphate receptor-channel molecule presumed to be located on the cytosolic aspect of the endoplasmic reticulum membrane (187).

The relation of these pulsatile calcium ion transients on one time scale to the need for pulsatile stimulation by hormones to retain cell responsiveness on a longer time scale is of interest. Some evidence from rat lactotropes indicates that desensitization of secretion may not relate to intracellular Ca^{2+} pulses. Pulses of TRH delivered every 10 min showed a desensitizing release of PRL but undiminished Ca^{2+} transients, indicating that desensitization is related neither to receptors nor to early transduction events (64). It has been suggested (14) that the necessity for brief spikes of intracellular calcium stimulated even in nonexcitable cells may be simply that prolonged elevation of calcium can be toxic; elevated Ca^{2+} can act on endonucleases in the nucleus to trigger programmed cell death. A similar reason for the need for intermittent pulsatile stimulation of these calcium spikes by hormones could be postulated.

ANALYSIS OF TIME SERIES OF HORMONE CONCENTRATIONS

What Is a Pulse?

A pulse is a discontinuity in quantity or perceived quality of an entity, which then returns to near its original state. That is, it is a rapid positive or negative change relative to the detected norm or basal variability.

Clearly, definitions of "discontinuities" and the rate of "rapid change" of a pulse are relative to "usual" variability or fluctuations and, therefore, to expectation of time in the observer, responsive system, or detecting system. The time span during which the baseline is defined may vary from split seconds to millennia. For example, a photon is absorbed in 10^{-15} s, a human lifetime may last 3×10^9 s, while the evolution of mammals, which has shaped the physical structures, mechanisms, and biochemicals of mammalian endocrine systems, has taken perhaps 4×10^{15} s. Our task here is comprehension of mechanism and function for both stimulatory endocrine pulses and response pulses from target tissue mainly in the region of $10^1 - 10^5$ s but also related to and influenced by all of the above factors and their dynamics.

All apparent pulses which can be measured may not be relevant to endocrine function. It is important that the definition of pulses does not depend on technological ability to measure differences which, for the biological system of interest, may constitute noise. For example, variations may be caused by irrelevant but

rhythmic fluctuations in blood flow or volume. A necessary criterion for defining pulses is biological relevance, that is, whether there is a biological mechanism underlying the fluctuations, or whether organisms or tissues alter their behavior in response to them. Also, historically, considerations of experimental convenience often have overridden dynamic aspects in measuring hormone concentrations so that valuable information may have been lost. For example, the tradition of taking a single blood sample, often at a fixed time of day, was used to determine whether a hormone level is outside a very broad "normal" range. This range would cover the full variation of pulse amplitude, thereby losing information on potentially pathological changes in other pulse characteristics. Alternatively, a measurement coinciding with a rare peak may be deemed to fall outside the "normal" range and, without knowledge of pulsatility, may lead to false conclusions and unnecessary intervention.

Considerations in Analyzing Biological Pulses

Methods for analysis of biological rhythms, and for describing and comparing endocrine pulses in particular, have evolved considerably. Such rhythms rarely conform to idealized deterministic mathematical models with neat and defined solutions, many of the latter being devised to describe physical models in closed or controlled circumstances (109). Special approaches tuned to the practical aspects of the measurement procedures as well as the large individual and group variabilities often found in biological systems have had to be devised. A collection of useful and comprehensive articles covering the practicalities of analyzing hormone pulses in blood is given in reference 80.

Some analytical considerations specific to hormonal rhythms, as opposed to some other biological rhythms, are discussed in the following listing. Time series analysis is particularly sensitive to small localized variations and trends in any aspect of blood collection and storage, assay reproducibility, randomization, quality control, etc., to which particular attention needs to be directed.

1. Noise in the pulse signal may arise from sampling procedures or variability in the physiological channel (for example, circulation) as opposed to the signal itself. Every dimension of the characteristics of rhythms is subject to noise and continuous modification; variable amplitudes occur above fluctuating baselines with changing frequencies, clearance, and initiation rates. For example, variable blood volume and pressure with time and external circumstances (such as lying down) add "noise" to the concentrations of hormones found

in the circulation (33). We have found that protein concentration in blood decreases by up to 14% when experimental subjects lie down. The neuroendocrine response to the stress of the experiment itself and of events which may occur during the experimental period may influence hormonal secretions or their processing in blood. Measurements of circadian rhythms in sex steroids in humans, for example, need to be continued beyond 24 h to allow initial disturbances to stabilize and to ensure that values return to near coincidence at the same time next day.

2. Assumptions behind traditional mathematical comparisons may not be appropriate. The sharp rise of many hormonal pulses followed by a relatively slow decline caused by clearance means that the use of descriptions based on sine waves (such as frequency analysis) is appropriate only occasionally, as in Figure 19.23. (Here, a regular frequency with a period of 27 days is evident by visual inspection of the changes in early morning body temperature which accompany variation in hormone levels during the menstrual cycle in women. A fitted sine curve adequately describes the similar rates of rise and decline in temperature and gives a precise frequency estimate, though a better model could probably be found.)

Parametric tests, such as the *t* test and analysis of variance, are designed to compare the means and dispersions of groups from independent, normally distributed measurements; this demands assumptions inappropriate to rhythms where the measurements in a time series are dependent on each other and may not show Gaussian distribution. For example, the lower limit of detection may skew or truncate the distribution of measurements.

3. Different forms of hormones may be measured inappropriately for their bioactivity or lack of it. Examples of such forms are those having variable glycosylation of proteins, isoforms, and metabolic products; those reacting with binding proteins; or those having access to more than one physiological compartment. Measurement and analysis of rhythms are influenced by hormones reacting strongly with binding proteins, which may occur for both steroids and protein hormones, for example, growth hormone (73, 157). An example of a hormone with different forms showing bioactivity is FSH (182, 209). The properties, rhythms, rates of interaction, and changes of form must be known to interpret rhythms and consequent tissue responses. For example, despite a long history of study of circulating steroid hormones and their binding proteins, aspects of testosterone binding and bioactivity in men remain undefined (33, 34).

Immunoassay is based on competition for binding of proteins to a particular antiserum; the unknown level of hormone protein in the sample competes with

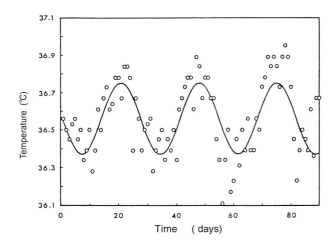

FIG. 19.23. Example of a hormonally controlled rhythm appropriate for analysis by methods based on a sine-wave model; pulsatile rhythms with relatively sharply rising edges and variable intervals between events are less suitable. Early morning *body temperature* was recorded *daily* in a normal woman with 27-day ovulatory cycles. *Smooth curve* represents results of fitting a sine curve model over data collected for 349 days. [Adapted from McIntosh and McIntosh (109) with permission from Springer-Verlag.]

a known concentration of added standard protein. The forms of hormone in the sample competing for antibody are assumed to be bioactive. In fact, bioactivity results from the binding of specific forms of hormone to a receptor and its subsequent activation. Antisera are raised to particular samples of extracted, purified hormone protein. Consequently, an antiserum may contain a range of immunoglobulins binding a selected distribution of epitopes on the purified hormone protein. Binding of these epitopes in a blood sample in competition with the standard purified protein may not reflect real changes in level of the bioactive form of hormone because variants of the hormone may bind antibody and tissue receptor differently. Hence, depending on the antiserum used, rates of metabolic clearance of the form of hormone detected in the blood from an individual and amplitudes of peaks may differ. Similarly, changes in bioactive forms within an individual in response to different conditions may not be detected. Comparisons may not be relevant between individuals where varying proportions of hormone forms are present or different antibodies are used.

Sometimes bioassays based on stimulation of cultured cells are used, for example, rat or mouse Leydig cells in the detection of gonadotropins. Although possibly more "biological" than immunoassays, in static cell culture, hormone forms cleared rapidly from the circulation may react for unnaturally long periods (114).

4. Parameters must be reassessed for each individual data set and cannot be carried over from one to the other. In early analysis of pulses of hormone in blood, clearance rates of hormones estimated in one or a few individuals were used to analyze pulses in other individuals (for example, 155). Experience has shown that clearance rates vary considerably and must be estimated from within the data in which pulse peaks are being detected. Further, general estimates of the precision of an assay used in determining characteristics of time series data were not sufficient to ensure accurate analyses, nor did mean values of duplicate assay measurements supply adequate information about the reliability of individual points. Precision varied greatly between assays, and bad duplicates capable of generating false peaks occurred randomly within assays. Hence, the more frequently the time series was sampled, the more false peaks would be detected.

5. There may be differences between measured concentration and biological effect. While it may be inferred that the concentration of a hormone in blood is a linear function of its secretion modified by clearance (114), its effect on the target tissue may not be proportional to its summed or meaned concentration. For example, as described above, the leading edge of pulses may be much more effective in eliciting a response than the remaining duration of hormone presence (42, 115, 199).

6. Interval of sampling is crucial. To define the frequency component of a pulsatile signal, the Nyquist theorem shows that the sampling rate must be at least twice that of the component with the highest frequency—for example, a rhythm with a periodicity of 1 h must be sampled at least every 30 min. This is too low for precision (126), and many more than two estimates of concentration are required to define a peak with noise. Figure 19.24 shows the phenomenon termed "aliasing," where if the system is sampled at longer intervals than the true period of the time series, a falsely long but apparently accurate impression of the period will be obtained. This misleading outcome arises whenever a rhythmical process is measured at intervals which happen to be similar to, or more widely spread than, the period of a dominant oscillation in the response. However, theoretical considerations must be secondary to limits on the number, and hence frequency, of blood samples that reasonably can be taken.

7. Combining results in order to distinguish norms from pathology can be misleading. It is particularly difficult to combine data on rhythms from individuals into meaningful averages; individual rhythms can thus be obscured by differences in phase, mean, amplitude, and frequency. In studying pulsatile and cyclic events, the study of an individual is essential and may need to be repetitive and extended. One example is shown by

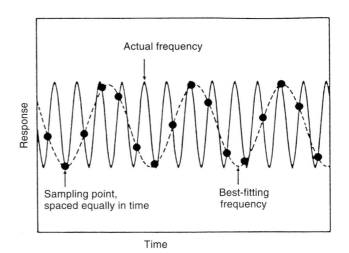

FIG. 19.24. Illustration of aliasing. If samples are taken at intervals longer than the period in a time series *(filled circles)*, a false picture will be obtained of its true period. [Adapted from McIntosh and McIntosh (109) with permission from Springer-Verlag.]

the variation in peak amplitude and interval during the same phases of repeated menstrual cycles in one normal ovulatory woman with regular cycles (Fig. 19.11). In another example, it was concluded that severe luteal defects can be diagnosed by a progesterone assay if the entire cycle is assayed but that single or even multiple progesterone assays are unreliable (81). The etiology is multifactorial and usually related to the hypothalamic–pituitary factors influencing the ovulatory luteinizing hormone surge, rather than to ovarian factors. Also, factors may vary from cycle to cycle, making it important to determine that the defect is repetitive. Nevertheless, substitution progesterone therapy is the most satisfactory treatment available (81).

Methods of Analyzing Pulses

Time series of peripheral concentrations of a hormone can give information on the physiological mechanisms underlying its production and indications of the significance of the hormone to broader physiological functions and in different experimental conditions. For pituitary hormones under hypothalamic control, pulses are generally assumed to reflect the appropriate neuronal pulse generator and feedback mechanisms (see earlier under *Pulses of Pituitary Hormones in Peripheral Blood*). Pulses in other systems (such as blood glucose regulation, placental hormone output, and cytokine production) seem to be an inherent part of their stable, regulated function.

One aim in analyzing time series data is to determine the times at which changes in hormone level can be distinguished from error in the measurement procedures, including experimental error and interval of sampling. Information can be sought on whether secretion of the hormone can be described as a continuous change in level over the time interval of interest or whether there are separate secretory events. Unravelling possible combinations of continuous and pulsatile secretions is a particularly difficult question mathematically because of strong dependence between solutions of the descriptive equations, yet this issue is fundamental to understanding mechanisms of secretion.

If there is a pulsatile component to the time series, it is of interest to determine the times of secretory events from the organ of origin, the intervals between events, the amplitude and shapes of the secretory pulses, and the clearance rate of the hormone. The regularity or instability of these characteristics is also informative. In some cases, there are multiple rhythms in the data, as with sex hormones, which show an ultradian and a circadian rhythm; in females, these hormones involve all of the rhythms depicted in Figure 19.1. Correlation in timing of pulses of different hormones in blood is also often of interest in questioning linkages between secretion mechanisms. Examples of some time series data of hormone concentrations in blood are shown in Figures 19.9–19.14.

The general trends in variation of secretory pulses of the various hormones in different endocrine states have become evident from the large literature available. However, the details reported can conflict because of differences between individual subjects, sampling procedures, and methods of measurement, as described earlier under *Considerations in Analyzing Biological Pulses.* Differences in methods of analysis also have played a role in these discrepancies as awareness of pitfalls has been developing and more comprehensive and sophisticated methods have evolved. Four common processes of analysis are described briefly below. (Detailed descriptions are given in reference 80.)

Moving Cluster Method.

The moving cluter method can be used to detect pulses in hormone blood levels or in perfusates of tissues in columns. A pulse is defined as a statistically significant increase in a "cluster" of several (typically two or three) successive values of hormone concentration, followed by a statistically significant decrease in a second cluster of values (178, 184). The significance of the changes is assessed in relation to actual experimental error expressed by the replicates in the tested nadir (low point) and peak data clusters. The cluster sizes of test peaks and pre- and post-peak nadirs may be chosen according to the data and the information required. Typical definitions of significance for a pulse may be if its maximum exceeds two to three times the local intraassay coefficient of variation.

Variable precision in the assay can be allowed for in this analysis. The method is not overly sensitive to fluctuating baseline hormone concentrations and is not concerned with varying pulse amplitudes, widths, or other characteristics. The simple statistical basis for this approach means that it is relatively independent of explicit or a priori assumptions about rates of hormonal secretion and metabolism or shapes of secretory episodes. The computer programs CLUSTER and DETECT (178, 184) which use this approach have been tested for the conditions under which they detect false peaks or miss real peaks in their analyses of large sets of simulated (computer-generated) time series data, constructed to include different sizes of "true" pulses and added measurement error.

Deconvolution.

A common method of analyzing hormone pulses in blood is deconvolution (114). This method aims at quantitative definition of secretory episodes of hormone. Two processes are assumed to occur: the hormone is secreted in discrete episodes; these are then distorted by mixing in the circulation and removed during metabolic clearance. At any time, the level of the hormone represents the sum of all previous episodes of secretion, each diminished due to clearance by an amount dependent on time since its secretion. If secretion episodes are infrequent, clearance ensures that concentrations decline to below the sensitivity of the assay and estimates of peak maxima, interpeak interval, and decay rates are simple to make. Frequently occurring overlapping episodes of release are more difficult to analyze. The simplest case is where secretory episodes are brief, less than the interval of sampling blood; this approximates the situation for luteinizing hormone. Figure 19.25 shows measurements of luteinizing hormone at intervals of 10 min in the peripheral blood (hatched lines) and a calculated optimized estimate of individual secretory episodes of hormone (heavy vertical lines) with their individual decay curves (light lines). The sum of the contributions from all previous peaks (medium line) is obtained by adjusting the parameters of a deconvolution model until the variance of the model about the experimental data is minimized. The optimization method used to minimize this variance was an iterative, least squares minimization computer program based on the Marquardt-Levenberg approach (109). The equation for such a model, summing the results of brief secretory episodes followed by a single exponential decay to describe clearance, is

$$[LH]_t = \sum_{i=1}^{n} (A_i e^{-\lambda(t-t_i)})$$

Where $[LH]_t$ is the concentration of hormone in blood at any time t since the beginning of sampling, n is

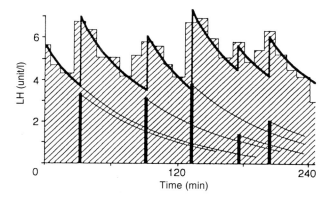

FIG. 19.25. Example of the result of deconvolution of hormone measurements in blood. Luteinizing hormone *(LH)* was measured at 10 min intervals in a woman 2 days after the start of menstruation. Secreted pulses of luteinizing hormone were assumed to be discrete and less than 10 min long; therefore, the summed equation in the text could be applied. Output of the model was estimated amplitude of peaks *(vertical bars)* and estimated single exponential decay of hormone clearance. Decays of individual secretory episodes *(thin curves)* are shown, and these when summed gave the best fitted description *(heavy curves)* of the stepped experimental data. [Adapted from Murray-McIntosh and McIntosh (128) with permission from Academic Press, Inc.]

the number of episodes analyzed, A_i is the maximum amplitude of the *i*th episode in blood occurring at time *t*, and λ is the mean exponential decay coefficient for the sampling session. The rate of clearance of luteinizing hormone from blood was one of the parameters in the model. In principle, it is possible to include more than one decay time (or clearance process) in the equation, but it was not necessary for measurements of luteinizing hormone secretion. In this case and as shown in Figure 19.10, several brief secretory episodes of luteinizing hormone secretion can approximate the data well, and it is not necessary to propose a baseline secretion of hormone (for example, at 3–4 units/l in Fig. 19.25) on which small pulses are superimposed, as had been done previously.

Further analysis of the peaks in Figures 19.10 and 19.11 indicates other mechanisms involved in their generation. Pulse amplitude correlates with the interval to the preceding peak, suggesting a recovery time controlling sensitivity of either the pituitary or the GnRH-secreting neurons after release. This effect is shown also in stimulated perifused pituitary cells, where longer intervals between stimulant pulses produce a greater output in the response pulse (Figs. 19.19*a*, 19.20).

Where the secretory episode is broader relative to the sampling interval, its shape can be estimated from treating the data as the sum of increments of the secretory pulse, each increment decaying at the opti-

mized rate (167). Convolution is illustrated in Figure 19.26. The secretion pattern is convoluted by dividing it into successive short time intervals, each of which decays. The sum of the decay function at any one time is represented by the measurement data. Deconvolution involves the reverse process of that shown in Figure 19.26 to estimate the secretion pattern from the data. Variations on this basic approach include the following. The computer program PULSE (176) allows determination of pulses independent of shape in which the approximate positions of peaks are not required to be supplied at the start of the fitting procedures. The half-life of the elimination function, however, must be assumed. The program PULSE2 includes a term for basal secretion and has been devised to allow more sensitive detection of small secretory events (43).

Simulation techniques can be used to considerable effect in testing such computer programs. "Data" are generated from choosing hypothetical secretory pulses with particular characteristics, assigning chosen clearance parameters to convolute to the "blood levels," and adding "experimental variance" within selected ranges. The ability of the program to extract the pulse characteristics used in simulating the data shows the limits and strengths of the analysis method.

Orderly Sine Wave Rhythms and Baseline Trends. Autocorrelation analysis (109) gives information on significant periodic components in the data. A correlation coefficient is calculated between the data and a copy of itself at increasing lag periods. If there is a period of, for example, 20 min between pulses, at time zero the correlation coefficient will be total and equal to 1, at 10 min it will be a negative minimum, and at 20 min a positive maximum. Significance can be calculated

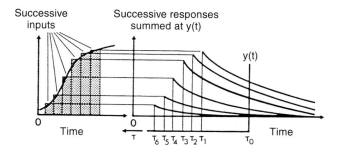

FIG. 19.26. Principles of convolution and deconvolution applied to a secretory episode broader than sampling intervals. At each time interval *(t)*, convolution sums successive decay curves (*y*, responses) calculated for each increment of the known or chosen secretory (input) pulse. Deconvolution takes the summed response *y(t)* (measured data) and, by the reverse process, selects the best fitted (unknown) secretory pulse. [Adapted from McIntosh and McIntosh (109) with permission from Springer-Verlag.]

with Z-values. Frequency or Fourier analysis describes the data as the sum of an arbitrary number of sine waves of different frequencies, phases, and amplitudes and is related to autocorrelation analysis by the Fourier transform. This method can detect periodicity within "noisy" data and indicates how "noisy" the data are. Both kinds of analysis require that baseline instability or low frequency trends are removed from the data before analysis.

Much hormonal data with sharply rising pulses and variable periods within the ultradian range cannot be analyzed usefully by these methods.

Analysis of Disorder in Rhythmic Data.
Another approach, mentioned earlier under *Pulses and Pathology*, also quantifies regularity or noisiness in endocrine time series but without necessarily precisely defining individual peaks (68, 140). The method quantifies the general disturbances in rhythmic secretions often seen intuitively in pathology when viewing time series of hormones in blood. Pincus (140) proposes that autonomy of endocrine systems is an indication of health; this is expressed as regular secretion little influenced by external disturbances. The results shown in Figure 19.14, however, suggest that in health there is an ability to respond rapidly and coherently to disturbances while maintaining a stable rhythmicity.

Analysis of disorder has been used to show effects of, for example, continuous versus pulsatile androgen replacement on orderliness of luteinizing hormone pulses in men (210a), and menopause on parathyroid secretion in women (154a).

Correlation of Peaks.
Correlations between rhythms of hormone pulses suggest some kind of causal relation. Correlation of pulses of pituitary hormones with delayed secretion from target organs suggests causation, while co-secretion or correlation of hormones from the same, or possibly, different glands suggests a common stimulation mechanism. Unless the clearance of hormones compared is rapid, deconvolution or some other analysis of the data may be needed to determine times of the initiation of peaks freed from clearance contributions. These values can then be used in cross-correlation analysis based on principles similar to those for autocorrelation described above. Examples are correlations detected between luteinizing hormone and progesterone in women, with maximum correlation at a 10 min lag (56), and between luteinizing hormone and testosterone in men (185).

Analysis of raw data to obtain meaningful biological information is an increasing challenge in biology. The techniques described here are part of the trend of increasing sophistication in analysis. Data need to be collected with more awareness of potential problems in interpretation, while new approaches and further effective developments in current approaches are required to elucidate mechanisms, correlations, and causations of pulsatility in health and disease.

CONCLUSION

Since the study of rhythmic events has become an important focus in endocrinology, several pulsatile systems have been described in detail and some ideas gained of the uses of pulses in the temporal organization of structural development, reproduction, and change. Within this fluid world of dynamics in which constant but organized, almost stable, change occurs, many interesting questions remain. What are the processes by which function is organized by pulses with frequencies covering orders of magnitude? How are pulses produced and by what mechanism? What is their importance to the receiver of the signal? Tantalizing hints of differential activation of gene transcription, of programmed apoptosis, and of the appearance of stimulated time- and space-differentiated intracellular waves of calcium have been given at the cellular level. Cells in a supportive structural and fluid environment individually programmed to sense the wider picture respond sensitively in a way that allows the whole organism to function, itself sensing and responding both internally to the many cells and externally to a larger environment. If we do not hear and respond to the dynamical interplay of this cellular life, we are deaf indeed.

The author thanks the Health Research Council of New Zealand for salary during the writing of this chapter and Professor Paul Harvey of the Zoology Department, University of Oxford, for hospitality and computing facilities.

REFERENCES

1. Abel, S., P. W. Oeller, and A. Theologis. Suppressed spontaneous and stimulated growth hormone secretion in patients with Cushing's disease before and after surgical cure. *J. Clin. Endocrinol. Metab.* 78: 131–137, 1994.
2. Adams, J. M., A. E. Taylor, D. A. Schoenfeld, W. F. Crowley, Jr., and J. E. Hall. The midcycle gonadotropin surge in normal women occurs in the face of an unchanging gonadotropin-releasing hormone pulse frequency. *J. Clin. Endocrinol. Metab.* 79: 858–864, 1994.
3. Akerman, S. N., R. Zorec, T. R. Cheek, R. B. Moreton, M. J. Berridge, and W. T. Mason. Fura-2 imaging of thyrotropin-releasing hormone and dopamine effects on calcium homeostasis of bovine lactotrophs. *Endocrinology* 129: 475–488, 1991.
4. Albanese, A., G. Hamill, J. Jones, D. Skuse, D. R. Matthews, and R. Stanhope. Reversibility of physiological growth hormone

secretion in children with psychosocial dwarfism. *Clin. Endocrinol. (Oxf.)* 40: 687–692, 1994.

5. Albers, N., M. Bettendorf, H. Herrmann, S. L. Kaplan, and M. M. Grumbach. Hormone ontogeny in the ovine fetus. XXVII. Pulsatile and copulsatile secretion of luteinizing hormone, follicle-stimulating hormone, growth hormone, and prolactin in late gestation: a new method for the analysis of copulsatility. *Endocrinology* 132: 701–709, 1993.

6. Anderson, L., J. Hoyland, W. T. Mason, and K. A. Eidne. Characterization of the gonadotrophin-releasing hormone calcium response in single alpha T3-1 pituitary gonadotroph cells. *Mol. Cell. Endocrinol.* 86: 167–175, 1992.

7. Antoni, F. A., J. Hoyland, M. D. Woods, and W. T. Mason. Glucocorticoid inhibition of stimulus-evoked adrenocorticotrophin release caused by suppression of intracellular calcium signals. *J. Endocrinol.* 133: R13–R16, 1992.

8. Apostolakis, E. M., L. D. Longo, and S. M. Yellon. Cortisol feedback regulation of pulsatile ACTH secretion in fetal sheep during late gestation. *Am. J. Physiol.* 267 (*Endocrinol. Metab.* 30): E521–E527, 1994.

9. Baird, D. T., and A. S. McNeilly. Gonadotrophic control of follicular development and function during the oestrous cycle of the ewe. *J. Reprod. Fertil. Suppl.* 30: 119–133, 1981.

10. Barnea, E. R., D. Feldman, and M. Kaplan. The effect of progesterone upon first trimester trophoblastic cell differentiation and human chorionic gonadotrophin secretion. *Hum. Reprod.* 6: 905–909, 1991.

11. Bauer Dantoin, A. C., J. Weiss, and J. L. Jameson. Gonadotropin-releasing hormone regulation of pituitary follistatin gene expression during the primary follicle-stimulating hormone surge. *Endocrinology* 137: 1634–1639, 1996.

12. Belchetz, P. E., T. M. Plant, Y. Nakai, E. J. Keogh, and E. Knobil. Hypophysial responses to continuous and intermittent delivery of hypothalamic gonadotropin-releasing hormone. *Science* 202: 631–633, 1978.

13. Bermann, M., C. A. Jaffe, W. Tsai, F. R. DeMott, and A. L. Barkan. Negative feedback regulation of pulsatile growth hormone secretion by insulin-like growth factor I. Involvement of hypothalamic somatostatin. *J. Clin. Invest.* 94: 138–145, 1994.

14. Berridge, M. J. The biology and medicine of calcium signalling. *Mol. Cell. Endocrinol.* 98: 119–224, 1994.

15. Berts, A., A. Ball, G. Dryselius, E. Gylfe, and B. Hellman. Glucose stimulation of somatostatin-producing islet cells involves oscillatory Ca^{2+} signaling. *Endocrinology* 137: 693–697, 1996.

16. Besser, G. M., A. S. McNeilly, D. C. Anderson, J. C. Marshall, P. Harsoulis, R. Hall, B. J. Ormston, L. Alexander, and W. P. Collins. Hormonal responses to synthetic luteinizing hormone and follicle stimulating hormone–releasing hormone in man. *BMJ* 3: 267– 271, 1972.

17. Best, E. N. Exploration of a menstrual cycle model. *Simulation Today* 25: 117–120, 1975.

18. Bogumil, R. J. *Computer simulation of endocrine control of the menstrual cycle.* Amsterdam: *Excerpta Med.,* 1976, p. 250–255. (Int. Congr. Ser. 402.)

19. Bogumil, R. J., M. Ferin, and R. L. Van de Wiele. Mathematical studies of the human menstrual cycle. II. Simulation performance of a model of the human menstrual cycle. *J. Clin. Endocrinol. Metab.* 35: 144–156, 1972.

20. Bremner, W. J., J. K. Findlay, I. A. Cumming, B. Hudson, and D. M. de Kretser. Pituitary–testicular responses in rams to prolonged infusion of LHRH. *Biol. Reprod.* 106: 329–336, 1976.

21. Brennemann, W., L. Sommer, W. B. Stoffel, F. Bidlingmaier, and D. Klingmueller. Secretion pattern of immunoreactive inhibin in men. *Acta Endocrinol.* 131: 273–279, 1994.

22. Brooks, A. N., A. S. McNeilly, and G. B. Thomas. Role of GnRH in the ontogeny and regulation of the fetal hypothalamo–pituitary–gonadal axis in sheep. *J. Reprod. Fertil. Suppl.* 49: 163–175, 1995.

23. Brown, D., A. E. Herbison, J. E. Robinson, R. W. Marrs, and G. Leng. Modelling the luteinizing hormone–releasing hormone pulse generator. *Neuroscience* 63: 869–879, 1994.

24. Campen, C. A., M. T. Lai, P. Kraft, T. Kirchner, A. Phillips, D. W. Hahn, and J. Rivier. Potent pituitary–gonadal axis suppression and extremely low anaphylactoid activity of a new gonadotropin releasing hormone (GnRH) receptor antagonist "azaline B." *Biochem. Pharmacol.* 49: 1313–1321, 1995.

25. Canny, B. J., L. G. Jia, and D. A. Leong. Corticotropin-releasing factor, but not arginine vasopressin, stimulates concentration-dependent increases in ACTH secretion from a single corticotrope. Implications for intracellular signals in stimulus–secretion coupling. *J. Biol. Chem.* 267: 8325–8329, 1992.

26. Cardenas, H., T. Ordog, K. T. O'Byrne, and E. Knobil. Growth hormone release evoked by electrical stimulation of the arcuate nucleus in anesthetized male rats. *Brain Res.* 623: 95–100, 1993.

27. Chen, L., J. D. Veldhuis, M. L. Johnson, and M. Straume. Systems-level analysis of physiological regulatory interactions controlling complex secretory dynamics of the growth hormone axis: a dynamical network model. In: *Quantitative Neuroendocrinology,* edited by M. L. Johnson and J. D. Veldhuis. San Diego: Academic, 1995, p. 270–335.

28. Chen, M. D., K. T. O'Byrne, S. E. Chiappini, J. Hotchkiss, and E. Knobil. Hypoglycemic "stress" and gonadotropin-releasing hormone pulse generator activity in the rhesus monkey: role of the ovary. *Neuroendocrinology* 56: 666–673, 1992.

29. Chen, M. D., T. Ordog, K. T. O'Byrne, J. R. Goldsmith, M. A. Connaughton, and E. Knobil. The insulin hypoglycemia-induced inhibition of gonadotropin-releasing hormone pulse generator activity in the rhesus monkey: roles of vasopressin and corticotropin-releasing factor. *Endocrinology* 137: 2012–2021, 1996.

30. Clarke, I. J., and J. T. Cummins. The temporal relationship between gonadotropin releasing hormone (GnRH) and luteinizing hormone (LH) secretion in ovariectomized ewes. *Endocrinology* 111: 1737–1739, 1982.

31. Conn, P. M., and W. F. Crowley, Jr. Gonadotropin-releasing hormone and its analogs. *Annu. Rev. Med.* 45: 391–405, 1994.

32. Conn, P. M., J. A. Janovick, D. Stanislaus, D. Kuphal, and L. Jennes. Molecular and cellular bases of gonadotropin-releasing hormone action in the pituitary and central nervous system. *Vitam. Horm.* 50: 151–214, 1995.

33. Cooke, R. R., J. E. McIntosh, and R. P. Murray-McIntosh. Circadian variations in free and non-SHBG-bound testosterone in normal men: measurement and simulation using a mass action model. *Clin. Endocrinol. (Oxf.)* 39: 163–171, 1993.

34. Cooke, R. R., J. E. McIntosh, and R. P. Murray-McIntosh. Effect of cortisol on percentage of non-sex-hormone-bound steroid: implications for distribution of steroids on binding proteins in serum. *Clin. Chem.* 42: 249–254, 1996.

35. Crowley, W. F., Jr., M. Filicori, D. I. Spratt, and N. F. Santoro. The physiology of gonadotropin-releasing hormone (GnRH) secretion in men and women. *Recent Prog. Horm. Res.* 41: 473–531, 1985.

36. Dalkin, A. C., D. J. Haisenleder, G. A. Ortolano, T. R. Ellis, and J. C. Marshall. The frequency of gonadotropin-releasing-hormone stimulation differentially regulates gonadotropin subunit messenger ribonucleic acid expression. *Endocrinology* 125: 917–924, 1989.

37. Dierschke, D. J., A. N. Bhattacharya, L. E. Atkinson, and E. Knobil. Circhoral oscillations of plasma LH levels in the

ovariectomized rhesus monkey. *Endocrinology* 87: 850–853, 1970.

38. Djahanbakhch, O., P. Warner, A. S. McNeilly, and D. T. Baird. Pulsatile release of LH and oestradiol during the periovulatory period in women. *Clin. Endocrinol. (Oxf.)* 20: 579–589, 1984.

39. Douglas, W. W. Mechanism of release of neurohypophysial hormones: stimulus-secretion coupling. In: *The Pituitary Gland,* edited by E. B. Astwood, R. O. Greep, E. Knobil, and W. H. Sawyer. Washington, D.C.: Am. Physiol. Soc., 1974, pt. 1, p. 191–224.

40. Engler, D., T. Pham, M. J. Fullerton, G. Ooi, J. W. Funder, and I. J. Clarke. Studies of the secretion of corticotropin-releasing factor and arginine vasopressin into the hypophysial-portal circulation of the conscious sheep. I. Effect of an audiovisual stimulus and insulin-induced hypoglycemia. *Neuroendocrinology* 49: 367–381, 1989.

41. Evans, M. J., J. T. Brett, R. P. McIntosh, J. E. McIntosh, J. L. McLay, J. H. Livesey, and R. A. Donald. Characteristics of the ACTH response to repeated pulses of corticotrophin-releasing factor and arginine vasopressin in vitro. *J. Endocrinol.* 117: 387–395, 1988.

42. Evans, M. J., J. T. Brett, R. P. McIntosh, J. E. McIntosh, H. K. Roud, J. H. Livesey, and R. A. Donald. The effect of various corticotropin-releasing factor trains on the release of adrenocorticotropin, beta-endorphin, and beta-lipotropin from perifused ovine pituitary cells. *Endocrinology* 117: 893–899, 1985.

43. Evans, W. S., M. J. Sollenberger, R. A. Booth, Jr., A. D. Rogol, R. J. Urban, E. C. Carlsen, M. L. Johnson, and J. D. Veldhuis. Contemporary aspects of discrete peak-detection algorithms. II. The paradigm of the luteinizing hormone pulse signal in women. *Endocr. Rev.* 13: 81–104, 1992.

44. Feng, L. J., D. Rodbard, R. Rebar, and G. T. Ross. Computer simulation of the human pituitary–ovarian cycle: studies of follicular phase estradiol infusions and the midcycle peak. *J. Clin. Endocrinol. Metab.* 45: 775–787, 1977.

45. Ferin, M. The antireproductive role of corticotropin releasing hormone and interleukin-1 in the female rhesus monkey. *Ann. Endocrinol. (Paris)* 56: 181–186, 1995.

46. Filicori, M., J. P. Butler, and W. F. Crowley, Jr. Neuroendocrine regulation of the corpus luteum in the human. Evidence for pulsatile progesterone secretion. *J. Clin. Invest.* 73: 1638–1647, 1984.

47. Filicori, M., M. Maresguerra, P. Mimmi, G. Bolelli, F. Franceschetti, G. Possati, and C. Flamigni. The pattern of LH and FSH pulsatile release: physiological and clinical significance. In: *The Gonadotrophins: Basic Science and Clinical Aspects in Females,* edited by C. Flamigni and J. R. Givens. London: Academic, 1982, p. 365–375.

48. Filicori, M., N. Santoro, G. R. Merriam, and W. F. Crowley, Jr. Characterization of the physiological pattern of episodic gonadotropin secretion throughout the human menstrual cycle. *J. Clin. Endocrinol. Metab.* 62: 1136–1144, 1986.

49. Fraser, H. M., and D. T. Baird. Clinical applications of LHRH analogues. *Baillieres Clin. Endocrinol. Metab.* 1: 43–70, 1987.

50. Friesen, W. O., T. R. Cheek, O. M. McGuiness, R. B. Moreton, and M. J. Berridge. Analysis of calcium fertilization transients in mouse oocytes. In: *Methods in Neuroscience,* edited by M. L. Johnson and J. D. Veldhuis. San Diego: Academic, 1995, p. 388–423.

51. Friesen, W. O., G. D. Block, and Hocker, C. G. Formal approaches to understanding biological oscillators. *Annu. Rev. Physiol.* 55: 661–681, 1993.

52. Frohman, L. A., T. R. Downs, I. J. Clarke, and G. B. Thomas. Measurement of growth hormone–releasing hormone and somatostatin in hypothalamic-portal plasma of unanesthetized

sheep. Spontaneous secretion and response to insulin-induced hypoglycemia. *J. Clin. Invest.* 86: 17–24, 1990.

53. Fujimoto, V. Y., S. J. Spencer, J. Rabinovici, S. Plosker, and R. B. Jaffe. Mechanisms of intracellular calcium release during hormone and neurotransmitter action investigated with flash photolysis. *J. Exp. Biol.* 184: 105–127, 1993.

54. Gambacciani, M., J. H. Liu, W. H. Swartz, V. S. Tueros, S. S. Yen, and D. D. Rasmussen. Intrinsic pulsatility of luteinizing hormone release from the human pituitary in vitro. *Neuroendocrinology* 45: 402–406, 1987.

55. Gay, V. L., and A. R. J. Midgeley. Response of the adult rat to orchidectomy and ovariectomy as determined by LH radioimmunoasay. *Endocrinology* 84: 1359–1365, 1969.

56. Genazzani, A. D., V. Guardabasso, F. Petraglia, and A. R. Genazzani. Specific concordance index defines the physiological lag between LH and progesterone in women during the midluteal phase of the menstrual cycle. *Gynecol. Endocrinol.* 5: 175–184, 1991.

57. Gevers, E. F., J. M. Wit, and I. C. Robinson. Growth, growth hormone (GH)–binding protein, and GH receptors are differentially regulated by peak and trough components of the GH secretory pattern in the rat. *Endocrinology* 137: 1013–1018, 1996.

58. Gluckman, P. D. Functional maturation of the neuroendocrine system in the perinatal period: studies of the somatotropic axis in the ovine fetus. *J. Dev. Physiol.* 6: 301–312, 1984.

59. Gluckman, P. D., M. M. Grumbach, and S. L. Kaplan. The neuroendocrine regulation and function of growth hormone and prolactin in the mammalian fetus. *Endocr. Rev.* 2: 363–395, 1981.

60. Goubillon, M. L., J. M. Kaufman, and J. C. Thalabard. Hypothalamic multiunit activity and pulsatile luteinizing hormone release in the castrated male rat. *Eur. J. Endocrinol.* 133: 585–590, 1995.

61. Greenwald, G. S. Role of follicle-stimulating hormone and luteinizing hormone in follicular development and ovulation. In: *The Pituitary Gland,* edited by E. B. Astwood, R. O. Greep, E. Knobil, and W. H. Sawyer. Washington, D.C.: Am. Physiol. Soc., 1974, pt. 2, p. 293–323.

62. Griffin, M. L., S. A. South, V. I. Yankov, R. J. Booth, C. M. Asplin, J. D. Veldhuis, and W. S. Evans. Insulin-dependent diabetes mellitus and menstrual dysfunction. *Ann. Med.* 26: 331–340, 1994.

63. Grosser, P. M., K. T. O'Byrne, C. L. Williams, J. C. Thalabard, J. Hotchkiss, and E. Knobil. Effects of naloxone on estrogen-induced changes in hypothalamic gonadotropin-releasing hormone pulse generator activity in the rhesus monkey. *Neuroendocrinology* 57: 115–119, 1993.

64. Guzick, D. S., R. Wing, D. Smith, S. L. Berga, and S. J. Winters. Calcium/calmodulin-dependent protein kinase-II activation in rat pituitary cells in the presence of thyrotropin-releasing hormone and dopamine. *Endocrinology* 134: 2245–2250, 1994.

65. Haisenleder, D. J., G. A. Ortolano, A. C. Dalkin, M. Yasin, and J. C. Marshall. Differential actions of thyrotropin (TSH)-releasing hormone pulses in the expression of prolactin and TSH subunit messenger ribonucleic acid in rat pituitary cells in vitro. *Endocrinology* 130: 2917–2923, 1992.

66. Haisenleder, D. J., M. Yasin, and J. C. Marshall. Enhanced effectiveness of pulsatile 3′,5′-cyclic adenosine monophosphate in stimulating prolactin and alpha-subunit gene expression. *Endocrinology* 131: 3027–3033, 1992.

67. Haisenleder, D. J., M. Yasin, A. Yasin, and J. C. Marshall. Regulation of prolactin, thyrotropin subunit, and gonadotropin subunit gene expression by pulsatile or continuous calcium signals. *Endocrinology* 133: 2055–2061, 1993.

68. Hartman, M. L., S. M. Pincus, M. L. Johnson, D. H. Matthews, L. M. Faunt, M. L. Vance, M. O. Thorner, and J. D. Veldhuis. Enhanced basal and disorderly growth hormone secretion distinguish acromegalic from normal pulsatile growth hormone release. *J. Clin. Invest.* 94: 1277–1288, 1994.

69. Hawes, B. E., and P. M. Conn. Development of gonadotrope desensitization to gonadotropin-releasing hormone (GnRH) and recovery are not coupled to inositol phosphate production or GnRH receptor number. *Endocrinology* 131: 2681–2689, 1992.

69a. Hindmarsh, P. C., C. H. Fall, P. J. Pringle, C. Osmond, and C. G. Brook. Peak and trough growth hormone concentrations have different associations with the insulin-like growth factor axis, body composition, and metabolic parameters. *J. Clin. Endocrinol. Metab.* 82: 2172–2176, 1997.

70. Hinney, B., C. Henze, and W. Wuttke. Regulation of luteal function by luteinizing hormone and prolactin at different times of the luteal phase. *Eur. J. Endocrinol.* 133: 701–717, 1996.

71. Ho, P. J., G. B. Kletter, N. J. Hopwood, F. R. DeMott, and A. L. Barkan. Age-related changes in the secretion of growth hormone in vivo and in vitro in infantile and prepubertal Holstein bull calves. *J. Endocrinol.* 139: 307–315, 1993.

72. Hochberg, Z., T. Amit, and Z. Zadik. Twenty-four-hour profile of plasma growth hormone–binding protein. *J. Clin. Endocrinol. Metab.* 72: 236–239, 1991.

73. Hochberg, Z., M. Phillip, M. B. Youdim, and T. Amit. Regulation of the growth hormone (GH) receptor and GH-binding protein by GH pulsatility. *Metabolism* 42: 1617–1623, 1993.

74. Hurban, P., and C. S. Thummel. Ontogenesis of the sexual dimorphism of growth hormone secretion by perifused rat hemipituitaries. *Neuroendocrinology* 57: 782–788, 1993.

75. Iberall, A. *Toward a General Science of Viable Systems.* New York: McGraw-Hill, 1972.

76. Irons, C. E., C. A. Sei, and C. C. Glembotski. Relationship of insulin secretory pulses to sex hormone–binding globulin in normal men. *J. Clin. Endocrinol. Metab.* 76: 279–282, 1993.

77. Janovick, J. A., and P. M. Conn. A cholera toxin–sensitive guanyl nucleotide binding protein mediates the movement of pituitary luteinizing hormone into a releasable pool: loss of this event is associated with the onset of homologous desensitization to gonadotropin-releasing hormone. *Endocrinology* 132: 2131–2135, 1993.

78. Janovick, J. A., and P. M. Conn. Progesterone diminishes the sensitivity of gonadotropin-releasing hormone–stimulated luteinizing hormone (LH) release and protects an LH pool from desensitization: actions opposed by cholera toxin. *Endocrinology* 137: 1823–1827, 1996.

79. Jarry, H., S. Leonhardt, and W. Wuttke. Gamma-aminobutyric acid neurons in the preoptic/anterior hypothalamic area synchronize the phasic activity of the gonadotropin-releasing hormone pulse generator in ovariectomized rats. *Neuroendocrinology* 53: 261–267, 1991.

80. Johnson, M. L., and J. D. Veldhuis. Quantitative neuroendocrinology. In: *Methods in Neurosciences,* edited by P. M. Conn. San Diego: Academic, 1995, p. 433.

81. Jones, G. S. Luteal phase defect: a review of pathophysiology. *Curr. Opin. Obstet. Gynecol.* 3: 641–648, 1991.

82. Kaiser, U. B., E. Sabbagh, R. A. Katzenellenbogen, P. M. Conn, and W. W. Chin. A mechanism for the differential regulation of gonadotropin subunit gene expression by gonadotropin-releasing hormone. *Proc. Natl. Acad. Sci. U.S.A.* 92: 12280–12284, 1996.

83. Karsch, F. J., G. E. Dahl, N. P. Evans, J. M. Manning, K. P. Mayfield, S. M. Moenter, and D. L. Foster. Seasonal changes in gonadotropin-releasing hormone secretion in the ewe: alteration in response to the negative feedback action of estradiol. *Biol. Reprod.* 49: 1377–1383, 1993.

84. Kato, M., J. Hoyland, S. K. Sikdar, and W. T. Mason. Imaging of intracellular calcium in rat anterior pituitary cells in response to growth hormone releasing factor. *J. Physiol. (Lond.)* 447: 171–189, 1992.

85. Katt, J. A., J. A. Duncan, L. Herbon, A. Barkan, and J. C. Marshall. The frequency of gonadotropin–releasing hormone stimulation determines the number of pituitary gonadotropin-releasing hormone receptors. *Endocrinology* 116: 2113–2115, 1985.

86. Kaufman, J. M., J. S. Kesner, R. C. Wilson, and E. Knobil. Electrophysiological manifestation of luteinizing hormone–releasing hormone pulse generator activity in the rhesus monkey: influence of alpha-adrenergic and dopaminergic blocking agents. *Endocrinology* 116: 1327–1333, 1985.

87. Kesner, J. S., J. M. Kaufman, R. C. Wilson, G. Kuroda, and E. Knobil. On the short-loop feedback regulation of the hypothalamic luteinizing hormone releasing hormone "pulse generator" in the rhesus monkey. *Neuroendocrinology* 42: 109–111, 1986.

88. Kirk, S. E., A. C. Dalkin, M. Yasin, D. J. Haisenleder, and J. C. Marshall. Gonadotropin-releasing hormone pulse frequency regulates expression of pituitary follistatin messenger ribonucleic acid: a mechanism for differential gonadotrope function. *Endocrinology* 135: 876–880, 1994.

89. Knobil, E. The neuroendocrine control of ovulation. *Hum. Reprod.* 3: 469–472, 1988.

90. Knobil, E. The GnRH pulse generator. *Am. J. Obstet. Gynecol.* 163: 1721–1727, 1990.

91. Knobil, E., T. M. Plant, L. Wildt, P. E. Belchetz, and G. Marshall. Control of the rhesus monkey menstrual cycle: permissive role of hypothalamic gonadotropin-releasing hormone. *Science* 207: 1371–1373, 1980.

92. Kruczynski, A., J. Astruc, E. Chazottes, and R. Kiss. Sex-dependent alteration in cortisol response to endogenous adrenocorticotropin. *J. Clin. Endocrinol. Metab.* 77: 234–240, 1993.

93. Kusano, K., S. Fueshko, H. Gainer, and S. Wray. Electrical and synaptic properties of embryonic luteinizing hormone–releasing hormone neurons in explant cultures. *Proc. Natl. Acad. Sci. U.S.A,* 92: 3918–3922, 1995.

94. Lederis, K. Neurosecretion and the functional structure of the neurohypophysis. In: *The Pituitary Gland,* edited by E. B. Astwood, R. O. Greep, E. Knobil, and W. H. Sawyer. Washington, D.C.: Am. Physiol. Soc., 1974, pt. 2, p. 81–102.

95. Leong, D. A., and M. O. Thorner. A potential code of luteinizing hormone–releasing hormone–induced calcium ion responses in the regulation of luteinizing hormone secretion among individual gonadotropes. *J. Biol. Chem.* 266: 9016–9022, 1991.

96. Levine, J. E., Pau, K.-Y. F., V. D. Ramirez, and G. L. Jackson. Simultaneous measurement of luteinising hormone–releasing hormone and luteinising hormone release in unanesthetized, ovariectomized sheep. *Endocrinology* 111: 1449–1455, 1982.

97. Li, Y. X., J. Keizer, S. S. Stojilkovic, and J. Rinzel. Ca^{2+} excitability of the ER membrane: an explanation for IP3–induced Ca^{2+} oscillations. *Am. J. Physiol.* 269 (*Cell Physiol.* 38): C1079–C1092, 1995.

98. Li, Y. X., J. Rinzel, L. Vergara, and S. S. Stojilkovic. Spontaneous electrical and calcium oscillations in unstimulated pituitary gonadotrophs. *Biophys. J.* 69: 785–795, 1996.

99. Licinio, J., M. L. Wong, M. Altemus, P. B. Bongiorno, A. Bernat, G. Brabant, L. Tamarkin, and P. W. Gold. Pulsatility of 24-hour concentrations of circulating interleukin-1-alpha in healthy women: analysis of integrated basal levels, discrete pulse properties, and correlation with simultaneous interleukin-2 concentrations. *Neuroimmunomodulation* 1: 242–250, 1994.

99a. Licinio, J., C. Mantzoros, A. B. Negrao, G. Cizza, M. L. Wong, P. B. Bongiorno, G. P. Chrousos, B. Karp, C. Allen, J. S. Flier, and P. W. Gold. Human leptin levels are pulsatile and inversely related to pituitary-adrenal function. *Nat. Med.* 3(5): 575–579, 1997.

100. Liu, Y. J., E. Grapengiesser, E. Gylfe, and B. Hellman. Glucose induces oscillations of cytoplasmic Ca^{2+}, Sr^{2+} and Ba^{2+} in pancreatic beta-cells without participation of the thapsigargin-sensitive store. *Cell Calcium* 18: 165–173, 1996.

101. Low, L. C. Growth hormone–releasing hormone: clinical studies and therapeutic aspects. *Neuroendocrinology* 1: 37–40, 1991.

102. Magiakou, M. A., G. Mastorakos, M. T. Gomez, S. R. Rose, and G. P. Chrousos. Pulse amplitude and frequency modulation of parathyroid hormone in early postmenopausal women before and on hormone replacement therapy. *J. Clin. Endocrinol. Metab.* 78: 48–52, 1994.

103. Mandiki, S. N., C. Piraux, J. L. Bister, and R. Paquay. Circadian variations in the amplitude of corticotropin-releasing hormone 41 (CRH41) episodic release measured in vivo in male rats: correlations with diurnal fluctuations in hypothalamic and median eminence CRH41 contents. *J. Biol. Rhythms* 8: 297–309, 1993.

104. Marshall, J. C., A. C. Dalkin, D. J. Haisenleder, M. L. Griffin, and R. P. Kelch. GnRH pulses—the regulators of human reproduction. *Trans. Am. Clin. Climatol. Assoc.* 104: 31–46, 1992.

105. Marshall, J. C., and M. L. Griffin. The role of changing pulse frequency in the regulation of ovulation. *Hum. Reprod.* 2: 57–61, 1993.

106. Martinez de la Escalera, G., A. L. Choi, and R. I. Weiner. Generation and synchronization of gonadotropin-releasing hormone (GnRH) pulses: intrinsic properties of the GT1–1 GnRH neuronal cell line. *Proc. Natl. Acad. Sci. U.S.A.* 89: 1852–1855, 1992.

107. May, R. M. Simple mathematical models with very complicated dynamics. *Nature* 261: 459–467, 1976.

108. McCann, S. M. Regulation of secretion of follicle-stimulating hormone and luteinizing hormone. In: *The Pituitary Gland*, edited by E. B. Astwood, R. O. Greep, E. Knobil, and W. H. Sawyer. Washington, D. C.: Am. Physiol. Soc., 1974, pt. 2, p. 489–517.

109. McIntosh, J.E.A., and R. P. McIntosh. *Mathematical Modelling and Computers in Endocrinology.* Berlin: Springer-Verlag, 1980.

110. McIntosh, J.E.A., and R. P. McIntosh. Varying the patterns and concentrations of gonadotrophin-releasing hormone stimulation does not alter the ratio of LH and FSH released from perifused sheep pituitary cells. *J. Endocrinol.* 109: 155–161, 1986.

111. McIntosh, J.E.A., R. P. McIntosh, and R. J. Kean. Microcomputer-controlled device for delivering hormone stimulation to cell suspensions in perifusion: release of luteinising hormone from sheep pituitary cells. *Med. Biol. Eng. Comput.* 22: 259–262, 1984.

112. McIntosh, R. P. The importance of timing in hormone and drug delivery. *Trends Pharmacol. Sci.* 5: 429–431, 1984.

113. McIntosh, R. P., and J.E.A. McIntosh. Influence of the characteristics of pulses of gonadotrophin releasing hormone on the dynamics of luteinizing hormone release from perifused sheep pituitary cells. *J. Endocrinol.* 98: 411–421, 1983.

114. McIntosh, R. P., and J.E.A. McIntosh. Amplitude of episodic release of LH as a measure of pituitary function analysed from the time-course of hormone levels in the blood: comparison of four menstrual cycles in an individual. *J. Endocrinol.* 107: 231–239, 1985.

115. McIntosh, R. P., and J.E.A. McIntosh. Dynamic characteristics of luteinizing hormone release from perifused sheep anterior pituitary cells stimulated by combined pulsatile and continuous gonadotropin-releasing hormone. *Endocrinology* 117: 169–179, 1985.

116. McIntosh, R. P., J.E.A. McIntosh, and L. Lazarus. A comparison of the dynamics of secretion of human growth hormone and luteinizing hormone. *J. Endocrinol.* 118: 339–345, 1988.

117. McIntosh, R. P., J.E.A. McIntosh, and L. Starling. Effects of modifiers of cytoskeletal structures on the dynamics of release of LH from sheep anterior pituitary cells stimulated with gonadotrophin-releasing hormone, K^+ or phorbol ester. *J. Endocrinol.* 112: 289–298, 1987.

118. McNeilly, A. S., D. C. Anderson, G. M. Besser, J. C. Marshall, P. Harsoulis, L. Alexander, B. J. Ormston, R. Hall, and W. Collins. The luteinizing hormone (LH) and follicle-stimulating hormone response to synthetic LH releasing factor in man. *J. Endocrinol.* 55: xxiv–xxv, 1972.

119. McNeilly, A. S., W. J. Crow, and H. M. Fraser. Suppression of pulsatile luteinizing hormone secretion by gonadotrophin-releasing hormone antagonist does not affect episodic progesterone secretion or corpus luteum function in ewes. *J. Reprod. Fertil.* 96: 865–874, 1992.

120. McNeilly, A. S., H. M. Picton, B. K. Campbell, and D. T. Baird. Gonadotrophic control of follicle growth in the ewe. *J. Reprod. Fertil. Suppl.* 43: 177–186, 1991.

121. McNeilly, A. S., C. C. Tay, and A. Glasier. Physiological mechanisms underlying lactational amenorrhea. *Ann. N. Y. Acad. Sci.* 709: 145–155, 1994.

122. McNeilly, J. R., P. Brown, A. J. Clark, and A. S. McNeilly. Gonadotrophin-releasing hormone modulation of gonadotrophins in the ewe: evidence for differential effects on gene expression and hormone secretion. *J. Mol. Endocrinol.* 7: 35–43, 1991.

123. Mershon, J. L., C. S. Sehlhorst, R. W. Rebar, and J. H. Liu. Evidence of a corticotropin-releasing hormone pulse generator in the macaque hypothalamus. *Endocrinology* 130: 2991–2996, 1992.

124. Mesiano, S., C. S. Hart, B. W. Heyer, S. L. Kaplan, and M. M. Grumbach. Hormone ontogeny in the ovine fetus. XXVI. A sex difference in the effect of castration on the hypothalamic–pituitary gonadotropin unit in the ovine fetus. *Endocrinology* 129: 3073–3079, 1991.

125. Midgley, A. R. Radioimmunoassay: a method for human chorionic gonadotrophin and human luteinizing hormone. *Endocrinology* 79: 10–18, 1966.

126. Midgley, A. R., R. M. Brand, P. A. Favreau, M. N. Boving, M. N. Ghazzi, V. Padmanabhan, E. Y. Young, and H. C. Cantor. *Monitoring Dynamic Responses of Perifused Neuroendocrine Tissues to Stimuli in Real Time.* San Diego: Academic, 1995.

127. Moenter, S. M., R. M. Brand, A. R. Midgley, and F. J. Karsch. Dynamics of gonadotropin-releasing hormone release during a pulse. *Endocrinology* 130: 503–510, 1992.

128. Murray-McIntosh, R. P., and J.E.A. McIntosh. Modeling pulsatile hormone stimulation of cell responses. In: *Pulsatility in Neuroendocrine Systems*, edited by J. E. Levine. San Diego: Academic, 1994, p. 423–442.

129. Nippoldt, T. B., N. E. Reame, R. P. Kelch, and J. C. Marshall. The roles of estradiol and progesterone in decreasing luteinizing hormone pulse frequency in the luteal phase of the menstrual cycle. *J. Clin. Endocrinol. Metab.* 69: 67–76, 1989.

130. O'Byrne, K. T., M. D. Chen, M. Nishihara, C. L. Williams, J. C. Thalabard, J. Hotchkiss, and E. Knobil. Ovarian control of gonadotropin hormone–releasing hormone pulse generator

activity in the rhesus monkey: duration of the associated hypo-thalamic signal. *Neuroendocrinology* 57: 588–592, 1993.

131. O'Byrne, K. T., and E. Knobil. Electrophysiological approaches to gonadotrophin releasing hormone pulse generator activity in the rhesus monkey. *Hum. Reprod.* 8 (Suppl. 2): 37–40, 1993.

132. O'Byrne, K. T., J. C. Thalabard, S. E. Chiappini, M. D. Chen, J. Hotchkiss, and E. Knobil. Ambient light modifies gonadotropin-releasing hormone pulse generator frequency in the rhesus monkey. *Endocrinology* 133: 1520–1524, 1993.

133. O'Byrne, K. T., J. C. Thalabard, P. M. Grosser, R. C. Wilson, C. L. Williams, M. D. Chen, D. Ladendorf, J. Hotchkiss, and E. Knobil. Radiotelemetric monitoring of hypothalamic gonadotropin-releasing hormone pulse generator activity throughout the menstrual cycle of the rhesus monkey. *Endocrinology* 129: 1207–1214, 1991.

134. O'Meara, N. M., J. Sturis, E. Van Cauter, and K. S. Polonsky. Lack of control by glucose of ultradian insulin secretory oscillations in impaired glucose tolerance and in non-insulin-dependent diabetes mellitus. *J. Clin. Invest.* 92: 262–271, 1993.

135. Ogden, D. C., K. Khodakhah, T. D. Carter, P. T. Gray, and T. Capiod. Timing of exposure to somatostatin relative to growth hormone–releasing factor dictates the rat anterior pituitary cell growth hormone response. *J. Endocrinol.* 138: 369–377, 1993.

136. Ono, M., N. Miki, and H. Demura. Effect of antiserum to rat growth hormone (GH)–releasing factor on physiological GH secretion in the female rat. *Endocrinology* 129: 1791–1796, 1991.

137. Pampori, N. A., A. K. Agrawal, and B. H. Shapiro. Renaturaliz-ing the sexually dimorphic profiles of circulating growth hor-mone in hypophysectomized rats. *Acta Endocrinol.* 124: 283–289, 1991.

138. Paolisso, G., A. J. Scheen, D. Giugliano, S. Sgambato, A. Albert, M. Varricchio, F. D'Onofrio, and P. J. Lefebvre. Pulsa-tile insulin delivery has greater metabolic effects than continu-ous hormone administration in man: importance of pulse fre-quency. *J. Clin. Endocrinol. Metab.* 72: 607–615, 1991.

139. Partsch, C. J., S. Abrahams, N. Herholz, M. Peter, J. D. Veldhuis, and W. G. Sippell. Variability of pulsatile luteinizing hormone secretion in young male volunteers. *Eur. J. Endocri-nol.* 131: 263–272, 1994.

140. Pincus, S. M. Quantification of evolution from order to ran-domness in practical time series analysis. *Methods Enzymol.* 240: 68–89, 1994.

141. Plant, T. M., E. Schallenberger, D. L. Hess, J. T. McCormack, L. Dufy Barbe, and E. Knobil. Influence of suckling on gonado-tropin secretion in the female rhesus monkey *(Macaca mulatta)*. *Biol. Reprod.* 23: 760–766, 1980.

142. Polonsky, K. S., B. D. Given, L. J. Hirsch, E. T. Shapiro, C. Beebe, B. H. Frank, J. A. Galloway, and E. Van Cauter. Abnormal patterns of insulin secretion in non-insulin-dependent diabetes mellitus. *N. Engl. J. Med.* 318: 1231–1239, 1988.

143. Polonsky, K. S., B. D. Given, and E. Van Cauter. Twenty-four-hour profiles and pulsatile patterns of insulin secretion in normal and obese subjects. *J. Clin. Invest.* 81: 442–448, 1988.

144. Prigogine, I., and G. Nicolis. Biological order, structure and instabilities. *Q. Rev. Biophys.* 4: 107–148, 1971.

145. Ram, P. A., S. H. Park, H. K. Choi, and D. J. Waxman. Growth hormone activation of Stat 1, Stat 3, and Stat 5 in rat liver. Differential kinetics of hormone desensitization and growth hormone stimulation of both tyrosine phosphorylation and serine/threonine phosphorylation. *J. Biol. Chem.* 271: 5929–5940, 1996.

146. Rapp, P. E., and M. J. Berridge. Oscillations in calcium–cyclic AMP control loops form the basis of pacemaker activity and other high frequency biological rhythms. *J. Theor. Biol.* 66: 497–525, 1977.

147. Rawlings, S. R., D. J. Berry, and D. A. Leong. Evidence for localized calcium mobilization and influx in single rat gonadotropes. *J. Biol. Chem.* 266: 22755–22760, 1991.

148. Rawlings, S. R., J. Hoyland, and W. T. Mason. Calcium homeo-stasis in bovine somatotrophs: calcium oscillations and calcium regulation by growth hormone–releasing hormone and somato-statin. *Cell Calcium* 12: 403–414, 1991.

149. Reiter, R. J. Circannual reproductive rhythms in mammals related to photoperiod and pineal function: a review. *Chronobi-ologia* 1: 365–395, 1974.

150. Rettori, V., M. F. Gimeno, A. Karara, M. C. Gonzalez, and S. M. McCann. Interleukin 1 alpha inhibits prostaglandin E2 release to suppress pulsatile release of luteinizing hormone but not follicle-stimulating hormone. *Proc. Natl. Acad. Sci. U.S.A.* 88: 2763–2767, 1991.

151. Rosen, R. The generation and recognition of patterns in biolog-ical systems. In: *Mathematics and the Life Sciences*, edited by D. E. Matthews. Berlin: Springer-Verlag, 1977, p. 222–341.

152. Russell, J., P. Gee, S. M. Liu, and R. H. Angeletti. Stoichiometry of the pulsating growth hormone (GH) binding to the GH-binding protein and the turnover of the GH-receptor. *Proc. Soc. Exp. Biol. Med.* 206: 249–253, 1994.

153. Samuels, M. H., J. D. Veldhuis, P. Henry, and E. C. Ridgway. Pathophysiology of pulsatile and copulsatile release of thyroid-stimulating hormone, luteinizing hormone, follicle-stimulating hormone, and alpha-subunit. *J. Clin. Endocrinol. Metab.* 71: 425–432, 1990.

154. Samuels, M. H., J. Veldhuis, and E. C. Ridgway. Copulsatile release of thyrotropin and prolactin in normal and hypothyroid subjects. *Thyroid* 5: 369–372, 1995.

154a. Samuels, M. H., J. D. Veldhuis, P. Kramer, R. J. Urban, R. Bauer, and G. R. Mundy. Episodic secretion of parathyroid hormone in postmenopausal women: assessment by deconvolu-tion analysis and approximate entropy. *J. Bone Miner. Res.* 12(4): 616–623, 1997.

155. Santen, R. J., and C. W. Bardin. Episodic luteinizing hormone secretion in man. Pulse analysis, clinical interpretation, physio-logic mechanisms. *J. Clin. Invest.* 52: 2617–2628, 1973.

156. Sarnyai, Z., J. D. Veldhuis, N. K. Mello, J. H. Mendelson, S. M. Eroes, G. Mercer, H. Gelles, and M. Kelly. The concor-dance of pulsatile ultradian release of adrenocorticotropin and cortisol in male rhesus monkeys. *J. Clin. Endocrinol. Metab.* 80: 54–59, 1995.

157. Schaefer, F., G. Baumann, D. Haffner, L. M. Faunt, M. L. Johnson, M. Mercado, E. Ritz, O. Mehls, and J. D. Veldhuis. Multifactorial control of the elimination kinetics of unbound (free) growth hormone (GH) in the human: regulation by age, adiposity, renal function, and steady state concentrations of GH in plasma. *J. Clin. Endocrinol. Metab.* 81: 22–31, 1996.

158. Schaefer, F., M. Daschner, J. D. Veldhuis, J. Oh, F. Qadri, and K. Scharer. Pulsatile fluctuations of plasma-gonadotropin-releasing hormone and corticotropin-releasing factor levels in healthy pregnant women. *Acta Obstet. Gynecol. Scand.* 73: 284–289, 1994.

159. Sharma, O. P., J. A. Flores, D. A. Leong, and J. D. Veldhuis. Cellular basis for follicle-stimulating hormone–stimulated cal-cium signaling in single rat Sertoli cells: possible dissociation from effects of adenosine 3′,5′-monophosphate. *Endocrinology* 134: 1915–1923, 1994.

160. Sharma, O. P., J. A. Flores, D. A. Leong, and J. D. Veldhuis. Mechanisms by which endothelin-1 stimulates increased cyto-solic free calcium ion concentrations in single rat Sertoli cells. *Endocrinology* 135: 127–134, 1994.

161. Shaw, R. W., W. R. Butt, D. R. London, and J. C. Marshall. Variation in response to synthetic luteinizing hormone–releasing hormone (LH-RH) at different phases of the same menstrual cycle in normal women. *J. Obstet. Gynaecol. Br. Commonw.* 81: 632–639, 1974.

162. Shupnik, M. A. Effects of gonadotropin-releasing hormone on rat gonadotropin gene transcription in vitro: requirement for pulsatile administration for luteinizing hormone-beta gene stimulation. *Mol. Endocrinol.* 4: 1444–1450, 1990.

163. Sikdar, S. K., R. P. McIntosh, and W. T. Mason. Differential modulation of Ca^{2+}-activated K^+ channels in ovine pituitary gonadotrophs by GnRH, Ca^{2+} and cyclic AMP. *Brain Res.* 496: 113–123, 1989.

164. Smith, W. R., G. C. Wake, J. E. McIntosh, R. P. McIntosh, M. Pettigrew, and R. Kao. Mathematical analysis of perifusion data: models predicting elution concentration. *Am. J. Physiol.* 261 (*Regulatory Integrative Comp. Physiol.* 32): R247–R256, 1991.

165. Soendoro, T., M. P. Diamond, J. R. Pepperell, and F. Naftolin. The in vitro perifused rat ovary: I. Steroid secretion in response to ramp and pulsatile stimulation with luteinizing hormone and follicle stimulating hormone. *Gynecol. Endocrinol.* 6: 229–238, 1992.

166. Soendoro, T., M. P. Diamond, J. R. Pepperell, and F. Naftolin. The in vitro perifused rat ovary: IV. Modulation of ovarian steroid secretion by insulin. *Gynecol. Endocrinol.* 7: 7–11, 1993.

167. Sollberger, A. *Biological Rhythm Research.* Amsterdam: Elsevier, 1965.

168. Stanislaus, D., V. Arora, W. M. Awara, and P. M. Conn. Biphasic action of cyclic adenosine 3',5'-monophosphate in gonadotropin-releasing hormone (GnRH) analog-stimulated hormone release from GH3 cells stably transfected with GnRH receptor complementary deoxyribonucleic acid. *Endocrinology* 137: 1025–1031, 1996.

169. Starling, L., R. P. McIntosh, and J. E. McIntosh. Effects of lithium and phorbol esters on the dynamics of LH release from dispersed sheep pituitary cells. *J. Endocrinol.* 111: 167–173, 1986.

170. Stojilkovic, S. S., L. Z. Krsmanovic, D. J. Spergel, M. Tomic, and K. J. Catt. Calcium signalling and episodic secretory responses of GnRH neurons. In: *Pulsatility in Neuroendocrine Systems,* edited by J. E. Levine. San Diego: Academic, 1994, p. 68–84.

171. Sturis, J., E. Mosekilde, and E. Van Cauter. Modeling modulatory effects on pulsatility. In: *Pulsatility in Neuroendocrine Systems,* edited by J. E. Levine. San Diego: Academic, 1994, p. 393–422.

172. Sturis, J., K. S. Polonsky, E. Mosekilde, and E. Van Cauter. Computer model for mechanisms underlying ultradian oscillations of insulin and glucose. *Am. J. Physiol.* 260 (*Endocrinol. Metab.* 23): E801–E809, 1991.

173. Sturis, J., A. J. Scheen, R. Leproult, K. S. Polonsky, and E. van Cauter. 24-hour glucose profiles during continuous or oscillatory insulin infusion. Demonstration of the functional significance of ultradian insulin oscillations. *J. Clin. Invest.* 95: 1464–1471, 1995.

174. Thomas, G. B., J. T. Cummins, B. Yao, K. Gordon, and I. J. Clarke. Release of prolactin is independent of the secretion of thyrotrophin-releasing hormone into hypophysial portal blood of sheep. *J. Endocrinol.* 117: 115–122, 1988.

175. Tse, A., and B. Hille. Patch-clamp studies on identified pituitary gonadotropes in vitro. In: *Pulsatility in Neuroendocrine Systems,* edited by J. E. Levine. San Diego: Academic, 1994, p. 95–99.

175a. Udy, G. B., R. P. Towers, R. G. Snell, R. J. Wilkins, S. H. Park, P. A. Ram, D. J. Waxman, and H. W. Davey. Requirement of STAT 5b for sexual dimorphism of body growth rates and liver gene expression. *Proc. Natl. Acad. Sci. U.S.A.* 94: 7239–7244, 1997.

176. Urban, R. J., W. S. Evans, A. D. Rogol, D. L. Kaiser, M. L. Johnson, and J. D. Veldhuis. Contemporary aspects of discrete peak-detection algorithms. I. The paradigm of the luteinizing hormone pulse signal in men. *Endocr. Rev.* 9: 3–37, 1988.

177. Vale, W., G. Grant, J. Rivier, M. Monahan, M. Amoss, R. Blackwell, R. Burgus, and R. Guillemin. Synthetic polypeptide antagonists of the hypothalamic luteinizing hormone releasing factor. *Science* 176: 933–934, 1972.

178. Van Cauter, E. Estimating false-positive and false-negative errors in analyses of hormonal pulsatility. *Am. J. Physiol.* 254 (*Endocrinol. Metab.* 17): E786–E794, 1988.

179. van den Berg, G., M. Frolich, J. D. Veldhuis, and F. Roelfsema. Combined amplification of the pulsatile and basal modes of adrenocorticotropin and cortisol secretion in patients with Cushing's disease: evidence for decreased responsiveness of the adrenal glands. *J. Clin. Endocrinol. Metab.* 80: 3750–3757, 1995.

180. Van Vugt, D. A., W. D. Diefenbach, E. Alston, and M. Ferin. Gonadotrophin-releasing hormone pulses in the third ventricular cerebrospinal fluid of ovariectomized rhesus monkeys: correlation with luteinizing hormone pulses. *Endocrinology* 117: 1550–1558, 1985.

181. Veldhuis, J. D. Gender differences in secretory activity of the human somatotropic (growth hormone) axis. *Eur. J. Endocrinol.* 134: 287–295, 1996.

182. Veldhuis, J. D., L. M. Faunt, and M. L. Johnson. Analysis of nonequilibrium dynamics of bound, free, and total plasma ligand concentrations over time following nonlinear secretory inputs: kinetics of two or more hormones pulsed into compartments containing multiple variable-affinity binding proteins. *Methods Enzymol.* 240: 349–377, 1994.

183. Veldhuis, J. D., A. Iranmanesh, M. L. Johnson, and G. Lizarralde. Twenty-four-hour rhythms in plasma concentrations of adenohypophyseal hormones are generated by distinct amplitude and/or frequency modulation of underlying pituitary secretory bursts. *J. Clin. Endocrinol. Metab.* 71: 1616–1623, 1990.

184. Veldhuis, J. D., and M. L. Johnson. Cluster analysis: a simple, versatile, and robust algorithm for endocrine pulse detection. *Am. J. Physiol.* 250 (*Endocrinol. Metab.* 13): E486–E493, 1986.

185. Veldhuis, J. D., J. C. King, R. J. Urban, A. D. Rogol, W. S. Evans, L. A. Kolp, and M. L. Johnson. Operating characteristics of the male hypothalamo–pituitary–gonadal axis: pulsatile release of testosterone and follicle-stimulating hormone and their temporal coupling with luteinizing hormone. *J. Clin. Endocrinol. Metab.* 65: 929–941, 1987.

186. Veldhuis, J. D., L. S. O'Dea, and M. L. Johnson. The nature of the gonadotropin-releasing hormone stimulus–luteinizing hormone secretory response of human gonadotrophs in vivo. *J. Clin. Endocrinol. Metab.* 68: 661–670, 1989.

187. Vergara, L. A., S. S. Stojilkovic, and E. Rojas. GnRH-induced cytosolic calcium oscillations in pituitary gonadotrophs: phase resetting by membrane depolarization. *Biophys. J.* 69: 1606–1614, 1996.

188. Waddington, C. H. ed. *Towards a Theoretical Biology,* vols. 1–4. Edinburgh: Edinburgh University Press, 1968–1972.

189. Waters, S. B., and P. M. Conn. Maintenance of gonadotropin-releasing hormone (GnRH)-stimulated luteinizing hormone release despite desensitization of GnRH-stimulated cytosolic calcium responses. *Endocrinology* 130: 2091–2100, 1992.

190. Waxman, D. J., N. A. Pampori, P. A. Ram, A. K. Agrawal, and B. H. Shapiro. Interpulse interval in circulating growth hormone patterns regulates sexually dimorphic expression of hepatic cytochrome P450. *Proc. Natl. Acad. Sci. U.S.A.* 88: 6868–6872, 1991.

191. Weill, J., A. Duhamel, M. Dherbomez, R. Beuscart, and C. Ponte. Pulsatility of growth hormone secretion and its relation to growth. *Horm. Res.* 38: 134–139, 1992.

192. Weiss, J., W. F. Crowley, Jr., and J. L. Jameson. Pulsatile gonadotropin-releasing hormone modifies polyadenylation of gonadotropin subunit messenger ribonucleic acids. *Endocrinology* 130: 415–420, 1992.

193. Weiss, J., P. E. Harris, L. M. Halvorson, W. F. Crowley, Jr., and J. L. Jameson. Dynamic regulation of follicle-stimulating hormone-beta messenger ribonucleic acid levels by activin and gonadotropin-releasing hormone in perifused rat pituitary cells. *Endocrinology* 131: 1403–1408, 1992.

194. Weiss, J., J. L. Jameson, J. M. Burrin, and W. F. Crowley, Jr. Divergent responses of gonadotropin subunit messenger RNAs to continuous versus pulsatile gonadotropin-releasing hormone in vitro. *Mol. Endocrinol.* 4: 557–564, 1990.

195. Westerlund, J., B. Hellman, and P. Bergsten. Pulsatile insulin release from mouse islets occurs in the absence of stimulated entry of Ca^{2+}. *J. Clin. Invest.* 97: 1860–1863, 1996.

196. Wildt, L., G. Marshall, and E. Knobil. Experimental induction of puberty in the infantile female rhesus monkey. *Science* 207: 1373–1375, 1980.

197. Williams, C. L., M. Nishihara, J. C. Thalabard, P. M. Grosser, J. Hotchkiss, and E. Knobil. Corticotropin-releasing factor and gonadotropin-releasing hormone pulse generator activity in the rhesus monkey. Electrophysiological studies. *Neuroendocrinology* 52: 133–137, 1990.

198. Williams, C. L., M. Nishihara, J. C. Thalabard, K. T. O'Byrne, P. M. Grosser, J. Hotchkiss, and E. Knobil. Duration and frequency of multiunit electrical activity associated with the hypothalamic gonadotropin releasing hormone pulse generator in the rhesus monkey: differential effects of morphine. *Neuroendocrinology* 52: 225–228, 1990.

199. Williams, C. L., J. C. Thalabard, K. T. O'Byrne, P. M. Grosser, M. Nishihara, J. Hotchkiss, and E. Knobil. Duration of phasic electrical activity of the hypothalamic gonadotropin-releasing hormone pulse generator and dynamics of luteinizing hormone pulses in the rhesus monkey. *Proc. Natl. Acad. Sci. U.S.A.* 87: 8580–8582, 1990.

200. Willoughby, J. O., and A. Medvedev. Opioid receptor activation resets the hypothalamic clock generating growth hormone secretory bursts in the rat. *J. Endocrinol.* 148: 149–155, 1996.

201. Winfree, A. T. Rotary chemical reactions. *Sci. Am.* 230: 82–95, 1974.

202. Wu, F. C., G. E. Butler, C. J. Kelnar, I. Huhtaniemi, and J. D. Veldhuis. Ontogeny of pulsatile gonadotropin releasing hormone secretion from midchildhood, through puberty, to adulthood in the human male: a study using deconvolution analysis and an ultrasensitive immunofluorometric assay. *J. Clin. Endocrinol. Metab.* 81: 1798–1805, 1996.

203. Yasin, M., A. C. Dalkin, D. J. Haisenleder, J. R. Kerrigan, and J. C. Marshall. Gonadotropin-releasing hormone (GnRH) pulse pattern regulates GnRH receptor gene expression: augmentation by estradiol. *Endocrinology* 136: 1559–1564, 1995.

204. Yates, F. E. Modeling periodicities in reproductive, adrenocortical, and metabolic systems. In: *Biorhythms and Human Reproduction,* edited by M. Ferin, F. Halberg, R. M. Richart, and R. L. Vande Wiele. New York: Wiley, 1974, p. 133–142.

205. Yates, F. E., D. J. Marsh, and A. S. Iberall. Integration of the whole organism—a foundation for a theoretical biology. In: *Challenging Biological Problems. Directions Toward Their Solution,* edited by J. A. Behnke. New York: Oxford University Press, 1972, p. 110–132.

206. Yen, S. S., D. Apter, T. Butzow, and G. A. Laughlin. Gonadotrophin releasing hormone pulse generator activity before and during sexual maturation in girls: new insights. *Hum. Reprod.* 8 (Suppl. 2): 66–71, 1993.

207. Yen, S. S., R. Rebar, F. Van den Berg, F. Naftolin, Y. Ehara, S. Engblom, K. J. Ryan, K. Benirschke, J. Rivier, M. Amoss, and R. Guillemin. Synthetic luteinizing hormone–releasing factor. A potent stimulator of gonadotropin release in man. *J. Clin. Endocrinol. Metab.* 34: 1108–1111, 1972.

208. Yen, S.S.C., C. C. Tsai, F. Naftolin, G. Vandenberg, and L. Ajabor. Pulsatile patterns of gonadotrophin release in subjects with and without ovarian function. *J. Clin. Endocrinol. Metab.* 34: 671–675, 1972.

208a. Yoo, M. J., M. Nishihara, and M. Takahashi. Tumor necrosis factor-α mediates endotoxin induced suppression of GnRH pulse generator activity in the rat. *Endocr. J.* 44: 141–148, 1997.

209. Zambrano, E., A. Olivares, J. P. Mendez, L. Guerrero, I. Diaz-Cueto, J. D. Veldhuis, and A. Ulloa-Aguirre. Dynamics of basal and gonadotrophin-releasing hormone–releasable serum follicle-stimulating hormone charge isoform distribution throughout the menstrual cycle. *J. Clin. Endocrinol. Metab.* 80: 1647–1656, 1995.

210. Zeeman, E. C. Catastrophe theory. *Sci. Am.* 234: 65–83, 1976.

210a. Zwart, A. D., A. Iranmanesh, and J. D. Veldhuis. Disparate serum free testosterone concentrations and degrees of hypothalamo-pituitary-luteinizing hormone suppression are achieved by continuous versus pulsatile intravenous androgen replacement in men: a clinical experimental model of ketoconazole-induced reversible hypoandrogenemia with controlled testosterone add-back. *J. Clin. Endocrinol. Metab.* 82(7): 2062–2069, 1997.

20. Apoptosis

SHEAU YU HSU
AARON J. W. HSUEH

*Division of Reproductive Biology, Department of Gynecology and Obstetrics,
Stanford University Medical School, Stanford, California*

APOPTOSIS IS AN ACTIVE CELL "SUICIDE" to eliminate superfluous tissues. Regulated cell death is essential during embryonic development, metamorphosis, tissue renewal, hormone-induced tissue atrophy, and many other physiological processes. As early as 1858, Virchow (262) defined two types of cell death that differ in their morphological characteristics. In 1885, Flemming (83) also made the clear distinction between natural cell death, as in regressing ovarian follicles, and other kinds of tissue degeneration. One type of cell death, *necrosis* or accidental cell death, occurs when cells are subjected to external insult. In contrast, the other type of cell death, *apoptosis*, is characterized usually by shrinkage and fragmentation of dying cells.

The term "apoptosis" was coined by Kerr and colleagues (131, 280, 282) in 1972 to describe the type of cell death they found in adrenal cells following ablation of the anterior pituitary gland, which leads to adrenocorticotropic hormone (ACTH) withdrawal. "Apoptosis" is derived from a Greek word describing the process of leaves falling from trees or petals falling from flowers, and the apoptotic mechanism is used to describe specifically the physiological nature of this process that permits cells to die in an active manner. It is generally believed that this form of cell death ensures the elimination of superfluous cells, including those that have *(1)* been generated in excess, *(2)* developed improperly, *(3)* already completed their specific functions, or *(4)* proved harmful to the whole organism. Apoptotic cell death is always accompanied by active phagocytosis of dying cells before rupture of their plasma membrane, thus protecting surrounding tissues from the potentially harmful inflammatory reactions that usually occur after necrosis (219, 281). Normally, apoptosis proceeds rapidly so that few apoptotic cells can be detected in most tissues in vivo (281); this helps explain the failure to appreciate apoptotic cell death in earlier studies.

The series of changes that occur during apoptosis are remarkably similar in a wide range of cell types responding to a diversity of stimuli. Three major processes commonly found during apoptosis are cell volume reduction, chromatin condensation, and recognition by phagocytic cells (169, 277, 278). During volume reduction, increases in cell density and blebbing of the cell surface are accompanied by compaction of cytoplasmic organelles and dilation of the endoplasmic reticulum. Studies on apoptotic thymocytes have shown that these cells lose up to one-third of their volume during apoptosis (277, 283). Apoptotic cells first show chromatin condensation, which is found as a continuous band of densely osmiophilic granules underlying the nuclear membrane, in the nucleus, and the condensed nucleus becomes fragmentated soon after (Fig. 20.1). Concomitant with these cytoplasmic and nuclear alterations, biochemical changes, such as endonuclease activation, internucleosomal cleavage of genomic DNA, and transglutaminase-catalyzed cross-linking of cellular proteins, also are observed in apoptotic cells (44, 79, 276, 281). In addition, it appears that apoptosis induced by a variety of agents requires the synthesis of new mRNA or protein, and involves cells with normal adenosine triphosphate (ATP) levels. Finally, dead cells are recognized by macrophages and phagocytosed while still intact (Table 20.1).

In contrast to apoptosis, necrotic death generally is associated with stressful or toxic stimuli, including severe hypoxia (224, 226), oxidative stress (27, 64), extreme pH and temperature (61, 150, 229), high concentrations of toxins, lytic virus infection, or exposure to agents that directly damage the membranes such as complement (254). Compared to apoptosis, which occurs in a sporadic manner and affects scattered individual cells, necrosis usually affects contiguous cells and is considered to be a passive response to noxious stimuli (129, 278). Necrotic cells usually exhibit severe swelling of all cytoplasmic compartments and disruption of the internal membranes. Their mitochondria

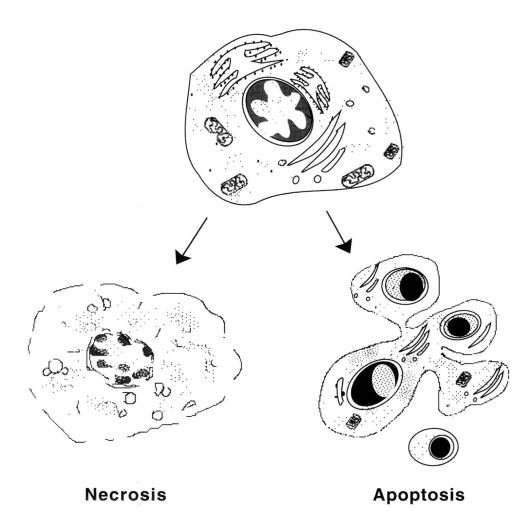

Necrosis   **Apoptosis**

FIG. 20.1. Diagrams illustrating sequences of structural changes during apoptosis and necrosis. *Lower left:* The nuclei of necrotic cells usually are associated with irregular chromatin clumping, and the plasma membrane dissolves following the loss of cell volume homeostasis. In addition, leakage of cellular contents to the environment leads to inflammatory reactions. *Lower right:* The nuclei of apoptotic cells are characterized by condensation and fragmentation of nuclear chromatin. Apoptotic cells also undergo volume shrinkage and become fragmented into membrane-bound apoptotic bodies. These apoptotic bodies are phagocytosed by macrophages or neighboring cells before degradation within their lysosomes.

TABLE 20.1. *Apoptosis vs. Necrosis*

Apoptosis	Necrosis
Chromatin and cytoplasmic condensation, cell shrinkage	Cell swelling and rupture of plasma membrane
Normal ATP* level	Decreased ATP level
Endonuclease activation and "ladder-like" internucleosomal DNA fragmentation	Activation of nonspecific DNAses leading to random DNA degradation
May require synthesis of RNA or proteins	Not dependent upon synthesis of macromolecules
Affects scattered individual cells	Affects tracts of contiguous cells
Engulfment by phagocytes before rupture of plasma membrane, no inflammation	Cell rupture elicits inflammatory reactions

* ATP, adenosine triphosphate.

characteristically appears as empty and distended vacuoles with aggregates of denatured matrix proteins. Due to loss of their capacity for volume homeostasis, necrotic cells undergo uncontrolled swelling and rupture of the plasma membrane (129). It is believed that damage to the plasma membrane leads to failure to exclude calcium ions from the cell interior. As a result, the calcium-dependent phospholipases and proteases are activated, leading to further destruction of the cell membrane, leakage of intracellular contents, inflammation, and extensive tissue damage (278). In addition, necrosis is associated with the activation of nonspecific DNAses and depleted ATP levels in cells. Unlike apoptosis, necrosis is not dependent on the synthesis of macromolecules (Table 20.1).

In a multicellular organism, apoptosis occur during diverse normal physiological states. It also occurs in specific pathological conditions, such as injuries incurred by certain exogenous noxious agents or during tumorigenesis. It has been postulated that, with the exception of blastomeres, all differentiated tissues in multicellular organisms are "programmed" to undergo apoptosis through an evolutionarily conserved "suicide" program (202, 203, 254). To stay alive, they presumably require signals provided by survival factors acting on the cell surface or intracellular receptors. Once the survival signals are absent, the accomplishment of cell "suicide" requires the participation of a set of "death genes" (203). Because the mechanism by which different cells maintain themselves over the life of the organism varies, extracellular signals and cellular receptors important for apoptosis and survival of different tissues are extremely diverse. Likewise, redundant genes in the apoptotic pathway may have developed during evolution, and different subsets of death and antideath genes may be responsible for apoptosis and survival of cells in a tissue-specific manner.

During embryonic development, apoptotic cell death is widespread and essential for the sculpturing of body shape (36, 256). For example, during the first embryonic cavitation process, the transformation of solid ectoderm into a columnar epithelium surrounding a proamniotic cavity is the result of selective apoptosis of inner ectodermal cells, while the columnar cells that line the cavity survive by contact with the basement membrane (48, 281). Massive apoptosis also is observed in embryonic neurons, and it is estimated that as much as 85% of embryonic neurons undergo apoptosis during development of the central nervous system (9, 190, 203). During metamorphosis, extensive apoptosis in the tail of tadpoles is necessary for the remodeling of body structure. Similarly, apoptosis in the alimentary tract of the tadpole is essential to accommodate the alteration of diet requirements during adult life (118, 195).

In adult tissues also, the occurrence of apoptosis is common and can be separated into three broad categories. The first group of tisssues, such as neuron, heart, liver, and kidney, are characterized by miminal cell proliferation and a low rate of cell turnover. Generally, very little apoptosis can be observed in these tissues (12, 13). The second group, including hemopoietic tissues, the epithelium lining intestinal crypts, and male germ cells (spermatogonia) in the testis, exhibit constant cell turnover and have high rates of stem cell proliferation accompanied by massive apoptosis (17, 278, 281). In the third type of tissue, such as the ovary, a high rate of follicular cell apoptosis continues during the reproductive life but with no replenishment of the original stockpile (115).

Regardless of the mechanism by which cell death is regulated, the maintenance of a balance between apoptosis and cell proliferation is crucial for the life of any multicellular organism that has reached maturity. When a high rate of proliferation is not counterbalanced by apoptosis, pathological conditions can develop. It is believed that certain forms of autoimmune disease are due to decreased levels of apoptosis in the immune system and the ensuing accumulation of autoreactive lymphoid cells. For example, the phenotype in some patients with system lupus erythematosus may be due to a failure to eliminate activated lymphocytes by the Fas antigen-based mechanism (29). In more extreme conditions, failure of cells to die could lead to tumorigenesis. Indeed, as many as 85% of follicular B-cell lymphomas are associated with the overexpression of a proto-oncogene, *bcl-2,* and the suppression of apoptosis (37). The development of B-cell lymphoma in these patients is presumably due to the enhanced survival of lymphoid cells, followed by secondary tumorigenic mutations (for example, *c-myc* mutation) during the prolonged life span of these cells (47, 164, 165). In addition, it has been shown that Bcl-2 expression is elevated in 90% of colorectal cancers, 30%–60% of prostate cancers, 20% of non-small-cell lung cancers, 70% of breast cancers, and 65% of lymphomas, suggesting that improper regulation of apoptosis predisposes diverse tissues to tumor development (206).

Like abnormal suppression of apoptosis, excessive cell death is found in different pathological states. Increased apoptosis has been associated with ischemic injury of vascular tissues and the development of neurodegenerative disorders, such as Alzheimer's disease, Parkinson's disease, Huntington's disease, Charcot-Marie-Tooth type 1A demyelinating neuropathy, and spinal muscular atrophies (67, 212, 254). Likewise, excessive apoptosis may be the cause of premature ovarian failure.

Many animal cells also undergo apoptosis when exposed to viruses. In an extreme example, the human immunodeficiency virus triggers massive apoptosis in host cells, leading to the eventual depletion of lymphoid cells and the acquired immunodeficiency syndrome (254). Of interest, apoptosis of virus-infected cells can be triggered not only by viruses but also by the host itself, and the active apoptosis of host cells following viral infection may have evolved as a body's defense mechanism to halt the production and spread of viral particles. To counter this type of host defense mechanism, some viruses have developed mechanisms that inhibit host cell apoptosis and allow viral particles to replicate (41). Thus, proper regulation of apoptosis also plays an important role in the defense of pathological agents, and too little cell death can lead to persistent viral infection. Understanding the mechanisms mediating apoptosis not only is important for the elucidation of basic mechanisms underlying diverse physiological processes but also, ultimately, may lead to new modalities to treat a wide range of diseases.

APOPTOTIC CELL DEATH SHOWS CONSERVED MORPHOLOGICAL AND BIOCHEMICAL CHANGES

Nuclear Condensation and Ladder Pattern of DNA Fragmentation

Apoptosis was first recognized as a type of cell death typified by morphological changes in the cell nucleus

and cytoplasm. The most distinct nuclear change is the appearance of heterochromatin aggregates, which form hemilunar caps or continuous circumferential zones underlying the nuclear membrane (278). Eventually, the nuclear membrane undergoes invagination and breakdown, and the nucleus dissociates into spherical fragments known as pyknotic nuclei. In contrast, the nucleus in necrotic cells usually exhibits only marginal clumping of loosely textured nuclear chromatin, which manifests as heterogenous nuclear staining.

In 1980, Wyllie (276) found that apoptosis is accompanied by fragmentation of the nuclear DNA between

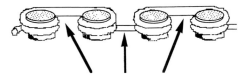

Super structure of chromatin : DNA string wrapped around nucleosomes

Endonucleases

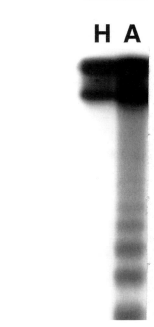

FIG. 20.2. Internucleosomal DNA fragmentation is a hallmark of apoptosis. Diagrams illustrate the superstructure of chromatin and sites cleaved during apoptosis *(upper)*. In the *lower panel*, an autoradiodiogram shows the "ladder-like" oligonucleosomal genomic DNA from ovarian cells undergoing apoptosis *(A)*. Generation of "ladder-like" DNA fragments in apoptotic cells is the result of activation of endonucleases which cleave DNA at internucleosomal sites. In contrast, DNA from healthy cells shows no sign of fragmentation *(H)*. Fragments of DNA are extracted from cells and labeled at 3' ends with ddATP using terminal transferase, followed by fractionation in agarose gels and autoradiographic analysis.

the nucleosomes, which appears as a "DNA ladder" following electrophoretic fractionation (Fig. 20.2). Since then the characteristic DNA ladder formation has been regarded as a biochemical hallmark of apoptosis. Apoptotic DNA fragmentation is presumably due to the activation of an endonuclease that degrades the genomic DNA into oligonucleosomal fragments containing DNA with size multiples of 185–200 base pairs. This endonuclease is calcium/magnesium-dependent and can be inhibited by $ZnCl_2$ (10, 86, 196). Although DNAse I and DNAse II have been implicated as the endonucleases responsible for internucleosomal DNA cleavage in apoptotic cells, the mechanism for activation of these enzymes during apoptosis remains unclear (279).

Generally, chromatin condensation found in the nucleus of apoptotic cells is accompanied by internucleosomal DNA fragmentation; however, these two events appear to be triggered through separate pathways (183, 240). While both processes can be induced by Ca^{2+}/Mg^{2+} in isolated nuclei, treatment with the endonuclease inhibitor $ZnCl_2$ blocks DNA fragmentation but not chromatin condensation (183). Furthermore, field inversion gel electrophoretic analysis of DNA fragments has revealed the cleavage of DNA into 300 and/or 50 kb fragments preceeding internucleosomal DNA fragmentation (142, 184). These long fragments might be formed following activation of topoisomerase II, which is important in the attachment of looped domains of DNA to the nuclear matrix via matrix attachment regions, an event important for chromatin condensation (11, 81, 184, 265). Unlike apoptotic cells, the nucleus of necrotic cells does not separate into discrete fragments and the DNA degradation is random, appearing as a diffuse smear following electrophoretic fractionation.

Cytoplasmic Shrinkage and Plasma Membrane Blebbing

In the cytoplasm of apoptotic cells, the endoplasmic reticulum dilates and forms a series of expanded vesicles, while various cytoplasmic organelles become aggregated, remaining structurally intact but disordered in their orientation. At the same time, shrinkage and blebbing of the plasma membrane takes place. Eventually, the cell divides into clusters of membrane-bound apoptotic bodies that are recognized by phagocytes.

Although the mechanism underlying cytoplasmic changes in apoptotic cells is not clear, the membrane budding and subsequent formation of apoptotic bodies can be inhibited by agents (such as cytochalasin B) that interfere with actin polymerization. Thus, cytoskeletal elements may be important for blebbing of the plasma membrane and apoptotic body formation.

Specific biochemical changes within the plasma membrane of apoptotic cells have been demonstrated. Tissue transglutaminase, an enzyme that catalyzes the formation of ϵ(r-glutamyl)lysine cross-linking between protein substrates, accumulates and becomes activated in apoptotic cells, resulting in decreased membrane permeability (79, 80). This process may maintain the plasma membrane integrity of dying cells and limit the leakage of cellular constituents before phagocytosis.

In healthy cells, low levels of phosphatidylserine are found on the external leaflet of the plasma membrane, and maintenance of this asymmetry is an energy-dependent process mediated by an aminophospholipid translocase situated within the plasma membrane (54). In contrast, the membrane phospholipid asymmetry is lost in apoptotic cells, resulting in exposure of phosphatidylserine on the outer leaflet of cellular membranes (69, 70, 166). As a consequence of apoptosis, cells undergo specific changes in surface carbohydrates, leading to loss of negative surface charges (57, 169, 219). Furthermore, there are increases of oxidatively modified proteins in the plasma membrane of dying cells.

Nuclear and Cytoplasmic Alterations

Because chromatin condensation and internucleosomal DNA fragmentation occur early in apoptotic cells, it was envisioned originally that nuclear changes may be pivotal in the initiation of apoptosis. However, cells without a nucleus show cytoplasmic shrinkage and apoptotic body formation during apoptosis. Studies using anucleated cytoplasts have demonstrated that morphological and biochemical changes found in the cytoplasm of apoptotic cells can be elicited in the absence of a nucleus, suggesting that cytoplasmic changes in apoptotic cells are independent of nuclear events (120, 143, 222). Likewise, nuclear changes in apoptotic cells, such as internucleosomal DNA cleavage, chromatin condensation, and pyknotic body formation, can be induced in isolated nuclei. The concept that nuclear and cytoplasmic alterations in apoptotic cells are independent events is reinforced by the finding that $ZnCl_2$ treatment blocks nuclear changes without affecting cytoplasmic condensation. Diverse apoptotic events in both isolated nuclei and anucleated cytoplasts can be prevented by an antiapoptosis protein, Bcl-2 (120, 179), suggesting that the morphological and biochemical alterations found in the cytoplasm or nucleus of apoptotic cells are parallel.

Phagocytosis

A key feature of apoptosis is the removal of dying cells by phagocytosis. Ordered phagocytosis is important for cell death in healthy organisms as it avoids the potential hazard of provoking detrimental inflammatory responses. Generally, macrophages are responsible for the engulfment of apoptotic bodies, but in some tissues, viable neighboring cells can participate (71). It has been postulated that biochemical changes at the plasma membrane of apoptotic cells provide signals to trigger phagocytosis, and at least three partially characterized mechanisms may be involved in the recognition of apoptotic cells by phagocytes. These mechanisms include *(1)* increases in phosphatidylserine in the outer leaf of cellular membranes, *(2)* loss of terminal sialic acid residues from glycoproteins in the plasma membrane (169), and *(3)* increases of oxidatively modified low-density lipoprotein in dying cells.

Recognition of these cell membrane changes appears to be mediated directly by receptors on phagocytes capable of binding specific moieties on the dying cell. For the recognition of phosphatidylserine and oxidatively modified low-density lipoprotein, a group of phagocyte receptors, jointly designated as "scavenger receptors," have been implicated; these receptors interact with a wide variety of negatively charged ligands, such as polyribonucleotides, polysaccharides, and anionic phospholipids (63, 68, 70, 84, 113, 138, 192, 213, 214, 219). For recognition of asialoglycoprotein and other amino sugar moieties on dying cells, receptors for glycosylation end products (57, 169), lectin, and vitronectin may be important (218, 219). In addition, the removal of damaged cells could be mediated partly by antibodies that recognize specific cell membrane domains in damaged cells. Presumably, following the binding of antibodies to the dying cell, the antibody–cell complex is recognized by the Fc receptor on phagocytes, leading to phagocytosis (1, 128).

CELLULAR MECHANISMS OF APOPTOSIS CONSERVED DURING EVOLUTION: NEMATODE AS A GENETIC MODEL

Studies on apoptosis have extended to almost every discipline of biology, and a variety of animal models have been used to elucidate molecular mechanisms. Among them, analysis of programmed cell death during *Caenorhabditis elegans* embryogenesis has contributed significantly to the understanding of genetic and molecular mechanisms underlying apoptosis. Programmed cell death in the nematode *C. elegans* shares morphological features with apoptosis commonly observed in both vertebrates and invertebrates. Normally, of the 1090 somatic cells formed during development of the nematode, 131 of them undergo programmed cell death shortly after birth, and the death of these cells is under stringent genetic control (59, 62).

Mutational analyses have shown that at least ten genes are essential for the regulation of programmed cell death in *C. elegans* (59) (Fig. 20.3). Among them, two genes, *ced-3* and *ced-4*, are necessary for apoptosis. Mutation of these genes prevents the cell death that normally occurs during embryogenesis, leading to the development of worms with excessive cells (62). The *ced-3* gene encodes a cysteine protease homologous to proteins of the caspase family in mammals (290) (Table 20.2). Because overexpression of cysteine proteases of the caspase gene family induces apoptosis in a variety of vertebrate cells, *ced-3* in the nematode also may promote apoptosis through proteolytic reactions. The nematode *ced-4* gene encodes a hydrophilic polypeptide containing two regions showing similarity to a Ca^{2+}-binding motif (289). Recently, a homologous protein Apaf-1 from mammals has been reported (291).

Another nematode gene, *ced-9*, encodes a protein that inhibits the cell death program (Table 20.3). Mutations that abnormally activate *ced-9* can prevent cell death during normal *C. elegans* development (104,

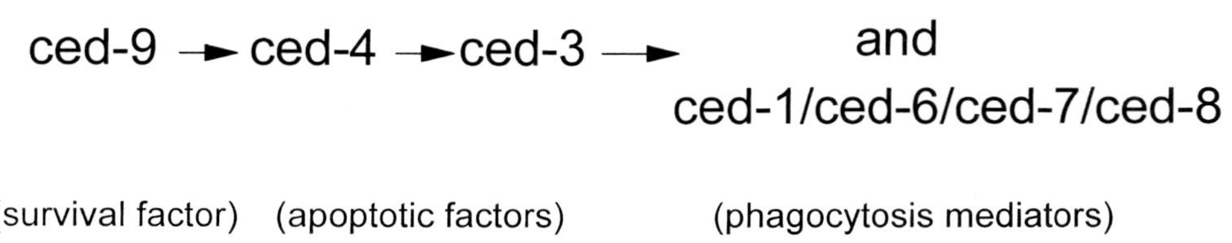

FIG. 20.3. Cellular regulators of apoptosis during *Caenorhabditis* elegans embryogenesis. Based on genetic analyses, genes designated as *ced-1* to *ced-10* have been shown to function at different points of the apoptotic pathway. These genes are indispensable for the normal procession of apoptosis during early development, and they can be categorized into three different groups: survival factors, apoptotic factors, and phagocytosis mediators.

TABLE 20.2. *The ced-3/Caspase Family*

	Characteristics	Method of Identification	Reference
Apoptosis-inducing proteins			
ced-3	*C. elegans* cell death gene	Mutation analysis	290
ICE (α, β, γ)	Interleukin-1β-converting enzyme (caspase-1)	Active site homologous to ced-3	3, 255
ICE$_{rel}$II	ICE/ced-3-related protease II (caspase-4)	Homologous cDNA screening	171
ICE$_{rel}$III	ICE/ced-3-related protease III (caspase-5)	Homologous cDNA screening	171
Ich-1$_L$/Nedd2	ICE and ced-3 homolog (caspase-2)	Homologous PCR* amplification; subtraction screening	140, 266
Ich-2/TX	ICE and ced-3 homolog (caspase-4)	Homologous PCR amplification	73, 123
Apopain/CPP32/YAMA	ced-3/ICE-related cysteine protease (caspase-3)	Substrate-specific enzyme purification; homologous cDNA screening; subtraction cloning	77, 180
Mch2	Mammalian ced-3 homolog (caspase-6)	Homologous PCR amplification	78
FLICE	Mammalian ced-3 homolog (caspase-6)	Protein–protein interaction assay	171a
Antiapoptosis proteins			
ICE (λ, σ)	Interleukin-1β-converting enzyme (caspase-1) splicing variants	Homologous cDNA screening	3
Ich-1$_S$	ICE and ced-3 homolog (caspase-2) splicing variant	Homologous PCR amplification	266

* PCR, polymerase chain reaction.

105). Conversely, if this gene is inactivated, most of the cells that would normally live now die and the animal dies early in development. Moreover, *ced-9* can function properly only if both *ced-3* and *ced-4* are functionally intact, suggesting that *ced-9* prevents cell death by suppressing the *ced-3/ced-4*–dependent death program in normal cells (103). The mammalian *bcl-2* gene is homologous to the *ced-9* gene, and its overexpression blocks apoptosis in nematode, insect, and mammalian cells (4, 104, 260). These findings suggest that a number of evolutionarily conserved genes could regulate a common cell death pathway in different organisms. Recent studies further demonstrated that the ced-9 protein binds directly to ced-4 (229a). In addition, over-expression of ced-4 in mammalian cells allowed co-precipitation of Bcl-XL and caspases (ICE and FLICE) (30a, 275a). It is becoming clear that ced-9, ced-4, and ced-3 or their mammalian homolog may form a large complex important in the regulation of apoptosis in diverse organisms (Fig. 20.3). Usually, the corpses of dead cells in developing embryos of the nematode are engulfed quickly and de-graded by neighboring cells. A third group of genes, which includes *ced-1, -2, -5, -6, -7, -8,* and *-10,* is important for efficient removal of dying cell corpses in developing worms (62, 100). Cells with mutation in these genes undergo apoptosis, exhibiting typical morphological changes, but the cell corpses are not removed efficiently. Although the identity of these genes has not been reported, they might encode specific molecules on the surface of dying cells or specific receptors on the surface of neighboring cells capable of engulfing the dying ones. These genes can be divided into two groups, and double mutant combinations of members of these two different sets *(ced-2, -5, -10* and *ced-1, -6, -7, -8)* exhibit greater accumulation of corpses, suggesting that there are at least two parallel, partially redundant pathways mediating phagocytosis in the nematode (59, 62). The existence of multiple mechanisms for apoptotic cell recognition in the nematode is similar to the system found in mammalian cells, in which multiple receptors have been implicated in the recognition of diverse plasma membrane changes of apoptotic cells.

TABLE 20.3. *The ced-9/Bcl-2 Protein Family*

	Characteristics	Method of Identification	Reference
Antiapoptosis proteins			
ced-9	*C. elegans* anti-cell death gene	Mutation analysis	104
Bcl-2	B-cell leukemia/lymphoma gene 2; overexpressed as the result of chromosomal translocation	Genetic screening	37
Bcl-x$_L$	bcl-2-related gene	Homologous cDNA screening	90
Mcl-1	Myeloid cell leukemia early-induction gene	Differential screening	136
A1	Granulocyte-macrophage colony-stimulating factor–inducible gene	Differential screening	151
BHRF-1	Epstein-Barr virus early lytic cycle protein	Viral genome analysis	101
LWHF-5 *	African swine fever virus gene	Viral genome analysis	178
NR-13 *	Rous sarcoma virus–inducible gene	Subtraction screening	87
Apoptosis-inducing proteins			
Bax	Bcl-2-associated X protein	Co-precipitation with Bcl-2	189
Bcl-X$_S$	bcl-2-related gene splicing variant	Homologous cDNA screening	90
Bad	bcl-XL/bcl-2-associated death promoter protein	Yeast two-hybrid protein–protein interaction assay; lambda expression cloning	285
Bak	bcl-2 homologous antagonist/killer	Yeast two-hybrid protein–protein interaction assay; homologous PCR† amplification	32, 72, 132
Bok	bcl-2-related ovarian killer	Yeast two-hybrid assay	114b

*Effects on apoptosis regulation have not been studied.   †PCR, polymerase chain reaction.

GENES REGULATING APOPTOSIS

The ced-9/bcl-2 *Gene Family*

Bcl-2 Overexpression Prevents Apoptosis. The *ced-9* gene of the nematode *C. elegans* and its mammalian homolog *bcl-2* protect cells from apoptosis. The *bcl-2* gene was isolated as a protooncogene at the breakpoint of a t(14,18) chromosomal translocation associated with follicular B-cell lymphoma (37). Close to the breakpoints are the immunoglobulin heavy chain locus, which is normally on chromosome 14, and the bcl-2 locus (B-cell leukemia/lymphoma 2), which is normally on chromosome 18 (37). This translocation leads to aberrant regulation of the *bcl-2* gene under the control of the immunoglobulin heavy chain gene promoter/

enhancer and overexpression of Bcl-2 in lymphoid cells. Owing to the survival advantage provided by Bcl-2, lymphoid cells become susceptible to other genetic alterations, leading to tumorigenesis.

The 26 kD membrane-associated Bcl-2 protein is localized to the mitochondria, perinuclear membrane, and smooth endoplasmic reticulum (30, 110, 168) and is topographically restricted to long-lived or proliferating cell zones in both embryonic and postnatal tissues (112). When overexpressed, the Bcl-2 protein suppresses apoptosis induced by a variety of agents both in vitro and in vivo (8, 181, 182) (Table 20.3). In transgenic mice, overexpression of Bcl-2 in the lymphoid system results in increased immunoglobulin-secreting cells, elevated serum immunoglobulins, exaggerated antibody response to immunization, development of spontaneous systemic autoimmune disease, and an increased incidence of malignant B-cell lymphoma in old age (164, 165, 181, 235, 236). In addition, immature thymocytes become resistant to apoptosis mediated by corticosteroids, calcium ionophore, and radiation (223, 227). In transgenic mice overexpressing Bcl-2 in their neurons or liver, Bcl-2 can prevent neonatal motoneurons from death induced by axotomy lesion (60) and lethal hepatic apoptosis induced by anti-Fas antibody (141), respectively. In transgenic mice over-expressing Bcl-2 in ovarian somatic cells, decreases in follicle cell apoptosis and increases in ovulatory potential were found. In aging mice, teratoma develops from the germ cells (114a).

However, the apoptosis-suppressing action of Bcl-2 is not universal, and this protein cannot prevent apoptosis in many circumstances (51, 258). For example, cell death incurred by withdrawal of trophic factors such as interleukin-2 (IL-2), IL-6 (182), or ciliary neurotrophic factor from dependent cells (2) is not altered by Bcl-2 overexpression. In transgenic mice overexpressing Bcl-2 in the lymphoid system, apoptosis induced by superantigens in immature thymocytes also is not suppressed (126, 223, 259). Likewise, mice deficient in Bcl-2 do not show an overt abnormality during development, and only cells in hair follicles, kidney, and lymphoid systems show defects in apoptosis (175, 261). Thus, suppression of apoptosis by Bcl-2 is restricted to selected apoptotic stimuli in certain tissues.

Susceptibility of Lymphoid Cells to Apoptosis and Bcl-2 Expression.

In the immune system of vertebrates, as many as 95% of B- and T-cell precursors die during development (43). The demise of lymphoid cells is a highly regulated process that selects cell populations bearing functional antigen receptors and removes cells that are no longer needed or are potentially autoreactive. Based on studies of Bcl-2–deficient mice, it has been postulated that Bcl-2 plays an important role in the maintenance of a balanced immune system. This view is supported by studies showing that overexpressed Bcl-2 can abolish the normal lymphoid cell selection process in transgenic mice, leading to the accumulation of autoreactive lymphoid cells (235, 236). During lymphoid development, expression of the bcl-2 gene is high at the earliest stages of maturation but decreases during later stages, which are associated with extensive apoptosis. Under in vitro conditions, the susceptibility of developing B cells to apoptosis induction also appears to correlate with levels of endogenous Bcl-2 (154). Thus, the Bcl-2 protein may

serve as a checkpoint to monitor incoming apoptotic signals.

Bcl-2-Related Genes in Vertebrates. Bcl-2 is only the first member to be identified of a growing family of homologous proteins (87, 269) (Table 20.3). All genes in this family have three to four conserved domains important for homodimerization or heterodimerization with other members of the family (19, 189, 217, 287). In addition, a C-terminal transmembrane domain is conserved. Of interest is the fact that not all members of the *bcl-2* gene family prevent apoptosis. They can be separated into three subgroups based on functional analysis. The first subgroup, including *Bcl-2, Mcl-1* (136, 207), *Bcl-w* (86a), *A1*, and *Bfl-1* (151), has anti-apoptosis properties. In contrast, the second subgroup, comprised of *Bax* (189), *Bad* (285), *Bid* (266a), *Bak* (32, 72, 132), *Bok* (114b), *Bik* (23a, 94a), and *Hrk* (115a), antagonizes the apoptosis-suppressing effect of Bcl-2. The third subgroup, including *Bcl-x*, encodes splicing variants with either anti-apoptosis or pro-apoptosis properties. While the long form of *Bcl-x*, $Bcl\text{-}x_L$, prevents apoptosis in transfected cells, the short form, $Bcl\text{-}x_S$, promotes cell death (90).

In addition to evolving into a family of homologous proteins with distinct functions, some of the *Bcl-2–* related genes encode different isoforms that vary in subcellular localization and levels of expression. For example, both *bcl-2* and *Bax* genes encode a dominant form containing a transmembrane domain and a short splicing variant lacking the transmembrane domain. The *bcl-2* variant, without the transmembrane domain, appears to have decreased antiapoptosis activity and a different subcellular localization (245).

Bcl-2 and Its Antagonistic Homologs Form Homo- and Heterodimers.

The mechanism by which Bcl-2 prevents apoptosis is not clear. Studies on the intracellular localization of several Bcl-2 homologs, including Bcl-2, Bax, Bcl-x, and Mcl-1, indicated that these proteins reside in the outer mitochondrial membrane suggesting that they act through similar pathways (286). It appears that both homo- and heterodimerization of these proteins, mediated by BH1 and BH2 domains, are important for the regulation of their biological activities (Fig. 20.4) (22, 135, 188, 189, 217, 287). Amino-acid substitutions in the binding domains of Bcl-2, which do not alter the ability of Bcl-2 to homodimerize with itself but impair its ability to heterodimerize with Bax, block the ability of Bcl-2 to suppress apoptosis (96). Thus, Bax, which counters Bcl-2 and promotes apoptosis, may act by heterodimerizing with Bcl-2. However, the complexity of homo- and heterodimeri-

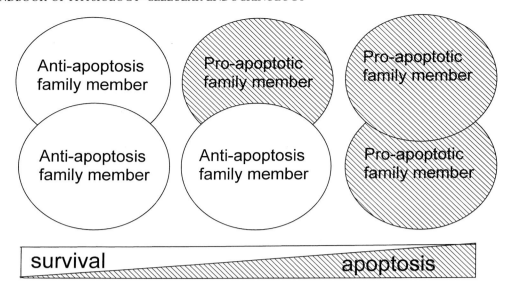

FIG. 20.4. hypothetical model for the regulation of functions of Bcl-2–related proteins. The antiapoptosis function of Bcl-2 could be mediated through interactions with other homologous proteins in the same family. A balance of the multiple pro-apoptotic and anti-apoptotic Bcl-2-proteins may determine a cell's susceptibility to apoptosis.

zations of this large family of proteins renders elucidation of their exact roles in apoptosis difficult.

In addition to interacting with proteins of the same family, *Bcl-2* interacts with a novel antiapoptosis protein, BAG-1 (Bcl-2–associated athanogene 1) (242). This protein shares no significant homology with the Bcl-2 family of proteins and prolongs cell survival in response to apoptotic stimuli in transfected cells. Because co-expression of Bcl-2 and BAG-1 provides synergistic protection from cell death, some of the anti-apoptosis effects of Bcl-2 may be attributed to the Bcl-2–BAG-1 complex.

Bcl-2 Genes Function in a Tissue-Specific Manner. Because multiple Bcl-2–related genes exist in vertebrates, they may represent a redundant system. The expression patterns of Bcl-2 homologs in different tissues appear to overlap and vary greatly; some are widely distributed, while others are restricted. For example, the Mcl-1 protein is expressed mainly in epithelial cells in the prostate, breast, endometrium, epidermis, stomach, intestine, colon, and respiratory tract, whereas expression of Bcl-x is restricted to bone marrow and thymus (19, 136). In contrast, Bax and Bak are found in most tissues (32, 72, 132, 137). Thus, the composition of different Bcl-2 homologs in any given cell type is likely to differ.

The notion that different Bcl-2 homologs regulate apoptosis in a tissue-specific manner is supported by studies on mice deficient in different members of the *bcl-2* gene family (Table 20.4). In *bcl-2*-deficient mice, most tissues develop normally, with only cells in hair follicles, kidney, and the lymphoid system showing apparent defects in apoptosis. During early life, lymphoid development in these mice appears normal but defects in lymphoid cell selection were observed at 1–2 weeks after birth. Thus, the role of Bcl-2 may be developmentally dependent. In contrast, targeted disruption of Bcl-x in mutant mice leads to lethality around embryonic day 13 (170). Histological studies have revealed excessive cell deaths in developing neurons and lymphoid cells of mutant embryos, suggesting that Bcl-x supports the viability of cells in the nervous and hematopoietic systems during fetal life. Likewise, mice deficient in Bax appear healthy, and only cells of lymphoid and gonadal lineages show aberrations in cell death. In these mice, hyperplasia in T and B cells results in enlarged thymus and spleen, whereas the accumulation of premeiotic germ cells in seminiferous tubules leads to male infertility (133).

Thus, multiple Bcl-2 homologs in vertebrates function in a tissue-specific manner. The evolution of such redundant systems for regulating apoptosis in different tissues may have survival advantages in higher organisms.

Viruses Prevent Apoptosis. Viral infection can trigger host cell apoptosis to limit viral propagation, and some

TABLE 20.4. *Phenotypes of Mice Deficient in Different Genes Regulating Apoptosis*

Genes	Major Affected Organs	Major Abnormalities	Reference
bcl-2	Kidney, hair follicle, and lymphoid system	Polycystic kidney, hypopigmented hair fulminant lymphoid apoptosis	175, 261
bcl-X	Neuron and lymphoid systems	Embryonic lethality	170
BAX	Lymphoid and gonadal systems	Enlarged thymus and spleen, male infertility	133
ICE	Lymphoid system	Defects in Fas antigen–mediated apoptosis in lymphocytes	139, 148
Granzyme B	Lymphoid system	Defects in cytotoxic T lymphocyte–mediated apoptosis	108
Fas antigen	Lymphoid system	Lymphoadenopathy and systemic autoimmune disease	173
Fas ligand	Lymphoid system	Lymphoadenopathy and systemic autoimmune disease	173

viruses have developed mechanisms to prevent host cell demise. The *bcl-2*-dependent pathway in host cells is one of the targets affected by viral genes. The Epstein Barr virus *BHRF-1* gene (101) and the African swine fever virus *LMW5-HL* gene (178) encode proteins homologous to the mammalian Bcl-2 (Table 20.3), and the BHRF-1-encoded protein prevents apoptosis when overexpressed (101). Furthermore, the adenovirus E1B 19K protein, which inhibits apoptosis induced by the adenovirus gene *E1A* and shares limited homology with Bcl-2 (268), is functionally interchangeable with Bcl-2 in dimerization with Bcl-2 homologs. Some viruses inhibit host cell apoptosis through the induction of apoptosis suppressors encoded by the host genome. For example, the Epstein Barr virus *LMP-1* and *EBNA-2* genes increase endogenous Bcl-2 expression in the host cell during latent stages of infection (82, 102). Similarly, the Rous sarcoma virus gene *p60^{v-src}* increases the expression of a Bcl-2 homolog, NR-13, in cells transfected with *p60^{v-src}* (87). Thus, the prevention of host cell demise by interfering with the Bcl-2–dependent pathway is a recurring scene during viral evolution.

The ced-3/caspase *Gene Family*

Cysteine Proteases. In both nematode and mammalian cells, proteins of the ced-3/caspase family are important for apoptosis (167, 290). ICE, the first of the caspase genes identified, was originally characterized as an IL-1β precursor processing enzyme which cleaves the inactive intracellular IL-1β precursor to generate the bioactive IL-1β from monocytic cells (255, 273). Mammalian ICE was found to have limited homology with the nematode *ced-3* gene and to enhance apoptosis following overexpression in cells transfected with this gene (167). Although introduction of practically any protease into cells in a deregulated manner is likely to damage and kill them (272), the *ced-3/caspase* family genes play a specific role in regulating apoptosis because apoptosis induced by a variety of agents can be blocked by viral inhibitors of the ced-3/caspase proteases or by specific synthetic substrates for these proteases (85, 155, 266, 284). Furthermore, levels of ICE transcript and other caspase activities increase during apoptosis in different cell types (23, 155).

Based on homologous gene amplification by polymerase chain reaction (PCR) or substrate-specific enzyme purification, several mammalian homologs of the ced-3/caspase family have been isolated (3, 73, 77, 78, 123, 140, 171, 180) (Table 20.3). This growing family of proteases encodes unique cytoplasmic cysteine proteases which require an Asp residue at the P1 site for cleavage (180, 266). In addition, the pentameric peptide QACRG surrounding the putative active site cysteine is conserved in all members of the family. These cysteine (C) proteases preferentially cleave aspartic acid (asp); they have been designated as members of the "Caspase" family of proteins (1a).

Proteolytic Activation. The mature proteins of these proteases are composed of two subunits derived from a precursor polypeptide following proteolytic modification at Asp sites. Activation of caspase family members involves heterocatalysis by Asp-specific proteases. For example, caspase-4 can process both pro-caspase-4 and pro-ICE (73) while ICE (caspase-1) is able to activate pro-caspase-3 (180, 273). In the mature ICE protein, the active site cysteine is located in the P20 subunit but both subunits are required for activity. Furthermore, studies on the crystal structure of recombinant ICE protein indicate that mature ICE proteins associate to form an active tetramer complex composed of two P20 and two P10 subunits (255).

Several *ced-3/caspase* family genes undergo complex post-transcriptional modifications to generate isoforms encoding proteins with distinct functions. Each of the caspase-2, -3, -6 genes encodes at least two major transcipts generated through alternative splicing. While the long form of caspase-2 induces apoptosis, the short form encodes a truncated protein and suppresses cell death. It is possible that the short form competes for the same substrate with the long form or oligomerizes with divergent full-length homologs to form inactive tetramers (255, 266). The human *ICE* gene encodes at least five different isoforms, designated as α, β, γ, δ, and ϵ, with distinct functions (153). When overexpressed, α, β, and γ, but not δ and ϵ, can induce apoptosis (78). In *ICE* δ, the cleavage site between the two subunits is missing, while most of the propeptide

and the P20 subunit are deleted in *ICE* ϵ. These two isoforms do not have proteolytic activities; however, *ICE* ϵ, which is homologous to the P10 subunit, retains its ability to bind the P20 subunit. Overexpression of *ICE* ϵ results in the suppression of apoptosis, probably by competing with the P10 subunit to form an inactive ICE complex (3). Thus, like genes of the *ced-9/caspase* family, genes of the *ced-3/ICE* family could encode splicing variants with divergent functions.

Proteolysis Triggers Apoptosis. The ced-3/caspases presumably mediate cell death by proteolytic cleavage of specific substrates (Fig. 20.5). Degradation of several cytoskeletal and nuclear proteins is associated with the onset of apoptosis in different cells, and proteolytic degradation of these proteins could lead to the characteristic morphological alterations found in the nucleus and cytoplasm of apoptotic cells (44, 85, 127, 216, 230). The cellular components that are degraded specifically during apoptosis include poly(ADP-ribose)

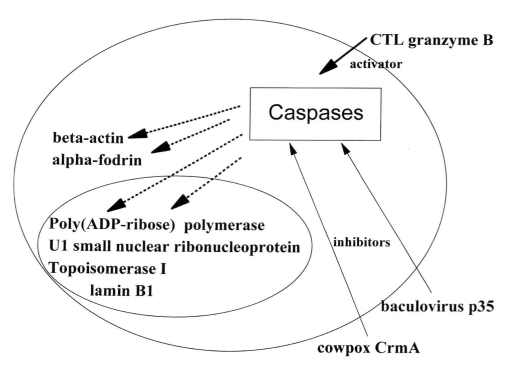

FIG. 20.5. Mechanism of action of ced-3/caspases in apoptosis. The ced-3/caspases promote apoptosis through degradation of specific cytoplasmic and nuclear components important for the maintenance of cellular homeostasis, and the multiple caspases present in different tissues may promote apoptosis in a collaborative or redundant manner. In a healthy cell, these enzymes are kept inactive by undefined mechanims, and the regulation of activities of these proteases may represent an important checkpoint for cellular control of apoptosis. These proteases may be kept inactive due to the lack of posttranscriptional modifications, and they become death promotors only after being activated. Alternatively, the function of these proteases may be blocked by endogenous inhibitors, for example, FLIP (116a), and proteins functionally similar to specific viral inhibitors for ICE-like proteases (for example, baculovirus p35 and cowpox virus CrmA). They become active when the inhibitor is removed.

polymerase (PARP) (127), the 70 kD protein component of the U1 small nuclear ribonucleoprotein (U1 SNRP) (28, 251), lamin B1 (145, 177, 263), topoisomerase I (263), β-actin (161), and α-fodrin (162). Because these proteins are essential for the integrity of the nuclear matrix, chromosome structure, cytoskeleton, and plasma membrane, their degradation would be detrimental to normal cellular functions, leading to apoptosis (161).

A chromatin-associated enzyme which catalyzes the poly(ADP-ribosyl)ation of nuclear proteins, PARP may be important in DNA repair and chromosome stability (5). Another nuclear protein, lamin B1, binds to matrix attachment regions and mediates the interaction of chromatin with the nuclear matrix (159). Degradation of these proteins may be important for nuclear condensation and dissolution of the nuclear membrane during apoptosis (177). However, U1 SNRP and the topoisomerases are important for the maintenance of a normal transcription process and chromosome structure, respectively, and their degradation may block cellular metabolism. In the cytoplasm, β-actin and α-fodrin are major components of the cytoskeleton of most eukaryotic cells; proteolysis of these proteins may contribute to the rearrangement of cellular membranes in apoptotic cells, leading to plasma membrane blebbing.

Among these cellular components degraded during apoptosis, PARP has specific substrate sites for caspases (93, 144, 180), and degradation of PARP and U1 SNRP during apoptosis can be inhibited by specific inhibitors for ced-3/caspases (180, 251). This suggests that caspases may act at the very proximal points of the apoptotic process and participate in the degradation of an array of proteins integral to the maintenance of cellular structures and functions (161). Alternatively, caspases may function as a group of specific "activators" to catalyze proteolysis of other apoptosis mediators. In this mode of action, they promote apoptosis by activating proenzymes. This hypothesis is supported by studies showing that the apoptosis-inducing activity of apopain caspase 3 on isolated nuclei requires other mediators in the apoptotic cascade (180).

Caspase Regulation and Apoptosis. Studies on ICE-deficient mice have shown that apoptosis proceeds normally during development and that only apoptosis triggered by Fas antigen activation in thymocytes is suppressed (Table 20.4). Thus, ICE is important for cell death only under specific conditions and does not have an obligatory role in apoptosis onset in most cells (139, 148). Furthermore, ICE, unlike caspase-2, -3, and -6, does not have the ability to degrade PARP (93, 180), suggesting that other caspases play a more

significant role in the induction of apoptosis or in the degradation of PARP and U1 SNRP during apoptosis (180).

Studies on the tissue distribution of the caspase family of proteins have shown that their expression is widespread but tissue-specific. However, because more than one homolog can be found in some cell types and these proteases vary in their substrate specificity, multiple caspases may function as redundant systems or contribute to apoptosis in a collaborative manner.

Another intriguing question regarding the role of ced-3/caspases in apoptosis is how the activities of these proteases are regulated in vivo. Apoptosis mediated through the activation of ced-3/caspases does not require the synthesis of macromolecules, and the ced-3/caspases can be expressed constitutively in many cell types. Therefore, the apoptosis-promoting effect of ced-3/caspases in these cells is likely to be regulated at posttranslational levels. These proteases may be maintained in an inactive state by an endogenous inhibitor(s). Recently, a specific endogenous inhibitor for FLICE (caspase-8) has been reported and named as FLIP (FLICE inhibitor protein, 116a).

Viral ced-3/Caspase Inhibitors. Specific inhibitors for caspases have been identified in the genome of different viruses. Viral mutants lacking such inhibitors are defective in their propagation, suggesting that these viruses have targeted the caspase pathway as a mechanism to suppress apoptosis and promote viral replication in infected cells (26, 38–41, 107, 193, 201, 204, 284). A cytokine response modifier found in cowpox virus, CrmA, is required to block cytotoxic T lymphocyte (CTL)–mediated killing of infected cells and to inhibit the development of an inflammatory response to virally infected cells (193, 204). The CrmA protein is a member of the serpin family of protease inhibitors and inhibits ICE by forming an active site–directed complex (Fig. 20.5) (134, 204). Such an inhibition dampens the apoptotic response of host cells and blocks production of the proinflammatory cytokine IL-1β to allow the replication of viruses (134, 204, 253).

Another viral inhibitor gene *P35*, derived from the baculovirus *Autographa californica*, encodes a protein that blocks apoptosis in nematode, insect, and mammalian cells (98, 238). It acts as an irreversible inhibitor of ced-3/caspases and is cleaved into two separate fragments after binding to these proteases (26, 284). Following cleavage, the large fragment of p35 protein remains associated with the protease and presumably inactivates it irreversibly. Thus, the ced-3/caspases not only serve as an important checkpoint for the regulation of apoptosis but also play an important role in the defense against viral infection.

Granzyme B. Studies on apoptosis induced by granzyme B from CTLs have provided a unique model to understand the potential mechanism regulating caspases during apoptosis. One major function of the lymphoid system is to defend against tumors, parasites, and virus-infected cells, and part of this function is carried out by CTL attack. The killing of target cells by CTL is mediated by apoptosis and is caused partly by the apoptotic "effectors" released from CTL granules by exocytosis. The CTL-mediated apoptosis of target cells proceeds rather fast and does not require the synthesis of macromolecules (106). During CTL attack, the secretion of perforin, a membrane pore-forming protein residing in the CTL granules, by CTL allows the insertion of a group of granular serine proteases known as granzymes into target cells (Fig. 20.5) (122, 153, 158, 225).

Studies on CTL granzymes have shown that two (granzymes A and B) are important for the induction of apoptosis in target cells (108, 228). Granzyme B, which is not related structurally to caspases, shares the rare Asp-X substrate specificity of the *ced-3/caspase* gene family and can be inhibited by CrmA, an inhibitor of caspases (199). In contrast, granzyme A has ICE activity (116). Furthermore, granzyme B has the ability to activate the caspase-3 precursor in vivo, while granzyme B–induced apoptosis can be inhibited by specific inhibitors for apopain, suggesting that CTL could trigger apoptosis by directly activating the ced-3/caspase pathway with granzyme B (52).

Death Domain–Containing Proteins

Death Domain. The death domain is a protein–protein interaction motif found in diverse genes associated with apoptotic signaling. This conserved region was characterized in the intracellular domain of two transmembrane receptors, Fas antigen and tumor necrosis factor receptor 1 (TNF-R1), and was named the "death domain" because it is essential for the transduction of apoptotic signals (172, 185, 249). Another gene, *reaper,* important for the regulation of apoptosis during *Drosophila* embryogenesis, also contains this domain, suggesting that functions of these genes have an ancient root (Table 20.5) (42, 74, 89). Unlike genes of the ced-9/Bcl-2 and ced-3/caspase families, genes with the death domain vary widely in their structures and belong to different protein families. Some are membrane-bound receptors (Fas antigen and TNF-R1), while others are cytoplasmic effectors (reaper, TRADD, FADD/MORT1, RIP, and DAP kinase; Table 20.5).

Reaper and *hid* are two adjacent genes, located in the third chromosome of *Drosophila,* that function as death initiators in many cells during embryogenesis

(270). Fly mutants with deletion in this region die late in embryogenesis with many extra cells in the nervous system due to the lack of programmed cell death (92, 270). Because some cells in these death-defective mutant embryos still undergo apoptosis after being treated with high doses of X rays, it is likely that the effector machinery of apoptosis is intact and that the *reaper* gene encodes a death initiator.

Several intracellular proteins of mammalian origin also contain the death domain (21, 31, 114, 232). The TRADD (TNF-R1-associated death domain protein), FADD/MORT1 (Fas-associated death domain protein/mediator of receptor-induced toxicity), and RIP (receptor-interacting protein) genes have been isolated based on their ability to bind the death domain in the Fas antigen or TNF-R1 in a yeast two-hybrid protein interaction assay. Binding of the death domain from Fas antigen or TNF-R1 to these molecules is mediated by interactions through similar death domains within these binding proteins. While FADD/MORT1 and RIP preferentially bind to the Fas antigen and, to a lesser extent, TNF-R1, TRADD interacts only with TNF-R1. All of these proteins also cause apoptosis when overexpressed in transfected cells, indicating that they

TABLE 20.5. *Functional Characteristics of Death Domain–Containing Genes*

Death Domain Proteins *	Characteristics	Interaction with Death Domain of Fas Antigen/ TNF-R1	Reference
Reaper	Intracellular effector, identified in *Drosophila*	?/?	270
Fas antigen	Membrane receptor, mediates antibody-induced lymphocyte apoptosis	+/?	20, 185
TNF receptor-1	Membrane receptor for TNF	?/+	20, 249
TRADD	Intracellular effector, induces apoptosis in transfected cells	−/+	114
FADD/MORT1	Intracellular effector, induces apoptosis in transfected cells	+/+	21, 31
RIP	Intracellular effector, induces apoptosis in transfected cells	+/+	232
DAP kinase	Intracellular effector essential for interferon-γ-induced cell death	?/?	53

* TNF, tumor necrosis factor; TRADD, TNF receptor-1–associated death domain; FADD/MORT1, Fas-associated death domain/mediator of receptor-induced toxicity; RIP, receptor-interacting protein; DAP, death-associated protein.

are potential intracellular transducers of apoptotic signals generated by the activation of plasma membrane–associated TNF-R1 or Fas antigen (Fig. 20.6) (21, 31, 114, 232).

Another gene, *DAP* kinase, is a positive mediator of programmed cell death, and its reduced expression confers resistance to cell killing (53). It contains multiple death domain-like sequences and a calmodulin-regulated serine/threonine kinase domain. Expression of this gene is indispensable for interferon-γ-induced cell death (53). Presumably, it signals apoptosis by associating with other death domain–containing proteins.

Inhibitors of Apoptosis Protein. Similar to the ced-3/ caspase inhibitor p35, the inhibitors of apoptosis protein (IAPs) were isolated as death-inhibiting genes from insect viruses (Table 20.6) (18, 40, 41, 50). Homologs to IAP from both *Drosophila* and mammals have been isolated. Overexpression of the *Drosophila* homologs

(DIAPs) suppresses normally occurring cell death as well as death due to overexpression of the death initiator, reaper, suggesting that the IAP function constitutes a checkpoint in the apoptotic pathway mediated by death domain–containing proteins (Fig. 20.6) (99). In addition, as gene inactivation of DIAPs results in cell death in different organs, DIAPs are likely to be required for normal cell survival. Several mammalian homologs of IAP also have been isolated (152, 209), two of which, designated c-IAP1 and c-IAP2 and isolated as TNF receptor 2 (TNF-R2)–associated proteins, interact with the TNF-R2 complex by binding to TNF-R2–associated factors (TRAFs) within the complex. Because TNF-R2 has been implicated in cell proliferation and survival instead of apoptosis (248, 250), TNF-R2–associated c-IAPs may be involved in protecting against apoptosis initiated by other events during receptor-triggered proliferation. In addition, a neuronal apoptosis inhibitory protein (NAIP), which has been implicated in human spinal muscular atrophy disorder

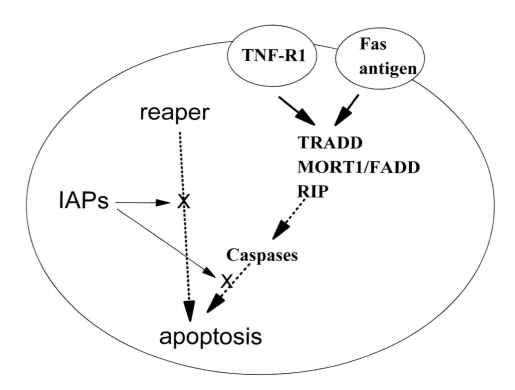

FIG. 20.6. Regulatory cascade mediating the apoptosis-promoting action of death domain–containing proteins. The death domain–containing receptors Fas antigen and tumor necrosis factor receptor 1 *(TNF-R1)* may promote apoptosis by interacting with intracellular death domain–containing effectors including TRADD, MORT1/FADD, and RIP, followed by activation of caspases. Furthermore, studies on *Drosophila* have shown that the action of intracellular death domain–containing effectors, such as reaper, could be suppressed by specific inhibitors of apoptosis proteins *(IAPs)*, suggesting that a balance between death domain–containing proteins and IAPs may serve as another checkpoint for the regulation of apoptosis.

TABLE 20.6. *Functional Characteristics of Inhibitors of Apoptosis Protein (IAP) Genes*

IAPs	Method of Identification	Reference
Orgyia pseudotsugata nuclear polyhedrosis virus IAP (OpIAP)	Genetic mutation screening	41
Cydia pomonella granulosis virus IAP (CpIAP)	Viral genome analysis	41
AcMNPV IAP (AcIAP)	Viral genome analysis	41
Drosophila IAP1, IAP2 (DIAP1, -2)	Genetic screening	99
Human cIAP-1, -2 (hc-IAP1, -2)	Yeast two-hybrid protein–protein interaction assay, homologous cDNA screening	152, 209
Neuronal apoptosis inhibitor protein (NAIP)	Genetic screening	152, 212
Human X-linked IAP (x-IAP)	Homologous cDNA screening	152

(212), and several homologous proteins, including hIAP-1, hIAP-2, xIAP (152), also share high homology with different IAPs and suppress apoptosis in transfected cells. These data indicate that IAP homologs play a pivotal role in apoptosis regulation in vertebrates and that these proteins regulate apoptosis in a tissue-specific manner.

Other Apoptosis Regulatory Genes

The cellular mechanisms leading to apoptosis are complicated. It is clear that a diversity of humoral and cell-bound factors are involved in the regulation of apoptosis in different tissues. In addition to the three major groups of apoptosis regulatory genes discussed above, a large number of intracellular effectors, many of them known to mediate other cellular functions, may be involved in the regulation of apoptosis in specific cells. As the fate of different cell types varies widely, the participation of diverse cellular effectors in apoptosis regulation is not unexpected. In the following section, regulation of apoptosis by some of these genes, which appears to have wide implications for the understanding of apoptosis regulation in diverse cell types, is discussed.

Dad-1 Gene. The *dad-1* gene was isolated from a hamster cell mutant which rapidly rounds up and comes off the culture at a nonpermissive temperature. The mutant cell line carries a mutation in the *dad-1* gene, and the mutated dad-1 protein disappears at the non-

permissive temperature, leading to apoptotic cell death (174). These data suggest that loss of the dad-1 protein triggers apoptosis. The *dad-1* gene encodes an evolutionarily conserved membrane protein expressed in many organs, and its counterparts in invertebrates and plants have been identified (7, 174). The function of these genes appears to be conserved as the mammalian *dad-1* is able to rescue cells from apoptosis in the nematode *C. elegans* (239). Although its mode of action has not been addressed, the importance of this gene in apoptosis regulation may be more than what has been recognized because its distribution is widespread; it is conserved across the plant and animal kingdoms (239).

Tumor-Suppressor Genes and Other Cellular Regulators. Among the tumor-suppressor genes that have been associated with the regulation of apoptosis in specific cells, *p53* may be one of the best characterized. The *p53* gene modulates DNA repair and growth arrest in many cells (109). Although most forms of apoptosis do not seem to be affected significantly in *p53* knock-out mice, radiation-induced apoptosis is suppressed (14, 157), suggesting that its expression is required for apoptosis resulting from radiation-induced DNA damage. In addition, loss of *p53* has been related to the resistance of tumor cells to undergo apoptosis in response to chemotherapeutic agents which affect chromosomal integrity (156). Thus, *p53* could be an essential component of the pathway leading from DNA damage to apoptosis, at least under specific conditions. Likewise, the protooncogene *c-myc* is associated with apoptosis under specific conditions. Usually, *c-myc* promotes cell proliferation; however, when the proliferation signals induced by constitutive expression of *c-myc* are combined with a block to cell proliferation (such as survival factor withdrawal), apoptosis ensues in response to the dysregulation of cell-cycle progression (66, 268). In addition to these better characterized factors, many cell cycle- or proliferation-associated genes have been associated with the progression of apoptosis under specific conditions (46, 65, 66).

EXTRACELLULAR SIGNALING OF APOPTOSIS

Apoptosis Induction Is Cell Type–Specific

To maintain homeostasis of an organism, the apoptotic processes in different tissues are coordinated by a variety of signaling mechanisms, including hormonal factors, cell-bound factors, and extracellular matrices. These signals not only vary among different cell types but also depend on the stage of tissue development.

Control of apoptosis by hormonal factors is exemplified by the regulation of cell turnover in a variety of endocrine tissues (115, 117, 125, 130, 160, 176, 208, 215) (Table 20.7), and the regulatory hormones could either suppress apoptosis or promote cell death. Many "trophic" hormones, previously known to be important for cell proliferation or differentiation, also play a role in the suppression of apoptosis or the maintenance of cell survival. In many tissues, hormonal factors initiate signaling pathways that protect cells from apoptosis, and apoptosis occurs by default when cells fail to receive the "trophic" signals required to suppress the death program.

Signals for apoptosis regulation also can be exerted by interactions between diverse cell-bound molecules on the surface of the plasma membrane. This mode of apoptosis regulation is best characterized by apoptosis mediated by Fas ligand and Fas antigen in lymphoid cells (25, 45, 119, 121).

The proper extracellular matrix environment is also important for the regulation of cell survival as well as apoptosis (24). Although massive apoptosis of the secretory epithelium in the mammary gland during postlactational involution originally was believed to be due to the withdrawal of lactogenic hormones, it is now known that loss of basement membrane extracellular matrices surrounding these cells also initiates apoptosis (23, 75, 76, 191, 234, 264). During mammary gland involution, the expression of matrix-degrading enzymes, including TRPM-2, stromelysin-1, stromelysin-3, and TIMP-1, increases in mammary tissues (56, 146, 149, 243). Treatment with antibodies to β1 integrin or overexpression of the extracellular matrix-degrading enzyme stromelysin-1 in the mammary gland epithelium induces apoptosis. Furthermore, extracellular ma-

trix proteins suppress apoptosis in the mammary gland epithelium by decreasing ICE enzyme expression (23).

The Mammalian Ovary Model

The death of a cell is usually under the control of multiple factors, and a balance of survival and apoptotic signals determines a cell's fate. The multifactorial mode of control is exemplified by the regulation of apoptosis in mammalian ovaries. In the ovary, apoptosis occurs at all stages of development, and more than 99% of ovarian follicles undergo atresia during reproductive life. Specifically, the massive loss of ovarian cells occurs during migration of the primordial germ cells from the yolk sac to the genital ridge, when germ cells enter meiosis, during development of antral follicles, and at luteolysis (49, 115, 197).

Morphological and biochemical studies have demonstrated that the death of both somatic and germ cells in the ovary is mediated by apoptosis and that distinct sets of hormones are involved in the regulation of apoptosis during different stages of ovarian development (15, 115, 194, 197). During fetal life, primordial germ cells undergo degeneration unless rescued by stem cell factor, leukemia-inhibiting factor, basic fibroblast growth factor (bFGF), or other related factors (58, 88, 197).

During postnatal life, follicular apoptosis is regulated by multiple hormones, including pituitary glycoprotein hormones, growth factors, cytokines, a diffusible gas (nitric oxide), and steroids (115). These hormones act through endocrine, paracrine, or autocrine mechanisms. In the vertebrate, pituitary gonadotropins are important trophic factors for the proliferation of follicular somatic cells and the development of preovulatory follicles. Decreases in circulating gonadotropins can lead to massive apoptosis of developing follicles, while treatment of cultured follicles with gonadotropins can prevent spontaneous onset of follicular apoptosis, suggesting that gonadotropins function as follicle survival factors in addition to their trophic actions (33, 34). The spontaneous onset of follicular cell apoptosis can be prevented by treatment with growth hormone or local factors, including insulin-like growth factor 1 (IGF-1), epidermal growth factor (EGF), transforming growth factor α (TGFα), bFGF, IL-1β, and nitric oxide, suggesting that these hormones also play important roles in the regulation of ovarian cell survival (115). In contrast, treatment with a gonadotropin-releasing hormone (GnRH) agonist TNF-α or IL-6 can directly induce apoptosis of ovarian cells (16, 91, 122a), suggesting that IL-6 and GnRH-like peptides act as in-

TABLE 20.7. *Hormonal Regulation of Apoptosis in Endocrine Tissues*

Endocrine Tissues	Survival Factor	Apoptotic Factor	Reference
Adrenal cortex	ACTH*	—	280, 282
Prostate	Androgens	—	117, 125, 130
Mammary gland	Prolactin	—	75, 76, 191, 234, 264
Uterus	Estrogens	Progesterones	160, 176, 208, 215
Testis	Gonadotropins, androgens	—	15, 17
Ovary	Gonadotropins, estrogens	Androgens	115

*ACTH, adrenocorticotropic hormone.

traovarian apoptotic factors. Furthermore, studies in vivo have implicated estrogens as antiapoptosis hormones in ovarian follicles, while androgens are apoptotic (15).

Gonadotropins appear to be the most important survival factors because gonadotropin treatment increases the expression of local survival factors in ovarian follicles. Specifically, the gonadotropins suppress ovarian cell apoptosis by activating the cyclic adenosine monophosphate (cAMP)–dependent pathway and increasing the production of paracrine and autocrine factors such as estrogens, IL-1, nitric oxide, and IGF-1 (Fig. 20.7). These factors in turn promote cell survival through the activation of nuclear estrogen receptor, the cyclic guanosine monophosphate (cGMP)–dependent pathway, and protein tyrosine phosphorylation, respectively (115). As the progression of apoptosis in ovarian follicles depends on the cooperative regulation of different paracrine and autocrine factors, it is likely that a balance of these different survival and apoptotic factors may decide whether a follicle will continue to develop or undergo apoptosis.

How the functions of various extracellular hormones and intracellular signal-transduction mediators are linked to the effectors in the apoptotic machinery remains, however, undefined. Elucidation of these links and identification of specific intracellular effectors re-

sponsible for the actions of different hormones is the challenge facing future studies.

Fas-Ligand/Fas Antigen and Apoptosis

Apoptosis induced by the activation of Fas antigen is one of the best examples of apoptosis regulation through a juxtacrine mechanism. The Fas antigen was discovered through its mediation of apoptosis triggered by monoclonal antibodies against lymphocyte cell surface proteins (257, 288). Isolation of Fas antigen indicates that it is a type I transmembrane receptor belonging to the TNF/nerve growth factor (NGF) receptor superfamily and has high homology to TNF-R1, TNF-R2, low-affinity NGF receptor, and several lymphocyte antigens (172). While most of these molecules are involved in the mediation of cell growth and differentiation, Fas antigen and TNF-R1 contain a unique death domain (Table 20.5) and are associated with apoptosis activation (172, 185, 246, 250).

Activation of Fas antigen requires interaction with the Fas ligand, a type II transmembrane protein of the TNF family (237). The Fas antigen is expressed mainly in the thymus, liver, heart, lung, and ovary (267), while the Fas ligand is expressed predominantly in activated T cells and nonlymphoid tissues, such as testis (237). This ligand–receptor coupling is involved in apoptosis

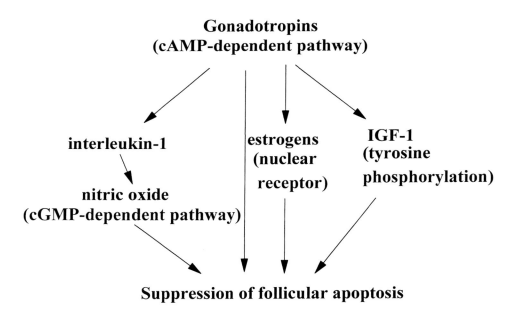

FIG. 20.7. Multifactorial regulation of apoptosis in ovarian follicles. Based on studies on rat ovarian follicles, gonadotropins are the major survival factors which suppress ovarian cell apoptosis through the activation of cyclic adenosine monophosphate (cAMP)–dependent pathways. In addition, the apoptosis-suppressing action of gonadotropins is augmented by multiple local factors, including interleukin-1, estrogens, and insulin-like growth factor-1 (IGF-1), which in turn promote cell survival by activating the cyclic guanosine monophosphate (cGMP)–dependent pathway, nuclear estrogen receptor, and tyrosine phosphorylation, respectively.

regulation in the immune system, liver, keratinocytes, and ovarian cells (94, 163, 186, 187, 200, 220). Other than the dominant membrane-bound form, there is also a soluble Fas antigen variant lacking the transmembrane domain. This variant acts as a competitive inhibitor, blocking apoptosis induced by Fas antigen activation (29, 237). With recent cloning of several genes related to the Fas ligand/Fas antigen, it is apparent that at least four pairs of ligand/receptor genes with overlapping specificity are present in this gene family (30b, 131a, 159a, 194a, 198a, 271a). Because Fas is also known as Apo-1, some of these new genes are named as Apo-2 and -3 or their ligands.

Although the physiological functions for Fas antigen are not fully understood, studies on mice deficient in either Fas antigen or its ligand suggest that this ligand–receptor coupling is important for the regulation of lymphoid cell apoptosis at specific stages of development (Table 20.4). Mutant lpr (lymphoproliferation) mice show decreased levels of full-length Fas mRNA in the thymus and liver due to the insertion of an early transposable element in intron 2 (173). These mice develop marked lymphadenopathy and systemic autoimmune disease as a result of the abnormal accumulation of lymphocytes. Another mutant mouse, gld (generalized lymphoproliferative disease), also develops lymphadenopathy and autoimmune disease similar to that of lpr mice (173, 210, 241). The gld mice carry a point mutation in the C-terminal region of the Fas ligand, which impairs the ability of the Fas ligand to bind Fas antigen. Dysfunction of the Fas antigen–Fas ligand system in these two mutant mice leads to impairment of the elimination of activated T and mature B cells, suggesting that this ligand–receptor system is important for apoptosis of lymphoid cells in the periphery (25, 55, 173, 205). In addition, Ca^{2+}-independent Fas ligand–receptor coupling is indispensable for normal CTL-mediated cytotoxicity in addition to the Ca^{2+}-dependent granzyme-based mechanism (6, 95, 122, 158, 211, 231).

Like Fas antigen, TNF-R1 mediates apoptosis induction in a variety of cells following activation by its ligand, TNF-α (147, 247, 274). It is expressed on most cell types and is responsible for most of the biological properties of TNF-α, including apoptosis induction, antiviral activity, and host defense against microorganisms (249, 275). Studies have shown that TNF-R1-deficient mice are defective in the clearance of bacterial pathogens and have an increased resistance toward lipopolysaccharide-mediated cytotoxicity, suggesting that the function of TNF-R1 is distinct from that of Fas antigen and is associated mainly with the mediation of cell death in response to foreign pathogens (198). Studies on signaling by Fas antigen and TNF-R1

have shown that these receptors can self-associate and that binding of these receptors to their respective ligands induces receptor oligomerization. In addition, the functional receptor for TNF-R1 is a trimer complex, and self-association of the receptor is sufficient to trigger signaling constitutively (20). Among the various signals triggered by the activation of Fas antigen or TNF-R1, the binding of the intracellular death domain within these receptors to the intracellular death domain–containing proteins, such as TRADD, FADD/MORT1, and RIP, is of particular interest (Fig. 20.6; 21, 31, 114, 221, 232). Recent studies have indicated that ligand binding to Fas/Apo-1 or to TNF receptor 1 recruits FLICE/MACH1/caspase-8 to the plasma membrane via interaction with FADD and/or TRADD. Formation of this large complex results in caspase-8 proteolytic activation (84a, 172a). Caspase-8, in turn, activates the downstream caspase-3 to initiate apoptosis.

In addition to the death domain interaction, the activation of sphingomyelinase(s) by Fas antigen or TNF-R1 may play a role in the initiation of apoptosis by these two receptors. Although sphingomyelin (N-acylsphingosin-1–phosphocholine), a phospholipid in the plasma membrane of mammalian cells, originally was considered a structural component, studies have demonstrated that it can participate in the signal transduction of apoptosis through the downstream effector ceramide, which triggers apoptosis in diverse cell types (35, 97, 233, 271).

Thus, several novel signal-transduction pathways could account for apoptosis mediated by TNF-R1 or Fas antigen.

CONCLUSION

Although the regulation of cell proliferation and differentiation traditionally has been regarded as the principal mechanism guiding the fate of a cell, recent studies have demonstrated the essential role of apoptosis. Studies of the extracellular regulatory factors and intracellular execution machinery of apoptosis have opened new avenues to understanding diverse physiological processes, and it is now widely accepted that apoptosis is of central importance for the development and homeostasis of metazoan animals (233). In most cells, the extracellular signals regulating apoptosis could act through endocrine, paracrine, autocrine, or juxtacrine mechanisms. These diverse signals ultimately may activate common intracellular programs, and at least four groups of proteins (the ced-9/Bcl-2, ced-4/Apaf-1, ced-3/caspases, and death domain–containing proteins) are important in the mediation of apoptosis.

Future studies of apoptotic pathways in different tissues will be important for an understanding of embryonic development, metamorphosis, tissue remodeling, hormone-induced tissue atrophy, and many other physiological processes involving cell turnover. Because of the important role of apoptosis in different disease states, such as cancer, viral infection, neurodegenerative disorders, and autoimmune diseases, the elucidation of tissue-specific mechanisms involved in apoptotic regulation will help to unravel the etiology of these diseases as well as to provide new therapeutic modalities.

This study was supported by NIH grant HD31566.

REFERENCES

1. Alderman, E. M., H. H. Fudenberg, and R. E. Lovins. Binding of immunoglobulin classes to subpopulations of human red blood cells separated by density-gradient centrifugation. *Blood* 55: 817–822, 1980.

1a. Alnemri, E. S., D. Livingston, D. Nicholson, G. Salvesen, N. Thornberry, W. Wong, and J. Yu. Human Ice/ced-3 protease nomenclature. *Cell* 87: 171, 1996.

2. Allsopp, T. E., S. Wyatt, H. F. Paterson, and A. M. Davies. The proto-oncogene bcl-2 can selectively rescue neurotrophic factor–dependent neurons from apoptosis. *Cell* 73: 295–307, 1993.

3. Alnemri, E. S., T. Fernandes-Alnemri, and G. Litwack. Cloning and expression of four novel isoforms of human interleukin-1 β converting enzyme with different apoptotic activities. *J. Biol. Chem.* 270: 4312–4317, 1995.

4. Alnemri, E. S., N. M. Robertson, T. F. Fernandes, C. M. Croce, and G. Litwack. Overexpressed full-length human Bcl2 extends the survival of baculovirus-infected Sf9 insect cells. *Proc. Natl. Acad. Sci. U.S.A.* 89: 7295–7299, 1992.

5. Althaus, F. R., and C. Richter. ADP-ribosylation of proteins. Enzymology and biological significance. *Mol. Biol. Biochem. Biophys.* 37: 1–237, 1987.

6. Apasov, S., F. Redegeld, and M. Sitkovsky. Cell-mediated cytotoxicity: contact and secreted factors. *Curr. Opin. Immunol.* 5: 404–410, 1993.

7. Apte, S. S., M. Marie-Genevieve, M. F. Seldin, and B. R. Olsen. The highly conserved defender against the death 1 (DAD1) gene maps to human chromosome 14q11–q12 and mouse chromosome 14 and has plant and nematode homologs. *FEBS Lett.* 363: 304–306, 1995.

8. Baffy, G., T. Miyashita, J. R. Williamson, and J. C. Reed. Apoptosis induced by withdrawal of interleukin-3 (IL-3) from an IL-3–dependent hematopoietic cell line is associated with repartitioning of intracellular calcium and is blocked by enforced Bcl-2 oncoprotein production. *J. Biol. Chem.* 268: 6511–6519, 1993.

9. Barres, B. A., I. K. Hart, H.S.R. Coles, J. F. Burne, J. T. Voyvodic, W. D. Richardson, and M. C. Raff. Cell death and control of cell survival in the oligodendrocyte lineage. *Cell* 70: 31–46, 1992.

10. Barry, M. A., and A. Eastman. Identification of deoxyribonuclease II as an endonuclease involved in apoptosis. *Arch. Biochem. Biophys.* 300: 440–450, 1993.

11. Beere, H. M., C. M. Chresta, A. Alejo-Herberg, A. Skladanowski, C. Dive, K. A. Larsen, and J. A. Hickman. Investigation of the mechanism of higher order chromatin fragmentation observed in drug-induced apoptosis. *Mol. Pharmacol.* 47: 986–996, 1995.

12. Benedetti, A., A. M. Jezequel, and F. Orlandi. A quantitative evaluation of apoptotic bodies in rat liver. *Liver* 8: 172–177, 1988.

13. Benedetti, A., A. M. Jezequel, and F. Orlandi. Preferential distribution of apoptotic bodies in acinar zone 3 of normal human and rat liver. *J. Hepatol.* 7: 319–324, 1988.

14. Berges, R. R., Y. Furuya, L. Remington, H. F. English, T. Jacks, and J. T. Issacs. Cell proliferation, DNA repair and p53 function are not required for programmed cell death of prostatic glandular cells induced by androgen ablation. *Proc. Natl. Acad. Sci. U.S.A.* 90: 8910–8914, 1993.

15. Billig, H., I. Furuta, and A. J. W. Hsueh. Estrogens inhibit and androgens enhance ovarian granulosa cell apoptosis. *Endocrinology* 133: 2204–2212, 1994.

16. Billig, H., I. Furuta, and A.J.W. Hsueh. Gonadotropin-releasing hormone directly induces apoptotic cell death in the rat ovary: biochemical and *in situ* detection of deoxyribonucleic acid fragmentation in granulosa cells. *Endocrinology* 134: 245–252, 1994.

17. Billig, H., I. Furuta, C. Rivier, J. Tapanainen, M. Parvinen, and A.J.W. Hsueh. Apoptosis in testis germ cells: developmental changes in gonadotropin dependence and localization to selective tubule stages. *Endocrinology* 136: 5–12, 1995.

18. Birnbaum, M. J., R. J. Clem, and L. K. Miller. An apoptosis-inhibiting gene from a nuclear polyhedrosis virus encoding a peptide with Cys/His sequence motifs. *J. Virol.* 68: 2521–2528, 1994.

19. Boise, L., M. Gonzalez-Garcia, C. Postema, L. Ding, T. Lindsten, L. Turka, X. Mao, G. Nunez, and C. Thompson. Bcl-x, a bcl-2 related gene that functions as a dominant regulator of apoptotic cell death. *Cell* 74: 597–608, 1993.

20. Boldin, M. P., I. L. Mett, E. E. Varfolomeev, I. Chumakov, Y. Shemer-Avni, J. H. Camonis, and D. Wallach. Self-association of the "death domain" of the p55 tumor necrosis factor (TNF) receptor and Fas/APO1 prompts signaling for TNF and Fas/APO1 effects. *J. Biol. Chem.* 270: 387–391, 1995.

21. Boldin, M. P., E. E. Varfolomeev, Z. Pancer, I. L. Met, J. H. Camonis, and D. Wallach. A novel protein that interacts with the death domain of Fas/APO1 contains a sequence motif related to the death domain. *J. Biol. Chem.* 270: 7795–7798, 1995.

22. Borner, C., I. Martinou, C. Mattmann, M. Irmler, E. Schaerer, J. Martinou, and J. Tschopp. The protein bcl-2α does not require membrane attachment, but two conserved domains to suppress apoptosis. *J. Cell Biol.* 126: 1059–1068, 1994.

23. Boudreau, N., C. J. Sympson, Z. Werb, and M. J. Bissell. Suppression of ICE and apoptosis in mammary epithelial cells by extracellular matrix. *Science* 267: 891–893, 1995.

23a. Boyd, J. M., G. J. Gallo, B. Elangovan, A. B. Houghton, S. Malstrom, B. J. Avery, R. G. Ebb, T. Subramanian, T. Chittenden, and R. J. Lutz. Bik, a novel death-inducing protein shares a distinct sequence motif with Bcl-2 family proteins and interacts with viral and cellular survival-promoting proteins. *Oncogene* 11: 1921–1928, 1995.

24. Brooks, P. C., A.M.P. Montagomery, M. Rosenfeld, R. A. Reisfeld, T. Hu, G. Klier, and D. A. Cheresh. Integrin $\alpha_v\beta_3$ antagonists promote tumor regression by inducing apoptosis of angiogenic blood vessels. *Cell* 79: 1157–1164, 1994.

25. Brunner, T., R. J. Mogil, D. LaFace, N. J. Yoo, A. Mahboubl, F. Echeverrl, S. J. Martin, W. R. Force, D. H. Lynch, C. F. Ware, and D. R. Green. Cell-autonomous Fas(CD95)/Fas-ligand interaction mediates activation-induced apoptosis in T-cell hybridomas. *Nature* 373: 441–444, 1995.

26. Bump, N. J., M. Hackett, M. Hugunin, S. Seshagiri, K. Brady, P. Chen, C. Ferenz, S. Franklin, T. Ghayur, P. Li, P. Licari, J. Mankovich, L. Shi, A. H. Greenberg, L. K. Miller, and W. W. Wong. Inhibition of ICE family proteases by baculovirus antiapoptotic protein p35. *Science* 269: 1885–1888, 1995.

27. Buttke, T. M., and P. A. Sandstrom. Oxidative stress as a mediator of apoptosis. *Immunol. Today* 15: 7–10, 1994.

28. Casciola-Rosen, L. A., D. K. Miller, G. J. Anhalt, and A. Rosen. Specific cleavage of the 70-kDa protein component of the U1 small nuclear ribonucleoprotein is a characteristic biochemical feature of apoptotic cell death. *J. Biol. Chem.* 269: 30757–30760, 1994.

29. Cheng, J., T. Zhou, C. Liu, J. P. Shapiro, M. J. Brauer, M. C. Kiefer, P. J. Barr, and J. D. Mountz. Protection from Fas-mediated apoptosis by a soluble form of the Fas molecule. *Science* 263: 1759–1762, 1994.

30. Chen-Levy, Z., and M. L. Cleary. Membrane topology of the Bcl-2 protooncogene protein demonstrated *in vitro*. *J. Biol. Chem.* 265: 4929–4933, 1989.

30a. Chinnaiyan A., K. O'Rourke, B. Lane, and V. Dixit. Interaction of ced-4 with ced-3 and ced-9: a molecular framework for cell-death. *Science* 275: 1122–1126, 1997.

30b. Chinnaiyan A. M., K. O'Rourke, G. L. Yu, R. H. Lyons, M. Garg, D. R. Duan, L. Xing, R. Gentz, J. Ni, and V. M. Dixit. Signal transduction by DR3, a death domain-containing receptor related to TNFR-1 and CD95. *Science* 274: 990–992, 1996.

31. Chinnaiyan, A. M., K. O'Rourke, M. Tewari, and V. M. Dixit. FADD, a novel death domain-containing protein, interacts with the death domain of Fas and initiates apoptosis. *Cell* 81: 505–512, 1995.

32. Chittenden, T., E. A. Harrington, R. O'Connor, C. Flemington, R. J. Lutz, G. I. Evan, and B. C. Guild. Induction of apoptosis by the Bcl-2 homologue Bak. *Nature* 374: 733–739, 1995.

33. Chun, S., H. Billig, J. L. Tilly, I. Furuta, A. Tsafriri, and A.J.W. Hsueh. Gonadotropin suppression of apoptosis in cultured pre-ovulatory follicles: mediatory role of endogenous insulin-like growth factor I. *Endocrinology* 135: 1845–1853, 1994.

34. Chun, S., K. M. Eisenhauer, M. Kubo, and A. J. W. Hsueh. Interleukin-1β suppresses apoptosis in rat ovarian follicles by increasing nitrix oxide production. *Endocrinology* 136: 3120–3127, 1995.

35. Cifone, M. G., P. Roncaioli, R. de Maria, G. Camarda, A. Santoni, G. Ruberti, and R. Testi. Multiple pathways originate at the Fas/APO-1 (CD95) receptor: sequential involvement of phosphatidylcholine-specific phospholipase C and acidic sphingomyelinase in the propagation of the apoptotic signal. *EMBO J.* 14: 5859–5868, 1995.

36. Clarke, P.G.H. Developmental cell death: morphological diversity and multiple mechanisms. *Anat. Embryol.* 181: 195–213, 1990.

37. Cleary, M. L., S. D. Smith, and J. Sklar. Cloning and structural analysis of cDNAs for bcl-2 and a hybrid bcl2/immunoglobulin transcript resulting from the t(14;18) translocation. *Cell* 47: 19–28, 1986.

38. Clem, R. J., M. Fechheimer, and L. K. Miller. Prevention of apoptosis by a baculovirus gene during infection of insect cells. *Science* 254: 1388–1390, 1991.

39. Clem, R. J., and L. K. Miller. Apoptosis reduces both the *in vitro* replication and the *in vivo* infectivity of a baculovirus. *J. Virol.* 67: 3730–3738, 1993.

40. Clem, R. J., and L. K. Miller. Control of programmed cell death by the baculovirus genes p35 and iap. *Mol. Cell. Biol.* 14: 5212–5222, 1994.

41. Clem, R. J., and L. K. Miller. Induction and inhibition of apoptosis by insect viruses. In: *Apoptosis II: The molecular basis of apoptosis in disease,* edited by L. D. Tomei and F. O. Cope. Cold Spring Harbor, NY: Cold Spring Harbor Laboratory Press, 1994, p. 89–110.

42. Cleveland, J. L., and J. N. Ihle. Contenders in FasL/TNF death signaling. *Cell* 81: 479–482, 1995.

43. Cohen, J. J. Programmed cell death in the immune system. *Adv. Immunol.* 50: 55–85, 1991.

44. Cohen, J. J., and R. C. Duke. Glucocorticoid activation of a calcium-dependent endonuclease in thymocyte nuclei leads to cell death. *J. Immunol.* 32: 38–42, 1984.

45. Cohen, J. J., R. C. Duke, V. A. Fadok, and K. S. Sellins. Apoptosis and programmed cell death in immunity. *Annu. Rev. Immunol.* 10: 267–293, 1992.

46. Colotta, F., N. Polentarutti, M. Sironi, and A. Mantovani. Expression and involvement of c-fos and c-jun protooncogenes in programmed cell death induced by growth factor deprivation in lymphoid cell lines. *J. Biol. Chem.* 267: 18278–18283, 1992.

47. Cory, S., A. W. Harris, and A. Strasser. Insights from transgenic mice regarding the role of bcl-2 in normal and neoplastic lymphoid cells. *Phil. Trans. R. Soc. Lond. [B]* 345: 289–295, 1994.

48. Coucouvanis, E., and G. R. Martin. Signals for death and survival: a two-step mechanism for cavitation in the vertebrate embryo. *Cell* 83: 279–287, 1995.

49. Coucouvanis, E. C., S. W. Sherwood, C. Carswell-Crumpton, E. G. Spack, and P. P. Jones. Evidence that the mechanism of prenatal germ cell death in the mouse is apoptosis. *Exp. Cell Res.* 209: 238–247, 1993.

50. Crook, N. E., R. J. Clem, and L. K. Miller. An apoptosis-inhibiting baculovirus gene with a zinc finger-like motif. *J. Virol.* 67: 2168–2174, 1993.

51. Cuende, E., J. E. Ales-Martinea, L. Ding, M. Gonzalez-Garcia, A. C. Martinez, and G. Nunez. Programmed cell death by bcl-2–dependent and independent mechanisms in B lymphoma cells. *EMBO J.* 12: 1555–1560, 1993.

52. Darmon, A. J., D. W. Nicholson, and R. C. Bleackley. Activation of the apoptotic protease CPP32 by cytotoxic T-cell-derived granzyme B. *Nature* 377: 446–448, 1995.

53. Deiss, L. P., E. Feinstein, H. Berissi, O. Cohen, and A. Kimchi. Identification of a novel serine/threonine kinase and a novel 15-kD protein as potential mediators of the γ interferon-induced cell death. *Genes Dev.* 9: 15–30, 1995.

54. Devaux, P. F. Protein involvement in transmembrane lipid asymmetry. *Annu. Rev. Biophys. Biomol. Struct.* 21: 417–439, 1992.

55. Dhein, J., H. Walczak, C. Baumler, K. Debatin, and P. H. Krammer. Autocrine T-cell suicide mediated by APO-1/(Fas/CD95). *Nature* 373: 438–441, 1995.

57. Dini, L., F. Autuori, A. Lentini, S. Oliverio, and M. Piacentini. The clearance of apoptotic cells in the liver is mediated by the asialoglycoprotein receptor. *FEBS Lett.* 296: 174–178, 1992.

58. Dolci, S., D. E. Williams, M. K. Ernst, J. L. Resnick, C. I. Brannan, L. F. Lock, S. D. Lyman, S. Boswell, and P. J. Donovan. Requirement for mast cell growth factor for primordial germ cell survival in culture. *Nature* 352: 809–811, 1991.

59. Driscoll, M. Molecular genetics of cell death in the nematode *Caenorhabditis elegans*. *J. Neurobiol.* 23: 1327–1351, 1992.

60. Dubois-Dauphin, M., H. Frankowski, Y. Tsujimoto, J. Huarte, and J. Martinou. Neonatal motoneurons overexpressing the bcl-2 protooncogene in transgenic mice are protected from axotomy-induced cell death. *Proc. Natl. Acad. Sci. U.S.A.* 91: 3309–3313, 1994.

61. Dyson, J.E.D., D. M. Simmons, J. Daniel, J. M. McLaughlin, P. Quirke, and C. C. Bird. Kinetic and physical studies of cell death induced by chemotherapeutic agents or hyperthermia. *Cell Tissue Kinet.* 19: 311–324, 1986.

62. Ellis, R. E., J. Yuan, and H. R. Horvitz. Mechanisms and functions of cell death. *Annu. Rev. Cell Biol.* 7: 663–698, 1991.

63. Endemann, G., L. W. Stanton, K. S. Madden, C. M. Bryant, R. T. White, and A. A. Protter. CD36 is a receptor for oxidized low density lipoprotein. *J. Biol. Chem.* 268: 11811–11816, 1993.

64. Enokido, Y., and H. Hatanaka. Apoptotic cell death occurs in hippocampal neurons cultured in a high oxygen atmosphere. *Neuroscience* 57: 965–972, 1993.

65. Evan, G. Integrated control of cell proliferation and cell death by the c-myc oncogene. *Proc. R. Soc. Lond. B Biol. Sci.* 345: 269–275, 1994.

66. Evan, G. I., A. H. Wyllie, C. S. Gilbert, T. D. Littlewood, H. Land, M. Brooks, C. M. Waters, L. Z. Penn, and D. C. Hancock. Induction of apoptosis in fibroblasts by c-myc protein. *Cell* 69: 119–128, 1992.

67. Fabbretti, E., P. Edomi, C. Brancolini, and C. Schneider. Apoptotic phenotype induced by overexpression of wild-type gas3/PMP22: its relation to the demyelinating peripheral neuropathy CMT1A. *Genes Dev.* 9: 1846–1856, 1995.

68. Fadok, V. A., D. J. Laszlo, P. W. Noble, L. Weinstein, D. W. Riches, and P. M. Henson. Particle digestibility is required for induction of the phosphatidylserine recognition mechanism used by murine macrophages to phagocytose apoptotic cells. *J. Immunol.* 151: 4274–4285, 1993.

69. Fadok, V. A., J. S. Savill, C. Haslett, D. L. Bratton, D. E. Doherty, P. A. Campbell, and P. M. Henson. Different populations of macrophages use either the vitronectin receptor or the phosphatidylserine receptor to recognize and remove apoptotic cells. *J. Immunol.* 149: 4029–4035, 1992.

70. Fadok, V. A., D. R. Voelker, P. A. Campbell, J. J. Cohen, D. A. Braton, and P. M. Henson. Exposure of phosphatidylserine on the surface of apoptotic lymphocytes triggers specific recognition and removal by macrophages. *J. Immunol.* 148: 2207–2216, 1992.

71. Farbman, A. I. Electron microscope study of palate fusion in mouse embryos. *Dev. Biol.* 18: 93–116, 1968.

72. Farrow, S. N., J.H.M. White, I. Martinou, T. Raven, K. Pun, C. J. Grinham, J. Martinou, and R. Brown. Cloning of a bcl-2 homologue by interaction with adenovirus E1B 19K. *Nature* 374: 731–736, 1995.

73. Faucheu, C., A. Diu, A.W.E. Chan, A. M. Blanchet, C. Miossec, F. Herve, V. Collard-Dutilleul, Y. Gu, R. A. Aldape, J. A. Lippke, C. Rocher, M. S. S. Su, D. J. Livingston, T. Hercend, and J. L. Lalanne. A novel human protease similar to the interleukin-1β converting enzyme induces apoptosis in transfected cells. *EMBO J.* 14: 1914–1922, 1995.

74. Feinstein, E., A. Kimchi, D. Wallach, M. Boldin, and E. Varfolomeev. The death domain: a module shared by proteins with diverse cellular functions. *Trends Biochem. Sci.* 20: 342–344, 1995.

74a. Han, J., P. Sabbatini, and E. White. Induction of apoptosis by human Nbk/Bik, a BH3-containing protein that interacts with E1B 19K. *Mol. Cell. Biol.* 16: 5857–5864, 1996.

75. Ferguson, D.J.P., and T. J. Anderson. Morphological evaluation of cell turnover in relation to the menstrual cycle in the "resting" human breast. *Br. J. Cancer* 44: 177–181, 1981.

76. Ferguson, D.J.P., and T. J. Anderson. Ultrastructural observation on cell death by apoptosis in the "resting" human breast. *Virchows Arch.* 393: 193–203, 1981.

77. Fernandes-Alnemri, T., G. Litwack, and E. S. Alnemri. CPP32, a novel human apoptotic protein with homology to *Caenorhabditis elegans* cell death protein Ced-3 and mammalian

interleukin-1β-converting enzyme. *J. Biol. Chem.* 269: 30761–30764, 1994.

78. Fernandes-Alnemri, T., G. Litwack, and E. S. Alnemri. Mch2, a new member of the apoptotic Ced-3/ICE cysteine protease gene family. *Cancer Res.* 55: 2737–2742, 1995.

79. Fesus, L., V. Thomazy, and A. Falus. Induction and activation of tissue transglutaminase during programmed cell death. *FEBS Lett.* 224: 104–108, 1987.

80. Fesus, L., P. J. Davies, and M. Piacentini. Apoptosis: molecular mechanisms in programmed cell death. *Eur. J. Cell. Biol.* 56: 170–177, 1991.

81. Filipski, J., J. Leblanc, T. Youdale, M. Sikorska, and P. R. Walker. Periodicity of DNA folding in higher order chromatin structures. *EMBO J.* 9: 1319–1327, 1990.

82. Finke, J., R. Fritzen, P. Ternes, P. Trivedi, K. J. Bross, W. Lange, R. Mertelsmann, and G. Dolken. Expression of bcl-2 in Burkitt's lymphoma cell lines: induction by latent Epstein-Barr virus genes. *Blood* 80: 459–469, 1992.

83. Flemming, W. Ueber die bildung von richtungsfiguren in saugethiereiern beim untergang graaf'scher follikel. *Arch. Anat. Physiol. Jahrgang.* 221–224, 1885.

84. Flora, P. K., and C. D. Gregory. Recognition of apoptotic cells by human macrophages: inhibition by a monocyte/macrophage-specific monoclonal antibody. *Eur. J. Immunol.* 24: 2625–2632, 1994.

84a. Fraser, A., and G. Evan. A license to kill. *Cell* 85: 781–784, 1996.

85. Gagliardini, V., P. Fernandez, R.K.K. Lee, H.C.A. Drexler, R. J. Rotello, M. C. Fishman, and J. Yuan. Prevention of vertebrate neuronal death by the crmA gene. *Science* 263: 826–828, 1994.

86. Gaido, M. L., and J. A. Cidlowski. Identification, purification, and characterization of a calcium-dependent endonuclease (NUC18) from apoptosis rat thymocytes, NUC18 is not Histone H₂B. *J. Biol. Chem.* 266: 18580–18585, 1991.

86a. Gibson, L., S. P. Holmgreen, D. C. Huang, O. Bernard, N. G. Copeland, N. A. Jenkins, G. R. Sutherland, E. Baker, J. M. Adams, and S. Cory. bcl-w, a novel member of the bcl-family, promotes cell survival. *Oncogene* 13: 665–675, 1996.

87. Gillet, G., M. Guerin, A. Trembleau, and G. Brun. A Bcl-2–related gene is activated in avian cells transformed by the Rous sarcoma virus. *EMBO J.* 14: 1372–1381, 1995.

88. Godin, I., R. Deed, J. Cooke, K. Zsebo, M. Dexter, and C. C. Wylie. Effects of the Steel gene product on mouse primordial germ cell culture. *Nature* 352: 807–809, 1991.

89. Golstein, P., D. Marguet, and V. Depraetere. Homology between reaper and the cell death domains of Fas and TNFR1. *Cell* 81: 185–186, 1995.

90. Gonzalez-Garcia, M., R. Perez-Ballestero, L. Ding, L. Duan, L. H. Boise, C. B. Thompson, and G. Nunez. Bcl-xL is the major bcl-x mRNA form expressed during murine development and its product localized to mitochondria. *Development* 120: 3033–3042, 1994.

91. Gorospe, W. C., and B. L. Spangelo. Interleukin 6: potential roles in neuronal, endocrine and ovarian functions. *Endocrinol. J.* 1: 3–9, 1993.

92. Grether, M. E., J. M. Abrams, J. Agapite, K. White, and H. Steller. The head involution defective gene of *Drosophila melanogaster* functions in programmed cell death. *Genes Dev.* 9: 1694–1708, 1995.

93. Gu, Y., C. Sarnecki, R. A. Aldape, D. J. Livingston, and M. S. Su. Cleavage of poly(ADP-ribose) polymerase by interleukin-1β converting enzyme and its homologs TX and Nedd2. *J. Biol. Chem.* 270: 18715–18718, 1995.

94. Guo, M. W., E. Mori, J. P. Xu, and T. Mori. Identification of Fas antigen associated with apoptotic cell death in murine ovary. *Biochem. Biophys. Res. Commun.* 203: 1438–1446, 1994.

95. Hanabuchi, S., M. Koyanagi, A. Kawasaki, N. Shinohara, A. Matsuzawa, Y. Nishimura, Y. Kobayashi, S. Yonehara, H. Yagita, and I. K. Okumura. Fas and its ligand in a general mechanism of T-cell-mediated cytotoxicity. *Proc. Natl. Acad. Sci. U.S.A.* 91: 4930–4934, 1994.

96. Hanada, M., C. Aime-Sempe, T. Sato, and J. C. Reed. Structure–function analysis of Bcl-2 protein, identification of conserved domains important for homodimerization with Bcl-2 and heterodimerization with Bax. *J. Biol. Chem.* 270: 11962–11969, 1995.

97. Hannun, Y. A., and L. M. Obeid. Ceramide: an intracellular signal for apoptosis. *Trends Biochem. Sci.* 20: 73–77, 1995.

98. Hay, B. A., T. Wolff, and G. M. Rubin. Expression of baculovirus p35 prevents cell death in *Drosophila*. *Development* 120: 2121–2129, 1994.

99. Hay, B. A., D. A. Wassarman, and G. M. Rubin. *Drosophila* homologs of baculovirus inhibitor of apoptosis proteins function to block cell death. *Cell* 83: 1253–1262, 1995.

100. Hedgecock, E., J. E. Sulston, and N. Thomson. Mutations affecting programmed cell deaths in the nematode *Caenorhabditis elegans*. *Science* 220: 1277–1280, 1983.

101. Henderson, S., D. Huen, M. Rowe, C. Dawson, G. Johnson, and A. Rickinson. Epstein-barr virus-coded BHRF1 protein, a viral homologue of Bcl-2, protects human B cells from programmed cell death. *Proc. Natl. Acad. Sci. U.S.A.* 90: 8479–8483, 1993.

102. Henderson, S., M. Rowe, C. Gregory, D. Croom-Carter, F. Wang, R. Longnecker, E. Lieff, and A. Richinson. Induction of bcl-2 expression by Epstein-Barr virus latent membrane protein 1 protects infected B cells from programmed cell death. *Cell* 65: 1107–1115, 1991.

103. Hengartner, M. O., R. E. Ellis, and H. R. Horvitz. *Caenorhabditis elegans* gene ced-9 protects cells from programmed cell death. *Nature* 356: 494–499, 1992.

104. Hengartner, M. O., and H. R. Horvitz. *C. elegans* cell survival gene ced-9 encodes a functional homolog of the mammalian proto-oncogene bcl-2. *Cell* 76: 665–676, 1994.

105. Hengartner, M. O., and H. R. Horvitz. Activation of *C. elegans* cell death protein CED-9 by an amino-acid substitution in a domain conserved in Bcl-2. *Nature* 369: 318–320, 1994.

106. Henkart, P. A., and M. V. Sitkovsky. Two ways to kill target cells. *Curr Biol.* 4: 923–925, 1994.

107. Hershberger, P. A., J. A. Dickson, and P. D. Friesen. Site-specific mutagenesis of the 35-kilodalton protein gene encoded by *Autographa californica* nuclear polyhedrosis virus: cell line-specific effects on virus replication. *J. Virol.* 66: 5525–5533, 1992.

108. Heusel, J. W., R. L. Wesselschmidt, S. Shresta, J. H. Russell, and T. J. Ley. Cytotoxic lymphocytes require granzyme B for the rapid induction of DNA fragmentation and apoptosis in allogenic target cells. *Cell* 76: 977–987, 1994.

109. Hinds, P. W., and R. A. Weinberg. Tumor suppressor genes. *Curr. Opin. Genet. Dev.* 4: 135–141, 1994.

110. Hockenberry, D., G. Nunez, C. Milliman, R. D. Schreiber, and S. J. Korsmeyer. Bcl-2 is an inner mitochondrial memebrane protein that blocks programmed cell death. *Nature* 348: 334–336, 1990.

111. Hockenbery, D. M., Z. N. Oltvai, X. M. Yin, C. L. Millman, and S. J. Korsmeyer. Bcl-2 functions in an antioxidant pathway to prevent apoptosis. *Cell* 75: 241–251, 1993.

112. Hockenbery, D. M., M. Zutter, W. Hickey, M. Nahm, and S. J. Korsmeyer. Bcl2 protein is topographically restricted in tissue characterized by apoptotic cell death. *Proc. Natl. Acad. Sci. U.S.A.* 88: 6961–6965, 1991.

113. Horn, S., J. Gopas, and N. Bashan. A lectin-like receptor on murine macrophage is involved in the recognition and phagocytosis of human red cells oxidized by phenylhydrazine. *Biochem. Pharmacol.* 39: 775–780, 1990.

114. Hsu, H., J. Xiong, and D. V. Goeddel. The TNF receptor 1–associated protein TRADD signals cell death and NF-kappa B activation. *Cell* 81: 495–504, 1995.

114a. Hsu, S. Y., R. J. Lai, M. Finegold, and A.J.W. Hsueh. Targeted over expression of Bcl-2 in ovaries of transgenic mice leads to decreased follicle apoptosis, enhanced folliculogenesis and increased germ cell tumorigenesis. *Endocrinology* 137: 4837–4843, 1996.

114b. Hsu, S. Y., A. Kaipia, E. McGee, M. Lomeli, and A.J.W. Hsueh. Bok is a pro-apototic Bcl-2 protein with restricted expression in reproductive tissues and heterodimerizes with selective anti-apoptotic Bcl-2 family members. *Proc. Natl. Acad. Sci. U.S.A.* (Nov) 1997.

115. Hsueh, A.J.W., H. Billig, and A. Tsafriri. Ovarian follicle atresia: a hormonally controlled apoptotic process. *Endocr. Rev.* 15: 1–18, 1994.

115a. Inohara, N., l. Ding, S. Chen, and G. Nunez. Harakiri, anovel regulator of cell death encodes a protein that activates apoptosis and interacts selectively with survival promotor proteins Bcl-2 and Bcl-XL. *EMBO J.* 16: 1686–1694, 1997.

116. Irmler, M., S. Hertig, H. R. MacDonald, R. Sadoul, J. D. Becherer, A. Proudfoot, R. Solari, and J. Tschopp. Granzyme A is an interleukin 1β-converting enzyme. *J. Exp. Med.* 181: 1917–1922, 1995.

116a. Irmler, M., M. Thome, M. Mahne, P. Schneider, K. Hofmann, V. Steiner, K. Burns, C. Mattmann, D. Rimold, L. E. French, and J. Tschopp. Inhibition of death receptor signals by cellular FLIP. *Nature* 388: 190–195, 1997.

117. Isaacs, J. T., Y. Furuya, and R. Berges. The role of androgen in the regulation of programmed cell death/apoptosis in normal and malignant prostatic tissue. *Semin. Cancer Biol.* 5: 391–400, 1994.

118. Ishizuya-Oka, A., and A. Shimozawa. Programmed cell death and heterolysis of larval epithelial cells by macrophage-like cells in the anuran small intestine *in vivo* and *in vitro*. *J. Morphol.* 213: 185–195, 1992.

119. Itoh, N., S. Yonehara, A. Ishii, M. Yonehara, S. Mizushima, M. Sameshima, A. Hase, Y. Seto, and S. Nagata. The polypeptide encoded by the cDNA for human cell surface antigen Fas can mediate apoptosis. *Cell* 66: 233–243, 1991.

120. Jacobson, M. D., J. F. Burne, and M. C. Raff. Programmed cell death and Bcl-2 protection in the absence of a nucleus. *EMBO J.* 13: 1899–1910, 1994.

121. Ju, S. T., D. J. Panka, H. Cul, R. Ettinger, M. El-Khatib, D. H. Sherr, B. Z. Stanger, and A. Marshak-Rothstein. Fas(CD95)/FasL interactions required for programmed cell death after T-cell activation. *Nature* 373: 444–448, 1995.

122. Kagi, D., F. Vignaux, B. Ledermann, K. Burki, V. Depraetere, S. Nagata, H. Hengartner, and P. Golstein. Fas and perforin pathways as major mechanisms of T cell-mediated cytotoxicity. *Science* 265: 528–530, 1994.

122a. Kaipia A., S. Y. Chun, K. Eisenhauer, and A. J. W. Hsueh. Tumor necrosis factor-α and its second messenger, ceramide, stimulate apoptosis in cultured ovarian follicles. *Endocrinology* 137: 4864–4870, 1996.

123. Kamens, J., M. Paskind, M. Hugunin, R. V. Talanian, H. Allen,

D. Banach, N. Bump, M. Hackett, C. G. Johnston, P. Li, J. A. Mankovich, M. Terranova, and T. Ghayur. Identification and characterization of ICH-2, a novel member of the interleukin-1β-converting enzyme family of cysteine proteases. *J. Biol. Chem.* 270: 15250–15256, 1995.

124. Kane, D. J., T. Ord, R. Anton, and D. E. Bredesen. Expression of bcl-2 inhibits necrotic neural cell death. *J. Neurosci. Res.* 40: 269–275, 1995.

125. Kaprianou, N., and J. T. Issacs. Activation of programmed cell death in the rat ventral prostate after castration. *Endocrinology* 122: 552–562, 1988.

126. Katsumata, M., R. M. Siegel, D. C. Louie, T. Miyashita, Y. Tsujimoto, P. C. Nowell, M. I. Greene, and J. C. Reed. Differential effects of bcl-2 on T and B cells in transgenic mice. *Proc. Natl. Acad. Sci. U.S.A.* 89: 11376–11380, 1992.

127. Kaufmann, S. H., S. Desnoyers, Y. Ottaviano, N. E. Davidson, and G. G. Poirier. Specific proteolytic cleavage of poly(ADP-ribose) polymerase: an early marker of chemotherapy-induced apoptosis. *Cancer Res.* 53: 3976–3985, 1993.

128. Kay, M.M.B., G. J. Bosman, S. S. Shapiro, A. Bendich, and P. S. Bassel. Oxidation as a possible mechanism of cellular aging: vitamin E deficiency causes premature aging and IgG binding to erythrocytes. *Proc. Natl. Acad. Sci. U.S.A.* 83: 2463–2467, 1986.

129. Kerr, J.F.R., and B. V. Harmon. Definition and incidence of apoptosis: an historical perspective. In: *Apoptosis: The Molecular Basis of Cell Death*, edited by L. D. Tomei and F. O. Cope. Cold Spring Harbor, NY: Cold Spring Harbor Laboratory Press, 1991, p. 5–29.

130. Kerr, J.F.R., and J. Searle. Deletion of cells by apoptosis during castration-induced involution of the rat prostate. *Virchows Arch. Zellpathol.* 13: 87–102, 1973.

131. Kerr, J.F.R., A. H. Wyllie, and A. R. Currie. Apoptosis: a basic biological phenomenon with wide-ranging implications in tissue kinetics. *Br. J. Cancer* 26: 239–257, 1972.

131a. Kitson, J., T. Raven, Y. P. Jiang, D. V. Goeddel, K. M. Giles, K. T. Pun, C. J. Grinham, R. Brown, and S. J. Farrow. A death-domain-containing receptor that mediates apoptosis. *Nature* 384: 372–375, 1996.

132. Klefer, M. C., M. J. Brauer, V. C. Powers, J. J. Wu, S. R. Umansky, L. D. Tomei, and P. J. Barr. Modulation of apoptosis by the widely distributed Bcl-2 homologue Bak. *Nature* 374: 736–739, 1995.

133. Knudson, C. M., K.S.K. Tung, W. G. Tourtellotte, G.A.J. Brown, and S. J. Korsmeyer. Bax-deficient mice with lymphoid hyperplasia and male germ cell death. *Science* 270: 96–99, 1995.

134. Komiyama, T., C. A. Ray, D. J. Pickup, A. D. Howard, N. A. Thornberry, E. P. Peterson, and G. Salvesen. Inhibition of interleukin-1β converting enzyme by the cowpox virus serpin crmA. An example of cross-class inhibition. *J. Biol. Chem.* 269: 19331–19337, 1994.

135. Korsmeyer, S. J., J. R. Shutter, D. J. Veis, D. E. Merry, and Z. N. Oltvai. Bcl-2/Bax: a rheostat that regulates an anti-oxidant pathway and cell death. *Semin. Cancer Biol.* 4: 327–332, 1993.

136. Kozopas, K. M., T. Yang, H. L. Buchan, P. Zhou, and R. W. Craig. MCL1, a gene expressed in programmed myeloid cell differentiation, has sequence similarity to BCL2. *Proc. Natl. Acad. Sci. U.S.A.* 90: 3516–3520, 1993.

137. Krajewski, S., M. Krajewska, A. Shabaik, T. Miyashita, H. G. Wang, and J. C. Reed. Immunohistochemical determination of *in vivo* distribution of Bax, a dominant inhibitor of Bcl-2. *Am. J. Pathol.* 145: 1323–1336, 1994.

138. Krieger, M., S. Acton, J. Ashkenas, A. Pearson, M. Penman, and D. Resnick. Molecular flypaper, host defense, and atherosclerosis. Structure, binding properties, and functions of macrophage scavenger receptors. *J. Biol. Chem.* 268: 4569–4572, 1993.

139. Kuida, K., J. A. Lippke, G. Ku, M. W. Harding, D. J. Livingston, M. S. Su, and R. A. Flavell. Altered cytokine export and apoptosis in mice deficient in interleukin-1β converting enzyme. *Science* 267: 2000–2003, 1995.

140. Kumar, S., M. Kinoshita, M. Noda, N. G. Copeland, and N. A. Jenkins. Induction of apoptosis by the mouse Nedd2 gene, which encodes a protein similar to the product of the *Caenorhabditis elegans* cell death gene ced-3 and the mammalian IL-1β-converting enzyme. *Genes Dev.* 8: 1613–1626, 1994.

141. Lacronique, V., A. Mignon, M. Fabre, B. Viollet, N. Rouquet, T. Molina, A. Porteu, A. Henrion, D. Bouscary, P. Varlet, V. Joulin, and A. Kahn. Bcl-2 protects from lethal hepatic apoptosis induced by an anti-Fas antibody in mice. *Nat. Med.* 2: 80–86, 1996.

142. Lagarkova, M. A., O. V. Iarovaia, and S. V. Razin. Large-scale fragmentation of mammalian DNA in the course of apoptosis preceeds via excision of chromosomal DNA loops and their liogomers. *J. Biol. Chem.* 270: 20239–20241, 1995.

143. Lazebnik, Y. A., S. Cole, C. A. Cooke, W. G. Nelson, and W. C. Earnshaw. Nuclear events of apoptosis *in vitro* in cell-free mitotic extracts: a model system for analysis of the active phase of apoptosis. *J. Cell Biol.* 123: 7–22, 1993.

145. Lazebnik, Y. A., A. Takahashi, R. D. Moir, R. D. Goldman, G. G. Poirier, S. H. Kaufmann, and W. C. Earnshaw. Studies of the lamin proteinase reveal multiple parallel biochemical pathways during apoptotic execution. *Proc. Natl. Acad. Sci. U.S.A.* 92: 9042–9046, 1995.

146. Lefebvre, O., C. Wolf, J. M. Limacher, P. Hutin, C. Wendling, M. LeMeur, P. Basset, and M. C. Rio. The breast cancer–associated stromelysin-3 gene is expressed during mouse mammary gland apoptosis. *J. Cell Biol.* 119: 997–1002, 1992.

147. Lewis, M., L. A. Tartaglia, A. Lee, G. L. Bennett, G. C. Rice, G. H. Wong, E. Y. Chen, and D. V. Goeddel. Cloning and expression of cDNAs for two distinct murine tumor necrosis factor receptors demonstrate one receptor is species specific. *Proc. Natl. Acad. Sci. U.S.A.* 88: 2830–2834, 1991.

148. Li, P., H. Allen, S. Banerjee, S. Franklin, L. Herzog, C. Johnston, J. McDowell, M. Paskind, L. Rodman, J. Salfeld, E. Towne, D. Tracey, S. Wardwell, F. Wei, W. Wong, R. Kamen, and T. Seshadri. Mice deficient in IL-1β-converting enzyme are defective in production of mature IL-1β and resistant to endotoxic shock. *Cell* 80: 401–411, 1995.

149. Li, P., R. Strange, R. R. Friis, V. Djonov, H. Altermatt, S. Saurer, H. Niemann, and A. Andres. Expression of stromelysin-1 and TIMP-1 in the involuting mammary gland and in early invasive tumors of the mouse. *Int. J. Cancer* 59: 560–568, 1994.

150. Liepins, A., and H. B. Younghusband. Low temperature–induced cell surface membrane vesicle shedding is associated with DNA fragmentation. *Exp. Cell Res.* 161: 525–532, 1985.

151. Lin, E. Y., A. Orlofsky, M. S. Berger, and M. B. Prysowsky. Characterization of A1, a novel hemopoietic-specific early-response gene with sequence similarity to bcl-2. *J. Immunol.* 151: 1979–1988, 1993.

152. Liston, P., N. Roy, K.Tamai, C. Lefebvre, S. Baird, G. Cherton-Horvat, R. Farahani, M. McLean, J. Ikeda, A. MacKenzie, and R. G. Korneluk. Suppression of apoptosis in mammalian cells by NAIP and a related family of IAP genes. *Nature* 379: 349–353, 1996.

153. Liu, C., C. M. Walsh, and J. D. Young. Perforin: structure and function. *Immunol. Today* 16: 194–201, 1995.

154. Liu, Y. J., D. Y. Mason, G. D. Johnson, S. Abbot, C. D. Gregory, D. L. Hardie, J. Gordon, and C. M. MacLennan. Germinal center cells express bcl-2 protein after activation by signals which prevent their entry into apoptosis. *Eur. J. Immunol.* 21: 1905–1910, 1991.

155. Los, M., M. van de Craen, L. C. Penning, H. Schenk, M. Westendorp, P. A. Baeuerle, W. Droge, P. H. Krammer, W. Fiers, and K. Schulzeosthoff. Requirement of an ICE/CED-3 protease for Fas/APO-1–mediated apoptosis. *Nature* 375: 81–83, 1995.

156. Lowe, S. W., S. Bodis, A. McClatchey, L. Remington, H. E. Ruley, D. E. Fisher, D. E. Housman, and T. Jacks. p53 status and the efficacy of cancer therapy *in vivo*. *Science* 266: 807–810, 1994.

157. Lowe, S. W., E. M. Schmitt, S. W. Smith, B. A. Osborne, and T. Jacks. p53 is required for radiation-induced apoptosis in mouse thymocytes. *Nature* 362: 847–849, 1993.

158. Lowin, B., M. Hahne, C. Mattmann, and J. Tschopp. Cytolytic T-cell cytotoxicity is mediated through perforin and Fas lytic pathways. *Nature* 370: 650–652, 1994.

159. Luderus, M. E., A. de Graaf, E. Mattia, J. L. den Blaauwen, M. A. Grande, L. de Jong, and R. van Driel. Binding of matrix attachment regions to lamin B$_1$. *Cell* 70: 949–959, 1992.

159a. Marsters, S. A., J. P. Sheridan, C. J. Donahue, R. M. Pitti, C. L. Gray, A. D. Goddard, K. D. Bauer, and A. Ashkenazi. Apo-3, a new member of the tumor necrosis factor receptor family, contains a death domain and activates apoptosis and NF-kappa B. *Current Biol.* 6: 1669–1676, 1996.

160. Martin, L., J. W. Pollard, and B. Fagg. Oestriol, oestradiol-17β and the proliferation and death of uterine cells. *J. Endocrinol.* 69: 103–115, 1976.

161. Martin, S. J., and D. R. Green. Protease activation during apoptosis: death by a thousand cuts? *Cell* 82: 349–352, 1995.

162. Martin, S. J., G. A. O'Brien, W. K. Nishioka, A. J. McGahon, A. Mahboubi, T. C. Saido, and D. R. Green. Proteolysis of fodrin (non-erythroid spectrin) during apoptosis. *J. Biol. Chem.* 270: 6425–6428, 1995.

163. Matsue, H., H. Kobayashi, T. Hosokawa, T. Akitaya, and A. Ohkawara. Keratinocytes constitutively express the Fas antigen that mediates apoptosis in IFN gamma-treated cultured keratinocytes. *Arch. Dermatol. Res.* 287: 315–320, 1995.

164. McDonnell, T. J., and S. J. Korsmeyer. Progression from lymphoid hyperplasia to high-grade malignant lymphoma in mice transgenic for the t(14;18). *Nature* 349: 254–256, 1991.

165. McDonnell, T. J., M. C. Marin, B. Hsu, S. M. Brisbay, K. McConnell, S. Tu, M. L. Cambell, and J. Rodriguez-Villanueva. Symposium: apoptosis/programmed cell death, the bcl-2 oncogene: apoptosis and neoplasia. *Radiat. Res.* 136: 307–312, 1991.

166. McEvoy, L., P. Williamson, and R. A. Schlegel. Membrane phospholipid asymmetry as a determinant of erythrocyte recognition by macrophages. *Proc. Natl. Acad. Sci. U.S.A.* 83: 3311–3315, 1986.

167. Miura, M., H. Zhu, R. Rotello, E. A. Hartwieg, and J. Yuan. Induction of apoptosis in fibroblasts by IL-1β-converting enzyme, a mammalian homolog of the *C. elegans* cell death gene ced-3. *Cell* 75: 653–660, 1993.

168. Monaghan, P., D. Robertson, T. A. Amos, M. J. Dyer, D. Y. Mason, and M. F. Greaves. Ultrastructural localization of bcl-2 protein. *J. Histochem. Cytochem.* 40: 1819–1825, 1992.

169. Morris, R. G., A. D. Hargreaves, E. Duvall, and A. H. Wyllie. Hormone-induced cell death, 2. Surface changes in thymocytes undergoing apoptosis. *Am. J. Pathol.* 115: 426–436, 1984.

170. Motoyama, N., F. Wang, K. A. Roth, H. Sawa, K. Nakayama, K. Nakayama, I. Negishi, S. Senju, Q. Zhang, S. Fujii, and D. Y. Loh. Massive cell death of immature hematopoietic cells and neurons in bcl-x-deficient mice. *Science* 267: 1506–1510, 1995.

171. Munday, N. A., J. P. Vaillancourt, A. Ali, F. J. Casano, D. K. Miller, S. M. Molineaux, T. Yamin, V. L. Yu, and D. W. Nicholson. Molecular cloning and pro-apoptotic activity of ICE$_{rel}$II and ICE$_{rel}$III, members of the ICE/CED-3 family of cysteine proteases. *J. Biol. Chem.* 270: 15870–15876, 1995.

171a. Muzio M., A. M. Chinnaiyan, F. C. Kischkel, K. O'Rourke, A. Shevchenko, J. Ni, C. Scaffidi, J. D. Bretz, M. Zhang, R. Gentz, M. Mann, P. H. Krammer, M. E. Peter, and V. M. Dixit. FLICE, a novel FADD-homologous ICE/CED-3-like protease, is recruited to the CD95 (Fas/APO-1) death-inducing signaling complex. *Cell* 85: 817–827, 1996.

172. Nagata, S., and P. Golstein. The Fas death factor. *Science* 267: 1449–1456, 1995.

172a. Nagata, S. Apoptosis by death factor. *Cell* 88: 355–356, 1977.

173. Nagata, S., and T. Suda. Fas and Fas ligand: lpr and gld mutations. *Immunol. Today* 16: 39–43, 1995.

174. Nakashima, T., T. Sekiguchi, A. Kuraoka, K. Fukushima, Y. Shibata, S. Komiyama, and T. Nishimoto. Molecular cloning of a human cDNA encoding a novel protein, DAD1, whose defect causes apoptotic cell death in hamster BHK21 cells. *Mol. Cell. Biol.* 13: 6367–6374, 1993.

175. Nakayama, K., K. Nakayama, I. Negishi, K. Kuida, H. Sawa, and D. Y. Loh. Targeted disruption of Bcl-2αβ in mice: occurrence of gray hair, polycystic kidney disease, and lymphocytopenia. *Proc. Natl. Acad. Sci. U.S.A.* 91: 3700–3704, 1994.

176. Nawaz, S., M. P. Lynch, and L. E. Gerschenson. Hormonal regulation of cell death in rabbit uterine epithelium. *Am. J. Pathol.* 127: 51–59, 1987.

177. Neamati, N., A. Fernandez, S. Wright, J. Kiefer, and D. J. McConkey. Degradation of lamin B1 precedes oligonucleosomal DNA fragmentation in apoptotic thymocytes and isolated thymocyte nuclei. *J. Immunol.* 154: 3788–3795, 1995.

178. Neilan, J. G., Z. Lu, C. L. Afonso, G. F. Kutish, M. D. Sussman, and D. L. Rock. An African swine fever virus gene with similarity to the proto-oncogene bcl-2 and the Epstein-Barr virus gene BHRF1. *J. Virol.* 67: 4391–4394, 1993.

179. Newmeyer, D. D., D. M. Farschon, and J. C. Reed. Cell-free apoptosis in *Xenopus* egg extracts: inhibition by Bcl-2 and requirement for an organelle fraction enriched in mitochondria. *Cell* 79: 353–364, 1994.

180. Nicholson, D. W., A. Ali, N. A. Thornberry, J. P. Vaillancourt, C. K. Ding, M. Gallant, Y. Gareau, P. R. Griffin, M. Labelle, Y. A. Lazebnik, N. A. Munday, M. R. Sayyaparaju, M. E. Smulson, T. Yamin, V. L. Yu, and D. K. Miller. Identification and inhibition of the ICE/CED-3 protease necessary for mammalian apoptosis. *Nature* 376: 37–43, 1995.

181. Nunez, G., D. Hockenbery, T. J. McDonnell, C. M. Sorensen, and S. J. Korsmeyer. Bcl-2 maintains B cell memory. *Nature* 353: 71–73, 1991.

182. Nunez, G., L. London, D. Hockenbery, M. Alexander, J. P. McKearn, and S. J. Korsmeyer. Deregulated Bcl-2 gene expression selectively prolongs survival of growth factor–deprived hemopoietic cell lines. *J. Immunol.* 144: 3602–3610, 1990.

183. Oberhammer, F., G. Fritsch, M. Schmied, M. Pavelka, D. Printz, T. Purchio, H. Lassmann, and R. Schulte-Hermann.

Condensation of the chromatin at the membrane of an apoptotic nucleus is not associated with activation of an endonuclease. *J. Cell Sci.* 104: 317–326, 1993.

184. Oberhammer, F., J. W. Wilson, C. Dive, I. D. Morris, J. A. Hickman, A. E. Wakeling, P. R. Walker, and M. Sikorska. Apoptotic death in epithelial cells: cleavage of DNA to 300 and/or 50 kb fragments prior to or in the absence of internucleosomal fragmentation. *EMBO J.* 12: 3679–3684, 1993.

185. Oehm, A., I. Behrmann, W. Falk, M. Pawlita, G. Maier, C. Klas, M. Li-Weber, S. Richards, J. Dhein, B. C. Trauth, H. Ponstingl, and P. H. Krammer. Purification and molecualr cloning of the APO-1 cell surface antigen, a member of the tumor necrosis factor/nerve growth factor receptor superfamily. *J. Biol. Chem.* 267: 10709–10715, 1992.

186. Ogasawara, J., R. Watanabe-Fukunaga, M. Adachi, A. Matsuzawa, T. Kasugal, Y. Kitamura, N. Itoh, T. Suda, and S. Nagata. Lethal effect of the anti-Fas antibody in mice. *Nature* 364: 806–809, 1993.

187. Oishi, M., K. Maeda, and S. Sugiyama. Distribution of apoptosis-mediating Fas antigen in human skin and effects of anti-Fas monoclonal antibody on human epidermal keratinocyte and squamous cell carcinoma cell lines. *Arch. Dermatol. Res.* 286: 396–407, 1994.

188. Oltvai, Z. N., and S. J. Korsmeyer. Checkpoints of dueling dimers foil death wishes. *Cell* 79: 189–192, 1994.

189. Oltvai, Z., C. Millman, and S. J. Korsmeyer. Bcl-2 Heterodimerizes *in vivo* with a conserved homolog, Bax, that accelerates programed cell death. *Cell* 74: 609–619, 1993.

190. Oppenheim, R. W. Cell death during development of the nervous system. *Annu. Rev. Neurosci.* 14: 453–501, 1991.

191. Ossowski, L., D. Biegel, and E. Reich. Mammary plasminogen activator: correlation with involution, hormonal modulation and comparison between normal and neoplastic tissues. *Cell* 16: 929–940, 1979.

192. Ottnad, E., S. Parthasarathy, G. R. Sambrano, M. P. Ramprasad, O. Quehenberger, N. Kondratenko, S. Green, and D. Steinberg. A macrophage receptor for oxidized low density lipoprotein distinct from the receptor for acetyl low density lipoprotein: partial purification and role in recognition of oxidatively damaged cells. *Proc. Natl. Acad. Sci. U.S.A.* 92: 1391–1395, 1995.

193. Palumbo, G. J., D. J. Pickup, T. N. Fredrickson, L. J. McIntyre, and R. M. Buller. Inhibition of an inflammatory response is mediated by a 38-kDa protein of cowpox virus. *Virology* 172: 262–273, 1989.

194. Palumbo, A., and J. Yeh. In situ localization of apoptosis in the rat ovary during follicle atresia. *Biol. Reprod.* 51: 888–895, 1994.

194a. Pan G., K. O'Rourke, A. M. Chinnaiyan, R. Gentz, R. Ebner, J. Ni, and V. M. Dixit. The receptor for the cytotoxic ligand TRAIL. *Science* 276: 111–113, 1997.

195. Patterton, D., W. P. Hayes, and Y. Shi. Transcriptional activation of the matrix metalloproteinase gene stromelysin-3 coincides with thyroid hormone-induced cell death during frog metamorphosis. *Dev. Biol.* 167: 252–262, 1995.

196. Peitsch, M. C., B. Polzar, H. Stephan, T. Crompton, H. R. MacDonald, H. G. Mannherz, and J. Tschopp. Characterization of the endogenous deoxyribonuclease involved in nuclear DNA degradation during apoptosis (programmed cell death). *EMBO J.* 12: 371–377, 1993.

197. Pesce, M., M. G. Farrace, M. Piacentini, S. Dolci, and M. De Felici. Stem cell factor and leukemia inhibitory factor promote primordial germ cell survival by suppressing programmed cell death (apoptosis). *Development* 118: 1089–1094, 1993.

198. Pfeffer, K., T. Matsuyama, T. M. Kundig, A. Wakeham, K. Kishihara, A. Shahinian, K. Wiegmann, P. S. Ohashi, M. Kronke, and T. W. Mak. Mice deficient for the 55 kd tumor necrosis factor receptor are resistant to endotoxic shock, yet succumb to *L. monocytogenes* infection. *Cell* 73: 457–467, 1993.

198a. Pitti, R. M., S. A. Marsters, S. Ruppert, C. J. Donahue, A. Moore, and A. Ashkenazi. Induction of apoptosis by Apo-2 ligand, a new member of the tumor necrosis factor cytokine family. *J. Biol. Chem.* 271: 12687–12690, 1996.

199. Quan, L. T., A. Caputo, R. C. Bleackley, D. J. Pickup, and G. S. Salvesen. Granzyme B is inhibited by the cowpox virus serpin cytokine response modifier A. *J. Biol. Chem.* 270: 10377–10379, 1995.

200. Quirk, S. M., R. G. Cowan, S. G. Joshi, and K. P. Kenrikson. Fas antigen-mediated apoptosis in human granulosa/luteal cells. *Biol. Reprod.* 52: 279–287, 1995.

201. Rabizadeh, S., D. J. LaCount, P. D. Friesen, and D. E. Bredesen. Expression of baculovirus p35 gene inhibits mammalian neural cell death. *J. Neurochem.* 61: 2318–2321, 1993.

202. Raff, M. C. Social controls on cell survival and cell death. *Nature* 356: 397–400, 1992.

203. Raff, M. C., B. A. Barres, J. F. Burne, H. S. Coles, Y. Ishizaki, and M. D. Jacobson. Programmed cell death and the control of cell survival: lessons from the nervous system. *Science* 262: 695–700, 1993.

204. Ray, C. A., R. A. Black, S. R. Kronheim, T. A. Greenstreet, P. R. Sleath, G. S. Salvesen, and D. J. Pickup. Viral inhibition of inflammation: cowpox virus encodes an inhibitor of the interleukin-1β converting enzyme. *Cell* 69: 597–604, 1992.

205. Reap, E. A., D. Leslie, M. Abrahams, R. A. Eisenberg, and P. L. Cohen. Apoptosis abnormalities of splenic lymphocytes in autoimmune lpr and gld mice. *J. Immunol.* 154: 936–943, 1995.

206. Reed, J. C. Bcl-2 and the regulation of programmed cell death. *J. Cell Biol.* 124: 1–6, 1994.

207. Reynolds, J. E., T. Yang, L. Qian, J. D. Jenkinson, P. Zhou, A. Eastman, and R. W. Craig. Mcl-1, a member of the Bcl-2 family, delays apoptosis induced by c-Myc overexpression in Chinese hamster ovary cells. *Cancer Res.* 54: 6348–6352, 1994.

208. Rotello, R. J., R. C. Lieberman, R. B. Lepoff, and L. E. Gerschenson. Characterization of uterine epithelium apoptotic cell death kinetics and regulation by progesterone and RU 486. *Am. J. Pathol.* 140: 449–456, 1992.

209. Rothe, M., M. Pan, W. J. Henzel, T. M. Ayres, and D. V. Goeddel. The TNFR2–TRAF signaling complex contains two novel proteins related to baculovirus inhibitor of apoptosis proteins. *Cell* 83: 1243–1252, 1995.

210. Roths, J. B., E. D. Murphy, and E. M. Eicher. A new mutation, gld, that produces lymphoproliferation and autoimmunity in C3H/HeJ mice. *J. Exp. Med.* 159: 1–20, 1984.

211. Rouvier, E., M. F. Luciani, and P. Golstein. Fas involvement in Ca^{++}-independent T cell-mediated cytotoxicity. *J. Exp. Med.* 177: 195–200, 1993.

212. Roy, N., M. S. Mahadevan, M. Mclean, G. Shutler, Z. Yaraghi, R. Farahani, S. Baird, A. Besner-Hohnston, C. Lefebvre, and X. Kang. The gene for neuronal apoptosis inhibitory protein is partially deleted in individuals with spinal muscular atrophy. *Cell* 80: 167–178, 1995.

213. Sambrano, G. R., S. Parthasarathy, and D. Steinberg. Recognition of oxidatively damaged erythrocytes by a macrophage receptor with specificity for oxidized low density lipoprotein. *Proc. Natl. Acad. Sci. U.S.A.* 91: 3265–3269, 1994.

214. Sambrano, G. R., and D. Steinberg. Recognition of oxidatively damaged and apoptotic cells by an oxidized low density lipoprotein receptor on mouse peritoneal macrophages: role of membrane phosphatidylserine. *Proc. Natl. Acad. Sci. U.S.A.* 92: 1396–1400, 1995.

215. Sandow, B. A., N. B. West, R. L. Norman, and R. M. Brenner. Hormonal control of apoptosis in hamster uterine luminal epithelium. *Am. J. Anat.* 156: 15–36, 1979.

216. Sarin, A., D. H. Adams, and P. A. Henkart. Protease inhibitors selectively block T cell receptor–triggered programmed cell death in a murine T cell hybridoma and activated peripheral T cells. *J. Exp. Med.* 178: 1693–1700, 1993.

217. Sato, T., M. Hanada, S. Bodrug, S. Irie, N. Iwama, L. H. Boise, C. B. Thompson, E. Golemis, L. Fong, H. G. Wang, and J. C. Reed. Interactions among members of the Bcl-2 protein family analyzed with a yeast two-hybrid system. *Proc. Natl. Acad. Sci. U.S.A.* 91: 9238–9242, 1994.

218. Savill, J., I. Dransfield, N. Hogg, and C. Haslett. Vitronectin receptor–mediated phagocytosis of cells undergoing apoptosis. *Nature* 343: 170–173, 1990.

219. Savill, J., V. Fadok, P. Henson, and C. Haslett. Phagocyte recognition of cells undergoing apoptosis. *Immunol. Today* 14: 131–136, 1993.

220. Sayama, K., S. Yonehara, Y. Watanabe, and Y. Miki. Expression of Fas antigen on keratinocytes *in vivo* and induction of apoptosis in cultured keratinocytes. *J. Invest. Dermatol.* 103: 330–334, 1994.

221. Schulze-Osthoff, K., P. H. Krammer, and W. Droge. Divergent signalling via APO-1/Fas and the TNF receptor, two homologous molecules involved in physiological cell death. *EMBO J.* 13: 4587–4596, 1994.

222. Schulze-Osthoff, K., H. Walczak, W. Droge, and P. H. Krammer. Cell nucleus and DNA fragmentation are not required for apoptosis. *J. Cell Biol.* 127: 15–20, 1994.

223. Sentman, C. L., J. R. Shutter, D. Hockenbery, O. Kanagawa, and S. J. Korsmeyer. bcl-2 inhibits multiple forms of apoptosis but not negative selection in thymocytes. *Cell* 67: 879–888, 1991.

224. Sheridan, J. W., C. J. Bishop, and R. J. Simmons. Effects of hypoxia on the kinetic and morphological characteristics of human melanoma cells grown as colonies in semi-solid agar medium. *Br. J. Exp. Pathol.* 65: 171–180, 1984.

225. Shi, L., C. M. Kam, J. C. Powers, R. Aebersold, and A. H. Greenberg. Purification of three cytotoxic lymphocyte granule serine proteases that induce apoptosis through distinct substrate and target cell interations. *J. Exp. Med.* 176: 1521–1529, 1992.

226. Shimizu, S., Y. Eguchi, H. Kosaka, W. Kamiike, H. Matsuda, and Y. Tsujimoto. Prevention of hypoxia-induced cell death by Bcl-2 and Bcl-xL. *Nature* 374: 811–816, 1995.

227. Siegel, R. M., M. Katsumata, T. Miyashita, D. C. Louie, M. I. Greene, and J. C. Reed. Inhibition of thymocyte apoptosis and negative antigenic selection in bcl-2 transgenic mice. *Proc. Natl. Acad. Sci. U.S.A.* 89: 7003–7007, 1992.

228. Smyth, M. J., and J. A. Trapani. Granzymes: exogenous proteinases that induce target cell apoptosis. *Immunol. Today* 16: 202–206, 1995.

229. Soloff, B. L., W. A. Nagle, A. J. Moss, Jr., K. J. Henle, and J. T. Crawford. Apoptosis induced by cold shock *in vitro* is dependent on cell growth phase. *Biochem. Biophys. Res. Commun.* 145: 876–883, 1987.

229a. Spector, M., S. Desnoyers, D. Hoeppner, and M. Hengartner. Interaction between the c-elegans cell-death regulators ced-9 and ced-4. *Nature* 385: 653–656, 1997.

230. Squier, M. K., A. C. Miller, A. M. Malkinson, and J. J. Cohen. Calpain activation in apoptosis. *J. Cell. Physiol.* 159: 229–237, 1994.

231. Stalder, T., S. Hahn, and P. Erb. Fas antigen is the major target molecule for CD4$^+$ T cell-mediated cytotoxicity. *J. Immunol.* 152: 1127–1133, 1994.

232. Stanger, B. Z., P. Leder, T. H. Lee, E. Kim, and B. Seed. RIP: a novel protein containing a death domain that interacts with Fas/APO-1 (CD95) in yeast and causes cell death. *Cell* 81: 513–523, 1995.

233. Steller, H. Mechanisms and genes of cellular suicide. *Science* 267: 1445–1449, 1995.

234. Strange, R., F. Li, S. Saurer, A. Burkhardt, and R. R. Friis. Apoptotic cell death and tissue remodelling during mouse mammary gland involution. *Development* 115: 49–58, 1992.

235. Strasser, A. S., A. W. Harris, and S. Cory. bcl2 transgene inhibits T cell death and perturbs thymic self-censorship. *Cell* 67: 889–899, 1991.

236. Strasser, A. S., S. Whittinghan, D. L. Vaux, M. L. Bath, J. M. Adams, S. Cory, and A. W. Harris. Enforced Bcl2 expression in B-lymphoid cells prolongs antibody responses and elicits autoimmune disease. *Proc. Natl. Acad. Sci. U.S.A.* 88: 8661–8665, 1991.

237. Suda, T., T. Takahashi, P. Golstein, and S. Nagata. Molecular cloning and expression of the Fas ligand, a novel member of the tumor necrosis factor family. *Cell* 75: 1169–1178, 1993.

238. Sugimoto, A., P. D. Friesen, and J. H. Rothman. Baculovirus p35 prevents developmentally programmed cell death and rescues a ced-9 mutant in the nematode *Caenorhabditis elegans*. *EMBO J.* 13: 2023–2028, 1994.

239. Sugimoto, A., R. R. Hozak, T. Nakashima, T. Nishimoto, and J. H. Rothman. Dad-1, an endogenous programmed celll death suppressor in *Caenorhabditis elegans* and vertebrates. *EMBO J.* 18: 4434–4441, 1995.

240. Sun, D. Y., S. Jiang, L. M. Zheng, D. M. Ojcius, and J. D. Young. Separate metabolic pathways leading to DNA fragmentation and apoptotic chromatin condensation. *J. Exp. Med.* 179: 559–568, 1994.

241. Takahashi, T., M. Tanaka, C. I. Brannan, N. A. Jenkins, N. G. Copeland, T. Suda, and S. Nagata. Generalized lymphoproliferative disease in mice, caused by a point mutation in the Fas ligand. *Cell* 76: 969–976, 1994.

242. Takayama, S., T. Sato, S. Krajewski, K. Kochel, S. Irie, J. A. Millan, and J. C. Reed. Cloning and functional analysis of BAG-1: a novel Bcl-2 binding protein with anti-cell death activity. *Cell* 80: 279–284, 1995.

243. Talhouk, R. S., M. J. Bissell, and Z. Werb. Coordinated expression of extracellular-matrix-degrading proteinases and their inhibitors regulates mammary epithelial function during involution. *J. Cell Biol.* 118: 1271–1282, 1992.

244. Talley, A. K., S. Dewhurst, S. W. Perry, S. C. Dollard, S. Gummuluru, S. M. Fine, D. New, L. G. Epstein, H. E. Gendelman, and H. A. Gelbard. Tumor necrosis factor alpha-induced apoptosis in human neuronal cells: protection by the antioxidant N-acetylcysteine and the genes bcl-2 and crmA. *Mol. Cell. Biol.* 15: 2359–2366, 1995.

245. Tanaka, S., K. Saito, and J. C. Reed. Structure–function analysis of the Bcl-2 oncoprotein: addition of a heterologous transmembrane domain to portions of the Bcl-2β protein restores function as a regulator of cell survival. *J. Biol. Chem.* 268: 10920–10926, 1993.

246. Tartaglia, L. A., T. M. Ayres, G. H. Wong, and D. V. Goeddel. A novel domain within the 55 kd TNF receptor signals cell death. *Cell* 74: 845–853, 1993.

247. Tartaglia, L. A., and D. V. Goeddel. Two TNF receptors. *Immunol. Today* 13: 151–153, 1992.

248. Tartaglia, L. A., D. V. Goeddel, C. Reynolds, I. S. Figari, R. F. Weber, B. M. Fendly, and M. A. Palladino. Stimulation of human T-cell proliferation by specific activation of the 75-kDa tumor necrosis factor receptor. *J. Immunol.* 151: 4637–4641, 1993.

249. Tartaglia, L. A., M. Rothe, Y. F. Hu, and D. V. Goeddel. Tumor necrosis factor's cytotoxic activity is signaled by the p55 TNF receptor. *Cell* 73: 213–216, 1993.

250. Tartaglia, L. A., R. F. Weber, I. S. Figari, C. Reynolds, M. A. Palladino, Jr., and D. V. Goeddel. The two different receptors for tumor necrosis factor mediate distinct cellular responses. *Proc. Natl. Acad. Sci. U.S.A.* 88: 9292–9296, 1991.

251. Tewari, M., D. R. Beidler, and V. M. Dixit. CrmA-inhibitable cleavage of the 70-kDa protein component of the U1 small nuclear ribonucleoprotein during Fas- and tumor necrosis factor–induced apoptosis. *J. Biol. Chem.* 270: 18738–18741, 1995.

252. Tewari, M., and V. M. Dixit. Fas- and tumor necrosis factor–induced apoptosis is inhibited by the poxvirus crmA gene product. *J. Biol. Chem.* 270: 3255–3260, 1995.

253. Tewari, M., W. G. Telford, R. A. Miller, and V. M. Dixit. CrmA, a poxvirus-encoded serpin, inhibits cytotoxic T-lymphocyte-mediated apoptosis. *J. Biol. Chem.* 270: 22705–22708, 1995.

254. Thompson, C. B. Apoptosis in the pathogenesis and treatment of disease. *Science* 267: 1456–1462, 1995.

255. Thornberry, N. A., H. G. Bull, J. R. Calaycay, K. T. Chapman, A. D. Howard, M. J. Kostura, D. K. Miller, S. M. Molineaux, J. R. Weidner, J. Aunins, K. O. Elliston, J. M. Ayala, F. J. Casano, J. Chin, G.J.F. Ding, L. A. Egger, E. P. Gaffney, G. Limjuco, O. C. Palyha, S. M. Raju, A. M. Ralando, J. P. Salley, T. T. Yamin, T. D. Lee, J. E. Shively, M. MacCross, R. A. Mumford, J. A. Schmidt, and M. J. Tocci. A novel heterodimeric cysteine protease is required for interleukin-1β processing in monocytes. *Nature* 356: 768–774, 1992.

256. Tomei, L. D., and F. O. Cope (eds.). *Apoptosis: The Molecular Basis of Cell Death.* Cold Spring Harbor, NY: Cold Spring Harbor Laboratory Press, 1991.

257. Trauth, B. C., C. Klas, A. M. Peters, S. Matzku, P. Moller, W. Falk, K. M. Debatin, and P. H. Krammer. Monoclonal antibody–mediated tumor regression by induction of apoptosis. *Science* 245: 301–305, 1989.

258. Vanhaesebroeck, B., J. C. Reed, J. De Valck, J. Grooten, T. Miyashita, S. Tanaka, R. Beyaert, F. Van Roy, and W. Fiers. Effect of bcl-2 proto-oncogene expression on cellular sensitivity to tumor necrosis factor–mediated cytotoxicity. *Oncogene* 8: 1075–1081, 1993.

259. Vaux, D. L., H. L. Aguila, and I. L. Weissman. Bcl-2 prevents death of factor-deprived cells but fails to prevent apoptosis in targets of cell mediated killing. *Int. J. Immunol.* 4: 821–824, 1992.

260. Vaux, D. L., I. L. Weissman, and S. K. Kim. Prevention of programmed cell death in *Caenorhabditis elegans* by human bcl-2. *Science* 258: 1955–1957, 1992.

261. Veis, D., C. Sorenson, J. Shutter, and S. J. Korsmeyers. Bcl2 deficient mice demonstrate fulminant lymphoid apoptosis, polycystic kidneys and hypopigmented hair. *Cell* 75: 229–240, 1993.

262. Virchow, R. *Die Cellularpathologoie in ihrer Begrundung auf Physiologische und Pathologische Gewebelehre* (4 Aufl.). Berlin, August Hirschwald Verlag, 1858.

263. Voelkel-Johnson, C., A. J. Entingh, W. S. Wold, L. R. Gooding, and S. M. Laster. Activation of intracellular proteases is an early event in TNF-induced apoptosis. *J. Immunol.* 154: 1707–1716, 1995.

264. Walker, N. I., R. E. Bennett, and J.F.R. Kerr. Cell death by apoptosis during involution of the lactating breast in mice and rats. *Am. J. Anat.* 185: 19–32, 1989.

265. Walker, P. R., C. Smith, T. Youdale, J. Leblanc, J. F. Whitfield, and M. Sikorska. Topoisomerase II-reactive chemotherapeutic drugs induce apoptosis in thymocytes. *Cancer Res.* 51: 1078–1085, 1991.

266. Wang, L., M. Miura, L. Bergeron, H. Zhu, and J. Yuan. Ich-1, an ICE/ced-3–related gene, encodes both positive and negative regulators of programmed cell death. *Cell* 78: 739–750, 1994.

266a. Wang, K., X. M. Yin, D. T. Chao, C. L. Milliman, and S. J. Korsmeyer. BID: a novel BH3 domain-only death agonist. *Genes Dev.* 10: 2859–2869, 1996.

267. Watanabe-Fukunaga, R., C. I. Brannan, N. Itoh, S. Yonehara, N. G. Copeland, N. A. Jenkins, and S. Nagata. The cDNA structure, expression, and chromosomal assignment of the mouse Fas antigen. *J. Immunol.* 148: 1274–1279, 1992.

268. White, E. Death-defying acts: a meeting review on apoptosis. *Genes Dev.* 7: 2277–2284, 1993.

269. White, E. Life, death, and the pursuit of apoptosis. *Genes Dev.* 10: 1–15, 1996.

270. White, K., M. E. Grether, J. M. Abrams, L. Young, K. Farrell, and H. Steller. Genetic control of programmed cell death in *Drosophila. Science* 264: 677–683, 1994.

271. Wiegmann, K., S. Schutze, T. Machleidt, D. Witte, and M. Kronke. Functional dichotomy of neutral and acidic sphingomyelinases in tumor necrosis factor signalling. *Cell* 78: 1005–1015, 1994.

271a. Wiley, S. R., K. Schooley, P. J. Smolak, W. S. Din, C. P. Huang, J. K. Nicholl, G. R. Sutherland, T. D. Smith, C. Rauch, C. A. Smith, et al. Identification and characterization of a new member of the TNF family that induces apoptosis. *Immunity* 3: 673–682, 1995.

272. William, M. S., and P. A. Henkart. Apoptotic cell death induced by intracellular proteolysis. *J. Immunol.* 153: 4247–4255, 1994.

273. Wilson, K. P., J. A. Black, J. A. Thompson, E. E. Kim, J. P. Griffith, M. A. Navia, M. A. Murcko, S. P. Chambers, R. A. Aldape, S. A. Raybuck, and D. J. Livingston. Structure and mechanism of interleukin-1β converting enzyme. *Nature* 370: 270–275, 1994.

274. Wong, G. H., and D. V. Goeddel. Fas antigen and p55 TNF receptor signal apoptosis through distinct pathways. *J. Immunol.* 152: 1751–1755, 1994.

275. Wong, G. H., L. A. Tartaglia, M. S. Lee, and D. V. Goeddel. Antiviral activity of tumor necrosis factor is signaled through the 55-kDa type I TNF receptor. *J. Immunol.* 149: 3350–3353, 1993.

275a. Wu, D. Y., H. Wallen, and G. Nunez. Interaction and regulation of subcellular-localization of ced-4 by ced-9. *Science* 275: 1126–1129, 1997.

276. Wyllie, A. H. Glucocorticoid-induced thymocyte apoptosis is associated with endogenous endonuclease activation. *Nature* 284: 555–556, 1980.

277. Wyllie, A. H. Apoptosis: cell death in tissue regulation. *J. Pathol.* 153: 313–316, 1987.

278. Wyllie, A. H. Cell death. *Int. Rev. Cytol.* 17(Suppl.): 755–785, 1987.

279. Wyllie, A. H., M. J. Arends, R. G. Morris, S. W. Walker, and G. Evan. The apoptosis endonuclease and its regulation. *Semin. Immunol.* 4: 389–397, 1992.

280. Wyllie, A. H., J.F.R. Kerr, and A. R. Currie. Cell death in the normal neonatal rat adrenal cortex. *J. Pathol.* 111: 255–261, 1973.

281. Wyllie, A. H., J.F.R. Kerr, and A. R. Currie. Cell death: the significance of apoptosis. *Int. Rev. Cytol.* 68: 251–306, 1980.

282. Wyllie, A. H., J.F.R. Kerr, I.A.M. Macaskill, and A. R. Currie. Adrenocortical cell deletion: the role of ACTH. *J. Pathol.* 111: 85–94, 1973.

283. Wyllie, A. H, and R. G. Morris. Hormone-induced cell death. Purification and properties of thymocytes undergoing apoptosis after glucocorticoid treatment. *Am. J. Pathol.* 109: 78–87, 1982.

284. Xue, D., and H. R. Horvitz. Inhibition of the *Caenorhabditis elegans* cell-death protease CED-3 by a CED-3 cleavage site in baculovirus p35 protein. *Nature* 377: 248–251, 1995.

285. Yang, E., J. Zha, J. Jockel, L. H. Boise, C. B. Thompson, and S. J. Korsmeyer. Bad, a heterodimeric partner for Bcl-x$_L$ and Bcl-2, displaces Bax and promotes cell death. *Cell* 80: 285–291, 1995.

286. Yang, T., K. M. Kozopas, and R. W. Craig. The intracellular distribution and pattern of expression of Mcl-1 overlap with, but are not identical to, those of Bcl-2. *J. Cell Biol.* 128: 1173–1184, 1995.

287. Yin, X., Z. N. Oltvai, and S. J. Korsmeyer. BH1 and BH2 domains of Bcl-2 are required for inhibition of apoptosis and heterodimerization with BAX. *Nature* 369: 321–323, 1994.

288. Yonehara, S., A. Ishii, and M. Yonehara. A cell-killing monoclonal antibody (anti-Fas) to a cell surface antigen co-downregulated with the receptor of tumor necrosis factor. *J. Exp. Med.* 169: 1747–1756, 1989.

289. Yuan, J., and H. R. Horvitz. The *Caenorhabditis elegans* cell death gene ced-4 encodes a novel protein and is expressed during the period of extensive programmed cell death. *Development* 116: 309–320, 1992.

290. Yuan, J., S. Shaham, S. Ledoux, H. M. Ellis, and H. R. Horvitz. The *C. elegans* cell death gene ced-3 encodes a protein similar to mammalian interleukin-1β-converting enzyme. *Cell* 75: 641–652, 1993.

291. Zou, H, W. J. Henzel, X. Liu, A. Lutschg, and X. Wang. Apaf-1, a human protein homologous to *C. elegans* CED-4, participates in cytochrome c-dependent activation of caspase-3. *Cell* 90: 401–413, 1997.

Index

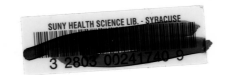

X